# Polyphenols for Cancer Treatment or Prevention

Special Issue Editors

**Karen Bishop**
**Lynnette Ferguson**
**Andrea Braakhuis**

MDPI • Basel • Beijing • Wuhan • Barcelona • Belgrade

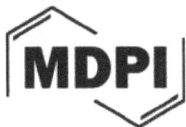

MDPI

*Special Issue Editors*

Karen Bishop
University of Auckland
New Zealand

Lynnette Ferguson
University of Auckland
New Zealand

Andrea Braakhuis
University of Auckland
New Zealand

*Editorial Office*
MDPI AG
St. Alban-Anlage 66
Basel, Switzerland

This edition is a reprint of the Special Issue published online in the open access journal *Nutrients* (ISSN 2072-6651) in 2016–2017 (available at: http://www.mdpi.com/journal/nutrients/special_issues/polyphenols_for_cancer).

For citation purposes, cite each article independently as indicated on the article page online and as indicated below:

Lastname, F.M.; Lastname, F.M. Article title. *Journal Name*. **Year**. *Article number*, page range.

**First Edition 2018**

**ISBN 978-3-03842-648-6 (Pbk)**
**ISBN 978-3-03842-649-3 (PDF)**

# Table of Contents

# About the Special Issue Editors

**Karen Bishop** received a PhD in Virology from the University of Natal, South Africa, in 2005. Karen joined the Auckland Cancer Society Research Centre, University of Auckland in 2010 and is currently employed as a Senior Research Fellow/Senior Lecturer in the Discipline of Nutrition and Dietetics. She lectures to undergrad and postgrad students on dietary interactions with genotype and epigenetics, and risk and progression of cancers. Her current research is focused on amelioration of cancer risk and progression via lifestyle changes, and the assessment of risk change through the application of biomarkers such as circulating tumour DNA and epigenetics. Karen has published more than 50 peer-reviewed research and review articles.

**Lynnette Ferguson** obtained her DPhil from Oxford University in the United Kingdom, working on DNA damage and DNA repair using yeast as a model system. After her return to New Zealand, she began working as part of the Auckland Cancer Society Research Centre (ACSRC), using mutagenicity testing as a predictor of carcinogenesis. In the year 2000, she became a full Professor and was invited to establish a new Nutrition department at The University of Auckland. Since that time, she has split her appointment 50/50 between the ACSRC and The University of Auckland. She has investigated the interplay between genes and diet in the development of chronic disease, with particular foci on inflammatory bowel disease and prostate cancer. She has supervised more than 50 students and has more than 500 peer-reviewed publications. Professor Ferguson has served on the editorial boards of several major cancer-related journals.

**Andrea Braakhuis** is a registered dietitian with a research interest in the clinical and health application of dietary antioxidants and phytochemicals. Andrea is currently employed by The University of Auckland lecturing to postgraduate Nutrition and Dietetic students. Andreas research team is currently investigating the effect of the dietary polyphenols on immune function, breast cancer and athletic performance. Andrea is an Associate Editor for the Nutrition & Dietetics journal. In future her research will focus on the mechanisms of dietary bioactives on athletic performance and efficacy of clinical nutrition interventions. She has published 30 peer-reviewed articles.

# Preface to "Polyphenols for Cancer Treatment or Prevention"

The current special issue book focuses on the impact of an important plant-based, dietary micronutrient, polyphenols, on cancer treatment and prevention. The range and type of research presented is wide and varied, including original research, a number of comprehensive review articles on specific polyphenols, polyphenol pharmacokinetics, specific cancer types, or polyphenols and cancer prevention and treatment in general.

This special issue was inspired by my students who, from time to time, expressed their frustration with the level of scientific evidence within the field of nutrition research with respect to health benefits of food bioactives. Although it is recognised that nutritional health is personal and is more than the sum of individual dietary components, it can be difficult to obtain interpretable results from a systemic approach, in part due to the number of variables that cannot be controlled for. Evidence of effect is more easily interpretable from tissue culture, animal model and human trials utilising individual dietary components or a limited combination of dietary components. For this reason these are the study types presented in this book.

Polyphenols are a broad group of plant-based chemical compounds. They are particularly well known for their inhibitory effects on cancer cells, and for their anti-oxidant activity. Polyphenols have been tested alone, in combination, and with conventional cancer drugs and are of interest as they have been found to induce apoptosis, inhibit proliferation, angiogenesis and metastasis, and modulate the immune system in cancer cells/tissues. Polyphenols are readily consumed in a diet rich in fresh fruit and vegetables and an increase in consumption could be encouraged by robust scientific evidence of health benefits.

Comprehensive reviews are presented on the use of polyphenols, both singularly and in combination, for the prevention and treatment of breast cancer (Braakhuis et al. 2016), as well as mechanism involved (Abdal Dayem et al. 2016), and for cancers in general (Zhou et al. 2016 and Niedzwiecki et al. 2016). In addition, the double edged sword of the influence of polyphenols on DNA damage, a reduction in damage in response to low doses and an increase in damage in response to high doses, is discussed in depth by Asqueta and Collins (2016). A review article of particular interest was that prepared by Benvenuto et al. 2016 on the response of asbestos induced malignant mesothelioma to the immune modulatory effects of polyphenols. Treatment options for malignant mesothelioma are limited, and in addition to providing a profile of up and down regulated cytokines, Benvenuto et al (2016) suggest ways in which the challenge of polyphenol bioavailability can be overcome. This article generated a high almetrix score and was widely publicised in the USA.

A number of articles have been included in this book that speak specifically to the anti-carcinogenic effects of specific polyphenols such as quercetin (Khan et al., 2016) and its glycoside form quercitrin (Truong et al. 2016), tea catechins (Xiang et al. 2015), resveratrol (Li et al. 2016; Pavan et al. 2016); curcumin (Pavan et al. 2016; Bimonte et al. 2016); mangiferin (Gold-smith et al. 2016); citrus extracts (Cirmi et al. 2016); olive leaf extract (oleurpein) (Boss et al. 2016); Elderflower extracts (Schrder et al. 2016), Chinese Bayberry Anthocyanin Extract (Wang et al. 2016); cuminaldehyde (Tsai et al. 2016); Punica granatum Juice (Tibulla et al. 2016); and rosemary extract (Moore et al. 2016).

Lastly, a number of articles included in this book include a discussion on polyphenol bioavailability, but Mandalari et al., Cao et al., Darag et al., Benvenuto et al. and Granja et al. specifically address polyphenol bioavailability, bioaccessibility, toxicology and nano-delivery.

**Karen Bishop, Lynnette Ferguson , Andrea Braakhuis**
*Special Issue Editors*

MDPI

*Article*

# SHP2, SOCS3 and PIAS3 Expression Patterns in Medulloblastomas: Relevance to STAT3 Activation and Resveratrol-Suppressed STAT3 Signaling

Cong Li [1], Hong Li [1], Peng Zhang [1], Li-Jun Yu [1], Tian-Miao Huang [1], Xue Song [1], Qing-You Kong [1], Jian-Li Dong [2], Pei-Nan Li [2] and Jia Liu [1,*]

[1]  Liaoning Laboratory of Cancer Genetics and Epigenetics and Department of Cell Biology, Dalian Medical University, Dalian 116044, China; goodluck_licong@163.com (C.L.); lihongmcn@dlmedu.edu.cn (H.L.); zhangpenggirl821@sina.com (P.Z.); yulijund1963@163.com (L.-J.Y.); huangtianmiao6688@aliyun.com (T.-M.H.); songxue0214@163.com (X.S.); kqydl@sina.com (Q.-Y.K.)
[2]  Department of Orthopedic Surgery, Second Hospital of Dalian Medical University, Dalian 116011, China; jldongdl@aliyun.com (J.-L.D.); delaho@126.com (P.-N.L.)
*  Correspondence: jialiudl@aliyun.com; Tel.: +86-411-8611-0317

Received: 12 September 2016; Accepted: 15 December 2016; Published: 27 December 2016

**Abstract:** Background: Activated STAT3 signaling is critical for human medulloblastoma cells. SHP2, SOCS3 and PIAS3 are known as the negative regulators of STAT3 signaling, while their relevance to frequent STAT3 activation in medulloblastomas remains unknown. Methods: Tissue microarrays were constructed with 17 tumor-surrounding noncancerous brain tissues and 61 cases of the classic medulloblastomas, 44 the large-cell medulloblastomas, and 15 nodular medulloblastomas, which were used for immunohistochemical profiling of STAT3, SHP2, SOCS3 and PIAS3 expression patterns and the frequencies of STAT3 nuclear translocation. Three human medulloblastoma cell lines (Daoy, UW228-2 and UW228-3) were cultured with and without 100 µM resveratrol supplementation. The influences of resveratrol in SHP2, SOCS3 and PIAS3 expression and SOCS3 knockdown in STAT3 activation were analyzed using multiple experimental approaches. Results: SHP2, SOCS3 and PIAS3 levels are reduced in medulloblastomas in vivo and in vitro, of which PIAS3 downregulation is more reversely correlated with STAT3 activation. In resveratrol-suppressed medulloblastoma cells with STAT3 downregulation and decreased incidence of STAT3 nuclear translocation, PIAS3 is upregulated, the SHP2 level remains unchanged and SOCS3 is downregulated. SOCS3 proteins are accumulated in the distal ends of axon-like processes of resveratrol-differentiated medulloblastoma cells. Knockdown of SOCS3 expression by siRNA neither influences cell proliferation nor STAT3 activation or resveratrol sensitivity but inhibits resveratrol-induced axon-like process formation. Conclusion: Our results suggest that (1) the overall reduction of SHP2, SOCS3 and PIAS3 in medulloblastoma tissues and cell lines; (2) the more inverse relevance of PIAS3 expression with STAT3 activation; (3) the favorable prognostic values of PIAS3 for medulloblastomas and (4) the involvement of SOCS3 in resveratrol-promoted axon regeneration of medulloblastoma cells.

**Keywords:** medulloblastoma; STAT3 signaling; STAT3 negative regulators; PIAS3; resveratrol

---

## 1. Introduction

Medulloblastoma is the most frequent primary brain malignancy in childhood and is characterized by rapid and aggressive intracranial growth and high recurrence incidence [1]. Although the combination of operation with adjuvant radiotherapy and/or chemotherapy has been adapted in clinical settings [2], the outcome of medulloblastomas remains poor due to the difficulty in removing the highly aggressive tumor radically and the long-term side effects of conventional anticancer therapies [3,4]. It is therefore urgently necessary to investigate the critical molecular alterations related with medulloblastoma formation and progression and to explore more effective therapeutic approaches with lesser toxicities for better management of medulloblastomas.

Several signaling pathways are known to be involved in the formation and progression of medulloblastomas [5–7], of which STAT3 signaling seems most crucial because selective inhibition of STAT3 activation suppresses growth and induces apoptosis of medulloblastoma cells [5,8,9]. However, the underlying mechanism by which STAT3 signaling is inhibited by resveratrol remains largely unknown. It has been found that several factors can negatively regulate STAT3 signal transduction. For instance, induction of SHP-1 and SHP-2 tyrosine phosphatases inhibit constitutive and inducible STAT3 activation and loss of protein tyrosine phosphatase leads to aberrant STAT3 activation and promotes gliomagenesis [10,11]. Similarly, PIAS3 down-regulation is associated with increased STAT3 activation and poor prognosis of malignant mesothelioma patients [12]. In some types of human malignancies, an interplay between STAT3 signaling and SOCS3 has been found in the form of feedback control [13,14]. Nevertheless, no comprehensive study is so far available concerning the statuses of those negative regulators in medulloblastoma tissues and their relevance with STAT3 activation.

Resveratrol (3,5,4′-trihydroxy-trans-stilbene), a naturally occurring polyphenol found in grapes, peanuts and the root of polygonum cuspidatum, has preventive and therapeutic effects on many kinds of human cancers including brain malignancies [15]. More importantly, the in vitro and in vivo anticancer doses of resveratrol have little toxic effect on the normal tissues and cells [16–18]. For example, resveratrol in 100 μM is sufficient to cause growth arrest and apoptosis of human medulloblastoma and glioblastoma cells in vitro [16,19] and rat orthotopic glioblastomas in vivo without affecting glial cells and neurons [18]. These findings thus suggest that resveratrol would be of potential practical value in improving the therapeutic outcome of medulloblastomas. Our previous studies demonstrate that STAT3 signaling is the critical molecular target of resveratrol although other signaling pathways are inhibited concurrently in resveratrol-treated medulloblastoma cells [19–21]. However, the reasons for resveratrol-caused STAT3 inactivation remain to be clarified. The current study aims to address these issues using medulloblastoma microarrays to profile SHP2, SOCS3 and PIAS3 expression patterns in medulloblastoma tissues and resveratrol-sensitive medulloblastoma cell lines to elucidate the impact(s) of resveratrol in SHP2, SOCS3 and PIAS3 expression when exerting its inhibitory effect on STAT3 signaling and cell proliferation.

## 2. Experimental Section

### 2.1. Medulloblastoma Specimens and Microarray Construction

The protocol of this study had been reviewed by the Ethics Committee of Dalian Medical University before conducting the experiments. The archived 120 paraffin-embedded medulloblastoma specimens were kindly provided by the Clinical Pathology Departments, the First Affiliated Hospital of Dalian Medical University and Shen-Jing Hospital of China Medical University at Shenyang. This study was approved by the hospital institution review board and the informed consent was obtained from all patients before tissue sample collection. The tissue microarrays were constructed in duplicate with 120 medulloblastoma and, where possible, the noncancerous tumor-surrounding brain tissue blocks by the method described previously [22].

### 2.2. Tissue Microarray-Based Immunohistochemical Staining

The expression levels and intracellular distribution patterns of STAT3, SHP2, SCOS1, SOCS3 and PIAS3 in the three subtypes (the classical, the large-cell and the nodular) of medulloblastomas were profiled immunohistochemically, using paraffin sections of the constructed medulloblastoma microarrays. The antibodies used were the rabbit anti-human p-STAT3 (Proteintech, Chicago, IL, USA), SCOS1, SCOS3, PIAS3 and SHP2 (Santa Cruz Biotechnology, Inc., Santa Cruz, CA, USA) antibodies at dilutions of 1:120, 1:100, 1:100, 1:120 and 1:100, respectively. Color reaction was developed using 3,

3'-diaminobenzidine tetrahydrochloride (DAB). The sections without the first antibody incubation were used as the background control. According to the labeling intensity, the staining results were evaluated by two researchers, and scored as negative (−) if no immunolabeling was observed in target cells, weakly positive (+) if the labeling was faint, moderately positive (++) if the labeling was stronger, and strongly positive (+++) if the labeling was distinctly stronger than (++).

### 2.3. Cell Culture and Resveratrol Treatments

Human medulloblastoma UW228-2 and UW228-3 cell lines were kindly provided by Dr. Keles GE, Department of Neurosurgery, Washington University at Seattle. Human medulloblastoma DAOY cell line was obtained from the Cell Culture Facility, Chinese Academy of Sciences Cell Bank, Shanghai. The three cell lines were cultured in DMEM (Gibco Life Science, Grand Island, NY, USA) supplemented with 10% fetal bovine serum (Gibco, Grand Island, NY, USA) under 37 °C and 5% $CO_2$ condition and were plated onto culture dishes (Nunc A/S, Roskilde, Denmark) at a density of $5 \times 10^4$/ml, and incubated for 24 h before further experiments. For paralleled H/E staining, Immunocytochemical (ICC) labeling and transferase-mediated deoxyuridine triphosphate-biotin nick end labeling TUNEL assay (Promega, Madison, WI, USA), dozens of cell-bearing coverslips were concurrently prepared under the exact same experimental conditions using Nest-Dishes (Nest Biotech., Inc., Wuxi, China; China invention patent No. ZL200610047607.0) and collected regularly during drug treatments. Resveratrol (Res; Sigma-Aldrich, St. Louis, MO, USA) was dissolved in dimethylsulfoxide (DMSO; Sigma-Aldrich, St. Louis, MO, USA) and diluted with culture medium to the optimal working concentration (100 μM) just before use. The cells were treated by 100 μM RA for 72 h, while the cells under normal culture condition and treated by 0.2% DMSO were used as normal and background controls, respectively. Cell numbers and viabilities were checked in 12 h intervals and the cell-bearing coverslips were fixed in cold acetone or 4% paraformaldehyde (pH 7.4) for morphological, immunocytochemical examinations and TUNEL assay. The experimental groups were set in triplicate and the experiments as well as the following examinations were repeated for three times to establish confidential conclusion.

### 2.4. Immunocytochemical Staining

Immunocytochemical (ICC) staining for p-STAT3, SOCS1, SOCS3, PIAS3 and SHP2 was performed on the coverslips of the three medulloblastoma cell lines collected from different experimental groups. The antibodies and their dilutions are the same as that used in immunohistochemical staining for tissue microarray sections. The cell-bearing coverslips without the first antibody incubation were used as the background control.

### 2.5. Protein Preparation and Western Blotting

Total cellular proteins were prepared from the cells under different culture conditions. The sample proteins (15 μg/lane) were separated by electrophoresis in 10% sodium dodecylsulfate–polyacrylamide gel electrophoresis and transferred to polyvinylidene difluoride membrane (Amersham, Buckinghamshire, UK). The membrane was blocked with 5% skimmed milk in TBS-T (10 mM Tris–Cl, pH 8.0, 150 mM NaCl and 0.5% Tween 20) at 4 °C overnight, rinsed three times with TBS-T and followed by 3 h incubation at room temperature with the first antibody, and 1 h incubation with HRP-conjugated anti-rabbit IgG (Zymed Lab Inc., San Francisco, CA, USA). The bound antibody was detected using the enhanced chemiluminescence system (Roche, Penzberg, Germany). After removing the labeling signal by incubation with stripping buffer (62.5 mM Tris–HCl, pH 6.7, 100 mM 2-mercaptoethanol, 2% SDS) at 55 °C for 30 min, the membrane was reprobed with other antibodies one-by-one until all of the parameters were examined.

### 2.6. RNA Isolation and RT-PCR

Total cellular RNAs of the experimental groups were extracted using Trizol solution (Life Technology, Grand Island, NY, USA). The sample RNAs were subjected to reverse transcription/RT and then polymerase chain reaction/PCR using the primers specific for STAT3, PTP, SOCS1, SOCS3 and PIAS3 according to producer's protocols (Takara Inc., Dalian Branch, Dalian, China). The sequences of PCR primers for each of the gene transcripts were listed in Table 1. The PCR products were resolved on ethidium bromide-stained 1.5% agarose gel and photographed under UV illumination (UVP, LLC, Upland, CA, USA). β-actin products generated from the same RT solutions were used as quantitative control.

**Table 1.** Sequences of PCR primers for SHP-2, SOCS3, PIAS3, β-actin amplifications.

|  | Primer Sequences | Annealing Temperature | Product Size | Reference |
|---|---|---|---|---|
| SHP-2 | F: 5′-CGAGTGATTGTCATGACAACG-3′<br>R: 5′-TGCTTCTGTCTGGACCATCC-3′ | 56 °C | 477 bp | [16] |
| SOCS3 | F: 5′-GAGCCCCCTCCTTCCCCTCGC-3′<br>R: 5′-GGTCCAGGAACTCCCGAATG-3′ | 56 °C | 264 bp | [21] |
| PIAS3 | F: 5′-ACGCTGTTGGCCCCTGGCAC-3′<br>R: 5′-GGGGCTCGGCCCCATTCTTGG-3′ | 56 °C | 411 bp | [22] |
| β-actin | F: 5′-GCATGGGAGTCCTGTGGCAT-3′<br>R: 5′-CTAGAAGCATTTGGGGTGG-3′ | 58 °C | 326 bp | [17] |

*2.7. siRNA Knockdown of SOCS3 Expression*

UW228-3 cells were selected to elucidate the impact(s) of SOCS3 down-regulation in cell growth, STAT3 activation and resveratrol sensitivity by SOCS3-specific siRNA transfection (siSOCS3-1: 5′-CCAAGAACCTGCGCATCCA-3′; siSOCS3-2: 5′-AGAGCCTATTACATCTACT-3′) [23]. The mock oligonucleotides (sense-50-UUCUCCGAACGUGUCACGUTT-30 and antisense-50-ACGUGACACGUUCGGAGA) and β-actin siRNAs (sense-50-UGAAGAUCAAGAUCAUUGCdTdT-30 and antisense-50-GCAAUGAUCUUGAUCUUCAdTdT-30) were used as negative and positive controls of transfection efficiency [24]. Those siRNAs were synthesized by Genepharma Company, Shanghai, China. Briefly, UW228-3 cells were conventionally cultured in 6-well plates to 60% to 70% confluence and then transfected with 0.3 nmol siRNA/well for 2 or 3 days using 4 mL X-tremeGENE siRNA transfection reagent according to manufacturer's manual (Roche, Penzberg, Germany). After confirming the efficiency of SOCS3 inhibition by RT-PCR, the transfectants were incubated in the medium without or with 100 μM resveratrol for 72 h; afterward, the cells were examined by morphological staining, viable and nonviable cell counting, STAT3- and SOCS3-oriented immunolabeling. The results were compared with those obtained from the normally cultured cells and the cells treated by mock oligonucleotides.

*2.8. Statistical Analyses*

The results obtained from tissue microarray based immunohistochemical profiling were evaluated with the independent-samples $t$-test and ANOVA. Data were presented as mean $\pm$ standard deviation (SD) of separate experiments ($n \geq 10$). When required, $p$-values are stated in the figure legends.

## 3. Results

*3.1. Frequent STAT3 Activation in Medulloblastomas*

According to the criteria of World Health Organization classification system [25], 120 medulloblastoma specimens were classified into three histological subtypes as classical (61 cases), large-cell (44 cases) and nodular (15 cases). The levels and intracellular distribution patterns of p-STAT3 in the three subtypes were analyzed according to the results of tissue microarray-based immunohistochemical staining. It was found that nuclear translocation of p-STAT3 could be observed in 63.9% (39/61) of the classical, 81.8% (36/44) of the large-cell, 53.3% (8/15) of the nodular medulloblastomas and 23.5% (4/17) of tumor-surrounding brain tissues (Figure 1). Statistical analyses (ANOVA) reveal that the staining densities and the frequencies of p-STAT3 nuclear translocation are significantly different between the three medulloblastoma subtypes and the tumor-surrounding brain tissues ($p = 0.000$).

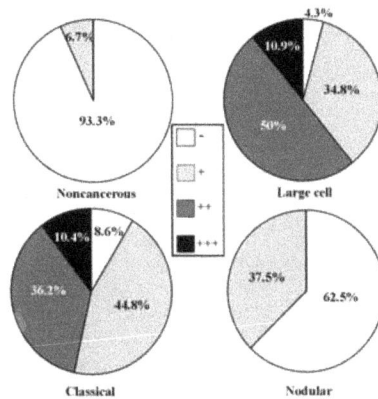

**Figure 1.** Incidences of p-STAT3 nuclear translocation in noncancerous brain tissues and the three histological subtypes of medulloblastomas.

## 3.2. Differential SHP2, SOCS3 and PIAS3 Expression Patterns

The results of immunohistochemical staining were summarized in Table 2 and shown in Figures 2 and 3. It was revealed that the frequencies of p-SHP2 cytoplasmic labeling were significantly different between the tumor-surrounding brain tissues (17/17; 100%) and the classical (32/61; 52.5%; $p = 0.016$), the large-cell (27/44; 61.4%; $p = 0.000$) or the nodular medulloblastomas (2/15; 13.3%; $p = 0.000$). The frequencies of SOCS3 cytoplasmic detection were 100% (17/17) in the tumor-surrounding brain tissues, 80.3% (49/61) in the classical, 90.9% (40/44) in the large-cell and 80.0% (12/15) in the nodular medulloblastomas (Figure 3). Statistical analyses showed no significant differences between the tumor-surrounding brain tissues and the classical ($p > 0.05$), the large-cell ($p > 0.05$) or the nodular medulloblastomas ($p > 0.05$). In the case of PIAS3, significant differences of nuclear PIAS3 detection were evidenced between the tumor-surrounding brain tissues (58.8%; 10/17) and the classical (21.3%; 13/61; $p = 0.000$), the large-cell (15.9%; 7/44; $p = 0.000$) or the nodular medulloblastomas (6.70%; 1/15; $p = 0.000$).

**Table 2.** p-STAT3, p-SHP2, SCOs3 and PIAS3 expression in three subtypes of medulloblastomas and cerebellum tissues.

| | $n$ | p-STAT3 | | | | p-SHP2 | | | | SOCS3 | | | | PIAS3 | | | |
|---|---|---|---|---|---|---|---|---|---|---|---|---|---|---|---|---|---|
| | | − | + | ≥++ | $p$ | − | + | ≥++ | $p$ | − | + | ≥++ | $p$ | − | + | ≥++ | $p$ |
| | | (%) | (%) | (%) | | (%) | (%) | (%) | | (%) | (%) | (%) | | (%) | (%) | (%) | |
| Noncancerous | 15 | 14 | 1 | 0 | | 0 | 4 | 11 | | 0 | 1 | 14 | | 5 | 7 | 3 | |
| | | (93.3) | (6.7) | (0.0) | | (0.0) | (26.7) | (73.3) | | (0.0) | (6.7) | (93.3) | | (33.3) | (46.7) | (20.0) | |
| MB | 112 | 12 | 45 | 55 | 0.000 [#] | 54 | 36 | 22 | 0.000 [#] | 17 | 37 | 58 | 0.003 [#] | 88 | 11 | 13 | 0.001 [#] |
| | | (10.7) | (40.2) | (49.1) | | (48.2) | (32.1) | (19.7) | | (15.2) | (33.0) | (51.8) | | (78.6) | (9.8) | (11.6) | |
| Large | 46 | 2 | 16 | 28 | 0.000 [*] | 18 | 15 | 13 | 0.001 [*] | 4 | 12 | 30 | 0.000 [*] | 35 | 6 | 5 | 0.000 [*] |
| | | (4.3) | (34.8) | (60.9) | | (39.1) | (32.6) | (28.3) | | (8.7) | (26.1) | (65.2) | | (76.1) | (13.0) | (10.9) | |
| Classic | 58 | 5 | 26 | 27 | 0.000 [&] | 29 | 21 | 8 | 0.001 [&] | 11 | 21 | 26 | 0.004 [&] | 45 | 5 | 8 | 0.000 [&] |
| | | (8.6) | (44.8) | (46.6) | | (50.0) | (36.2) | (13.8) | | (19.0) | (36.2) | (44.8) | | (77.6) | (8.6) | (13.8) | |
| Nodular | 8 | 5 | 3 | 0 | | 7 | 1 | 0 | | 2 | 4 | 2 | | 8 | 0 | 0 | |
| | | (62.5) | (37.5) | (0.0) | | (87.5) | (12.5) | (0.0) | | (25.0) | (75.0) | (25.0) | | (100) | (0.0) | (0.0) | |

[#]: Noncancerous vs. Large; [*]: Noncancerous vs. Classic; [&]: Noncancerous vs. Nodular.

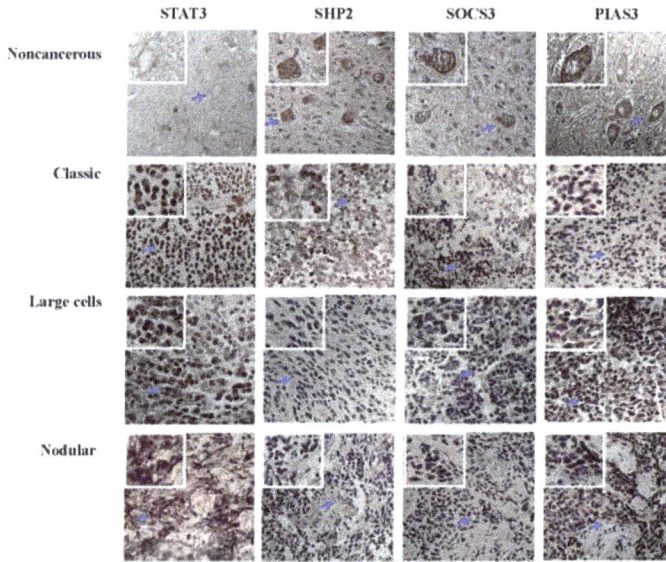

**Figure 2.** Immunohistochemical illustration (20×) of expression levels and intracellular distribution patterns of STAT3, SHP2, SOCS3 and PIAS3 in the three medulloblastoma subtypes and the tumor-surrounding cerebellum tissues. The arrows indicate the regions shown in the insets with higher magnification (40×).

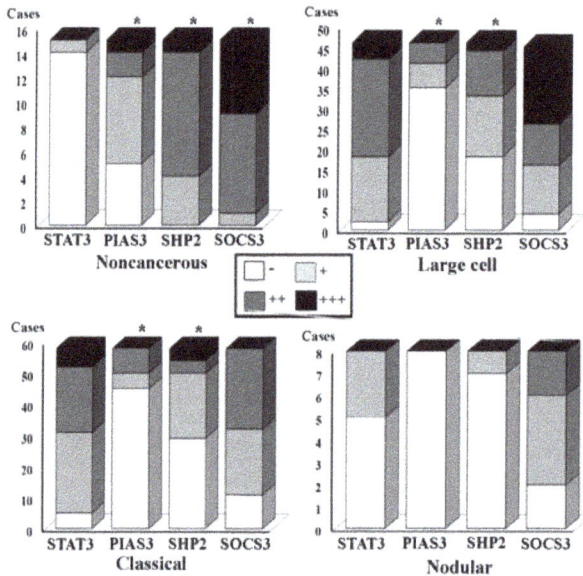

**Figure 3.** Fractionation of STAT3 nuclear translocation and SHP2, SOCS3 and PIAS3 expression levels in the tumor-surrounding noncancerous brain tissues (Upper left) and the large-cell (Upper right), classical (Low left) and nodular medulloblastomas (Low right). * Statistical analyses show significant reduction of their detection rates in comparison with that of the tumor-surrounding brain tissues ($p = 0.000$).

### 3.3. STAT3 Activation and SOCS3 and PIAS3 Down-Regulation

The concurrent p-STAT3 nuclear translocation and p-SHP2, SOCS3 and/or PIAS3 down-regulation are summarized in Figure 3, followed by correlative analyses to elucidate the relevance of p-STAT3 nuclear translocation and the expression levels of p-SHP2, SOCS3 and PIAS3, respectively. Statistical correlations were established between p-STAT3 nuclear translocation and the level of SOCS3 ($R = 0.333$; $p = 0.047$) or PIAS3 expression ($R = -0.494$; $p = 0.002$) but not p-SHP2 down-regulation ($R = 0.02$; $p > 0.05$) in the large-cell medulloblastomas. Inverse correlation could be established between p-SHP2 ($R = -0.35$; $p = 0.029$), SOCS3 ($R = 0.495$; $p = 0.001$) or PIAS3 expression ($R = -0.352$; $p = 0.020$) and p-STAT3 nuclear translocation in the classic medulloblastomas. The corresponding data of the nodular group were not analyzed due to the limited case number.

### 3.4. Inhibited STAT3 Signaling in Resveratrol-Suppressed Cells

Growth suppression, remarkable morphological alteration and frequent cell death were observed in UW228-2, UW228-3 and DAOY cells in a time-related fashion after 100 μM resveratrol treatment, and the majority of resveratrol-treated cells died of apoptosis at the 72-h time point [9,16]. As shown in Figure 4, high levels of STAT3 expression and distinct STAT3 nuclear translocation were observed in the three normally cultured medulloblastoma cell lines; the inhibitory effects of resveratrol on STAT3 signaling were evidenced in terms of reduction of STAT3 nuclear immunostaining (Figure 4) and down-regulated STAT3 expression (Figure 5).

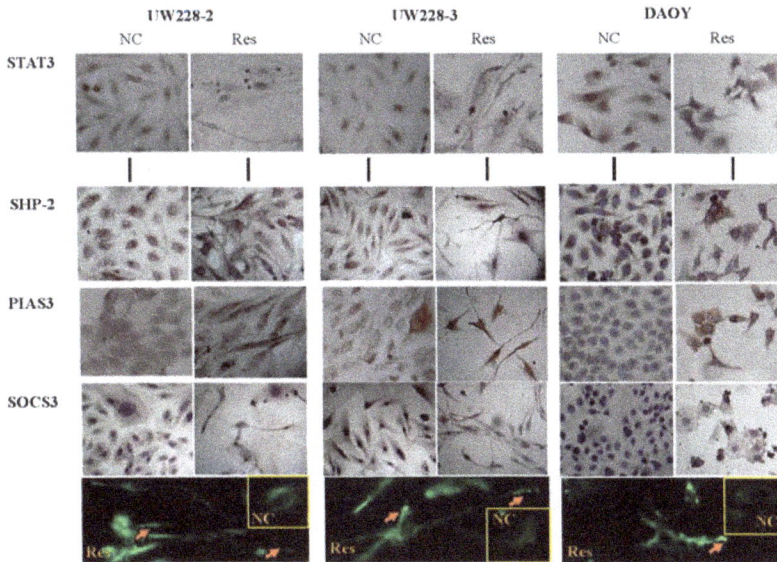

**Figure 4.** Immunocytochemical demonstration of STAT3, p-SHP2, SOCS3 and PIAS3 expression in three human medulloblastoma cell lines without (NC) and with 100 μM resveratrol treatment (Res) for 48 h (20×). Arrows in the immunofluorescent images (40×) indicate SOCS3 accumulation in the distal end of the axon-like processes of the three resveratrol-treated medulloblastoma cell lines. The inset images are the normally cultured cells.

### 3.5. Differential Responses of PIAS3, SOCS3 and SHP2 to Resveratrol

The results of immunocytochemical staining (Figure 4), RT-PCR (Figure 5A) and Western blotting (Figure 5B) demonstrated that the level of PIAS3 was low in normally cultured UW228-2, UW228-3 and DAOY cells, which became increased with distinct nuclear labeling after resveratrol treatment for

48 h. SOCS3 levels were reduced in resveratrol-treated cells (Figure 5), accompanied with preferable accumulation of SOCS3 proteins in the distal end of the axon-like long process (Figure 4). SHP2 was expressed in the three cell lines and its level remained almost unchanged in resveratrol-treated cells.

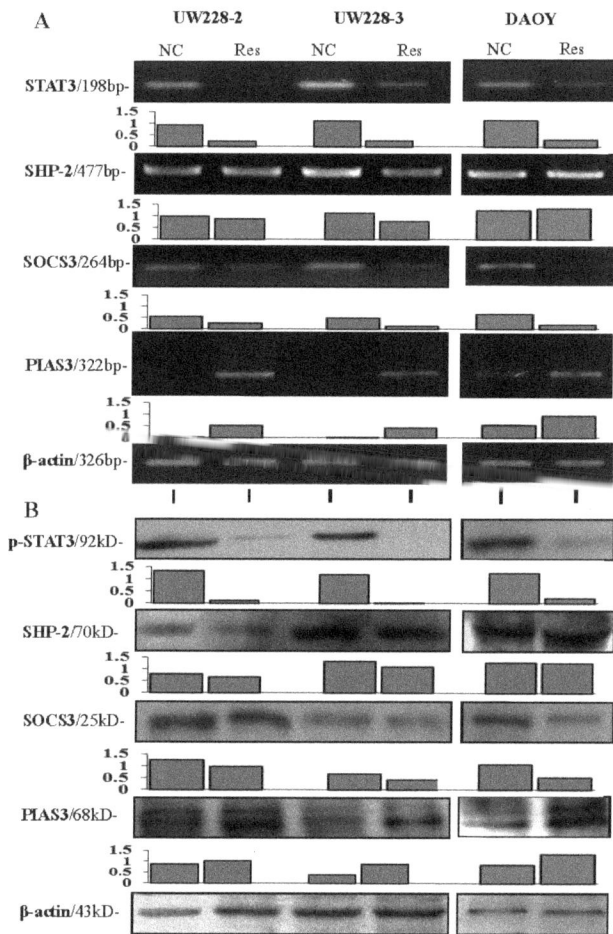

**Figure 5.** The results of RT-PCR (**A**) and Western blotting (**B**) and their grayscale analyses for STAT3, p-SHP2, SOCS3 and PIAS3 expression in three human medulloblastoma cell lines without and with 100 μM resveratrol treatment for 48 h.

### 3.6. SOCS3 Knockdown Caused Process Shortening

The results of RT-PCR demonstrate that the level of SOCS3 transcription is remarkably suppressed (Figure 6A), accompanied with decreased SOCS3 immuno-labeling in SOCS3 siRNA transfected cells (Figure 6B). H/E staining (data not shown) and viable:nonviable cell counting (Figure 6C) reveal that neither morphological alteration nor distinct cell death are found in the transfected population. p-STAT3-oriented immunocytochemical staining demonstrates p-STAT3 nuclear translocation in normally cultured transfectants and its remarkable reduction after resveratrol treatment (Figure 6D). After being treated by 100 μM resveratrol, the SOCS3 siRNA transfectants show distinct growth arrest in a time-related fashion (Figure 6C) without forming long axon-like processes (Figure 6B,D). SOCS3 level and growth of UW228-3 cells treated by 10 µM mock oligonucleotides are similar to those of normally cultured cells (Figure 6A,B).

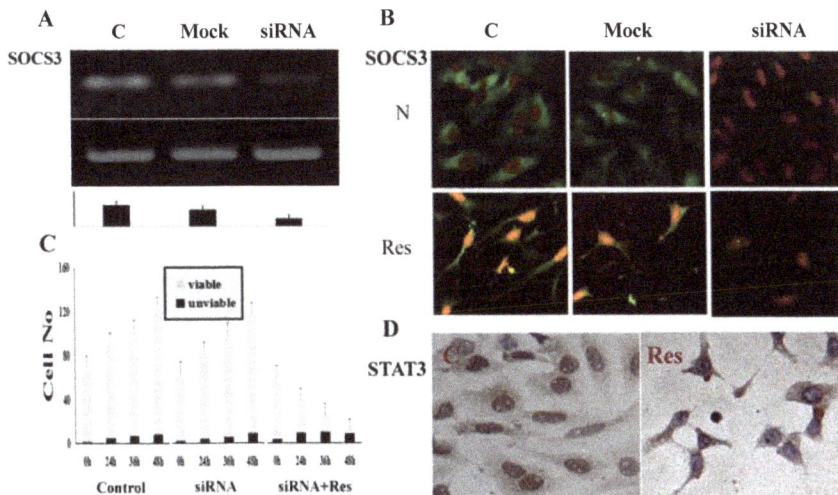

**Figure 6.** Knockdown of SOCS3 expression and its influence in STAT3 activation, resveratrol-sensitivity and axon-like process regeneration of medulloblastoma UW228-3 cells. (**A**) RT-PCR demonstration of SOCS3 downregulation in SOCS3-specific siRNA transfected UW228-3 cells (siRNA). The normally cultured (C), and mock RNA transfected (mock) cells are used as controls; (**B**) Immunofluorescent illustration (20×) of SOCS3 expression and intracellular distribution in normally cultured (C), mock RNA transfected (mock) and SOCS3-specific siRNA transfected UW228-3 cells (siRNA) before (N) and after resveratrol treatment (Res); (**C**) Viable:nonviable cell counting (mean cell number/visual field) reveals no influence of SOCS3 knockdown in the proliferation and resveratrol sensitivity of UW228-3 cells. N, UW228-3 cells without siRNA transfection; siRNA, normally cultured SOCS3 siRNA transfected UW228-3 cells; siRNA+Res, 100 µM resveratrol-treated UW228-3 cells with SOCS3 siRNA transfection; (**D**) SOCS3 knockdown exerts little effect on STAT3 activation in normally cultured cells (C) and resveratrol-caused STAT3 inactivation of UW228-3 cells (Res).

## 4. Discussion

Severe short- and long-term adverse effects and frequent drug resistance are the major therapeutic dilemma in the management of childhood medulloblastomas [2–4]. It is therefore necessary to explore safer and more effective anti-medulloblastoma drugs. Our previous studies demonstrate that resveratrol efficiently suppresses growth and induces neuronal-like differentiation and extensive apoptosis of human medulloblastoma cells [9,19–21]. More importantly, this polyphenol compound has little harmful effect on rat glial cells and neurons in vitro and in vivo [16,18], suggesting its suitability for treating this sort of pediatric malignancy and the need to investigate the molecular event(s) occurring in resveratrol-treated medulloblastoma cells.

STAT3 signaling plays a pivotal role in regulating differentiation and proliferation of neuronal cells [26] and its activation is closely related with brain cancer formation [27,28]. Accordingly, our current study reveals that STAT3 nuclear translocation is frequently observed in classical and large-cell medulloblastomas in comparison with the tumor-surrounding brain tissues. According to the clinical data, the prognoses of medulloblastomas vary in a subtype-related manner. For instance, the patients with nodular tumors usually have relatively better prognoses, while the fates of the patients with classic and especially large-cell tumors are extremely poor [29]. Because some cancer prognostic factors such as VEGF, Bcl-2 and survivin are the downstream genes of STAT3 signaling, the constitutive

STAT3 activation may lead to unfavorable outcomes for the large-cell and classic medulloblastomas. In this context, it would be worthwhile to elucidate the statuses of STAT3 regulatory factors and their correlations with STAT3 activation in medulloblastomas.

It has been recognized that STAT3 signaling can be regulated positively [28,29] or negatively [10–14]. Multiple factors have been identified as STAT3 signaling promoters, including IL-6 [30] and LIF [31] which are over expressed in medulloblastomas [32]. Nevertheless, we found that LIF was up-regulated in resveratrol-treated medulloblastoma cells with STAT3 inactivation presumably due to the feedback loop of STAT3 and LIF in those cells [9]. Alternatively, this finding suggests the presence of additional factor(s) that might negatively regulate STAT3 signaling. However, no report is so far available concerning the statuses of intrinsic STAT3 inhibitory factors in medulloblastomas and the impacts of resveratrol in their expression.

Several molecular factors are supposed to negatively regulate STAT3 signaling in different manners. PIAS3 inhibits STAT3 signaling by interrupting the interaction of p-STAT3 with its target genes [12]; SHP2 is a non-receptor type protein tyrosine phosphatases and its phosphorylated form (p-SHP2) interferes STAT-3 activation by dephosphorylating the active STAT-3 complexes in the cytoplasm and in nucleus [10]. SOCS3 works in a classic negative feedback loop to attenuate STAT3 activity by suppressive binding with phosphorylated JAK [14] and/or facilitating ubiqitination of JAK in the cytoplasm [33]. To shed light on the potential link(s) of these three negative regulators to STAT3 activation, their expression patterns in the three subtypes of medulloblastomas were profiled by tissue microarray-based immunohistochemical staining. The results revealed the general reductions of p-SHP2, SOCS3 and especially PIAS3 levels in the three medulloblastoma subtypes with frequent p-STAT3 nuclear translocation. It was also found that p-SHP2 downregulation was inversely correlated with STAT3 activation in classic but not large-cell medulloblastomas, suggesting differential regulation of STAT3 signaling in the histological subtypes of medulloblastomas. It would be therefore necessary to clarify whether the downregulation of those negative regulators is directly linked to or merely the paralleled molecular events with STAT3 activation. Alternatively, it would be more convincing if the levels of SHP2, SOCS1/SOCS3 and/or PIAS3 are altered accordingly in medulloblastoma cells with suppressed STAT3 signaling.

Our previous results clearly demonstrated that resveratrol can attenuate STAT3 activation of medulloblastoma cells via inhibiting STAT3 transcription and nuclear translocation [9]. Therefore, the resveratrol-treated medulloblastoma cells would be an ideal model to evaluate the role of SHP2, SOCS3 or PIAS3 in regulating STAT3 signaling. It is found that upon resveratrol treatment, PIAS3 is up-regulated and translocalized in nuclei, SOCS3 level is reduced and SHP2 remains unchanged in the three medulloblastoma cells so far checked. These findings thus suggest that of the three so-called STAT3 negative regulators examined here, PIAS3 rather than the other two proteins may be more correlated with resveratrol-caused STAT3 inactivation.

It has been proposed that SOCS3 is up-regulated as a feedback response to STAT3 activation [13,14]. Therefore, it would be possible that SOCS3 level is reduced in resveratrol-treated medulloblastoma cells with suppressed STAT3 signaling. The maintenance of STAT3 activation in SCOS3 siRNA transfected UW228-3 cells is in accordance with this notion. It has been evidenced that resveratrol inhibits growth and induces neuronal-like differentiation of human medulloblastoma cells [9]. Our finding of preferable accumulation and intracellular rearrangement of SOCS3 to the synapse-like end of the long processes indicates the involvement of this protein in axon regeneration [34]. This speculation is elucidated and proved by treating SOCS3 siRNA transfected UW228-3 cells with resveratrol, because the transfectants remain sensitive to resveratrol but fail to form axon-like long processes. These findings also suggest SOCS3 as a potential indicator of resveratrol-promoted neuronal differentiation of medulloblastoma cells.

## 5. Conclusions

Taken together, the expression patterns of three STAT3 negative regulators and their correlation with STAT3 activation in human medulloblastomas are investigated in this study. The results reveal that PIAS3 downregulation is more reversely correlated with STAT3 activation. PIAS3 upregulation and nuclear translocation in resveratrol-treated medulloblastoma cells with suppressed STAT3 signaling further suggests the negative regulatory effects of PIAS3 on STAT3 signaling and the potential value of PIAS3 in evaluating the prognosis of medulloblastoma patients. Inhibition of resveratrol-induced long process formation by SOCS3 siRNA transfection suggests the active role of SOCS3 in axon regeneration. In the future, we will further elucidate the influence of PIAS3 manipulation in the survival and resveratrol sensitivities of medulloblastoma cells.

**Acknowledgments:** This work was supported by grants from National Natural Science Foundation of China (No. 81272786) and the special research fund for outstanding scholar of Dalian Medical University to Jia Liu. We thank the doctors in the Department of Clinical Pathology of Sheng-Jing Hospital, China Medical University for their cooperation in sample collection and pathological consultation.

**Author Contributions:** Hong Li and Jia Liu carried out experiments, data analyses and manuscript writing; Cong Li, Peng Zhang, Li-Jun Yu and Tian-Miao Huang performed experiments; Xue Song cultured cells; Qing-You Kong constructed tissue microarrays; Jian-Li Dong and Pei-Nan Li collected surgical specimens. All authors read and approved the final manuscript.

**Conflicts of Interest:** The authors declare no conflict of interest.

## References

1. Gottardo, N.G.; Hansford, J.R.; McGlade, J.P.; Alvaro, F.; Ashley, D.M.; Bailey, S.; Baker, D.L.; Bourdeaut, F.; Cho, Y.; Clay, M.; et al. Medulloblastoma down under 2013: A report from the third annual meeting of the International Medulloblastoma Working Group. *Acta Neuropathol.* **2014**, *127*, 189–201. [CrossRef] [PubMed]
2. Ramaswamy, V.; Remke, M.; Bouffet, E.; Faria, C.C.; Perreault, S.; Cho, Y.J.; Shih, D.J.; Lu, B.; Dubuc, A.M.; Northcott, P.A.; et al. Recurrence patterns across medulloblastoma subgroups: An integrated clinical and molecular analysis. *Lancet Oncol.* **2013**, *14*, 1200–1207. [CrossRef]
3. Pritchard, J.R.; Lauffenburger, D.A.; Hemann, M.T. Understanding resistance to combination chemotherapy. *Drug Resist. Updates* **2012**, *15*, 249–257. [CrossRef] [PubMed]
4. Cox, M.C.; Kusters, J.M.; Gidding, C.E.; Schieving, J.H.; van Lindert, E.J.; Kaanders, J.H.; Janssens, G.O. Acute toxicity profile of craniospinal irradiation with intensity-modulated radiation therapy in children with medulloblastoma: A prospective analysis. *Radiat. Oncol.* **2015**, *10*, 241. [CrossRef] [PubMed]
5. Yang, F.; Jove, V.; Xin, H.; Hedvat, M.; Van Meter, T.E.; Yu, H. Sunitinib induces apoptosis and growth arrest of medulloblastoma tumor cells by inhibiting STAT3 and AKT signaling pathways. *Mol. Cancer Res.* **2010**, *8*, 35–45. [CrossRef] [PubMed]
6. Ellison, D.W.; Dalton, J.; Kocak, M.; Nicholson, S.L.; Fraga, C.; Neale, G.; Kenney, A.M.; Brat, D.J.; Perry, A.; Yong, W.H.; et al. Medulloblastoma: Clinicopathological correlates of SHH, WNT, and non-SHH/WNT molecular subgroups. *Acta Neuropathol.* **2011**, *121*, 381–396. [CrossRef] [PubMed]
7. Hatton, B.A.; Villavicencio, E.H.; Pritchard, J.; LeBlanc, M.; Hansen, S.; Ulrich, M.; Ditzler, S.; Pullar, B.; Stroud, M.R.; Olson, J.M. Notch signaling is not essential in sonic hedgehog-activated medulloblastoma. *Oncogene* **2010**, *29*, 3865–3872. [CrossRef] [PubMed]
8. Xiao, H.; Bid, H.K.; Jou, D.; Wu, X.; Yu, W.; Li, C.; Houghton, P.J.; Lin, J. A novel small molecular STAT3 inhibitor, LY5, inhibits cell viability, cell migration, and angiogenesis in medulloblastoma cells. *J. Biol. Chem.* **2015**, *290*, 3418–3429. [CrossRef] [PubMed]
9. Yu, L.-J.; Wu, M.-L.; Li, H.; Chen, X.-Y.; Wang, Q.; Sun, Y.; Kong, Q.Y.; Liu, J. Inhibition of STAT3 expression and signaling in resveratrol-differentiated medulloblastoma cells. *Neoplasia* **2008**, *10*, 736–744. [CrossRef] [PubMed]
10. Phromnoi, K.; Prasad, S.; Gupta, S.C.; Kannappan, R.; Reuter, S.; Limtrakul, P.; Aggarwal, B.B. Dihydroxypentamethoxyflavone down-regulates constitutive and inducible signal transducers and activators of transcription-3 through the induction of tyrosine phosphatase SHP-1. *Mol. Pharmacol.* **2011**, *80*, 889–899. [CrossRef] [PubMed]

11. Siveen, K.S.; Nguyen, A.H.; Lee, J.H.; Li, F.; Singh, S.S.; Kumar, A.P.; Low, G.; Jha, S.; Tergaonkar, V.; Ahn, K.S.; et al. Negative regulation of signal transducer and activator of transcription-3 signalling cascade by lupeol inhibits growth and induces apoptosis in hepatocellular carcinoma cells. *Br. J. Cancer* **2014**, *111*, 1327–1337. [CrossRef] [PubMed]

12. Dabir, S.; Kluge, A.; Dowlati, A. The association and nuclear translocation of PIAS3-STAT3 complex is ligand and time dependent. *Mol. Cancer Res.* **2009**, *7*, 1854–1860. [CrossRef] [PubMed]

13. Zhang, W.N.; Wang, L.; Wang, Q.; Luo, X.; Fang, D.F.; Chen, Y.; Pan, X.; Man, J.H.; Xia, Q.; Jin, B.F.; et al. CUEDC2 (CUE Domain-containing 2) and SOCS3 (Suppressors of Cytokine Signaling 3) cooperate to negatively regulate janus kinase 1/signal transducers and activators of transcription 3 signaling. *J. Biol. Chem.* **2012**, *287*, 382–392. [CrossRef] [PubMed]

14. Jiang, C.; Kim, J.H.; Li, F.; Qu, A.; Gavrilova, O.; Shah, Y.M.; Gonzalez, F.J. Hypoxia-inducible factor 1α regulates a SOCS3-STAT3-adiponectin signal transduction pathway in adipocytes. *J. Biol. Chem.* **2013**, *288*, 3844–3857. [CrossRef] [PubMed]

15. Jiao, Y.M.; Li, H.; Liu, Y.D.; Guo, A.C.; Xu, X.X.; Qu, X.J.; Wang, S.; Zhao, J.Z.; Li, Y.; Cao, Y. Resveratrol inhibits the invasion of glioblastoma-initiating cells via down-regulation of the PI3K/Akt/NF-kappa B signaling pathway. *Nutrients* **2015**, *7*, 4383–4402. [CrossRef] [PubMed]

16. Shu, X.H.; Li, H.; Sun, X.X.; Wang, Q.; Sun, Z.; Wu, M.L.; Chen, X.Y.; Li, C.; Kong, Q.Y.; Liu, J. Metabolic patterns and biotransformation activities of resveratrol in human glioblastoma cells: Relevance with therapeutic efficacies. *PLoS ONE* **2011**, *6*, e27484. [CrossRef] [PubMed]

17. Wu, M.L.; Li, H.; Yu, L.J.; Chen, X.Y.; Kong, Q.Y.; Song, X.; Shu, X.H.; Liu, J. Short-term resveratrol exposure causes in vitro and in vivo growth inhibition and apoptosis of bladder cancer cells. *PLoS ONE* **2014**, *9*, e89806. [CrossRef] [PubMed]

18. Shu, X.H.; Wang, L.L.; Li, H.; Song, X.; Shi, S.; Gu, J.Y.; Wu, M.L.; Chen, X.Y.; Kong, Q.Y.; Liu, J. Diffusion efficiency and bioavailability of resveratrol administered to rat brain by different routes: Therapeutic implications. *Neurotherapeutics* **2015**, *12*, 491–501. [CrossRef] [PubMed]

19. Shu, X.H.; Li, H.; Sun, Z.; Wu, M.L.; Ma, J.X.; Wang, J.M.; Wang, Q.; Sun, Y.; Fu, Y.S.; Chen, X.Y.; et al. Identification of metabolic pattern and bioactive form of resveratrol in human medulloblastoma cells. *Biochem. Pharmacol.* **2010**, *79*, 1516–1525. [CrossRef] [PubMed]

20. Wang, Q.; Li, H.; Liu, N.; Chen, X.Y.; Wu, M.L.; Zhang, K.L.; Kong, Q.Y.; Liu, J. Correlative analyses of notch signaling with resveratrol-induced differentiation and apoptosis of human medulloblastoma cells. *Neurosci. Lett.* **2008**, *438*, 168–173. [CrossRef] [PubMed]

21. Wen, S.; Li, H.; Wu, M.L.; Fan, S.H.; Wang, Q.; Shu, X.H.; Kong, Q.Y.; Chen, X.Y.; Liu, J. Inhibition of NF-κB signaling commits resveratrol-treated medulloblastoma cells to apoptosis without neuronal differentiation. *J. Neuro-Oncol.* **2011**, *104*, 169–177. [CrossRef] [PubMed]

22. Li, H.; Chen, X.Y.; Kong, Q.Y.; Liu, J. Cytopathological evaluations combined RNA and protein analyses on defined cell regions using single frozen tissue block. *Cell Res.* **2002**, *12*, 117–121. [CrossRef] [PubMed]

23. Liu, Y.X.; Dong, X.; Gong, F.; Su, N.; Li, S.; Zhang, H.T.; Liu, J.L.; Xue, J.H.; Ji2, S.P.; Zhang, Z.W. Promotion of erythropoietic differentiation in hematopoietic stem cells by SOCS3 knock-down. *PLoS ONE* **2015**, *10*, e0135259. [CrossRef] [PubMed]

24. Fu, Y.S.; Wang, Q.; Ma, J.X.; Yang, X.H.; Wu, M.L.; Zhang, K.L.; Kong, Q.Y.; Chen, X.Y.; Sun, Y.; Chen, N.N.; et al. CRABP-II methylation: A critical determinant of retinoic acid resistance of medulloblastoma cells. *Mol. Oncol.* **2012**, *6*, 48–61. [CrossRef] [PubMed]

25. Ellison, D. Classifying the medulloblastoma: Insights from morphology and molecular genetics. *Neuropathol. Appl. Neurobiol.* **2002**, *1*, 257–282. [CrossRef]

26. Wen, S.; Li, H.; Liu, J. Epigenetic background of neuronal fate determination. *Prog. Neurobiol.* **2009**, *87*, 98–117. [CrossRef] [PubMed]

27. Sherry, M.M.; Reeves, A.; Wu, J.K.; Cochran, B.H. STAT3 is required for proliferation and maintenance of multipotency in glioblastoma stem cells. *Stem Cells* **2009**, *27*, 2383–2392. [CrossRef] [PubMed]

28. Gu, D.; Fan, Q.; Zhang, X.; Xie, J. A role for transcription factor STAT3 signaling in oncogene smoothened-driven carcinogenesis. *J. Biol. Chem.* **2012**, *287*, 38356–38366. [CrossRef] [PubMed]

29. MacDonald, T.J.; Aguilera, D.; Castellino, R.C. The rationale for targeted therapies in medulloblastoma. *Neuro Oncol.* **2014**, *16*, 9–20. [CrossRef] [PubMed]

30. Rodriguez-Barrueco, R.; Yu, J.; Saucedo-Cuevas, L.P.; Olivan, M.; Llobet-Navas, D.; Putcha, P.; Castro, V.; Murga-Penas, E.M.; Collazo-Lorduy, A.; Castillo-Martin, M.; et al. Inhibition of the autocrine IL-6–JAK2–STAT3–calprotectin axis as targeted therapy for HR$^-$/HER2$^+$ breast cancers. *Genes Dev.* **2015**, *29*, 1631–1648. [CrossRef] [PubMed]
31. Liu, X.; Tseng, S.C.; Zhang, M.C.; Chen, S.Y.; Tighe, S.; Lu, W.J.; Zhu, Y.T. LIF-JAK1-STAT3 signaling delays contact inhibition of human corneal endothelial cells. *Cell Cycle* **2015**, *14*, 1197–1206. [CrossRef] [PubMed]
32. Liu, J.; Li, J.W.; Gang, Y.; Guo, L.; Li, H. Expression of leukemia inhibitory factor (LIF) as an autocrinal growth factor in human medulloblastomas. *J. Cancer Res. Clin. Oncol.* **1999**, *125*, 475–480. [CrossRef] [PubMed]
33. Gao, Y.; Cimica, V.; Reich, N.C. Suppressor of cytokine signaling 3 inhibits breast tumor kinase activation of STAT3. *J. Biol. Chem.* **2012**, *287*, 20904–20912. [CrossRef] [PubMed]
34. Liu, X.; Williams, P.R.; He, Z. SOCS3: A common target for neuronal protection and axon regeneration after spinal cord injury. *Exp. Neurol.* **2015**, *263*, 364–367. [CrossRef] [PubMed]

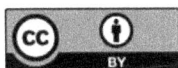

*nutrients*

MDPI

*Article*

# Effects of Phytoestrogen Extracts Isolated from Elder Flower on Hormone Production and Receptor Expression of Trophoblast Tumor Cells JEG-3 and BeWo, as well as MCF7 Breast Cancer Cells

Lennard Schroder [1], Dagmar Ulrike Richter [2], Birgit Piechulla [3], Mareike Chrobak [3], Christina Kuhn [1], Sandra Schulze [1], Sybille Abarzua [3], Udo Jeschke [1,*] and Tobias Weissenbacher [1]

[1] Department of Obstetrics and Gynaecology, Ludwig-Maximilians-University of Munich, Munich 80337, Germany; lennard.schroeder@med.uni-muenchen.de (L.S.); Christina.kuhn@med.uni-muenchen.de (C.K.); sandra.schulze@med.uni-muenchen.de (S.S.); tobias.weissenbacher@med.uni-muenchen.de (T.W.)
[2] Department of Obstetrics and Gynaecology, University of Rostock, Rostock 18059, Germany; dagmar.richter@kliniksued-rostock.de
[3] Department of Biological Sciences, University of Rostock, Rostock 18059, Germany; birgit.piechulla@uni-rostock.de (B.P.); chrobak@bni-hamburg.de (M.C.); sybille.abarzua@uni-rostock.de (S.A.)
* Correspondence: udo.jeschke@med.uni-muenchen.de; Tel.: +49-89-51604240, Fax: +49-89-51604916

Received: 15 July 2016; Accepted: 22 September 2016; Published: 8 October 2016

**Abstract:** Herein we investigated the effect of elderflower extracts (EFE) and of enterolactone/enterodiol on hormone production and proliferation of trophoblast tumor cell lines JEG-3 and BeWo, as well as MCF7 breast cancer cells. The EFE was analyzed by mass spectrometry. Cells were incubated with various concentrations of EFE. Untreated cells served as controls. Supernatants were tested for estradiol production with an ELISA method. Furthermore, the effect of the EFE on ERα/ERβ/PR expression was assessed by immunocytochemistry. EFE contains a substantial amount of lignans. Estradiol production was inhibited in all cells in a concentration-dependent manner. EFE upregulated ERα in JEG-3 cell lines. In MCF7 cells, a significant ERα downregulation and PR upregulation were observed. The control substances enterolactone and enterodiol in contrast inhibited the expression of both ER and of PR in MCF7 cells. In addition, the production of estradiol was upregulated in BeWo and MCF7 cells in a concentration dependent manner. The downregulating effect of EFE on ERα expression and the upregulation of the PR expression in MFC-7 cells are promising results. Therefore, additional unknown substances might be responsible for ERα downregulation and PR upregulation. These findings suggest potential use of EFE in breast cancer prevention and/or treatment and warrant further investigation.

**Keywords:** lignans; isoflavones; elder flower; breast cancer; trophoblast tumor

---

## 1. Introduction

A growing body of data points to health benefits of phytoestrogens in diet and to possible pharmaceutical applications [1]. The two main groups of phytoestrogens, isoflavones and lignans, are polyphenolic compounds derived from plants with a molecular structure that closely resembles mammalian estrogens [2]. Due to their molecular structure, these compounds can bind and interact with human estrogen receptors (ER) resulting in both estrogen and anti-estrogen effects [3]. Thus, it is assumed that some phytoestrogens can be classified as selective estrogen receptor modulators (SERM) [4,5].

Isoflavones are mostly found in legumes, with the most common representative being soy and its derivative products [6], making them more common in Asian diets, whereas lignans, more common in occidental diets, are usually found in seeds and fiber-rich cereals [7,8]. Their role in the pathogenesis of hormone-dependent malignancies, especially breast cancer, has been investigated using chemically pure isolates or product extracts in several in vitro or in vivo models [9–11]. Their effects as hormonally-active diet components have been excessively and controversially discussed [12,13]. Isoflavone extracts and supplements are often used for the treatment of menopausal symptoms and for the prevention of age-associated conditions, such as cardiovascular diseases and osteoporosis in postmenopausal women [12].

In humans the most important lignans are secoisolariciresinol and matairesinol [14].

After oral intake they are transformed by intestinal aerobe and anerobe flora into bioavailable enterolignans enterodiol and enterolactone [15].

Clinical studies proved that a high exposition to enterolignans reduced the risk of breast cancer by 16% [16]. Moreover, increased blood concentrations of enterolactone in postmenopausal women are related with a significant reduction of breast cancer mortality [17].

With the goal of identifying potential sources of phytoestrogens and selecting those with beneficial functions, our group has tested, in prior trials, the phytoestrogen properties of pumpkin and flax seed lignan and isoflavone extracts on the proliferation of trophoblast and breast cancer cell lines [18,19]. Moreover, the effect of the phytoestrogens genistein and daidzein on human term trophoblasts and their influence on fertility was investigated [20].

Elder flower (*Sambucus nigra*) is a historically-significant herbal medicinal plant used for centuries as a cold remedy. It is used as a general nutritive tonic and due to its strong taste as a flavor enhancer in meals and beverages. Elder extracts possess significant antioxidant activity and have been shown to impair angiogenesis. The anthocyanins present in elderberries protect vascular epithelial cells against oxidative insult, and reduce low-density lipoprotein (LDL) and cholesterol, therefore, preventing vascular disease [21]. Elder extracts boost cytokine production [22]. The influenza A virus subtype H1N1 inhibition activities of the elder flavonoids compare favorably to the known anti-influenza activities of oseltamivir and amantadine [23]. The terpenes extracted from elder flower show notably strong antimicrobial effects in vitro upon methicillin-resistant *Staphylococcus aureus* [24]. Moreover elder flower could improve bone properties by inhibiting the process of bone resorption and stimulating the process of bone formation [25].

Due to the interesting characteristics of elder flower described above, this in vitro study aims to identify the distribution of lignans and isoflavones in elder flower extracts (EFE) and evaluate the potential phytoestrogen effects of EFE on tumor trophoblast BeWo and JEG-3 cells and the ER-positive MCF7 breast cancer cell lines, and compare those with the effects of enterodiol and enterolactone.

## 2. Materials and Methods

### 2.1. Preparation of the EFE

In total six EFE from the species *Sambucus nigra* were produced. Three lignan-isolations were prepared as previously described [26] and, afterwards, dissolved in 100% ethanol. In the aim to verify the previously-reported increased lignan concentration in elder flowers [27] the molecular–chemical composition of the extract was further analyzed by pyrolysis-field ionization mass spectrometry by using an LCQ-Advantage (Thermo Finnigan's, Arcade, NY, USA). The peaks were identified by ion trap technology in electrospray ionisation (ESI) mode. The source voltage was set at 4.5 kV, while the mass detection range was 150–2000 amu. For the production of the three flavonoid extracts, the method previously described by Franz and Koehler was used [28].

## 2.2. Cell Lines

For the current work the chorion carcinoma cell lines JEG-3 and BeWo, and the breast carcinoma cell line MCF7, were used. All cell lines were obtained from the European Collection of Cell Cultures (ECACC, Salisbury, UK). The cells were grown in Dulbecco's Modified Eagle Medium (DMEM) without phenol red (Biochrom AG, Berlin, Germany) supplemented with 10% heat-inactivated fetal calf serum (PAA Laboratories GmbH, Pasching, Austria), 100 µg/mL Penicillin/Streptomycin (Biochrom AG) and 2.5 µg/mL Amphotericin B (Biochrom AG). Cultures were maintained in a humidified incubator at 37 °C with a 5% $CO_2$ atmosphere. Prior to cell culture, the levels of estrogen or progesterone in the medium were measured, using an automated Immulite (DPC Biermann, Freiburg, Germany) hormone analyzer, in order to exclude their presence.

## 2.3. Effect of EFE on Cell Lines

For all experiments, the cells were seeded on Quadriperm tissue slides with or without added lignan and flavonoid EFE separately. In brief, cells were seeded at a concentration of 400,000 cells per slide. The cells were left to attach for 24 h. Then, the medium was replaced by medium supplemented with lignan and flavonoid EFE separately at final effective concentrations of 10, 50, and 100 µg/mL. Since the original EFE was diluted in 100% ethanol, medium supplemented with 100% ethanol at a concentration of 5 µg/mL (this being the maximum ethanol concentration achieved during these experiments) served as the internal control. In addition, enterolactone and enterodiol (Sigma Aldrich Taufkirchen, Germany) were added to the same cell cultures as used for EFE in concentrations of 10, 50, and 100 µg/mL, respectively. After the cells were cultured for 72 h, 1 mL from each supernatant was stored at −80 °C for estradiol analysis. The remaining supernatant was then discarded and the slides were washed in phosphate-buffered saline (PBS), fixed in acetone for 10 min, and left to dry at room temperature. Cells treated with equal concentrations of estradiol (10, 50, and 100 µg/mL) served as external controls.

## 2.4. Estradiol Determination in the Cell Culture Medium

For the determination of estradiol in the culture medium, a competitive enzyme immuno-assay (EIA) was applied as described previously [29]. The measurements were performed using an automated Immulite 2000 (DPC Biermann, Freiburg, Germany) hormone analyzer.

## 2.5. Immunocytochemistry for the ERα, ERβ, and Progesterone Receptor (PR)

For immuno-detection of the steroid receptors ERα, ERβ, and PR, the Vectastain R Elite Avidin/Biotin Complex (ABC) Kit (Vector Laboratories, Burlingame, CA, USA) was used according to the manufacturer's protocol. After being air dried, the slides were rinsed in PBS for 5 min and incubated with the ABC normal serum for 60 min in a humidified environment. The slides were then washed and incubated with the respective primary antibodies. Salient features of the antibodies used are presented in Table 1. The slides were then incubated with the diluted biotinylated secondary antibody (30 min), followed by incubation with the ABC reagent (30 min), and the ABC substrate (15 min). A PBS wash (5 min) was applied between steps. Finally, the slides were counterstained with Mayer's acidic hematoxylin (30 s), rinsed with water, and covered with Aquatex. The intensity and distribution patterns of the specific immunocytochemical staining was evaluated using a semi-quantitative method (IRS score) as previously described [30]. Briefly, the IRS score was calculated as the product of the optical staining intensity (0 = no staining; 1 = weak staining; 2 = moderate staining; and 3 = strong straining) multiplied by staining extent (0 = no staining; 1% ≤ 10% staining; 2 = 11%–50% staining; 3 = 51%–80% staining and 4 ≥ 80% staining). The percentage of positively-stained cells was estimated by counting approximately 100 cells.

**Table 1.** Antibodies used for expression analysis of steroid hormone receptors.

| Salient Features of the Antibodies Used in the Present Study | | | | |
|---|---|---|---|---|
| Antibody | (Source) | Origin | Dilution in PBS | Temperature |
| Anti-ERcr | (Dako, Germany) | Mouse monoclonal | 1:150 | 1 h RT |
| Anti-ERβ | (Serotec, Germany) | Mouse monoclonal | 1:600 | O/N 4 °C |
| Anti-PR | (Dako, Germany) | Mouse monoclonal | 1:50 | 1 h RT |

ER = estrogen receptor; PR = progesterone receptor; O/N = overnight; RT = room temperature.

## 2.6. Statistical Analysis

The results are presented as mean ± sem of three independent experiments. Statistical analysis was performed using the Wilcoxon's signed rank tests for pairwise comparisons. Each observation with $p < 0.05$ was considered statistically significant.

## 3. Results

### 3.1. EFE Contains Phytoestrogen Compounds

Mass spectrometry was performed to identify the different substrates and to determine their proportions in EFE. The results showed that the EFE contains phytoestrogen compounds. Lignan dimers (LDIM) were found with a total intensity of 2.6%, lignans (LIGNA) with 1.3%, isoflavones (ISOFL) with 0.6%, and flavones (FLAVO) with 0.1%. Figure 1 demonstrates the distribution of the different substance classes found in EFE. With a total intensity of 18.1% the most abundant substance class in EFE were lipids, including alcanes, alcenes, fatty acids, waxes, and fats (LIPID). Monolignoles (PHLM) were found with an intensity of 13.4% and carbohydrates (CHYDR) with 11.1%. Nitrogen (NCOMP) compounds were found with a total intensity of 6%, amino acids and peptides with 5.4% (PEPTI), isoprenoid compounds (ISOPR) with 1.5%, other polyphenolic (POLYO) with 5.2%, and low molecular compounds (LOWMW) with 4.7%.

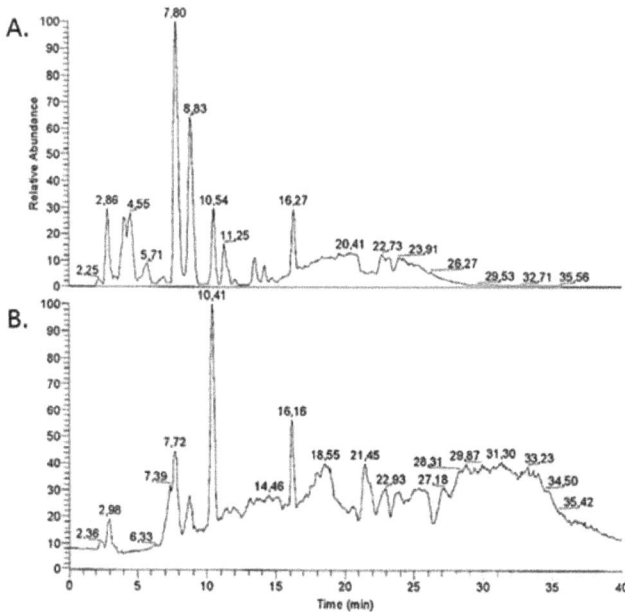

**Figure 1.** *Cont.*

C.

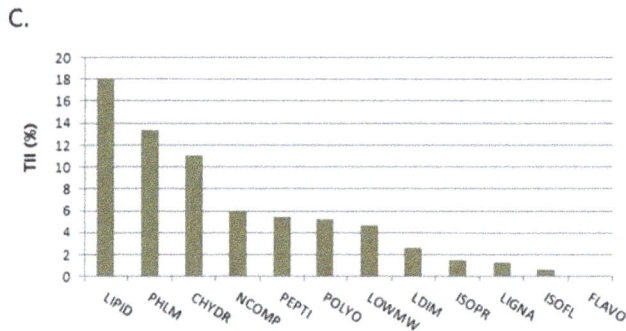

**Figure 1.** Characteristic diagram of mass spectrometry analysis results of the EFE using both the microwave extraction (**A**) and the extraction method modified from Luyengi et al. [26] (**B**); moreover, the different substances extracted are presented (**C**).

*3.2. EFE Lignan and Flavonoid Extracts Induce the Inhibition of Estradiol Secretion in JEG-3, BeWo, and MCF7 Cells in a Dose-Response Pattern and the Inhibition of Progesterone Secretion in JEG-3 Cells*

To assess the estradiol and progesterone secretion, all three cell lines were cultured for 72 h in the presence of different EFE concentrations. An automated hormone analyzer was used to determine the estradiol and progesterone concentration in the medium by applying a competitive EIA. All cell lines were incubated with elder flower flavonoid and lignan extracts. The EFE lignan and flavonoid extracts demonstrated a statistical significant inhibition in estradiol secretion in a dose-response pattern in all three cell lines (Figure 2). Only statistical significant data is demonstrated in the figures. The cell culture medium with 10% FCS did not contain any measurable amounts of estrogen and progesterone, as determined with the automated hormone analyzer Immulite (DPC Biermann, Freiburg, Germany).

In JEG-3 cells, the estradiol production was inhibited from $5634.96 \pm 235.77$ pg/mL in the control to $4547.48 \pm 145.89$ pg/mL, $1283.88 \pm 29.78$ pg/mL, and $1030.43 \pm 24.50$ pg/mL when the EFE lignan concentration was 10 µg/mL, 50 µg/mL, and 100 µg/mL, $p = 0.018$, respectively (Figure 2A). EFE flavonoids had a similar effect using the same concentrations, as the estradiol production was inhibited from $5634.97 \pm 235.77$ pg/mL in the control to $5049 \pm 187.28$ pg/mL, $1264.5 \pm 151.26$ pg/mL, and $1137 \pm 138.08$ pg/mL (Figure 2B).

In JEG-3 cell lines progesterone secretion was also significantly inhibited using EFE lignan extracts from $87.95 \pm 1.36$ pg/mL in the control to $84.88 \pm 1.98$ pg/mL, $66.22 \pm 2.25$ pg/mL, and $45.98 \pm 1.92$ pg/mL when the EFE concentration was 10 µg/mL, 50 µg/mL and 100 µg/mL.

The cultivation of the BeWo cell line with EFE lignan extracts resulted again in an inhibition of estradiol secretion from $245.25 \pm 16.25$ pg/mL in the control to $230.85 \pm 8.17$ pg/mL, $231.95 \pm 6.1$ pg/mL, and $206.81 \pm 5.69$ pg/mL when the EFE concentration was 10 µg/mL, 50 µg/mL, and 100 µg/mL (Figure 2C). The differences between the stimulated cells and the control were only significant at a concentration of 100 µg/mL, with $p = 0.05$.

In MCF7 cell lines the EFE flavonoid concentrations of 10 µg/mL and 50 µg/mL first provoked a transient increased secretion of estradiol from $146.37 \pm 9.91$ pg/mL in the control to $185.44 \pm 4.28$ pg/mL at 10 µg/mL and $164.07 \pm 3.16$ pg/mL at 50 µg/mL (Figure 2D). Then, at 100 µg/mL, the estradiol secretion was inhibited to $140.21 \pm 2.22$ pg/mL, $p = 0.08$ respectively.

Using the same concentrations with EFE flavonoid-extracts, progesterone secretion was also significantly inhibited in JEG-3 cells (Figure 2E) from $104.83 \pm 5.13$ pg/mL in the control to $77.94 \pm 1.32$ pg/mL, $56.18 \pm 1.7$ pg/mL, and $47.76 \pm 1.56$ pg/mL ($p = 0.043$).

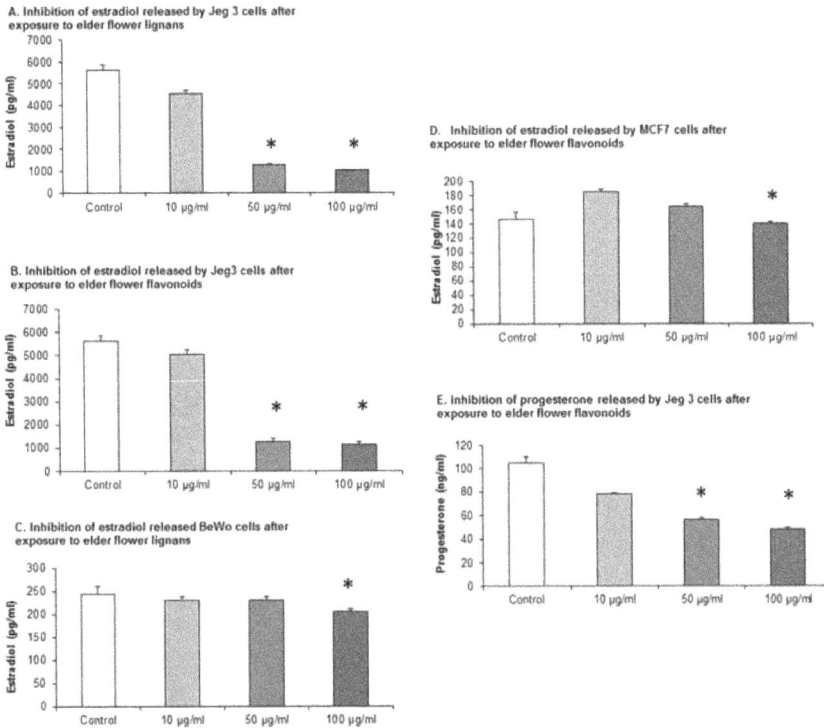

**Figure 2.** Estradiol and progesterone concentration in the tissue culture medium of JEG-3, BeWo, and MCF7 cells in the absence or presence of EFE. The effective EFE concentrations were 10 µg/mL, 50 µg/mL, and 100 µg/mL. Significantly different observations are highlighted with an asterisk.

### 3.3. EFE Flavonoid Extracts up Regulates ERα in JEG-3 Cells

JEG-3 cell lines that were cultivated with EFE flavonoid in the concentrations of 10 µg/mL, 50 µg/mL, and 100 µg/mL an upregulation of ERα was demonstrated. The IRS score of ERα was increased from $1 \pm 0$ in the control to $1.33 \pm 0.23$, $1.67 \pm 0.54$, and $2.167 \pm 0.44$. At 100 µg/mL statistical significance was demonstrated, $p = 0.015$, respectively (Figure 3A).

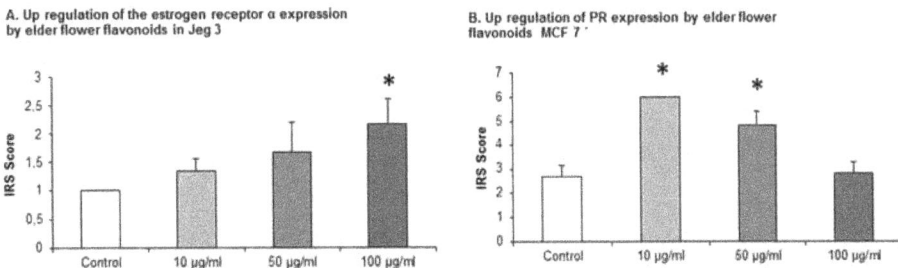

**Figure 3.** Upregulation of ER α and progesterone receptor by elder flower flavonoids in JEG-3 and MCF7 cells. The effective EFE concentrations were 10 µg/mL, 50 µg/mL, and 100 µg/mL. Significantly different observations are highlighted with an asterisk.

### 3.4. EFE Flavonoids Downregulate ER α and EFE Lignans and Flavonoids Upregulate the PR in a Dose-Response Pattern Predominantly in Lower Concentrations in MCF7 Cells

MCF7 cells that were exposed to EFE flavonoids with the concentrations of 10 µg/mL, 50 µg/mL, and 100 µg/mL responded significantly with a downregulation of ER α at the concentrations of 10 µg/mL (3.5 ± 0.55) and 50 µg/mL (6.3 ± 0.88) compared to the control (11.33 ± 0.73, $p$ = 0.002 and 0.004), (Figure 4A).

MCF7 cells that were exposed to EFE lignan and flavonoid extracts with the concentrations of 10 µg/mL, 50 µg/mL, and 100 µg/mL responded significantly in an upregulation of the PR in a dose-response pattern (Figure 4B). The upregulation of the progesterone IRS score significantly reached a peak at the EFE lignan concentration of 10 µg/mL (8 ± 0.98) compared to the control (3.3 ± 0.36, $p$ = 0.002). As the EFE concentration increased, the IRS score decreased at 50 µg/mL to 7.66 ± 1.04, and at 100 µg/mL to 5.83 (Figure 4B).

The same phenomenon was observed using EFE flavonoids where the IRS score increased from 2.66 ± 0.46 in the control to 6 ± 0 at 10 µg/mL ($p$ = 0.002), and then decreased to 4.83 ± 0.59 ($p$ = 0.026) at 50 µg/mL, and to 2.83 ± 0.44 at 100 µg/mL (Figure 3B).

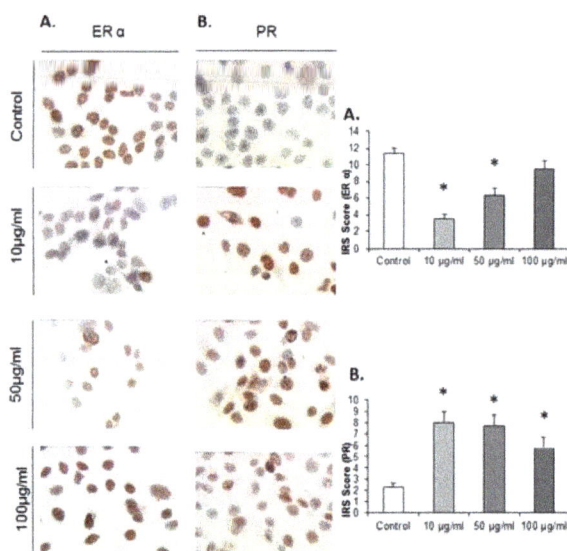

**Figure 4.** Representative microphotographs of MCF7 cells grown in the absence or presence of elder flower extract (at effective EFE concentrations of 10 µg/mL, 50 µg/mL, and 100 µg/mL), after immuno-detection of ER-α (**A**) and PR (**B**); and presentation of the immunocytochemistry results by the semi-quantitative immunoreactivity score (IRS). Significantly different observations are highlighted with an asterisk.

### 3.5. Enterolactone Downregulates Expression of ERα and PR in a Dose-Response Pattern in MCF7 Cells

MCF7 cells that were exposed to enterolactone at concentrations of 10 µg/mL, 50 µg/mL, and 100 µg/mL responded significantly with a downregulation of ER α at concentrations of 50 µg/mL (IRS score 2.5) and 100 µg/mL (IRS score 0) compared to the control (IRS score 5, $p$ = 0.027 and 0.024) (see Figure 5). MCF7 cells that were exposed to enterolactone at concentrations of 10 µg/mL, 50 µg/mL, and 100 µg/mL responded with a dose-response-related downregulation of the PR. The downregulation of the PR was significant at enterolactone concentrations of 50 µg/mL (IRS score 4) and 100 µg/mL downregulation (IRS score 2) compared to the control (IRS score 9, $p$ = 0.028 for both concentrations).

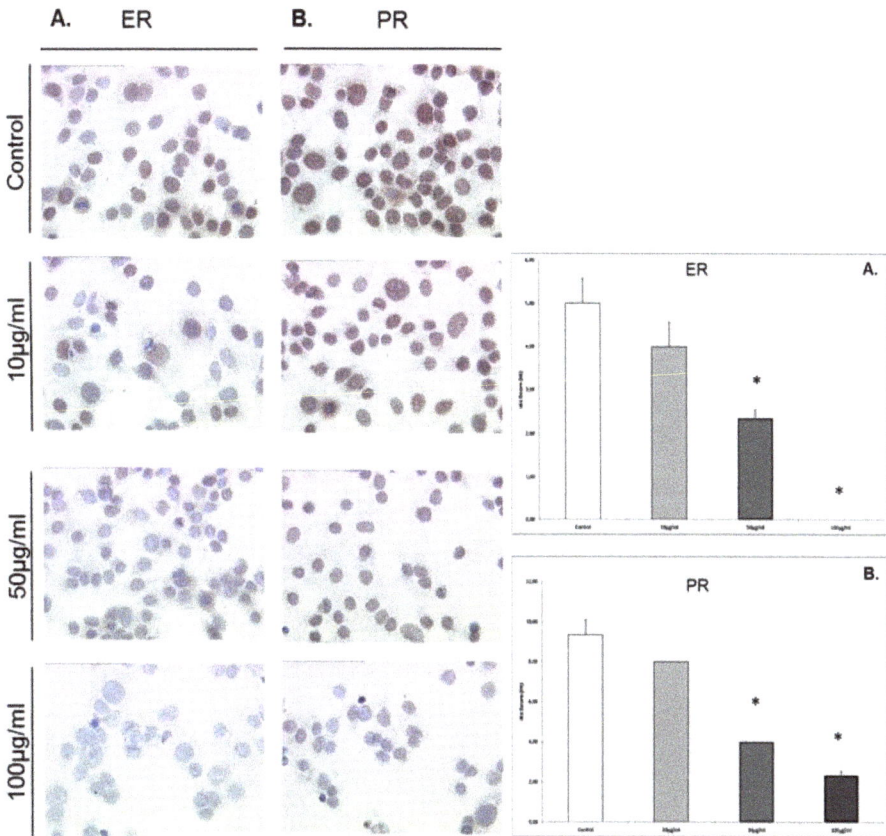

**Figure 5.** Representative microphotographs of MCF7 cells grown in the absence or presence of enterolactone at concentrations of 10 µg/mL, 50 µg/mL, and 100 µg/mL), after immuno-detection of ER-α (**A**) and PR (**B**); and presentation of the immunocytochemistry results by the semi-quantitative immunoreactivity score (IRS). Significantly different observations are highlighted with an asterisk.

### 3.6. Enterodiol Downregulates Expression of ERα and PR Only at High Concentrations in MCF7 Cells

MCF7 cells that were exposed to enterodiol at concentrations of 10 µg/mL, 50 µg/mL, and 100 µg/mL responded with a significant downregulation of ERα only at 100 µg/mL (IRS score 0) compared to the control (IRS score 5, $p = 0.023$) (Figure 6). MCF7 cells that were exposed to enterodiol at concentrations of 10 µg/mL, 50 µg/mL, and 100 µg/mL responded with a significant downregulation of the PR at 100 µg/mL (IRS score 0) compared to the control (IRS score 5.5, $p = 0.023$).

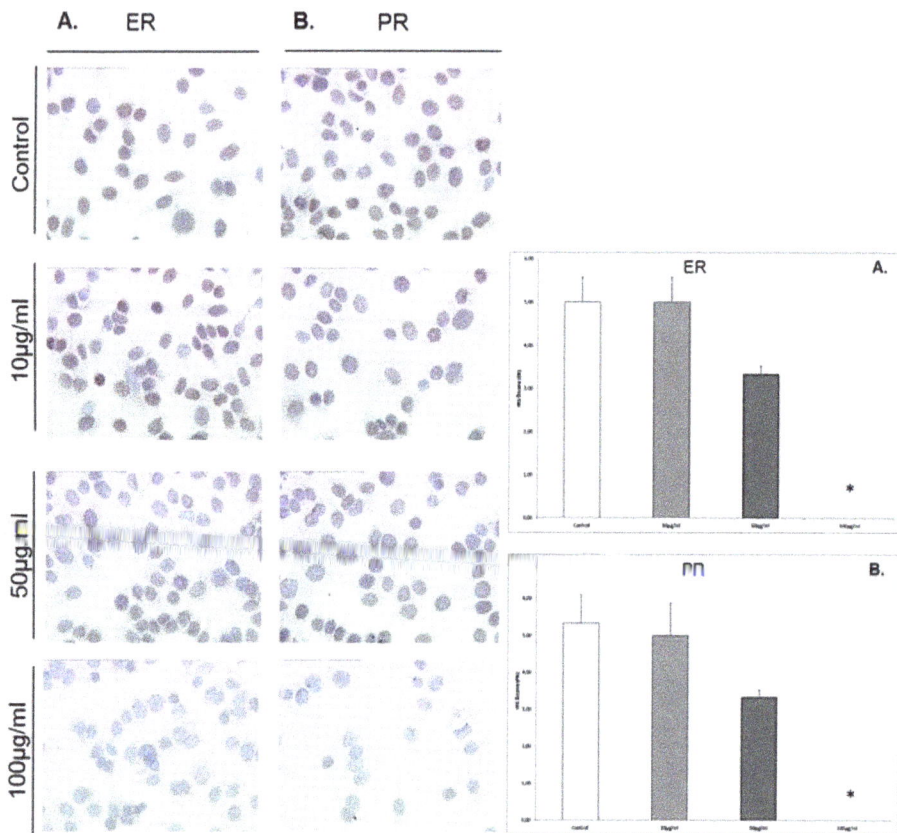

**Figure 6.** Representative microphotographs of MCF7 cells grown in the absence or presence of enterodiol at concentrations of 10 μg/mL, 50 μg/mL, and 100 μg/mL), after immuno-detection of ER-α (**A**) and PR (**B**) ; and presentation of the immunocytochemistry results by the semi-quantitative immunoreactivity score (IRS). Significantly observations are highlighted with an asterisk.

*3.7. Enterolactone Inhibits Estradiol Secretion in JEG-3 Cells and Induce Estradiol Secretion in BeWo and MCF7 Cells in a Dose-Response Pattern*

In JEG-3 cells, the estradiol production was inhibited from 211.8 ± 8.88 pg/mL in the control to 190.9 ± 7.9 pg/mL, and 149.59 ± 7 pg/mL at enterolactone concentrations of 10 μg/mL and 50 μg/mL, $p = 0.028$, respectively (Figure 7).

The cultivation of the BeWo cell line with enterolactone resulted again in an upregulation of estradiol secretion from 75.07 ± 2.33 pg/mL in the control to 94.66 ± 6.39 pg/mL, 137.66 ± 10.04 pg/mL, and 173.53 ± 9.56 pg/mL when the enterolactone concentration was 10 μg/mL, 50 μg/mL, and 100 μg/mL. The differences between the stimulated cells and the control were significant at all concentration levels of enterolactone, $p = 0.028$, respectively.

In MCF7 cells the concentrations of 10 μg/mL, 50 μg/mL and 100 μg/mL provoked an increased secretion of estradiol from 52.65 ± 7.90 pg/mL in the control to 75.22 ± 2.11 pg/mL at 10 μg/mL, 123.93 ± 3.93 pg/mL at 50 μg/mL, and 172.12 ± 10.05 pg/mL at 100 μg/mL, $p = 0.028$, respectively.

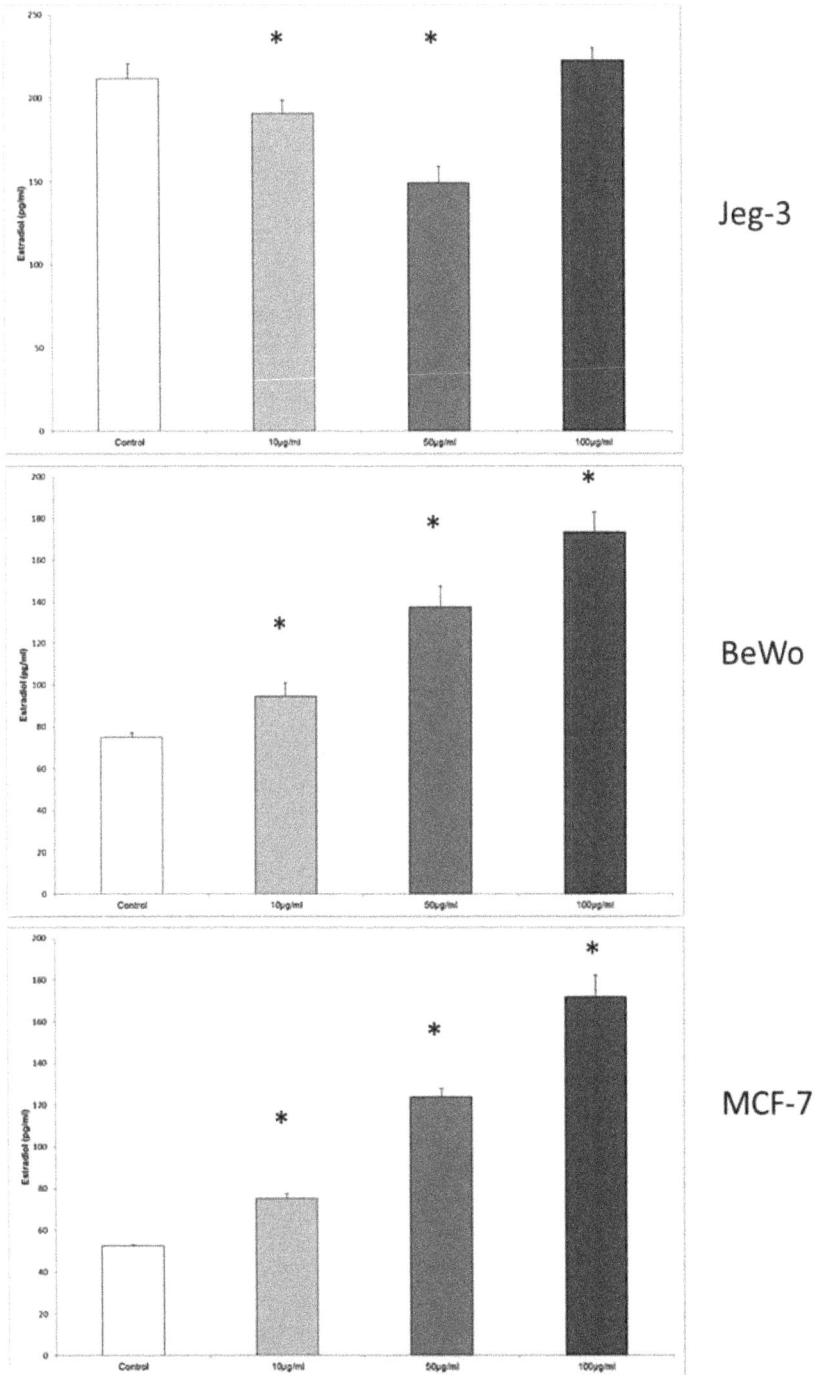

**Figure 7.** Estradiol concentration in the tissue culture medium of JEG-3, BeWo and MCF7 cells in the absence or presence of enterolactone. The effective enterolactone concentrations were 10 μg/mL, 50 μg/mL, and 100 μg/mL. Significantly different observation are highlighted with an asterisk.

### 3.8. Enterodiol Induces Estradiol Secretion in JEG-3, BeWo, and MCF7 Cells at Distinct Concentrations

In JEG-3 cells, the estradiol secretion was significantly enhanced from $79.85 \pm 1.14$ pg/mL in the control to $86.37 \pm 1.07$ pg/mL, when the concentration was 50 µg/mL enterodiol, $p = 0.028$ (Figure 8).

The cultivation of the BeWo cell line with enterodiol resulted again in a significant upregulation of estradiol secretion from $63.71 \pm 0.68$ pg/mL in the control to $72.71 \pm 0.79$ pg/mL, and $84.37 \pm 4.63$ pg/mL at the enterodiol concentrations of 50 µg/mL and 100 µg/mL, respectively. The differences between the stimulated cells and the control were significant at both concentration of enterodiol, $p = 0.028$, respectively.

In MCF7 cells the concentrations of 50 µg/mL and 100 µg/mL provoked an increased secretion of estradiol from $35.64 \pm 1.32$ pg/mL in the control to $53.28 \pm 0.39$ pg/mL at 50 µg/mL, and $56.94 \pm 2.54$ pg/mL at 100 µg/mL, $p = 0.028$, respectively.

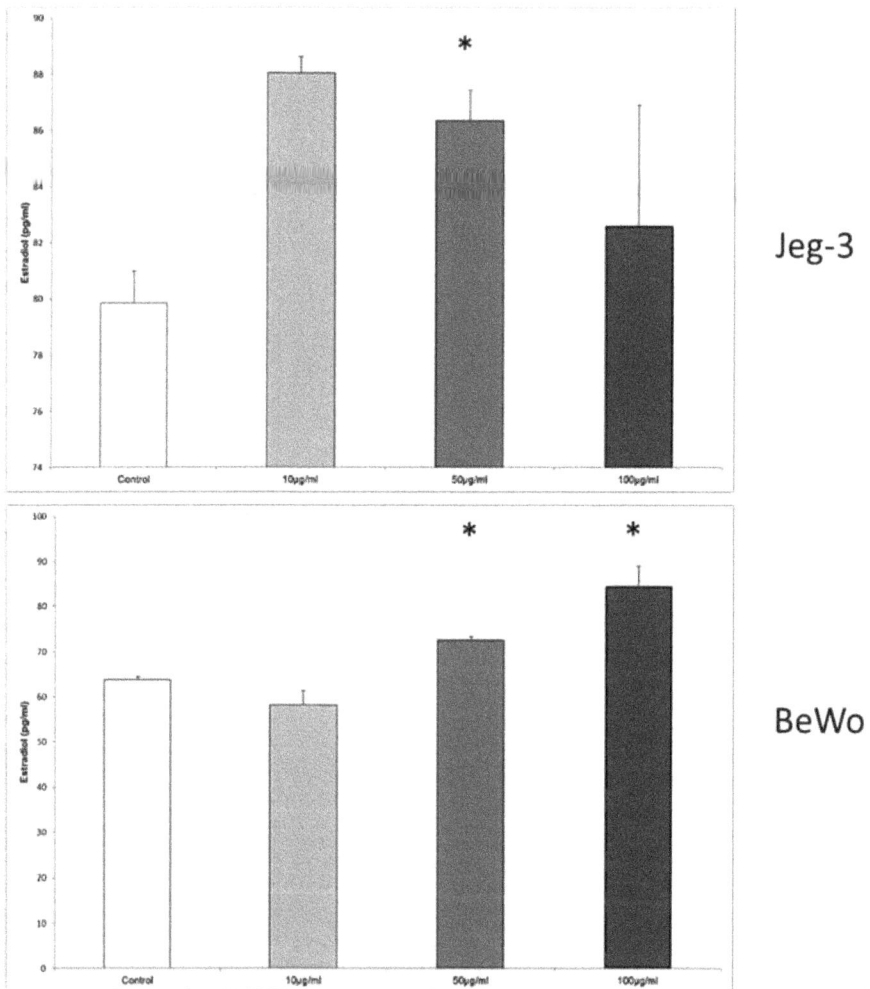

**Figure 8.** *Cont.*

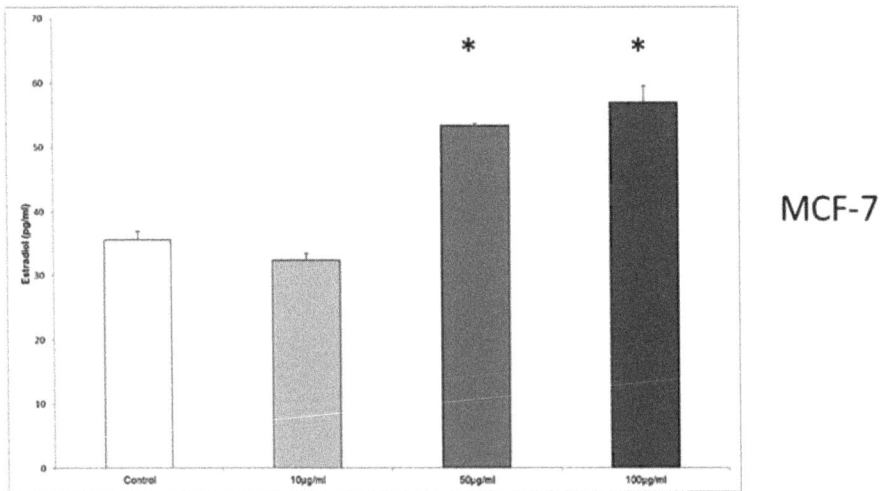

**Figure 8.** Estradiol concentration in the tissue culture medium of JEG-3, BeWo and MCF7 cells in the absence or presence of enterodiol. The effective enterodiol concentrations were 50 μg/mL and 100 μg/mL. Significantly different observation are highlighted with an asterisk.

## 4. Discussion

To our knowledge, this is the first study evaluating the phytoestrogen properties of EFE on BeWo, JEG-3, and MCF7 cells regarding the estrogen and progesterone response. Prior to this study it was uncertain if EFE contains phytoestrogen compounds. Although mass spectrometry proved that EFE contains lignans and isoflavones, the subgroups of each class were not identified and, thus, precision is lacking. EFE proved to be richer in lignans than in isoflavones (presented in Figure 1). This may explain why more significant results were found using the lignan EFE. However, further studies with isolated fractions of the subgroups of EFE lignans and isoflavones could clarify if one subgroup is more potent than the other. Therefore, it would be interesting to isolate and identify the different lignans and isoflavones in the EFE that cause phytoestrogen activity for further characterization. Before further evaluation in an animal model, in vitro evaluation of the various components' effects as single substances is required.

In a previous study of our group, the phytoestrogen properties of pumpkin seed extract were tested on the same cells, which resulted in an unexpected estrogen secretion in all cell lines [18]. As hormone-dependent tumors react with proliferation when exposed to estrogens, pumpkin seeds, thus, could provoke carcinogenic effects.

In contrast, EFE was the first of the potential phytoestrogens previously tested by our group, which had an inhibitory effect on the estradiol secretion of all three cell lines.

The effect on JEG-3 and BeWo cells was observed to be dose-dependent. Interestingly, in MCF7 cells, estrogen secretion was higher following the administration of intermediate phytoestrogen concentrations than in controls or with the highest EFE concentration tested. The degree to which the inhibition of estrogen secretion results in a decreased cell proliferation has to be tested in further investigations using EFE. In addition, it is possible that at the highest EFE concentration estrogen secretion was decreased due to cytotoxic effects of the extract itself, as other studies suggest that phytoestrogens cause cytotoxicity and decrease growth in MCF7 tumors. For example, in a study by Bergman et al. [31] ovariectomized mice were treated with continuous release of estrogen. MCF7 tumors were established and mice were fed with basal diet or 10% flaxseed, and two groups that were fed basal diet received daily injections with enterodiol or enterolactone (15 mg/kg body weight).

The regimens containing flax seeds or enterodiol or enterolactone injections resulted in decreased estrogen-induced growth and angiogenesis in solid tumors by decreasing the secretion of VEGF.

It is of interest that EFE induces not only an inhibition of estradiol secretion, but also an upregulation of the ERα in JEG-3 cells. It could be assumed that, if EFE causes an inhibition on the trophoblast estrogen secretion, the cells react by increasing ERα expression in order to obtain stimulation even in a low-estrogen environment. A recent study by Lim et al. [32] outlined that the flavonoid apigenin reduces survival of JEG-3 cells by inducing apoptosis via the PI3K/AKT and ERK1/2 MAPK pathways. Therefore, it seems likely that the phytoestrogens also found in EFE could trigger non-genomic estradiol receptor signal transduction causing apoptosis in JEG-3 cells. In contrast to the effects of EFE on JEG-3 cells, another study by our group [33] demonstrated that the two well-known phytoestrogens genistein and daidzein provoked a reduced progesterone production and a stimulation of the estrogen production in JEG-3 cells. Therefore, regarding the other extracts investigated by our group, the characteristics of EFE seem to be favorable for further research due to the properties of decreased estrogen secretion and increased ERα expression in JEG-3 cells.

MCF7 cells that were exposed to EFE extracts responded with a significant downregulation of ERα and an upregulation of PR, both predominantly in lower concentrations of EFE. Why the lower concentrations provoked a stronger effect on receptor expression remains unknown. Although it is, again, possible that higher concentrations of EFE resulted in cytotoxic effects leading to cell damage and, therefore, to decreased cellular function. Nevertheless, the fact that lower EFE concentrations resulted in a decreased expression of the ERα receptor and an increase in the progesterone receptor could be beneficial for clinical use as low blood concentrations of phytoestrogens are easier to achieve by dietary intake alone. It is important to mention that the concentrations used in this study were extremely high (non-physiological). The highest level of enterolactone that has been measured in serum/plasma in humans is 2 μmol/L (over 16 times less than the enterolactone concentration used). Furthermore, estradiol levels in adult females reach levels only as high as 300 pg/mL in the luteal phase (30,000 times less than the external control). Therefore, before realistic interpretation, our findings must be reevaluated in further studies using more physiologically relevant doses.

Our current findings partially concur with a previously-described downregulation of ERα and upregulation of PR on the MCF7 cells when treated with other potential phytoestrogen compounds such as flax and pumpkin isoflavone and lignan extracts or mixtures [19,34]. Interestingly, it has been demonstrated that estradiol has similar effects on the MCF7 ERα and on PR, as it causes a downregulation of ERα and an upregulation of PR [35,36]. Therefore, whether EFE causes MCF7 cell proliferation or inhibition has to be tested in future investigations. In a study by Stendahl et al., it was demonstrated that high progesterone receptor expression correlates with a better effect of adjuvant tamoxifen in premenopausal breast cancer patients [37]. This suggests clinical trial evaluation of elderflower as a combination partner for tamoxifen.

It is unclear whether the lignans present in the EFE require any metabolic processing prior to exerting biological effects and whether the cell culture systems used are capable of completing this conversion. For example secoisolariciresinol diglycoside (SDG) is the primary lignan in flaxseed; however, in vitro studies use bioavailabile enterodiol and enterolactone when investigating effects of flaxseed lignans. This is because in vitro systems do not have the components necessary to convert SDG to enterodiol and enterolactone. Therefore, additional in vivo studies could provide valuable information regarding EFE metabolism prior to the conduction of further in vitro studies. Nevertheless, the pattern of hormone secretion and receptor expression of enerolactone and enterodiol tested on JEG-3, BeWo, and MCF7 cells were different to those of EFE. Therefore, it is probable that the lignans in EFE are not related to the enterolignans. Enterolactone and enterodiol in contrast to EFE inhibited not only the expression of the ER but also PR in MCF7 cells. Moreover contrary to EFE, both control substances upregulated estradiol production in BeWo and MCF7 cells in a concentration-dependent manner.

## 5. Conclusions

Our results clearly demonstrate beneficial features of EFE in the setting of hormone receptor-positive breast cancer MCF7 cells by inhibition of estrogen secretion, downregulation of Erα, and upregulation of PR. Decreased local and circulating estrogen concentrations are certainly considered an advantage in treating breast cancer. In that view, EFE could be related to reduced tumor cell proliferation, possibly suggesting a protective effect on breast cancer. Nevertheless, the results and the conclusions made must be interpreted with caution as this is an in vitro cell culture study. In this setting, the use of plant extracts instead of chemically pure agents may be advantageous as it may more accurately reflect the effects of phytoestrogen-rich diets.

If the effects of EFE can be attributed solely to potential phytoestrogen activity remains unsolved. To which degree other non-estrogenic pathways play a role can currently not be clarified. For example, mass spectrometry demonstrated a high amount of lipids in EFE. Lipids can inhibit cell proliferation through activation of PPARα and PPARγ (peroxisome proliferator-activated receptors) which bind as transcription factors to the retinoid X receptors and, thus, regulate the expression of various genes [38,39]. In MCF7 breast cancer cells PPARγ activates p53 by stimulating the transcription factor NFkB (nuclear factor kappa-light-chain-enhancer of activated B-cells), which is a gene promoter of p53 and, thus, induces apoptosis [40]. Therefore, the following additional investigations are necessary to obtain further insight of the promising anti-carcinogenic effects of EFE: the results of hormone secretion and receptor expression of EFE should be correlated with DNA synthesis performance (BRDU proliferation assay), metabolic activity (MTT assay), and cytotoxicity (LDH assay) tests. Cytotoxicity could be evaluated in detail by immunohistochemistry or reverse transcriptase quantitative (RTQ)-PCR quantification of apoptosis-induced markers (for example, p53, p21, BCL2, Caspase 8/9). Then, as a possibility to determine the role of hormone receptor-mediated cell response, EFE could be tested on malignant ER-negative cells (e.g., BT-20). Furthermore, fractional chromatography could provide information of the individual substances and their impact on breast cancer cells. Finally, after further in vitro investigations, properly designed animal studies could highlight a potential role of EFE in trophoblast and breast cancer prevention and/or treatment.

**Acknowledgments:** The authors thank S. Hofmann for technical support. The study was founded by the Department of Obstetrics & Gynecology of the LMU Munich and by the "Deutsche Krebshilfe" for D.U. Richter.

**Author Contributions:** L.S. and D.U.R. conceived and designed the experiments; M.C., C.K. and S.S. performed the experiments; B.P. and S.A. analyzed the data; T.W. contributed analysis tools; L.S. and U.J. wrote the paper.

**Conflicts of Interest:** The authors declare no conflict of interest.

## References

1. Tham, D.M.; Gardner, C.D.; Haskell, W.L. Clinical review 97: Potential health benefits of dietary phytoestrogens: A review of the clinical, epidemiological, and mechanistic evidence. *J. Clin. Endocrinol. Metab.* **1998**, *83*, 2223–2235. [PubMed]
2. Usui, T. Pharmaceutical prospects of phytoestrogens. *Endocr. J.* **2006**, *53*, 7–20. [CrossRef] [PubMed]
3. Setchell, K.D. Phytoestrogens: The biochemistry, physiology, and implications for human health of soy isoflavones. *Am. J. Clin. Nutr.* **1998**, *68*, 1333S–1346S. [PubMed]
4. Setchell, K.D. Soy isoflavones—Benefits and risks from nature's selective estrogen receptor modulators (SERMs). *J. Am. Coll. Nutr.* **2001**, *20*, 354S–362S. [CrossRef] [PubMed]
5. Riggs, B.L.; Hartmann, L.C. Selective estrogen-receptor modulators—Mechanisms of action and application to clinical practice. *N. Engl. J. Med.* **2003**, *348*, 618–629. [PubMed]
6. Shu, X.O.; Zheng, Y.; Cai, H.; Gu, K.; Chen, Z.; Zheng, W.; Lu, W. Soy food intake and breast cancer survival. *JAMA* **2009**, *302*, 2437–2443. [CrossRef] [PubMed]
7. Saarinen, N.M.; Wärri, A.; Airio, M.; Smeds, A.; Mäkelä, S. Role of dietary lignans in the reduction of breast cancer risk. *Mol. Nutr. Food Res.* **2007**, *51*, 857–866. [CrossRef] [PubMed]
8. Fletcher, R.J. Food sources of phyto-oestrogens and their precursors in Europe. *Br. J. Nutr.* **2003**, *89*, S39–S43. [CrossRef] [PubMed]

9. Chi, F.; Wu, R.; Zeng, Y.C.; Xing, R.; Liu, Y.; Xu, Z.G. Post-diagnosis soy food intake and breast cancer survival: A meta-analysis of cohort studies. *Asian Pac. J. Cancer Prev.* **2013**, *14*, 2407–2412. [CrossRef] [PubMed]

10. Ingram, D.; Sanders, K.; Kolybaba, M.; Lopez, D. Case-control study of phyto-oestrogens and breast cancer. *Lancet* **1997**, *350*, 990–994. [CrossRef]

11. Limer, J.L.; Speirs, V. Phyto-oestrogens and breast cancer chemoprevention. *Breast Cancer Res.* **2004**, *6*, 119–127. [CrossRef] [PubMed]

12. Andres, S.; Abraham, K.; Appel, K.E.; Lampen, A. Risks and benefits of dietary isoflavones for cancer. *Crit. Rev. Toxicol.* **2011**, *41*, 463–506. [CrossRef] [PubMed]

13. Park, E.J.; John, M.P. Flavonoids in Cancer Prevention. *Anti Cancer Agents Med. Chem.* **2012**, *12*, 836–851. [CrossRef]

14. Adlercreutz, H.; Fotsis, T.; Heikkinen, R.; Dwyer, J.T.; Woods, M.; Goldin, B.R.; Gorbach, S.L. Excretion of the lignans enterolactone and enterodiol and of equol in omnivorous and vegetarian postmenopausal women and in women with breast cancer. *Lancet* **1982**, *2*, 1295–1298. [CrossRef]

15. Heinonen, S.; Nurmi, T.; Liukkonen, K.; Poutanen, K.; Wähälä, K.; Deyama, T.; Nishibe, S.; Adlercreutz, H. In vitro metabolism of plant lignans: New precursors of mammalian lignans enterolactone and enterodiol. *J. Agric. Food Chem.* **2001**, *49*, 3178–3186. [CrossRef] [PubMed]

16. Buck, K.; Vrieling, A.; Zaineddin, A.K.; Becker, S.; Hüsing, A.; Kaaks, R.; Linseisen, J.; Flesch-Janys, D.; Chang-Claude, J. Serum enterolactone and prognosis of postmenopausal breast cancer. *J. Clin. Oncol.* **2011**, *29*, 3730–3738. [CrossRef] [PubMed]

17. Buck, K.; Zaineddin, A.K.; Vrieling, A.; Linseisen, J.; Chang-Claude, J. Meta-analyses of lignans and enterolignans in relation to breast cancer risk. *Am. J. Clin. Nutr.* **2010**, *92*, 141–153. [CrossRef] [PubMed]

18. Richter, D.; Abarzua, S.; Chrobak, M.; Vrekoussis, T.; Weissenbacher, T.; Kuhn, C.; Schulze, S.; Kupka, M.S.; Friese, K.; Briese, V.; et al. Effects of phytoestrogen extracts isolated from pumpkin seeds on estradiol production and ER/PR expression in breast cancer and trophoblast tumor cells. *Nutr. Cancer* **2013**, *65*, 739–745. [CrossRef] [PubMed]

19. Richter, D.U.; Abarzua, S.; Chrobak, M.; Scholz, C.; Kuhn, C.; Schulze, S.; Kupka, M.S.; Friese, K.; Briese, V.; Piechulla, B.; et al. Effects of phytoestrogen extracts isolated from flax on estradiol production and ER/PR expression in MCF7 breast cancer cells. *Anti-Cancer Res.* **2010**, *30*, 1695–1699.

20. Jeschke, U.; Briese, V.; Richter, D.U.; Bruer, G.; Plessow, D.; Waldschläger, J.; Mylonas, I.; Friese, K. Effects of phytoestrogens genistein and daidzein on production of human chorionic gonadotropin in term trophoblast cells in vitro. *Gynecol. Endocrinol.* **2005**, *21*, 180–184. [CrossRef] [PubMed]

21. Youdim, K.A.; Martin, A.; Joseph, J.A. Incorporation of the elderberry anthocyanins by endothelial cells increases protection against oxidative stress. *Free Radic. Biol. Med.* **2000**, *29*, 51–60. [CrossRef]

22. Barak, V.; Birkenfeld, S.; Halperin, T.; Kalickman, I. The effect of herbal remedies on the production of human inflammatory and anti-inflammatory cytokines. *Isr. Med. Assoc. J.* **2002**, *4*, 919–922. [PubMed]

23. Zakay-Rones, Z.; Varsano, N.; Zlotnik, M.; Manor, O.; Regev, L.; Schlesinger, M.; Mumcuoglu, M. Inhibition of Several Strains of Influenza Virus in vitro and Reduction of Symptoms by an Elderberry Extract (*Sambucus Nigra* L.) during an Outbreak of Influenza B Panama. *J. Altern. Complement. Med.* **1995**, *4*, 361–369. [CrossRef] [PubMed]

24. Hearst, C.; Mccollum, G.; Nelson, D.; Ballard, L.M.; Millar, B.C.; Goldsmith, C.E.; Rooney, P.J.; Loughrey, A.; Moore, J.E.; Rao, J.R. Antibacterial activity of elder (*Sambucus nigra* L.) flower or berry against hospital pathogens. *J. Med. Plants Res.* **2010**, *4*, 1805–1809.

25. Zhang, Y.; Li, Q.; Wan, H.Y.; Xiao, H.H.; Lai, W.P.; Yao, X.S.; Wong, M.S. Study of the mechanisms by which Sambucus williamsii HANCE extract exert protective effects against ovariectomy-induced osteoporosis in vivo. *Osteoporos. Int.* **2011**, *22*, 703–709. [CrossRef] [PubMed]

26. Luyengi, L.; Suh, N.; Fong, H.H.S.; Pezzuto, J.M.; Kinghorn, A.D. A lignan and four terpenoids from Brucea javanica that induce differentiation with cultured HL-60 promyelocytic leukemia cells. *Phytochemistry* **1996**, *43*, 409–412. [CrossRef]

27. Sicilia, T.; Niemeyer, H.B.; Honig, D.M.; Metzler, M. Identification and stereochemical characterization of lignans in flaxseed and pumpkin seeds. *J. Agric. Food Chem.* **2003**, *51*, 1181–1188. [CrossRef] [PubMed]

28. Franz, G.; Köhler, H. Allgemeine Nachweismethoden für Flavonoide in Drogen. In *Drogen und Naturstoffe: Grundlagen und Praxis der Chemischen Analyse*; Springer: Berlin/Heidelberg, Germany, 1992; p. 129.

29. Matscheski, A.; Richter, D.U.; Hartmann, A.M.; Effmert, U.; Jeschke, U.; Kupka, M.S.; Abarzua, S.; Briese, V.; Ruth, W.; Kragl, U.; et al. Effects of phytoestrogen extracts isolated from rye, green and yellow pea seeds on hormone production and proliferation of trophoblast tumor cells Jeg3. *Horm. Res.* **2006**, *65*, 276–288. [CrossRef] [PubMed]

30. Remmele, W.; Stegner, H.E. Recommendation for uniform definition of an immunoreactive score (IRS) for immunohistochemical estrogen receptor detection (ER-ICA) in breast cancer tissue. *Pathology* **1987**, *8*, 138–140.

31. Bergman, J.M.; Thompson, L.U.; Dabrosin, C. Flaxseed and its lignans inhibit estradiol-induced growth, angiogenesis, and secretion of vascular endothelial growth factor in human breast cancer xenografts in vivo. *Clin. Cancer Res.* **2007**, *13*, 1061–1067. [CrossRef] [PubMed]

32. Lim, W.; Park, S.; Bazer, F.W.; Song, G. Apigenin Reduces Survival of Choriocarcinoma Cells by Inducing Apoptosis via the PI3K/AKT and ERK1/2 MAPK Pathways. *J. Cell. Physiol.* **2016**, *231*, 2690–2699. [CrossRef] [PubMed]

33. Richter, D.U.; Mylonas, I.; Toth, B.; Scholz, C.; Briese, V.; Friese, K.; Jeschke, U. Effects of phytoestrogens genistein and daidzein on progesterone and estrogen (estradiol) production of human term trophoblast cells in vitro. *Gynecol. Endocrinol.* **2009**, *25*, 32–38. [CrossRef] [PubMed]

34. Taxvig, C.; Elleby, A.; Sonne-Hansen, K.; Bonefeld-Jørgensen, E.C.; Vinggaard, A.M.; Lykkesfeldt, A.E.; Nellemann, C. Effects of nutrition relevant mixtures of phytoestrogens on steroidogenesis, aromatase, estrogen, and androgen activity. *Nutr. Cancer* **2010**, *62*, 122–131. [CrossRef] [PubMed]

35. Horwitz, K.B.; McGuire, W.L. Estrogen control of progesterone receptor in human breast cancer. Correlation with nuclear processing of estrogen receptor. *J. Biol. Chem.* **1978**, *253*, 2223–2228. [PubMed]

36. Umans, R.S.; Weichselbaum, R.R.; Johnson, C.M.; Little, J.B. Effects of estradiol concentration on levels of nuclear estrogen receptors in MCF7 breast tumor cells. *J. Steroid Biochem.* **1984**, *20*, 605–609. [CrossRef]

37. Stendahl, M.; Rydén, L.; Nordenskjöld, B.; Jönsson, P.E.; Landberg, G.; Jirström, K. High progesterone receptor expression correlates to the effect of adjuvant tamoxifen in premenopausal breast cancer patients. *Clin. Cancer Res.* **2006**, *12*, 4614–4618. [CrossRef] [PubMed]

38. Dionisi, M.; Alexander, S.P.H.; Bennett, A.J. Oleamide activates peroxisome proliferator-activated receptor gamma (PPARγ) in vitro. *Lipids Health Dis.* **2012**, *11*, 51. [CrossRef] [PubMed]

39. Thoennes, S.R.; Tate, P.L.; Price, T.M.; Kilgore, M.W. Differential transcriptional activation of peroxisome proliferator-activated receptor gamma by omega-3 and omega-6 fatty acids in MCF7 cells. *Mol. Cell. Endocrinol.* **2000**, *160*, 67–73. [CrossRef]

40. Bonofiglio, D.; Aquila, S.; Catalano, S.; Gabriele, S.; Belmonte, M.; Middea, E.; Qi, H.; Morelli, C.; Gentile, M.; Maggiolini, M.; et al. Peroxisome proliferator-activated receptor-gamma activates p53 gene promoter binding to the nuclear factor-kappaB sequence in human MCF7 breast cancer cells. *Mol. Endocrinol.* **2006**, *20*, 3083–3092. [CrossRef] [PubMed]

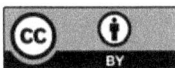

**nutrients**

MDPI

Article

# Antiproliferative and Antiangiogenic Effects of *Punica granatum* Juice (PGJ) in Multiple Myeloma (MM)

Daniele Tibullo [1,2], Nunzia Caporarello [3], Cesarina Giallongo [1,3], Carmelina Daniela Anfuso [3], Claudia Genovese [2,4], Carmen Arlotta [2,4], Fabrizio Puglisi [1], Nunziatina L. Parrinello [1], Vincenzo Bramanti [3], Alessandra Romano [1], Gabriella Lupo [3], Valeria Toscano [4], Roberto Avola [3], Maria Violetta Brundo [2,*], Francesco Di Raimondo [1,†] and Salvatore Antonio Raccuia [2,4,†]

[1]   Section of Hematology, Department of Surgery and Medical Specialties, University of Catania, Catania 95125, Italy; d.tibullo@unict.it (D.T.); cesarinagiallongo@yahoo.it (C.G.); puglisi.fabri@gmail.com (F.P.); lauraparrinello@tiscali.it (N.L.P.); alessandraromano@google.it (A.R.); diraimon@unict.it (F.D.R.)

[2]   Department of Biological, Geological and Environmental Sciences, University of Catania, Catania 95125, Italy; claudia.genovese@cnr.it (C.G.); carmen.arlotta@isafom.cnr.it (C.A.); salvatore.raccuia@cnr.it (S.A.R.)

[3]   Department of Biomedical and Biotechnological Sciences, University of Catania, Catania 95125, Italy; nunzia.caporarello@gmail.com (N.C.); anfudan@unict.it (C.D.A.); V.bramanti@unict.it (V.B.); lupogab@unict.it (G.L.); alessandraromano@google.it (R.A.)

[4]   Institute for Agricultural and Forest Systems in the Mediterranean, National Research Council, Catania 95125, Italy; valeria.toscano@cnr.it

*   Correspondence: mvbrundo@unict.it; Tel.: +39-095-730-6040

†   These authors contributed equally to this work.

Received: 15 July 2016; Accepted: 13 September 2016; Published: 1 October 2016

**Abstract:** Multiple myeloma (MM) is a clonal B-cell malignancy characterized by an accumulation of clonal plasma cells (PC) in the bone marrow (BM) leading to bone destruction and BM failure. Despite recent advances in pharmacological therapy, MM remains a largely incurable pathology. Therefore, novel effective and less toxic agents are urgently necessary. In the last few years, pomegranate has been studied for its potential therapeutic properties including treatment and prevention of cancer. Pomegranate juice (PGJ) contains a number of potential active compounds including organic acids, vitamins, sugars, and phenolic components that are all responsible of the pro-apoptotic effects observed in tumor cell line. The aim of present investigation is to assess the antiproliferative and antiangiogenic potential of the PGJ in human multiple myeloma cell lines. Our data demonstrate the anti-proliferative potential of PGJ in MM cells; its ability to induce G0/G1 cell cycle block and its anti-angiogenic effects. Interestingly, sequential combination of bortezomib/PGJ improved the cytotoxic effect of the proteosome inhibitor. We investigated the effect of PGJ on angiogenesis and cell migration/invasion. Interestingly, we observed an inhibitory effect on the tube formation, microvessel outgrowth aorting ring and decreased cell migration and invasion as showed by wound-healing and transwell assays, respectively. Analysis of angiogenic genes expression in endothelial cells confirmed the anti-angiogenic properties of pomegranate. Therefore, PGJ administration could represent a good tool in order to identify novel therapeutic strategies for MM treatment, exploiting its anti-proliferative and anti-angiogenic effects. Finally, the present research supports the evidence that PGJ could play a key role of a future therapeutic approach for treatment of MM in order to optimize the pharmacological effect of bortezomib, especially as adjuvant after treatment.

**Keywords:** *Punica granatum* juice; multiple myeloma; proliferation; angiogenesis

## 1. Introduction

Multiple myeloma (MM) is a clonal B-cell malignancy characterized by accumulation of clonal plasma cells (PC) in the bone marrow (BM) leading to bone destruction and BM failure [1–3]. MM encompasses a spectrum of clinical variants ranging from benign Monoclonal Gammopathies of Undetermined Significance (MGUS) and smoldering/indolent MM, to more aggressive, disseminated forms of MM and plasma cell leukemia. Despite recent advances in proteasome inhibitor and immunomodulatory drug-based therapies [4,5], and MM remains largely incurable [2,6]. The genetic complexity of myeloma is due to intraclonal heterogeneity in the myeloma-propagating cell [7,8]. Multiple mutations in different pathways trigger a deregulation of the intrinsic biology of the PC, leading to the features of myeloma [7–9]. The sequential acquisition of multiple genetic events can lead to disease progression and the development of treatment-resistant disease [8,9]. Therefore, novel effective and less toxic agents are urgently necessary in order to treat patients affected by multiple myeloma. The development of novel therapeutic compounds without significant adverse side effects is considered an important area for immunopharmacological studies. A wide variety of natural compounds possesses significant cytotoxic as well as chemopreventive activity, through induction of cancer cell apoptosis [10]. Over 60% of currently used anticancer agents are derived from natural sources, including plants, marine organisms and microorganisms.

*Punica granatum* L., also known as pomegranate, belonging to the Punicaceae family, has been gaining popularity as a nutraceutical food having potential beneficial effects on health, including prevention and/or treatment of oncologic diseases, cardiovascular and neurological disorders, metabolic diseases [11,12]. Moreover, pomegranate has been studied for its potential therapeutic properties including treatment and prevention of cancer [13,14]. Pomegranate fruit is widely consumed fresh as well as in processed forms, such as juice, jams, sauce, and wine. The pharmacological effects of PGJ are related to a large number of phytochemicals, including hydrolyzable tannins and related compounds (ellagitanin, punicalagin, pedunculagin, punicalin, gallagic acid, ellagic acid and gallic acid), flavonoids (anthocyanins and catechins), flavonols (quercetin and kaempferol), flavones (apigenin and luteolin), and conjugated fatty acids (punicic acid), present in discrete anatomical parts, such as peel (pericarp or husk), juice, and seeds [13,15]. PGJ, extracts, and phytoconstituents have been extensively studied preclinically for their anticarcinogenic and cancer chemopreventive effects in colon, lung, skin, and prostate cancer [16].

Based on numerous in vitro studies, several pomegranate products and phytoconstituents exhibited cytotoxic, antiproliferative, proapoptotic, antiangiogenic, antiinvasive, and antimetastatic effects against estrogen receptor-positive and -negative breast carcinoma cells [17–25].

Pomegranate seed oil and fermented juice concentrate suppressed 7,12-dimethyl benz(*a*)anthracene (DMBA)-induced precancerous mammary gland lesions ex vivo [26] and pomegranate extract inhibited the growth of xenografted BT-474 tumors in vivo [23].

Recently, some authors reported for the first time that a pomegranate formulation (emulsion) containing the most bioactive phytochemicals present in the whole fruit affords a remarkable chemopreventive effect against DMBA-induced mammary tumorigenesis in rats [27].

The aim of the present investigation is to assess the antiproliferative and antiangiogenic potential of PGJ in human multiple myeloma cell lines.

## 2. Experimental Section

### 2.1. Reagents and Compounds

Recombinant human VEGF-A (VEGF-A$_{165}$ isoform) was obtained from Peprotech (Rocky Hill, NJ, USA). The serum-free endothelial cell basal medium (EBM) was obtained from ScienceCell Research Laboratories (San Diego, CA, USA). The proteosome inhibitor bortezomib (BTZ) was used at 30 nM (Takeda, Italy).

## 2.2. Pomegranate Juice

Pomegranate juice (PGJ) was extracted by plants of five-year-old Wonderful varieties. The plants were produced under organic agricultural practices in an experimental farmland of the section of National Research Council—Institute for Agricultural and Forest Systems in the Mediterranean (ISAFOM).

Pomegranate fruits were harvested at physiological maturity in October 2014 and randomly collected from each of four geographical orientation of tree. The fruits were stored at 4 °C for three days. After manual separations of the arils, the PGJ was obtained by mechanical press. Subsequently, the PGJ was centrifuged at 5000 rpm for 5 min at room temperature and then filtered by sterile syringe with filters 0.22 μm (Invitrogen, Paisley, UK). Afterwards, each aliquot (20 mL) of the juice was collected into specific vials and stored at −20 °C.

## 2.3. Phenolic Compounds by HPLC Analysis

After being thawed at room temperature, the sample of the PGJ was analyzed using a liquid chromatography system Dionex UltiMate 3000 (Thermo Fisher Scientific, Waltham, MA, USA), including a solvent rack, a quaternary pump with an integrated four-channel degasser, a thermostatted column compartment, an autosampler and a four wavelength UV-Vis detector. Separation was performed on a column Dionex Acclaim 120, C18, 3 μm (4.6 × 150 mm) (Thermo Fisher Scientific, Waltham, MA, USA) with a gradient program at a flow rate of 0.8 mL·min$^{-1}$. Column temperature was maintained at 30 °C and the injection volume was 20 μL. The mobile phases consisted of water and formic acid (95:5, v/v) (eluent A) and methanol (eluent B). The gradient started with 1% B to reach 20% B at 20 min, 40% B at 30 min, 95% B at 35 min and 1% B after 41 min. The chromatograms were recorded simultaneously at 280, 360 and 520 nm. Calculation of concentrations was based on the external standard method. The HPLC analysis was replicated three times and the average values are reported in Table 1.

**Table 1.** Phenolic compounds composition (mg·L$^{-1}$) of pomegranate juice (Wonderful variety).

| Compound | Concentration (mg·L$^{-1}$) |
|---|---|
| gallic acid | 18.2 |
| ellagic acid | 97.5 |
| ellagic acid glucoside | 11.7 |
| α-punicalagin | 3.1 |
| β-punicalagin | 6.5 |
| delphinidin 3,5-diglucoside | 110.5 |
| cyanidin 3,5-diglucoside | 242.8 |
| pelargonidin 3,5-diglucoside | 9.3 |
| delphinidin 3-diglucoside | 60.4 |
| cyanidin 3-diglucoside | 180.6 |
| pelargonidin 3-diglucoside | 12.1 |

## 2.4. Cell Cultures and Cell Viability Assay

MM cell lines KMS26, MM1S and U266 (established from peripheral blood of a multiple myeloma patients in refractory and terminal stage) were cultured in suspension using RPMI1640 medium supplemented with 10% or 20% fetal bovine serum (FBS) and 1% penicillin/streptomycin at 37 °C and 5% $CO_2$. Human lymphocytes and monocytes were isolated, after informed consent, from fresh buffy coat of healthy volunteers provided by the Transfusional Centre of E. Muscatello Hospital—Augusta (SR). Monocytes and lymphocytes then were purified from the lymphomonocytic population by positive isolation using magnetic beads coated with goat anti-mouse CD14+ IgG and anti-mouse CD3+ IgG respectively (MiltenyiBiotec GmbH, Bergisch Gladbach, Germany) [28].

Human Brain Microvascular Endothelial Cells (HBMEC) (Innoprot, Elexalde Derio, Spain) were grown in monolayer in EBM supplemented with 5% fetal bovine serum (FBS), 1% endothelial cell growth supplement (ECGS), 100 U/mL penicillin and 100 mg/mL streptomycin. In studies involving serum-starvation, serum was reduced at 1% v/v.

Cell viability was assessed using ATPlite 1step assay (PerkinElmer, Milan, Italy) according to the manufacturers' protocol. ATPlite TM 1step is an Adenosine TriPhosphate (ATP) monitoring system based on firefly (Photinus pyralis) luciferase. ATP is a marker for cell viability because it is present in all metabolically active cells. Because ATP concentration declines rapidly when cells undergo necrosis or apoptosis, monitoring ATP is a good indicator of proliferation effects [29–31].

This analysis is a patented luminescence test that analyzes cell proliferation and cytotoxicity in mammalian cells considering the light release induced by ATP-luciferase-D-luciferin reaction.

This luminescence assay is an alternative to colorimetric, fluorometric and radioisotopic assays for the quantitative evaluation of proliferation and cytotoxicity of cultured mammalian cells. ATP monitoring can be used to assess the cytocidal, cytostatic and proliferative effects of a wide range of drugs, biological response modifiers and biological compounds.

ATPlite 1 step (PerkinElmer, Waltham, Massachusetts MA, USA) is a true homogeneous high sensitivity ATP monitoring 1-step addition assay kit for the quantification of viable cells. Because the kit needs no stabilization of the luminescence signal, high throughput is preserved. Briefly, the 96-well black culture plate was taken from the incubator and equilibrated at room temperature for 30 min. Subsequently, to each well containing 100 µL of the cell suspension (5 × 105 cells/mL), 100 µL of reconstituted reagent was added and the plate was shaken for 20 min at 700 rpm using orbital shaker (Stuart Scienti c, Staffordshire, UK). The luminescence was measured using Victor3 (PerkinElmer, Milan, Italy). Viability of the cells was expressed as percentage of vitality of untreated cells.

MTT assay: To quantify cell viability in endothelial cells, the 3-[4,5-dimethylthiazol-2-yl]-2,5-diphenyl tetrasodium bromide (MTT) assay was used (Chemicon, Temecula, CA, USA). 10,000 cells/well were plated in 96-well plates and grown in complete medium, in the absence or in the presence of PGJ (3%, 6% or 12% v/v) for 24–48 or 72 h. At the end of treatment, the cells were incubated with MTT for 4 h; then, 100 µL dimethyl sulfoxide was added and the absorbance was read at 590 nm, as previously described [32].

*2.5. Cell Cycle Analysis*

Cells were washed and resuspended in cold 80% ethanol to obtain a final concentration of $0.5 \times 10^6$ cells/mL for 1 h at 4 °C. The ethanol-fixed cells were centrifuged to remove ethanol and the pellet was resuspended in propidium iodide-staining reagent (0.1% Triton X-100), 0.1 mm Ethylenediaminetetraacetic acid (EDTA), 0.05 mg/mL RNase A and 50 mg/mL propidium iodide). Cells were stored in the dark at room temperature for about 3 h. Cells were then analyzed with a flow cytometer (FC500 Beckman Coulter; Beckman Coulter S.p.A., Milano, Italy) and the data were processed by the ModFit program (Verity Software House, version 4.0, Topsham ME 04086, US).

*2.6. Cell Invasion Assay*

In order to perform cell invasion/migration experiments, harvested cells ($1 \times 10^6$ cells/mL) were seeded into 8.0-µm-pore transwell inserts (Corning Life Sciences, Lowell, MA, USA) coated with Matrigel in the absence (control cells) or in the presence of PGJ (3% or 6% v/v) in medium containing 1% FBS. Cells migration was stimulated by addition of VEGF (50 ng/mL) to the lower well of the Boyden chamber. After 24 h, the cells were fixed with 95% ethanol and the invading cells were stained with 1× crystal violet. Invaded cells were stained with 0.1% crystal violet and counted after scanning membranes (×100 total magnification) by using ImageJ software (ImageJ 1.50e, National Institutes of Health, NIH, Bethesda, MD, USA). The membranes were also dissolved in acetic acid the density of invading cells was measured by reading the absorbance at 590 nm using a plate reader (Synergy 2-BioTek, Winooski, VT, USA).

## 2.7. Tube Formation Assay

The ability of cells to migrate and organize into capillary-like structures was carried out by using Matrigel (BD, Franklin Lakes, NJ, USA). Briefly, the cells were shifted to medium containing 1% serum for the 24 h. Next, the cells at $1 \times 10^4$ were suspended in 200 μL of the same medium containing either PGJ at different concentrations or PGJ plus VEGF (50 ng/mL). The mixtures were seeded in 96-well plates covered with polymerized growth factor-reduced Matrigel matrix (BD, Franklin Lakes, NJ, USA), incubated for 4 h (37 °C, 5% $CO_2$) and photographed at 100× magnification using an inverted Leica DM IRB microscope (Leica, Buffalo Grove, IL, USA) equipped with a Charge-Coupled Device (CCD) camera as previously described [33].

## 2.8. Aortic Ring Assay

Aortic rings were obtained by cross-sectioning the thoracic aorta of New Zealand white male rabbits at 1-mm intervals. Rings were placed individually on the bottom of 24-well plates, pre-coated with 150 μL of Matrigel. After 10 min, wells were rinsed with 150 μL of endothelial cell basal medium and incubated with the same medium containing 1% FBS in the absence or in the presence of VEGF-A (50 ng/mL) and the compound under test. The medium was changed in control and treated cells three times a week starting from day two. Aortic rings were observed daily for signs of angiogenic sprouting. The angiogenic response was measured by counting the length of neovessels sprouting out of the rings after 14 days. PGJ was renewed every two days during the assay.

## 2.9. Wound Healing Assay

Twenty-four well tissue culture plates were seeded with HBMEC to a final density of 150,000 cells per well, and these were maintained at 37 °C and 5% $CO_2$. Cells were cultured in 1% serum medium supplemented or not with 3% or 6% PGJ, or with PGJ added to VEGF-A (50 ng/mL)-stimulated cells. As described before, VEGF-A alone was used as a positive control, and 1% serum medium was a negative control. Wound closure was monitored within 24 h to 48 h of seeding. Confluent HBMEC monolayer was scratched with a p200 pipet tip. The wounds were photographed at 40× using phase-contrast microscope. After 24 h and 48 h, endothelial cells invading the wound were quantified by computerized analysis of the digitalized images. For each image acquired, areas of scratch were measured using ImageJ tools. The migration of cells toward the wounds was expressed as percentage of wound closure, as previously described [34].

## 2.10. Gene Expression Analysis

RNA was extracted by Trizol reagent (Invitrogen, Carlsbad, CA, USA). First strand cDNA was then synthesized with Applied Biosystem (Foster City, CA, USA) reverse transcription reagent [29]. PPARγ mRNA expression was assessed by TaqMan Gene Expression, Applied Biosystem and quantified using a fluorescence-based real-time detection method by 7900HT Fast Real Time PCR System (Life Technologies, Carlsbad, CA, USA). For each sample, the relative expression level of PPARγ (Hs01115514_m1) mRNA was normalized using Glyceraldehyde 3-phosphate dehydrogenase (GAPDH) (Hs02758991_g1) as an invariant control [35]. Analysis of angiogenic genes was performed using TaqMan Low Density Array Human Angiogenic Panel (Life Technologies, Carlsbad, CA, USA) that contains assays for 93 human genes in addition to three endogenous controls (18S, ACTB, GAPDH).

## 2.11. Statistical Analysis

Statistical significance between two groups was analyzed by Student's *t*-test. One-way and two-way analysis of variance (ANOVA), followed by Tukey's post hoc test, was used for multiple comparisons. *p* values < 0.05 were considered statistically significant.

## 3. Results

### 3.1. Effect of Pomegranate Juice on Multiple Myeloma Cell Viability

The anticancer activity of the PGJ was tested in U266, KMS26 and MM1S cell lines at different concentrations (3%, 6% and 12% of juice). After 24 h of treatment, we observed the inhibition of cell proliferation in a dose-dependent manner ($p < 0.0001$) (Figure 1A). The KMS26 cells showed a major sensitivity to the 12% PGJ exposure with 20% of proliferation only ($p < 0.001$). As showed in Figure 1B for U266 cell line, 6% and 12% PGJ induced G0/G1 cell cycle arrest in a dose-dependent manner (untreated: 50.58% ± 7%; 6% PGJ: 65.8% ± 5.2%; 12% PGJ: 73% ± 3%; $p < 0.05$), with a decrease of the percentage of cells in G(2)/M and S phase. In healthy lymphocytes and monocytes, the PGJ treatment did not show any effects (Figure 1A).

### 3.2. Pomegranate Juice Induces PPARγ Expression in Multiple Myeloma Cells

PGJ polyphenols can regulate the activation of PPARγ in several cancer cells [36]. It has been reported that this protein induces inhibition of cell proliferation in MM [37]. We observed a significant increase of PPARγ mRNA expression in U266 cells after treatment con PGJ in a dose-dependent manner. PGJ induced up-regulation of PPARγ of about 20 and 30 fold, respectively, at 6% and 12% ($p < 0.0001$) (Figure 1C), suggesting that this molecular mechanism may contribute to a PGJ anti-proliferative effect on MM cells.

### 3.3. Pomegranate Juice Inhibits Angiogenesis

Since angiogenesis is associated with progression of MM [38], we first examined the effect of PGJ on HBMEC cell viability. As shown in Figure 2A, PGJ inhibited cell proliferation in a dose- and time-dependent manner by 18% and 19% at 48 h and 72 h, respectively, in the presence of 3% PGJ. Moreover, inhibitions by 29%, 31% and 32% at 24 h, 48 h, and 72 h, respectively, in the presence of 6% PGJ, were found. Since PGJ significantly reduced cell viability at 12%, this dose was not used for the subsequent tests. The direct effect of PGJ on angiogenesis was tested by using the tube formation and ex vivo rabbit aortic ring assays. We studied the effect of VEGF-A alone or in combination with 3% or 6% PGJ, on tubule formation of HBMEC by using the Matrigel assay. The results in Figure 2B show that the tubular networks formed on Matrigel vary in the different environments. The number of the interconnections between the tubes provides information on the way the HBMEC organize them and grow. In panel a (control), some cells are joined by projections or direct cell contact. Cellular projections that do not result in contact with other cells are also visible (arrows). In the presence of VEGF-A (panel b) the cells show sprouts which connect with similar projections originating from other cells to form a cell–cell contact. Some cells forming polygon structures are also visible (arrowheads). In the presence of 3% (panel c) or 6% (panel e) PGJ, the cells show few sprouts. Both 3% and 6% PGJ suppressed the formation of tube-like structures in presence of VEGF-A (panels d and f). As expected, the VEGF-A treatment significantly induced an enhancement of both tube length and number of branch points by 1.7 and 2.0 fold, respectively, in comparison to control unstimulated cells (Figure 2C,D). The total length and the number of branch points were significantly reduced by both concentrations of PGJ respect to VEGF-A-treated cells ($p < 0.0001$). The incubation of the cells with 3% or 6% PGJ in the presence of VEGF-A significantly reduced tube total length by 1.7 fold after both treatments in comparison to VEGF-A-treated cells. Moreover, fewer branch points between cells incubated with 3% or 6% PGJ plus VEGF-A was observed, with a reduction by 2.2- and 2.3-fold, respectively, in comparison to growth factor stimulated cells. Moreover, PGJ in the presence or not of VEGF-A totally inhibited the formation of enclosed spaces in Matrigel (mesh number, panel e). The ex vivo rabbit aortic ring assay (Figure 3) showed an evident new vessel sprouting of endothelial tubes from aorta rings when the incubations were carried out in presence of VEGF (panel d). Total length was about 6 fold greater with VEGF-A than controls cells (panel a) or 3% and 6% PGJ treated cells (panels b and c). Panels e and f show the effects of both 3% and 6% PGJ, respectively, on VEGF-treated cells. As shown in the bar graph inset, there is a dose-dependent effect, with a higher concentration of PGJ leading to a greater reduction of outgrowth of vascular shoots.

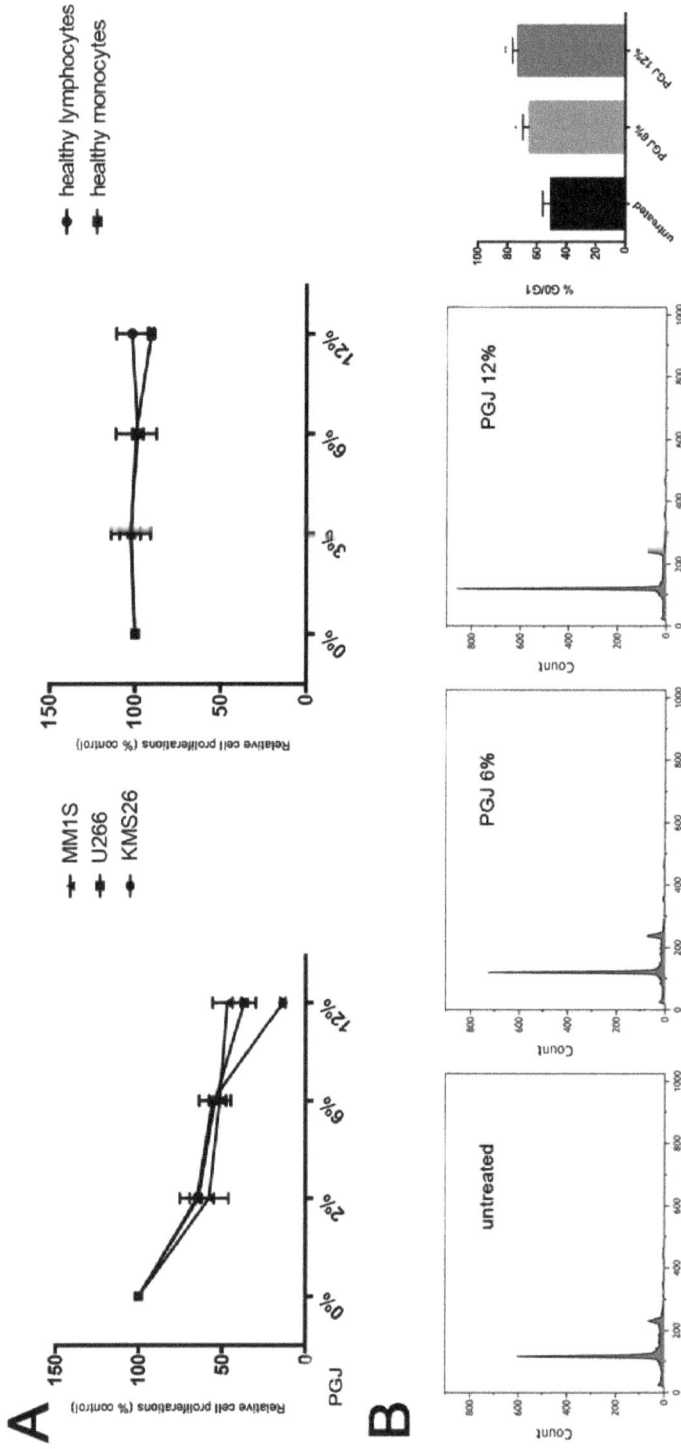

Figure 1. *Cont.*

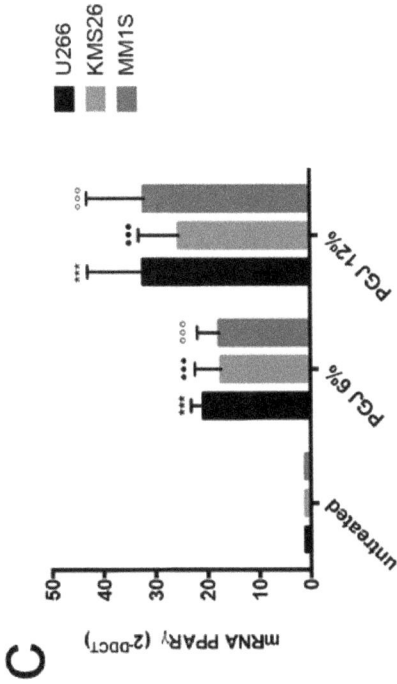

**Figure 1.** (**A**) the survival assay in U266, KMS26 and MM1S cell lines treated with PGJ. *Bars* represent the mean ± SEM of four independent experiments. \*\*\*/ ●●●/ ○○○ $p < 0.0001$ versus untreated cells; (**B**) the effect of PGJ treatment on G0/G1 phase in U266 cells. Cell cycle analysis was performed by the ModFit program ((Verity Software House, version 4.0, Topsham ME 04086, US). Results represent three independent experiments in triplicate ($p < 0.002$); (**C**) mRNA expression of PPARγ in MM cells treated with PGJ. *Bars* represent the mean ± SEM of four independent experiments. \*\*\* (U266 cells), ●●● (KMS26 cells), ○○○ (MM1S cells) $p < 0.0001$ versus untreated cells. (Calculated value of $2^{-\Delta\Delta Ct}$ in U266, KMS26, MM1S untreated was 1).

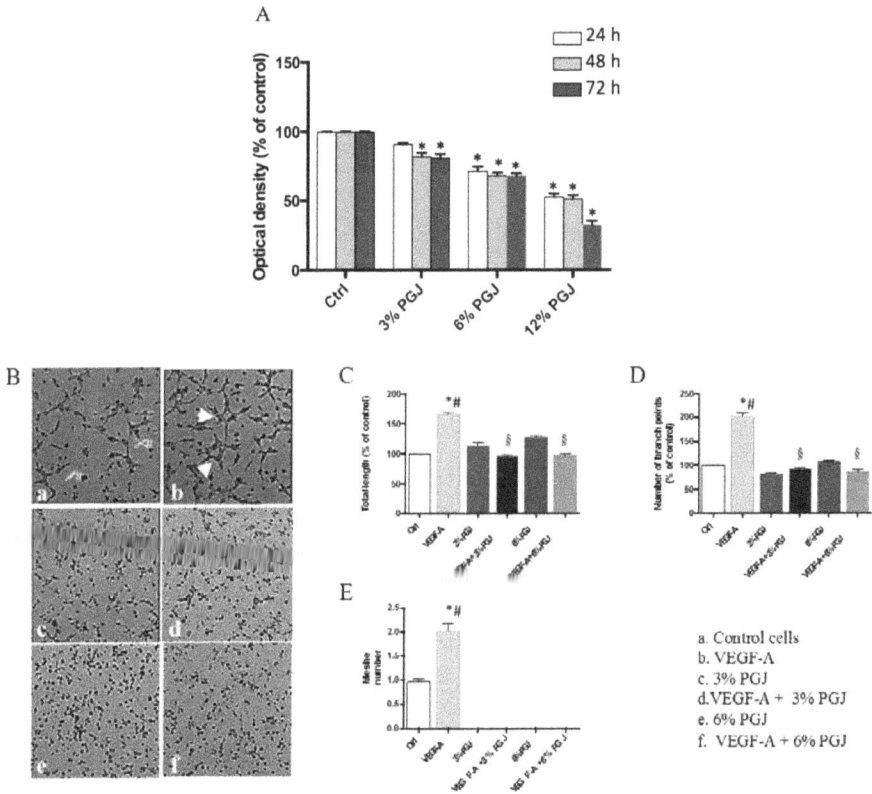

**Figure 2.** (**A**) Effect of PGJ on HBMEC viability. Cells ($1 \times 10^4$ cells/well) were cultured in complete medium in the absence or in the presence of PGJ at 3% or 6% or 12% (v/v). Cell viability was assessed by MTT assay. Values are expressed as mean ± SD of three independent experiments, each involving six different wells per condition. (* $p < 0.05$ vs. respective control); (**B**) Effect of PGJ on VEGF-A-induced HBMEC in vitro angiogenesis. Tube formation was evaluated with light microscopy and representative fields are shown. Panel (**a**): Control cells; panel (**b**): VEGF-A stimulated cells; panels (**c**) and (**e**): Cells treated with 3% and 6% PGJ, respectively; panels (**d**) and (**f**): Cells treated with 3% and 6% PGJ, respectively, in the presence of VEGF-A; Quantitative analysis of tube formation was indicated as tube length (**C**) and number of branch points (**D**) expressed as percentage of control cells. Image analysis of the total length and the number of branch points in the whole photographed area (representing central 70% of the well) were carried out by using Angiogenesis Analyzer tool for ImageJ (ImageJ 1.50e, National Institutes of Health, NIH, Bethesda, MD, USA). Values are expressed as a mean ± SD of three independent experiments performed in duplicate. Statistically significant differences by one-way analysis of variance (ANOVA) followed by Tukey's test ($p < 0.05$) are indicated: (*) VEGF-A-stimulated cells vs. control; (§) 3% and 6% PGJ plus VEGF-A-treated cells vs. VEGF-A-stimulated cells.

### 3.4. Effect of Pomegranate Juice on Cell Invasion and Migration

Since endothelial cell migration is essential for the formation of new blood vessels during neo-angiogenesis, we evaluated the effects of PGJ treatment on the migratory and invasive properties of endothelial cells by using, respectively, the wound-healing and the transwell assays (Figure 4). As shown in panel A, the presence of VEGF-A in the medium increased HBMEC migration in comparison to control cells. Quantitative analysis showed in panel b revealed a VEGF-dictated increase of cell migration by almost 1.7- and 2.0-fold after 24 h and 48 h, respectively, compared with control cells. The incubation with VEGF-A plus 3% and 6% PGJ reduced the cell migration (panel a); this reduction was estimated at almost 6.0 fold when both 3% or 6% PGJ, respectively, were added to VEGF-A-treated cells for both 24 h and 48 h.

The effect of PGJ on HBMEC migration was also assessed by using transwell migration assays (panels c, d and e). A reduction of the number of invaded cells by 30% and 40% after 3% or 6% PGJ, respectively, was found in comparison to VEGF-treated cells.

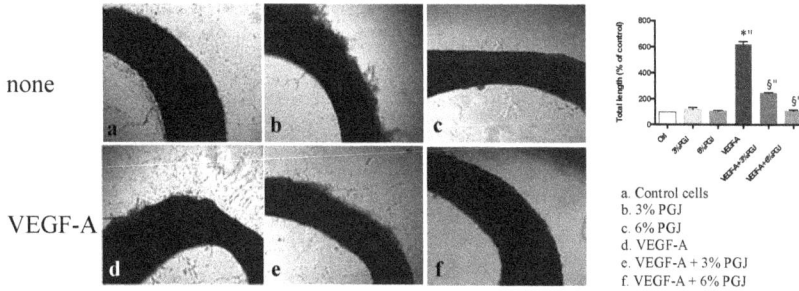

a. Control cells
b. 3% PGJ
c. 6% PGJ
d. VEGF-A
e. VEGF-A + 3% PGJ
f. VEGF-A + 6% PGJ

**Figure 3.** Developing microvessels from the intimal/subintimal layers of the aortic wall. Rabbit thoracic aortic rings were isolated and embedded on Matrigel, in the absence of VEGF-A ((**a**): untreated; (**b**): 3% PGJ; (**c**): 6% PGJ) or in the presence of 50 ng/ml VEGF-A ((**d**): VEGF-A alone; (**e**): 3% PGJ; (**f**): 6% PGJ). After 14 days, the angiogenic response was measured by counting the lenght of neovessels sprouting out of the rings. Representative photographs from a single experiment that was performed three times are shown. Statistically significant differences by one-way ANOVA followed by Tukey's test ($p < 0.05$) are indicated: (*) VEGF-A-stimulated cells vs. control; (§) 3% and 6% PGJ plus VEGF-A-treated cells vs. VEGF-A-stimulated cells.

### 3.5. Effect of Pomegranate Juice on Angiogenic Genes Expression

To confirm the anti-angiogenic properties of PGJ, we analyzed the expression of mRNA angiogenic genes in HBMEC cells after treatment with VEGF-A alone or in combination with 3% and 6% PGJ. Compared to cells exposed to VEGF-A alone, we observed that several angiogenic genes were downregulated in cells treated with VEGF-A in combination with PGJ (Table 2).

### 3.6. Combination of Pomegranate Juice with Proteosome Inhibitor Bortezomib

For its anti-proliferative and anti-angiogenic properties, we tested in vitro the combination of PGJ with the proteasome inhibitor BTZ, a first-line drug used for MM therapy. We observed that combination of PGJ (6%) with BTZ inhibited the cytotoxicity of the drug in MM cells (Figure 5A). It may be linked to the G0/G1 cell cycle arrest induced by PGJ that could protect MM cells from BTZ cytotoxic effects. For this reason, we used alternating BTZ/PGJ or PGJ/BTZ combinations for treatment of 24 h each one. Before the addition of the second compound, cells were washed and resuspended in drug-free medium. Pre-treatment with PGJ inhibited cytotoxic effect of BTZ (Figure 5B), probably for the same mechanism that led to the failure of concurrent combination PGJ-BTZ. On the contrary, treatment with PGJ after BTZ improved the cytotoxic effect in MM cell lines ($p < 0.0001$).

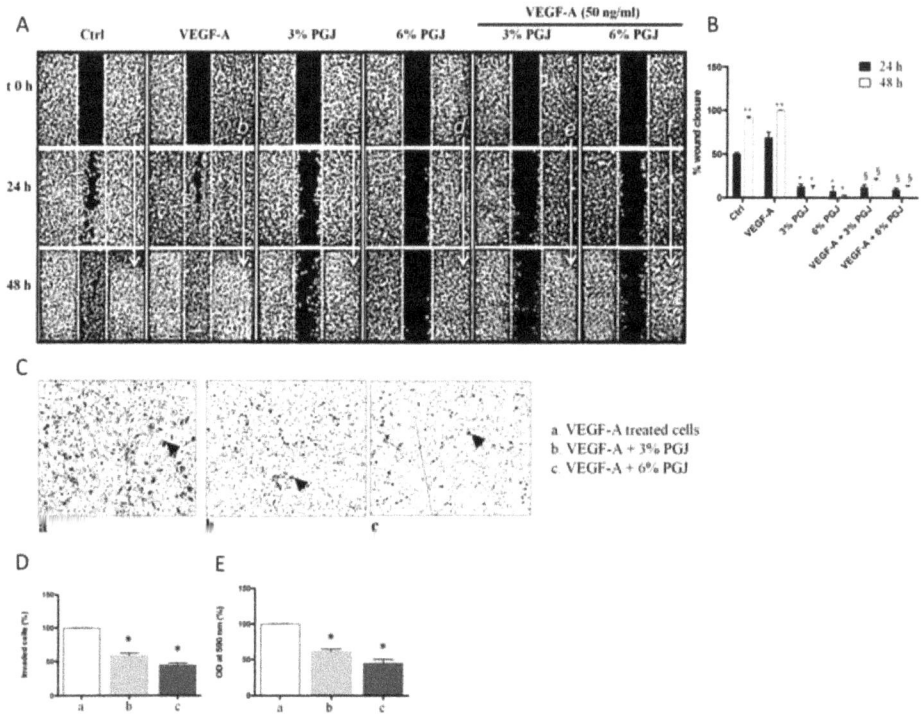

**Figure 4.** (**A″**) Effect of PGJ on VEGF induced HBMEC migration (wound healing assay). Images of scratch photographed with at ×40 using phase-contrast microscope at different time point, 0, 24 and 48 h. (**a**) Control cells, 1% serum; (**b**) VEGF-A + 1% serum; (**c**) 3% PGJ; (**d**) 6% PGJ; (**e**) VEGF-A + 3% PGJ; (**f**) VEGF-A + 6% PGJ; (**B″**) migration of HBMEC cells after wounding evaluated as percentage of wound closure respect to 48 h VEGF-A treated cells considered as 100% wound closure. The results are expressed as mean ± standard deviation. Statistically significant differences by one-way ANOVA followed by Tukey's test ($p < 0.05$) are indicated: (#) non stimulated cells vs. control at 24 h; (*) 3% and 6% PGJ vs. control at 24- and 48 h; (**) VEGF-A-stimulated cells vs. respective control at at 24- and 48 h; (§) 3% and 6% PGJ plus VEGF-A-treated cells vs. VEGF-A-stimulated cells at 24- and 48 h; (**C″**) effect of PGJ on VEGF-A induced HBMEC invasion. Harvested HBMEC ($1 \times 10^6$ cells/mL) were allowed to migrate through transwell membranes towards 50 ng/mL VEGF in the absence or in the presence of PGJ for 24 h. Cells that had migrated to the underside of the transwell membrane were fixed and evaluated with light microscopy. Representative fields are shown at 100× magnification; (**D″**) average number (displayed as percentage of control) of HREC migrated in three different wells in each condition ($n = 5$ different fields of the same membrane); and (**E″**) quantitative analysis of invaded cells, which were eluted using 10% acetic acid and measured optical density value at 590 nm. Data are the mean ± SD of three independent experiments. Statistically significant differences by one-way ANOVA followed by Tukey's test ($p < 0.05$) are indicated: (*) 3% and 6% PGJ plus VEGF-A-treated cells vs. VEGF-A-stimulated cells.

**Table 2.** Effect of 6% PGJ on the expression levels of angiogenic genes in HBMEC. Reported data are expressed by relative quantification (fold change) using a $2^{-\Delta\Delta Ct}$ method. VEGF-A treated cells was of the control.

| Genes | VEGF | PGJ + VEGF | *p* Value |
|---|---|---|---|
| VEGF | 43 | 0.036 | $p < 0.001$ |
| ADAMST1 | 23 | 0.041 | $p < 0.001$ |
| CXCL12 | 16 | 0.136 | $p < 0.001$ |
| CXCL2 | 9 | 0.038 | $p < 0.001$ |
| FGF2 | 32 | 0.011 | $p < 0.001$ |
| FIGF | 12 | 0.065 | $p < 0.05$ |
| IL12A | 9 | 0.030 | $p < 0.001$ |
| IL8 | 21 | 0.007 | $p < 0.01$ |
| MMP2 | 5 | 0.031 | $p < 0.001$ |
| PDGFB | 15 | 0.116 | $p < 0.001$ |
| VEGFB | 19 | 0.028 | $p < 0.001$ |
| VEGFC | 18 | 0.008 | $p < 0.001$ |

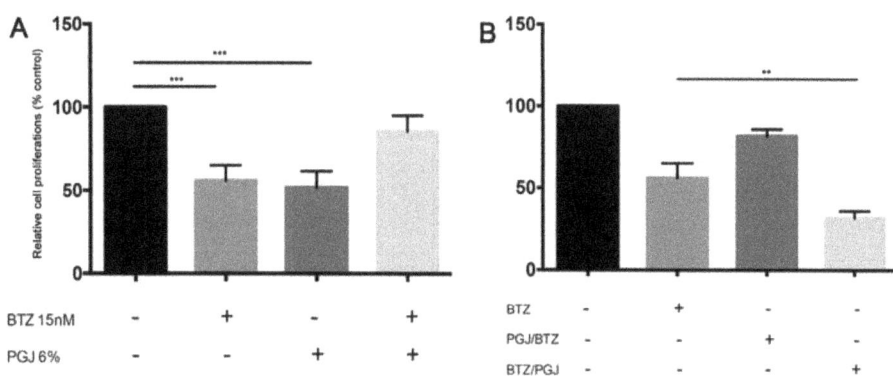

**Figure 5.** (**A**) the survival assay in U266 cell line treated with Bortezomib (BTZ) alone and in combination with PGJ. *Bars* represent the mean ± SEM of four independent experiments. *** $p < 0.0001$ versus untreated cells; and (**B**) the survival assay in U266 cell line treated alternating BTZ/PGJ or PGJ/BTZ combinations for treatment of 24 h each one. *Bars* represent the mean ± SEM of four independent experiments. * $p < 0.05$; ** $p < 0.001$; *** $p < 0.0001$.

## 4. Discussion

It is well-known that *Punica granatum* extracts contain bioactive compounds with anti-cancer actions leading to their use in a number of randomized clinical trials for prostate cancer [39]. Accumulated experimental evidence demonstrates that PGJ inhibits tumor proliferations [40] and induces apoptosis through a nuclear factor-kB-dependent mechanism in vitro and in mice [41]. Previous studies in vitro have also shown that pomegranate metabolites were able to inhibit prostate cancer cell proliferation [42]. The treatment with PGJ showed anticancer effects also in some cancer lines of colon (HT29 and HCT116), liver (HepG2 and Huh7), and breast (MCF-7 and MDA-MB-231) [43]. Our data demonstrated the anti-proliferative potential of PGJ in MM cells and its ability to improve the cytotoxic effect of the proteosome inhibitor BTZ. PGJ contains a number of potential active compounds including organic acids, vitamins, sugars, and phenolic components that are all responsible of the pro-apoptotic effects of PGJ observed in tumor cell lines. The phenolic components include phenolic acids: principally, hydroxybenzoic acids (such as gallic acid and ellagic acid) [44], hydroxycinnamic acids (such as caffeic acid and chlorogenic acid) [45], anthocyanins, including glycosylated forms of cyanidin, delphinidin, and pelargonidin [46], gallotannins and ellagitannins [44]. However, the concentration and the contents of these compounds vary due to growing region, climate, cultivation practice, and storage conditions [45,47]. In particular, it has been reported that the anthocyanins, which are major components of PGJ, were found to have binding affinity against eicosanoid receptors (e.g., peroxisome proliferator-activated receptors α and γ), by this way regulating gene expression and suppressing chemically induced carcinogenesis [48]. Several data demonstrated that the pomegranate leaves, stem and flower extracts modulate cell cycle progression and induce apoptosis in human MM cells through G2/M and S phase cell cycle arrest and mitochondrial membrane permeabilization [49]. It has also been reported that pomegranate induces apoptosis in leukemia cell lines and its polyphenols are responsible for these pro-apoptotic properties [50]. Our results confirm the anti-proliferative effect of PGJ in MM cell lines with a block of cell cycle in G0/G1 phase. Moreover, it upregulated PPARγ mRNA expression, which has been reported to induce apoptosis in MM cells [51,52] and be involved in the induction of G0/G1 phase cell cycle arrest [53]. In addition, accumulated evidence demonstrated that PGJ inhibits tumor angiogenesis and cell invasion [40] Angiogenesis is a constant hallmark of MM progression with prognostic potential [38,54]. In the bone marrow, increased vascularization correlated with a poor prognosis for MM patient [38]. Moreover, it has been reported that MM tumor progression is dependent on endothelial progenitor cells-trafficking (*targeting vasculogenesis to prevent progression in multiple myeloma*). For this reason, we investigated the effect of PGJ on angiogenesis and cell migration/invasion. Interestingly, we observed an inhibitory effect on the tube formation, microvessel outgrowth aorting ring and decreased cell migration and invasion as showed by wound-healing and transwell assays, respectively. Analysis of angiogenic genes expression in endothelial cells confirmed the anti-angiogenic properties of pomegranate. Therefore, PGJ administration could represent a good tool in order to identify novel therapeutic strategies for MM treatment, exploiting its anti-proliferative and anti-angiogenic effects.

Furthermore, we assessed the effect of PGJ treatment in combination with the proteosome inhibitor BTZ. Our results demonstrated that the concurrent administration of PGJ-BTZ on MM cells in vitro reduced the cytotoxic effect of proteosome inhibitor. We hypothesized that block of cell cycle in GO/G1 induced by PGJ could protect MM cells from bortezomib activity. We therefore evaluated sequential exposure of MM cells to the two compounds and found that the sequence of PGJ followed by BTZ did not add any cytotoxic effect to BTZ alone, thus confirming our hypothesis. On the contrary, by exposing MM cells to BTZ followed by PGJ, we observed an increase cytotoxic effect.

This is a pre-clinical model of potential benefits of bortezomib-PGJ combination. We propose using the entire pomegranate juice as a nutraceutical means, able to induce a modulation of the well-known pharmacological function of bortezomib in multiple myeloma, due to the metabolic relationships of individual components present in the whole pomegranate juice and not to a single one. Indeed, several previous studies have well shown that the single phytochemical agents are not able to induce the same effects of the entire pomegranate juice [55,56].

A phase 1 study has been planned to verify potential side effects in patients undergoing treatment, since the effect of PGJ on CYP450 or biochemical interactions is unknown. Most recently, it has been reported that the proteasome-inhibitory and anticancer activity of bortezomib can be blocked by green tea polyphenols, quercetin, myricetin and ascorbic acid through their interaction with the structure of a boronic acid to form boronic ester complexes [57,58]. It is worth noting that the drug has been administered in combination with a variety of antitumor agents in patients with cancer without significant alterations to its pharmacokinetic or pharmacodynamic profile (as reviewed by [4]).

## 5. Conclusions

In conclusion, the current work supports the evidence that PGJ could play a key role of a future nutraceutical approach for treatment of multiple myeloma in order to optimize the pharmacological effect of BTZ, especially as an adjuvant after treatment. Other stimulating studies are necessary in this field in order to better clarify all of the biochemical mechanisms that supervise these interesting antiproliferative and antiangiogenic effects. Future and stimulating studies of PGJ in combination with BTZ or other anti-MM agents are warranted.

*Nutrients* **2016**, *8*, 611

**Author Contributions:** All authors had full access to all of the data in the study and take responsibility for the integrity of the data and the accuracy of the data analysis. Conception and design: Daniele Tibullo, Cesarina Giallongo, Vincenzo Bramanti, Maria Violetta Brundo, and Salvatore Antonio Raccuia; Production and assembly of data: Daniele Tibullo, Nunzia Caporarello, Cesarina Giallongo, Carmelina Daniela Anfuso, Gabriella Lupo, Fabrizio Puglisi, and Nunziatina L. Parrinello; Analysis and interpretation of data: Daniele Tibullo, Carmelina Daniela Anfuso, Gabriella Lupo, Vincenzo Bramanti, Claudia Genovese, and Alessandra Romano; Drafting of the manuscript: Daniele Tibullo, Vincenzo Bramanti, Carmelina Daniela Anfuso, and Maria Violetta Brundo; Critical revision of the manuscript for important intellectual content: Daniele Tibullo, Carmelina Daniela Anfuso, Gabriella Lupo, Vincenzo Bramanti, and Maria Violetta Brundo; Statistical analysis: Carmen Arlotta, and Valeria Toscano; Study supervision: Roberto Avola, Francesco Di Raimondo, Carmelina Daniela Anfuso, and Salvatore Antonio Raccuia; Final approval of manuscript: All authors.

**Conflicts of Interest:** The authors declare no conflict of interest.

## References

1. Tibullo, D.; Di Rosa, M.; Giallongo, C.; La Cava, P.; Parrinello, N.L.; Romano, A.; Conticello, C.; Brundo, M.V.; Saccone, S.; Malaguarnera, L.; et al. Bortezomib modulates CHIT1 and YKL40 in monocyte-derived osteoclast and in myeloma cells. *Front. Pharmacol.* **2015**, *6*, 226. [CrossRef] [PubMed]

2. Gozzetti, A.; Candi, V.; Papini, G.; Bocchia, M. Therapeutic advancements in multiple myeloma. *Front. Oncol.* **2014**, *4*, 241. [CrossRef] [PubMed]

3. Giallongo, C.; Tibullo, D.; Parrinello, N.L.; La Cava, P.; Di Rosa, M.; Bramanti, V.; Di Raimondo, C.; Conticello, C.; Chiarenza, A.; Palumbo, G.A.; et al. Granulocyte-like myeloid derived suppressor Cells (G-MDSC) are increased in multiple myeloma and are driven by dysfunctional mesenchymal stem cells (MSC). *Oncotarget* **2016**. [CrossRef]

4. Romano, A.; Conticello, C.; Di Raimondo, F. Bortezomib for the treatment of previously untreated multiple myeloma. *Immunotherapy* **2013**, *5*, 327–352. [CrossRef] [PubMed]

5. Gambella, M.; Rocci, A.; Passera, R.; Gay, F.; Omede, P.; Crippa, C.; Corradini, P.; Romano, A.; Rossi, D.; Ladetto, M.; et al. High XBP1 expression is a marker of better outcome in multiple myeloma patients treated with bortezomib. *Haematologica* **2014**, *99*, e14–e16. [CrossRef] [PubMed]

6. Botta, C.; Gulla, A.; Correale, P.; Tagliaferri, P.; Tassone, P. Myeloid-derived suppressor cells in multiple myeloma: Pre-clinical research and translational opportunities. *Front. Oncol.* **2014**, *4*, 348. [CrossRef] [PubMed]

7. Kryukov, F.; Nemec, P.; Dementyeva, E.; Kubiczkova, L.; Ihnatova, I.; Budinska, E.; Jarkovsky, J.; Sevcikova, S.; Kuglik, P.; Hajek, R. Molecular heterogeneity and centrosome-associated genes in multiple myeloma. *Leuk. Lymphoma* **2013**, *54*, 1982–1988. [CrossRef] [PubMed]

8. Tibullo, D.; Barbagallo, I.; Giallongo, C.; Vanella, L.; Conticello, C.; Romano, A.; Saccone, S.; Godos, J.; Di Raimondo, F.; Volti, L.G. Heme oxygenase-1 nuclear translocation regulates bortezomibinduced cytotoxicity and mediates genomic instability in myeloma cells. *Oncotarget* **2016**, *7*, 28868–28880. [CrossRef] [PubMed]

9. Chung, T.H.; Mulligan, G.; Fonseca, R.; Chng, W.J. A novel measure of chromosome instability can account for prognostic difference in multiple myeloma. *PLoS ONE* **2013**, *8*, e66361. [CrossRef] [PubMed]

10. Safarzadeh, E.; Sandoghchian, S.S.; Baradaran, B. Herbal medicine as inducers of apoptosis in cancer treatment. *Adv. Pharm. Bull.* **2014**, *4*, 421–427. [PubMed]

11. Syed, D.N.; Chamcheu, J.C.; Adhami, V.M.; Mukhtar, H. Pomegranate extracts and cancer prevention: Molecular and cellular activities. *Anticancer Agents Med. Chem.* **2013**, *13*, 1149–1161. [CrossRef] [PubMed]

12. Turrini, E.; Ferruzzi, L.; Fimognari, C. Potential effects of pomegranate polyphenols in cancer prevention and therapy. *Oxid. Med. Cell. Longev.* **2015**, *2015*, 938475. [CrossRef] [PubMed]

13. Lansky, E.P.; Newman, R.A. *Punica granatum* (pomegranate) and its potential for prevention and treatment of inflammation and cancer. *J. Ethnopharmacol.* **2007**, *109*, 177–206. [CrossRef] [PubMed]

14. Katz, S.R.; Newman, R.A.; Lansky, E.P. *Punica granatum*: Heuristic treatment for diabetes mellitus. *J. Med. Food* **2007**, *10*, 213–217. [CrossRef] [PubMed]

15. Heber, D. Pomegranate ellagitannins. In *Herbal Medicine: Biomolecular and Clinical Aspects*, 2nd ed.; Benzie, I.F.F., Wachtel-Galor, S., Eds.; CRC Press: Boca Raton, FL, USA, 2011.

16. Adhami, V.M.; Khan, N.; Mukhtar, H. Cancer chemoprevention by pomegranate: Laboratory and clinical evidence. *Nutr. Cancer* **2009**, *61*, 811–815. [CrossRef] [PubMed]

17. Kim, N.D.; Mehta, R.; Yu, W.; Neeman, I.; Livney, T.; Amichay, A.; Poirier, D.; Nicholls, P.; Kirby, A.; Jiang, W.; et al. Chemopreventive and adjuvant therapeutic potential of pomegranate (*Punica granatum*) for human breast cancer. *Breast Cancer Res. Treat.* **2002**, *71*, 203–217. [CrossRef] [PubMed]

18. Toi, M.; Bando, H.; Ramachandran, C.; Melnick, S.J.; Imai, A.; Fife, R.S.; Carr, R.E.; Oikawa, T.; Lansky, E.P. Preliminary studies on the anti-angiogenic potential of pomegranate fractions in vitro and in vivo. *Angiogenesis* **2003**, *6*, 121–128. [CrossRef] [PubMed]

19. Adams, L.S.; Zhang, Y.; Seeram, N.P.; Heber, D.; Chen, S. Pomegranate ellagitannin-derived compounds exhibit antiproliferative and antiaromatase activity in breast cancer cells in vitro. *Cancer Prev. Res.* **2010**, *3*, 108–113. [CrossRef] [PubMed]

20. Dai, Z.; Nair, V.; Khan, M.; Ciolino, H.P. Pomegranate extract inhibits the proliferation and viability of MMTV-WNT-1 mouse mammary cancer stem cells in vitro. *Oncol. Rep.* **2010**, *24*, 1087–1091. [PubMed]

21. Dikmen, M.; Ozturk, N.; Ozturk, Y. The antioxidant potency of *Punica granatum* L. Fruit peel reduces cell proliferation and induces apoptosis on breast cancer. *J. Med. Food* **2011**, *14*, 1638–1646. [CrossRef] [PubMed]

22. Joseph, M.M.; Aravind, S.R.; Varghese, S.; Mini, S.; Sreelekha, T.T. Evaluation of antioxidant, antitumor and immunomodulatory properties of polysaccharide isolated from fruit rind of *Punica granatum*. *Mol. Med. Rep.* **2012**, *5*, 489–496. [PubMed]

23. Banerjee, N.; Talcott, S.; Safe, S.; Mertens-Talcott, S.U. Cytotoxicity of pomegranate polyphenolics in breast cancer cells in vitro and vivo: Potential role of MIRNA-27a and MIRNA-155 in cell survival and inflammation. *Breast Cancer Res. Treat.* **2012**, *136*, 21–34. [CrossRef] [PubMed]

24. Sreeja, S.; Santhosh Kumar, T.R.; Lakshmi, B.S.; Sreeja, S. Pomegranate extract demonstrate a selective estrogen receptor modulator profile in human tumor cell lines and in vivo models of estrogen deprivation. *J. Nutr. Biochem.* **2012**, *23*, 725–732. [CrossRef] [PubMed]

25. Shirode, A.B.; Kovvuru, P.; Chittur, S.V.; Henning, S.M.; Heber, D.; Reliene, R. Antiproliferative effects of pomegranate extract in MCF-7 breast cancer cells are associated with reduced DNA repair gene expression and induction of double strand breaks. *Mol. Carcinog.* **2014**, *53*, 458–470. [CrossRef] [PubMed]

26. Mehta, R.; Lansky, E.P. Breast cancer chemopreventive properties of pomegranate (*Punica granatum*) fruit extracts in a mouse mammary organ culture. *Eur. J. Cancer Prev.* **2004**, *13*, 345–348. [CrossRef] [PubMed]

27. Bishayee, A.; Mandal, A.; Bhattacharyya, P.; Bhatia, D. Pomegranate exerts chemoprevention of experimentally induced mammary tumorigenesis by suppression of cell proliferation and induction of apoptosis. *Nutr. Cancer* **2016**, *68*, 120–130. [CrossRef] [PubMed]

28. Di Rosa, M.; Tibullo, D.; Vecchio, M.; Nunnari, G.; Saccone, S.; Di Raimondo, F.; Malaguarnera, L. Determination of chitinases family during osteoclastogenesis. *Bone* **2014**, *61*, 55–63. [CrossRef] [PubMed]

29. Wang, P.; Henning, S.M.; Heber, D. Limitations of MTT and MTS-based assays for measurement of antiproliferative activity of green tea polyphenols. *PLoS ONE* **2010**, *5*, e10202. [CrossRef] [PubMed]

30. Cree, I.A.; Andreotti, P.E. Measurement of cytotoxicity by ATP-based luminescence assay in primary cell cultures and cell lines. *Toxicol. In Vitro* **1997**, *11*, 553–556. [CrossRef]

31. Petty, R.D.; Sutherland, L.A.; Hunter, E.M.; Cree, I.A. Comparison of MTT and ATP-based assays for the measurement of viable cell number. *J. Biolumin. Chemilumin.* **1995**, *10*, 29–34. [CrossRef] [PubMed]

32. Motta, C.; D'Angeli, F.; Scalia, M.; Satriano, C.; Barbagallo, D.; Naletova, I.; Anfuso, C.D.; Lupo, G.; Spina-Purrello, V. Pj-34 inhibits parp-1 expression and erk phosphorylation in glioma-conditioned brain microvascular endothelial cells. *Eur. J. Pharmacol.* **2015**, *761*, 55–64. [CrossRef] [PubMed]

33. Lupo, G.; Motta, C.; Salmeri, M.; Spina-Purrello, V.; Alberghina, M.; Anfuso, C.D. An in vitro retinoblastoma human triple culture model of angiogenesis: A modulatory effect of TGF-beta. *Cancer Lett.* **2014**, *354*, 181–188. [CrossRef] [PubMed]

34. Giurdanella, G.; Motta, C.; Muriana, S.; Arena, V.; Anfuso, C.D.; Lupo, G.; Alberghina, M. Cytosolic and calcium-independent phospholipase a(2) mediate glioma-enhanced proangiogenic activity of brain endothelial cells. *Microvasc. Res.* **2011**, *81*, 1–17. [CrossRef] [PubMed]

35. Giallongo, C.; Tibullo, D.; La Cava, P.; Branca, A.; Parrinello, N.; Spina, P.; Stagno, F.; Conticello, C.; Chiarenza, A.; Vigneri, P.; et al. Brit1/mcph1 expression in chronic myeloid leukemia and its regulation of the g2/m checkpoint. *Acta Haematol.* **2011**, *126*, 205–210. [CrossRef] [PubMed]

36. Khateeb, J.; Gantman, A.; Kreitenberg, A.J.; Aviram, M.; Fuhrman, B. Paraoxonase 1 (pon1) expression in hepatocytes is upregulated by pomegranate polyphenols: A role for ppar-gamma pathway. *Atherosclerosis* **2010**, *208*, 119–125. [CrossRef] [PubMed]

37. Aouali, N.; Broukou, A.; Bosseler, M.; Keunen, O.; Schlesser, V.; Janji, B.; Palissot, V.; Stordeur, P.; Berchem, G. Epigenetic activity of peroxisome proliferator-activated receptor gamma agonists increases the anticancer effect of histone deacetylase inhibitors on multiple myeloma cells. *PLoS ONE* **2015**, *10*, e0130339. [CrossRef] [PubMed]

38. Vacca, A.; Ria, R.; Reale, A.; Ribatti, D. Angiogenesis in multiple myeloma. *Chem. Immunol. Allergy* **2014**, *99*, 180–196. [PubMed]

39. Paller, C.J.; Ye, X.; Wozniak, P.J.; Gillespie, B.K.; Sieber, P.R.; Greengold, R.H.; Stockton, B.R.; Hertzman, B.L.; Efros, M.D.; Roper, R.P.; et al. A randomized phase II study of pomegranate extract for men with rising psa following initial therapy for localized prostate cancer. *Prostate Cancer Prostatic Dis.* **2013**, *16*, 50–55. [CrossRef] [PubMed]

40. Sartippour, M.R.; Seeram, N.P.; Rao, J.Y.; Moro, A.; Harris, D.M.; Henning, S.M.; Firouzi, A.; Rettig, M.B.; Aronson, W.J.; Pantuck, A.J.; et al. Ellagitannin-rich pomegranate extract inhibits angiogenesis in prostate cancer in vitro and in vivo. *Int. J. Oncol.* **2008**, *32*, 475–480. [CrossRef] [PubMed]

41. Rettig, M.B.; Heber, D.; An, J.; Seeram, N.P.; Rao, J.Y.; Liu, H.; Klatte, T.; Belldegrun, A.; Moro, A.; Henning, S.M.; et al. Pomegranate extract inhibits androgen-independent prostate cancer growth through a nuclear factor-kappab-dependent mechanism. *Mol. Cancer Ther.* **2008**, *7*, 2662–2671. [CrossRef] [PubMed]

42. Seeram, N.P.; Aronson, W.J.; Zhang, Y.; Henning, S.M.; Moro, A.; Lee, R.P.; Sartippour, M.; Harris, D.M.; Rettig, M.; Suchard, M.A.; et al. Pomegranate ellagitannin-derived metabolites inhibit prostate cancer growth and localize to the mouse prostate gland. *J. Agric. Food Chem.* **2007**, *55*, 7732–7737. [CrossRef] [PubMed]

43. Costantini, S.; Rusolo, F.; De Vito, V.; Moccia, S.; Picariello, G.; Capone, F.; Guerriero, E.; Castello, G.; Volpe, M.G. Potential anti-inflammatory effects of the hydrophilic fraction of pomegranate (*Punica granatum* L.) seed oil on breast cancer cell lines. *Molecules* **2014**, *19*, 8644–8660. [CrossRef] [PubMed]

44. Amakura, Y.; Okada, M.; Tsuji, S.; Tonogai, Y. High-performance liquid chromatographic determination with photodiode array detection of ellagic acid in fresh and processed fruits. *J. Chromatogr. A* **2000**, *896*, 87–93. [CrossRef]

45. Elfalleh, W.; Tlili, N.; Nasri, N.; Yahia, Y.; Hannachi, H.; Chaira, N.; Ying, M.; Ferchichi, A. Antioxidant capacities of phenolic compounds and tocopherols from tunisian pomegranate (*Punica granatum*) fruits. *J. Food Sci.* **2011**, *76*, C707–C713. [CrossRef] [PubMed]

46. Fanali, C.; Dugo, L.; D'Orazio, G.; Lirangi, M.; Dacha, M.; Dugo, P.; Mondello, L. Analysis of anthocyanins in commercial fruit juices by using nano-liquid chromatography-electrospray-mass spectrometry and high-performance liquid chromatography with UV-Vis detector. *J. Sep. Sci.* **2011**, *34*, 150–159. [CrossRef] [PubMed]

47. Pande, G.; Akoh, C.C. Antioxidant capacity and lipid characterization of six georgia-grown pomegranate cultivars. *J. Agric. Food Chem.* **2009**, *57*, 9427–9436. [CrossRef] [PubMed]

48. Kohno, H.; Suzuki, R.; Yasui, Y.; Hosokawa, M.; Miyashita, K.; Tanaka, T. Pomegranate seed oil rich in conjugated linolenic acid suppresses chemically induced colon carcinogenesis in rats. *Cancer Sci.* **2004**, *95*, 481–486. [CrossRef] [PubMed]

49. Kiraz, Y.; Neergheen-Bhujun, V.S.; Rummun, N.; Baran, Y. Apoptotic effects of non-edible parts of *Punica granatum* on human multiple myeloma cells. *Tumour Biol.* **2016**, *37*, 1803–1815. [CrossRef] [PubMed]

50. Dahlawi, H.; Jordan-Mahy, N.; Clench, M.; McDougall, G.J.; Maitre, C.L. Polyphenols are responsible for the proapoptotic properties of pomegranate juice on leukemia cell lines. *Food Sci. Nutr.* **2013**, *1*, 196–208. [CrossRef] [PubMed]

51. Aouali, N.; Palissot, V.; El-Khoury, V.; Moussay, E.; Janji, B.; Pierson, S.; Brons, N.H.; Kellner, L.; Bosseler, M.; Van Moer, K.; et al. Peroxisome proliferator-activated receptor gamma agonists potentiate the cytotoxic effect of valproic acid in multiple myeloma cells. *Br. J. Haematol.* **2009**, *147*, 662–671. [CrossRef] [PubMed]

52. Eucker, J.; Bangeroth, K.; Zavrski, I.; Krebbel, H.; Zang, C.; Heider, U.; Jakob, C.; Elstner, E.; Possinger, K.; Sezer, O. Ligands of peroxisome proliferator-activated receptor gamma induce apoptosis in multiple myeloma. *Anticancer Drugs* **2004**, *15*, 955–960. [CrossRef] [PubMed]

53. Liu, X.; Malki, A.; Cao, Y.; Li, Y.; Qian, Y.; Wang, X.; Chen, X. Glucose- and triglyceride-lowering dietary penta-*O*-galloyl-alpha-D-glucose reduces expression of ppargamma and c/ebpalpha, induces p21-mediated g1 phase cell cycle arrest, and inhibits adipogenesis in 3t3-l1 preadipocytes. *Exp. Clin. Endocrinol. Diabetes* **2015**, *123*, 308–316. [PubMed]

54. Di Raimondo, F. Angiogenesis in hematology: A field of active research. *Leuk. Res.* **2003**, *27*, 571–573. [CrossRef]

55. Wang, L.; Martins-Green, M. Pomegranate and its components as alternative treatment for prostate cancer. *Int. J. Mol. Sci.* **2014**, *15*, 14949–14966. [CrossRef] [PubMed]

56. Faria, A.; Calhau, C. The bioactivity of pomegranate: Impact on health and disease. *Crit. Rev. Food Sci. Nutr.* **2011**, *51*, 626–634. [CrossRef] [PubMed]

57. Glynn, S.J.; Gaffney, K.J.; Sainz, M.A.; Louie, S.G.; Petasis, N.A. Molecular characterization of the boron adducts of the proteasome inhibitor bortezomib with epigallocatechin-3-gallate and related polyphenols. *Org. Biomol. Chem.* **2015**, *13*, 3887–3899. [CrossRef] [PubMed]

58. Jia, L.; Liu, F.T. Why bortezomib cannot go with 'green'? *Cancer Biol. Med.* **2013**, *10*, 206–213. [PubMed]

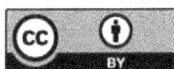

*nutrients*

MDPI

Article

# The Growth of SGC-7901 Tumor Xenografts Was Suppressed by Chinese Bayberry Anthocyanin Extract through Upregulating *KLF6* Gene Expression

Yue Wang [1], Xia-nan Zhang [1], Wen-hua Xie [1], Yi-xiong Zheng [2], Jin-ping Cao [3], Pei-rang Cao [4], Qing-jun Chen [5], Xian Li [1] and Chong-de Sun [1,*]

[1]   Laboratory of Fruit Quality Biology/The State Agriculture ministry Laboratory of Horticultural Plant Growth, Development and Quality Improvement, Zhejiang University, Zijingang Campus, Hangzhou 310058, China; fruit@zju.edu.cn (Y.W.); xiananzhang@zju.edu.cn (X.-n.Z.); 21516063@zju.edu.cn (W.-h.X.); xianli@zju.edu.cn (X.L.)
[2]   Department of Surgery, Second Affiliated Hospital, School of Medicine, Zhejiang University, Hangzhou 310009, China; zyx_xxn@126.com
[3]   Taizhou Academy of Agricultural Sciences, Linhai 317000, China; caojinpingabc@126.com
[4]   State Key Laboratory of Food Science and Technology, School of Food Science and Technology, Jiangnan University, Wuxi 214122, China; prcao@jiangnan.edu.cn
[5]   National Light Industry Food Quality Inspection Hangzhou Station, Hangzhou 310009, China; chenqj@zzytech.com
*   Correspondence: adesun2006@zju.edu.cn; Tel.: +86-571-8898-2229

Received: 14 July 2016; Accepted: 20 September 2016; Published: 27 September 2016

**Abstract:** To investigate the antitumor effect of anthocyanins extracted from Chinese bayberry fruit (*Myrica rubra* Sieb. et Zucc.), a nude mouse tumor xenograft model was established. Treatments with C3G (cyanidin-3-glucoside, an anthocyanin) significantly suppressed the growth of SGC-7901 tumor xenografts in a dose-dependent manner. Immunohistochemical staining showed a significant increase in p21 expression, indicating that the cell cycle of tumor xenografts was inhibited. qPCR screening showed that C3G treatment up-regulated the expression of the *KLF6* gene, which is an important tumor suppressor gene inactivated in many human cancers. Western blot showed that C3G treatments markedly increased KLF6 and p21 protein levels, inhibited CDK4 and Cyclin D1 expression, but did not notably change the expression of p53. These results indicated that KLF6 up-regulates p21 in a p53-independent manner and significantly reduces tumor proliferation. This study provides important information for the possible mechanism of C3G-induced antitumor activity against gastric adenocarcinoma in vivo.

**Keywords:** Chinese bayberry; anthocyanin; SGC-7901 cell; tumor xenograft; *KLF6* gene

## 1. Introduction

Anthocyanins are the most abundant water-soluble pigment found in fruit, vegetables and beans. It has been well established that anthocyanins from different sources exhibit multiple functional properties including antioxidant [1], anticancer [2], anti-obesity [3] and anti-diabetic effects [4]. It has been demonstrated in our laboratory that the proliferation of human SGC-7901, BGC-823 and AGS gastric cancer cells in vitro was inhibited by anthocyanins from Chinese bayberry fruit [5].

Gastric cancer, also called stomach cancer, is the fourth most frequently diagnosed cancer in humans and the third leading cause of cancer death worldwide [6]. It ranks second as the most frequently diagnosed cancer and is the leading cause of cancer death in China today, second only to lung cancer [7]. Further epidemiological and experimental studies showed that diet pattern variations play an important role in the etiology of gastric cancer [8,9], and a reverse association between fruit intake and gastric cancer risk has been widely reported [10–13].

Chinese bayberry (*Myrica rubra* Sieb. et Zucc.) is a subtropical native Chinese fruit with high nutrient and health values. The red-colored Chinese bayberry pulp is a rich source of anthocyanins, especially cyanidin-3-glucoside (C3G) [14], which has been well characterized as having anticancer activity in vitro [15] and in vivo [16]. Previous studies have demonstrated that the in vitro anticancer activities of anthocyanins are exerted through mechanisms of promotion of apoptosis [17], inhibition of cell cycle [18] and cell invasion [5,19]. However, the antitumor effects of C3G in vivo have been less clearly demonstrated.

Krüppel-like transcription factor 6 (*KLF6*) is a novel tumor suppressor gene and is involved in the pathogenesis of many cancers [20]. In addition to gastric cancer [21], functional inactivation of *KLF6* was observed in a number of other human cancers including prostate [20], colorectal [22,23], ovarian [24], liver [25,26], and breast cancer [27]. With different cell types and contexts, *KLF6* exhibits growth inhibition activity through several major cancer pathways such as p53-independent up-regulation of p21 [20], disruption of Cyclin D1 and CDK4 interaction [28] and induction of apoptosis [23]. Although the tumor-suppressing activity of the *KLF6* gene is well known, it has not been reported whether natural nutrients such as anthocyanins could affect *KLF6* expression.

In this study, it was first discovered that C3G, a major component of anthocyanins from Chinese bayberry, could suppress the growth of SGC-7901 tumor xenografts through up-regulating *KLF6* gene expression.

## 2. Materials and Methods

### 2.1. Materials and Chemicals

Chinese bayberry (*Myrica rubra* Sieb. et Zucc c.v. Dongkui) fruits were harvested at commercial maturity from Xianju County, Zhejiang Province, China. The SGC-7901 gastric cancer cell line was obtained from the Department of Surgery, Second Affiliated Hospital, School of Medicine, Zhejiang University.

C3G standards were purchased from Sigma-Aldrich Co. LLC (Shanghai, China). RIPA (Radio Immunoprecipitation Assay) lysis buffer was purchased from the Beyotime Institute of Biotechnology (Hangzhou, China). Anti-KLF6, anti-caspase3, anti-p21, anti-p53, anti-Cyclin D1, anti-CDK4 antibodies were obtained from Proteintech (Chicago, IL, USA). All the other reagents were of analytical grade and purchased from Sinopharm Chemical Reagent Co., Ltd. (Shanghai, China). Double-distilled water (ddH$_2$O) was used in all experiments. All samples for HPLC (High Performance Liquid Chromatography) analyses were filtered through a 0.22 μm membrane before injection.

### 2.2. Purification and Identification of C3G from Chinese Bayberry Fruit

Fifty grams of fresh Chinese bayberry fruit pulp was extracted ultrasonically with 80% aqueous methanol (1% formic acid) in a material-to-solvent ratio of 1:10 (*w/v*) three times. The supernatants from three extractions were combined and evaporated under reduced pressure at 36 °C to remove the methanol. A phenolic-rich extract (PRE) was obtained by solid-phase extraction (SPE) using a Sep-pak C$_{18}$ cartridge (12 cc, 2 g sorbent; Waters Corp., Milford, MA, USA). Sugars and organic acids were removed by eluting with ddH$_2$O. Phenolics were eluted with 10% aqueous methanol after eluting with 5% aqueous methanol.

The purity of C3G was determined by HPLC (2695 pump, 2996 diode array detector; Waters Corp., Milford, MA, USA) coupled with a Waters SunFire C$_{18}$ analytical column (4.6 × 250 mm) at a column temperature of 25 °C. The HPLC analyses were performed as per previously published procedures [29] with some modifications. The mobile phase consisted of 0.1% (*v/v*) formic acid in water (eluent A) and of acetonitrile: 0.1% formic acid (1:1, *v/v*) (eluent B). The gradient program was as follows: 0 to 40 min, 10% to 38% of B; 40 to 60 min, 38% to 48% of B; 60 to 70 min, 48% to 100% of B; 70 to 75 min, 100% to 10% of B; 75 to 80 min, 10% of B. Then 10 μL samples were injected and were detected from 200 to 600 nm. Anthocyanins were calculated as C3G equivalent at 515 nm.

LC-MS (Liquid Chromatograph-Mass Spectrometer) experiments were performed according to our previous publication [5]. Briefly, an Agilent 6430 Triple Quadrupole LC/MS system (Agilent Technologies Inc., Santa Clara, CA, USA) was used for LC-MS. Multiple reaction monitoring (MRM) was used for analytical identification and electrospray ionization (ESI) was in positive mode. The operation conditions were as follows: capillary 4000 V, nebulizer 35 psi, dry gas flow rate 9 L/min at 350 °C. An Agilent MassHunter Workstation was used to carry out data acquisition and processing.

The $^1$H-NMR (Hydrogen-Nuclear Magnetic Resonance) (500.18 MHz) spectra were obtained on a Bruker Avance 500 instrument (Bruker Biospin, Fallanden, Switzerland). Extracts (15 mg) were dissolved in 0.5 mL deuterated methanol ($CD_3OD$) in a 5 mm $\Phi$ tube at variable temperatures; $\delta$ (parts per million) and the coupling constants ($J$) in Hertz were presented as chemical shifts.

## 2.3. Animal and Tumor Xenograft Studies

Balb/c nude mice (weighing 19–21 g) were used for building a model and were maintained at 23–25 °C and 50%–60% humidity in the Laboratory Animal Center of Zhejiang University (Hangzhou, China). Balb/c-nu mice were randomly allocated to four groups: a model group (drinking water), low-dose group (C3G, 25 mg·kg$^{-1}$·bw$^{-1}$·day$^{-1}$), high-dose group (C3G, 125 mg·kg$^{-1}$·bw$^{-1}$·day$^{-1}$) and positive control group (tegafur, 10 mg·kg$^{-1}$·bw$^{-1}$·day$^{-1}$) (three mice in each group). Mice were s.c. injected with $2 \times 10^6$ SGC-7901 cells on the right groin and were housed under a regular 12 h light/12 h dark cycle. After 18 days, the mice were sacrificed for the assay of tumorigenicity (e.g., body weight and tumor volume). All experiments were carried out in accordance with the ethical guidelines of the Animal Experimentation Committee in the College of Medicine, Zhejiang University. Our experiment ethic approval code is ZJU20160443.

## 2.4. Immunohistochemical Staining

The tumor tissues were removed from each mouse and the samples were subsequently fixed in 4% ($v/v$) paraformaldehyde/PBS (Phosphate Buffer Saline) and embedded in paraffin for staining. The paraffin sections were deparaffinized in xylene, rehydrated in a 10 mM citrate buffer (pH 6.0), and heated in a microwave oven for 15 min to restore the antigens. To suppress endogenous peroxidase within the tissues, the samples were treated with 3% peroxide for 5 min and then with a blocking solution for 30 min. Slides were incubated with the primary antibody and secondary antibody in a humid chamber for 60 min. Tissue staining was visualized with a 3,3′-diaminobenzidine substrate chromogen solution and the images were taken by using a microscope set (Zeiss, Germeny) at a 200× magnification.

## 2.5. Quantitative Real-Time PCR and Western Blot Assay

Total RNA was isolated from tumor tissues using Trizol reagent (Invitrogen, Waltham, MA, USA) according to the manufacturer's protocol. Equal amounts of total RNA (1.0 μg) were used to synthesize cDNA with the iScriptTM cDNA Synthesis kit (Bio-Rad, Hercules, CA, USA). Quantitative real-time PCR was performed in triplicate using a SYBR Green Master I kit (Roche, Basel, Switzerland) and the LightCycler480 real-time PCR System (Roche, Basel, Switzerland). Gene-specific primers were used as mentioned in Table 1. The RNA quality was detected by OD$_{260}$/OD$_{280}$ and gel electrophoresis. The fold change of the treatment group versus control group for each target gene was calculated using the $2^{-\Delta\Delta Ct}$ method and was evaluated as the effect of treatment on relative gene expression. Expression was normalized against expression of the housekeeping gene *β-actin*.

Tumor tissues were lysed using RIPA buffer containing 1% PMSF (Phenylmethanesulfonyl Fluoride), and protein inhibitor (cOmplete mini, Roche, Los Angeles, CA, USA). The protein concentration was determined using the Pierce BCA Protein Assay Kit (Thermo Scientific, Waltham, MA, USA). The concentration was adjusted to 1 μg/μL using PBS and 5× loading buffer. Equal amounts (40 μg) of protein were separated on a 10% SDS (Sodium Dodecyl Sulfate)-polyacrylamide gel and transferred onto PVDF (Polyvinylidene Fluoride) membranes. After blocking the membrane with 5% nonfat dried milk for 1.5 h, the protein abundance was detected with antibodies against KLF6 (1:1000 dilutions), p21 (1:1000 dilutions), p53 (1:1000 dilutions), Cyclin D1 (1:1000 dilutions), CDK4.

(1:1000 dilutions), followed by incubation with peroxide-conjugated anti-rabbit immunoglobulin. β-*actin* was used as a loading control.

**Table 1.** Primer sequences used in quantitative real-time PCR.

| Gene | Forward Primer (5′ to 3′) | Reverse Primer (3′ to 5′) |
| --- | --- | --- |
| *p53* | AGGCCTTGGAACTCAAGGAT | CCCTTTTTGGACTTCAGGTG |
| *KLF6* | GACAGCTCCGAGGAACTTTCT | CACGCAACCCCACAGTTGA |
| *P21* | TGGAGACTCTCAGGGTCGAAAA | GGCGTTTGGAGTGGTAGAAATCT |
| *CDK4* | ACAGTTCGTGAGGTGGCTTTA | TCAGATCCTTGATCGTTTCG |
| *Cyclin D1* | GAACACGGCTCACGCTTACC | GCCCAGACCCTCAGACTTGC |
| β-*actin* | TGACGTGGACATCCGCAAAG | CTGGAAGGTGGACAGCGAGG |

## 2.6. Statistics

Statistical analyses were carried out using SPSS version 19.0 (IBM, Armonk, NY, USA). Data were analyzed by one-way ANOVA. Multiple comparison between the groups was performed using the LSD (Least Significant Difference) method, OriginPro 8.0 software packages (OriginLab Corporation, Northampton, MA, USA) was used for plotting the experimental data. Values were expressed as the mean ± standard deviation.

## 3. Results

### 3.1. Purification of C3G Extracted from Chinese Bayberry

The identification and quantification of C3G extracted and purified from Chinese bayberry was accomplished by HPLC, LC-MS and $^1$H-NMR (Figure 1). HPLC identification was carried out according to the retention time and peak area compared with those of standard C3G. HPLC analysis of the identified anthocyanin compounds showed that the retention time of cyanidins-3-glucoside was 15.6 to 17.9 min. The HPLC chromatograms of Chinese bayberry pulp showed impurity peaks (Figure 1A), while purified C3G extracts did not have any other significant peaks (Figure 1B). The purity was determined with a standard curve chart and C3G with a purity of 88.81% was achieved.

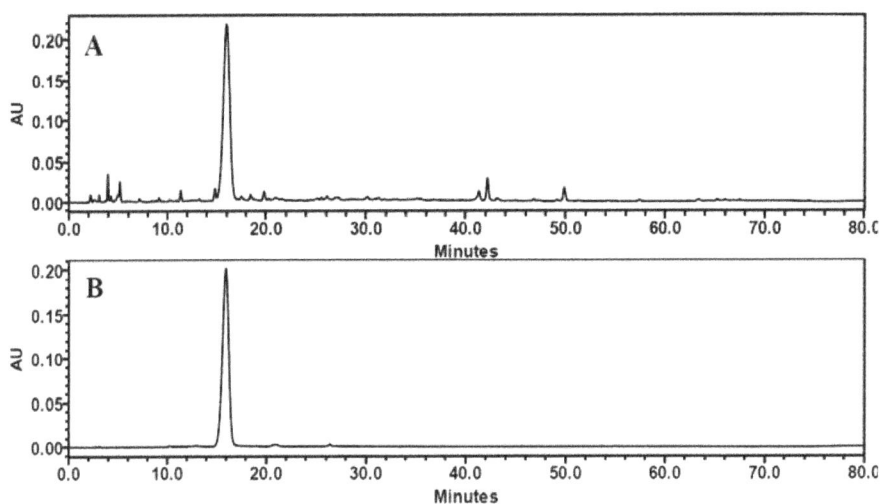

**Figure 1.** *Cont.*

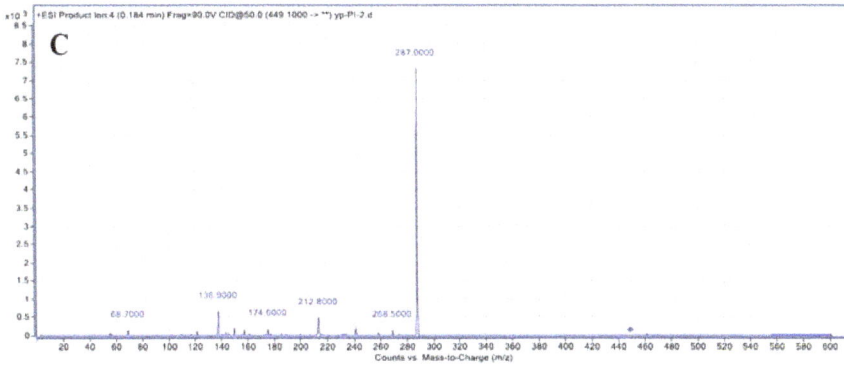

**Figure 1.** HPLC chromatograms of Chinese bayberry pulp (**A**) and purified C3G from Chinese bayberry (**B**) ($\lambda$ = 280 nm) and LC-MS$^2$ spectrum of purified C3G (**C**).

Further identification of C3G was confirmed by LC-MS (Figure 1C) and $^1$H-NMR (Table 2). Among all the LC-MS$^2$ products, ions at $m/z$ 287.0 were present in great abundance which was related to the loss of one hexose ([M − 162]$^+$) molecule, furnishing the cyanidin aglycone, the main body structure of C3G. The ions at $m/z$ 136.9 and 240.6 resulted from the ring-cross cleavage of cyanidin. The $^1$H-NMR spectrum showed the presence of one cyaniding nucleus and one hexose (Table 2). Therefore, all HPLC, LC-MS and $^1$H-NMR data confirmed the purified extract was C3G.

**Table 2.** $^1$H spectral data (ppm) for purified C3G.

| Cyanidin-3-Glucoside | $^1$H |
|:---:|:---:|
| *Aglycone* | |
| 4 | 9.02 (s) |
| 6 | 6.63 (d, $J$ = 2.5 Hz) |
| 8 | 7.06 (d, $J$ = 2 Hz) |
| 2' | 8.08 (s) |
| 5' | 7.10 (s) |
| 6' | 8.26 (s) |
| *Glucose* | |
| 1'' | 5.30 (d, $J$ = 16 Hz) |
| 2'' | 3.70 (m) |
| 3'' | 3.66 (br, s) |
| 4'' | 3.54 (m) |
| 5'' | 3.63 (s) |
| 6''A | 4.02 (s) |
| 6''B | 3.83 (s) |

*3.2. C3G Suppressed the Growth of SGC-7901 Tumor Xenografts*

A tumor xenograft model was established to study the inhibition effects of C3G on tumor growth in vivo. Through preliminary tests (data not shown), we chose 25 mg·kg$^{-1}$·bw$^{-1}$·day$^{-1}$ and 125 mg·kg$^{-1}$·bw$^{-1}$·day$^{-1}$ as our C3G treatment doses and selected 18 days as the duration of this experiment. The effects of C3G on tumor size were monitored every alternate day. After eight days of cancer cell injection treatment, the average tumor volume in the control group began to appear significantly different from that of other treatment groups, reaching up to 230.8 mm$^3$ (Figure 2A). At 18 days before the sacrifice, the average tumor volume in the control group had increased to 771.5 mm$^3$, while the C3G treatment groups with low dose and high dose grew to 384.1 mm$^3$ and 276.0 mm$^3$, respectively, compared to the tegafur-treated group (positive control), which was 211.7 mm$^3$ (Figure 2A).

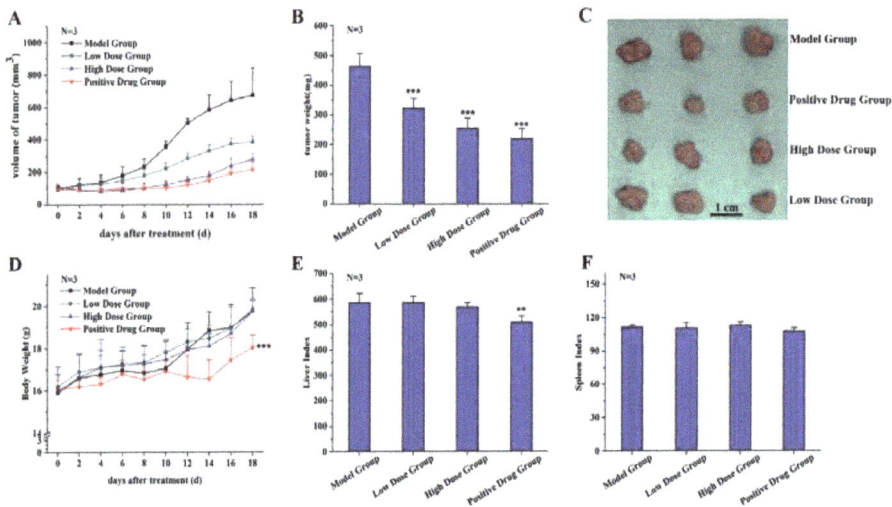

**Figure 2.** Effects of purified C3G on tumorigenesis in vivo. (**A**) The volumes of tumors were monitored at the indicated times; (**B**) tumor weights were measured after rats were sacrificed; (**C**) photographs of individual tumor xenografts removed from mice; (**D**) the body weights were monitored every alternate day after treatments; (**E**) the liver index and (**F**) the spleen index. The index was calculated as liver weight (mg)/body weight (g); and spleen weight (mg)/body weight (g), respectively. Values are mean ± SEM of three mice. ** $p < 0.01$, *** $p < 0.001$.

The inhibitory effect of C3G on tumor growth was evaluated based on tumor xenograft size when tumor tissues were removed and weighed after sacrifice. The tumor weight and size of treatment groups were significantly lower than those of the control group (Figure 2B,C). Inhibition rates of the low C3G dose group, the high dose group and the drug group were 30.4%, 45.1% and 53.0%, respectively.

Experimental results showed no significant changes in body weight, liver index and spleen index between the control group and C3G treatment groups (Figure 2D–F), indicating that C3G extracted from Chinese bayberry has little toxicity to mice. However, compared with the control group and C3G treatment groups, the body weight and liver index of the tegafur group was significant decreased (Figure 2D,E), showing the positive drug had some toxic effects or side effects on the liver and whole body of mice.

### 3.3. C3G Inhibited the Cell Cycle of SGC-7901 Tumor Xenografts

Expressions of caspase 3 and p21 in tumor tissues were determined by immunohistochemistry staining. The negative cellular nuclei were stained blue, while the positive nuclei were stained dark brown. Immunohistochemical studies showed clear positive p21 staining in cell nuclei in C3G treatment groups with a dose-dependent manner. In contrast, the positive caspase 3 staining, which appeared in the cytoplasm, showed no marked change among different treatments (Figure 3). These results indicated that anthocyanin C3G from Chinese bayberry could suppress the growth of tumor xenografts by inhibiting the cell cycle but with less induction of apoptosis.

| Model Group | Low Dose Group | High Dose Group |
|---|---|---|

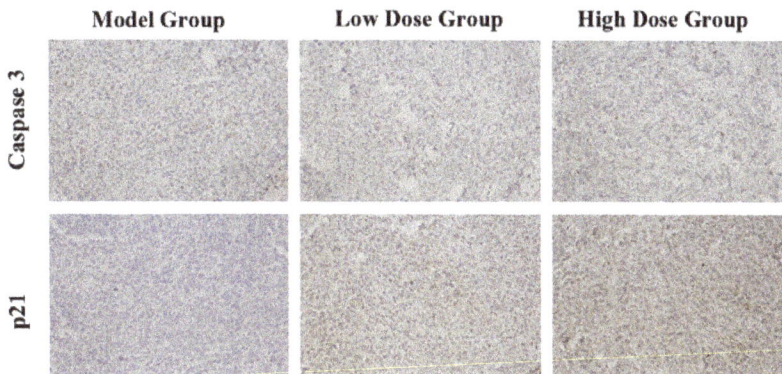

**Figure 3.** Caspase 3 and p21 immunochemical staining of tumor xenografts sections (200× magnification) (*n* = 3).

### 3.4. Gene Expression Analysis

To elucidate the in vivo mechanism of C3G inhibition of the cell cycle in SGC-7901 cell tumor xenografts, the effects of C3G on expression of cancer-related genes, including *KLF6, p21, Cyclin D1, CDK4* and *p53*, were further evaluated. Both mRNA levels, measured by quantitative real-time PCR, and protein levels, measured by Western blot, were analyzed to determine these effects. As indicated in Figure 4A, results showed that the *KLF6* and *p21* genes were up-regulated in a dose-dependent manner in C3G treatment groups. The relative mRNA expression of *KLF6* in the low dose and high dose groups was about 1.61- and 2.06-fold higher than in the control group. Similarly, *p21* was up-regulated 2.19- and 3.48-fold in the low dose group and high dose group, respectively. Both *Cyclin D1* and *CDK4* gene expressions in C3G treatment groups were inhibited significantly. In comparison with the control group (Figure 4A), *Cyclin D1* gene expression was decreased 0.62- and 0.26-fold and the *CDK4* gene was down-regulated 0.69- and 0.32-fold, respectively. However, there were no obvious changes in the expression of *p53*, the master tumor suppressor gene, between the treatment groups and the control (Figure 4A). The protein expressions of various genes as measured by Western blot analysis were in accordance with their qPCR analysis (Figure 4B). KLF6 and p21 protein levels were significantly increased, indicating the critical role of KLF6 in the tumor xenograft suppression in vivo. However, the p53 protein did not change significantly, whereas CDK4 and Cyclin D1 proteins were decreased with C3G treatments.

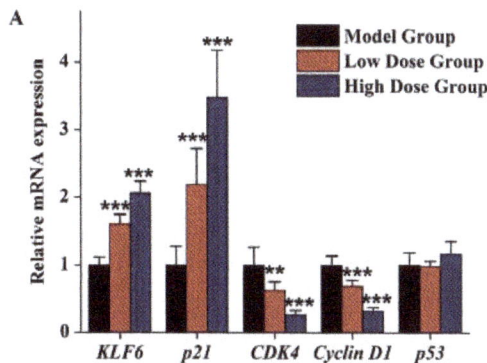

**Figure 4.** *Cont.*

**B**

MG  MG  MG  HDG  HDG  HDG  LDG  LDG  LDG

KLF6

p21

Cyclin D1

CDK4

p53

ACTIN

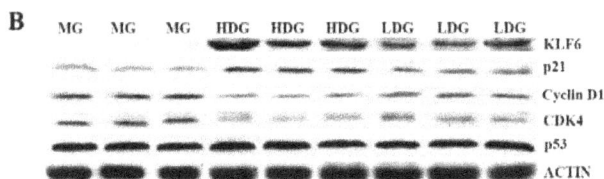

**Figure 4.** Effects of purified C3G on gene expression and protein expression in tumor xenografts. (**A**) Relative mRNA expression of *KLF6*, *p21*, *CDK4*, *Cyclin D1*, *p53* after C3G treatments; (**B**) protein expression of KLF6, p21, CDK4, Cyclin D1, p53 after C3G treatments. Values are mean ± SEM of measurements from three mice. ** $p < 0.01$, *** $p < 0.001$.

## 4. Discussion

A nude mouse tumor xenograft model was established to study the in vivo anticancer effect of high-purity anthocyanin C3G from Chinese bayberry. Results showed that C3G inhibited the growth of SGC-7901 cell tumor xenografts in a dose-dependent manner. The inhibition rates of low dose and high dose groups were 30.4% and 45.1%, respectively. Compared with the positive drug tegafur treatment, the C3G treatment did not show any toxic effects or other side effects. Immunohistochemical staining indicated that the tumor-suppressing effect was due to cell cycle inhibition but lower apoptosis induction. Through qPCR and Western blot, it was established that C3G treatment could up-regulate *KLF6* gene expression and the downstream effector *p21* in a *p53*-independent manner. As a consequence, it is concluded that C3G activity on tumor growth inhibition was probably through KLF6-mediated p21 induction, by disruption of the Cyclin D1 and CDK4 interaction, thus blocking the cell cycle.

The Krüppel-like family (KLF) of transcription factors is characterized by three contiguous C2H2-type zinc finger motifs at the carboxy terminus which comprise the DNA-binding domain [30, 31]. *KLF6* is a member of the KLF family that consists of four exons and encodes a nuclear core promoter element-binding protein [32]. *KLF6* is a tumor suppressor based on its inactivation and somatic mutations in a variety of cancers such as prostate [20], gastric [21], ovarian [24], breast [27], liver [25,26], and colorectal cancer [22,23]. *KLF6*'s growth-suppressive activity is linked to p53-independent transactivation of p21 [20] and inhibition of the Cyclin D1/CDK4 complex [28]. This study could be the first report that *KLF6* can be up-regulated by anthocyanin C3G extracted from Chinese bayberry, thus reducing the mouse tumor growth burden.

In vitro effects of C3G are well studied and it is known that C3G can suppress tumor cell proliferation by various mechanisms such as apoptosis induction [17], cell cycle inhibition [18], peroxidation inhibition [33] and migration inhibition [5,19], etc. Several signaling pathways have been implicated, such as inhibiting Ras signaling [16], down-regulating the expressions of CDKs [34], abolishing ethanol-mediated p130[Cas]/JNK interaction [19], elevating the Bax/Bcl-2 ratio [17], and inducing signaling by p38/p53 and c-jun [35]. Mulberry anthocyanins containing 46.13% of cyanidine-3-gluoside induce apoptosis in gastric cancer cell AGS by up-regulating *p53* and other apoptosis-mediated gene expression [35]. However, the in vivo experiment from this study did not show any significant change of *p53* expression in tumor tissues, either at the mRNA or protein level, illustrating that the mechanism of the antitumor effect of C3G in vitro and in vivo might be different. There have been multiple reports about antitumor effects of anthocyanins extracted from natural products. Baked purple-fleshed potato reduced the colon CSCs number via induction of apoptosis [36]. Anthocyanins extracted from Korean wild berry, Meoru, could inhibit hepato-carcinoma cell metastasis via the AMPK pathway [37]. Delphinidin-3-glucoside suppressed breast carcinogenesis in vivo through decreasing HOX transcript antisense RNA (HOTAIR) transcript [38]. Pomegranate polyphenolics showed cytotoxicity in vitro and in vivo through the PI3K/AKT pathway [39]. A diet containing anthocyanins from black raspberries inhibited NMBA-induced rat esophagus tumor development by reducing NF-κB and COX-2 expression [40]. Anthocyanin-rich extract from roselle could inhibit

*N*-Nitrosomethylurea–induced leukemia in vivo [41]. A diet with anthocyanin-enriched potato P40 prevented rats from colorectal cancer [42]. Furthermore, although its tumor inhibition capacities are clearly indicated [16,35,43,44], the reported in vivo C3G antitumor mechanisms are nuanced in different animal models and different purities of C3G. However, reports expatiating the mechanism of C3G suppressing tumor growth in vivo are limited [16,35,43,44], which is partly due to the difficulty of separating and purifying high-purity C3G.

In this study, by using high-purity C3G and a tumor xenograft model, it was demonstrated that C3G treatment could up-regulate *KLF6* gene expression and *KLF6* exhibited tumor growth–suppressing activity by cell cycle inhibition with a p53-independent up-regulation of p21 and disrupted the Cyclin D1 and CDK4 interaction. However, further progress could be made by studying the oral administration of C3G, its metabolism and digestion in mice to investigate the target points of C3G. Since the *KLF6* gene belongs to the transcription factor Krüppel-like family, the antitumor function of other KLF family members could also be studied.

## 5. Conclusions

In conclusion, C3G treatment showed in vivo antitumor effects in dose-dependent manner, where significantly tumor growth inhibition was observed in nude mouse xenograft model. C3G treatments also showed no toxic effects or other side effects compared with the positive drug tegafur treatment. The tumor-suppressing effect was due to cell cycle inhibition but lower apoptosis induction through Immunohistochemical staining test. Further q-PCR and Western blot results showed that C3G treatment could up-regulate the *KLF6* gene expression and the downstream effector *p21* in a *p53*-independent manner. These results might provide important information concerning the possible mechanism of C3G-induced antitumor activity against gastric adenocarcinoma in vivo and shed light on the potential application of food anthocyanins in cancer prevention.

**Acknowledgments:** The work was supported by the National Natural Science Foundation of China (31171668; 31571838), the Special Scientific Research Fund of Agricultural Public Welfare Profession of China (201203089) and the Agricultural Outstanding Talents and Innovation Team of the State Agricultural ministry on Health and Nutrition of Fruit. The authors would like to thank Don Grierson from the University of Nottingham (UK) for discussions, suggestions, and efforts in language editing.

**Author Contributions:** Yue Wang carried out the experiments and wrote the original manuscript. Xia-nan Zhang participated in the animal experiments. Wen-hua Xie assisted with the extraction experiment. Jin-ping Cao helped with data mining. Pei-rang Cao edited and revised the manuscript. Yi-xiong Zheng, Pei-rang Cao and Xian Li, Qing-jun Chen offered experiment advice and suggestions. Chong-de Sun conceived and designed the study. All authors approved the final manuscript.

**Conflicts of Interest:** The authors declare no conflict of interest.

## Abbreviations

The following abbreviations are used in this manuscript:

| | |
|---|---|
| C3G | Cyanidin-3-glucoside |
| CDK4 | Cyclin-dependent kinase 4 |
| RIPA | Radio Immunoprecipation Assay |
| HPLC | High Performance Liquid Chromatography |
| LC-MS | Liquid Chromatograph-Mass Spectrometer |
| $^1$H-NMR | Hydrogen-Nuclear Magnetic Resonance |
| PBS | Phosphate Buffer Saline |
| PMSF | Phenylmethanesulfonyl Fluoride |
| SDS | Sodium Dodecyl Sulfate |
| PVDF | Polyvinylidene Fluoride |
| KLF6 | Krueppel-Like Factor 6 |
| LSD | Least Significant Difference |
| CSCs | Cancer stem cells |

## References

1. Bräunlich, M.; Slimestad, R.; Wangensteen, H.; Brede, C.; Malterud, K.E.; Barsett, H. Extracts, anthocyanins and procyanidins from aronia melanocarpa as radical scavengers and enzyme inhibitors. *Nutrients* **2013**, *5*, 663–678. [CrossRef] [PubMed]

2. Chen, P.N.; Chu, S.C.; Chiou, H.L.; Kuo, W.H.; Chiang, C.L.; Hsieh, Y.S. Mulberry anthocyanins, cyanidin 3-rutinoside and cyanidin 3-glucoside, exhibited an inhibitory effect on the migration and invasion of a human lung cancer cell line. *Cancer Lett.* **2006**, *235*, 248–259. [CrossRef] [PubMed]

3. Meydani, M.; Hasan, S.T. Dietary polyphenols and obesity. *Nutrients* **2010**, *2*, 737–751. [CrossRef] [PubMed]

4. Zhang, X.; Lv, Q.; Jia, S.; Chen, Y.; Sun, C.; Li, X.; Chen, K. Effects of flavonoids-rich chinese bayberry (*Morella rubra* Sieb. et Zucc.) fruits extract on regulating glucose and lipids metabolism in diabetic KK-Ay mice. *Food Funct.* **2016**, *7*, 3130–3140. [CrossRef] [PubMed]

5. Sun, C.; Zheng, Y.; Chen, Q.; Tang, X.; Jiang, M.; Zhang, J.; Li, X.; Chen, K. Purification and anti-tumour activity of cyanidin-3-*O*-glucoside from Chinese bayberry fruit. *Food Chem.* **2012**, *131*, 1287–1294. [CrossRef]

6. Torre, L.A.; Bray, F.; Siegel, R.L.; Ferlay, J.; Lortet-Tieulent, J.; Jemal, A. Global cancer statistics, 2012. *CA Cancer J. Clin.* **2015**, *65*, 87–108. [CrossRef] [PubMed]

7. Chen, W.; Zheng, R.; Baade, P.D.; Zhang, S.; Zeng, H.; Bray, F.; Jemal, A.; Yu, X.Q.; He, J. Cancer statistics in China, 2015. *CA Cancer J. Clin.* **2016**, *66*, 115–132. [CrossRef] [PubMed]

8. Liu, C.; Russell, R.M. Nutrition and gastric cancer risk: An update. *Nutr. Rev.* **2008**, *66*, 237–249. [CrossRef] [PubMed]

9. Song, P.; Wu, L.; Guan, W. Dietary nitrates, nitrites, and nitrosamines intake and the risk of gastric cancer: A meta-analysis. *Nutrients* **2015**, *7*, 9872–9895. [CrossRef] [PubMed]

10. Lunet, N.; Lacerda-Vieira, A.; Barros, H. Fruit and vegetables consumption and gastric cancer: A systematic review and meta-analysis of cohort studies. *Nutr. Cancer* **2005**, *53*, 1–10. [CrossRef] [PubMed]

11. Nouraie, M.; Pietinen, P.; Kamangar, F.; Dawsey, S.M.; Abnet, C.C.; Albanes, D.; Virtamo, J.; Taylor, P.R. Fruits, vegetables, and antioxidants and risk of gastric cancer among male smokers. *Cancer Epidem. Biomark.* **2005**, *14*, 2087–2092. [CrossRef] [PubMed]

12. González, C.A.; Pera, G.; Agudo, A.; Bueno-de-Mesquita, H.B.; Ceroti, M.; Boeing, H.; Schulz, M.; Del Giudice, G.; Plebani, M.; Carneiro, F. Fruit and vegetable intake and the risk of stomach and oesophagus adenocarcinoma in the European prospective investigation into cancer and nutrition (EPIC–EURGAST). *Int. J. Cancer* **2006**, *118*, 2559–2566. [CrossRef] [PubMed]

13. Vauzour, D.; Rodriguez-Mateos, A.; Corona, G.; Oruna-Concha, M.J.; Spencer, J.P. Polyphenols and human health: Prevention of disease and mechanisms of action. *Nutrients* **2010**, *2*, 1106–1131. [CrossRef] [PubMed]

14. Zhang, W.; Li, X.; Zheng, J.; Wang, G.; Sun, C.; Ferguson, I.B.; Chen, K. Bioactive components and antioxidant capacity of Chinese bayberry (*Myrica rubra* Sieb. and Zucc.) fruit in relation to fruit maturity and postharvest storage. *Eur. Food Res. Technol.* **2008**, *227*, 1091–1097. [CrossRef]

15. Sorrenti, V.; Vanella, L.; Acquaviva, R.; Cardile, V.; Giofre, S.; Di Giacomo, C. Cyanidin induces apoptosis and differentiation in prostate cancer cells. *Int. J. Oncol.* **2015**, *47*, 1303–1310. [CrossRef] [PubMed]

16. Fukamachi, K.; Imada, T.; Ohshima, Y.; Xu, J.; Tsuda, H. Purple corn color suppresses ras protein level and inhibits 7,12-dimethylbenz[a]anthracene-induced mammary carcinogenesis in the rat. *Cancer Sci.* **2008**, *99*, 1841–1846. [PubMed]

17. Shih, P.H.; Yeh, C.T.; Yen, G.C. Effects of anthocyanidin on the inhibition of proliferation and induction of apoptosis in human gastric adenocarcinoma cells. *Food Chem. Toxicol.* **2005**, *43*, 1557–1566. [CrossRef] [PubMed]

18. Malik, M.; Zhao, C.W.; Schoene, N.; Guisti, M.M.; Moyer, M.P.; Magnuson, B.A. Anthocyanin-rich extract from Aronia meloncarpa E induces a cell cycle block in colon cancer but not normal colonic cells. *Nutr. Cancer* **2003**, *46*, 186–196. [CrossRef] [PubMed]

19. Xu, M.; Bower, K.A.; Wang, S.; Frank, J.A.; Chen, G.; Ding, M.; Wang, S.; Shi, X.; Ke, Z.; Luo, J. Cyanidin-3-glucoside inhibits ethanol-induced invasion of breast cancer cells overexpressing ErbB2. *Mol. Cancer* **2010**, *9*, 1. [CrossRef] [PubMed]

20. Narla, G.; Heath, K.E.; Reeves, H.L.; Li, D.; Giono, L.E.; Kimmelman, A.C.; Glucksman, M.J.; Narla, J.; Eng, F.J.; Chan, A.M.; et al. *KLF6*, a candidate tumor suppressor gene mutated in prostate cancer. *Science* **2001**, *294*, 2563–2566. [CrossRef] [PubMed]

21. Sangodkar, J.; Shi, J.; DiFeo, A.; Schwartz, R.; Bromberg, R.; Choudhri, A.; McClinch, K.; Hatami, R.; Scheer, E.; Kremer-Tal, S. Functional role of the *KLF6* tumour suppressor gene in gastric cancer. *Eur. J. Cancer* **2009**, *45*, 666–676. [CrossRef] [PubMed]

22. Miyaki, M.; Yamaguchi, T.; Iijima, T.; Funata, N.; Mori, T. Difference in the role of loss of heterozygosity at 10p15 (*KLF6* locus) in colorectal carcinogenesis between sporadic and familial adenomatous polyposis and hereditary nonpolyposis colorectal cancer patients. *Oncol. Basel* **2007**, *71*, 131–135. [CrossRef] [PubMed]

23. Mukai, S.; Hiyama, T.; Tanaka, S.; Yoshihara, M.; Arihiro, K.; Chayama, K. Involvement of kruppel-like factor 6 (*KLF6*) mutation in the development of nonpolypoid colorectal carcinoma. *World J. Gastroenterol.* **2007**, *13*, 3932–3938. [CrossRef] [PubMed]

24. DiFeo, A.; Narla, G.; Hirshfeld, J.; Camacho-Vanegas, O.; Narla, J.; Rose, S.L.; Kalir, T.; Yao, S.; Levine, A.; Birrer, M.J. Roles of *KLF6* and *KLF6*-SV1 in ovarian cancer progression and intraperitoneal dissemination. *Clin. Cancer Res.* **2006**, *12*, 3730–3739. [CrossRef] [PubMed]

25. Song, J.; Kim, C.J.; Cho, Y.G.; Kim, S.Y.; Nam, S.W.; Lee, S.H.; Yoo, N.J.; Lee, J.Y.; Park, W.S. Genetic and epigenetic alterations of the *KLF6* gene in hepatocellular carcinoma. *J. Gastroenterol. Hepatol.* **2006**, *21*, 1286–1289. [CrossRef] [PubMed]

26. Yea, S.; Narla, G.; Zhao, X. Ras promotes growth by alternative splicing-mediated inactivation of the *KLF6* tumor suppressor in hepatocellular carcinoma. *Gastroenterology* **2008**, *135*, 326. [CrossRef] [PubMed]

27. Ozdemir, F.; Koksal, M.; Ozmen, V.; Aydin, I.; Buyru, N. Mutations and kruppel-like factor 6 (*KLF6*) expression levels in breast cancer. *Tumor Biol.* **2014**, *35*, 5219–5225. [CrossRef] [PubMed]

28. Benzeno, S.; Narla, G.; Allina, J.; Cheng, G.Z.; Reeves, H.L.; Banck, M.S.; Odin, J.A.; Diehl, J.A.; Germain, D.; Friedman, S.L. Cyclin-dependent kinase inhibition by the *KLF6* tumor suppressor protein through interaction with *Cyclin D1*. *Cancer Res.* **2004**, *64*, 3885–3891. [CrossRef] [PubMed]

29. Schieber, A.; Keller, P.; Carle, R. Determination of phenolic acids and flavonoids of apple and pear by high-performance liquid chromatography. *J. Chromatogr. A* **2001**, *910*, 265–273. [CrossRef]

30. Schuh, R.; Aicher, W.; Gaul, U.; Côte, S.; Preiss, A.; Maier, D.; Seifert, E.; Nauber, U.; Schröder, C.; Kemler, R. A conserved family of nuclear proteins containing structural elements of the finger protein encoded by krüppel, a drosophila segmentation gene. *Cell* **1986**, *47*, 1025–1032. [CrossRef]

31. Pearson, R.; Fleetwood, J.; Eaton, S.; Crossley, M.; Bao, S. Krüppel-like transcription factors: A functional family. *Int. J. Biochem. Cell Biol.* **2008**, *40*, 1996–2001. [CrossRef] [PubMed]

32. Koritschoner, N.P.; Bocco, J.L.; Panzetta-Dutari, G.M.; Dumur, C.I.; Flury, A.; Patrito, L.C. A novel human zinc finger protein that interacts with the core promoter element of a tata box-less gene. *J. Biol. Chem.* **1997**, *272*, 9573–9580. [PubMed]

33. Reddy, M.K.; Alexander-Lindo, R.L.; Nair, M.G. Relative inhibition of lipid peroxidation, cyclooxygenase enzymes, and human tumor cell proliferation by natural food colors. *J. Agric. Food Chem.* **2005**, *53*, 9268–9273. [CrossRef] [PubMed]

34. Chen, P.N.; Chu, S.C.; Chiou, H.L.; Chiang, C.L.; Yang, S.F.; Hsieh, Y.S. Cyanidin 3-glucoside and peonidin 3-glucoside inhibit tumor cell growth and induce apoptosis in vitro and suppress tumor growth in vivo. *Nutr. Cancer* **2005**, *53*, 232–243. [CrossRef] [PubMed]

35. Huang, H.P.; Chang, Y.C.; Wu, C.H.; Hung, C.N.; Wang, C.J. Anthocyanin-rich mulberry extract inhibit the gastric cancer cell growth in vitro and xenograft mice by inducing signals of p38/p53 and c-jun. *Food Chem.* **2011**, *129*, 1703–1709. [CrossRef]

36. Charepalli, V.; Reddivari, L.; Radhakrishnan, S.; Vadde, R.; Agarwal, R.; Vanamala, J.K.P. Anthocyanin-containing purple-fleshed potatoes suppress colon tumorigenesis via elimination of colon cancer stem cells. *J. Nutr. Biochem.* **2015**, *26*, 1641–1649. [CrossRef] [PubMed]

37. Song, Y.P.; Lee, Y.K.; Lee, W.S.; Park, O.J.; Kim, Y.M. The involvement of AMPK/GSK3-beta signals in the control of metastasis and proliferation in hepato-carcinoma cells treated with anthocyanins extracted from Korea wild berry Meoru. *BMC Complement. Altern. Med.* **2014**, *14*, 109.

38. Yang, X.; Luo, E.; Liu, X.; Han, B.; Yu, X.; Peng, X. Delphinidin-3-glucoside suppresses breast carcinogenesis by inactivating the Akt/HOTAIR signaling pathway. *BMC Cancer* **2016**, *16*, 423. [CrossRef] [PubMed]

39. Banerjee, N.; Talcott, S.; Safe, S.; Mertens-Talcott, S.U. Cytotoxicity of pomegranate polyphenolics in breast cancer cells in vitro and vivo: Potential role of miRNA-27a and miRNA-155 in cell survival and inflammation. *Breast Cancer Res. Treat.* **2012**, *136*, 21–34. [CrossRef] [PubMed]

40. Wang, L.S.; Hecht, S.S.; Carmella, S.G.; Yu, N.; Larue, B.; Henry, C.; McIntyre, C.; Rocha, C.; Lechner, J.F.; Stoner, G.D. Anthocyanins in black raspberries prevent esophageal tumors in rats. *Cancer Prev. Res. (Phila)* **2009**, *2*, 84–93. [CrossRef] [PubMed]

41. Tsai, T.C.; Huang, H.P.; Chang, Y.C.; Wang, C.J. An anthocyanin-rich extract from hibiscus sabdariffa linnaeus inhibits N-nitrosomethylurea-induced leukemia in rats. *J. Agric. Food Chem.* **2014**, *62*, 1572–1580. [CrossRef] [PubMed]

42. Lim, S.; Xu, J.T.; Kim, J.; Chen, T.Y.; Su, X.Y.; Standard, J.; Carey, E.; Griffin, J.; Herndon, B.; Katz, B.; et al. Role of anthocyanin-enriched purple-fleshed sweet potato p40 in colorectal cancer prevention. *Mol. Nutr. Food Res.* **2013**, *57*, 1908–1917. [CrossRef] [PubMed]

43. Duthie, S.J.; Gardner, P.T.; Morrice, P.C.; Wood, S.G.; Pirie, L.; Bestwick, C.C.; Milne, L.; Duthie, G.G. DNA stability and lipid peroxidation in vitamin e-deficient rats in vivo and colon cells in vitro—Modulation by the dietary anthocyanin, cyanidin-3-glycoside. *Eur. J. Nutr.* **2005**, *44*, 195–203. [CrossRef] [PubMed]

44. Chang, H.; Yu, B.; Yu, X.P.; Yi, L.; Chen, C.Y.; Mi, M.T.; Ling, W.H. Anticancer activities of an anthocyanin-rich extract from black rice against breast cancer cells in vitro and in vivo. *Nutr. Cancer* **2010**, *62*, 1128–1136.

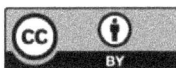

*nutrients*

MDPI

*Article*

# YAP Inhibition by Resveratrol via Activation of AMPK Enhances the Sensitivity of Pancreatic Cancer Cells to Gemcitabine

Zhengdong Jiang [1], Xin Chen [1], Ke Chen [1], Liankang Sun [1], Luping Gao [1], Cancan Zhou [1], Meng Lei [1], Wanxing Duan [1], Zheng Wang [1], Qingyong Ma [1,*] and Jiguang Ma [2,*]

[1]   Department of Hepatobiliary Surgery, First Affiliated Hospital of Xi'an Jiaotong University,
      Xi'an 710061, China; jiang.19900708@stu.xjtu.edu.cn (Z.J.); chenxin.77@stu.xjtu.edu.cn (X.C.);
      ck532128@stu.xjtu.edu.cn (K.C.); sunliankang@stu.xjtu.edu.cn (L.S.); gaoluping@stu.xjtu.edu.cn (L.G.);
      trytofly@stu.xjtu.edu.cn (C.Z.); leimeng7@stu.xjtu.edu.cn (M.L.); 0556029@fudan.edu.cn (W.D.);
      zheng.wang11@mail.xjtu.edu.cn (Z.W.)
[2]   Department of Anesthesiology, First Affiliated Hospital of Xi'an Jiaotong University, Xi'an 710061, China
*    Correspondence: qyma56@xjtu.edu.cn (Q.M.); jgma86@xjtu.edu.cn (J.M.);
      Tel.: +86-29-8532-3899 (Q.M. & J.M.)

Received: 15 July 2016; Accepted: 30 August 2016; Published: 23 September 2016

**Abstract:** Resveratrol, a natural polyphenol present in most plants, inhibits the growth of numerous cancers both in vitro and in vivo. Aberrant expression of YAP has been reported to activate multiple growth-regulatory pathways and confer anti-apoptotic abilities to many cancer cells. However, the role of resveratrol in YES-activated protein (YAP) expression and that of YAP in pancreatic cancer cells' response to gemcitabine resistance remain elusive. In this study, we found that resveratrol suppressed the proliferation and cloning ability and induced the apoptosis of pancreatic cancer cells. These multiple biological effects might result from the activation of AMP-activation protein kinase (AMPK) (Thr172) and, thus, the induction of YAP cytoplasmic retention, Ser127 phosphorylation, and the inhibition of YAP transcriptional activity by resveratrol. YAP silencing by siRNA or resveratrol enhanced the sensitivity of gemcitabine in pancreatic cancer cells. Taken together, these findings demonstrate that resveratrol could increase the sensitivity of pancreatic cancer cells to gemcitabine by inhibiting YAP expression. More importantly, our work reveals that resveratrol is a potential anticancer agent for the treatment of pancreatic cancer, and YAP may serve as a promising target for sensitizing pancreatic cancer cells to chemotherapy.

**Keywords:** pancreatic cancer; resveratrol; AMPK; YAP; gemcitabine

## 1. Introduction

Pancreatic ductal adenocarcinoma (PDAC) is one of the most malignant and lethal tumors, with an overall five-year survival rate less than 7% [1]. Over recent decades, the prognosis of patients with this malignancy has not improved due to aggressive local invasion, metastases, and resistance to chemotherapy [2]. Currently, surgical resection is the only opportunity for curing pancreatic cancer at an early stage. Unfortunately, only approximately 20% of patients are eligible for surgical resection at the time of diagnosis, with most patents losing the opportunity for radical surgery. At present, gemcitabine is the first-line chemotherapeutic agent for pancreatic cancer patients. However, a low response rate to gemcitabine is common in the clinic, and less than 20% of patients experience the ideal effects of gemcitabine [3]. In recent years, FOLFIRINOX (oxaliplatin, irinotecan, fluorouracil, and leucovorin) has become the recommended frontline chemotherapeutic regimen for metastatic pancreatic cancer patients [4]. However, the seriously adverse reaction and acquired drug resistance associated with FOLFIRINOX limits its cytotoxic efficacy. Therefore, a novel target for enhancing current chemotherapy is clearly needed to improve the outcomes of patients with pancreatic cancer.

The Hippo pathway was first discovered by genetic mosaic screens in *Drosophila melanogaster* [5,6], and increasing evidence has demonstrated that the Hippo pathway also limits organ size in mammalian systems [7,8]. The YES-associated protein (YAP), a main component of the Hippo pathway, has been proved to be overexpressed and to participate in the tumorigenesis of a variety of cancers, including breast cancer [9], lung cancer [10], ovarian cancer [11], liver cancer [12], and pancreatic cancer [13,14]. YAP functions as an oncogene and promotes the survival of cancer cells by regulating cancer cell proliferation and apoptosis. The abnormal overexpression of YAP has also been reported to be linked to disease progression and poor prognosis in breast cancer patients [15]. However, whether aberrant YAP expression causes resistance of pancreatic cancer cells to chemotherapy is currently unclear. We hypothesized that overexpression of YAP might be closely correlated to the sensitivity of gemcitabine treatment in pancreatic cancer cells.

Resveratrol (*trans-3,4',5-trihydroxystilbene*, Res) is a natural polyphenolic phytoalexin that was first isolated by Takaoka from the roots of white helebore in 1939. Since then, resveratrol has been widely found in plants (such as grape skin, red wine, berries, and peanuts) and in traditional Chinese medicines (such as Rheum officinale Baill and Polygonum cuspidatum) [16,17]. Numerous studies have shown that resveratrol exhibits antioxidant activity, anti-inflammatory activity, and protective activity against cardiac diseases and metabolic disorders [18]. Over the past several years, many reports have demonstrated that resveratrol acts as a cancer chemo-preventive agent to induce growth inhibition, cell cycle arrest, apoptosis, and changes in biomarker expression in several human cancer cell lines [19–21]. Our previous study showed that resveratrol plays an important role in suppressing the proliferation of pancreatic cancer cells via the PI-3K/Akt/NF-κB signaling pathway [22] and the hedgehog signaling pathway [23,24]. However, whether resveratrol can inhibit YAP expression and its molecular mechanism have not been elucidated.

In the present study, we tested the hypothesis that resveratrol is able to inhibit YAP expression via activation of the AMP-activated protein kinase (AMPK) pathway and inhibit the proliferation ability of pancreatic cancer cells. YAP is associated with resistance to gemcitabine chemotherapy and targeting YAP via resveratrol can enhance the sensitivity of pancreatic cancer cells to gemcitabine. Our findings indicate that YAP is a novel molecular target for improving the efficacy of current chemotherapeutic regimens for patients with pancreatic cancer and improving their long-term outcomes.

## 2. Materials and Methods

All experimental protocols were approved by the Ethical Committee of the First Affiliated Hospital of Medical College, Xi'an Jiaotong University, Xi'an, China.

### 2.1. Reagents

Resveratrol (>99% pure) and MTT (3-(4,5-dimethyl-2-thiazolyl)-2,5-diphenyl-2-H-tetrazolium bromide) were purchased from Sigma-Aldrich (St. Louis, MO, USA), and gemcitabine was purchased from Selleck Chemicals (Houston, TX, USA). Resveratrol and gemcitabine were initially dissolved in Dimethyl Sulfoxide (DMSO) at stock concentrations of 50 mM and 10 mM, respectively. Working dilutions for resveratrol and gemcitabine were prepared in culture medium immediately before use, and DMSO was used as control in all experiments. The antibodies used in this study are listed in Supplementary Materials Table S1.

### 2.2. Cell Lines and Cell Culture

The human pancreatic cancer cell lines Panc-1 and BxPC-3 were purchased from the Type Culture Collection of the Chinese Academy of Sciences (Shanghai, China). Panc-1 and BxPC-3 were cultured in Dulbecco's Modified Eagle Medium (DMEM) or RPMI-1640, respectively, containing 10%

dialyzed heat-inactivated fetal bovine serum (FBS) (HyClone, Logan, UT, USA), 100 U/mL penicillin and 100 µg/mL streptomycin in a humidified atmosphere containing 5% $CO_2$ at 37 °C.

## 2.3. Cell Viability Assay

Cancer cell lines (Panc-1, BxPC-3) were plated into 96-well plates at a density of 5000 cells/well and treated with various concentrations (0, 25, 50, 100, and 200 µM) of resveratrol and various concentrations (0, 1, 2, 5, 10, and 20 µM) of gemcitabine for designated lengths of time (24, 48, and 72 h). After being transfected with siRNA for 48 h, cells were plated in 96-well plates at a density of 5000 cells/well and treated with 2 µM gemcitabine for 72 h. Cell viability was assessed by the MTT assay. Ten microliters of 5 mg/mL MTT was added into each well after media were removed and incubated at 37 °C for 4 h. Then, 100 µL DMSO was added to each well, and the optical density (OD) was measured at 490 nm on a multifunction microplate reader (POLARstar OPTIMA; BMG, Offenburg, Germany). The proliferation inhibition rate was calculated according to the following equation: Proliferation inhibition rate = (1 − OD sample/OD control) × 100%.

## 2.4. Apoptosis Assay

Cell apoptosis was assessed by flow cytometry with an Annexin V-FITC/7-AAD apoptosis detection kit from Becton, Dickinson and Company (BD) (Franklin Lakes, NJ, USA) according to the manufacturer's instructions. Briefly, cancer cells were seeded into 6-well plates at a density of $1 \times 10^5$ cells per well, after being starved overnight, and each treatment was applied for 48 h. Then, cells were trypsinized, washed with phosphate buffered saline (PBS) and stained with Annexin V and 7-AAD. The percentage of apoptotic cells was quantified by flow cytometry using a FACSCalibur (BD Biosciences, San Diego, CA, USA) instrument. The total apoptosis rate was calculated by summing the rate of populations stained with Annexin V-FITC+/7-AAD- (early apoptotic cells) and Annexin V-FITC+/7-AAD+ (late apoptotic cells).

## 2.5. Immunofluorescence Staining

Cells were fixed in 4% formaldehyde diluted in phosphate buffered saline (PBS) for 15 min, permeabilized with 0.3% Triton X-100, treated with blocking buffer (5% BSA in PBS), and then incubated overnight with the primary antibody at 4 °C. Cells were then incubated with the Red conjugated secondary antibody from Jackson Immunoresearch Laboratories (West Grove, PA, USA) for 1 h at room temperature. Slides were mounted and examined using a Zeiss Instruments confocal microscope.

## 2.6. Gene Silencing by Small Interfering RNA

Loss-of-function analysis was performed using siRNAs targeting AMPK and YAP, which were purchased from GenePharm (Shanghai, China). The siRNA sequences are provided in Supplementary Materials Table S2. Each siRNA (100 nM) was transfected into pancreatic cancer cells using Lipofectamine 2000 according to the manufacturer's instructions. The knockdown of each target gene was confirmed by Western blot analysis. The cells were used for subsequent experiments 48 h after transfection.

## 2.7. Western Blot Analysis

Total proteins were extracted by RIPA lysis buffer (Beyotime, Guangzhou, China), and the concentration of proteins was determined using the BCA protein assay kit (Pierce, Rockford, IL, USA) according to the manufacturer's instruction. The proteins were then subjected to SDS-PAGE using a 10% polyacrylamide gel with a 5% stacking gel. The proteins were subsequently transferred to polyvinylidene difluoride (PVDF) membranes. The membranes were blocked with 5% fat-free milk in Tris-buffered saline-Tween (TBS-T) for 2 h and then incubated with the primary antibodies (listed in Supplementary Materials Table S1) at 4 °C overnight. Then, the membranes were incubated with a secondary antibody (diluted 1:10,000) for 2 h at room temperature. Chemiluminescence detection of bound antibodies was performed using an enhanced chemiluminescence (ECL) PLUS system and a Molecular Imager ChemiDoc XRS System (Bio-Rad Laboratories, Hercules, CA, USA).

*2.8. Real-Time PCR*

Total RNA was extracted using the Fastgen1000 RNA isolation system (Fastgen, Shanghai, China) according to the manufacturer's protocol. Total RNA was reverse-transcribed into cDNA using the Prime Script RT reagent kit (TaKaRa, Dalian, China). Real-time PCR was used to quantitatively examine the expression of YAP, CTGF and CYR61 at the mRNA level. Real-time PCR was conducted according to a previous report [25]. The PCR primer sequences for YAP, CTGF, CYR61, and β-actin are shown in Supplementary Materials Table S3. The expression of each target gene was determined using β-actin as the normalization control. Relative gene expression was calculated using the $2^{-\Delta\Delta Ct}$ method [26].

*2.9. Colony Formation Assay*

One thousand cells were seeded into a 35-mm petri dish and allowed to adhere overnight. The next day, a different treatment was applied to the dishes for 24 h, after which the medium was replaced with drug free medium. Cells were further cultured for two weeks to allow colonies to form. At the indicated time point, colonies were fixed with 4% paraformaldehyde and then stained with 0.1% crystal violet solution, rinsed, and then imaged. The number of colonies larger than 0.5 mm in diameter was counted using a microscope (Nikon Eclipse Ti-S, Tokyo, Japan) at a magnification of 400×.

*2.10. Statistical Analysis*

Each experiment was performed at least three times. Data are presented as means ± standard deviation. Differences were evaluated using Student's *t*-test, with $p < 0.05$ considered to be statistically significant.

## 3. Results

*3.1. Resveratrol Inhibits the Proliferation of Pancreatic Cancer Cells*

First, we examined the effects of resveratrol on the viability of cancer cells. Pancreatic cancer cells Panc-1 and BxPC-3 were treated with increasing doses of resveratrol (0, 25, 50, 100, and 200 μM). At the indicated time points (24, 48, and 72 h), the cell viability was assessed by the MTT assay. As shown in Figure 1, resveratrol decreased the growth of cancer cell lines in a dose- and time-dependent manner. The 50% inhibitory concentration (IC50) for both BxPC-3 and Panc-1 cells was approximately 50 μM resveratrol, which exhibited no cytotoxic effects on the BxPC-3 and Panc-1 cells. These results were in accord with our previous results. Therefore, cells were treated with 50 μM resveratrol in subsequent experiments.

*3.2. Resveratrol Inhibits Clone Formation and Induces Apoptosis of Pancreatic Cancer Cells*

To address the underlying mechanism governing the inhibitory effect of resveratrol (Res) on pancreatic cancer cell viability, we measured Res-induced apoptosis in BxPc-3 and Panc-1 cells by flow cytometry. The flow cytometric analyses were conducted after Panc-1 and BxPC-3 cells were treated with or without resveratrol (50 μM) for 48 h. As shown in Figure 2A,B, treatment of cancer cells with resveratrol caused an increase in the apoptotic population compared with that of the untreated control cells. Next, we detected the effect of resveratrol on the clone formation ability of cancer cells Panc-1 and BxPC-3. As shown in Figure 2C,D, treatment with 50 μM resveratrol markedly decreased the number of colonies compared with the untreated control cells. These results demonstrate that Res has a potent effect against clone formation and induces apoptosis of cancer cells.

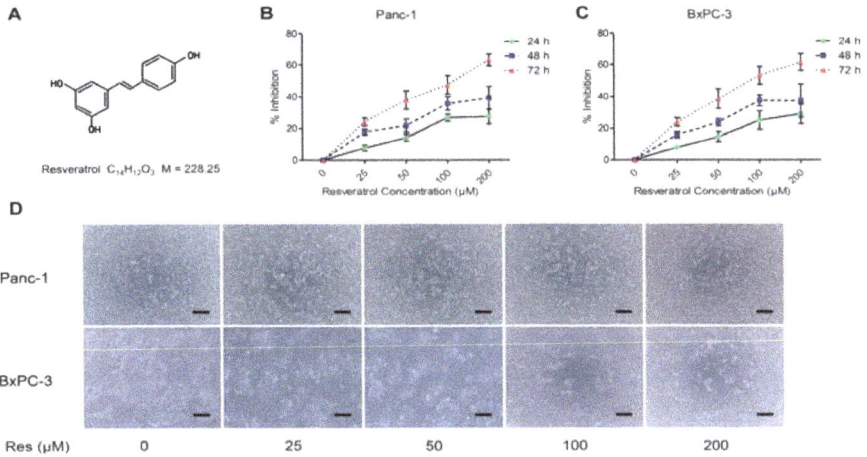

**Figure 1.** Resveratrol inhibits the proliferation of pancreatic cancer cells. (**A**) The structure of resveratrol (Res); (**B,C**) Panc-1 and BxPC-3 pancreatic cancer cells were treated with increasing concentrations of resveratrol (0, 25, 50, 100, and 200 μM) for 24 h, 48 h, or 72 h to analyze the inhibition ratio for cancer cell proliferation; (**D**) Micrographs of Panc-1 and BxPC-3 cells after being treated with the indicated concentrations of resveratrol for 48 h; representative images were captured (magnification, 100×; Scar bar: 100 μm).

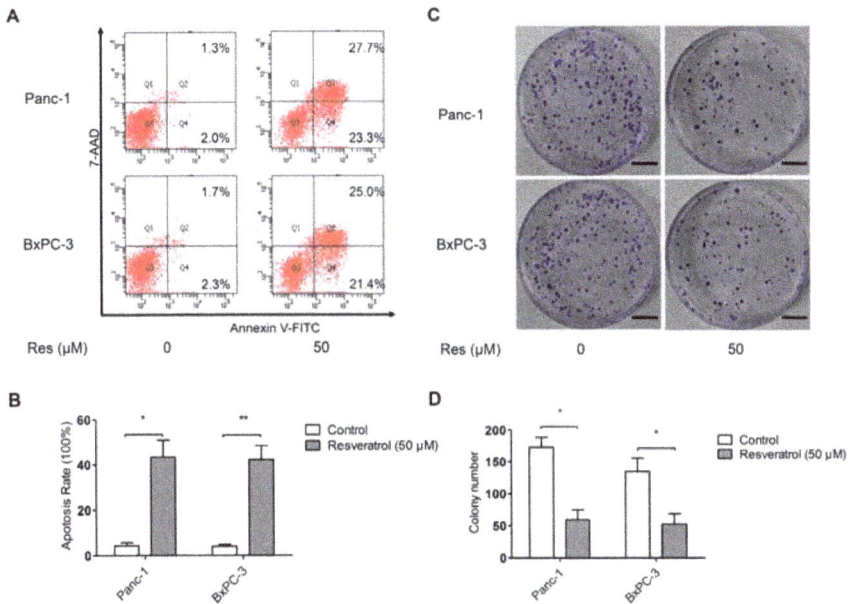

**Figure 2.** Resveratrol inhibits clone formation and induces apoptosis of pancreatic cancer cells. (**A,B**) The effects of resveratrol on Panc-1 and BxPC-3 cells apoptosis were detected by flow cytometry; (**C,D**) The effects of resveratrol on the colony-forming ability of Panc-1 and BxPC-3 cells. Images are representative of three independent experiments (Scale bar: 1 cm). Column: Mean, bar: SD, * $p < 0.05$, ** $p < 0.01$.

### 3.3. Resveratrol Inhibits YAP Expression of Pancreatic Cancer Cells

Increasing evidence has suggested that overexpression of YAP plays a key role in cancer cell survival and progression [27]. In particular, YAP can be phosphorylated at Ser127 and forms a more stable complex with the 14-3-3 proteins; therefore, it is retained in the cytoplasm and subject to degradation [28]. To determine whether resveratrol affects the YAP expression of cancer cells, Panc-1 and BxPC-3 cells were treated with resveratrol (0, 25, 50, and 100 µM) for 24 h. The protein expression of YAP and p-YAP (Ser127) in the pancreatic cancer cells exposed to resveratrol was evaluated by Western blot analysis. As shown in Figure 3A,B, resveratrol treatment up-regulated the level of p-YAP (Ser127), and the total level of YAP was significantly inhibited by resveratrol in a dose-dependent manner. Connective tissue growth factor (CTGF) and cysteine-rich angiogenic inducer 61 (CYR61) are two YAP-mediated downstream effectors that play an important role in tumor progression [29,30]. We therefore examined the expression of YAP, CTGF and CYR61 in response to treatment with resveratrol. The results showed that the mRNA levels of YAP, CTGF, and CYR61 were downregulated upon treatment with resveratrol (50 µM) (Figure 3C,D). Additionally, the nuclear translocation of YAP was decreased due to the effect of resveratrol, as demonstrated by immunofluorescence (Figure 3E). Together, these data indicate that resveratrol inhibits YAP expression of cancer cells via YAP phosphorylation at Ser127.

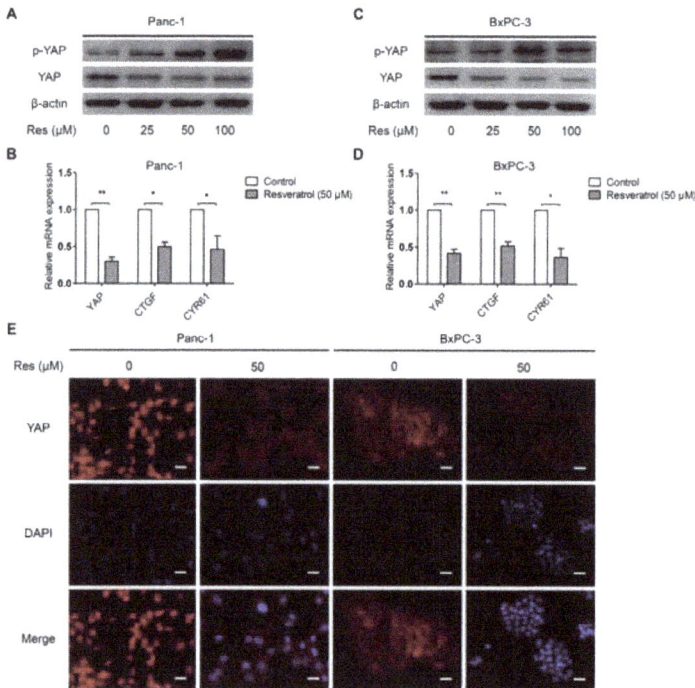

**Figure 3.** Resveratrol inhibits YAP expression of pancreatic cancer cells. (**A,B**) The effects of resveratrol on the protein expression of YAP and p-YAP (Ser127) were examined by Western blot analysis using β-actin as an internal loading control; (**C,D**) The effects of resveratrol on the mRNA expression of YAP, connective tissue growth factor (CTGF) and CYR61 were examined by real-time PCR with β-actin as the normalized reference gene. The data represent the results of three independent experiments; (**E**) Immunofluorescence staining of YAP in Panc-1 and BxPC-3 cells after treatment with resveratrol (50 µM) for 24 h. YAP staining is shown in red, and nuclear DNA staining by DAPI is shown in blue. (Magnification, 400×; Scale bar: 20 µm). Column: mean, bar: SD, * $p < 0.05$, ** $p < 0.01$.

### 3.4. Knockdown of AMPK Rescues Resveratrol Induced Suppression of YAP in Pancreatic Cancer Cells

Previous studies have established that resveratrol can activate the AMPK pathway [31]. The activation of AMPK leads to the suppression of YAP expression [32]. Based on the abovementioned promising findings, we speculated that the effect of resveratrol on cancer cell YAP inhibition may be mediated by AMPK signaling. To test this hypothesis, we further examined the effect of resveratrol on the activity of AMPK signaling. Immunoblotting results revealed that the phosphorylation level of AMPK (p-AMPK) in pancreatic cancer cells was significantly increased in response to resveratrol treatment in a dose-dependent manner (Figure 4A,B). To verify that resveratrol-inhibited YAP expression in cancer cells is mediated by AMPK signaling, siRNA technology was developed to knock down AMPK expression. We found that knocking down AMPK expression alone did not affect the expression of YAP or the phosphorylation level of p-YAP in Panc-1 and BxPC-3 cells (Figure 4C,D). However, resveratrol induced the activation of p-AMPK and p-YAP, and inhibition of YAP was restored by AMPK knockdown (Figure 4C,D). Additionally, the immunofluorescence results indicated that the nuclear translocation and total level of YAP was inhibited by resveratrol and that this inhibition effect was restored by AMPK knockdown (Figure 4E). Together, these data suggest that AMPK signaling is involved in resveratrol-suppressed YAP expression in pancreatic cancer cells.

### 3.5. Knockdown of YAP Increased Gemcitabine Sensitivity in Pancreatic Cancer Cells

First, we used the MTT assay to examine the effects of gemcitabine on the proliferation of the Panc-1 and BxPC-3 cell lines. As shown in Figure 5A,B, we found that BxPC-3 was sensitive whereas Panc-1 was resistant to gemcitabine, in accord with previous findings [33]. Therefore, we used Panc-1 in further experiments. To evaluate the effects of YAP on cell survival and resistance to chemotherapy, we treated Panc-1 cells, which express high levels of YAP natively and are resistant to gemcitabine, with 2 μM gemcitabine in the presence of either siControl or siYAP and confirmed the silencing of YAP in the cells using Western blot analysis (Figure 5H). MTT assay results showed that the proliferation capacity was lower in siYAP cells than in siControl cells after treating them with gemcitabine (Figure 5C). Furthermore, silencing of YAP increased the apoptotic response to treatment with gemcitabine (2 μM) in Panc-1 cells (Figure 5D,E). The clone ability was significantly decreased after silencing YAP, and siYAP enhanced the gemcitabine inhibition effect on clone ability (Figure 5F,G). Together, these data suggest that YAP silencing enhances the sensitivity of gemcitabine in gemcitabine-resistant pancreatic cancer cells.

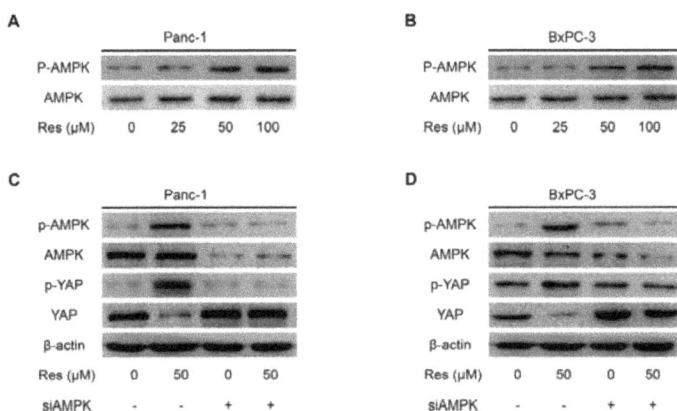

**Figure 4.** *Cont.*

65

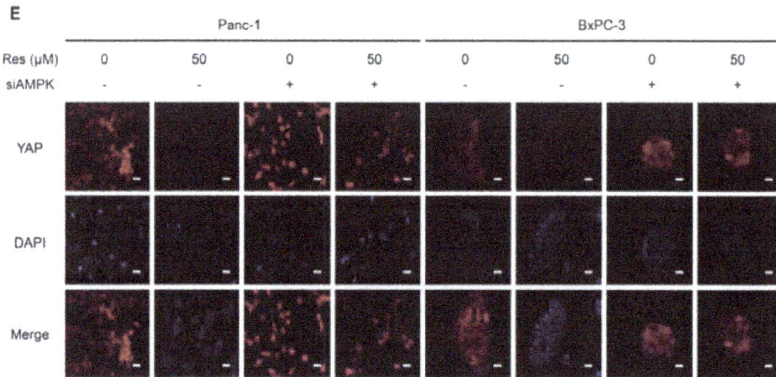

**Figure 4.** Knockdown of AMP-activated protein kinase (AMPK) rescues resveratrol-induced suppression of YES-associated protein (YAP) of pancreatic cancer cells. (**A,B**) The effects of resveratrol on the activation of AMPK (Thr172) in Panc-1 and BxPC-3 cells were measured by Western blot analysis; (**C,D**) After transfection with siAMPK or siControl for 48 h, Panc-1 and BxPC-3 cells were treated with resveratrol (50 μM) for 24 h. The protein expression levels of YAP, p YAP (Ser127), AMPK and p AMPK (Thr172) were examined by Western blot analysis using β-actin as an internal loading control; (**E**) YAP in Panc-1 and BxPC-3 cells was stained for immunofluorescence after transfection with siAMPK or siControl for 48 h and then treated with resveratrol (50 μM) for 24 h. YAP staining is shown in red, and nuclear DNA staining by DAPI is shown in blue (Magnification, 400×; Scale bar: 20 μm).

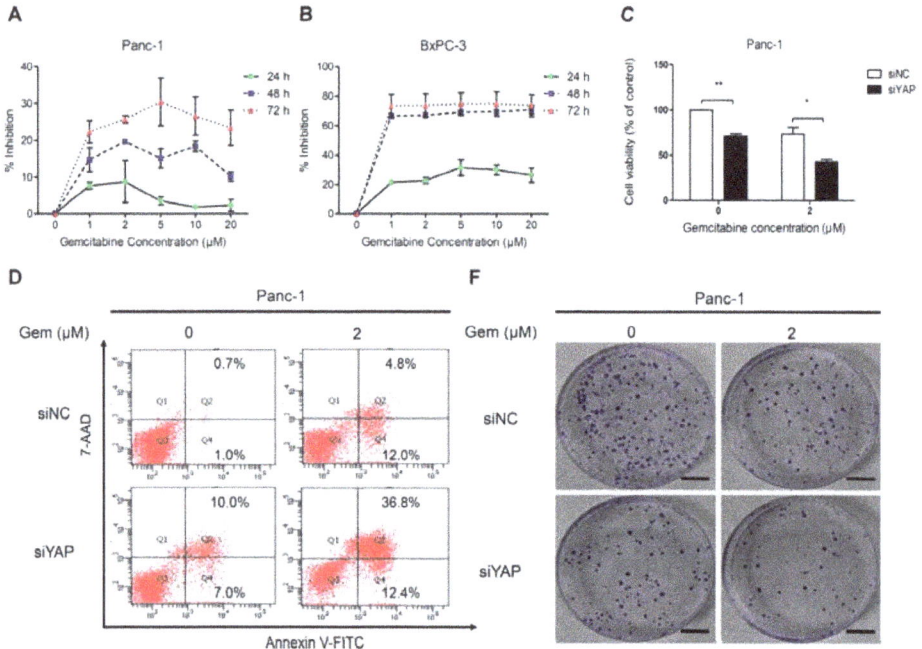

**Figure 5.** *Cont.*

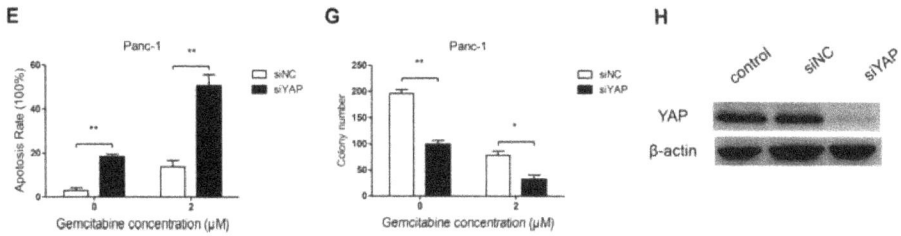

**Figure 5.** Knockdown of YAP increases gemcitabine sensitivity in pancreatic cancer cells. (**A,B**) Panc-1 and BxPC-3 cells were treated with increasing concentrations of gemcitabine (0, 1, 2, 5, 10, and 20 μM) for 24 h, 48 h, or 72 h to analyze the inhibition ratio for cancer cell proliferation; (**C**) After being transfected with siControl or siYAP for 48 h, cells were plated in 96-well plates and treated with 2 μM gemcitabine for 72 h. Cell viability was assessed by the MTT assay; (**D,E**) The effects of siControl or siYAP on Panc-1 cancer cells apoptosis after treatment with 2 μM gemcitabine for 48 h was detected by flow cytometry; (**F,G**) The effects of siControl or siYAP combined with gemcitabine on the colony-forming ability of Panc-1 cells. Images are representative of three independent experiments (Scale bar: 1 cm); (**H**) The efficiency of siRNAs targeting YAP in Panc-1cells was evaluated by Western blot analysis. Column: Mean, bar: SD, * $p < 0.05$, ** $p < 0.01$.

### 3.6. Inhibition of YAP Activity by Resveratrol Enhanced the Sensitivity of Pancreatic Cancer Cells to Gemcitabine

To determine whether resveratrol increases the susceptibility of Panc-1 cells to gemcitabine, we treated Panc-1 cells with 50 μM resveratrol and 2 μM gemcitabine. The MTT assay results showed that the proliferation capacity was significantly lower in the resveratrol and gemcitabine therapy group than in the resveratrol alone or gemcitabine alone group (Figure 6A). The protein expression of YAP and p-YAP (Ser127) in Panc-1 exposed to resveratrol and gemcitabine was evaluated by Western blot analysis. As shown in Figure 6B, resveratrol treatment up-regulated the level of p-YAP (Ser127), and the total level of YAP was significantly inhibited by resveratrol. However, gemcitabine had no effect on YAP expression. Next, we measured the apoptosis rate in Panc-1 cells by flow cytometry. Flow cytometric analyses were conducted after Panc-1 cells were treated with or without resveratrol (50 μM) and gemcitabine (2 μM) for 48 h. As shown in Figure 6C,D, treatment of cancer cells with resveratrol caused an increase in apoptotic population compared with the untreated control cells, but almost all cells underwent apoptosis in the resveratrol and gemcitabine combined therapy group. Next, we detected the clone formation ability of Panc-1 cancer cells after treatment with resveratrol and gemcitabine. As shown in Figure 6E,F, treatment with resveratrol and gemcitabine markedly decreased the number of colonies compared with the number measured for the gemcitabine or resveratrol alone cells. Taken together, these results demonstrate that resveratrol has a potent effect in enhancing the sensitivity of pancreatic cancer cells to gemcitabine by inhibiting YAP expression.

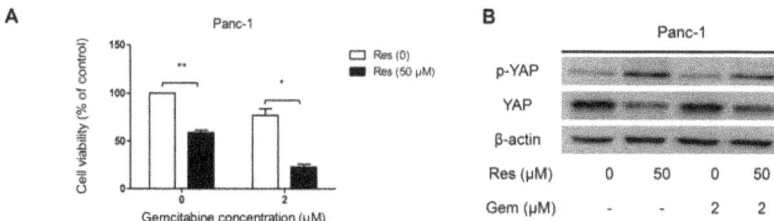

**Figure 6.** *Cont.*

C

D

E

F

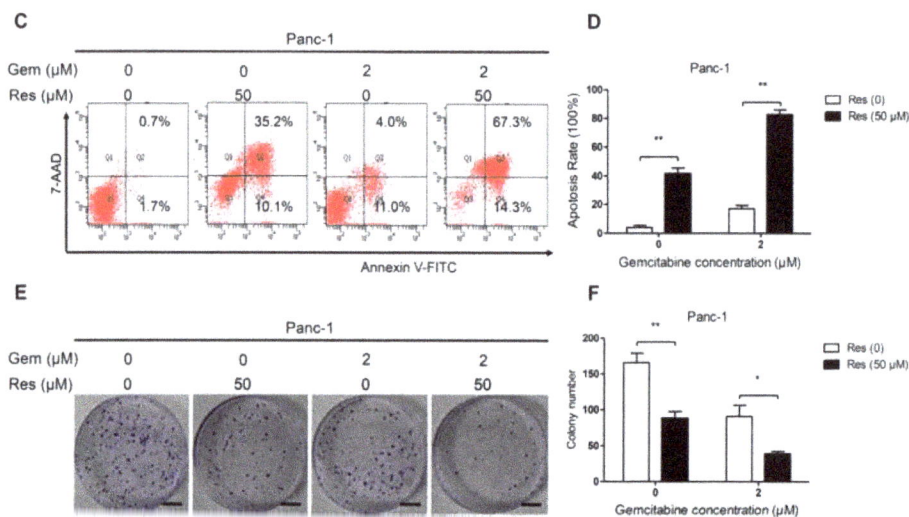

**Figure 6.** Inhibition of YAP activity by resveratrol enhances the sensitivity of pancreatic cancer cells to gemcitabine. (**A**) Panc-1 cells were treated with gemcitabine (2 μM) and resveratrol (50 μM) for 72 h. Cell viability was assessed by the MTT assay; (**B**) Panc-1 cells were treated with gemcitabine (2 μM) and resveratrol (50 μM) for 24 h. The protein expression levels of YAP and p-YAP (Ser127) were examined by Western blot analysis using β-actin as an internal loading control; (**C,D**) Panc-1 cells were treated with gemcitabine (Gem) (2 μM) and resveratrol (50 μM) for 48 h. Apoptosis was detected by flow cytometry; (**E,F**) The combined effects of Res and Gem on Panc-1 cell clones' colony-forming ability was detected. Images are representative of three independent experiments (Scale bar: 1 cm). Column: Mean, bar: SD, * $p < 0.05$, ** $p < 0.01$.

## 4. Discussion

In this study, we observed that resveratrol inhibited pancreatic cancer cell proliferation and clone formation and induced cell apoptosis, which was accompanied by the activation of p-AMPK and p-YAP and a decreased level of YAP in BxPc-3 and Panc-1 cells. Moreover, the results suggest that AMPK signaling is essential in resveratrol-suppressed YAP expression in pancreatic cancer cells. Furthermore, we found that YAP silencing enhances the sensitivity of gemcitabine in gemcitabine-resistant Panc-1 cancer cells. Resveratrol has a synergistic effect with gemcitabine in Panc-1 cells by inhibiting YAP expression. Our findings suggest that resveratrol is a potential drug for adjuvant therapy or a complementary alternative medicine for the management of pancreatic cancers via activation of AMPK and inhibition of YAP.

Despite great advances in modern medicine over the past several years, pancreatic cancer is still associated with an extremely high mortality rate [1]. Currently, gemcitabine [3] and FOLFIRINOX [4] are considered first-line drugs for treating pancreatic cancer, but their efficacy is still low because of a seriously adverse reaction and because acquired drug resistance limits their cytotoxic efficacy. Therefore, we must find a novel target for enhancing current chemotherapy to improve the outcomes of patients with pancreatic cancer.

Resveratrol is a natural polyphenolic phytoalexin that is widely found in plants and in traditional Chinese medicines [16,17]. Resveratrol has been shown to directly inhibit the proliferation and viability of human pancreatic cancer cells in vitro in a dose- and time-dependent manner [22]. Accordingly, our results demonstrated that resveratrol inhibited cell proliferation and clone formation and induced cell apoptosis. Interestingly, we found that Panc-1 and BxPC-3 cells respond differently to gemcitabine (BxPC-3 being more sensitive). But their biochemical and functional response to resveratrol appears to be the same. As we know, BxPC-3 and Panc-1 cells have many differences such as K-*ras* mutation types (BxPC-3 is a K-*ras* wild cell while Panc-1 is a K-*ras* mutant cell) [34] and epithelial-mesenchymal transition (EMT) regulated genes (E-cadherin and Zeb-1) [35] which could affect gemcitabine sensitivity in pancreatic cancer cells. Our previous reports have shown that resveratrol could inhibit the EMT of pancreatic cancer cells via suppression of the PI3K/Akt/NF-kappaB pathway in Panc-1 and BxPC-3 cells [22]. Furthermore, resveratrol could also inhibit pancreatic cancer stem cell characteristics in human and Kras (G12D) transgenic mice by inhibiting pluripotency maintaining factors and epithelial-mesenchymal transition [36]. However, the specific mechanism needs to be further explored.

The AMPK system is traditionally considered a sensor of cellular energy status and a regulator of metabolism [37]. Recent studies have provided novel evidence that AMPK may function as a suppressor of cell proliferation. Indeed, activation of AMPK has been shown to benefit a variety of malignant tumors by inhibiting the proliferation of tumor cells [38,39]. In this respect, our results demonstrated that resveratrol could activate AMPK (Thr172) and suppress the proliferation of pancreatic cancer cells, indicating the anti-proliferative action of AMPK in pancreatic cancer cells. The effect of AMPK on cell proliferation appears to be mediated through multiple mechanisms, mainly the regulation of cell cycle progression, inhibition of protein synthesis, and de novo fatty acid biosynthesis [40,41]. Previous reports have suggested that AMPK activation stabilizes and increases AMOTL1 steady-state protein levels, contributing to YAP inhibition [42]. Accordingly, our results demonstrated that resveratrol induces YAP cytoplasmic retention and S127 phosphorylation and inhibits YAP transcriptional activity and YAP-dependent transformation via activation of AMPK. Knockdown of AMPK rescues resveratrol-induced suppression of YAP in pancreatic cancer cells. Some reports have suggested that glucose starvation and energy stress could result in phosphorylation of YAP and contribute to its inactivation [43]. Harris et al. [44] demonstrated that resveratrol could inhibit glycogen synthesis, which may serve as the underlying mechanism in the inhibition of YAP. However, Jung-Soon Mo [32] and his colleagues also found that AMPK inhibits YAP activity through phosphorylation of serine 94. Whether resveratrol could induce YAP phosphorylation at serine 94 need further investigation.

As an oncogene, YAP is abundantly expressed in many types of cancers [15,27], and tremendous progress has been made toward our understanding of the roles of YAP in tumorigenesis, size control, and stem cell renewal and differentiation [45,46]. However, YAP's function in chemotherapeutic drug response is largely unknown in pancreatic cancer cells. Ciamporcero et al. [47] demonstrated that YAP overexpression protected, whereas YAP knockdown sensitized, urothelial cell carcinoma (UCC) cells to chemotherapy and radiation effects by increasing the accumulation of DNA damage and apoptosis. Verteporfin, a pharmacological YAP inhibitor, could inhibit tumor cell proliferation and restore sensitivity to cisplatin. In our study, we found that the chemotherapeutic sensitivity of pancreatic cancer to gemcitabine can be increased by YAP inhibition in vitro. YAP may participate in regulating the chemosensitivity of pancreatic cancer to chemotherapy. As a dietary and synthetic agent that is a pharmacological YAP inhibitor, resveratrol may exhibit greater efficacy and lower toxicity for the prevention and treatment of pancreatic cancer. However, its more specific mechanisms and safety require further investigation.

## 5. Conclusions

In conclusion, the present study demonstrated that resveratrol suppressed the proliferation and cloning ability and induced the apoptosis of pancreatic cancer cells. These multiple biological effects might result from the activation of AMPK (Thr172), thus, inducing YAP cytoplasmic retention and S127 phosphorylation, and inhibiting YAP transcriptional activity by resveratrol. YAP silencing by siRNA or resveratrol could enhance the sensitivity of gemcitabine in pancreatic cancer cells. These results suggest that resveratrol is a potential anticancer agent for the treatment of pancreatic cancer. However, whether other mechanisms are involved in the anti-tumor effects of resveratrol and its safety in humans warrant further study.

**Supplementary Materials:** The following are available online at http://www.mdpi.com/2072-6643/8/10/546/s1, Table S1: A list of the utilized primary antibodies, Table S2: The siRNA sequences, Table S3: Primers sequences for real-time PCR analysis.

**Acknowledgments:** This study was supported by grants from the National Natural Science Foundation of China (No. 81402971) and the Clinical Innovation Funds of the 1st Affiliated Hospital of XJTU (No. 14ZD05, No. 14ZD06, No. 15ZD02, No. 15ZD03, No. 15ZD07 and No. 15ZD15).

**Author Contributions:** Z.J. designed and performed the experiments, analyzed and interpreted the data, and wrote the manuscript. X.C. and K.C. participated in the design of the study and performed the statistical analysis. C.Z., M.L., L.S., L.G., W.D., and Z.W. contributed to the conception of the study and the revision of the article. J.M. and Q.M. contributed to the conception and design of the study, the revision of the manuscript, and the final approval of the version to be published. All authors read and approved the final manuscript.

**Conflicts of Interest:** The authors declare no conflict of interest.

## References

1. Siegel, R.L.; Miller, K.D.; Jemal, A. Cancer statistics, 2016. *CA Cancer J. Clin.* **2016**, *66*, 7–30. [CrossRef] [PubMed]
2. Bosetti, C.; Bertuccio, P.; Negri, E.; La Vecchia, C.; Zeegers, M.P.; Boffetta, P. Pancreatic cancer: Overview of descriptive epidemiology. *Mol. Carcinog.* **2012**, *51*, 3–13. [CrossRef] [PubMed]
3. Tamburrino, A.; Piro, G.; Carbone, C.; Tortora, G.; Melisi, D. Mechanisms of resistance to chemotherapeutic and anti-angiogenic drugs as novel targets for pancreatic cancer therapy. *Front. Pharmacol.* **2013**, *4*, 56. [CrossRef] [PubMed]
4. Conroy, T.; Desseigne, F.; Ychou, M.; Bouche, O.; Guimbaud, R.; Becouarn, Y.; Adenis, A.; Raoul, J.L.; Gourgou-Bourgade, S.; de la Fouchardiere, C.; et al. FOLFIRINOX versus gemcitabine for metastatic pancreatic cancer. *N. Engl. J. Med.* **2011**, *364*, 1817–1825. [CrossRef] [PubMed]
5. Edgar, B.A. From cell structure to transcription: Hippo forges a new path. *Cell* **2006**, *124*, 267–273. [CrossRef] [PubMed]
6. Huang, J.; Wu, S.; Barrera, J.; Matthews, K.; Pan, D. The Hippo signaling pathway coordinately regulates cell proliferation and apoptosis by inactivating Yorkie, the Drosophila Homolog of YAP. *Cell* **2005**, *122*, 421–434. [CrossRef] [PubMed]
7. Yimlamai, D.; Christodoulou, C.; Galli, G.G.; Yanger, K.; Pepe-Mooney, B.; Gurung, B.; Shrestha, K.; Cahan, P.; Stanger, B.Z.; Camargo, F.D. Hippo pathway activity influences liver cell fate. *Cell* **2014**, *157*, 1324–1338. [CrossRef] [PubMed]
8. Yu, F.X.; Zhao, B.; Guan, K.L. Hippo Pathway in Organ Size Control, Tissue Homeostasis, and Cancer. *Cell* **2015**, *163*, 811–828. [CrossRef] [PubMed]
9. Von, E.B.; Jaenicke, L.A.; Kortlever, R.M.; Royla, N.; Wiese, K.E.; Letschert, S.; McDuffus, L.A.; Sauer, M.; Rosenwald, A.; Evan, G.I.; et al. A MYC-Driven Change in Mitochondrial Dynamics Limits YAP/TAZ Function in Mammary Epithelial Cells and Breast Cancer. *Cancer Cell* **2015**, *28*, 743–757.
10. Dubois, F.; Keller, M.; Calvayrac, O.; Soncin, F.; Hoa, L.; Hergovich, A.; Parrini, M.C.; Mazieres, J.; Vaisse-Lesteven, M.; Camonis, J.; et al. RASSF1A Suppresses the Invasion and Metastatic Potential of Human Non-Small Cell Lung Cancer Cells by Inhibiting YAP Activation through the GEF-H1/RhoB Pathway. *Cancer Res.* **2016**, *76*, 1627–1640. [CrossRef] [PubMed]
11. Yagi, H.; Asanoma, K.; Ohgami, T.; Ichinoe, A.; Sonoda, K.; Kato, K. GEP oncogene promotes cell proliferation through YAP activation in ovarian cancer. *Oncogene* **2016**, *35*, 4471–4480. [CrossRef] [PubMed]
12. Wang, J.; Ma, L.; Weng, W.; Qiao, Y.; Zhang, Y.; He, J.; Wang, H.; Xiao, W.; Li, L.; Chu, Q.; et al. Mutual interaction between YAP and CREB promotes tumorigenesis in liver cancer. *Hepatology* **2013**, *58*, 1011–1020. [CrossRef] [PubMed]
13. Yuan, Y.; Li, D.; Li, H.; Wang, L.; Tian, G.; Dong, Y. YAP overexpression promotes the epithelial-mesenchymal transition and chemoresistance in pancreatic cancer cells. *Mol. Med. Rep.* **2016**, *13*, 237–242. [CrossRef] [PubMed]
14. Morvaridi, S.; Dhall, D.; Greene, M.I.; Pandol, S.J.; Wang, Q. Role of YAP and TAZ in pancreatic ductal adenocarcinoma and in stellate cells associated with cancer and chronic pancreatitis. *Sci. Rep.* **2015**, *5*, 16759. [CrossRef] [PubMed]

15. Zhao, Y.; Khanal, P.; Savage, P.; She, Y.M.; Cyr, T.D.; Yang, X. YAP-induced resistance of cancer cells to antitubulin drugs is modulated by a Hippo-independent pathway. *Cancer Res.* **2014**, *74*, 4493–4503. [CrossRef] [PubMed]

16. Borriello, A.; Bencivenga, D.; Caldarelli, I.; Tramontano, A.; Borgia, A.; Pirozzi, A.V.; Oliva, A.; Della, R.F. Resveratrol and cancer treatment: Is hormesis a yet unsolved matter. *Curr. Pharm. Des.* **2013**, *19*, 5384–5393. [CrossRef] [PubMed]

17. Xu, Q.; Zong, L.; Chen, X.; Jiang, Z.; Nan, L.; Li, J.; Duan, W.; Lei, J.; Zhang, L.; Ma, J.; et al. Resveratrol in the treatment of pancreatic cancer. *Ann. N. Y. Acad. Sci.* **2015**, *1348*, 10–19. [CrossRef] [PubMed]

18. Zhang, H.; Morgan, B.; Potter, B.J.; Ma, L.; Dellsperger, K.C.; Ungvari, Z.; Zhang, C. Resveratrol improves left ventricular diastolic relaxation in type 2 diabetes by inhibiting oxidative/nitrative stress: in vivo demonstration with magnetic resonance imaging. *Am. J. Physiol. Heart Circ. Physiol.* **2010**, *299*, H985–H994. [CrossRef] [PubMed]

19. Hu, F.W.; Tsai, L.L.; Yu, C.H.; Chen, P.N.; Chou, M.Y.; Yu, C.C. Impairment of tumor-initiating stem-like property and reversal of epithelial-mesenchymal transdifferentiation in head and neck cancer by resveratrol treatment. *Mol. Nutr. Food Res.* **2012**, *56*, 1247–1258. [CrossRef] [PubMed]

20. Buhrmann, C.; Shayan, P.; Popper, B.; Goel, A.; Shakibaei, M. Sirt1 Is Required for Resveratrol-Mediated Chemopreventive Effects in Colorectal Cancer Cells. *Nutrients* **2016**, *8*, 145. [CrossRef] [PubMed]

21. Roy, S.K.; Chen, Q.; Fu, J.; Shankar, S.; Srivastava, R.K. Resveratrol inhibits growth of orthotopic pancreatic tumors through activation of FOXO transcription factors. *PLoS ONE* **2011**, *6*, e25166. [CrossRef] [PubMed]

22. Li, W.; Ma, J.; Ma, Q.; Li, B.; Han, L.; Liu, J.; Xu, Q.; Duan, W.; Yu, S.; Wang, F.; et al. Resveratrol inhibits the epithelial-mesenchymal transition of pancreatic cancer cells via suppression of the PI-3K/Akt/NF-kappaB pathway. *Curr. Med. Chem.* **2013**, *20*, 4185–4194. [CrossRef] [PubMed]

23. Li, W.; Cao, L.; Chen, X.; Lei, J.; Ma, Q. Resveratrol inhibits hypoxia-driven ROS-induced invasive and migratory ability of pancreatic cancer cells via suppression of the Hedgehog signaling pathway. *Oncol. Rep.* **2016**, *35*, 1718–1726. [CrossRef] [PubMed]

24. Qin, Y.; Ma, Z.; Dang, X.; Li, W.; Ma, Q. Effect of resveratrol on proliferation and apoptosis of human pancreatic cancer MIA PaCa-2 cells may involve inhibition of the Hedgehog signaling pathway. *Mol. Med. Rep.* **2014**, *10*, 2563–2567. [PubMed]

25. Ma, Q.; Zhang, M.; Wang, Z.; Ma, Z.; Sha, H. The beneficial effect of resveratrol on severe acute pancreatitis. *Ann. N. Y. Acad. Sci.* **2011**, *1215*, 96–102. [CrossRef] [PubMed]

26. Schmittgen, T.D.; Livak, K.J. Analyzing real-time PCR data by the comparative C(T) method. *Nat. Protoc.* **2008**, *3*, 1101–1108. [CrossRef] [PubMed]

27. Hall, C.A.; Wang, R.; Miao, J.; Oliva, E.; Shen, X.; Wheeler, T.; Hilsenbeck, S.G.; Orsulic, S.; Goode, S. Hippo pathway effector Yap is an ovarian cancer oncogene. *Cancer Res.* **2010**, *70*, 8517–8525. [CrossRef] [PubMed]

28. Basu, S.; Totty, N.F.; Irwin, M.S.; Sudol, M.; Downward, J. Akt phosphorylates the Yes-associated protein, YAP, to induce interaction with 14–3-3 and attenuation of p73-mediated apoptosis. *Mol. Cell* **2003**, *11*, 11–23. [CrossRef]

29. Dong, J.; Feldmann, G.; Huang, J.; Wu, S.; Zhang, N.; Comerford, S.A.; Gayyed, M.F.; Anders, R.A.; Maitra, A.; Pan, D. Elucidation of a universal size-control mechanism in Drosophila and mammals. *Cell* **2007**, *130*, 1120–1133. [CrossRef] [PubMed]

30. Lu, L.; Li, Y.; Kim, S.M.; Bossuyt, W.; Liu, P.; Qiu, Q.; Wang, Y.; Halder, G.; Finegold, M.J.; Lee, J.S.; et al. Hippo signaling is a potent in vivo growth and tumor suppressor pathway in the mammalian liver. *Proc. Natl. Acad. Sci. USA* **2010**, *107*, 1437–1442. [CrossRef] [PubMed]

31. Yi, C.O.; Jeon, B.T.; Shin, H.J.; Jeong, E.A.; Chang, K.C.; Lee, J.E.; Lee, D.H.; Kim, H.J.; Kang, S.S.; Cho, G.J.; et al. Resveratrol activates AMPK and suppresses LPS-induced NF-kappaB-dependent COX-2 activation in RAW 264.7 macrophage cells. *Anat. Cell Biol.* **2011**, *44*, 194–203. [CrossRef] [PubMed]

32. Mo, J.S.; Meng, Z.; Kim, Y.C.; Park, H.W.; Hansen, C.G.; Kim, S.; Lim, D.S.; Guan, K.L. Cellular energy stress induces AMPK-mediated regulation of YAP and the Hippo pathway. *Nat. Cell Biol.* **2015**, *17*, 500–510. [CrossRef] [PubMed]

33. Cao, J.; Yang, J.; Ramachandran, V.; Arumugam, T.; Deng, D.; Li, Z.; Xu, L.; Logsdon, C.D. TM4SF1 Promotes Gemcitabine Resistance of Pancreatic Cancer in vitro and in vivo. *PLoS ONE* **2015**, *10*, e0144969. [CrossRef] [PubMed]

34. Shao, T.; Zheng, Y.; Zhao, B.; Li, T.; Cheng, K.; Cai, W. Recombinant expression of different mutant K-ras gene in pancreatic cancer Bxpc-3 cells and its effects on chemotherapy sensitivity. *Sci. China Life Sci.* **2014**, *57*, 1011–1017. [CrossRef] [PubMed]

35. Arumugam, T.; Ramachandran, V.; Fournier, K.F.; Wang, H.; Marquis, L.; Abbruzzese, J.L.; Gallick, G.E.; Logsdon, C.D.; McConkey, D.J.; Choi, W. Epithelial to mesenchymal transition contributes to drug resistance in pancreatic cancer. *Cancer Res.* **2009**, *69*, 5820–5828. [CrossRef] [PubMed]

36. Shankar, S.; Nall, D.; Tang, S.N.; Meeker, D.; Passarini, J.; Sharma, J.; Srivastava, R.K. Resveratrol inhibits pancreatic cancer stem cell characteristics in human and KrasG12D transgenic mice by inhibiting pluripotency maintaining factors and epithelial-mesenchymal transition. *PLoS ONE* **2011**, *6*, e16530. [CrossRef] [PubMed]

37. Foretz, M.; Taleux, N.; Guigas, B.; Horman, S.; Beauloye, C.; Andreelli, F.; Bertrand, L.; Viollet, B. Regulation of energy metabolism by AMPK: A novel therapeutic approach for the treatment of metabolic and cardiovascular diseases. *Med. Sci.* **2006**, *22*, 381–388.

38. Ming, M.; Sinnett-Smith, J.; Wang, J.; Soares, H.P.; Young, S.H.; Eibl, G.; Rozengurt, E. Dose-Dependent AMPK-Dependent and Independent Mechanisms of Berberine and Metformin Inhibition of mTORC1, ERK, DNA Synthesis and Proliferation in Pancreatic Cancer Cells. *PLoS ONE* **2014**, *9*, e114573. [CrossRef] [PubMed]

39. Hadad, S.M.; Hardie, D.G.; Appleyard, V.; Thompson, A.M. Effects of metformin on breast cancer cell proliferation, the AMPK pathway and the cell cycle. *Clin. Transl. Oncol.* **2014**, *16*, 746–752. [CrossRef] [PubMed]

40. Ma, J.; Duan, W.; Han, S.; Lei, J.; Xu, Q.; Chen, X.; Jiang, Z.; Nan, L.; Li, J.; Chen, K.; et al. Ginkgolic acid suppresses the development of pancreatic cancer by inhibiting pathways driving lipogenesis. *Oncotarget* **2015**, *6*, 20993–21003. [CrossRef] [PubMed]

41. Lin, V.C.; Tsai, Y.C.; Lin, J.N.; Fan, L.L.; Pan, M.H.; Ho, C.T.; Wu, J.Y.; Way, T.D. Activation of AMPK by pterostilbene suppresses lipogenesis and cell-cycle progression in p53 positive and negative human prostate cancer cells. *J. Agric. Food Chem.* **2012**, *60*, 6399–6407. [CrossRef] [PubMed]

42. De Ran, M.; Yang, J.; Shen, C.H.; Peters, E.C.; Fitamant, J.; Chan, P.; Hsieh, M.; Zhu, S.; Asara, J.M.; Zheng, B.; et al. Energy stress regulates hippo-YAP signaling involving AMPK-mediated regulation of angiomotin-like 1 protein. *Cell Rep.* **2014**, *9*, 495–503. [CrossRef] [PubMed]

43. Wang, W.; Xiao, Z.D.; Li, X.; Aziz, K.E.; Gan, B.; Johnson, R.L.; Chen, J. AMPK modulates Hippo pathway activity to regulate energy homeostasis. *Nat. Cell Biol.* **2015**, *17*, 490–499. [CrossRef] [PubMed]

44. Harris, D.M.; Li, L.; Chen, M.; Lagunero, F.T.; Go, V.L.; Boros, L.G. Diverse mechanisms of growth inhibition by luteolin, resveratrol, and quercetin in MIA PaCa-2 cells: A comparative glucose tracer study with the fatty acid synthase inhibitor C75. *Metabolomics* **2012**, *8*, 201–210. [CrossRef] [PubMed]

45. Hong, W.; Guan, K.L. The YAP and TAZ transcription co-activators: Key downstream effectors of the mammalian Hippo pathway. *Semin. Cell Dev. Biol.* **2012**, *23*, 785–793. [CrossRef] [PubMed]

46. Yu, F.X.; Guan, K.L. The Hippo pathway: Regulators and regulations. *Genes Dev.* **2013**, *27*, 355–371. [CrossRef] [PubMed]

47. Ciamporcero, E.; Shen, H.; Ramakrishnan, S.; Yu, K.S.; Chintala, S.; Shen, L.; Adelaiye, R.; Miles, K.M.; Ullio, C.; Pizzimenti, S.; et al. YAP activation protects urothelial cell carcinoma from treatment-induced DNA damage. *Oncogene* **2016**, *35*, 1541–1553. [CrossRef] [PubMed]

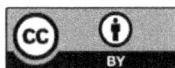

*nutrients*

MDPI

*Article*

# Food Matrix Effects of Polyphenol Bioaccessibility from Almond Skin during Simulated Human Digestion

Giuseppina Mandalari [1,2,*], Maria Vardakou [2], Richard Faulks [2], Carlo Bisignano [1], Maria Martorana [1], Antonella Smeriglio [1] and Domenico Trombetta [1]

[1] Dipartimento di Scienze Chimiche, Biologiche, Farmaceutiche ed Ambientali, University of Messina, Sal. Sperone 31, 98166 Messina, Italy; cbisignano@unime.it (C.B.); mmartorana@live.it (M.M.); asmeriglio@unime.it (A.S.); dtrombetta@unime.it (D.T.)

[2] The Model Gut, Institute of Food Research, Norwich Research Park, Colney Lane, Norwich NR4 7UA, UK; M.Vardakou@uea.ac.uk (M.V.); r.faulks147@btinternet.com (R.F.)

* Correspondence: gmandalari@unime.it; Tel.: +39-90-676-6593

Received: 11 July 2016; Accepted: 18 August 2016; Published: 15 September 2016

**Abstract:** The goal of the present study was to quantify the rate and extent of polyphenols released in the gastrointestinal tract (GIT) from natural (NS) and blanched (BS) almond skins. A dynamic gastric model of digestion which provides a realistic simulation of the human stomach was used. In order to establish the effect of a food matrix on polyphenols bioaccessibility, NS and BS were either digested in water (WT) or incorporated into home-made biscuits (HB), crisp-bread (CB) and full-fat milk (FM). Phenolic acids were the most bioaccessible class (68.5% release from NS and 64.7% from BS). WT increased the release of flavan-3-ols ($p < 0.05$) and flavonols ($p < 0.05$) from NS after gastric plus duodenal digestion, whereas CB and HB were better vehicles for BS. FM lowered the % recovery of polyphenols, the free total phenols and the antioxidant status in the digestion medium, indicating that phenolic compounds could bind protein present in the food matrix. The release of bioactives from almond skins could explain the beneficial effects associated with almond consumption.

**Keywords:** almond skin; food matrix; simulated human digestion; polyphenols; bioaccessibility

## 1. Introduction

The presence of polyphenols in almond skin has been related to several health benefits associated with almond (Prunus dulcis Miller D.A. Webb) consumption [1–3]. The antioxidant and free-radical scavenging activity of almond skin polyphenols has been reported [4]. It has been shown that flavonoids and phenolic acids, including flavonols, flavanols, flavanones and simple phenolic acids identified in almond skins may play a role in reducing risk factors against chronic inflammatory diseases and ageing disorders [5,6]. A range of biological effects of flavonoids, including anticancer, antiviral, antimutagenic and anti-inflammatory activities, have been reported [7,8]. Nevertheless, one of the major limiting factors affecting the beneficial effects of polyphenols is their bioaccessibility and subsequent absorption in the gastrointestinal tract (GIT), together with their bio-transformation by the gut microbiota enzymes [9].

This process depends on the physico-chemical properties of the food matrix and its changes during digestion. We refer to bioaccessibility as the proportion of a nutrient or phytochemical compound 'released' from a complex food matrix during digestion and therefore becoming potentially available for absorption in the GIT. A number of studies have reported that food matrix affects polyphenol release in the gut as well as the efficacy by which they are transported across the mucosal epithelium [10,11]. The presence of a food matrix (muffin) decreased the bioaccessibility of certain bioactive compounds, such as protocatechuic acid and luteolin, from raw shelled and roasted salted pistachios during simulated human digestion [12]. Interaction with other food nutrients and the formation of complexes mainly with protein and fat is also known to affect bioaccessibility of phenolic acids [13]. The influence of digestion conditions, such as pH, temperature, bile salts, gastric and pancreatic enzymes on the bioaccessibility of certain polyphenols has been reported [14,15]. Milk has been found to affect bioaccessibility of epicatechin metabolites [16]. We have previously identified a combination of flavonols, flavan-3-ols, hydroxybenzoic acids and flavanones present in almond skin [1]: the major flavonoids were (+)-catechin, (−)-epicatechin, kaempferol and isorhamnetin, both as aglycones or conjugated with rhamnose (Rha) and glucose (Glc). The total phenolic content, expressed as mg gallic acid equivalents (GAE) per 100 g of fresh skin, was higher in natural almond skin (NS, 3474.1 ± 239.8) than blanched almond skin (BS, 278.9 ± 12.0). The blanching process is known to remove most of the water-soluble flavonoids and other polyphenols [1]. BS, obtained by industrial blanching, currently represents a commercially available product. Our previous investigation on the release of almond skin polyphenols during simulated human digestion using a static model demonstrated higher percentages of polyphenols released from NS compared to BS [17].

The aim of the present study was to assess the effect of a range of food matrices on the rate and extent of polyphenol bioaccessibility from NS and BS during simulated human digestion. A dynamic gastric model (DGM) was used to simulate the human stomach [12,18]. Gastric digesta were then subjected to a duodenal phase in order to simulate the full human upper GIT.

## 2. Materials and Methods

### 2.1. Production of Test Meals

Natural almonds with intact skin were kindly provided by the Almond Board of California and stored in the dark. NS was removed using liquid-nitrogen as previously reported and milled [17]. BS, provided by ABCO laboratories, was obtained by hot water blanching, dried and powdered. Home-made biscuits (HB) containing NS or BS were prepared using the following ingredients: white flour (200 g), butter at room temperature (100 g), sugar (sucrose, 100 g), eggs (one standard egg) and baked at 180 °C for 12 min. For the digestion experiments, 25 g of HB containing 2 g of either NS or BS were used. Home-made crisp-bread (CB) containing NS or BS was prepared using the following ingredients: baking soda (5 g), hot water (400 mL), salt (1.2 g), fennel seed (1 g), white flour (250 g) and baked at 230 °C for 2–4 min. For the digestion experiments, 34 g of CB containing 2 g of either NS or BS were used.

### 2.2. Chemicals and Enzymes

Egg L-α-phosphatidylcholine (PC, lecithin grade 1, 99% purity) was obtained from Lipid Products (South Nutfield, Surrey, UK). Porcine gastric mucosa pepsin, bovine α-chymotrypsin, pancreatic α-amylase, porcine colipase, porcine pancreatic lipase and bile salts were obtained from Sigma (Poole, Dorset, UK). Lipase for the gastric phase of digestion was a gastric lipase analogue of fungal origin (F-AP15) from Amano Enzyme Inc. (Nagoya, Japan). All flavonoid and other phytochemical standards were obtained from either Sigma-Aldrich (Poole, UK) or Extrasynthese (Genay, France). All solvents were HPLC grade, water was ultra-pure grade, and other chemicals were of AR quality.

### 2.3. Simulated Human Digestion

Eight meals were prepared as follows and subjected to in vitro gastric and gastric plus duodenal digestion: WT (200 mL) containing either NS (2 g) or BS (2 g), HB (25 g) containing either NS (2 g) or BS (2 g) added to water (240 mL), CB (34 g) containing either NS (2 g) or BS (2 g) added to water (240 mL), FM (200 mL) containing either NS (2 g) or BS (2 g).

## 2.4. Gastric Digestion

Individual meals were fed onto the DGM in the presence of priming acid (20 mL), as previously reported [18]. In order to replicate the conditions found in the human stomach, samples were processed in two zones: within the fundus/main body of the DGM, where the meals were subjected to inhomogeneous mixing while gastric acid and enzyme secretions were added; in the antrum, where physiological shear and grinding forces were applied in order to mimic the antral shearing and rate of delivery to the duodenum. The composition of the simulated gastric acid solution has also been previously reported [12]. The simulated gastric enzyme solution was prepared by dissolving porcine gastric mucosa pepsin and a gastric lipase analogue from *Rhizopus oryzae* in the above described salt mixture (no acid) at a final concentration of 9000 U/mL and 60 U/mL for pepsin and lipase, respectively. A suspension of single-shelled lecithin liposomes was added to the gastric enzyme solution at a final concentration of 0.127 mM.

A total of six samples (G1–G6) were ejected from the antrum of the DGM at regular intervals during each run (see Table 1 for sampling details) in order to replicate the predicted gastric emptying regimes under physiological conditions. Samples digested in WT were ejected from the antrum of the DGM every 4 min: the amount of gastric acid secretion was $1.5 \pm 0.1$ mL and $1.6 \pm 0.1$ mL for NS and BS respectively; the amount of gastric enzyme secretion was $2.8 \pm 0.1$ mL and $2.7 \pm 0.1$ mL for NS and BS respectively. Samples digested in HB were ejected from the antrum of the DGM every 4 min: the amount of gastric acid secretion was $6.4 \pm 0.1$ mL and $6.3 \pm 0.1$ mL for NS and BS respectively; the amount of gastric enzyme secretion was $11.2 \pm 0.2$ mL and $11.4 \pm 0.1$ mL for NS and BS respectively. Samples digested in CB were ejected from the antrum of the DGM every 5 min: the amount of gastric acid secretion was $17.6 \pm 0.2$ mL and $18.2 \pm 0.2$ mL for NS and BS respectively; the amount of gastric enzyme secretion was $13.8 \pm 0.1$ mL and $14.2 \pm 0.2$ mL for NS and BS respectively. Samples digested in FM were ejected from the antrum of the DGM every 6 min: the amount of gastric acid secretion was $4.4 \pm 0.2$ mL and $4.6 \pm 0.2$ mL for NS and BS respectively; the amount of gastric enzyme secretion was $13.1 \pm 0.3$ mL and $13.8 \pm 0.2$ mL for NS and BS respectively. A control digestion without addition of gastric enzymes was performed for each meal. Each gastric sample was weighed, its pH recorded and adjusted to 7.0 with NaOH (1 M) in order to inhibit gastric enzyme activity.

**Table 1.** Simulated human digestion parameters.

| Matrix | DGM 1 | DGM 2 | DGM 3 | DGM 4 | DGM 5 | DGM 6 | DD | TDT |
|---|---|---|---|---|---|---|---|---|
| | Sampling Time (min) | | | | | | | |
| Water | 4 | 8 | 12 | 16 | 20 | 24 | 120 | 144 |
| Home-made biscuit | 4 | 8 | 12 | 16 | 20 | 24 | 120 | 144 |
| Crisp bread | 5 | 10 | 15 | 20 | 25 | 30 | 120 | 150 |
| Full-fat milk | 6 | 12 | 18 | 24 | 30 | 36 | 120 | 156 |

DGM = Gastric sample; DD = Duodenal digestion; TDT = Total digestion time.

## 2.5. Duodenal Digestion

Individual gastric samples (23 g, G1 to G6) were transferred upon ejection, to a Sterilin plastic tube for duodenal digestion with the addition of simulated bile solution (2.5 mL) and pancreatic enzyme solution (7.0 mL) and incubated at 37 °C under shaking conditions (170 rpm) for 2 h. Simulated bile was prepared fresh daily. It contained lecithin (6.5 mM), cholesterol (4 mM), sodium taurocholate (12.5 mM), and sodium glycodeoxycholate (12.5 mM) in a solution containing NaCl (146.0 mM), CaCl2 (2.6 mM) and KCl (4.8 mM).

Pancreatic enzyme solution contained NaCl (125.0 mM), $CaCl_2$ (0.6 mM), $MgCl_2$ (0.3 mM), and $ZnSO_4 \cdot 7H_2O$ (4.1 µM). Porcine pancreatic lipase (590 U/mL), porcine colipase (3.2 µg/mL), porcine trypsin (11 U/mL), bovine α-chymotrypsin (24 U/mL) and porcine α-amylase (300 U/mL) were added to the pancreatic solution.

### 2.6. Poliphenols Extraction from Samples before and after Dynamic in Vitro Digestion

All original samples (WT, HB, CB and FM containing NS or BS) and aliquotes obtained from each sample subjected to a dynamic in vitro gastric digestion (NSWT G, NSHB G, NSCB G, NSFM G, BSWT G, BSHB G, BSCB G, BSFM G) and gastric plus duodenal digestion (NSWT G + D, NSHB G + D, NSCB G + D, NSFM G + D, BSWT G + D, BSHB G + D, BSCB G + D, BSFM G + D), were harvested and centrifuged to separate the residual material from the supernatant. The volume of each supernatant was measured; the residues were dried in a forced air heated oven (T °C < 40 °C) and brought to constant weight.

Each residue was extracted with hexane (1:5, w/v) to remove the lipid fraction. The procedure was repeated 3 times. Afterwards it was extracted with a methanol/water mixture (70:30) (1:10, w/v) by shaking for 5 min and sonicating for 10 min. After centrifugation at 12,074 rcf for 10 min, the supernatant was collected. The procedure was repeated 3 times. The supernatants were pooled. In order to precipitate proteins, MeOH (8 mL) and 2M NaOH (600 µL) were added in 10 mL extract. Samples were stirred vigorously and after centrifugation at 5916 rcf for 5 min the supernatant was brought to dryness in a rotavapor. Finally, the residue was correspouded with 10 mL of 1% HCl in MeOH and extracted, using a separatory funnel, with the same volume of ethyl acetate. The extraction was repeated 4 times. The ethyl acetate fractions were combined and evaporated to dryness in a rotavapor. The residue was weighed, solubilised in MeOH, filtered through a Nalgene 0.22 µM nylon filter and subjected to total phenol, radical scavenging activity and HPLC analysis.

For NS and BS digested in water no protein precipitation step was performed, given that they were not incorporated into any food matrix.

### 2.7. Polyphenols Release and Radical Scavenging Activity

Total phenol content was determined colorimetrically by the Folin-Ciocalteu method as modified by Singleton, Orthofer and Lamuela-Raventos [19] using gallic acid as a reference compound. Total phenol content was expressed as mg of gallic acid equivalents (GAE) per 100 g of sample. The anti-radical activity was determined using the stable 2,2-diphenyl-1-picrylhydrazyl radical (DPPH) and the procedure previously described [20]. Results were expressed as mg of extract needed to scavenge 50 µmol of the initial DPPH concentration (SE50). The determination of phenolics and flavonoids was carried out using a Shimadzu high performance liquid chromatography system equipped with an UV–Vis photodiode-array detector (DAD) (SPD-M10AVP, Shimadzu, Kyoto, Japan) and a fluorescence detector (1046A Hewlett Packard, Palo Alto, CA, USA), as previously reported [17].

### 2.8. Statistical Analysis

All assays were performed in triplicate and expressed as means ± standard deviation (SD). Data analysis was performed using ANOVA tests using SigmaPlot software version 12.0 for Windows (SPSS Inc., Hong Kong, China). To isolate the group or groups that differ from the others, a multiple comparison procedure (*Tukey* Test) was used. Results were considered statistically significant at $p < 0.05$.

## 3. Results

### 3.1. Polyphenols Release during Simulated Digestion

The polyphenolic content of the baseline meals (NS WT, NS HB, NS CB and NS FM, BS WT, BS HB, BS CB and BS FM) is reported in Table 2. As expected, the NS meals had a total phenol content nearly ten times higher than the BS meals.

The release of polyphenols as a percentage of the original amount present in each meal (Table 2) after simulated gastric plus duodenal digestion is reported in Figure 1. No polyphenols were detected in blank samples of each meal not containing almond skin. As expected, a high release of bioactive compounds was observed from both NS and BS in WT (Figure 1A).

**Table 2.** Baseline polyphenols content of natural skins and blanched skins in water (W); home-made biscuits (HB); crisp-bread (CB) and full-fat milk (FM). Values were given as μg/g and represent averages (±SD) of triplicate measurements.

| Natural Skin | | | | | |
|---|---|---|---|---|---|
| Sample | Phenolic acids | Flavonols | Flavan-3-ols | Flavanones | Total phenols |
| W | 2.15 ± 0.11 | 14.31 ± 1.05 | 2.37 ± 0.18 | 3.43 ± 0.22 | 22.26 |
| HB | 17.85 ± 1.02 | 115.30 ± 8.32 | 20.82 ± 1.65 | 30.44 ± 2.21 | 184.41 |
| CB | 12.53 ± 0.89 | 83.89 ± 4.22 | 14.72 ± 1.12 | 21.78 ± 1.44 | 132.92 |
| FM | 2.07 ± 0.12 | 13.95 ± 1.22 | 2.15 ± 0.12 | 3.22 ± 0.17 | 21.39 |
| Blanched Skin | | | | | |
| Sample | Phenolic acids | Flavonols | Flavan-3-ols | Flavanones | Total phenols |
| W | 0.31 ± 0.02 | 1.28 ± 0.05 | 0.62 ± 0.03 | 0.22 ± 0.02 | 2.43 |
| HB | 2.25 ± 0.14 | 9.82 ± 0.59 | 5.18 ± 0.21 | 1.73 ± 0.102 | 18.98 |
| CB | 1.78 ± 0.12 | 7.24 ± 0.35 | 3.65 ± 0.25 | 1.31 ± 0.09 | 13.98 |
| FM | 0.29 ± 0.01 | 1.19 ± 0.08 | 0.60 ± 0.02 | 0.19 ± 0.01 | 2. 27 |

The % release from NS and BS in WT during the gastric phase of digestion was higher for phenolic acids (47.1% from NS and 45.3% from BS) compared with the other classes of polyphenols, with a further increase in the duodenal phase of digestion (68.5% from NS and 64.7% from BS). Lower % release from BS in WT was observed with flavanones after both gastric (29.3%) and gastric plus duodenal incubation (48.2%). Higher release of flavonols (65.6%) and phenolic acids (59.4%) was observed after in vitro gastric plus duodenal digestion from NS (Figure 1A). The % of recovery, calculated from the amount of polyphenols present in the medium at the end of each step of digestion, confirmed the data obtained from the % of release (Figure 2). This data demonstrated a different bioaccessibility across the various classes of polyphenols in the absence of an interfering food matrix. In accordance with our previous investigation [1], high release of polyphenols was detected when NS and BS were incubated in WT. However, the static and dynamic digestion models used affected the rate and extent of bioactives potentially available for absorption in the gut.

The % of release and recovery of polyphenols from NS and BS incorporated into HB are reported in Figures 1B and 2, respectively. Phenolic acids were the class of polyphenols mostly released from NS in the gastric phase, followed by flavonols and flavanones, with an average % release of 40.72 in the gastric compartment. Flavonols had the highest % release from BS in the gastric phase (48.5), followed by flavanones and phenolic acids. For both NS and BS, the gastric + duodenal digestion (G + D) produced only a slight increase in polyphenol release over that observed in the gastric compartment. In addition, higher percentages of phenolic acids and flavonols were released from NSHB G + D.

Higher % of release of phenolic acids, flavonols, flavan-3-ols and flavanones were observed in BSCB G compared with NSCB G, whereas the opposite behaviour was detected in the duodenal phase (Figure 1C). A higher release of phenolic acids was observed in BSCB G (52.7%) compared with BSWT G (45.3%), as well as flavonols both in the gastric (51.4 in BSCB G vs. 33.9 in BSWT G) and in the duodenal phase (63.9 in BSCB G + D vs. 52.3 in BSWT G + D) and flavanones both in the gastric (47.6 in BSCB G vs. 29.3 in BSWT G) and in the duodenal phase (59.8 in BSCB G + D vs. 48.2 in BSWT G + D). The % release data were confirmed by % recovery values (Figure 2).

The % of release and recovery of flavonoids and phenolic acids from NS and BS incorporated into FM are reported in Figures 1D and 2, respectively. The highest % release from NS was detected with flavonols after gastric plus duodenal digestion, followed by flavanones and phenolic acids. About 60% of phenolic acids and flavanones were released from BS in FM after simulated digestion.

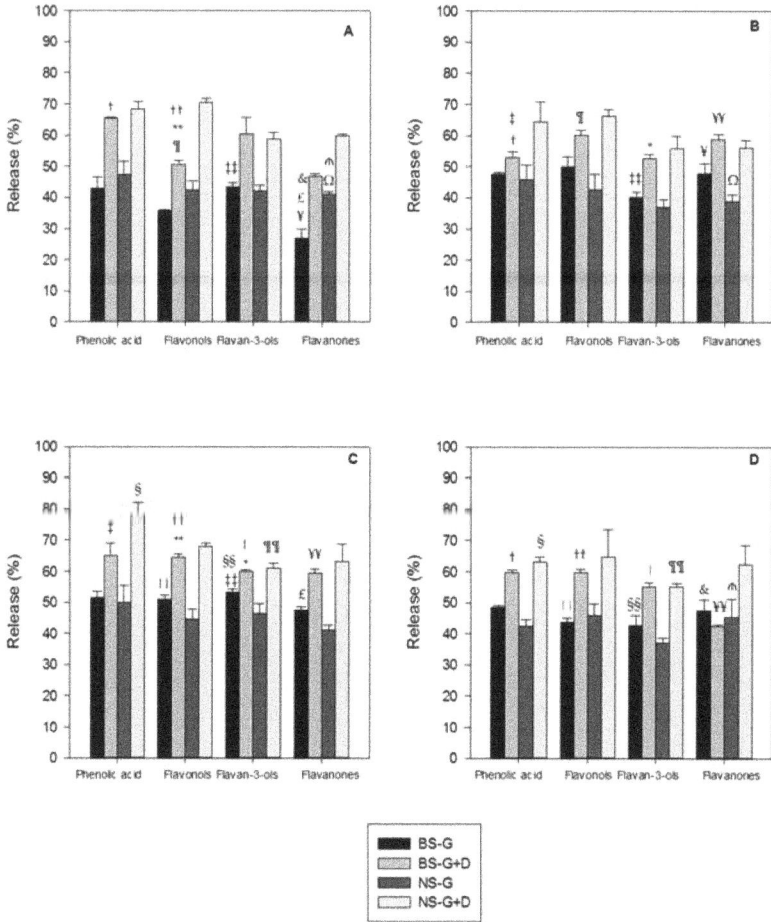

**Figure 1.** Release of flavonoids and phenolic acids from natural almond skin (NS) and blanched almond skin (BS) in water (**A**); home-made biscuits (**B**); crisp-bread (**C**) and full-fat milk (**D**). Values are given as % phenolic acids, flavanols, flavan-3-ols and flavanones released from the initial amounts presents in the meals (Table 2) during in vitro gastric (G) and gastric + duodenal (G + D) digestion. Values represent averages (±SD) of triplicate measurements. Matching symbols across the four panels indicate significantly different (*p* < 0.01) samples. [†] Phenolic acid release in BS-G + D significantly different between A, B and D; [††] Flavonols release in BS-G + D significantly different between A, C and D; [**] Flavonols release in BS-G + D significantly different between A and C; [¶] Flavonols release in BS-G + D significantly different between A and B; [‡‡] Flavan-3-ols release in BS-G significantly different between A, B and C; [&] Flavanones release in BS-G significantly different between A and D; [¥] Flavanones release in BS-G significantly different between A and B; [Ѫ] Flavanones release in NS-G significantly different between A and D; [Ω] Flavanones release in NS-G significantly different between A and B; [‡] Phenolic acid release in BS-G + D significantly different between B and C; [*] Flavan-3-ols release in BS-G + D significantly different between B and C; [¥¥] Flavanones release in BS-G + D significantly different between B, C and D; [§] Phenolic acid release in NS-G + D significantly different between C and D; [ǀǀ] Flavonols release in BS-G significantly different between C and D. [§§] Flavan-3-ols release in BS-G significantly different between C and D; [ǀ] Flavan-3-ols release in BS-G + D significantly different between C and D; [¶¶] Flavan-3-ols release in NS-G+D significantly different between C and D.

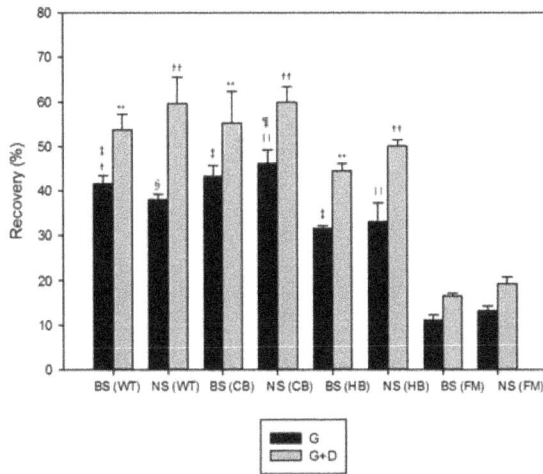

**Figure 2.** Recovery of total phenolic compounds in the digestion medium from natural almond skin (NS) and blanched almond skin (BS) in water (WT), home-made biscuits (HB), crisp-bread (CB) and full-fat milk (FM). Values are given as % of total phenolic compounds calculated from the amount of polyphenols present in the medium at the end of each step of digestion. Values represent averages (±SD) of triplicate measurements. [†] $p < 0.01$ vs. BS (CB); [‡] $p < 0.01$ vs. BS (FM); [§] $p < 0.01$ vs. NS (CB); [||] $p < 0.01$ vs. NS (FM); [¶] $p < 0.01$ vs. NS (HB); [**] $p < 0.01$ vs. BS (FM); [††] $p < 0.01$ vs. NS (FM).

Statistical analysis of Figure 1 showed significant differences in the % of bioactives released from the tested meals: higher release ($p < 0.05$) of phenolic acid was detected from NS in CB vs. FM after G + D, flavan-3-ols from NS in WT vs. FM after G + D and flavonols from NS in WT vs. HB after G + D; higher release ($p < 0.01$) of flavan-3-ols was also observed from NS in CB vs. FM after G + D; higher release ($p < 0.05$) of flavan-3-ols was found from NS in CB vs. FM after G; higher release ($p < 0.01$) of flavanones from BS in HB vs. WT after G and vs. FM after G + D and flavan-3-ols from BS in CB vs. HB after G + D; higher release ($p < 0.01$) of flavanones from BS in FM, CB and HB vs. WT after G + D and of flavonols in CB vs. FM after G; higher release ($p < 0.05$) of phenolic acids from BS in CB vs. WT after G. This data confirmed the presence of a food matrix affected the release of bioactives from almond skin during simulated digestion. Overall WT and CB were good vehicles for the release of polyphenols from NS, whereas HB and CB were optimal for polyphenols bioaccessibility from BS. This could be due to the previous loss of water soluble polyphenols from BS during the industrial blanching process.

Statistical analysis of Figure 2 showed significant differences in the % recovery of polyphenols from the tested meals: higher recovery was observed from both NS and BS in CB vs. HB ($p < 0.05$) and vs. FM ($p < 0.01$) after G + D; higher recovery was also detected from NS in CB vs. WT ($p < 0.01$), FM ($p < 0.01$) and HB ($p < 0.01$) after G, as well as NS in WT vs. HB ($p < 0.05$); lower recovery ($p < 0.01$) was observed with BS in WT vs. CB and FM vs. HB after G. The recovery data also confirmed WT was a good vehicle for bioactives bioaccessibility from NS, whereas CB was optimal for BS.

Significantly ($p < 0.01$) lower % recoveries were obtained with FM from both NS and BS after gastric plus duodenal digestion. We believe the % recovery demonstrated that milk protein were able to bind the free polyphenols present in the digestion medium and the interaction between phenolic compounds and proteins was more pronounced in milk rather than biscuits [21]. Furthermore, complexes made by protein and tannin are less well digested and the amino acid profile may be damaged.

The same trend was also detected when comparing the kinetics (%) of release for flavan-3-ols from NS in WT and FM during the full digestion process (Figure 3). When NS was digested in WT, a steady release of flavan-3-ols over time was observed, corresponding to a significant increase detected for the initial 5 gastric digestion samples. In the presence of FM, the dynamics of release were very similar to WT but at a significantly slower rate.

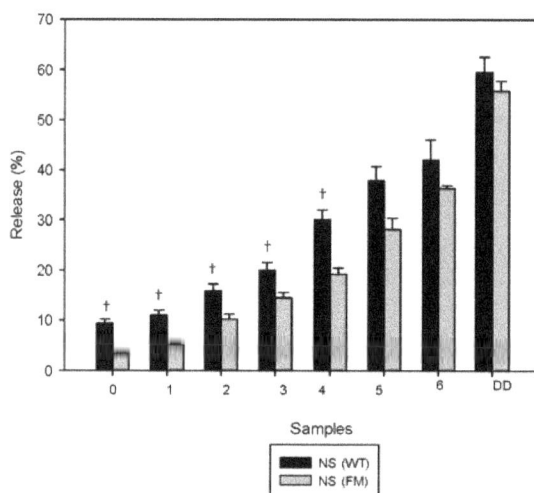

**Figure 3.** Kinetic of release of flavan-3-ols from natural almond skin (NS) in water and full-fat milk. Values are given as % of flavan-3-ols released from the initial amounts of flavan-3-ols in the meals (Table 2) during in vitro gastric (samples 0 to 6, see Table 1 for sampling time) and gastric + duodenal (DD) digestion. Values represent averages (±SD) of triplicate measurements. SD were always <10%. Water (WT), full-fat milk (FM). [†] $p < 0.01$ vs. NS (FM).

### 3.2. Antioxidant Profile during Digestion

The total phenolic content, measured by the Folin-Ciocalteu method, from all the tested meals during digestion is reported in Figure 4A,B. A decrease in the total phenols was observed post in vitro gastric and gastric plus duodenal digestion for both NS and BS in WT, HB, CB and FM. In agreement with the polyphenols release data, significant differences were observed across the four food matrices. A corresponding increase in free total phenols in the digestion medium, expressed as mg GAE/200 mL medium, was observed for WT, HB and CB (Figure 5). However, much lower than expected values of free total phenols were detected in FM, in agreement with the polyphenols recovery data. This data demonstrated that phenolic compounds could bind protein present in the food matrix, thus hindering the antioxidant potential in vitro [21].

In agreement with the total phenolic content, the radical scavenging activity, measured by DPPH, was lower after digestion (Figure 6). As shown in panel A, no statistically significant difference was observed in NS across all matrices; however in panel B, a statistically significant difference in WT vs. CB, HB and FM for sample 6 (last gastric sample) was observed. A corresponding increase of the antioxidant status was detected in the digestion medium, with the exception of FM; a statistically significant difference ($p < 0.01$) was observed in BS digestion media when comparing FM vs. WT, CB and HB and in NS when comparing FM vs. WT and CB (Figure 7).

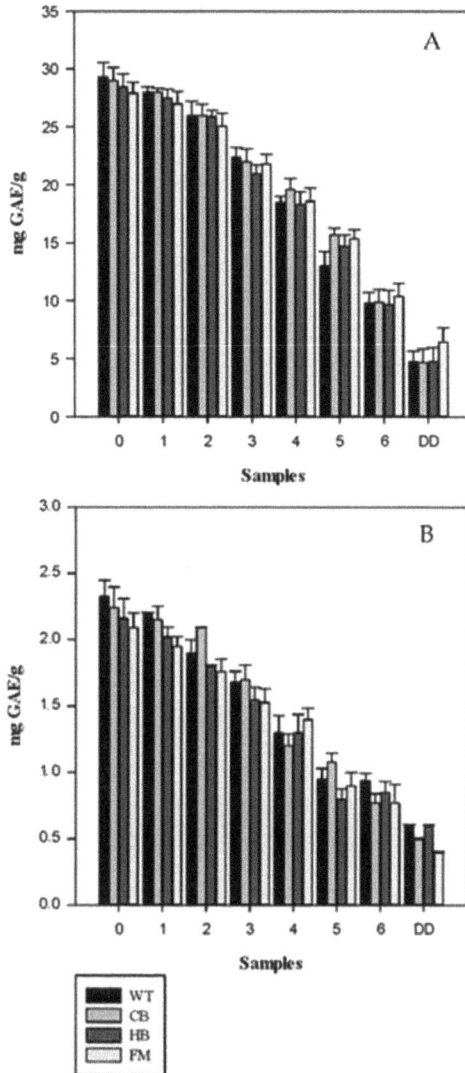

**Figure 4.** Total phenolic content in natural (NS, panel (**A**)) and blanched (BS, panel (**B**)) almond skin before and after simulated human digestion. Values are expresses in mg GAE/g and they represent mean ± SD of three different experiments. 0 to 6: gastric samples (see Table 1 for sampling time). DD: sample post in vitro gastric + duodenal digestion. Water (WT), home-made biscuits (HB), crisp-bread (CB) and full-fat milk (FM).

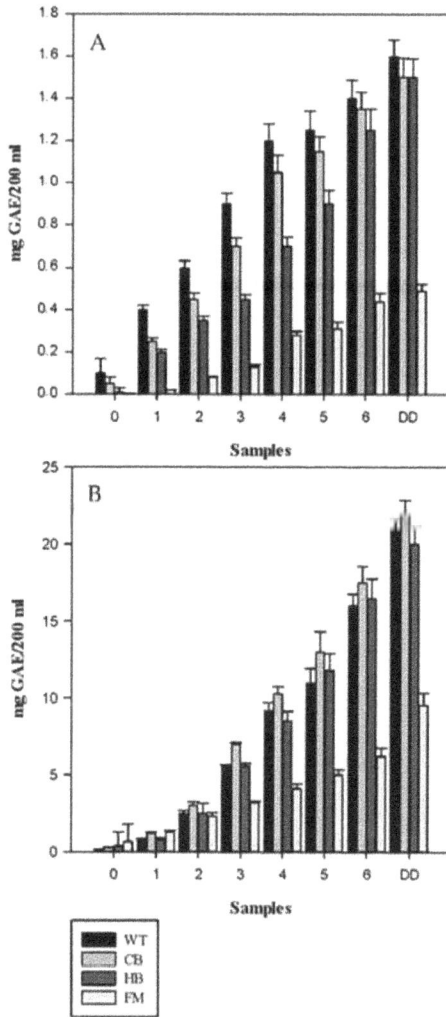

**Figure 5.** Free total phenols measured in the digestion medium of natural almond skin (**A**) and blanched almond skin (**B**) after in vitro gastric and gastric + duodenal digestion. Values are expressed as mg GAE/200 mL medium. 0 to 6: gastric samples (see Table 1 for sampling time). DD: sample post in vitro gastric + duodenal digestion. Water (WT), home-made biscuits (HB), crisp-bread (CB) and full-fat milk (FM).

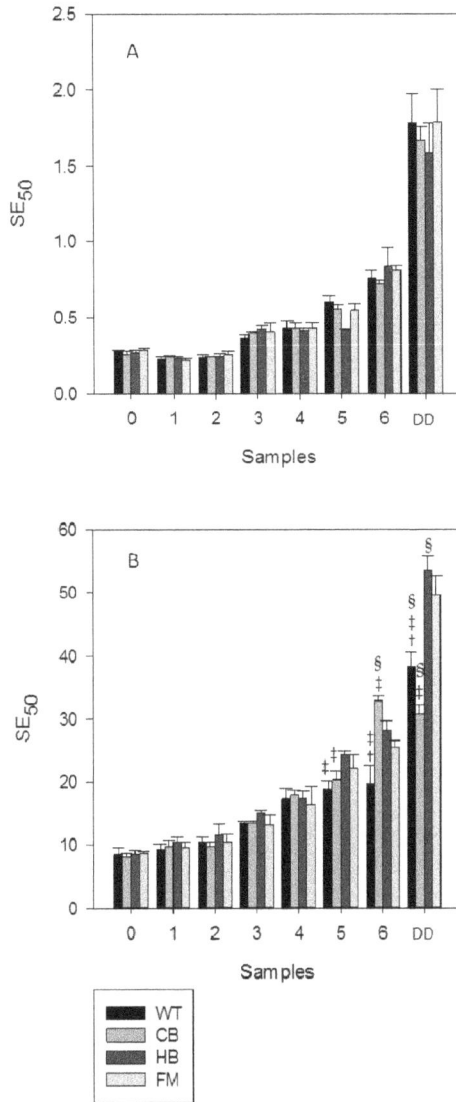

**Figure 6.** Radical scavenging activity measured in natural (NS, panel (**A**)) and blanched (BS, panel (**B**)) almond skin before and after simulated human digestion. Values are expresses as mg of sample containing the amount needed to scavenge 50 µmol of the initial DPPH solution (SE50) and they represent mean ± SD of three different experiments. 0 to 6: gastric samples (see Table 1 for sampling time). DD: sample post in vitro gastric + duodenal digestion. Water (WT), home-made biscuits (HB), crisp-bread (CB) and full-fat milk (FM). [†] $p < 0.01$ vs. CB at the same sampling time; [‡] $p < 0.01$ vs. HB at the same sampling time; [§] $p < 0.01$ vs. FM at the same sampling time.

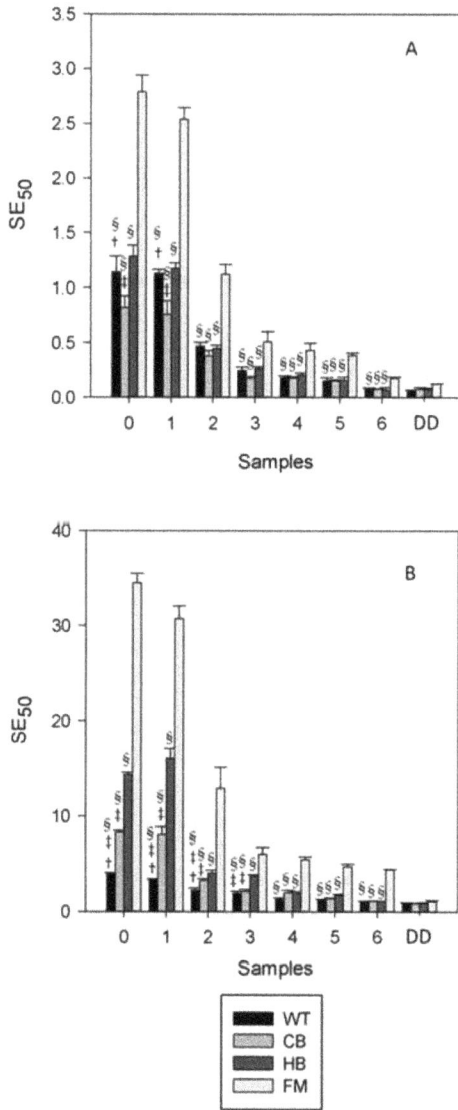

**Figure 7.** Radical scavenging activity measured in the natural almond skin digestion medium (panel (**A**)) and the blanched almond skin (BS) digestion medium (panel (**B**)) after in vitro gastric and gastric + duodenal digestion. Values are expressed as mg of extract needed to scavenge 50 μmol of the initial DPPH• concentration (SE50). 0 to 6: gastric samples (see Table 1 for sampling time). DD: sample post in vitro gastric + duodenal digestion. Water (WT), home-made biscuits (HB), crisp-bread (CB) and full-fat milk (FM). [†] $p < 0.01$ vs. CB at the same sampling time; [‡] $p < 0.01$ vs. HB at the same sampling time; [§] $p < 0.01$ vs. FM at the same sampling time.

## 4. Discussion

The data presented here has demonstrated that bioaccessibility of polyphenols from almond skin was significantly affected by the type of food matrix used. Given the lack of understanding of the fate of antioxidant compounds in the human body, research focused on the bioaccessibility of polyphenols from solid matrices are extremely important in order to better understand the beneficial effect on the host.

We have previously shown that polyphenols from almond skin were bioaccessible in the upper GIT during simulated human digestion in a static system and most of the release occurred in the gastric phase of digestion [1]. However, in the present study, a considerable further loss of polyphenols was observed during the duodenal phase over that detected in the gastric environment across all the food matrices used (Figure 1). The amount of individual polyphenols released from NS and BS are quite different, although a similar rate was detected across the two skin samples. The use of a dynamic model of digestion (DGM), where the digestion products are removed during the time course of the experiment, has likely affected the rate and release of almond skin polyphenols. A similar trend was observed with lipid bioaccessibility from natural raw and roasted almonds after mastication [22]. A study on polyphenols bioaccessibility from apples indicated the release was mainly achieved during the gastric phase (65% of phenolics and flavonoids), with a slight increase (<10%) during intestinal digestion [23].

In vitro digestion of the cocoa insoluble water fraction, source of polyphenols, lead to a 51% release of the total phenols from the insoluble material, without a reduction of the total antioxidant capacity [24].

In our previous study investigating bioaccessibility of bioactives from pistachios, more of 90% of polyphenols were released in the gastric compartment, with little or no increase in the duodenal phase [12]. The lower % of bioaccessibility in almonds (Figure 1) could be due to the properties of their cell walls, which is known to affect lipid and protein bioaccessibility in the gut [22,25]. Almond skins contain high amount of dietary fiber and several cell wall bound phenolics, including *p*-hydroxybenzoic acid, vanillic acid and *t*-ferulic acid [17]. We have previously shown that complex carbohydrates present in dietary fiber can directly interact with antioxidants and therefore interfere with their bioaccessibility in the gut [26,27]. Furthermore, the polyphenols structure plays a crucial role in relation to their adsorption, which was improved by low degree of hydroxylation and reduced by methylation or methoxylation. An increased degree of polymerization determined enhanced absorption for certain polyphenolic classes, including procyanidins [28]. However, the role of glycosylation still remains controversial [13,28]. Dietary fiber can reduce fat bioaccessibility in the GIT and pectin was found to strongly lower β-carotene bioavailability [29].

The high dietary fiber content in almond skin, as well as the significant amounts of lipids, could have affected the release of phytochemicals, especially in the absence of a food matrix. Dietary fiber could also reduce the rate of antioxidant absorption by physically trapping the bioactive compounds within its matrix in the chyme, thus restricting enzyme diffusion [30]. Therefore, it is hypothesised that certain polyphenols, mainly phenolic acids which are bound to dietary fiber, are not released in the upper GIT but reach the large bowel where they can be metabolised by the gut microbiota. This could also be due to a dietary fiber specific effect on gastrointestinal physiology (e.g., motility and/or secretion) [28]. The polyphenols-carbohydrates interaction could exert positive effects on lipid metabolism and increase the antioxidant activity in the large intestine [13,28].

A number of studies have reported on the effects of a food matrix in a simulated gastrointestinal environment: the findings demonstrated that green tea polyphenols were protected more by the interaction with dairy products, which could help maintain their antioxidant activity during digestion [31] and cheese was identified as an effective matrix for polyphenols protection during gastrointestinal digestion [32]. Stanisavljevic et al. [11] have investigated the changes in polyphenols content and antioxidant activity of chokeberry juice subjected to in vitro gastric digestion in the presence of a food matrix: the results demonstrated a decrease in the total phenolic content, anthocyanin content and DPPH radical scavenging activity immediately after addition of the food matrix. However, the fat content in cocoa samples increased the released of phenolic compounds during duodenal digestion [33]. Lesser et al. [34] have shown that high fat content in meals could either enhance or reduce the absorption of certain flavonoids; polyphenols could also affect the fat adsorption process at the emulsification stage by a direct interaction with phosphatidylcholine or by incorporation within the lipid layer, thus leading to physicochemical property changes of emulsions directly related to lipase activity and fat adsorption decrease, as suggested for tea polyphenols [28]. Moreover, several studies suggested that polyphenols were able to create a positive antioxidant environment at the gastrointestinal level fighting the harmful products of lipid peroxidation [28]. All these interactions could contribute to the well-known beneficial effects of polyphenols.

Another important aspect to discuss is the polyphenols ability to bind proteins, thus affecting the amino acids availability and leading in some cases to protein denaturation (e.g., $\alpha$-amylase, trypsin, lysozyme) or to their lower digestibility (e.g., $\beta$-lactoglobulin) [28,35]. This often affects enzyme activity in a positive way ($\alpha$-amylase inhibition which could be connected to the prevention of dental injuries) or negative way (when digestive enzymes are involved). It is known, in fact, that protein-polyphenol interactions might influence their adsorption, even though proteins could be carriers of polyphenols through the gastrointestinal tract, thus protecting them from oxidative reactions and increasing their availability at the large intestine [28,35].

In the present study, the fat and protein content in the milk matrix have significantly lowered the release of phenolic acids and flavan-3-ols after simulated human digestion from both NS and DO compared with water, whereas the home made biscuits decreased bioaccessibility of flavonols (Figure 3). In a recent study [36] the addition of milk decreased the total phenolic, flavonoid and anthocyanin content, although it had no effect on the polyphenols being absorbed in vitro.

It has also been suggested, with respect to what is mentioned above, that the presence of digestible carbohydrates, lipids and other antioxidant compounds may have a beneficial impact on polyphenols bioaccessibility [37]. This could explain the high bioaccessibility detected when almond skins were incorporated in bread.

Even if the bioaccessibility of each antioxidant differs greatly, the potential synergistic effect amongst polyphenols could affect their bioactivity and influence on glycoprotein transporters across the mucosal epithelium. It is well established that a variety of factors, including chemical structure, food matrix, digestion enzymes and interaction with the gut microbiota can directly influence polyphenols bioaccessibility and rate of absorption [38]. A number of studies have indicated some unique technological strategies, including micro-encapsulation, which increase polyphenols bioavailability and therefore increase their beneficial health benefits [39–41].

## 5. Conclusions

In summary, the results of the present study indicate that the presence of a food matrix had a significant effect on polyphenol bioaccessibility from almond skin in both the gastric and duodenal environments. The dietary fiber present in almond skin may act as barrier to prevent a total release of phytochemicals during digestion. Further studies are warranted in order to investigate absorption of bioactives, which could explain the beneficial health effects associated with almond consumption.

**Acknowledgments:** We wish to dedicate the present study to our friend and colleague Antonio Tomaino, whose memory will always remain alive in our hearts. This research was funded by the Almond Board of California and the University of Messina (Research & Mobility 2015 Project, project code: RES_AND_MOB_2015_DE_LUCA). We gratefully thank Karen Lapsley from the Almond Board of California for providing the almond samples.

**Author Contributions:** All authors contributed to the study design. D.T. is the Principal Investigator responsible for study design. G.M. designed the study and wrote the paper. M.V. and R.F. were responsible and performed the experiments of simulated gastric and duodenal digestion. M.M. and A.S. performed instrumental assessment and were responsible for data collection and data analysis; C.B. contributed to interpretation data. All authors approved the final version.

**Conflicts of Interest:** The work was partially funded by the Almond Board of California.

*Nutrients* **2016**, *8*, 568

## Abbreviations

The following abbreviations are used in this manuscript:

| | |
|---|---|
| NS | natural almond skin |
| BS | blanched almond skin |
| CB | crisp bread water |
| WT | water |
| FM | full-fat milk |
| HB | home-made biscuits |
| NSWT G | natural almond skin in water post in vitro gastric digestion |
| NSHB G | natural almond skin in home-made biscuits post in vitro gastric digestion |
| NSCB G | natural almond skin in crisp-bread post in vitro gastric digestion |
| NSFM G | natural almond skin in full-fat milk post in vitro gastric digestion |
| NSWT G + D | natural almond skin in water post in vitro gastric plus duodenal digestion |
| NSHB G + D | natural almond skin in home-made biscuits post in vitro gastric plus duodenal digestion |
| NSCB G + D | natural almond skin in crisp-bread post in vitro gastric plus duodenal digestion |
| NSFM G + D | natural almond skin in full-fat milk post in vitro gastric plus duodenal digestion |
| BSWT G | blanched almond skin in water post in vitro gastric digestion |
| BSHB G | blanched almond skin in home-made biscuits post in vitro gastric digestion |
| BSCB G | blanched almond skin in crisp-bread post in vitro gastric digestion |
| BSFM G | blanched almond skin in full-fat milk post in vitro gastric digestion |
| BSWT G + D | blanched almond skin in water post in vitro gastric plus duodenal digestion |
| BSHB G + D | blanched almond skin in home-made biscuits post in vitro gastric plus duodenal digestion |
| BSCB G + D | blanched almond skin in crisp-bread post in vitro gastric plus duodenal digestion |
| BSFM G + D | blanched almond skin in full-fat milk post in vitro gastric plus duodenal digestion |

## References

1. Mandalari, G.; Tomaino, A.; Rich, G.T.; Lo Curto, R.B.; Arcoraci, T.; Martorana, M.; Martorana, M.; Bisignano, C.; Saija, A.; Parkerd, M.L.; et al. Polyphenol and nutrient release from skin of almonds during simulated human digestion. *Food Chem.* **2010**, *122*, 1083–1088. [CrossRef]

2. Mandalari, G.; Bisignano, C.; Genovese, T.; Mazzon, E.; Wickham, M.S.J.; Paterniti, I.; Cuzzocrea, S. Natural almond skin reduced oxidative stress and inflammation in an experimental model of inflammatory bowel disease. *Int. Immunopharm.* **2011**, *11*, 915–924. [CrossRef] [PubMed]

3. Mandalari, G.; Genovese, T.; Bisignano, C.; Mazzon, E.; Wickham, M.S.J.; di Paola, R.; Bisignano, G.; Cuzzocrea, S. Neuroprotective effects of almond skins in experimental spinal cord injury. *Clin. Nutr.* **2011**, *30*, 221–233. [CrossRef] [PubMed]

4. Chen, C.Y.O.; Blumberg, J.B. In vitro activity of almond skin polyphenols for scavenging free radicals and inducing quinine reductase. *J. Agric. Food Chem.* **2008**, *56*, 4427–4434. [CrossRef] [PubMed]

5. Milbury, P.E.; Chen, C.Y.; Dolnikowski, G.G.; Blumberg, J.B. Determination of flavonoids and phenolics and their distribution in almonds. *J. Agric. Food Chem.* **2006**, *54*, 5027–5033. [CrossRef] [PubMed]

6. Garrido, I.; Monagas, M.; Gómez-Cordovés, C.; Bartolomé, B. Polyphenols and antioxidant properties of almond skins: Influence of industrial processing. *J. Food Sci.* **2008**, *73*, C106–C115. [CrossRef] [PubMed]

7. Benavente-García, O.; Castillo, J. Update on uses and properties of citrus flavonoids: New findings in anticancer, cardiovascular, and anti-inflammatory activity. *J. Agric. Food Chem.* **2008**, *56*, 6185–6205. [CrossRef] [PubMed]

8. Vuorela, S.; Kreander, K.; Karonen, M.; Nieminen, R.; Hämäläinen, M.; Galkin, A.; Laitinen, L.; Salminen, J.P.; Moilanen, E.; Pihlaja, K.; et al. Preclinical evaluation of rapeseed, raspberry, and pine bark phenolics for health related effects. *J. Agric. Food Chem.* **2005**, *53*, 5922–5931. [CrossRef] [PubMed]

9. Stevens, J.F.; Maier, C.S. The chemistry of gut microbial metabolism of polyphenols. *Phytochem. Rev.* **2016**, *15*, 425–444. [CrossRef] [PubMed]

10. Tagliazucchi, D.; Verzelloni, E.; Bertolini, D.; Conte, A. In vitro bioaccessibility and antioxidant activity of grape polyphenols. *Food Chem.* **2010**, *120*, 599–606. [CrossRef]

11. Stanisavljevic, N.; Samardzic, J.; Jankovic, T.; Šavikin, K.; Mojsin, M.; Topalovic, V. Antioxidant and antiproliferative activity of chokeberry juice phenolics during in vitro simulated digestion in the presence of food matrix. *Food Chem.* **2015**, *175*, 516–522. [CrossRef] [PubMed]
12. Mandalari, G.; Bisignano, C.; Filocamo, A.; Chessa, S.; Saro, M.; Torre, G.; Faulks, R.M.; Dugo, P. Bioaccessibility of pistachio polyphenols, xanthophylls, and tocopherols during simulated human digestion. *Nutrition* **2013**, *29*, 338–344. [CrossRef] [PubMed]
13. D'Archivio, M.; Filesi, C.; Varì, R.; Scazzocchio, B.; Masella, R. Bioavailability of the polyphenols: Status and controversies. *J. Mol. Sci.* **2010**, *11*, 1321–1342. [CrossRef] [PubMed]
14. D'Antuono, I.; Garbetta, A.; Linsalata, V.; Minervini, F.; Cardinali, A. Polyphenols from artichoke heads (*Cynara cardunculus* L. subsp. scolymus Hayek): In vitro bio-accessibility, intestinal uptake and bioavailability. *Food Funct.* **2015**, *6*, 1268–1277. [CrossRef] [PubMed]
15. Perez-Vicente, A.; Gil-Izquierdo, A.; Garcia-Viguera, C. In vitro gastrointestinal digestion study of pomegranate juice phenolic compounds, anthocyanins, and vitamin C. *J. Agric. Food Chem.* **2002**, *50*, 2308–2312. [CrossRef] [PubMed]
16. Roura, E.; Andres-Lacueva, C.; Estruch, R.; Mata-Bilbao, M.L.; Izquierdo-Pulido, M.; Waterhouse, A.L.; Lamuela-Raventós, R.M. Milk does not affect the bioavailability of cocoa powder flavonoid in healthy human. *Ann. Nutr. Met.* **2007**, *51*, 493–498. [CrossRef] [PubMed]
17. Mandalari, G.; Tomaino, A.; Arcoraci, T.; Martorana, M.; Lo Turco, V.; Cacciola, F.; Richa, G.T.; Bisignano, C.; Saija, A.; Dugo, P.; et al. Characterization of polyphenols, lipids and dietary fibre from skins of almonds (*Amygdalus communis* L.). *J. Food Comp. Anal.* **2010**, *23*, 166–174. [CrossRef]
18. Pitino, I.; Randazzo, C.L.; Mandalari, G.; Lo Curto, A.; Faulks, R.M.; le Marc, Y.; Bisignano, C.; Caggia, C.; Wickham, M.S. Survival of *Lactobacillus rhamnosus* strains in the upper gastrointestinal tract. *Food Microbiol.* **2010**, *27*, 1121–1127. [CrossRef] [PubMed]
19. Singleton, V.L.; Orthofer, R.; Lamuela-Raventos, R.M. Analysis of total phenols and other oxidation substrates and antioxidants by means of Folin-Ciocalteu reagents. *Methods Enzymol.* **1999**, *299*, 152–178.
20. Bonina, F.; Saija, A.; Tomaino, A.; Lo Cascio, R.; Rapisarda, P.; Dederen, J.C. In vitro antioxidant activity and in vivo photoprotective effect of a red orange extract. *Int. J. Cosmet. Sci.* **1998**, *20*, 331–342.
21. Xu, L.; Diosady, L.L. Removal of phenolic compounds in the production of high-quality canola protein isolates. *Food Res. Int.* **2002**, *35*, 23–30. [CrossRef]
22. Mandalari, G.; Grundy, M.M.; Grassby, T.; Parker, M.L.; Cross, K.L.; Chessa, S.; Bisignano, C.; Barreca, D.; Bellocco, E.; Laganà, G.; et al. The effects of processing and mastication on almond lipid bioaccessibility using novel methods of in vitro digestion modelling and micro-structural analysis. *Br. J. Nutr.* **2014**, *112*, 1521–1529. [CrossRef] [PubMed]
23. Bouayed, J.; Hoffmann, L.; Bohn, T. Total phenolics, flavonoids, anthocyanins and antioxidant activity following simulated gastro-intestinal digestion and dialysis of apple varieties: Bioaccessibility and potential uptake. *Food Chem.* **2011**, *128*, 14–21. [CrossRef] [PubMed]
24. Fogliano, V.; Corollaro, M.L.; Vitaglione, P.; Napolitano, A.; Ferracane, R.; Travaglia, F.; Arlorio, M.; Costabile, A.; Klinder, A.; Gibson, G. In vitro bioaccessibility and gut biotransformation of polyphenols present in the water-insoluble cocoa fraction. *Mol. Nutr. Food Res.* **2011**, *55*, S44–S55. [CrossRef] [PubMed]
25. Grassby, T.; Picout, D.R.; Mandalari, G.; Faulks, R.M.; Kendall, C.W.; Rich, G.T.; Wickham, M.S.; Lapsley, K.; Ellis, P.R. Modelling of nutrient bioaccessibility in almond seeds based on the fracture properties of their cell walls. *Food Funct.* **2014**, *5*, 3096–3106. [CrossRef] [PubMed]
26. Faulks, R.M.; Southon, S. Challenges to understanding and measuring carotenoid bioavailability. *Biochim. Biophys. Acta* **2005**, *1740*, 95–100. [CrossRef] [PubMed]
27. Del Rio, D.; Costa, L.G.; Lean, M.E.; Crozier, A. Polyphenols and health: What compounds are involved? *Nutr. Metab. Cardiovasc. Dis.* **2010**, *20*, 1–6. [CrossRef] [PubMed]
28. Jakobek, L. Interactions of polyphenols with carbohydrates, lipids and proteins. *Food Chem.* **2015**, *175*, 556–567. [CrossRef] [PubMed]
29. Rock, C.L.; Swendseid, M.E. Plasma beta-carotene response in humans after meals supplemented with dietary pectin. *Am. J. Clin. Nutr.* **1992**, *55*, 96–99. [PubMed]
30. Palafox-Carlos, H.; Ayala-Zavala, J.F.; González-Aguilar, G.A. The role of dietary fiber in the bioaccessibility and bioavailability of fruit and vegetable antioxidants. *J. Food Sci.* **2011**, *76*, R6–R15. [CrossRef] [PubMed]

31. Lamothe, S.; Langlois, A.; Bazinet, L.; Couillard, C.; Britten, M. Antioxidant activity and nutrient release from polyphenol-enriched cheese in a simulated gastrointestinal environment. *Food Funct.* **2016**, *7*, 1634–1644. [CrossRef] [PubMed]

32. Lamothe, S.; Azimy, N.; Bazinet, L.; Couillard, C.; Britten, M. Interaction of green tea polyphenols with dairy matrices in a simulated gastrointestinal environment. *Food Funct.* **2014**, *5*, 2621–2631. [CrossRef] [PubMed]

33. Ortega, N.; Reguant, J.; Romero, M.P.; Macià, A.; Motilva, M.J. Effect of fat content on the digestibility and bioaccessibility of cocoa polyphenol by an in vitro digestion model. *J. Agric. Food Chem.* **2009**, *57*, 5743–5749. [CrossRef] [PubMed]

34. Lesser, S.; Cermak, R. Wolffram S. Bioavailability of quercetin in pigs is influenced by the dietary fat content. *J. Nutr.* **2004**, *134*, 1508–1511. [PubMed]

35. Ozdal, T.; Capanoglu, E.; Altay, F. A review on protein–phenolic interactions and associated changes. *Food Res. Int.* **2013**, *51*, 954–970. [CrossRef]

36. Cebeci, F.; Şahin-Yeşilçubuk, N. The matrix effect of blueberry, oat meal and milk on polyphenols, antioxidant activity and potential bioavailability. *Int. J. Food Sci. Nutr.* **2014**, *65*, 69–78. [CrossRef] [PubMed]

37. Bohn, T. Dietary factors affecting polyphenol bioavailability. *Nutr. Rev.* **2014**, *72*, 429–452. [CrossRef] [PubMed]

38. Smeriglio, A.; Barreca, D.; Bellocco, E.; Trombetta, D. Chemistry, pharmacology and health benefits of anthocyanins. *Phytother. Res.* **2016**, *30*, 1265–1286. [CrossRef] [PubMed]

39. Lopez-Rubio, A.; Gavara, R.; Lagaron, J.M. Bioactive packaging: Turning foods into healthier foods through biomaterials. *Trends Food Sci. Technol.* **2006**, *17*, 567–575. [CrossRef]

40. Koga, C.C.; Lee, S.Y.; Lee, Y. Consumer acceptance of bars and gummies with unencapsulated and encapsulated resveratrol. *J. Food Sci.* **2016**, *81*, S1222–S1229. [CrossRef] [PubMed]

41. Neves, A.R.; Martins, S.; Segundo, M.A.; Reis, S. Nanoscale delivery of resveratrol towards enhancement of supplements and nutraceuticals. *Nutrients* **2016**, *8*, 131. [CrossRef] [PubMed]

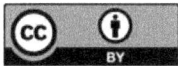

*nutrients*

MDPI

*Article*

# Quercitrin from *Toona sinensis* (Juss.) M.Roem. Attenuates Acetaminophen-Induced Acute Liver Toxicity in HepG2 Cells and Mice through Induction of Antioxidant Machinery and Inhibition of Inflammation

Van-Long Truong [1,†], Se-Yeon Ko [1,†], Mira Jun [2] and Woo-Sik Jeong [1,*]

[1] Department of Smart Food and Drug, College of Biomedical Science & Engineering, Inje University, Gimhae 50834, Korea; truonglongpro@gmail.com (V.-L.T.); kose91@daum.net (S.-Y.K.)
[2] Department of Food and Science & Nutrition, Dong-A University, Busan 49315, Korea; mjun@dau.ac.kr
[*] Correspondence: jeongws@inje.ac.kr; Tel.: +82-55-320-3238; Fax: +82-55-321-0691
[†] These authors contributed equally to this work.

Received: 30 May 2016; Accepted: 11 July 2016; Published: 15 July 2016

**Abstract:** Quercitrin is found in many kinds of vegetables and fruits, and possesses various bioactive properties. The aim of the present study was to elucidate hepatoprotective mechanisms of quercitrin isolated from *Toona sinensis* (Juss.) M.Roem. (syn. *Cedrela sinensis* Juss.), using acetaminophen (APAP)-treated HepG2 cell and animal models. In an in vitro study, quercitrin suppressed the production of reactive oxygen species and enhanced expression of nuclear factor E2-related factor 2 (Nrf2), activity of antioxidant response element (ARE)-reporter gene, and protein levels of NADPH: quinone oxidoreductase 1 (NQO1), catalase (CAT), glutathione peroxidase (GPx), and superoxide dismutase 2 (SOD-2) in APAP-treated HepG2 cells. In an in vivo study, Balb/c mice were orally administered with 10 or 50 mg/kg of quercitrin for 7 days and followed by the injection with single dose of 300 mg/kg APAP. Quercitrin decreased APAP-caused elevation of alanine aminotransferase and aspartate aminotransferase levels, liver necrosis, the expression of pro-inflammatory factors including inducible nitric oxide synthase, cyclooxygenase 2 and inerleukin-1β, and phosphorylation of kinases including c-Jun N-terminal kinase and p38. Quercitrin restored protein levels of Nrf2, NQO1 and activities and expressions of CAT, GPx, SOD-2. The results suggested that quercitrin attenuates APAP-induced liver damage by the activation of defensive genes and the inhibition of pro-inflammatory genes via the suppressions of JNK and p38 signaling.

**Keywords:** quercitrin; acetaminophen; hepatoprotection; Nrf2/ARE; antioxidant

## 1. Introduction

Acetaminophen (APAP, marketed as Paracetamol® or Tylenol®), a widely used over-the-counter analgesic and antipyretic drug, is safe and effective at therapeutic dose. However, it can cause acute liver failures such as serve hepatic necrosis, hepatic lesions and cirrhosis, and even death when taken in high doses. APAP-induced hepatotoxicity is initiated by formation of excess reactive intermediate *N*-acetyl-p-benzoquinone imine (NAPQI), which is produced by metabolism of liver cytochrome P450s (CYPs) including CYP2E1, CYP3A4 and CYP1A2 [1]. NAPQI depletes cellular glutathione (GSH) and adenosine triphosphate (ATP), causes mitochrondrial dysfunction and damage, and finally causes DNA fragmentation and apoptosis. Acetaminophen also contributes to overproduction of reactive oxygen species (ROS) [2]. In addition, lipid peroxidation resulting from oxidative stress has been demonstrated to contribute to the initiation and progression of APAP-induced liver damage [3]. Furthermore, accumulating evidence indicates that acetaminophen overdose triggers the transcriptional activation of pro-inflammatory mediators and cytokines such as inducible nitric oxide (iNOS), cyclooxygenase 2 (COX-2), tumor necrosis factor $\alpha$ (TNF-$\alpha$), and interleukin 1$\beta$ (IL-1$\beta$) [2,4].

*N*-acetylcysteine (NAC) is used as a clinical antidote for APAP poisoning [5,6]. NAC protects liver from APAP-induced injury by restoring hepatic glutathione and scavenging free radicals [7]. However, NAC therapy has considerable limitations because the therapeutic effect of this drug is quite narrow and it could cause some side-effects such as nausea, anaphylactic reaction, headaches and diarrhea [7,8]. Thus, alternative and effective agents are needed to prevent APAP-induced hepatotoxicity.

*Toona sinensis* (Juss.) M.Roem. (syn. *Cedrela sinensis* Juss.), a member of the Meliaceae family, is an upland tree that has been used as traditional medicine and nutritious food for a long time in China and Korea. *T. sinensis* leaves contain a variety of bioactive compounds such as gallic acid, methyl gallte, kaemferol, quercetin, rutin, quercitrin, palmitic acid and linoleic acid, etc. [9–12]. Of these compounds, quercitrin (3-rhamnosyl quercetin) (Figure 1), a glycoside of quercetin, has been found as a main bioactive constituent in *T. sinensis* leaves [13,14]. The sugar portion bound to the aglycone in quercitrin has been demonstrated to increase solubility of quercitrin and consequently improve the absorption by interacting with the sodium dependent glucose transport receptor in the small intestine [15,16]. Pharmacological studies have shown that quercitrin has antioxidant [17,18], anti-inflammatory [19,20], and anti-allergic [21] activities. Quercitrin has been demonstrated to exert a protective effect against UV-induced cell death and apoptosis [22,23]. Furthermore, quercitrin has been studied as an anti-cancer agent against non-small cell lung cancer through the modulation of immune response [24]. Our group previously reported that quercitrin from *T. sinensis* leaves potently scavenged free radicals and induced antioxidant enzymes in $H_2O_2$-treated HepG2 cells [9]. However, the protective mechanisms of quercitrin against APAP-induced hepatotoxicity have not been investigated.

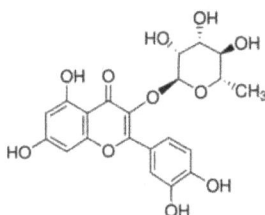

**Figure 1.** Chemical structure of quercitrin.

In the present study, we examined the hepatoprotective effects of quercitrin in both cell line and animal models of hepatotoxicity challenged by APAP. The stimulating activity of quercitrin on cellular defensive genes including transcription factor nuclear factor E2-related factor 2 (Nrf2), antioxidant response element (ARE)-reporter gene and antioxidant enzymes was determined. The inhibitory effects of quercitrin on liver damage markers of alanine aminotransferase (ALT) and aspartate aminotransferase (AST) as well as inflammatory targets of iNOS, COX-2 and IL-1$\beta$ were evaluated in APAP-induced hepatotoxic mice. In addition, the modulation of mitogen activated protein kinases (MAPKs) by quercitrin was examined.

## 2. Materials and Methods

### 2.1. Chemicals

Acetaminophen, silymarin, MTT [3-(4,5-dimethylthiazol-2-yl)-2,5-diphenyltetrazolium bromide], dimethyl sulphoxide (DMSO), polyethylene glycol (PEG), and triton X-100 were purchased from Sigma-Aldrich (St. Louis, MO, USA). 2′,7′-dichlorodihydrofluorescein diacetate (DCFH-DA) was purchased from Molecular Probe Inc. (Eugene, OR, USA). The colorimetric ALT and AST assay kits were supplied by Young-Dong Co. (Seoul, Korea). Anti-Nrf2 (sc-13032), anti-NQO1 (sc-25591), anti-SOD-2 (sc-18504), anti-GPx (sc-30147), anti-COX-2 (sc-1745), anti-iNOS (sc-651), anti-IL-1β (sc-7884), anti-β-actin (sc-1616), and horseradish peroxidase-conjugated anti-goat immunoglobulin IgG (sc-2350) antibodies were purchased from Santa Cruz Biotechnology Inc. (Santa Cruz, CA, USA). Anti-p-ERK (9101), anti-p-JNK (9251), anti-p-p38 MAPK (9211), anti-CAT (14097), and horseradish peroxidase-conjugated anti-rabbit immunoglobulin IgG (7074) were purchased from Cell Signaling Technology (Beverly, MA, USA). All other reagents used in this study were of the highest grade commercially available.

## 2.2. Preparation of Quercitrin

Quercitrin from powder of *T. sinensis* (Juss.) M.Roem. leaves, kindly provided by Slow-life Chamjook Farm Corporation (Hamyang, Korea), was isolated according to previous literature [9]. A voucher specimen (Jeong, W.S. 001) of the raw material was deposited at the Herbarium of Kyungpook National University (KNU), Daegu, Korea. Briefly, the powder of *T. sinensis* was extracted three times with 95% ethanol (EtOH) for 24 h in room temperature and concentrated by rotary evaporation at 40 °C. After concentration, the concentrate was suspended in 10% EtOH and then fractionated with a series of organic solvents, including h-hexane, DCM, ethylacetate (EtOAc), n-butanol, and water in sequence. The EtOAc-solution fraction, the most potent antioxidant fraction to both scavenging radicals and antioxidant enzyme activity, was applied onto a silica gel open column. The column was eluted with solvent mixtures of DCM/methanol under gradient conditions to yield 17 fractions. The most potent subfraction (Fr. 10) was purified by recycling preparatory high-performance liquid chromatography (HPLC) and structural analyses were performed using 1H- and 13C-nuclear magnetic resonance (NMR) analysis.

## 2.3. Cell Culture

Human hepatoma cell line HepG2, obtained from American Type Culture Collection (ATCC, Rockville, MD, USA), was maintained DMEM containing 10% fetal bovine serum (FBS), 100 units/mL penicillin, 100 µg/mL streptomycin, 1% essential amino acids, 1% glutamax in humidified atmosphere of 5% $CO_2$ at 37 °C. The medium was renewed once every two days.

## 2.4. Cell Viability Assay

Cell viability was examined using MTT assay. Briefly, HepG2 cells were cultured in a 24-well plate at density of $1 \times 10^5$ cells/well. After starvation, cells were treated with a series of various concentrations of quercitrin in the presence of 10 mM APAP for 24 h and then incubated with 5 mg/mL MTT for additional 4 h. The dark blue formazan crystal was solubilized in DMSO and followed by measurement of absorbance at 570 nm with a microplate reader (BioTek Instruments, Winooski, VT, USA).

## 2.5. ROS Formation Assay

Level of intracellular ROS was measured using DCFH-DA. In viable cells, the DCFH-DA is cleaved by esterase to DCFH and followed oxidizing by ROS to form a highly florescent molecule, DCF. Briefly, HepG2 cells were seeded onto 96-well plates at density of $2 \times 10^4$ cells/well and then treated either vehicle (DMSO, 0.1%) or various concentrations of quercitrin in the presence of 10 mM APAP for 24 h. After washing twice with phosphate-buffered saline (PBS), the cells were incubated with 20 µM DCF-DA for 1 h at 37 °C in darkness. The fluorescence that is representative of intracellular reactive oxygen species level was measured at 485/20 nm excitation and 528/20 nm emission using a fluorescence multidetection reader (Synergy HT, BioTek, VT, USA).

*2.6. Assay of Reporter Gene Activity*

HepG2-C8 cell line, kindly donated by Ah-Ng Tony Kong (Rutgers University, New Brunswick, NJ, USA), was established by the table transfection of HepG2 cells with p-ARE-T1-luciferase reporter gene as previously described [25]. After starvation, the HepG2-C8 cells were treated with various concentrations of quercitrin for 24 h and then ARE-luciferase activity was measured using a luciferase kit from Promega (Promega Corp., Madison, WI, USA) according to the manufacturer's instructions. Luciferase activity was normalized against total protein concentration, determined by a BCA protein assay kit (Pierce, Rockford, IL, USA), and expressed as a fold induction over that in vehicle-treated cells.

*2.7. Animals and Experimental Design*

Thirty male Balb/c mice (6 weeks old, 20–25 g) were obtained from Hyochang Science (Daegu, Korea) and allowed free access to standard laboratory diet and distilled water *ad libitum* for at least one week prior to the experiment. The animal room was environmentally controlled at $25 \pm 2$ °C, 55%–60% humidity, 12 h light/dark cycle. This animal experiment was approved by the Animal Care and Used Committee of Inje University with protocol number 2013-50 (Gimhae, Korea). The mice were randomly divided into six groups with five mice each. Group I (control group) received 50% PEG as a vehicle for 7 days. Group II (quercitrin group) was only administered 50 mg/kg quercitrin for 7 days. Group III (APAP group) received 50% PEG for 7 days. Group IV and V (quercitrin + APAP group) were orally gavaged with 10 or 50 mg/kg of quercitrin, respectively, for 7 consecutive days. Group VI (APAP + silymarin group) was orally administered 50 mg/kg of silymarin (SIL), which is frequently used as a natural hepatoprotectant by its antioxidant and anti-inflammatory properties [26] for 7 days. After 1 h last administration, a single dose of APAP (300 mg/kg) was injected to mice in groups III-VI. After 24 h APAP challenge, all mice were sacrificed to obtain blood and livers for further biochemical analysis.

*2.8. Measurement of Plasma ALT and AST Levels*

Blood samples from mice were centrifuged at $3000 \times g$, 4 °C for 10 min to obtain serum supernatant. The ALT and AST activities in serum were measured using commercially available kits (Young-dong Pharm, Seoul, Korea).

*2.9. Assay for Antioxidant Enzymes Activity*

Liver tissues were collected and homogenized in phosphate buffer (pH 7.0) and then tissue homogenates were centrifuged at $10,000 \times g$, 4 °C for 10 min to obtain separately supernatant and pellet for further experiments. The protein concentration was determined using a BCA protein assay kit (Pierce, Rockford, IL, USA). CAT activity was determined by the method of Aebi [27]. GPx activity was performed according to the method of Bongdanska et al. [28]. SOD activity was determined by the method of Oyanagui [29]. Enzyme activities were expressed in relation to the vehicle-treated control.

*2.10. Western Blot Analysis*

Cells and liver tissues were homogenized in RIPA buffer and then centrifuged at $10,000 \times g$, 4 °C for 10 min to obtain supernatant. Total protein concentration of each sample was determined using a BCA protein assay kit (Pierce, Rockford, IL, USA) according to the manufacturer's instructions. Equal amounts of protein were resolved on SDS-PAGE gels and then transferred onto PVDF membranes (Millipore, Bedford, MA, USA) using a semidry transfer system (Bio-rad, Hercules, CA, USA). After blocking with 5% non-fat milk in PBST (0.1% Tween 20 in PBS) for 2 h at 4 °C, the membranes were incubated overnight with appropriate primary antibodies at 4 °C. Then, the membranes were washed five times with PBST and hybridized with horseradish peroxidase-conjugated anti-rabbit or anti-goat immunoglobulin IgG secondary antibodies for 3 h at 4 °C. After washing five times with

PBST, blots were visualized using enhanced chemiluminescence western blotting reagent (Santa Cruz Biotechnology, Santa Cruz, CA, USA).

### 2.11. Statistical Analysis

Data were expressed as means $\pm$ SD. Statistical comparisons were evaluated using analysis of variance (ANOVA) followed by Tukey's test. $p < 0.05$ was considered as significant.

## 3. Results

### 3.1. Protective Effect of Quercitrin against Oxidative Stress in APAP-Induced HepG2 Cells

To investigate the effect of quercitrin on the APAP-induced ROS formation, we measured the intracellular level of ROS using a redox-sensitive fluorescence reagent, DCF-DA. As shown in Figure 2A, exposure of HepG2 cells to APAP remarkably elevated the ROS production by over 2-fold at 24 h when compared to the control. Pre-treatment of quercitrin, however, inhibited the increase of APAP-induced ROS level. The presence of 10, 25, 50 µg/mL quercitrin significantly decreased the ROS formation in HepG2 cells by 0.5-, 0.5-, and 1.3-fold, respectively, compared to APAP-treated cells alone. Enhanced oxidative stress can result in apoptosis and cell death; thus, we tested whether quercitrin rescue APAP induced cell death using MTT assay. Consequently, 10 mM APAP reduced 30% cell viability, which was restored by quercitrin (Figure 2B).

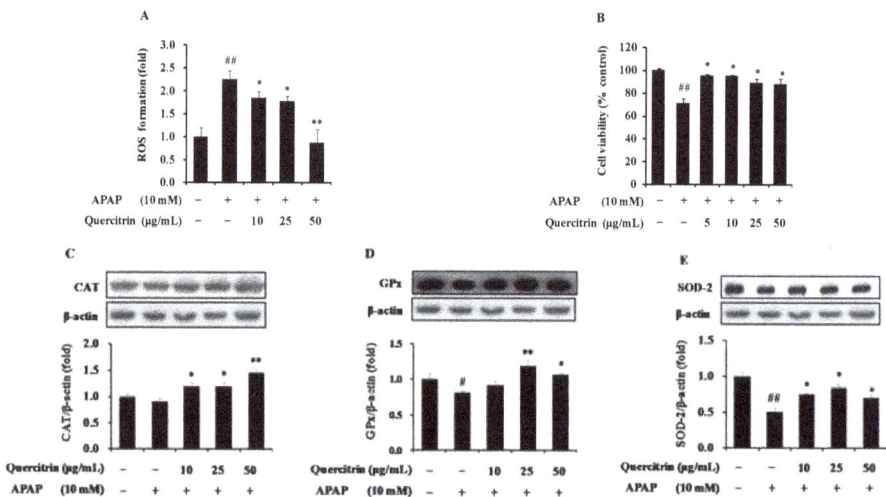

**Figure 2.** Protective effects of quercitrin on acetaminophen (APAP)-treated HepG2 cells. (**A**) Effect of quercitrin on APAP-mediated reactive oxygen species (ROS) formation; (**B**) Effect of quercitrin on cell viability using MTT assay at 24 h. Effect of quercitrin on protein expressions of (**C**) catalase (CAT); (**D**) glutathione peroxidase (GPx); and (**E**) superoxide dismutase 2 (SOD-2) in APAP-treated HepG2 cells. ROS was presented as the fold induction of vehicle-treated control. Cell viability was normalized as 100% for control (without any treatments). Protein expression levels were normalized with β-actin. All data represent means $\pm$ SD of at least three independent experiments. Significant differences were (##) $p < 0.01$ or (#) $p < 0.05$ as compared with the control; (**) $p < 0.01$ or (*) $p < 0.05$ as compared with the APAP group.

Antioxidant enzymes including CAT, GPx, and SOD constitute the primary part of enzymatic antioxidant defense system against oxidative stress via directly eliminating ROS. Thus, the effects of quercitrin on expression levels of antioxidant enzymes were examined. The results showed that

APAP significantly reduced protein expressions of GPx and SOD but not CAT compared with control (Figure 2C–E). However, pretreatment with quercitrin for 1 h blocked the effect of APAP on the decreased expression of antioxidant enzymes. Overall, these results obviously suggested that quercitrin prevents APAP-induced ROS formation and cell death through the induction of antioxidant enzymes in HepG2 cells.

### 3.2. Upregulation of Nrf2/ARE-Mediated Phase II Detoxifying Enzymes by Quercitrin in APAP-Treated HepG2 Cells

To further confirm the role of quercitrin in protection of cells from APAP toxicity, the activation of Nrf2/ARE pathway was evaluated. Nrf2 is considered as a key transcriptional factor responsible for the regulation of phase II detoxifying and/or antioxidant enzymes, which protect cells from cell death-induced APAP toxicity. The basal levels of protein expression of Nrf2 were detected in HepG2 cells. Compared with untreated control, APAP was able to significantly decrease the Nrf2 protein level for up to 24 h (Figure 3A). Further, we investigated the inhibitory effect of quercitrin on APAP-induced the reduction of Nrf2 expression. Results showed that quercitrin has the potential to induce Nrf2 for 24 h. The quercitrin concentration at $\geqslant 25$ µg/mL caused a significant increase in protein level of Nrf2. In particular, quercitrin concentration at 50 µg/mL resulted in a strong up-regulation of Nrf2 at 24 h by 1.6-fold compared to control and 2.0-fold compared with APAP alone. In addition, in order to elucidate whether the activation of Nrf2 induces ARE-mediated phase II detoxifying and/or antioxidant enzymes using ARE-reporter gene activity assay, HepG2-C8 cells, stably transfected with a pARE-TI-luciferase reporter gene were exposed to quercitrin for 24 h. As illustrated in Figure 3B, quercitrin enhanced the ARE-luciferase activity. The luciferase activity by quercitrin at the highest concentration of 50 µg/mL reached 2.6-fold compared with that by vehicle-treated control. This result demonstrated the role of Nrf2 in up-regulation of ARE-mediated phase II enzymes. Furthermore, the effect of quercitrin on protein level of a phase II detoxifying enzyme, NQO1, was examined in APAP-treated HepG2 cells. The result showed that treatment with APAP resulted in the decrease of NQO1 protein level; however, pre-treatment of quercitrin restored the APAP-reduced expression level of NQO1, even more than in the control at quercitrin concentration of 25 µg/mL (Figure 3C). These data suggest that quercitrin promotes hepatoprotective system through the activation of Nrf2 and Nrf2/ARE-mediated antioxidant defense mechanism.

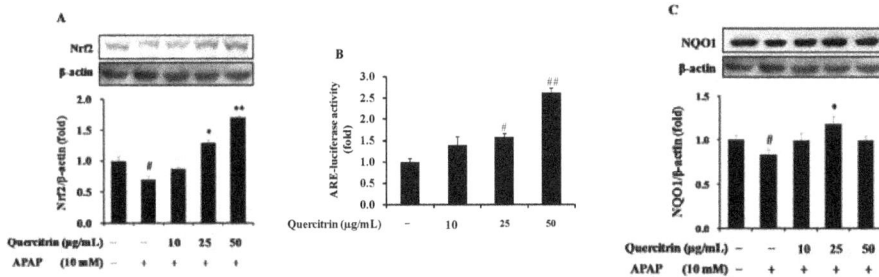

**Figure 3.** Up-regulation of nuclear factor E2-related factor 2 (Nrf2)/antioxidant response element (ARE)-mediated phase II detoxifying enzyme in APAP-treated HepG2 cells. (**A**) Effect of quercitrin on protein expression of Nrf2; (**B**) Effect of quercitrin on ARE-luciferase activity; (**C**) Effect of quercitrin on protein level of quinone oxidoreductase 1 (NQO1). Luciferase activity was normalized with total protein content and expressed as fold induction of normal control. Protein expression levels were normalized with β-actin. All data represent means ± SD of at least three independent experiments. Significant differences were ($^{\#\#}$) $p < 0.01$ or ($^{\#}$) $p < 0.05$ as compared with the control; (**) $p < 0.01$ or (*) $p < 0.05$ as compared with APAP group.

### 3.3. Protective Effect of Quercitrin against APAP-Induced Hepatotoxicity in Vivo

To further investigate the role of quercitrin in protecting liver from APAP-induced toxicity, Balb/c mice were administered quercitrin at a dose of 10 and 50 mg/kg before injection of 300 mg/kg APAP. As shown in Table 1, APAP significantly increased liver weight within 24 h compared with the control and quercitrin alone groups, whereas body weights were comparable among all experimental groups. Oral pre-administration of quercitrin (10 and 50 mg/kg) or SIL (50 mg/kg) reduced the APAP-induced increase of liver weight. In addition, injection of 300 mg/kg APAP highly elevated 14- and 3-fold of serum ALT and AST activities, respectively, compared to the vehicle-treated group, implying that a high dose of APAP caused liver toxicity (Figure 4A,B). Quercitrin treatment significantly prevented the APAP-induced elevation of ALT and AST levels. Similarly, 50 mg/kg of SIL, considered as a positive control in this study, was found to attenuate the ALT and AST activities. Further, the administration of 50 mg/kg quercitrin alone was unlikely to significantly alter the basal activity of these transaminases, suggesting no liver damage caused by quercitrin. Histological (H&E) analysis further revealed that APAP-induced severe hepatic lesions such as hydropic degeneration, inflammation, and hemorrhage were improved by quercitrin pretreatment. Also, a similar result was observed in the positive control group, SIL (Figure 4C). These results prove that quercitrin may be a potential agent in the prevention of APAP-induced liver injury in a mouse model.

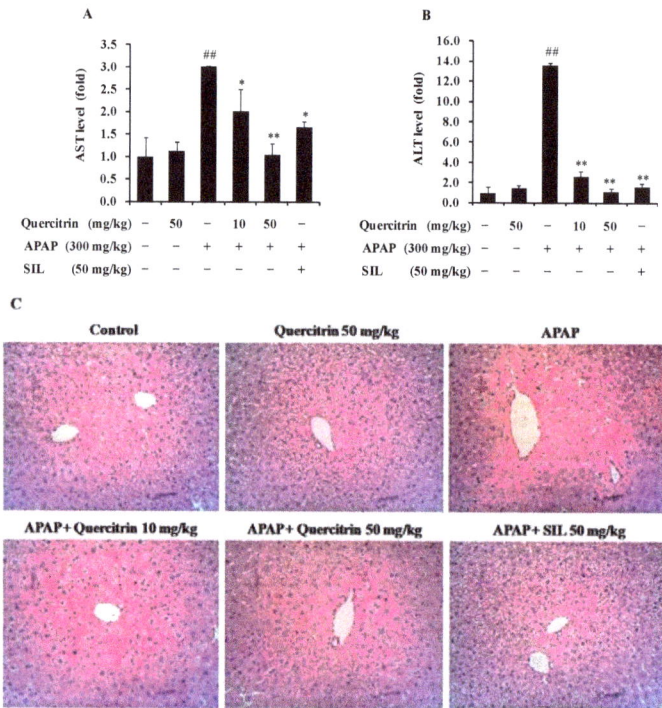

**Figure 4.** Protective effects of quercitrin on APAP intoxicated mice. Mice were orally administered quercitrin of 10 or 50 mg/kg once a day for seven days. The control group received the same volume of saline. After the seventh gavage of quercitrin or saline, animals received a single injection of APAP (300 mg/kg). All mice were sacrificed at 24 h after APAP injection to obtain blood and liver. Serum ALT (**A**) and AST (**B**) levels; and H&E staining (**C**). All data represent means $\pm$ SD of five mice in each group. Significant differences were ($^{\#\#}$) $p < 0.01$ as compared with the control; (\*\*) $p < 0.01$ or (\*) $p < 0.05$ as compared with APAP group.

**Table 1.** Effect of quercitrin on body weight and liver weight/body weight (%) in APAP intoxicated mice.

| Groups | Treatment | Initial Body Weight (g) | Final Body Weight (g) | Liver Weight (g) | Relative Liver Weight (Percentage Ratio) |
|--------|-----------|-------------------------|-----------------------|------------------|-------------------------------------------|
| I | Control | 20.12 ± 0.49 | 23.02 ± 1.36 | 1.42 ± 0.09 | 6.19 ± 0.30 |
| II | Quercitrin (50 mg/kg) | 19.62 ± 0.59 | 23.40 ± 0.45 | 1.53 ± 0.11 | 6.55 ± 0.53 |
| III | APAP (300 mg/kg) | 19.68 ± 0.40 | 23.37 ± 0.90 | 1.65 ± 0.11 | 7.21 ± 0.36 [#] |
| IV | Quercitrin (10 mg/kg) + APAP | 20.20 ± 0.34 | 24.1 ± 0.41 | 1.50 ± 0.10 | 6.20 ± 0.31 * |
| V | Quercitrin (50 mg/kg) + APAP | 19.92 ± 0.38 | 23.02 ± 0.97 | 1.47 ± 0.09 | 6.40 ± 0.28 * |
| VI | Silymarin (50 mg/kg) + APAP | 19.68 ± 0.85 | 23.42 ± 0.92 | 1.50 ± 0.10 | 6.38 ± 0.19 * |

([#]) $p < 0.05$ as compared with the control, (*) $p < 0.05$ as compared with APAP group.

### 3.4. Protective Effect of Quercitrin against APAP-Induced Hepatotoxicity through Enhancement of Activity and Expression of Antioxidant Enzymes

To examine whether quercitrin activates antioxidant defense system in APAP-treated mouse models, we measured activity and protein level of antioxidant enzymes including CAT, GPx, and SOD-2, which importantly contribute to the protection of cells/tissues from oxidative stress through directly neutralizing and eliminating ROS. The results indicated that injection of mice to 300 mg/kg APAP resulted in the reduction in activities of three antioxidant enzymes. Quercitrin pre-administration, however, prevented the APAP-induced decrease of CAT, GPx, and SOD-2 enzyme activities (Figure 5A–C). It is likely that quercitrin, SIL (50 mg/kg), also significantly increased the activities of these enzymes when compared to APAP-treated mice. Interestingly, oral administration of 50 mg/kg quercitrin alone was shown to enhance the CAT and SOD-2 activities but not GPx activity compared to the vehicle-treated control. In order to further confirm the inductive effect as well as the role of quercitrin on liver protection against APAP-induced oxidative stress, protein expression levels of antioxidant enzymes including CAT, GPx, and SOD-2 were determined. The results showed that treatment of 300 mg/kg APAP caused slightly reduced protein expressions of these antioxidant enzymes. However, as expected, quercitrin significantly induced the APAP-abolished CAT, GPx, and SOD-2 proteins, even more than those in the control group (Figure 5D–F). This result is consistent with SIL, which also enhanced the expressions of antioxidant enzymes in APAP-treated mice. Overall, our study supports the use of quercitrin in preventing APAP-mediated liver toxicity.

### 3.5. Upregulation of NQO1 Expression by Nrf2-Mediated Quercitrin in APAP-Treated Mice

As demonstrated, quercitrin up-regulated Nrf2-mediated phase II detoxifying enzyme in HepG2 cells, thus we confirmed the inductive effect of quercitrin on protein levels of NQO1 in an APAP-treated mouse model. Similar to the in vitro result, exposure of mice to APAP caused a significant attenuate of NQO1 protein level (Figure 6B) but was unlikely to suppress protein expression of Nrf2 after 24 h challenge (Figure 6A) when compared to the untreated control. The presence of quercitrin restored the APAP-reduced protein expression of both Nrf2 and NQO1. Further, the levels of Nrf2 and NQO1 expression induced by quercitrin were even higher than those induced by a positive control, SIL (50 mg/kg) (Figure 6A,B). These results demonstrate the role of quercitrin in the activation of Nrf2/ARE-mediated phase II detoxifying enzyme, implying protection of cells/tissues against APAP-induced toxicity.

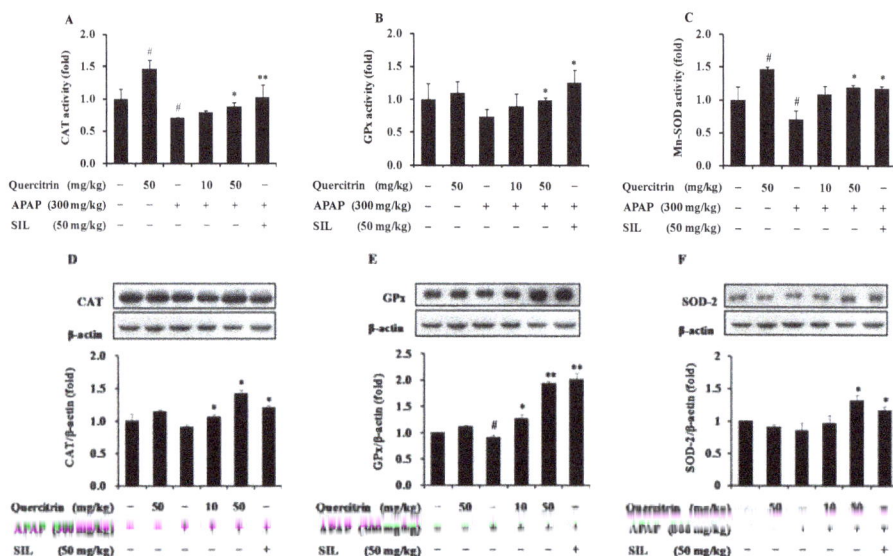

**Figure 5.** Effects of quercitrin on activities and protein expressions of hepatic antioxidant enzymes in APAP intoxicated mice. The hepatic activities of CAT (**A**); GPx (**B**) and SOD-2 (**C**) were measured as described in Materials and Methods section. The protein levels of CAT (**D**); GPx (**E**) and SOD-2 (**F**) were determined using Western blot analysis. Protein expression levels were normalized with β-actin. All data represent means ± SD of five mice in each group. Significant differences were ($^{\#}$) $p < 0.05$ as compared with the control; (**) $p < 0.01$ or (*) $p < 0.05$ as compared with APAP group.

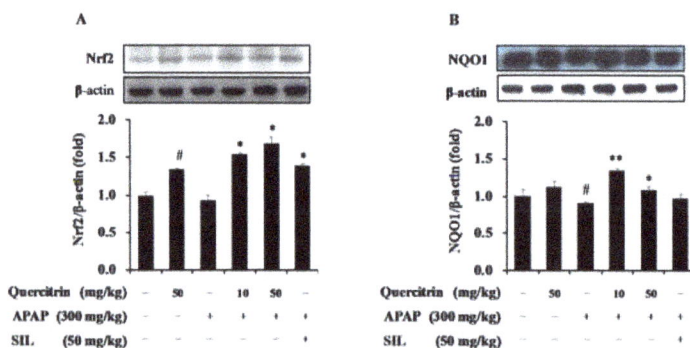

**Figure 6.** Effects of quercitrin on expressions of Nrf2 and NQO1 in APAP intoxicated mice. The protein levels of Nrf2 (**A**) and NQO1 (**B**) were measured by Western blot analysis as described in Materials and Methods section. Protein expression levels were normalized with β-actin. All data represent means ± SD of five mice in each group. Significant differences were ($^{\#}$) $p < 0.05$ as compared with the control; (**) $p < 0.01$ or (*) $p < 0.05$ as compared with APAP group.

### 3.6. Quercitrin Attenuates Inflammatory Response in APAP-Treated Mice

In further studies, we evaluated the effects of quercitrin on APAP-induced expression of pro-inflammatory mediators and cytokines implicated in hepatotoxicity. APAP treatment significantly increased protein expression for the pro-inflammatory mediators and cytokine such as iNOS, COX-2 and IL-1β compared to vehicle-treated control, whereas animals receiving quercitrin alone did not show elevated levels of these hepatic inflammatory factors (Figure 7A–C). APAP-enhanced protein expression of iNOS, the enzyme mediating production of nitric oxide, was also inhibited by the presence of quercitrin (Figure 7A). Expression of pro-inflammatory mediator COX-2 that was up-regulated in mice exposing APAP intoxication was reduced in mice pre-treated with quercitrin (Figure 7B). Additionally, quercitrin administration resulted in a decrease in the APAP-induced IL-1β protein level (Figure 7C).

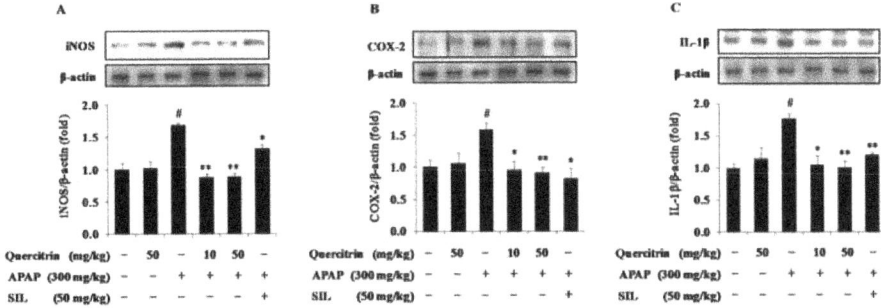

**Figure 7.** Effects of quercitrin on inflammatory response in APAP intoxicated mice. The hepatic inducible nitric oxide (iNOS) (**A**); cyclooxygenase 2 (COX-2) (**B**) and interleukin 1β (IL-1β) (**C**) levels were evaluated by Western blot analysis. Protein expression levels were normalized with β-actin. All data represent means ± SD of five mice in each group. Significant differences were (#) $p < 0.05$ as compared with the control; (**) $p < 0.01$ or (*) $p < 0.05$ as compared with APAP group.

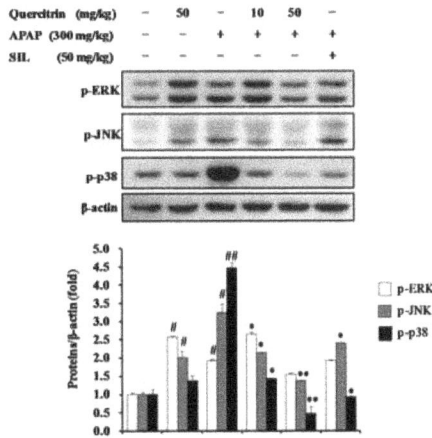

**Figure 8.** Effects of quercitrin on MAP kinases in APAP intoxicated mice. The phosphorylations of ERK, JNK and p38 MAPK were analyzed by Western blotting. Protein expression levels were normalized with β-actin. All data represent means ± SD of five mice in each group. Significant differences were (##) $p < 0.01$ or (#) $p < 0.05$ as compared with the control; (**) $p < 0.01$ or (*) $p < 0.05$ as compared with APAP group.

*3.7. Activation of Cytoprotective Mechanisms by Quercitrin through Regulation of MAPK Pathways in APAP-Treated Mice*

To investigate role of quercitrin on the modulation of MAPKs in APAP-treated mice, phosphorylation levels of MAPKs including ERK, JNK, and p38 MAPK were determined using western blotting. As shown in Figure 8, exposure of APAP (300 mg/kg) increased the phosphorylation levels of ERK, JNK, and p38 MAPK in the liver by 2-, 3-, and 4-fold, respectively, when compared to the control group. This suggested that MAPKs involved in APAP-caused hepatotoxicity. On other hand, treatment of quercitrin (50 mg/kg) alone resulted in a significant elevation of phosphorylated ERK and JNK but not phosphorylated p38. Oral administration of quercitrin or SIL, however, strongly inhibited the JNK and p38 MAPK phosphorylations, whereas ERK phosphorylation was slightly decreased at 50 mg/kg quercitrin and there was no change at 50 mg/kg SIL. Overall, our results indicate that the inhibition of APAP-induced phosphorylation levels of JNK and p38 MAPK by quercitrin contributes to protection of liver from toxicity.

## 4. Discussion

The present study demonstrated the role of quercitrin from *T. sinensis* in the protection of cells/tissues from APAP-induced toxicity. Quercitrin attenuated the ROS formation and cell death induced by APAP overdose through the restoration of antioxidant enzymes as well as enhancement of Nrf2/ARE pathway-mediated cytoprotecive enzymes in HepG2 cells. Moreover, oral administration of quercitrin exhibited protective effects against APAP-caused liver injury in mice, which is consistent with an in vitro test. Indeed, quercitrin pretreatment prevented APAP toxicity, as evidenced by much less liver injury and decreased serum ALT and AST levels. Quercitrin restored the APAP-induced reduction of activities and protein expressions of antioxidant enzymes, including CAT, GPx, and SOD-2 as well as protein level of phase II enzyme NQO1 through the activation of transcription factor Nrf2. In addition, quercitrin exerted the anti-inflammatory property through inhibiting the expression of pro-inflammatory mediators and cytokine such as iNOS, COX-2, IL-1β in APAP-treated liver. Furthermore, inhibition of APAP-mediated phosphorylation levels of JNK and p38 MAPK were considered as a protective mechanism of quercitrin from APAP toxicity in liver. These results, for the first time, demonstrate that antioxidant and anti-inflammatory properties of quercitrin potently contribute to the prevention of APAP-induced liver injury.

Reactive oxygen species (ROS) including free radicals such as superoxide ($O_2 \cdot^-$), hydroxyl radical ($\cdot OH$), peroxyl radical ($RO_2 \cdot$) and non-radical species such as hydrogen peroxide ($H_2O_2$) are implicated in the development of various diseases such as aging, cancer, atherosclerosis, fibrosis, and inflammation [30–32]. The accumulation of ROS results in oxidative stress, lipid peroxidation, protein inactivation, DNA damage, loss of cell function, and finally apoptosis and necrosis [33]. Increased oxidative stress and massive impairment of antioxidant defense systems are well-known as the main mechanisms of APAP-caused hepatotoxicity [34]. The major reactive oxygen species generated by APAP toxicity is superoxide ($O_2 \cdot^-$), which dismutates to molecular oxygen and hydrogen peroxide or reacts with nitric oxide (NO) to produce peroxynitrite ($ONOO^-$), a potent oxidant and nitrating species [35]. A variety of phenomena such as lipid peroxidation, increased ALT and AST, reduced levels of cellular antioxidant enzymes, and DNA damages was observed in APAP toxicity. In this study, we confirmed that ROS levels were dramatically increased, whereas protein expressions and activities of CAT, GPx, and SOD-2 in HepG2 cells and mouse livers significantly decreased after APAP treatment. In addition, HepG2 cell death and liver necrosis were elevated, suggesting that APAP-induced ROS formation results in loss of cell function and ultimately apoptosis. However, quercitrin could inhibit ROS formation and consequently reduce hepatic cell death as well as liver necrosis caused by APAP toxicity. Quercitrin also remarkably abolished plasma ALT and AST levels, which coincided with the decrease of APAP-mediated oxidative damage. Furthermore, the levels of antioxidant enzymes including CAT, GPx, and SOD-2 were restored by pretreatment of quercitrin in APAP-treated HepG2 cells and livers of mice. These results indicate that quercitrin protects cells/livers from APAP-induced oxidative stress through the suppression of ROS production and enhancement of an antioxidant defense system.

Recent studies have demonstrated that transcription factor Nrf2 importantly contributes to cellular defense mechanisms from APAP toxicity [36,37]. Treatment of Nrf2 knockout mice (Nrf2-/-) with APAP results in enhanced hepatotoxicity and mortality compared to wild-type [36]. NAC treatment produced a low efficacy in Nrf2-/- mice, although NAC still exhibited the effective protection against APAP toxicity in wild-type mice [37,38]. Additionally, hepatocyte-specific Kelch-like ECH-associated protein-1 (*keap1*) gene knockout mice that highly express detoxifying enzymes are significantly more resistant to APAP toxicity than wild-type animals [39]. Consequently, up-regulation of phase II antioxidant/detoxifying enzymes by Nrf2/ARE pathway plays a critical role in preventing hepatic damage caused by APAP. To clarify the underlying hepatoprotective mechanism of quercitrin, we investigated the inductive effect of quercitrin on the Nrf2/ARE pathway. The results suggested that protein level of Nrf2 was enhanced by the pre-treatment of quercitrin in both in vitro and in vivo models. Quercitrin also significantly increased the ARE-reporter gene activity in HepG2-C8 cells. Furthermore, quercitrin restored the APAP-induced reduction of phase II enzyme NQO1, which are capable of scavenging oxidative stress and detoxifying/eliminating toxic chemicals. NQO1 has been demonstrated to be capable of lowering NAPQI availability by the conversion of NAPQI back to the parent APAP, prevent adenosine triphosphate (ATP) depletion as well as mitochondrial dysfunction caused by APAP [40,41]. Our findings strongly indicate that quercitrin enhances the hepatic defense system through the activation of Nrf2/ARE-mediated phase II detoxifying/ antioxidant enzymes.

Uncontrolled inflammation initiates the progression of tissue damage and results in the development of many diseases such as Alzheimer's disease, cardiovascular disease, atherosclerosis and cancer [42,43]. During the inflammatory response, pro-inflammatory mediators and cytokines such as iNOS, COX-2, IL-1$\beta$, and TNF-$\alpha$ were up-regulated and accumulated in the liver [44]. Numerous evidence has showed that APAP causes early damage, which triggers an inflammatory response with the production of pro-inflammatory factors and innate immune cell infiltration in the liver [45–48]. Thus, inhibition of these mediators and cytokines production is an important mechanism for treatment of inflammation, contributing to preventing APAP-induced hepatotoxicity. In the current study, we confirmed that APAP intoxication resulted in increased expression levels of iNOS, COX-2 as well as IL-1$\beta$ in the liver. However, mice pre-administered quercitrin exhibited the inhibitory effect on protein expressions of iNOS, COX-2, and IL-1$\beta$. These results, for the first time, imply that the hepatoprotective effect of quercitrin may be due to its anti-inflammatory property.

MAP kinases including ERK, JNK, and p38 MAPK play a crucial role in transduction extracellular signals to cellular responses including cellular proliferation, differentiation, development, inflammation and apoptosis in response to various signals produced by growth factors, hormones, cytokines, and xenobiotics as well as oxidative stress [49,50]. A massive study demonstrated that MAP kinases directly implicate in the mechanism of APAP-caused hepatocellular injury. During APAP overdose, JNK is phosphorylated and translocates into mitochondria early in APAP hepatotoxicity in mice, resulting in an initial oxidative stress, induction of mitochorial permeability transition, and inhibition of bioenergetics [35,51]. Additionally, activated JNK can trigger Bax activation, which is responsible for the initial apoptosis-inducing factor (AIF) and endonuclease G release from the mitochondria and early DNA damage, as well as induce iNOS expression, which promotes peroxynitrite formation [52,53]. Furthermore, inhibition of JNK activation or *jnk* gene knockout in mice decreased the liver injury, nuclear DNA fragmentation, and prevented the development of mitochondrial oxidative stress after APAP overdose [51,52,54]. Different from JNK inhibitor, the inhibitors of ERK and p38 MAPK exhibited no protection against APAP toxicity either in vitro or in vivo [52]. Although activations of ERK and p38 MAPK were observed, the roles of ERK and p38 MAPK in APAP-caused heptotoxic mechanism have not been clearly investigated. Overall, the inhibition of JNK phosphorylation contributes to reduction of liver injury induced by APAP challenge. In the present study, we also investigated the inhibition of JNK phosphorylation and concluded it could play a part in the hepatoprotective mechanism of quercitrin against APAP-mediated damage.

## 5. Conclusions

In conclusion, quercitrin protects against APAP-induced liver injury by enhancing the cellular defense system and lowering inflammatory response. Activation of Nrf2/ARE pathway-mediated cytoprotective proteins by quercitrin may contribute to neutralizing ROS, eliminating toxicants and finally preventing cell death and liver necrosis. Quercitrin also exhibits anti-inflammatory properties through the inhibition of pro-inflammatory mediators including iNOS and COX-2 as well as a cytokine IL-1β in APAP-caused inflammation. Furthermore, the suppression of JNK phosphorylation by quercitrin was identified as a protective mechanism against apoptosis. Our study revealed that quercitrin may have safe therapeutic potential in protecting cell/liver from APAP toxicity.

**Acknowledgments:** This research was supported by Basic Science Research Program through the National Research Foundation of Korea (NRF) funded by the Ministry of Science, ICT and Future Planning (NRF-2014R1A2A1A11050006).

**Author Contributions:** Woo-Sik Jeong designed the study and revised the manuscript, Van-Long Truong and Se-Yeon Ko contributed equally to this work, performed experiments and prepared the manuscript, Mira Jun analyzed data.

**Conflicts of Interest:** The authors declare no conflict of interest.

## Abbreviations

The following abbreviations are used in this manuscript:

| | |
|---|---|
| APAP | Acetaminophen |
| ALT | Alanine transaminase |
| ARE | Antioxidant response element |
| AST | Aspartate aminotransferase |
| CAT | Catalase |
| COX-2 | Cyclooxygenase-2 |
| CYP | Cytochrome P450 |
| ERK | Extracellular signal regulated kinase |
| GSH | Glutathione |
| GPx | Glutathione peroxidase |
| iNOS | Inducible nitric oxide synthase |
| JNK | c-Jun N-terminal kinase |
| Keap 1 | Kelch-like ECH-associated protein 1 |
| MAPK | Mitogen activated protein kinase |
| NAC | *N*-acetylcysteine |
| NQO1 | NADPH:quinone oxidoreductase 1 |
| Nrf2 | Nuclear factor erythroid-2-related factor-2 |
| ROS | Reactive oxygen species |
| SOD | Superoxide dismutase |

## References

1. Slitt, A.M.L.; Dominick, P.K.; Roberts, J.C.; Cohen, S.D. Effect of ribose cysteine pretreatment on hepatic and renal acetaminophen metabolite formation and glutathione depletion. *Basic Clin. Pharmacol. Toxicol.* **2005**, *96*, 487–494. [CrossRef] [PubMed]
2. Song, E.; Fu, J.; Xia, X.; Su, C.; Song, Y. Bazhen decoction protects against acetaminophen induced acute liver injury by inhibiting oxidative stress, inflammation and apoptosis in mice. *PLoS ONE* **2014**, *9*, e107405. [CrossRef] [PubMed]
3. Noh, J.-R.; Kim, Y.-H.; Hwang, J.H.; Choi, D.-H.; Kim, K.-S.; Oh, W.-K.; Lee, C.-H. Sulforaphane protects against acetaminophen-induced hepatotoxicity. *Food Chem. Toxicol.* **2015**, *80*, 193–200. [CrossRef] [PubMed]
4. Jaeschke, H.; Williams, C.D.; Ramachandran, A.; Bajt, M.L. Acetaminophen hepatotoxicity and repair: The role of sterile inflammation and innate immunity. *Liver Int.* **2012**, *32*, 8–20. [CrossRef] [PubMed]
5. Buckley, N.A.; Whyte, I.M.; O'Connell, D.L.; Dawson, A.H. Oral or intravenous *N*-acetylcysteine: Which is the treatment of choice for acetaminophen (paracetamol) poisoning? *J. Toxicol. Clin. Toxicol.* **1999**, *37*, 759–767. [CrossRef] [PubMed]

6.  Flanagan, R.J.; Meredith, T.J. Use of *N*-acetylcysteine in clinical toxicology. *Am. J. Med.* **1991**, *91*, 131S–139S. [CrossRef]

7.  Heard, K.J. Acetylcysteine for acetaminophen poisoning. *N. Engl. J. Med.* **2008**, *359*, 285–292. [CrossRef] [PubMed]

8.  Sandilands, E.A.; Bateman, D.N. Adverse reactions associated with acetylcysteine. *Clin. Toxicol.* **2009**, *47*, 81–88. [CrossRef] [PubMed]

9.  Bak, M.-J.; Jeong, J.-H.; Kang, H.-S.; Jin, K.-S.; Jun, M.; Jeong, W.-S. Stimulation of activity and expression of antioxidant enzymes by solvent fractions and isolated compound from *Cedrela sinensis* leaves in HepG2 cells. *J. Med. Food* **2011**, *14*, 405–412. [CrossRef] [PubMed]

10. Chia, Y.-C.; Rajbanshi, R.; Calhoun, C.; Chiu, R.H. Anti-neoplastic effects of gallic acid, a major component of *Toona sinensis* leaf extract, on oral squamous carcinoma cells. *Molecules* **2010**, *15*, 8377–8389. [CrossRef] [PubMed]

11. Hsiang, C.-Y.; Hseu, Y.-C.; Chang, Y.-C.; Kumar, K.J.S.; Ho, T.-Y.; Yang, H.-L. *Toona sinensis* and its major bioactive compound gallic acid inhibit LPS-induced inflammation in nuclear factor-κB transgenic mice as evaluated by in vivo bioluminescence imaging. *Food Chem.* **2013**, *136*, 426–434. [CrossRef] [PubMed]

12. Su, Y.-F.; Yang, Y.-C.; Hsu, H.-K.; Hwang, S.-L.; Lee, K.-S.; Lieu, A.-S.; Chan, T.-F.; Lin, C.-L. *Toona sinensis* leaf extract has antinociceptive effect comparable with non-steroidal anti-inflammatory agents in mouse writhing test. *BMC Complement. Altern. Med.* **2015**, *15*, 70. [CrossRef] [PubMed]

13. Da Silva, E.R.; Maquiaveli, C.D.C.; Magalhães, P.P. The leishmanicidal flavonols quercetin and quercitrin target *Leishmania* (*Leishmania*) *amazonensis* arginase. *Exp. Parasitol.* **2012**, *130*, 183–188. [CrossRef] [PubMed]

14. Wagner, C.; Fachinetto, R.; Dalla Corte, C.L.; Brito, V.B.; Severo, D.; de Oliveira Costa Dias, G.; Morel, A.F.; Nogueira, C.W.; Rocha, J.B.T. Quercitrin, a glycoside form of quercetin, prevents lipid peroxidation in vitro. *Brain Res.* **2006**, *1107*, 192–198. [CrossRef] [PubMed]

15. Ader, P.; Block, M.; Pietzsch, S.; Wolffram, S. Interaction of quercetin glucosides with the intestinal sodium/glucose co-transporter (SGLT-1). *Cancer Lett.* **2001**, *162*, 175–180. [CrossRef]

16. Gee, J.M.; DuPont, M.S.; Rhodes, M.J.C.; Johnson, I.T. Quercetin glucosides interact with the intestinal glucose transport pathway 1. *Free Radic. Biol. Med.* **1998**, *25*, 19–25. [CrossRef]

17. Babujanarthanam, R.; Kavitha, P.; Mahadeva Rao, U.S.; Pandian, M. Quercitrin a bioflavonoid improves the antioxidant status in streptozotocin: Induced diabetic rat tissues. *Mol. Cell. Biochem.* **2011**, *358*, 121–129. [CrossRef] [PubMed]

18. Ham, Y.-M.; Yoon, W.-J.; Park, S.-Y.; Song, G.-P.; Jung, Y.-H.; Jeon, Y.-J.; Kang, S.-M.; Kim, K.-N. Quercitrin protects against oxidative stress-induced injury in lung fibroblast cells via up-regulation of Bcl-xl. *J. Funct. Foods* **2012**, *4*, 253–262. [CrossRef]

19. Camuesco, D.; Comalada, M.; Rodríguez-Cabezas, M.E.; Nieto, A.; Lorente, M.D.; Concha, A.; Zarzuelo, A.; Gálvez, J. The intestinal anti-inflammatory effect of quercitrin is associated with an inhibition in iNOS expression. *Br. J. Pharmacol.* **2004**, *143*, 908–918. [CrossRef] [PubMed]

20. Choi, S.-J.; Tai, B.; Cuong, N.; Kim, Y.-H.; Jang, H.-D. Antioxidative and anti-inflammatory effect of quercetin and its glycosides isolated from mampat (*Cratoxylum formosum*). *Food Sci. Biotechnol.* **2012**, *21*, 587–595. [CrossRef]

21. Cruz, E.A.; Da-Silva, S.A.G.; Muzitano, M.F.; Silva, P.M.R.; Costa, S.S.; Rossi-Bergmann, B. Immunomodulatory pretreatment with *Kalanchoe pinnata* extract and its quercitrin flavonoid effectively protects mice against fatal anaphylactic shock. *Int. Immunopharmacol.* **2008**, *8*, 1616–1621. [CrossRef] [PubMed]

22. Yang, H.-M.; Ham, Y.-M.; Yoon, W.-J.; Roh, S.W.; Jeon, Y.-J.; Oda, T.; Kang, S.-M.; Kang, M.-C.; Kim, E.-A.; Kim, D.; et al. Quercitrin protects against ultraviolet B-induced cell death in vitro and in an in vivo zebrafish model. *J. Photochem. Photobiol. B* **2012**, *114*, 126–131. [CrossRef] [PubMed]

23. Yin, Y.; Li, W.; Son, Y.-O.; Sun, L.; Lu, J.; Kim, D.; Wang, X.; Yao, H.; Wang, L.; Pratheeshkumar, P.; et al. Quercitrin protects skin from UVB-induced oxidative damage. *Toxicol. Appl. Pharmacol.* **2013**, *269*, 89–99. [CrossRef] [PubMed]

24. Cincin, Z.B.; Unlu, M.; Kiran, B.; Bireller, E.S.; Baran, Y.; Cakmaglu, B. Molecular mechanisms of quercitrin-induced apoptosis in non-small cell lung cancer. *Arch. Med. Res.* **2014**, *45*, 445–454. [CrossRef] [PubMed]

25. Yu, R.; Chen, C.; Mo, Y.-Y.; Hebbar, V.; Owuor, E.D.; Tan, T.-H.; Kong, A.-N.T. Activation of mitogen-activated protein kinase pathways induces antioxidant response element-mediated gene expression via a Nrf2-dependent mechanism. *J. Biol. Chem.* **2000**, *275*, 39907–39913. [CrossRef] [PubMed]

26. Bektur, N.E.; Sahin, E.; Baycu, C.; Unver, G. Protective effects of silymarin against acetaminophen-induced hepatotoxicity and nephrotoxicity in mice. *Toxicol. Ind. Health* **2016**, *32*, 589–600. [CrossRef] [PubMed]

27. Aebi, H. Catalase in vitro. *Methods Enzymol.* **1984**, *105*, 121–126. [PubMed]

28. Bogdanska, J.J.; Korneti, P.; Todorova, B. Erythrocyte superoxide dismutase, glutathione peroxidase and catalase activities in healthy male subjects in republic of macedonia. *Bratisl. Lek. Listy* **2003**, *104*, 108–114. [PubMed]

29. Oyanagui, Y. Reevaluation of assay methods and establishment of kit for superoxide dismutase activity. *Anal. Biochem.* **1984**, *142*, 290–296. [CrossRef]

30. Hybertson, B.M.; Gao, B.; Bose, S.K.; McCord, J.M. Oxidative stress in health and disease: The therapeutic potential of Nrf2 activation. *Mol. Aspects Med.* **2011**, *32*, 234–246. [CrossRef] [PubMed]

31. Lessig, J.; Fuchs, B. Plasmalogens in biological systems: Their role in oxidative processes in biological membranes, their contribution to pathological processes and aging and plasmalogen analysis. *Curr. Med. Chem.* **2009**, *16*, 2021–2041. [CrossRef] [PubMed]

32. Mena, S.; Ortega, A.; Estrela, J.M. Oxidative stress in environmental-induced carcinogenesis. *Mutat. Res.* **2009**, *674*, 36–44. [CrossRef] [PubMed]

33. Valko, M.; Leibfritz, D.; Moncol, J.; Cronin, M.T.D.; Mazur, M.; Telser, J. Free radicals and antioxidants in normal physiological functions and human disease. *Int. J. Biochem. Cell Biol.* **2007**, *39*, 44–84. [CrossRef] [PubMed]

34. Jaeschke, H.; McGill, M.R.; Williams, C.D.; Ramachandran, A. Current issues with acetaminophen hepatotoxicity—A clinically relevant model to test the efficacy of natural products. *Life Sci.* **2011**, *88*, 737–745. [CrossRef] [PubMed]

35. McGill, M.R.; Williams, C.D.; Xie, Y.; Ramachandran, A.; Jaeschke, H. Acetaminophen-induced liver injury in rats and mice: Comparison of protein adducts, mitochondrial dysfunction, and oxidative stress in the mechanism of toxicity. *Toxicol. Appl. Pharmacol.* **2012**, *264*, 387–394. [CrossRef] [PubMed]

36. Enomoto, A.; Itoh, K.; Nagayoshi, E.; Haruta, J.; Kimura, T.; O'Connor, T.; Harada, T.; Yamamoto, M. High sensitivity of Nrf2 knockout mice to acetaminophen hepatotoxicity associated with decreased expression of ARE-regulated drug metabolizing enzymes and antioxidant genes. *Toxicol. Sci.* **2001**, *59*, 169–177. [CrossRef] [PubMed]

37. Chan, K.; Han, X.-D.; Kan, Y.W. An important function of Nrf2 in combating oxidative stress: Detoxification of acetaminophen. *Proc. Natl. Acad. Sci. USA* **2001**, *98*, 4611–4616. [CrossRef] [PubMed]

38. Aleksunes, L.M.; Manautou, J.E. Emerging role of Nrf2 in protecting against hepatic and gastrointestinal disease. *Toxicol. Pathol.* **2007**, *35*, 459–473. [CrossRef] [PubMed]

39. Okawa, H.; Motohashi, H.; Kobayashi, A.; Aburatani, H.; Kensler, T.W.; Yamamoto, M. Hepatocyte-specific deletion of the *keap1* gene activates Nrf2 and confers potent resistance against acute drug toxicity. *Biochem. Biophys. Res. Commun.* **2006**, *339*, 79–88. [CrossRef] [PubMed]

40. Hwang, J.; Kim, Y.-H.; Noh, J.-R.; Gang, G.-T.; Kim, K.-S.; Chung, H.; Tadi, S.; Yim, Y.-H.; Shong, M.; Lee, C.-H. The protective role of NAD(P)H:Quinone oxidoreductase 1 on acetaminophen-induced liver injury is associated with prevention of adenosine triphosphate depletion and improvement of mitochondrial dysfunction. *Arch. Toxicol.* **2015**, *89*, 2159–2166. [CrossRef] [PubMed]

41. Moffit, J.S.; Aleksunes, L.M.; Kardas, M.J.; Slitt, A.L.; Klaassen, C.D.; Manautou, J.E. Role of NAD(P)H:Quinone oxidoreductase 1 in clofibrate-mediated hepatoprotection from acetaminophen. *Toxicology* **2007**, *230*, 197–206. [CrossRef] [PubMed]

42. Lu, H.; Ouyang, W.; Huang, C. Inflammation, a key event in cancer development. *Mol. Cancer Res.* **2006**, *4*, 221–233. [CrossRef] [PubMed]

43. Reddy, S.A.; Shelar, S.B.; Dang, T.-M.; Lee, B.N.-C.; Yang, H.; Ong, S.-M.; Ng, H.-L.; Chui, W.-K.; Wong, S.-C.; Chew, E.-H. Sulforaphane and its methylcarbonyl analogs inhibit the LPS-stimulated inflammatory response in human monocytes through modulating cytokine production, suppressing chemotactic migration and phagocytosis in a NF-κB- and MAPK-dependent manner. *Int. Immunopharmacol.* **2015**, *24*, 440–450. [CrossRef] [PubMed]

44. Chung, H.Y.; Cesari, M.; Anton, S.; Marzetti, E.; Giovannini, S.; Seo, A.Y.; Carter, C.; Yu, B.P.; Leeuwenburgh, C. Molecular inflammation: Underpinnings of aging and age-related diseases. *Ageing Res. Rev.* **2009**, *8*, 18–30. [CrossRef] [PubMed]

45. Dragomir, A.-C.; Sun, R.; Mishin, V.; Hall, L.B.; Laskin, J.D.; Laskin, D.L. Role of galectin-3 in acetaminophen-induced hepatotoxicity and inflammatory mediator production. *Toxicol. Sci.* **2012**, *127*, 609–619. [CrossRef] [PubMed]

46. Hong, S.-W.; Lee, H.-S.; Jung, K.; Lee, H.; Hong, S.-S. Protective effect of fucoidan against acetaminophen-induced liver injury. *Arch. Pharm. Res.* **2012**, *35*, 1099–1105. [CrossRef] [PubMed]

47. Tai, M.; Zhang, J.; Song, S.; Miao, R.; Liu, S.; Pang, Q.; Wu, Q.; Liu, C. Protective effects of luteolin against acetaminophen-induced acute liver failure in mouse. *Int. Immunopharmacol.* **2015**, *27*, 164–170. [CrossRef] [PubMed]

48. Williams, C.D.; Farhood, A.; Jaeschke, H. Role of caspase-1 and interleukin-1β in acetaminophen-induced hepatic inflammation and liver injury. *Toxicol. Appl. Pharmacol.* **2010**, *247*, 169–178. [CrossRef] [PubMed]

49. Chen, C.; Kong, A.-N.T. Dietary cancer-chemopreventive compounds: From signaling and gene expression to pharmacological effects. *Trends Pharmacol. Sci.* **2005**, *26*, 318–326. [CrossRef] [PubMed]

50. Kim, E.K.; Choi, E.-J. Pathological roles of MAPK signaling pathways in human diseases. *Biochim. Biophys. Acta* **2010**, *1802*, 396–405. [CrossRef] [PubMed]

51. Hanawa, N.; Shinohara, M.; Saberi, B.; Gaarde, W.A.; Han, D.; Kaplowitz, N. Role of JNK translocation to mitochondria leading to inhibition of mitochondria bioenergetics in acetaminophen-induced liver injury. *J. Biol. Chem.* **2008**, *283*, 13565–13577. [CrossRef] [PubMed]

52. Gunawan, B.K.; Liu, Z.X.; Han, D.; Hanawa, N.; Gaarde, W.A.; Kaplowitz, N. C-jun n-terminal kinase plays a major role in murine acetaminophen hepatotoxicity. *Gastroenterology* **2006**, *131*, 165–178. [CrossRef] [PubMed]

53. Saito, C.; Lemasters, J.J.; Jaeschke, H. C-jun n-terminal kinase modulates oxidant stress and peroxynitrite formation independent of inducible nitric oxide synthase in acetaminophen hepatotoxicity. *Toxicol. Appl. Pharmacol.* **2010**, *246*, 8–17. [CrossRef] [PubMed]

54. Henderson, N.C.; Pollock, K.J.; Frew, J.; Mackinnon, A.C.; Flavell, R.A.; Davis, R.J.; Sethi, T.; Simpson, K.J. Critical role of c-jun (NH2) terminal kinase in paracetamol-induced acute liver failure. *Gut* **2007**, *56*, 982–990. [CrossRef] [PubMed]

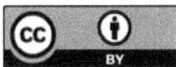

*nutrients*

MDPI

*Article*

# Cuminaldehyde from *Cinnamomum verum* Induces Cell Death through Targeting Topoisomerase 1 and 2 in Human Colorectal Adenocarcinoma COLO 205 Cells

Kuen-daw Tsai [1,2,3], Yi-Heng Liu [1], Ta-Wei Chen [1], Shu-Mei Yang [1,2], Ho-Yiu Wong [1], Jonathan Cherng [4], Kuo-Shen Chou [5] and Jaw-Ming Cherng [6,7,*]

[1] Department of Internal Medicine, China Medical University Beigang Hospital, Yunlin 65152, Taiwan; d4295@yahoo.com.tw (K.-d.T.); yeeheng6061@gmail.com (Y.-H.L.); slowfish1234@yahoo.com.tw (T.-W.C.); kd2624@yahoo.com.tw (S.-M.Y.); pk1977wong@gmail.com (H.-Y.W.)
[2] School of Chinese Medicine, College of Chinese Medicine, China Medical University, Taichung 40402, Taiwan
[3] Institute of Molecular Biology, National Chung Cheng University, Chiayi 62102, Taiwan
[4] Faculty of Medicine, Medical University of Lublin, Lublin 20-059, Poland; jcherngca@yahoo.com.tw
[5] Department of Family Medicine, Saint Mary's Hospital Luodong, Yilan 26546, Taiwan; smh01002@smh.org.tw
[6] Department of Internal Medicine, Saint Mary's Hospital Luodong, Yilan 26546, Taiwan
[7] St. Mary's Junior College of Medicine, Nursing and Management, Yilan 26644, Taiwan
* Correspondence: happy.professor@yahoo.com; Tel.: +886-3-938-8652; Fax: +886-3-957-5653

Received: 14 February 2016; Accepted: 18 May 2016; Published: 24 May 2016

**Abstract:** *Cinnamomum verum*, also called true cinnamon tree, is employed to make the seasoning cinnamon. Furthermore, the plant has been used as a traditional Chinese herbal medication. We explored the anticancer effect of cuminaldehyde, an ingredient of the cortex of the plant, as well as the molecular biomarkers associated with carcinogenesis in human colorectal adenocarcinoma COLO 205 cells. The results show that cuminaldehyde suppressed growth and induced apoptosis, as proved by depletion of the mitochondrial membrane potential, activation of both caspase-3 and -9, and morphological features of apoptosis. Moreover, cuminaldehyde also led to lysosomal vacuolation with an upregulated volume of acidic compartment and cytotoxicity, together with inhibitions of both topoisomerase I and II activities. Additional study shows that the anticancer activity of cuminaldehyde was observed in the model of nude mice. Our results suggest that the anticancer activity of cuminaldehyde *in vitro* involved the suppression of cell proliferative markers, topoisomerase I as well as II, together with increase of pro-apoptotic molecules, associated with upregulated lysosomal vacuolation. On the other hand, *in vivo*, cuminaldehyde diminished the tumor burden that would have a significant clinical impact. Furthermore, similar effects were observed in other tested cell lines. In short, our data suggest that cuminaldehyde could be a drug for chemopreventive or anticancer therapy.

**Keywords:** cuminaldehyde; antiproliferative; topoisomerase I; topoisomerase II; lysosomal vacuolation; xenograft

## 1. Introduction

Colorectal cancer is one of the most common malignancies [1]. Nevertheless, it is not sensitive to conventional chemotherapeutic drugs and there is a need for better management of the disease.

Over the past three decades, various approaches have been used for prevention and treatment of cancer, such as traditional Chinese medicine (TMC). The therapeutic usage described in classic books of Chinese materia medica are still informative even the present-day; for example, *Artemisia annua*. Artemisinin, an ingredient of the plant, was discovered by Tu Youyou, a Chinese scientist, who was awarded half of the 2015 Nobel Prize in Medicine for her discovery of its effect against *Plasmodium falciparum* malaria.

Moreover, contemporary epidemiological and experimental studies have unremittingly suggested a correlation between regularly eating vegetables and fruits and avoidance of lifestyle disorders, including tumors and heart disorders [2,3]. Phytochemicals, e.g., flavonoids and polyphenols of which plants are rich sources, appear to possess desirable characters required for avoiding malignancy and may have great possibility as antiproliferative drugs [4–9]. Indeed, the common seasoning cinnamon is manufactured from the true cinnamon tree. In addition, the plant has been applied for the treatment of dyspepsia, circulatory disorders, and inflammation, such as gastroenteritis [2,3]. Cuminaldehyde, an ingredient of true cinnamon tree's bark, may be the compound that has this effect. Cuminaldehyde exists in the true cinnamon tree in a high concentration, and it is also found in the shoot of *Artemisia salsoloides*, leaf of *Aegle marmelos,* and essential oil from cumin [10]. The chemical is stable, soluble in ethanol, and available commercially. Until now, very little research on cuminaldehyde has been published. Therefore, the current study intended to explore the anticancer activity of cuminaldehyde and clarify its mechanisms in human colorectal adenocarcinoma COLO 205 cells.

Malignancy is a hyperproliferative disease. Various genetic and epigenetic aberrations are needed to convert normal cells into transformed ones. These abnormalities regulate different pathways which collaborate to enable malignant cells endowed with an extensive capabilities needed for proliferating, metastating, and killing their host [11]. Although antiproliferative drugs are possibly able to act through various mechanisms, apoptosis has been shown to be the most common and preferred mechanism through which many anticancer agents kill and eradicate cancer cells [12].

Apoptosis-inducing antiproliferative agents may act by targeting mitochondria. The drugs may alter mitochondria through various mechanisms. They may cause the development of pores on membranes, leading to swelling of mitochondria, or increase membrane permeability, resulting in the discharge of pro-apoptotic cytochrome from the organelle into the cytosolic compartment. Cytochrome *c* interacts with protease activating factor-1 together with deoxyadenosine triphosphate, which then interacts with pro-caspase-9 resulting in the formation of apoptosome. Then the inactive pro-caspase-9 is activated by the formed apoptosome into active caspase-9. Next, the active form caspase-9 acuates caspase-3, resulting in a proteolytic cascade [13–15].

Topoisomerases, enzymes controlling the DNA's topological status, are involved in conserving the integrity of the genome [16]. They relax intertwined DNA by transitory protein-linked breaks of only one (topoisomerase I) or two (topoisomerase II) strands of the double-stranded DNA [17]. Topoisomerase I plays a role in DNA processing by engaging systems of tracking and being involved in conserving the integrity of the genome [16]. Upregulated enzyme's catalytic activity, protein, and mRNA have been demonstrated across human cancers [18]. Indeed, topoisomerase I is involved in the chromosomal instability of colorectal cancer (CRC) and the expression levels of the enzyme has been suggested as prognostic markers [19–21] in CRC. Topoisomerase II is upregulated during cell growth and peaks at G2/M. Topoisomerase II gene copy number is also elevated in CRC and considered as a potential predictive biomarker for anticancer treatment [20]. In addition to cell cycle regulation, the enzyme has been demonstrated to be another main target of antiproliferative agents [22–25]. What is more, apoptotic cell death was shown to be the ultimate effective pathway of death in cancer subsequent to suppression of topoisomerase [26].

This diversification of machineries of carcinogenesis implies that there could be various processes that are crucially objective for avoidance of cancer. In an effort to investigate the activities and latent machineries of cuminaldehyde in human colorectal adenocarcinoma COLO 205 cell, we performed a series of tests to study the effects of cuminaldehyde on growth as well as activities of topoisomerase I and II in human colorectal COLO 205 cells. Our results prove that cuminaldehyde suppressed the activities of both topoisomerase I and II and increased lysosomal vacuolation with upregulated volume of acidic compartment together with cytotoxicity. Lastly, cuminaldehyde induced apoptosis, resulting in the suppression of cell proliferation, *in vitro* as well as *in vivo*.

## 2. Materials and Methods

### 2.1. Materials

We purchased RPMI-1640 and fetal bovine serum (FBS) from GIBCO BRL (Gaithersburg, MD, USA), together with dimethyl sulfoxide and cuminaldehyde from Sigma-Aldrich, Inc. (St. Louis, MO, USA).

### 2.2. Cell Culture

Human colorectal adenocarcinoma COLO 205 cells (American Type Culture Collection CCL-222, American Type Culture Collection, Manassas, VA, USA) were purchased via BCRC (Bioresource Collection and Research Center, Hsinchu, Taiwan) on 27 July 2010 and stored in liquid nitrogen until usage. The cells were incubated in the medium of RPMI-1640, complemented with penicillin 10 U/mL, amphotericin B 0.25 μg/mL, streptomycin 10 μg/mL, and FBS 10% (*v*/*v*) at 37 °C with 5% carbon dioxide.

### 2.3. Cell Viability XTT Test

We incubated the cells in the culture plate with 96 wells at the concentration of ten thousand cells per well. After being incubated for 24 h, we treated the cells with cuminaldehyde at the concentration of 10, 20, 40, 80, or 160 μM for 12, 24, or 48 h. We determined cell viability using the Cell Proliferation Kit II (XTT) (Roche Applied Science, Mannheim, Germany) according to the supplier's instructions. The value of absorbance was evaluated by a spectrophotometer (Tecan infinite M200, Tecan, Männedorf, Switzerland) using 492 nm wavelength with a reference of 650 nm wavelength.

### 2.4. Lactate Dehydrogenase Cytotoxicity Test

We incubated the cells in the culture plate with 96 wells at the concentration of ten thousand cells per well. After being incubated for 24 h, cells were incubated with various cuminaldehyde's concentrations for 48 h. Lactate dehydrogenase's activity was evaluated by LDH-Cytotoxicity Kit (BioVision, Milpitas, CA, USA) according to the supplier's instructions. The samples' absorbance at 490 nm wavelength was evaluated by a spectrophotometer (Tecan infinite M200, Tecan, Männedorf, Switzerland). Data are presented as the percent of activity's variation relative to untreated control.

### 2.5. Test for Nuclear Fragmentation

Nuclear fragmentation test using acridine orange was performed to investigate the possible mechanism of suppressive effect of cuminaldehyde on growth in human colorectal COLO 205 cells. We cultured the cells with various cuminaldehyde concentrations for 48 h and stained the cells with acridine orange (5 μg per mL) at 25 °C. The cells were then examined by the Nikon ECLIPSE T*i* fluorescence microscope [27].

### 2.6. Comet Test

Comet test is an electrophoretic assay and has been employed to study the injury of DNA in eukaryotic cells individually. The assay is comparatively easy to achieve, versatile, and sensitive. The sensitivity' limit is approximately 50 strand breakages per diploid cell. This test was achieved following Olive's alkaline protocol (with 4′,6-diamidino-2-phenylindole staining) [28]. The cells were then observed using the Nikon ECLIPSE T*i* fluorescence microscope with C-FL Epi-Fl Filter Cube and analyzed with automated analytical software (Comet Assay 2.0, Perceptive Instruments, Bury St. Edmunds, UK) following the manufacturer's instructions.

*2.7. Test for Volume of Acidic Compartments*

Increase of the volume of acidic compartment is a general phenomenon of the cells subjected to necrotic or apoptotic death of the cell. Moreover, upregulated volume of the acidic compartment may be an implication of cells that are about to die [29]. To investigate the activities of cuminaldehyde in the cell, the volume of acidic compartment test for lysosomes was achieved as reported formerly [27] with modification. Briefly, human colorectal COLO 205 cells were seeded in 6 cm dishes at the density of $6000/cm^2$ (instead of $6250/cm^2$) 24 h before cuminaldehyde was added. After incubation with cuminaldehyde for another 48 h (instead of 24 h), the cells were washed twice with PBS (phosphate-buffered saline) and incubated for 4 min with 4 mL staining solution. The rest of the experiment was performed similarly. The optical density (OD) at 540 nm of samples was determined by a spectrophotometer (Tecan infinite M200, Tecan, Männedorf, Switzerland). All tests were performed in triplicate.

*2.8. Mitochondrial Membrane Potential Test*

Mitochondrial dysfunction plays a crucial role in the initiation of apoptotic cell death. Actually, the opening of the transition pore creates depolarization of the mitochondrial membrane potential and releasing of apoptogenic factors [30]. To investigate the mitochondria's role of in cuminaldehyde-caused apoptotic cell death, we observed the variations in mitochondrial membrane potential.

The potential of mitochondrial membrane was determined by the reagent JC-1, a mitochondrial-specific fluorescent compound (Invitrogen, Carlsbad, CA, USA.) according to the protocol described previously [31]. The JC-1 reagent is monomer and the mitochondrial membrane potential is less than 120 millivolt. Under such a condition, the dye emits green fluorescence (wavelength of 540 nm) after excitement by blue light (wavelength of 490 nm). In addition, the dye becomes dimmer (J-aggregate) at a mitochondrial membrane potential of more than 180 millivolt and emits red fluorescence (590 nm) after excitation by green light (540 nm). Human colorectal COLO 205 cells were treated with various cuminaldehyde concentrations for 48 h, harvested, and then stained with JC-1 at the concentration of 25 µM at 37 °C for 30 min. Finally, the samples were examined using a spectrophotometer and a fluorescence microscope. Changes in the percentage of red (wavelength of 590-nm)/green (wavelength of 540-nm) fluorescence represent the variations of membrane potential [32].

*2.9. Caspase Activity Test*

Proteins of mitochondrial called SMACs (second mitochondria-derived activator of caspases) are discharged into the cytosolic compartment after the increased membranes' permeability. Then, SMAC interacts with the inhibitor of apoptosis proteins (IAPs), thereby making IAPs inactive, which then abolishes IAPs from inhibiting caspases [33,34] that demolish the cell subsequently.

To farther explore the details in cuminaldehyde-caused apoptotic cell death, the variations in activities of the crucial caspases implicated in apoptotic cell death were determined. The assay is established on the evaluation of the AFC chromophore following division from DEVD- and LEHD-AFC through caspase-3 and -9, respectively. The released AFC emits a yellow-green fluorescence. Human colorectal COLO 205 cells were treated with various concentrations of cuminaldehyde for 48 h and activities of the caspases were measured by Fluorometric Assay Kit (BioVision, Milpitas, CA, USA) according to the supplier's instructions. The light emission was determined by a spectrophotometer (Tecan infinite M200, Tecan, Männedorf, Switzerland). Data are presented as the percent of activity's variation relative to control.

*2.10. Test for Topoisomerase I and II Activities*

Topoisomerase I and II extracts from the cells were prepared according to the methods of TopoGEN (Port Orange, FL, USA). Briefly, cells from two 100 mm dishes were pelleted at $800 \times g$ for 3 min at 4 °C, resuspended in 3 ml of ice cold TEMP buffer (10 mM Tris-HCl, pH 7.5, 1 mM EDTA, 4 mM $MgCl_2$, 0.5 mM PMSF). The sample was then pelleted as described above, resuspended in 3 mL of TEMP and kept on ice for 10 min. The sample was then homogenized using tight fitting homogenizer with eight strokes. Nuclei were pelleted by centrifugation at $1500 \times g$ for 10 min at 4 °C, resuspended in 1 mL of cold TEMP, transferred to a microfuge tube, and pelleted in Microfuge at $1500 \times g$ at 4 °C for 2 min, sequentially. The nuclear pellet was resuspended in a small volume (no more than 4 pellet volumes) of TEP (same as TEMP but lacking $MgCl_2$). An equal volume of 1 M NaCl was added. The sample was then vortexed, kept on ice for 60 min, and centrifuged at $100,000 \times g$ for 1 h at 4 °C. Tests for topoisomerase I as well as II activities were performed according to the methods described by Har-Vardi *et al.* [35].

*2.11. In Vivo Tumor Xenograft Study*

The study has been approved by the Institutional Animal Care and Use Committee (IACUC) of China Medical University that conforms to the provisions of the Declaration of Helsinki (the animal ethical approval number: 97-108-N). Nude mice (male, 6 weeks old, BALB/c Nude) were from the National Science Council Animal Center (Taipei City, Taiwan, Republic of China). The animals were raised under pathogen-free conditions under China Medical University's regulations and ethical guidelines for the use and care of laboratory animals. Human colorectal COLO 205 cells ($5 \times 10^6$ cells in 200 µL of culture medium) were subcutaneously injected into the mice's flanks. Treatment was started when the tumors reached about 75 mm$^3$. Thirty-two mice were divided randomly into four groups (eight mice/group). Cuminaldehyde-treated mice received intratumoral injection of 5, 10, or 20 mg/kg/day of cuminaldehyde in a 200 µL volume (the solutions were prepared from stock solution of cuminaldehyde in dimethyl sulfoxide and diluted into appropriate concentrations in PBS) daily. The mice in the control group were treated with an equal volume of vehicle. After transplantation, body weight as well as tumor size were monitored at weekly intervals. Tumor size was measured using calipers, and tumor volume was calculated using the hemiellipsoid model formula (1):

$$\text{tumor volume} = 1/2(4\pi/3) \times (l/2) \times (w/2) \times h \tag{1}$$

where $l$ = length, $w$ = width, and $h$ = height.

Specimens (tumor masses) at the end of the experiment (42 days after the treatment) were investigated by terminal deoxynucleotidyl transferase dUTP nick end labeling test using the Quick Apoptotic DNA Ladder Detection Kit (Chemicon, Temecuba, CA, USA) according to the supplier's instructions.

*2.12. Statistical Analysis*

Results are presented by means plus/minus standard error. The statistical significance was determined by ANOVA (one-way analysis of variance), followed by the Bonferroni *t*-test for multiple comparisons. A *p* value lower than 0.05 was regarded as statistically significant.

## 3. Results

*3.1. Cuminaldehyde's Effects on Cell Morphological Changes*

When human colorectal COLO 205 cells were incubated with 20 µM of cuminaldehyde for 48 h, blebbing of the plasma membrane was found. In addition, cell shrinkage and cell detachment also occurred (Figure 1C).

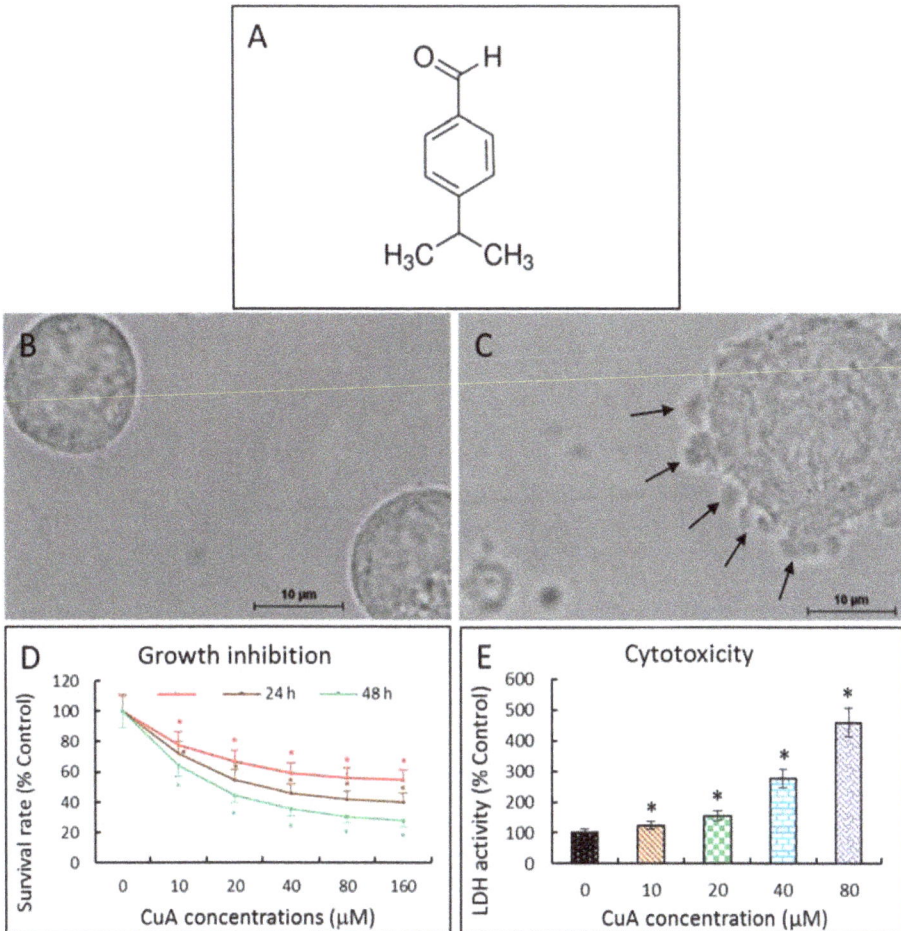

**Figure 1.** Cuminaldehyde's chemical structure and effects on cellular morphology, proliferation, as well as lactate dehydrogenase releasing in human colorectal COLO 205 cells. (**A**) Chemical structure; (**B**) and (**C**) Cuminaldehyde's effect on cellular morphology; Cells were treated without (**B**) and with 20 μM (**C**) cuminaldehyde for 48 h. Cell detachment, shrinkage, and blebbing of plasma membrane (arrows) were found when the cells were incubated with 20 μM of cuminaldehyde; (**D**) Cuminaldehyde's effect on growth. Human colorectal COLO 205 cells were treated with cuminaldehyde at the specified circumstances. Proliferation suppressive effect was determined using the XTT test; (**E**) Cuminaldehyde's effect on the lactate dehydrogenase releasing in the cells. The supernatant was gathered after 48 h of incubation with the indicated cuminaldehyde concentrations. Absorptions of light were determined by a spectrophotometer (Tecan infinite M200, Tecan, Männedorf, Switzerland). Results are shown by means plus/minus standard error of the mean, *n* equal to 3. *, Statistically significant ($p$ less than 0.05) from the control group. CuA, cuminaldehyde.

## 3.2. Cuminaldehyde Inhibited Human Colorectal COLO 205 Cell Proliferation

Different methods have been used for quantifying cell growth; for instance, DNA synthesis as well as metabolic activity. Although radioactive labelling of synthesized DNA is the most accurate assay for DNA quantification, the disadvantages of this assay are the hazards and hassle of using radioactivity. An alternative method quantifying growth is the metabolic activity. The assay is established on the cleavage of a salt (the tetrazolium, e.g., XTT and MTT) into formazan by cell's dehydrogenases which then modifies culture medium's color. This assay is easier, faster, and does not require the use of radioactive materials.

We investigated cuminaldehyde's potential cell proliferation inhibitory activity in human colorectal COLO 205 cells by the XTT test. As demonstrated in Figure 1D, cuminaldehyde inhibited cell proliferation in a dose- as well as time-dependent manner. The $IC_{50}$ value following 48 h of treatment was 16.31 μM.

### 3.3. Cuminaldehyde Caused Cytotoxicity in Human Colorectal COLO 205 Cells

The first morphological evidence of apoptotic phenomenon is retraction of the cell, loss of adherence, followed by convolution of cytoplasm and membrane of the plasma, together with blebbing. Finally, the cell disintegrated into small particles called apoptotic bodies, leading to the release of the cell's content into the bathing medium [36]. One way of studying loss of integrity of the membrane is determining the releasing of enzyme lactate dehydrogenase into the supernatant medium [37]. The assay was initially employed to test cellular death developed through necrosis [38]. Then, the assay was shown to accurately quantify apoptosis [39–41].

Cuminaldehyde was cytotoxic, as proved by the elevation of lactate dehydrogenase activity in the bathing medium (Figure 1E).

### 3.4. Cuminaldehyde Caused Nuclear Fragmentation In Human Colorectal COLO 205 Cells

Apoptosis is the most frequent and preferred mechanism through which various anticancer drugs kill cancer cells [12]. Moreover, apoptosis also has been shown to be the major machinery of the death of cancer caused by several polyphenols [42–45]. In the nucleus, apoptosis is characterized by endonuclease activation, resulting in cleavage of nucleic acid into fragments.

Acridine orange is a dye with nucleic acid-selective metachromatic characteristic and valuable for quantifying apoptosis, determinations of cell cycle, proton-pump activity, and pH gradients [46]. When acridine orange inserts into double-stranded DNA, it fluoresces green. In addition, when interacting with RNA or single-stranded DNA, acridine orange fluoresces orange. Apoptotic cells which contain a high fraction of the nucleic acid in the denatured status exhibit an orange fluorescence along with a diminished green one relative to interphase non-apoptotic cells. In addition, when acridine orange are in an acidic environment (e.g., cellular lysosomes), the dye becomes protonated as well as sequestered. Under such an acidic environment, when excited by the blue light, the dye fluoresces orange [47]. The test of nuclear fragmentation is established on acridine orange's characters and examined microscopically.

When human colorectal COLO 205 cells were treated with cuminaldehyde at the concentration of 20 μM for 48 h, the result of staining using acridine orange demonstrated that COLO cells demised partially through apoptosis, along with fragmentation and nuclear condensation. In addition, orange-stained lysosomal vacuoles were observed. On the other hand, no significant chromosomal fragmentation was found in the control group (Figure 2A).

DNA strand breakage was also explored using the comet test after treatment with various cuminaldehyde concentrations. As demonstrated in Figure 2C,D, treatment with cuminaldehyde led to increased tail intensity as well as moment.

Given that nuclear condensation, fragmentation, blebbing of the plasma membrane and the formation of apoptotic body are apoptosis's morphologic characteristics [48], the morphological changes observed in the study prove that treatment with cuminaldehyde did lead to apoptosis in human colorectal COLO 205 cells (Figures 1C and 2B).

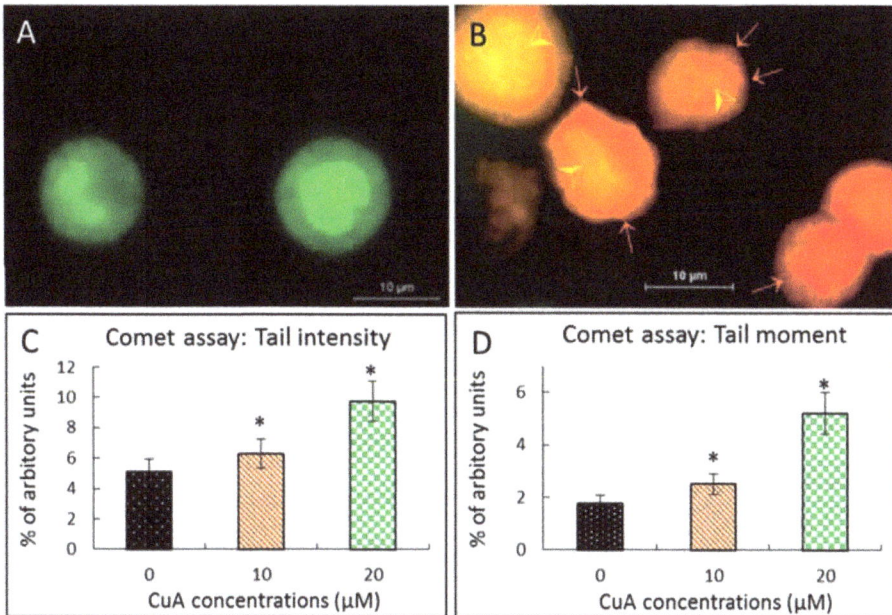

**Figure 2.** Cuminaldehyde caused nuclear fragmentation in human colorectal COLO 205 cells. (**A** and **B**) Acridine orange staining; COLO 205 cells were incubated without (**A**) with 20 μM (**B**) cuminaldehyde, respectively, for 48 h, then stained using acridine orange. The orange vacuoles in COLO cells demonstrate that they existed acidic; (**A**) Typical picture of control cells accompanying intact nucleus with green fluorescence that implicates a good cell viability; (**B**) Typical picture of test cells incubated with cuminaldehyde with lysosomal vacuolation (arrows) and nuclear fragmentation (arrow heads) were found; (**C** and **D**) Comet test. Cuminaldehyde's effect on intensities of tail (**C**) as well as moment (**D**). Human colorectal COLO 205 cells were incubated with cuminaldehyde at the indicated concentrations for 48 h. Data are shown as means plus/minus standard error of the mean, $n = 125$. *, Significant difference ($p < 0.05$) from the control. CuA, cuminaldehyde.

*3.5. Cuminaldehyde Increased Volume of Acidic Compartment in Human Colorectal COLO 205 Cells*

Neutral Red has been used to stain lysosomes and quantify the volume of acidic compartment in cells [27,49,50]. As demonstrated in Figure 3A,B, positive neutral red staining suggests that incubation with cuminaldehyde resulted in acidic vacuoles in human colorectal COLO 205 cells. Moreover, Figure 3C shows that the treatment increased the volume of the acidic compartment in a quantity-dependent manner in the cells.

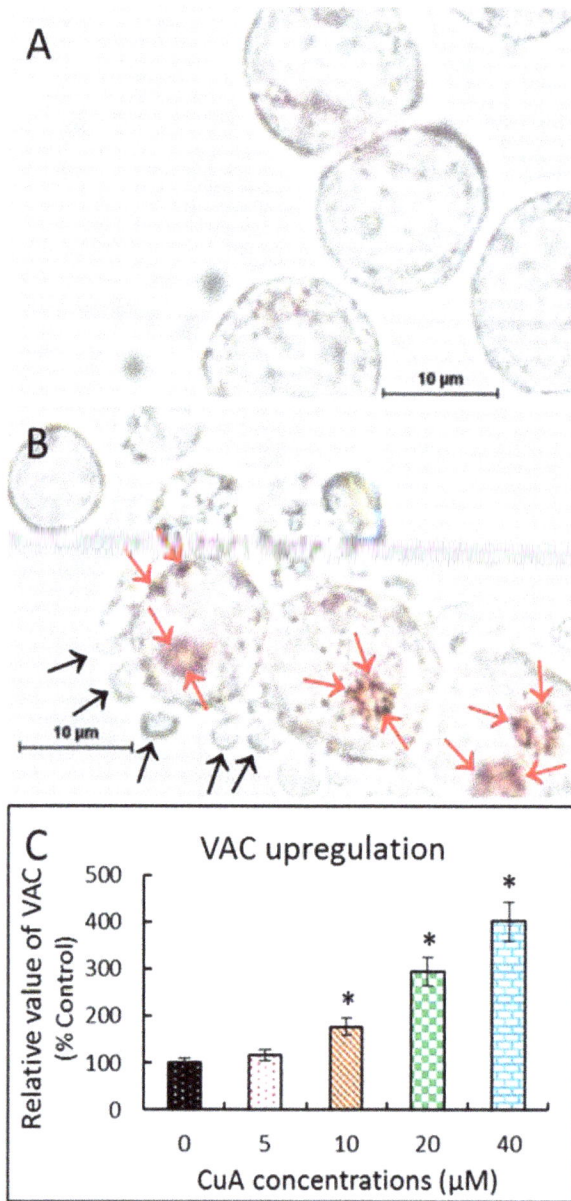

**Figure 3.** Cuminaldehyde increased the volume of the acidic compartment in human colorectal COLO 205 cells. After treatment without and with 20 μM cuminaldehyde, respectively, for 48 h, human colorectal COLO 205 cells were stained using neutral red. (**A**) Human colorectal COLO 205 cells without treatment: There were no observable vacuoles in the cell; (**B**) Human colorectal COLO 205 cells treated with cuminaldehyde at the concentration of 20 μM for 48 h. The blebbing (black arrows) and acidic red-stained vacuoles (red arrows) in cells happened; (**C**) Cuminaldehyde increased volume of acidic compartment in a quantity-dependent manner. After treating the cells using the specified concentrations of cuminaldehyde for 48 h, results were evaluated by a spectrophotometer. Results are shown by means plus/minus standard error of the mean, *n* equal to 3. *, Statistically significant (*p* less than 0.05) from the control group. CuA, cuminaldehyde.

### 3.6. Cuminaldehyde Caused Apoptosis via the Mitochondrial Pathway in Human Colorectal COLO 205 Cells

We then investigated the mitochondria's role of in the cuminaldehyde-caused apoptosis in human colorectal COLO 205 cells. Initial apoptotic cell death frequently involves mitochondrial depolarization, followed by releasing of mitochondrial apoptogenic molecules into cytosol. Therefore, we explored mitochondrial dysfunction by determining mitochondrial membrane potential in cuminaldehyde-treated human colorectal COLO 205 cells using the mitochondria-specific dye JC-1 with a spectrophotometer. Figure 4A shows that cuminaldehyde caused the loss of mitochondrial membrane potential, as suggested by downregulation of mitochondrial membrane potential in a quantity-dependent manner.

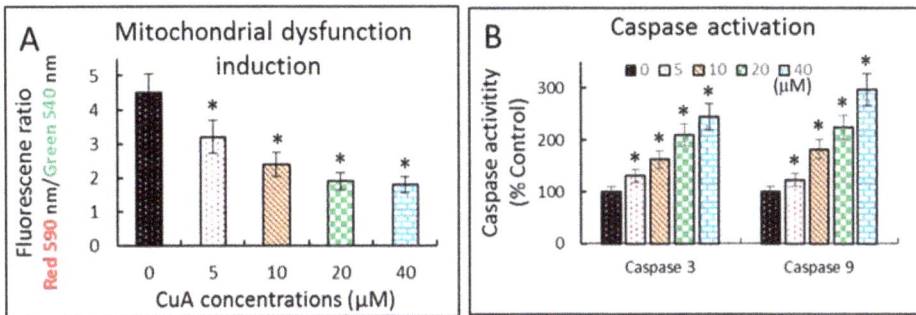

**Figure 4.** Cuminaldehyde caused apoptosis via the mitochondrial pathway in human colorectal COLO 205 cells. (**A**) Cells were treated with the specified cuminaldehyde concentrations for 48 h and mitochondrial membrane potential was evaluated using JC-1 spectrophotometrically; (**B**) Activations of caspase-3 as well as -9. After treating the cells using the specified concentrations of cuminaldehyde for 48 h, activities of caspases-3 and -9 were determined using a spectrophotometer. Results are expressed by means plus/minus standard error of the mean, *n* equal to 3. \*, Statistically significant (*p* less than 0.05) from the control group. CuA, cuminaldehyde.

Caspases are cysteine proteases that play critical roles in apoptosis. Figure 4B shows that the activities of caspase-3 and -9 elevated in a quantity-dependent manner in cuminaldehyde-treated human colorectal COLO 205 cells.

### 3.7. Cuminaldehyde Suppressed Topoisomerase I Activity in Human Colorectal COLO 205 Cells

The effect of cuminaldehyde on activity of topoisomerase I in human colorectal COLO 205 cells was performed with increasing cuminaldehyde concentration (Figure 5A, lane 3–5) or camptothecin (a known specific suppressor of type I topoisomerase and used as a positive control, lane 6) [51]. Figure 5A shows the transformation of the intertwined plasmid pUC 19 into the unrestrained form declined in a quantity-dependent manner under the existence of cuminaldehyde or camptothecin (please correlate lane 3–6 to lane 2). These data suggest that cuminaldehyde suppressed the DNA loosening activity topoisomerase I the human colorectal COLO 205 cell nuclear proteins.

Topoisomerase inhibition

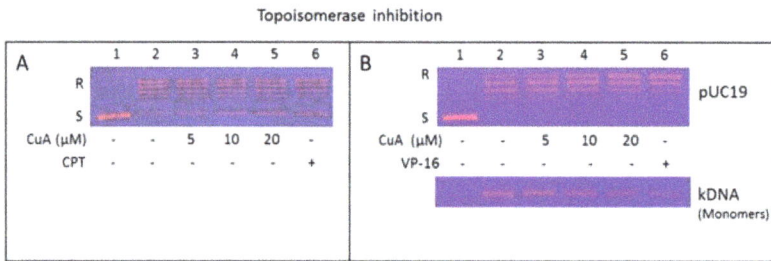

**Figure 5.** Cuminaldehyde inhibited topoisomerase I as well as II activities in human colorectal COLO 205 cells. (**A**) Cuminaldehyde inhibited topoisomerase I activity. Nuclear proteins of COLO 205 cells interacted with the indicated cuminaldehyde concentrations in a topoisomerase I's specific reaction mixture (lanes 3–5), or 60 µM of camptothecin (CPT, a specific topoisomerase I inhibitor and used as positive control, lane 6), or the vehicle (1% dimethyl sulfoxide, lane 2). Lane 1, pUC19 DNA only; (**B**) Cuminaldehyde inhibited topoisomerase II activity. DNA relaxation test (upper panel) and decatenation test (lower panel). Nuclear proteins of COLO 205 cells were added to a specific topoisomerase II reaction mixture with the specified cuminaldehyde concentrations (lanes 3–5) or 60 µM of camptothecin (a specific suppressor of topoisomerase II and used as positive control, lane 6), or the vehicle (one percent dimethyl sulfoxide, lane 2). Lane 1, Interwined pUC 19 DNA (upper panel) or kinetoplast DNA (lower panel) only. kinetoplast DNA is an extensive chain of plasmids. When kinetoplast DNA is examined using electrophoretic analysis, it gets the gel only a lightly (figure not demonstrated). Consequent to topoisomerase II's decatenation, small monomeric circles of nucleic acid were produced (lower panel, lane 2–6). This is the representative of six experiments. CPT, camptothecin; CuA, cuminaldehyde; kDNA, kinetoplast; S & R, Interwined and the unrestrained forms of the pUC 19 plasmid, respectively; VP-16, etoposide.

## 3.8. Cuminaldehyde Suppressed Activity of Topoisomerase II in Human Colorectal COLO 205 Cells

The effect of cuminaldehyde on topoisomerase II activity in human colorectal COLO 205 cells was investigated using increasing concentration of cuminaldehyde (Figure 5B, lane 3–5) or etoposide (a known inhibitor of topoisomerase II and used as a positive control, lane 6) [52]. Figure 5B, upper panel, shows transformation of the interwined plasmid pUC 19 into the unrestrained form declined in a quantity-dependent manner under the existence of cuminaldehyde or etoposide (please correlate lane 3–6 to lane 2). The data suggest that cuminaldehyde suppressed DNA relaxation activity of topoisomerase II in the human colorectal COLO 205 cell nuclear proteins. In addition, this effect was further evaluated using the decatenation test. The decatenation effect involves the releasing of mini circular DNA (monomers) from the kinetoplast, an extensive chain of plasmids. Nuclear proteins in human colorectal COLO 205 cells enclosed type II topoisomerase that transformed kinetoplast to monomeric DNA (Figure 5B, lower panel, please correlate lane 2 to lane 1). The transformation of kinetoplast into monomeric DNA declined in a quantity-dependent manner under the existence of cuminaldehyde (please correlate lane 3–5 to lane 2) or etoposide (please correlate lane 6 to lane 2). The data suggest cuminaldehyde suppressed the topoisomerase II's decatenation activity in the human colorectal COLO 205 cell nuclear proteins.

## 3.9. Cuminaldehyde Suppressed Growth of Human Colorectal COLO 205 Xenograft in a Nude Mice Model

To investigate if cuminaldehyde suppresses proliferation of the human colorectal COLO 205 xenograft, $5 \times 10^6$ human colorectal COLO 205 cells in 200 µL of culture medium were used for subcutaneous injection. Figure 6A, left panel, shows that, in comparison with tumors of control mice (orange arrows), obvious tumor burden reduction was found in the tumors of the mice injected with 20 mg/kg/day of cuminaldehyde (blue arrows). Tumor growth inhibition was found in all groups with cuminaldehyde injection (5, 10, and 20 mg/kg/day of cuminaldehyde, respectively). On the other hand, significant growth inhibition was observed only in mice injected with 10 and 20 mg/kg/day of cuminaldehyde, where about 48.9% and 69.4%, respectively, decreases in tumor volume were found (Figure 6B,C). None of the cuminaldehyde injections resulted in any significant decrease in body weight and/or diet consumption relative to the control group. The mechanism of cuminaldehyde's antiproliferative effect *in vivo* was explored. We gathered the human colorectal COLO 205 xenograft from vehicle and cuminaldehyde-treated mice, then investigated the cause of the death by the terminal deoxynucleotidyl transferase dUTP nick end labeling assay. Figure 6A, right panel, demonstrates that, in comparison with tumors of control mice (white arrows), elevated terminal deoxynucleotidyl transferase dUTP nick end labeling-positive cells that suggest apoptotic death were found in the cancers of the cuminaldehyde-injected mice (yellow arrows).

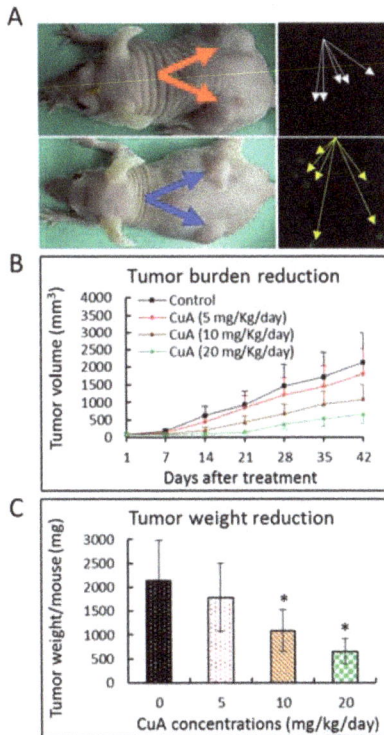

**Figure 6.** Cuminaldehyde suppressed growth and caused apoptosis in human colorectal COLO 205 xenograft. The mice with pre-established cancers (*n* = 8 per group) were treated using intratumoral injection with the specified cuminaldehyde concentrations. Tumor volumes were recorded by calipers and apoptosis was evaluated by terminal deoxynucleotidyl transferase dUTP nick end labeling test. (**A**) Left panel, Representative of tumor-bearing mice from the control (orange arrows) and 20 mg/kg/day of cuminaldehyde-injected (blue arrows) groups; (**A**) Right panel, cuminaldehyde caused apoptosis in human colorectal COLO 205 xenograft using terminal deoxynucleotidyl transferase dUTP nick end labeling test. Representative of terminal deoxynucleotidyl transferase dUTP nick end labeling test of tumors from the control (white arrows) and 20 mg/kg/day of cuminaldehyde-injected (yellow arrows) groups; (**B**) Mean of tumor volume observed at the specified number of days after the start of treatment; (**C**) Cuminaldehyde's effects on tumor weight observed at the endpoint of the experiment. Tumor weight per mouse was collected and analyzed. Results are shown by means plus/minus standard error of the mean, *n* = 8. *, Statistically significant (*p* less than 0.05) from the control group. CuA, cuminaldehyde.

## 4. Discussion

In addition to providing taste and flavor to foods, certain spices have been used as remedies in traditional medicine [53]. True cinnamon tree is used to manufacture the seasoning cinnamon and has been used for more than 5000 years by both of the two most ancient forms of medicine in the words: Ayurveda and traditional Chinese herbal medicines for various applications such as adenopathy, rheumatism, dermatosis, dyspepsia, stroke, tumors, elephantiasis, trichomonas, yeast, and virus infections [54]. Cuminaldehyde, an ingredient of the cortex of the plant, possesses various activities, including: (i) suppressions of melanin formation (through inhibiting the oxidation of L-3,4-dihydroxyphenylalanine catalyzed by tyrosinase) [55], lipoxygenase [56], aldose reductase, α-glucosidase [57], alpha-synuclein fibrillation (possibly by the interaction with amine groups through cuminaldehyde's aldehyde group as a Schiff base reaction) [58]; and (ii) insulinotropic and β-cell protective action (through the closure of the ATP-sensitive K channel and the increase in intracellular $Ca^{2+}$ concentration) [59].

Although cuminaldehyde exists in true cinnamon tree in a high concentration (100 PPM), it is also found in the shoot of *Artemisia salsoloides* (1000 PPM), leaf of *Aegle marmelos* (300 PPM), and essential oil from cumin [10]. Essential oil from cumin with the major constituents of cuminaldehyde, cymene, and terpenoids has been reported to possess: (i) antibacterial, antifungal, and insecticidal [60] activities; (ii) antioxidant capacity; (iii) anticancer activity [61,62] with glutathione-*S*-transferase activating, β-glucuronidase and mucinase inhibiting properties [60].

In this research, we initially explored the effects of cuminaldehyde on the proliferation of human colorectal COLO 205 cells. We observed that cuminaldehyde suppressed the growth of human colorectal COLO 205 cells in a concentration- as well as time-dependent manner (Figure 1D). Although cells may die through necrotic or other mechanisms, apoptosis is the preferred and most common mechanism through which different anticancer drugs kill as well as remove cancer cells [12]. Moreover, apoptosis was demonstrated to be the main machinery of tumor cell demise caused by several polyphenols [42–45].

Our data demonstrate that cuminaldehyde caused apoptotic cell death, as suggested by loss of mitochondrial membrane potential, increase of caspase-3 and -9 (Figure 4), along with morphological features of apoptosis, including apoptotic body formation, fragmentation, and nuclear condensation as demonstrated in different stainings as well as comet assay (Figures 1–3).

Our data also suggest that cuminaldehyde generated vacuolation associated increased volume of the acidic compartment. Increase of volume of the acidic compartment has been demonstrated to be an ordinary event observed in cells that are subjected to apoptotic or necrotic cell demise and could be an indication of failing cells [29]. Because apoptotic cell death is an ordered process, an upregulated volume of acidic compartment could cause the self-digestion in the course of cell death [29].

In addition to cell cycle control, topoisomerase has been demonstrated to be another main target of anticancer drugs [22–25]. The chemotherapeutic agent etoposide kills tumor cells by stabilizing the transient intermediate division complex. The resulting accumulation of division complexes may lead to the development of permanent DNA strand divisions that fragment the chromosome leading to the stimulation of death pathways [63]. Furthermore, apoptosis has been demonstrated to be the most efficient death-pathway in cancer cells subsequent to the suppression of topoisomerase II [26]. Clinically, topoisomerase has been suggested as a potential predictive biomarker in CRC [20,64]. Topoisomerase I seems to be involved in the chromosomal instability pathway of sporadic CRC [21] and high frequency of gene gain of the topoisomerase I and II genes in CRC [20,65]. CRC patients with low topoisomerase I expression were statistically favorably associated with overall survival [19].

Our findings prove that cuminaldehyde inhibited activities of topoisomerase I and II in a quantity-dependent manner (Figure 5), which, in part, could be a machinery causing the cells to move toward apoptosis. Although most of inhibitors of topoisomerase are specifically targeting either type I or II topoisomerase [66], our results clearly show that cuminaldehyde inhibited activities of topoisomerase I along with II in human colorectal COLO 205 cells.

Our results clearly demonstrated that cuminaldehyde possesses antiproliferative activity in human colorectal COLO 205 cells. Furthermore, cuminaldehyde thiosemicarbazone has been shown to possess antiproliferative with anti-topoisomerase II activity in U937 cells [67]. However, some other tumor cell lines did not show the same negative effect of the plant extracts containing cuminaldehyde on cell proliferation [58]. Possible explanation for these contradictory phenomena could be the extracts also possess antioxidant [61] and/or other activities. Therefore, further research is needed to clarify the specific latent mechanisms of the suppression, possible mutagenic effects, as well as other side effects for clinical usage of cuminaldehyde as an anticancer and/or chemopreventive drug against human colorectal adenocarcinoma and/or other malignancies.

Treatment-associated cytotoxicity and other side effects of antiproliferative drugs are the main concerns of anticancer therapy. Consequently, the perfect anticancer agent would discriminatorily destroy malignant cells but not the healthy ones. Our results show that none of the therapy with cuminaldehyde caused any observable decline in body weight or consumption of diet relative to the control mice. Our data present persuasive evidence of the protecting activity of cuminaldehyde against human colorectal COLO 205 xenograft growth in the current study using nude mice model without any detectable side effect; this implies that cuminaldehyde has an antiproliferative effect in human colorectal COLO 205 cells and this agent may potentially serve as an anticancer and/or chemopreventive drug.

## 5. Conclusions

Collectively, our data clearly suggest that the antiproliferative effect of cuminaldehyde in human colorectal COLO 205 cells *in vitro* involved inhibition of cell growth markers, topoisomerase I and II, together with upregulation of proapoptotic molecules, associated with increased lysosomal vacuolation. *In vivo*, cuminaldehyde diminished the tumor burden and may have significant clinical impact.

The present study provides fundamental knowledge on the cancer inhibitory activity of cuminaldehyde in human colorectal COLO 205 cells that implicates a model for the exploration of possible antiproliferative drugs against human colorectal adenocarcinoma. Indeed, similar effects were observed in other tested cell lines, including human hepatocellular carcinoma SK-Hep-1 and Hep 3B, lung squamous cell carcinoma NCI-H520 and adenocarcinoma A549, and T-lymphoblastic MOLT-3. Our results present a rationalization for further developing cuminaldehyde as an effective and safe anticancer and/or chemopreventive drug. A future direction would be to synthesize the derivatives of cuminaldehyde and examine the protective effects of cuminaldehyde and their derivatives *in vitro*. We would then extend the study to examine the effects of these agents in a mouse model and use these systems for new drug design and discovery based on parental compound cuminaldehyde as a lead for safer and potent chemopreventive and/or anticancer usage.

**Acknowledgments:** We thank Alice Y. Yu for her excellent technical assistance. This work was supported by grants from St. Mary's Hospital Luodong (grant # SMHRF104001) and China Medical University Beigang Hospital (grant # CMUBH R103-002 and CMUBH R103-006).

**Author Contributions:** Jaw-Ming Cherng and Kuen-daw Tsai conceived and designed the study; Jonathan Cherng, Yi-Heng Liu, and Ta-Wei Chen performed the experiment; Shu-mei Yang and Ho-Yiu Wong analyzed the data and evaluated the literature. All authors have contributed to the interpretation of results and the writing of the manuscript.

**Conflicts of Interest:** The authors declare no conflict of interest.

## References

1. Tanzer, M.; Liebl, M.; Quante, M. Molecular biomarkers in esophageal, gastric, and colorectal adenocarcinoma. *Pharmacol. Ther.* **2013**, *140*, 133–147. [CrossRef] [PubMed]
2. Tanaka, S.; Yoon, Y.H.; Fukui, H.; Tabata, M.; Akira, T.; Okano, K.; Iwai, M.; Iga, Y.; Yokoyama, K. Antiulcerogenic compounds isolated from chinese cinnamon. *Planta Medica* **1989**, *55*, 245–248. [CrossRef] [PubMed]

3. Reddy, A.M.; Seo, J.H.; Ryu, S.Y.; Kim, Y.S.; Kim, Y.S.; Min, K.R.; Kim, Y. Cinnamaldehyde and 2-methoxycinnamaldehyde as NF-κB inhibitors from *Cinnamomum cassia*. *Planta Medica* **2004**, *70*, 823–827. [CrossRef] [PubMed]

4. Shukla, S.; Meeran, S.M.; Katiyar, S.K. Epigenetic regulation by selected dietary phytochemicals in cancer chemoprevention. *Cancer Lett.* **2014**, *355*, 9–17. [CrossRef] [PubMed]

5. Priyadarsini, R.V.; Nagini, S. Cancer chemoprevention by dietary phytochemicals: Promises and pitfalls. *Curr. Pharm. Biotechnol.* **2012**, *13*, 125–136. [CrossRef] [PubMed]

6. Surh, Y.J. Cancer chemoprevention with dietary phytochemicals. *Nat. Rev. Cancer* **2003**, *3*, 768–780. [CrossRef] [PubMed]

7. Yang, C.S.; Landau, J.M.; Huang, M.T.; Newmark, H.L. Inhibition of carcinogenesis by dietary polyphenolic compounds. *Annu. Rev. Nutr.* **2001**, *21*, 381–406. [CrossRef] [PubMed]

8. Watson, W.H.; Cai, J.; Jones, D.P. Diet and apoptosis. *Annu. Rev. Nutr.* **2000**, *20*, 485–505. [CrossRef] [PubMed]

9. Middleton, E., Jr.; Kandaswami, C.; Theoharides, T.C. The effects of plant flavonoids on mammalian cells: Implications for inflammation, heart disease, and cancer. *Pharmacol. Rev.* **2000**, *52*, 673–751. [PubMed]

10. Duke, J.A. Dr. Duke's Phytochemical and Ethnobotanical Databases. Available online: https://phytochem. nal.usda.gov/phytochem/chemicals/show/6429?et=C (accessed on 21 May 2016).

11. Artandi, S.E.; DePinho, R.A. Telomeres and telomerase in cancer. *Carcinogenesis* **2010**, *31*, 9–18. [CrossRef] [PubMed]

12. Aleo, E.; Henderson, C.J.; Fontanini, A.; Solazzo, B.; Brancolini, C. Identification of new compounds that trigger apoptosome-independent caspase activation and apoptosis. *Cancer Res.* **2006**, *66*, 9235–9244. [CrossRef] [PubMed]

13. Pop, C.; Timmer, J.; Sperandio, S.; Salvesen, G.S. The apoptosome activates caspase-9 by dimerization. *Mol. Cell* **2006**, *22*, 269–275. [CrossRef] [PubMed]

14. Zou, H.; Henzel, W.J.; Liu, X.; Lutschg, A.; Wang, X. Apaf-1, a human protein homologous to C. elegans CED-4, participates in cytochrome c-dependent activation of caspase-3. *Cell* **1997**, *90*, 405–413. [CrossRef]

15. Li, P.; Nijhawan, D.; Budihardjo, I.; Srinivasula, S.M.; Ahmad, M.; Alnemri, E.S.; Wang, X. Cytochrome c and dATP-dependent formation of Apaf-1/caspase-9 complex initiates an apoptotic protease cascade. *Cell* **1997**, *91*, 479–489. [CrossRef]

16. McClendon, A.K.; Osheroff, N. DNA topoisomerase II, genotoxicity, and cancer. *Mutat. Res.* **2007**, *623*, 83–97. [CrossRef] [PubMed]

17. Heck, M.M.; Earnshaw, W.C. Topoisomerase II: A specific marker for cell proliferation. *J. Cell Biol.* **1986**, *103*, 2569–2581. [CrossRef] [PubMed]

18. Husain, I.; Mohler, J.L.; Seigler, H.F.; Besterman, J.M. Elevation of topoisomerase I messenger RNA, protein, and catalytic activity in human tumors: Demonstration of tumor-type specificity and implications for cancer chemotherapy. *Cancer Res.* **1994**, *54*, 539–546. [PubMed]

19. Negri, F.V.; Azzoni, C.; Bottarelli, L.; Campanini, N.; Mandolesi, A.; Wotherspoon, A.; Cunningham, D.; Scartozzi, M.; Cascinu, S.; Tinelli, C.; *et al.* Thymidylate synthase, topoisomerase-1 and microsatellite instability: Relationship with outcome in mucinous colorectal cancer treated with fluorouracil. *Anticancer Res.* **2013**, *33*, 4611–4617. [PubMed]

20. Sonderstrup, I.M.; Nygard, S.B.; Poulsen, T.S.; Linnemann, D.; Stenvang, J.; Nielsen, H.J.; Bartek, J.; Brunner, N.; Norgaard, P.; Riis, L. Topoisomerase-1 and -2A gene copy numbers are elevated in mismatch repair-proficient colorectal cancers. *Mol. Oncol.* **2015**, *9*, 1207–1217. [CrossRef] [PubMed]

21. Azzoni, C.; Bottarelli, L.; Cecchini, S.; Ziccarelli, A.; Campanini, N.; Bordi, C.; Sarli, L.; Silini, E.M. Role of topoisomerase I and thymidylate synthase expression in sporadic colorectal cancer: Associations with clinicopathological and molecular features. *Pathol. Res. Pract.* **2014**, *210*, 111–117. [CrossRef] [PubMed]

22. Naowaratwattana, W.; De-Eknamkul, W.; De Mejia, E.G. Phenolic-containing organic extracts of mulberry (*Morus alba* L.) leaves inhibit HepG2 hepatoma cells through G2/M phase arrest, induction of apoptosis, and inhibition of topoisomerase IIα activity. *J. Med. Food* **2010**, *13*, 1045–1056. [CrossRef] [PubMed]

23. Baikar, S.; Malpathak, N. Secondary metabolites as DNA topoisomerase inhibitors: A new era towards designing of anticancer drugs. *Pharmacogn. Rev.* **2010**, *4*, 12–26. [PubMed]

24. Bandele, O.J.; Clawson, S.J.; Osheroff, N. Dietary polyphenols as topoisomerase II poisons: B ring and C ring substituents determine the mechanism of enzyme-mediated DNA cleavage enhancement. *Chem. Res. Toxicol.* **2008**, *21*, 1253–1260. [CrossRef] [PubMed]

25. Sudan, S.; Rupasinghe, H.P. Flavonoid-enriched apple fraction AF4 induces cell cycle arrest, DNA topoisomerase II inhibition, and apoptosis in human liver cancer HepG2 cells. *Nutr. Cancer* **2014**, *66*, 1237–1246. [CrossRef] [PubMed]

26. El-Awady, R.A.; Ali, M.M.; Saleh, E.M.; Ghaleb, F.M. Apoptosis is the most efficient death-pathway in tumor cells after topoisomerase II inhibition. *Saudi Med. J.* **2008**, *29*, 558–564. [PubMed]

27. Fan, C.; Wang, W.; Zhao, B.; Zhang, S.; Miao, J. Chloroquine inhibits cell growth and induces cell death in A549 lung cancer cells. *Bioorg. Med. Chem.* **2006**, *14*, 3218–3222. [CrossRef] [PubMed]

28. Olive, P.L.; Banath, J.P. The comet assay: A method to measure DNA damage in individual cells. *Nat. Protoc.* **2006**, *1*, 23–29. [CrossRef] [PubMed]

29. Ono, K.; Wang, X.; Han, J. Resistance to tumor necrosis factor-induced cell death mediated by PMCA4 deficiency. *Mol. Cell Biol.* **2001**, *21*, 8276–8288. [CrossRef] [PubMed]

30. Ly, J.D.; Grubb, D.R.; Lawen, A. The mitochondrial membrane potential ($\Delta\psi$m) in apoptosis; an update. *Apoptosis* **2003**, *8*, 115–128. [CrossRef] [PubMed]

31. Reers, M.; Smiley, S.T.; Mottola-Hartshorn, C.; Chen, A.; Lin, M.; Chen, L.B. Mitochondrial membrane potential monitored by JC-1 dye. *Methods Enzymol.* **1995**, *260*, 406–417. [PubMed]

32. Martin, E.J.; Forkert, P.G. Evidence that 1,1-dichloroethylene induces apoptotic cell death in murine liver. *J. Pharmacol. Exp. Ther.* **2004**, *310*, 33–42. [CrossRef] [PubMed]

33. Fesik, S.W.; Shi, Y. Controlling the caspases. *Science* **2001**, *294*, 1477–1478. [CrossRef] [PubMed]

34. Deveraux, Q.L.; Reed, J.C. Iap family proteins—Suppressors of apoptosis. *Genes Dev.* **1999**, *13*, 239–252. [CrossRef] [PubMed]

35. Har-Vardi, I.; Mali, R.; Breiteman, M.; Sonin, Y.; Albotiano, S.; Levitas, E.; Potashnik, G.; Priel, E. DNA topoisomerases I and II in human mature sperm cells: Characterization and unique properties. *Hum. Reprod.* **2007**, *22*, 2183–2189. [CrossRef] [PubMed]

36. Andrade, R.; Crisol, L.; Prado, R.; Boyano, M.D.; Arluzea, J.; Arechaga, J. Plasma membrane and nuclear envelope integrity during the blebbing stage of apoptosis: A time-lapse study. *Biol. Cell* **2010**, *102*, 25–35. [CrossRef] [PubMed]

37. Lobner, D. Comparison of the LDH and MTT assays for quantifying cell death: Validity for neuronal apoptosis? *J. Neurosci. Methods* **2000**, *96*, 147–152. [CrossRef]

38. Koh, J.Y.; Choi, D.W. Quantitative determination of glutamate mediated cortical neuronal injury in cell culture by lactate dehydrogenase efflux assay. *J. Neurosci. Methods* **1987**, *20*, 83–90. [CrossRef]

39. Gwag, B.J.; Lobner, D.; Koh, J.Y.; Wie, M.B.; Choi, D.W. Blockade of glutamate receptors unmasks neuronal apoptosis after oxygen-glucose deprivation *in vitro*. *Neuroscience* **1995**, *68*, 615–619. [CrossRef]

40. Koh, J.Y.; Gwag, B.J.; Lobner, D.; Choi, D.W. Potentiated necrosis of cultured cortical neurons by neurotrophins. *Science* **1995**, *268*, 573–575. [CrossRef] [PubMed]

41. Li, J.; Zhang, J. Inhibition of apoptosis by ginsenoside RG1 in cultured cortical neurons. *Chin. Med. J. (Engl.)* **1997**, *110*, 535–539. [PubMed]

42. Miura, T.; Chiba, M.; Kasai, K.; Nozaka, H.; Nakamura, T.; Shoji, T.; Kanda, T.; Ohtake, Y.; Sato, T. Apple procyanidins induce tumor cell apoptosis through mitochondrial pathway activation of caspase-3. *Carcinogenesis* **2008**, *29*, 585–593. [CrossRef] [PubMed]

43. Liu, J.R.; Dong, H.W.; Chen, B.Q.; Zhao, P.; Liu, R.H. Fresh apples suppress mammary carcinogenesis and proliferative activity and induce apoptosis in mammary tumors of the sprague-dawley rat. *J. Agric. Food Chem.* **2009**, *57*, 297–304. [CrossRef] [PubMed]

44. Yoon, H.; Liu, R.H. Effect of selected phytochemicals and apple extracts on NF-κB activation in human breast cancer MCF-7 cells. *J. Agric. Food Chem.* **2007**, *55*, 3167–3173. [CrossRef] [PubMed]

45. Zheng, C.Q.; Qiao, B.; Wang, M.; Tao, Q. Mechanisms of apple polyphenols-induced proliferation inhibiting and apoptosis in a metastatic oral adenoid cystic carcinoma cell line. *Kaohsiung J. Med. Sci.* **2013**, *29*, 239–245. [CrossRef] [PubMed]

46. White, K.; Grether, M.E.; Abrams, J.M.; Young, L.; Farrell, K.; Steller, H. Genetic control of programmed cell death in drosophila. *Science* **1994**, *264*, 677–683. [CrossRef] [PubMed]

47. Darzynkiewicz, Z. Differential staining of DNA and RNA in intact cells and isolated cell nuclei with acridine orange. *Methods Cell Biol.* **1990**, *33*, 285–298. [PubMed]

48. Wyllie, A.H.; Kerr, J.F.; Currie, A.R. Cell death: The significance of apoptosis. *Int. Rev. Cytol.* **1980**, *68*, 251–306. [PubMed]

49. Cover, T.L.; Puryear, W.; Perez-Perez, G.I.; Blaser, M.J. Effect of urease on HeLa cell vacuolation induced by Helicobacter pylori cytotoxin. *Infect. Immun.* **1991**, *59*, 1264–1270. [PubMed]

50. Patel, H.K.; Willhite, D.C.; Patel, R.M.; Ye, D.; Williams, C.L.; Torres, E.M.; Marty, K.B.; MacDonald, R.A.; Blanke, S.R. Plasma membrane cholesterol modulates cellular vacuolation induced by the Helicobacter pylori vacuolating cytotoxin. *Infect. Immun.* **2002**, *70*, 4112–4123. [CrossRef] [PubMed]

51. Pommier, Y. Diversity of DNA topoisomerases I and inhibitors. *Biochimie* **1998**, *80*, 255–270. [CrossRef]

52. Li, T.K.; Liu, L.F. Tumor cell death induced by topoisomerase-targeting drugs. *Annu. Rev. Pharmacol. Toxicol.* **2001**, *41*, 53–77. [CrossRef] [PubMed]

53. Srinivasan, K. Role of spices beyond food flavoring: Nutraceuticals with multiple health effects. *Food Rev. Int.* **2005**, *21*, 167–188. [CrossRef]

54. Duke, J.A.; Duke, P.-A.K.; duCellier, J.L. *Duke's Handbook of Medicinal Plants of the Bible*; CRC Press: Boca Raton, NY, USA, 2008.

55. Nitoda, T.; Fan, M.D.; Kubo, I. Effects of cuminaldehyde on melanoma cells. *Phytother. Res.* **2008**, *22*, 809–813. [CrossRef] [PubMed]

56. Tomy, M.J.; Dileep, K.V.; Prasanth, S.; Preethidan, D.S.; Sabu, A.; Sadasivan, C.; Haridas, M. Cuminaldehyde as a lipoxygenase inhibitor: *In vitro* and *in silico* validation. *Appl. Biochem. Biotechnol.* **2014**, *174*, 388–397. [CrossRef] [PubMed]

57. Lee, H.S. Cuminaldehyde: Aldose reductase and α-glucosidase inhibitor derived from *Cuminum cyminum* L. seeds. *J. Agric. Food Chem.* **2005**, *53*, 2446–2450. [CrossRef] [PubMed]

58. Morshedi, D.; Aliakbari, F.; Tayaranian-Marvian, A.; Fassihi, A.; Pan-Montojo, F.; Perez-Sanchez, H. Cuminaldehyde as the major component of *Cuminum cyminum*, a natural aldehyde with inhibitory effect on alpha-synuclein fibrillation and cytotoxicity. *J. Food Sci.* **2015**, *80*, 2336–2345. [CrossRef] [PubMed]

59. Patil, S.B.; Takalikar, S.S.; Joglekar, M.M.; Haldavnekar, V.S.; Arvindekar, A.U. Insulinotropic and β-cell protective action of cuminaldehyde, cuminol and an inhibitor isolated from *Cuminum cyminum* in streptozotocin-induced diabetic rats. *Br. J. Nutr.* **2013**, *110*, 1434–1443. [CrossRef] [PubMed]

60. Aruna, K.; Sivaramakrishnan, V.M. Anticarcinogenic effects of the essential oils from cumin, poppy and basil. *Phytother. Res.* **1996**, *10*, 577–580. [CrossRef]

61. Allahghadri, T.; Rasooli, I.; Owlia, P.; Nadooshan, M.J.; Ghazanfari, T.; Taghizadeh, M.; Astaneh, S.D. Antimicrobial property, antioxidant capacity, and cytotoxicity of essential oil from cumin produced in Iran. *J. Food Sci.* **2010**, *75*, 54–61. [CrossRef] [PubMed]

62. Chen, Q.; Hu, X.; Li, J.; Liu, P.; Yang, Y.; Ni, Y. Preparative isolation and purification of cuminaldehyde and p-menta-1,4-dien-7-al from the essential oil of *Cuminum cyminum* L. by high-speed counter-current chromatography. *Anal. Chim. Acta* **2011**, *689*, 149–154. [CrossRef] [PubMed]

63. Baldwin, E.L.; Osheroff, N. Etoposide, topoisomerase II and cancer. *Curr. Med. Chem. Anticancer Agents* **2005**, *5*, 363–372. [CrossRef] [PubMed]

64. Gilbert, D.C.; Chalmers, A.J.; El-Khamisy, S.F. Topoisomerase I inhibition in colorectal cancer: Biomarkers and therapeutic targets. *Br. J. Cancer* **2012**, *106*, 18–24. [CrossRef] [PubMed]

65. Smith, D.H.; Christensen, I.J.; Jensen, N.F.; Markussen, B.; Romer, M.U.; Nygard, S.B.; Muller, S.; Nielsen, H.J.; Brunner, N.; Nielsen, K.V. Mechanisms of topoisomerase I (TOP1) gene copy number increase in a stage III colorectal cancer patient cohort. *PLoS ONE* **2013**, *8*, e60613. [CrossRef] [PubMed]

66. Denny, W.A.; Baguley, B.C. Dual topoisomerase I/II inhibitors in cancer therapy. *Curr. Top. Med. Chem.* **2003**, *3*, 339–353. [CrossRef] [PubMed]

67. Bisceglie, F.; Pinelli, S.; Alinovi, R.; Goldoni, M.; Mutti, A.; Camerini, A.; Piola, L.; Tarasconi, P.; Pelosi, G. Cinnamaldehyde and cuminaldehyde thiosemicarbazones and their copper(II) and nickel(II) complexes: A study to understand their biological activity. *J. Inorg. Biochem.* **2014**, *140*, 111–125. [CrossRef] [PubMed]

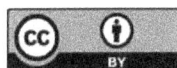

*nutrients*

MDPI

*Review*

# Effect of Tea Polyphenol Compounds on Anticancer Drugs in Terms of Anti-Tumor Activity, Toxicology, and Pharmacokinetics

Jianhua Cao [1], Jie Han [2], Hao Xiao [1], Jinping Qiao [1,*] and Mei Han [1,*]

[1]  Key Laboratory of Radiopharmaceuticals, Ministry of Education, College of Chemistry,
    Beijing Normal University, Beijing 100875, China; caojianhua0303@163.com (J.H.C.);
    201521150080@mail.bnu.edu.cn (H.X.)
[2]  Analytical Center, Beijing Normal University, Beijing 100875, China; 13701290930@139.com
*   Correspondence: qiao_jinping@bnu.edu.cn (J.Q.); hanmei@bnu.edu.cn (M.H.); Tel.: +86-10-6220-07786 (J.Q.)

Received: 1 August 2016; Accepted: 21 November 2016; Published: 14 December 2016

**Abstract:** Multidrug resistance and various adverse side effects have long been major problems in cancer chemotherapy. Recently, chemotherapy has gradually transitioned from mono-substance therapy to multidrug therapy. As a result, the drug cocktail strategy has gained more recognition and wider use. It is believed that properly-formulated drug combinations have greater therapeutic efficacy than single drugs. Tea is a popular beverage consumed by cancer patients and the general public for its perceived health benefits. The major bioactive molecules in green tea are catechins, a class of flavanols. The combination of green tea extract or green tea catechins and anticancer compounds has been paid more attention in cancer treatment. Previous studies demonstrated that the combination of chemotherapeutic drugs and green tea extract or tea polyphenols could synergistically enhance treatment efficacy and reduce the adverse side effects of anticancer drugs in cancer patients. In this review, we summarize the experimental evidence regarding the effects of green tea-derived polyphenols in conjunction with chemotherapeutic drugs on anti-tumor activity, toxicology, and pharmacokinetics. We believe that the combination of multidrug cancer treatment with green tea catechins may improve treatment efficacy and diminish negative side effects.

**Keywords:** tea polyphenol; anticancer agent; synergistic anticancer activity; toxicology; pharmacokinetics

---

## 1. Introduction

Tea made from the plant species *Camellia sinensis* is the most widely consumed beverage other than water. Tea is divided into three subtypes based on fermentation levels: green (unfermented), oolong (partially fermented), and black (highly to fully fermented). Among the various types of tea, green tea is believed to have better antioxidant and health benefits than black and oolong teas [1]. Previous studies reported that green tea could lower the risk of cardiovascular disease, improve brain function, promote fat loss, and combat cancer and type II diabetes, among many other health benefits [2–5]. Green tea is also associated with many therapeutic effects, including anti-blood coagulation, the reduction of hypertension, oxidative damage repair, HIV treatment, and cancer prevention and treatment [6–9]. Green tea contains substantial amounts of polyphenols, caffeine, theanine, polysaccharides, and other compounds. Caffeine is a functional alkaloid in tea products. Medicinally it can be used as a cardiac, cerebral, and respiratory stimulant, among other uses. Tea polyphenols are a class of bioactive molecules in green tea, categorized as epistructured catechins or nonepistructured catechins. Epistructured catechins include epicatechin (EC), epicatechin gallate (ECG), epigallocatechin (EGC), and epigallocatechin gallate (EGCG). Nonepistructured catechins include catechin (C), catechin gallate (CG), gallocatechin (GC), and gallocatechin gallate (GCG). EGCG is the most abundant polyphenol in green tea; a typical catechin profile in an extract from green tea leaf is comprised of 10%–15% EGCG, 6%–10% EGC, 2%–3% ECG, and 2% EC. Figure 1 shows the chemical structures of the main polyphenol ingredients in green tea [1,10].

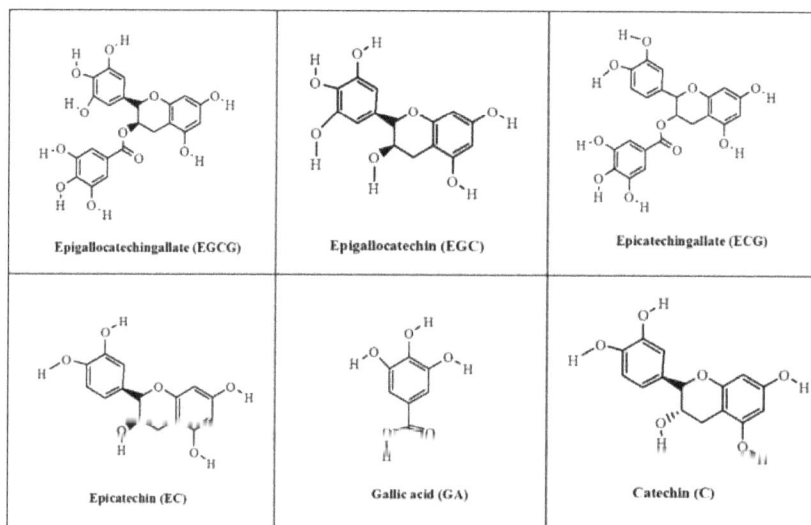

**Figure 1.** The chemical structures of the main polyphenols in green tea.

Nutritional supplements are commonly integrated into chemotherapeutic strategies for cancer treatment. Combination chemotherapy is an approach to cancer treatment that utilizes multiple medications. This approach can overcome the disadvantages of monotherapy and enhance therapeutic effects in cancer treatment [11]. Due to their various health benefits, green tea polyphenols are increasingly used for cancer prevention or as an adjuvant in chemotherapy. Previous studies have demonstrated that combining chemotherapeutic drugs with green tea could reduce cancer risk, improve survival rates among cancer patients, and decrease chemotherapy-associated side effects [12–15].

In this paper, we mainly reviewed the experimental data regarding the effects of tea polyphenols in conjunction with chemotherapeutic drugs on anti-tumor activity, toxicology, and pharmacokinetics. We believe that the combination of green tea catechins and anticancer drugs may enhance cancer treatment efficacy and diminish negative side effects.

## 2. Synergistic Anticancer Activity of Tea Polyphenols and Chemotherapeutic Agents

The combination of green tea catechins and anticancer drugs is a new treatment strategy that has been widely accepted by cancer researchers [11]. Although anticancer drugs and tea polyphenols are very different in terms of structure and function, tea polyphenols can synergistically enhance the effects of anticancer drugs and make them 10–15 times more effective than monotherapy [11]. Some studies have also reported beneficial effects of EGCG or green tea extract with anticancer drugs, such as bleomycin, cisplatin, tamoxifen, and bortezomib [16–19]. We have also studied the effect of green tea extract on 5-fluorouracil (5-FU) in cancer cells and animals. Our results demonstrated that green tea catechins with anticancer agents are more effective than monotherapy [15]. The effects of tea polyphenols or tea extracts on the therapeutic efficacy of anticancer agents are listed in Table 1.

## 2.1. Combination of Tea Polyphenols and Bleomycin

Bleomycin is frequently used in the treatment of various cancers [10]. However, the monotherapy strategy has often failed to produce therapeutic benefit due to multidrug-resistant cancer. Green tea polyphenols have been used as an adjuvant in bleomycin therapy. Alshatwi et al. [10] reported a synergistic anticancer effect with a combination of tea polyphenols and bleomycin. Various concentrations of tea polyphenols, bleomycin, or tea polyphenols combined with bleomycin were added to cervical cancer cells (SiHa), and then the cell growth, intracellular reactive oxygen species, poly-caspase activity, early apoptosis and expression of caspase-3, caspase-8, caspase-9, Bcl-2, and p53 were observed. This study showed that tea polyphenols combined with bleomycin synergistically inhibited cervical cancer cell viability and proliferation through the induction of apoptosis. Other studies have also suggested that tea polyphenols may increase antitumor activity of bleomycin [18].

## 2.2. Combination of Tea Polyphenols and Cisplatin

Cisplatin is often the first chemotherapeutic agent used to treat many forms of cancer. Unfortunately, cisplatin resistance often develops during the course of treatment. Both preclinical and clinical studies have shown that multiple mechanisms drive tumor resistance to cisplatin. The synergistic effect of cisplatin and tea polyphenols has been studied in vitro and in vivo [20–22]. Tea polyphenols combined with cisplatin can decrease proliferation and induce apoptosis in breast cancer cells. Additionally, tea polyphenols plus cisplatin may minimize or slow the development of drug resistance, which may also reduce drug toxicity and improve therapeutic efficacy [18]. The combination of EGCG with cisplatin has increased beneficial effects on cell cycle arrest, modulation of ROS- and apoptosis-related gene expression and potent antioxidant activity when compared with monotherapy. EGCG may also reduce oxidative stress, inhibit proliferation, and sensitize ovarian cancer cells to cisplatin. The combination of tea polyphenols and cisplatin can synergistically inhibit the growth of various cancer cells, such as MCF-7 breast cancer cells and non-small cell lung cancer (NSCLC) A549 cells. Additionally, we found that, compared with cisplatin monotherapy, the combination of cisplatin and EGCG can significantly decrease tumor size in animal models—the data will be reported in the near future.

## 2.3. Combination of Tea Polyphenols and Ibuprofen

Ibuprofen is a non-selective nonsteroidal anti-inflammatory drug (NSAID) [23], which may inhibit the growth of prostate cancer cells in both in vitro and in vivo xenograft models. The synergistic effect of EGCG and ibuprofen (EGCG+ibuprofen) treatment on DU-145 prostate cancer cells has been investigated. This study showed that EGCG + ibuprofen treatment resulted in greater growth inhibition than ibuprofen or EGCG alone. EGCG + ibuprofen treatment acts synergistically to block proliferation and promote apoptosis in DU-145 prostate cancer cells [23].

## 2.4. Combination of Tea Polyphenols and Tamoxifen

Tamoxifen is an anti-estrogenic compound used for the prevention of breast cancer. Green tea is often used as a supplement in breast cancer treatment and prevention [4]. Co-administration of green tea and tamoxifen improves experimental outcomes in breast cancer cell lines and animal models. Green tea increased the inhibitory effect of tamoxifen on the proliferation of estrogen receptor-positive MCF-7, ZR75, and T47D human breast cancer cells in vitro [24,25]. The combination of EGCG (75 and 100 μM) and tamoxifen (5–200 μM) significantly increased apoptosis in PC-9 cells compared to EGCG or tamoxifen alone [26]. When MCF-7 xenograft-bearing mice were treated with both green tea and tamoxifen, their tumor sizes were significantly diminished, and more cancer cell apoptosis occurred in tumor tissue [27,28].

### 2.5. Combination of Tea Polyphenols and Bortezomib

Bortezomib exerts its antitumor effects by reversibly blocking the 26S proteasome [29]. EGCG interferes with bortezomib's anticancer activity [30]. EGCG's negative impact on bortezomib efficacy was concentration-dependent in CWR22 xenograft-bearing breast cancer mice. Only very high levels of EGCG antagonized bortezomib's antitumor activity, while low levels of EGCG had no adverse effects in CWR22 mice [31]. This example demonstrates the negative interaction of EGCG and an anticancer drug.

### 2.6. Combination of Tea Polyphenols and Other Anticancer Drugs

Tea extract or tea polyphenols also synergistically enhance the anticancer activity of other chemotherapy drugs, such as Paclitaxel, sulindac, celecoxib, curcumin, luteolin, docetaxel, retinoids, and so on [32–35]. Our group has studied the effects of green tea extract and 5-fluorouracil treatment in SW480, BIU-87, and BGC823 human cancer cell lines; a daily dose of green tea (equivalent to <6 cups daily in humans) did not alter the cytotoxicity of 5-FU treatment in these cells [15].

**Table 1.** The effects of green tea catechins on anticancer compounds in anti-tumor activity.

| Anticancer Drugs | Experiment | Effects | Reference |
|---|---|---|---|
| Bleomycin | SiHa cervical cancer cells or uterine cervical cancer cells were treated with tea polyphenol and bleomycin; poly-caspase activity, early apoptosis, and the expression of caspase-3, caspase-8, caspase-9, Bcl-2, and p53 were assessed. | Synergistic increase in antitumor effects. | [10] |
| 5-Fluorouracil (5-FU) | Some cancer cells—such as human SW480, BIU-87, BGC823, and Hep3B—were treated with green tea and 5-FU; the cytotoxicity, cell apoptosis, and proliferation were studied. | Increase in cell apoptosis; synergistic inhibition of cell proliferation; no reduction in antitumor activity. | [15,35] |
| Cisplatin | Cancer cells YCU-N861, YCU-H891, Hep3B, SW480, BIU-87, BGC823, et al. were coadministered cisplatin with tea polypnenols; the cell apoptosis and proliferation were studied. | Synergistic inhibition of cell proliferation; induction of apoptosis. | [20–22] |
| Ibuprofen | DU-145 cells were treated with EGCG and ibuprofen; cell death analysis, immunoblotting, RT-PCR analysis, and caspase activity assay were used. | Synergistic effect on the anti-proliferative and pro-apoptotic action. | [23] |
| Tamoxifen | Cancer cells PC-9, MCF-7, and MDA-MB-231were treated with tea polyphenols and tamoxifen; some factors such as EGFR, MMP-2, MMP-9, and EMMPRIN were assessed. | Induction of apoptosis; enhanced expression of apoptotic genes; synergistic increase in antitumor effects. | [24–26] |
| Sulindac | PC-9 cancer cells were treated with sulindac and tea polyphenols; gene expression was assessed. | Induction of apoptosis; enhanced expression of apoptotic genes. | [27,28] |

**Table 1.** *Cont.*

| Anticancer Drugs | Experiment | Effects | Reference |
|---|---|---|---|
| Bortezomib | Cancer cells 26S and CWR22 were treated with bortezomib and tea polyphenols; cell apoptosis and proliferation were assessed. | Antagonized antitumor activity. | [29–31] |
| Celecoxib | A549 and MCF-7 cancer cells were treated with celecoxib and tea polyphenols; the cell activity and gene expression were assessed. | Increased cell apoptosis; enhanced expression of GADD153 gene | [32] |
| Luteolin | Cancer cells H292, A549, H460, and Tu212 were treated with luteolin and EGCG; phosphorylation of p53 was studied. | Induction of caspase-8 and caspase-3 cleavage; increase in cell apoptosis. | [33] |
| Docetaxel | PC-3ML cancer cells were treated with docetaxel and tea polyphenols; hTERT and Bcl-2 were studied. | Increase in the expression of apoptotic genes; reduction in growth rate of cancer cells. | [34] |
| Curcumin | Cancer cells PC-9, A549, NCI-H460, and ER alpha-breast cancer cells were treated with curcumin and tea polyphenols; the cell activity and cell cycle were assessed. | Induction of apoptosis; enhancement of cell cycle arrest at G1 and S/G2 phases. | [36–38] |
| Quercetin | Cancer cells PC-3, LNCaP, and CWR22Rv1 were treated with quercetin and tea polyphenols; the cell growth and gene expression were assessed. | Synergistic expression of androgen receptor; inhibition of cancer cell growth. | [39,40] |
| Paclitaxel | PC-3ML cancer cells were treated with paclitaxel and tea polyphenols; the cell growth and apoptotic gene expression were assessed. | Increase in the expression of apoptotic genes; reduction in growth rate of cancer cells. | [34,41] |
| Doxorubicin | Cancer cells BEL-7404/DOX, PC-3ML, IBC-10a, and PCa-20a were treated with doxorubicin and tea; the cell proliferation and apoptosis were assessed. | Enhanced sensitivity to doxorubicin; synergistic increase in antitumor effects. | [42] |
| Resveratrol | Cancer cells ALVA-41, PC-3, and MCF-7 were treated with resveratrol and green tea; the cell growth and apoptosis were assessed. | Inhibition of cell growth; induction of apoptosis | [19,43] |
| Sulforaphane | Cancer cells PC-3 AP-1, HT-29, SKOV-ip1, SKOVTR-ip2 were treated with sulforaphane and EGCG; the cell activity and gene expression were assessed. | Diminished induction of cancer cell activity; inhibition of cell viability; increase in apoptosis. | [34,44] |

EGFR (epidermal growth factor receptor); MMP-2, MMP-9 (a family of matrix metalloproteinases); EMMPRIN (extracellular matrix metalloproteinase inducer); hTERT (human telomerase reverse transcriptase); ER (estrogen receptor).

## 2.7. Combination of Caffeine and Anticancer Drugs

Caffeine is another ingredient in tea. Caffeine can inhibit the activities of both ATM and ATR—two important protein kinases involved in DNA damage-induced cell cycle arrest and apoptosis. It has been reported that caffeine increased the cisplatin-induced apoptosis in both HTB182 and CRL5985 lung cancer cells by inhibiting ATR and inducing ATM activation [45]. Caffeine could enhance the antitumor effect of cisplatin; when the dosing period of caffeine was increased, the synergistic effect was increased in osteosarcoma-bearing rats [46]. Significant inhibition of tumor growth and prolongation of survival time were also found in sarcoma-bearing mice [47]. Caffeine significantly decreased mutagenicity of the anticancer aromatic drugs daunomycin, doxorubicin, and mitoxantrone. Caffeine decreased the anticancer drug vinblastine-induced chromosomal aberrations and mitotic index in bone marrow cells [48].

## 3. Ameliorating Toxicity Induced by Chemotherapeutic Agents

Two major problems in cancer chemotherapy are adverse side effects and multidrug resistance. Chemotherapy can cause fatigue, nausea, vomiting, and more serious side effects in cancer patients. Previous studies found that anticancer drugs caused serious adverse effects via antioxidant defense abnormalities against reactive oxygen species (ROS) [5,49]. Antioxidants may protect against chemotherapy-induced toxicity. Due to their antioxidant and ROS-scavenging properties, green tea polyphenols could circumvent the adverse effects of ROS and chemotherapy and enhance treatment efficacy (Table 2). Additionally, P-glycoprotein (P-gp) plays an important role in multidrug resistance [50]. EGCG was found to inhibit the transport activity of P-gp and may be an effective P-gp modulator [51]. EGCG also increased chemotherapy drug accumulation in multidrug resistant cells.

Doxorubicin is a potent broad-spectrum chemotherapeutic agent. However, the clinical use of doxorubicin has been seriously limited by its undesirable side effects, especially dose-dependent myocardial injury, which can lead to lethal congestive heart failure [52]. Treatment with green tea ameliorated the cardiotoxicity of doxorubicin. Doxorubicin-induced oxidative stress, heart and liver morphological changes, and metabolic disorders were also mitigated by green tea in male Wistar rats [53]. The mechanism underlying these effects is currently unknown, but it may involve the modulation of enzymes required for lipid synthesis, such as HMG-CoA (3-hydroxy-3-methylglutary-coenzyme A) reductase [54].

**Table 2.** A combination of green tea catechins and anticancer compounds ameliorating the toxicity induced by chemotherapeutic agents.

| Anticancer Drugs | Experiment | Effects | Reference |
| --- | --- | --- | --- |
| Doxorubicin | Wistar albino rats with cardiotoxicity induced by doxorubicin were treated with green tea. AST, CK, LDH, LPO, cytochrome P450, blood glutathione, tissue glutathione, and enzymatic and non-enzymatic antioxidants were evaluated along with histopathological studies. | Oral administration of green tea prevented doxorubicin-induced cardiotoxicity by accelerating heart antioxidant defense mechanisms and downregulating the LPO levels to the normal levels. | [52] |
| Doxorubicin (DOX) | Neonatal Rats with cardiotoxicity induced by doxorubicin were treated with EGCG; LDH, MnSOD, catalase, and glutathione peroxidase were detected. | EGCG could protect cardiomyocytes from DOX-induced oxidative stress by attenuating ROS production and apoptosis, and increasing activities and protein expression of endogenous antioxidant enzymes. | [53] |

Table 2. *Cont.*

| Anticancer Drugs | Experiment | Effects | Reference |
|---|---|---|---|
| Doxorubicin | Rats were treated with doxorubicin and different doses of EGCG. Cardiac enzymes (creatine kinase isoenzyme-MB and lactate dehydrogenase) and histopathological changes were studied. | EGCG possesses cardioprotective action against doxorubicin-induced cardiotoxicity by suppressing oxidative stress, inflammation, and apoptotic signals, as well as the activation of pro-survival pathways. | [54] |

AST (aspartate transaminase); CK (creatine kinase); LDH (lactate dehydrogenase); LPO (lipid peroxidation); MnSOD (superoxide dismutase).

## 4. Pharmacokinetic Effect on Chemotherapeutic Agents

Based on food–drug interactions, green tea polyphenols may affect the expression or activities of drug-metabolizing enzymes and drug transporters [55,56]. It is currently unknown whether green tea consumption will alter the pharmacokinetics and bioavailability of a chemotherapeutic agent in cancer patients. Alterations in the pharmacokinetic parameters may also alter the drug's efficacy or toxicity [57]. Therefore, anticancer drugs should contain warnings on the potential pharmacokinetic interaction of drugs and EGCG.

In our previous study, we reported that green tea extracts increase the bioavailability of 5-FU in rats [15]. The maximum plasma concentrations ($C_{max}$) and the area under the plasma concentration-time curves (AUC) of 5-FU in rats increased significantly following administration of green tea extract for 14 days. The half-life of 5-FU in plasma was also substantially prolonged [19]. Green tea may decrease the activity of dihydropyrimidine dehydrogenase (DPD)—the initial and rate-limiting enzyme of 5-FU metabolism. Reduced DPD activity may result in decreased 5-FU metabolism, leading to higher plasma concentrations.

Co-administration of EGCG and irinotecan (CPT-11) altered the pharmacokinetics of CPT-11 and its metabolite, SN-38, in Sprague–Dawley rats [58]. When the animals were pretreated with EGCG, the CPT-11 and SN-38 AUC in plasma were increased by 57.7% and 18.3%, respectively, while the AUC in bile were decreased by 15.8% and 46.8%, respectively. Therefore, the plasma-to-bile distribution ratio ($AUC_{bile}/AUC_{plasma}$) was significantly reduced, while the half-lives of CPT-11 and SN-38 in plasma were substantially prolonged. EGCG may inhibit the transport of CPT-11 and SN-38 into the biliary tract by modulating P-gp and reduce hepatobiliary excretion of CPT-11 and SN-38. The increased plasma concentrations of CPT-11 and SN-38 may be associated with enhanced pharmacological effects or toxicity.

Sunitinib is a novel oral antitumor agent. Plasma concentrations of sunitinib in rats significantly decreased with co-administration of EGCG [59]. The related pharmacokinetic parameters of plasma sunitinib (such as $AUC_{0-\infty}$ and $C_{max}$) were markedly reduced by the co-administration of EGCG. In the sunitinib with EGCG group, the mean $C_{max}$ decreased by 47.7% compared with the sunitinib with water group, while $AUC_{0-\infty}$ significantly decreased by 51.5%. These results indicate that EGCG markedly reduced the bioavailability of sunitinib. Therefore, it is necessary for patients receiving sunitinib therapy to avoid consuming green tea or EGCG dietary supplements.

## 5. Human Trials

The aims of the clinical trials are to study the effectiveness of green tea extract in treating cancer patients. A total of 100 clinical trials involving both green tea and cancer are listed in clinicalTrials.gov [60]. Some results proved that green tea contains ingredients that may prevent or slow the growth of certain cancers. For example, in the clinicalTrial NCT00685516 (a multicenter, randomized, phase II trial), 113 men diagnosed with prostate cancer were randomized to consume six cups daily of brewed green tea, black tea, or water (control) prior to radical prostatectomy. The prostate tumor markers of cancer development and progression were determined by tissue immunostaining of proliferation (Ki67), apoptosis (Bcl-2, Bax, Tunel), inflammation (nuclear and cytoplasmic nuclear factor kappa B (NFκB)) and oxidation (8-hydroxydeoxy-guanosine (8OHdG)). Blood and urine samples, as well as tissue from diagnostic biopsy and radical prostatectomy specimens were evaluated by high performance liquid chromatography and ELISA analysis; the concentrations of total and free tea polyphenols (i.e., EGCG, EC, EGC, and ECG), theaflavins, and conjugated/colonic tea metabolites were also detected [61]. The estimated study completion date is August 2017; some primary data have been published [62]. The results showed that green tea can change NFκB and systemic oxidation, and future longer-term studies are warranted to further examine the role of green tea for prostate cancer prevention and treatment.

## 6. Conclusions

The benefits of combining tea polyphenols with anticancer compounds are now widely accepted by cancer researchers. Previous studies have demonstrated that a combination of chemotherapeutic drugs and green tea extract could enhance therapeutic effects and reduce the adverse side effects of anticancer drugs most of the time. Several papers have also reported the potential for negative interactions between tea polyphenols and anticancer drugs. In this article, we provided a brief overview of the pharmacodynamics, toxicology, and pharmacokinetic interactions between green tea and anticancer drugs. We believe that the combination of green tea and anticancer drugs may be important in enhancing therapeutic efficacy while diminishing negative side effects.

**Acknowledgments:** The authors appreciate the Open Foundation of the Key Laboratory of Radiopharmaceuticals, Ministry of Education, College of Chemistry, Beijing Normal University.

**Conflicts of Interest:** The authors declare no conflict of interest.

## References

1. Qiao, J.; Kong, X.; Kong, A.; Han, M. Pharmacokinetics and biotransformation of tea polyphenols. *Curr. Drug Metab.* **2014**, *15*, 30–36. [CrossRef] [PubMed]
2. Fujiki, H.; Suganuma, M.; Imai, K.; Nakachi, K. Green tea: Cancer preventive beverage and/or drug. *Cancer Lett.* **2002**, *188*, 9–13. [CrossRef]
3. Afzal, M.; Safer, A.M.; Menon, M. Green tea polyphenols and their potential role in health and disease. *Inflammopharmacology* **2015**, *23*, 151–161. [CrossRef] [PubMed]
4. Hara, Y. Tea catechins and their applications as supplements and pharmaceutics. *Pharmacol. Res.* **2011**, *64*, 100–104. [CrossRef] [PubMed]
5. Fujiki, H. Green tea: Health benefits as cancer preventive for humans. *Chem. Rec.* **2005**, *5*, 119–132. [CrossRef] [PubMed]
6. Lambert, J.D.; Yang, C.S. Mechanisms of cancer prevention by tea constituents. *J. Nutr.* **2003**, *133*, 3262S–3267S. [PubMed]
7. Higdon, J.V.; Frei, B. Tea catechins and polyphenols: Health effects, metabolism, and antioxidant functions. *Crit. Rev. Food Sci. Nutr.* **2003**, *43*, 89–143. [CrossRef] [PubMed]
8. Yang, C.S.; Maliakal, P.; Meng, X. Inhibition of carcinogenesis by tea. *Annu. Rev. Pharmacol. Toxicol.* **2002**, *42*, 25–54. [CrossRef] [PubMed]
9. Fujiki, H.; Imai, K.; Nakachi, K.; Shimizu, M.; Moriwaki, H.; Suganuma, M. Challenging the effectiveness of green tea in primary and tertiary cancer prevention. *J. Cancer Res. Clin. Oncol.* **2012**, *138*, 1259–1270. [CrossRef] [PubMed]
10. Alshatwi, A.A.; Periasamy, V.S.; Athinarayanan, J.; Elango, R. Synergistic anticancer activity of dietary tea polyphenols and bleomycin hydrochloride in human cervicalcancer cell: Caspase-dependent and independent apoptotic pathways. *Chem. Biol. Interact.* **2016**, *247*, 1–10. [CrossRef] [PubMed]
11. Suganuma, M.; Saha, A.; Fujiki, H. New cancer treatment strategy using combination of green tea catechins and anticancer drugs. *Cancer Sci.* **2011**, *102*, 317–323. [CrossRef] [PubMed]

12. Morre, D.J.; Morre, D.M.; Sun, H.; Cooper, R.; Chang, J.; Janle, E.M. Tea catechin synergies in inhibition of cancer cell proliferation and of a cancer specific cell surface oxidase (ECTO-NOX). *Pharmacol. Toxicol.* **2003**, *92*, 234–241. [CrossRef] [PubMed]

13. Fujiki, H.; Sueoka, E.; Watanabe, T.; Suganuma, M. Synergistic enhancement of anticancer effects on numerous human cancer cell lines treated with thecombination of EGCG, other green tea catechins, and anticancer compounds. *J. Cancer Res. Clin. Oncol.* **2015**, *141*, 1511–1522. [CrossRef] [PubMed]

14. Adhami, V.M.; Malik, A.; Zaman, N.; Sarfaraz, S.; Siddiqui, I.A.; Syed, D.N.; Afaq, F.; Pasha, F.S.; Saleem, M.; Mukhtar, H. Combined inhibitory effects of green tea polyphenols and selective cyclooxygenase-2 inhibitors on the growth of human prostate cancer cells both in vitro and in vivo. *Clin. Cancer Res.* **2007**, *13*, 1611–1619. [CrossRef] [PubMed]

15. Qiao, J.; Gu, C.; Shang, W.; Du, J.; Yin, W.; Zhu, M.; Wang, W.; Han, M.; Lu, W. Effect of green tea on pharmacokinetics of 5-fluorouracil in rats and pharmacodynamics in human cell lines in vitro. *Food Chem. Toxicol.* **2011**, *49*, 1410–1415. [CrossRef] [PubMed]

16. Sriram, N.; Kalayarasan, S.; Sudhandiran, G. Epigallocatechin-3-gallate exhibits anti-fibrotic effect by attenuating bleomycin-induced glycoconjugates, lysosomal hydrolases and ultrastructural changes in rat model pulmonary fibrosis. *Chem. Biol. Interact.* **2009**, *180*, 271–280. [CrossRef] [PubMed]

17. Periasamy, V.S.; Alshatwi, A.A. Tea polyphenols modulate antioxidant redox system on cisplatin-induced reactive oxygen species generation in a human breast cancer cell. *Basic Clin. Pharmacol. Toxicol.* **2013**, *112*, 374–384. [CrossRef] [PubMed]

18. Chen, S.Z.; Zhen, Y.S. Molecular targets of tea polyphenols and its roles of anticancer drugs in experimental therapy. *Yao Xue Xue Bao* **2013**, *48*, 1–7. [PubMed]

19. Ahmad, K.A.; Harris, N.H.; Johnson, A.D.; Lindvall, H.C.; Wang, G.; Ahmed, K. Protein kinase CK2 modulates apoptosis induced by resveratrol and epigallocatechin-3-gallate in prostate cancer cells. *Mol. Cancer Ther.* **2007**, *6*, 1006–1012. [CrossRef] [PubMed]

20. Mazumder, M.E.; Beale, P.; Chan, C.; Yu, J.Q.; Huq, F. Epigallocatechin gallate acts synergistically in combination with cisplatin and designed trans-palladiums in ovarian cancer cells. *Anticancer Res.* **2012**, *32*, 4851–4860. [PubMed]

21. Chan, M.M.; Soprano, K.J.; Einstein, K.; Fong, D. Epigallocatechin-3-gallate delivers hydrogen peroxide to induce death of ovarian cancer cells and enhancestheir cisplatin susceptibility. *J. Cell Physiol.* **2006**, *207*, 389–396. [CrossRef] [PubMed]

22. Chan, M.M.; Fong, D.; Soprano, K.J.; Holmes, W.F.; Heverling, H. Inhibition of growth and sensitization to cisplatin-mediated killing of ovarian cancer cells by polyphenolic chemopreventive agents. *J. Cell Physiol.* **2003**, *194*, 63–70. [CrossRef] [PubMed]

23. Kim, M.H.; Chung, J. Synergistic cell death by EGCG and ibuprofen in DU-145 prostate cancer cell line. *Anticancer Res.* **2007**, *27*, 3947–3956. [PubMed]

24. Farabegoli, F.; Papi, A.; Orlandi, M. (−)-Epigallocatechin-3-gallate down-regulates EGFR, MMP-2, MMP-9 and EMMPRIN and inhibits the invasion of MCF-7 tamoxifen-resistant cells. *Biosci. Rep.* **2011**, *31*, 99–108. [CrossRef] [PubMed]

25. Scandlyn, M.J.; Stuart, E.C.; Somers-Edgar, T.J.; Menzies, A.R.; Rosengren, R.J. A new role for tamoxifen in oestrogen receptor-negative breast cancer when it is combined with epigallocatechin gallate. *Br. J. Cancer* **2008**, *99*, 1056–1063. [CrossRef] [PubMed]

26. Chisholm, K.; Bray, B.J.; Rosengren, R.J. Tamoxifen and epigallocatechin gallate are synergistically cytotoxic to MDA-MB-231 human breast cancer cells. *Anticancer Drugs* **2004**, *15*, 889–897. [CrossRef] [PubMed]

27. Suganuma, M.; Okabe, S.; Kai, Y.; Sueoka, N.; Sueoka, E.; Fujiki, H. Synergistic effects of (−)-epigallocatechin gallate with (−)-epicatechin, sulindac, or tamoxifen on cancer-preventive activity in the human lung cancer cell line PC-9. *Cancer Res.* **1999**, *59*, 44–47. [PubMed]

28. Fujiki, H.; Suganuma, M.; Kurusu, M.; Okabe, S.; Imayoshi, Y.; Taniguchi, S.; Yoshida, T. New TNF-α releasing inhibitors as cancer preventive agents from traditional herbal medicine and combination cancer prevention study with EGCG and sulindac or tamoxifen. *Mutat. Res.* **2003**, *524*, 119–125. [CrossRef]

29. Bannerman, B.; Xu, L.; Jones, M.; Tsu, C.; Yu, J.; Hales, P.; Monbaliu, J.; Fleming, P.; Dick, L.; Manfredi, M.; et al. Preclinical evaluation of the antitumor activity of bortezomib in combination with vitamin C or with epigallocatechin gallate, a component of green tea. *Cancer Chemother. Pharmacol.* **2011**, *68*, 1145–1154. [CrossRef] [PubMed]

30. Golden, E.B.; Lam, P.Y.; Kardosh, A.; Kardosh, A.; Gaffney, K.J.; Cadenas, E.; Louie, S.G.; Petasis, N.A.; Chen, T.C.; Schönthal, A.H. Green tea polyphenols block the anticancer effects of bortezomib and other boronic acid-based proteasome inhibitors. *Blood* **2009**, *113*, 5927–5937. [CrossRef] [PubMed]

31. Glynn, S.J.; Gaffney, K.J.; Sainz, M.A.; Louie, S.G.; Petasis, N.A. Molecular characterization of the boron adducts of the proteasome inhibitor bortezomib with epigallocatechin-3-gallate and related polyphenols. *Org. Biomol. Chem.* **2015**, *13*, 3887–3899. [CrossRef] [PubMed]

32. Suganuma, M.; Kurusu, M.; Suzuki, K.; Tasaki, E.; Fujiki, H. Green tea polyphenol stimulates cancer preventive effects of celecoxib in human lung cancer cells by upregulation of GADD153 gene. *Int. J. Cancer* **2006**, *119*, 33–40. [CrossRef] [PubMed]

33. Amin, A.R.; Wang, D.; Zhang, H.; Peng, S.; Shin, H.J.; Brandes, J.C.; Tighiouart, M.; Khuri, F.R.; Chen, Z.G.; Shin, D.M. Enhanced anti-tumor activity by the combination of the natural compounds (−)-epigallocatechin-3-gallate and luteolin: Potential role of p53. *J. Biol. Chem.* **2010**, *285*, 34557–34565. [CrossRef] [PubMed]

34. Chen, H.; Landen, C.N.; Li, Y.; Alvarez, R.D.; Tollefsbol, T.O. Epigallocatechin gallate and sulforaphane combination treatment induce apoptosis in paclitaxel-resistant ovarian cancer cells through hTERT and Bcl-2 down-regulation. *Exp. Cell Res.* **2013**, *319*, 697–706. [CrossRef] [PubMed]

35. Yang, X.W.; Wang, X.L.; Cao, L.Q.; Jiang, X.F.; Peng, H.P.; Lin, S.M.; Xue, P.; Chen, D. Green tea polyphenol epigallocatechin-3-gallate enhances 5-fluorouracil-induced cell growth inhibition of hepatocellular carcinoma cells. *Hepatol. Res.* **2012**, *42*, 494–501. [CrossRef] [PubMed]

36. Saito, A.; Kurahara, T.; Echigo, N.; Suganuma, M.; Fujiki, H. New role of (−)-epicatechin in enhancing the induction of growth inhibition and apoptosis in human lung cancer cells by curcumin. *Cancer Prev. Res.* **2010**, *3*, 953–962. [CrossRef] [PubMed]

37. Ghosh, A.K.; Kay, N.E.; Secreto, C.R.; Shanafelt, T.D. Curcumin inhibits prosurvival pathways in chronic lymphocytic leukemia B cells and may overcome their stromal protection in combination with EGCG. *Clin. Cancer Res.* **2009**, *15*, 1250–1258. [CrossRef] [PubMed]

38. Somers-Edgar, T.J.; Scandlyn, M.J.; Stuart, E.C.; Le Nedelec, M.J.; Valentine, S.P.; Rosengren, R.J. The combination of epigallocatechin gallate and curcumin suppresses ER alpha-breast cancer cell growth in vitro and in vivo. *Int. J. Cancer* **2008**, *122*, 1966–1971. [CrossRef] [PubMed]

39. Tang, S.N.; Singh, C.; Nall, D.; Meeker, D.; Shankar, S.; Srivastava, R.K. The dietary bioflavonoid quercetin synergizes with epigallocatechin gallate (EGCG) to inhibit prostate cancer stem cell characteristics, invasion, migration and epithelial-mesenchymal transition. *J. Mol. Signal.* **2010**, *5*, 14. [CrossRef] [PubMed]

40. Hsieh, T.C.; Wu, J.M. Targeting CWR22Rv1 prostate cancer cell proliferation and gene expression by combinations of the phytochemicals EGCG, genistein and quercetin. *Anticancer Res.* **2009**, *29*, 4025–4032. [PubMed]

41. Stearns, M.E.; Wang, M. Synergistic effects of the green tea extract epigallocatechin-3-gallate and taxane in eradication of malignant human prostate tumors. *Transl. Oncol.* **2011**, *4*, 147–156. [CrossRef] [PubMed]

42. Liang, G.; Tang, A.; Lin, X.; Li, L.; Zhang, S.; Huang, Z.; Tang, H.; Li, Q.Q. Green tea catechins augment the antitumor activity of doxorubicin in an in vivo mouse model for chemoresistant liver cancer. *Int. J. Oncol.* **2010**, *37*, 111–123. [PubMed]

43. Hsieh, T.C.; Wu, J.M. Suppression of cell proliferation and gene expression by combinatorial synergy of EGCG, resveratrol and gamma-tocotrienol in estrogen receptor-positive MCF-7 breast cancer cells. *Int. J. Oncol.* **2008**, *33*, 851–859. [PubMed]

44. Nair, S.; Hebbar, V.; Shen, G.; Gopalakrishnan, A.; Khor, T.O.; Yu, S.; Xu, C.; Kong, A.N. Synergistic effects of a combination of dietary factors sulforaphane and (−)-epigallocatechin-3-gallate in HT-29 AP-1 human colon carcinoma cells. *Pharm. Res.* **2008**, *25*, 387–399. [CrossRef] [PubMed]

45. Wang, G.; Bhoopalan, V.; Wang, D.; Wang, L.; Xu, X. The effect of caffeine on cisplatin-induced apoptosis of lung cancer cells. *Exp. Hematol. Oncol.* **2015**, *4*. [CrossRef] [PubMed]

46. Tsuchiya, H.; Mori, Y.; Ueda, Y.; Okada, G.; Tomita, K. Sensitization and caffeine potentiation of cisplatin cytotoxicity resulting from introduction of wild-type p53 gene in human osteosarcoma. *Anticancer Res.* **2000**, *20*, 235–242. [PubMed]

47. Karita, M.; Tsuchiya, H.; Kawahara, M.; Kasaoka, S.; Tomita, K. The antitumor effect of liposome-encapsulated cisplatin on rat osteosarcoma and its enhancement by caffeine. *Anticancer Res.* **2008**, *28*, 1449–1457. [PubMed]

48. Geriyol, P.; Basavanneppa, H.B.; Dhananjaya, B.L. Protecting effect of caffeine against vinblastine (an anticancer drug) induced genotoxicity in mice. *Drug Chem. Toxicol.* **2015**, *38*, 188–195. [CrossRef] [PubMed]

49. Dudka, J.; Gieroba, R.; Korga, A.; Burdan, F.; Matysiak, W.; Jodlowska-Jedrych, B.; Mandziuk, S.; Korobowicz, E.; Murias, M. Different effects of resveratrol on dose-related doxorubicin-induced heart and liver toxicity. *Evid.-Based Complement. Altern. Med.* **2012**, *2012*, 606183. [CrossRef] [PubMed]

50. Chari, N.S.; Pinaire, N.L.; Thorpe, L.; Medeiros, L.J.; Routbort, M.J.; McDonnell, T.J. The p53 tumor suppressor network in cancer and the therapeutic modulation of cell death. *Apoptosis* **2009**, *14*, 336–347. [CrossRef] [PubMed]

51. Weijl, N.I.; Elsendoorn, T.J.; Lentjes, E.G.; Hopman, G.D.; Wipkink-Bakker, A.; Zwinderman, A.H. Supplementation with antioxidant micronutrients and chemotherapy-induced toxicity in cancer patients treated with cisplatin-based chemotherapy: A randomised, double-blind, placebo-controlled study. *Eur. J. Cancer* **2004**, *40*, 1713–1723. [CrossRef] [PubMed]

52. Li, W.; Nie, S.; Xie, M.; Chen, Y.; Li, C.; Zhang, H. A major green tea component, (−)-epigallocatechin-3-gallate ameliorates doxorubicin-mediated cardiotoxicity in cardiomyocytes of neonatal rats. *J. Agric. Food Chem.* **2010**, *58*, 8877. [CrossRef] [PubMed]

53. Khan, G.; Haque, S.E.; Anwer, T.; Ahsan, M.N.; Safhi, M.M.; Alam, M.F. Cardioprotective effect of green tea extract on doxorubicin-induced cardiotoxicity in rats. *Acta Pol. Pharm.* **2014**, *71*, 861–867. [PubMed]

54. Saeed, N.M.; El-Naga, R.N.; El-Bakly, W.M.; Abdel-Rahman, H.M.; Salah El-Din, R.A.; El-Demerdash, E. Epigallocatechin-3-gallate pretreatment attenuates doxorubicin-induced cardiotoxicity in rats: A mechanistic study. *Biochem. Pharmacol.* **2015**, *95*, 145–155. [CrossRef] [PubMed]

55. Fleisher, B.; Unum, J.; Shao, J.; An, G. Ingredients in fruit juices interact with dasatinib through inhibition of BCRP: A new mechanism of beverage-drug interaction. *J. Pharm. Sci.* **2015**, *104*, 266–275. [CrossRef] [PubMed]

56. Knop, J.; Misaka, S.; Singer, K.; Hoier, E.; Müller, F.; Glaeser, H.; König, J.; Fromm, M.F. Inhibitory Effects of Green Tea and (−)-Epigallocatechin Gallate on Transport by OATP1B1, OATP1B3, OCT1, OCT2, MATE1, MATE2-K and P-Glycoprotein. *PLoS ONE* **2015**, *10*, e0139370. [CrossRef] [PubMed]

57. Shang, W.; Lu, W.; Han, M.; Qiao, J. The interactions of anticancer agents with tea catechins: Current evidence from preclinical studies. *Anticancer Agents Med. Chem.* **2014**, *14*, 1343–1450. [CrossRef] [PubMed]

58. Mirkov, S.; Komoroski, B.J.; Ramírez, J.; Graber, A.Y.; Ratain, M.J.; Strom, S.C.; Innocenti, F. Effects of green tea compounds on irinotecan metabolism. *Drug Metab. Dispos.* **2007**, *35*, 228–233. [CrossRef] [PubMed]

59. Zhou, Y.; Tang, J.; Du, Y.; Ding, J.; Liu, J.Y. The green tea polyphenol EGCG potentiates the antiproliferative activity of sunitinib in human cancer cells. *Tumor Biol.* **2016**, *5*, 1–12. [CrossRef] [PubMed]

60. ClinicalTrials gov. Available online: https://clinicaltrials.gov/ (accessed on 26 September 2016).

61. Jonsson Comprehensive Cancer Center. Available online: https://clinicaltrials.gov/ct2/show/NCT00685516 (accessed on 22 May 2008).

62. Henning, S.M.; Wang, P.; Said, J.W.; Huang, M.; Grogan, T.; Elashoff, D.; Carpenter, C.L.; Heber, D.; Aronson, W.J. Randomized clinical trial of brewed green and black tea in men with prostate cancer prior to prostatectomy. *Prostate* **2015**, *75*, 550–559. [CrossRef] [PubMed]

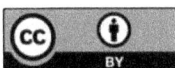

*nutrients*

MDPI

*Review*

# Polyphenols and DNA Damage: A Mixed Blessing

**Amaya Azqueta [1,2,*] and Andrew Collins [3]**

[1] Department of Pharmacology and Toxicology, Faculty of Pharmacy, University of Navarra, C/Irunlarrea 1, 31009 Pamplona, Spain
[2] IdiSNA, Navarra Institute for Health Research
[3] Department of Nutrition, Institute of Basic Medical Sciences, University of Oslo, PB 1046 Blindern, 0316 Oslo, Norway; a.r.collins@medisin.uio.no
* Correspondence: amazqueta@unav.es; Tel.: +34-948-425-600 (ext. 806-343)

Received: 11 October 2016; Accepted: 23 November 2016; Published: 3 December 2016

**Abstract:** Polyphenols are a very broad group of chemicals, widely distributed in plant foods, and endowed with antioxidant activity by virtue of their numerous phenol groups. They are widely studied as putative cancer-protective agents, potentially contributing to the cancer preventive properties of fruits and vegetables. We review recent publications relating to human trials, animal experiments and cell culture, grouping them according to whether polyphenols are investigated in whole foods and drinks, in plant extracts, or as individual compounds. A variety of assays are in use to study genetic damage endpoints. Human trials, of which there are rather few, tend to show decreases in endogenous DNA damage and protection against DNA damage induced ex vivo in blood cells. Most animal experiments have investigated the effects of polyphenols (often at high doses) in combination with known DNA-damaging agents, and generally they show protection. High concentrations can themselves induce DNA damage, as demonstrated in numerous cell culture experiments; low concentrations, on the other hand, tend to decrease DNA damage.

**Keywords:** polyphenols; flavonoids; human studies; in vitro; in vivo; DNA damage; DNA protection

## 1. Introduction

For many years now it has been recognised that fruits and vegetables play an important role in preventing or alleviating the effects of various chronic diseases, notably cardiovascular disease and various cancers. The mechanism(s) of this protection is still not clear. A common explanation is the so-called antioxidant hypothesis; oxidative stress is a factor in many diseases; fruits and vegetables contain various phytochemicals with antioxidant properties, and so these are likely to be the agents of protection. This is clearly a simplistic hypothesis; phytochemicals have been shown to have a wide array of influences on the physiological processes of human cells, and reducing them to sources of antioxidant activity is misguided and misleading. A meta-analysis of clinical trials indicates that antioxidant phytochemicals taken as supplements have no beneficial effect on mortality and may even increase it [1]. In natural plant foods, of course, phytochemicals of different kinds are present, acting in concert, often in all likelihood synergistically, and so studies of whole foods or extracts are particularly valuable. The reductionist approach (looking at individual components) is still popular, however, as evidenced by the large number of studies of individual phytochemicals, and by the growing catalogue of plant species that have been extracted and tested for potential health-promoting effects using a range of molecular markers. DNA damage is one of the most commonly employed such markers, in the reasonable belief that a decrease in DNA damage—as the initiating event of carcinogenesis—must signify a decrease in cancer risk.

Currently, the most popular assay for DNA damage at the cellular level is single cell gel electrophoresis, or the comet assay [2]. It is based on the ability of a strand break (SB) to relax supercoiling in a loop of DNA, thus allowing the DNA to extend to the anode during electrophoresis forming a comet-like image in which the relative intensity of the comet tail reflects the break frequency. Strand breakage is a feature of some but not all kinds of DNA-damaging agent. Reactive oxygen species, in particular, tend to cause damage to DNA bases. An example of base oxidation is 8-oxo–7,8-dihydroguanine (8-OH–Gua). This is converted to a SB by the action of formamidopyrimidine DNA glycosylase (Fpg)—a bacterial repair enzyme, and a simple modification of the comet assay, incorporating an enzymic digestion of the DNA after lysis of cells in agarose—allows the detection of oxidised purines. An analogous enzyme, endonuclease III (or Nth) converts oxidised pyrimidines to SBs. In the search for antioxidant protection of cells against such damage, it is surprising that so few published studies actually use the enzyme-modified comet assay.

The measurement of resistance to $H_2O_2$-induced damage is a good marker of cellular antioxidant status. Typically, cells are exposed in vitro to 50–100 μM $H_2O_2$ for a brief period, and the yield of SBs is measured with the basic comet assay; the lower the break frequency, the higher the antioxidant status.

The base 8-OH–Gua and the nucleosides 8-OH–Guo and 8-OH–dGuo can be detected in tissues, but are more commonly measured in urine, plasma or serum, using high performance liquid chromatography (often linked with mass spectrometry) and antibody-based techniques (ELISA or immunohistochemistry). In the tables and text that follow, we use the abbreviation 8-OH–G to cover all three compounds, as the oxidised base is the common factor. They are markers of oxidative stress [3,4]; free 8-OH–Gua can arise through cellular DNA base excision repair, though the origin of the oxidised nucleosides is not certain.

γ-H2AX is the phosphorylated form of histone H2AX, which appears at the site of DNA damage (particularly double SBs); it is detected by immunocytochemistry [5], or sometimes by immunofluorescence combined with flow cytometry [6], and is a sensitive damage indicator.

Unrepaired DNA damage can result in alterations at the level of chromosomes. Classically, chromosome aberrations (chrom abs) were studied as an index of genomic instability, but now the presence of micronuclei (MN: fragments of chromosomes or whole chromosomes that segregate as discrete bodies at mitosis) is a more common marker [7]. Both chrom abs and MN have been confirmed—in long-term human clinical studies—as prospective markers of cancer risk [8,9].

Here, we summarise the results of recent investigations of effects of polyphenols—a very broad class of phytochemicals—on DNA damage, at the level of humans, in animal experiments, and in in vitro studies using cultured (usually human) cells.

## 2. Methods

In this review, we have concentrated on papers published from 2010 to the present. We used PubMed with the followings terms in the title or abstract: polyphenols/polyphenol/flavonoids/ flavonoid combined with DNA damage/DNA protection/DNA repair. We found a total of 386 papers. We have concentrated on papers where the effect of polyphenols, in the form of real food, plant extract or pure compound, is tested in cell culture, animals and humans. We have excluded papers where only gene expression was studied, papers specifically focused on other diseases than cancer, and papers, for example, with deficient experimental design. Papers in which the main interest is in the induction of apoptosis were also excluded.

The reports are summarised in tables according to whether they deal with whole foods (or drinks) (Table 1), with extracts of plants (Table 2), or with single phytochemicals (Table 3). Studies are further classified as 'in humans', 'in vivo' (animal studies), or 'in vitro' (experiments with cultured cells). Extracts and phytochemicals are, where possible, grouped according to functional, chemical or botanical relationships (such as 'tea and coffee related compounds', or 'flavonoids', or '*Lamiaceae*'). We have generally excluded in vitro experiments with plants or compounds appearing in just one or two publications, unless they fall into one of these groups.

**Table 1.** Effects of whole foods or drinks on various genetic damage endpoints, in humans, in animals ('in vivo'), and in cultured cells ('in vitro').

| Reference | Material Tested | Analysis | Assays | System | Concentration/Dose | Result |
|---|---|---|---|---|---|---|
| | | | | **In Humans** | | |
| [10] | Orange juice | Polyphenols | 8-OH-G in urine by ELISA | Overweight/obese humans | 300 or 745 mg/day (12 weeks) | 8-OH-G ↓ |
| [11] | Aronia-citrus juice | Flavonones, flavones, antocyanins etc. | 8-OH-G in plasma by UHPLC-MS/MS | Triathletes (supplemented and placebo groups) | 200 mL/day 45 days) | Inconclusive—levels of DNA damage products too low |
| [12] | Dark chocolate | Polyphenols | Comet assay | Healthy subjects: PBMN cells | 860 mg/day 2 weeks) | $H_2O_2$-induced SBs ↓ (short-term—2 h—only) |
| [13] | De-alcoholised wine | Anthocyanins, flavonols etc. | Comet assay with Fpg | Post-menopausal women; peripheral blood lymphocytes | 500 mL/day (1 month) | No effect |
| [14] | Wild blueberry drink | Phenolic acids and anthocyanins | Comet assay + Fpg; $H_2O_2$ resistance (comet assay); DNA repair (in vitro comet assay) | Subjects with cardiovascular risk factors: PBMN cells | 375 mg anthocyanins/day (6 weeks) | No effect on DNA SBs. Fpg-sensitive sites ↓; $H_2O_2$ resistance ↑; no effect on repair |
| [15] | Green tea | | Comet assay | Healthy subjects: PBMN cells 30, 60, 90 min after ingestion, exposed ex vivo to UV(A)/VIS radiation | Single 540 mL dose | Protection against UV(A)/VIS-induced DNA SBs seen in 'responders' |
| [16] | Honey | Phenolic compounds | Comet assay with EndoIII, Fpg | Pesticide-exposed humans | 2-week honey supplementation (50 g/day) | DNA repair ↑, EndoIII and Fpg sites ↓ |
| | | | | **In Vivo** | | |
| [17] | *Chrysobalanus icaco* fruit | Polyphenols, Mg, Se | Comet assay on blood and MN assay on bone marrow and PBMN | Rats + Dox | Up to 0.4 g/kg/day for 14 days | Blood cells; DNA SBs ↓. Bone marrow, blood cells; MN ↓ |
| [18] | Green and black teas | | 8-OH-G on liver by HPLC | Swiss albino mice + Na arsenite | 2.5% o. 0.5 g dry leaves/5 mL of boiled water equivalent to human consumption of 1 cup). 22 days. | Protection (8-OH-G ↓) |
| [19] | Piquia pulp | Phenolic compounds, carotenoids | Comet assay on liver, kidney, heart cells MN on bone marrow and PBMN cells | Rats + Dox | 75, 150, 300 mg/kg/day for 14 days | Protection against DNA SBs and MN formation: lowest dose tends to be most effective |
| [20] | Açai pulp | Phenolic compounds, carotenoids | Comet assay on liver, kidney and PBMN cells; MN on bone marrow and PBMN cells | Mice + Dox | 3.33, 10, 5.7 g/kg/day for 1 or 14 days | Protection against DNA SBs and MN formation: 14 days pretreatment more effective |
| [21] | Cloudy apple juice | Polyphenols | Comet assay on liver cells | Rats | 10 mL/kg/day for 28 days | DNA SBs ↑ and no effect on N-nitrosodiethylamine-induced damage |

**Table 1.** *Cont.*

| Reference | Material Tested | Analysis | Assays | System | Concentration/Dose | Result |
|---|---|---|---|---|---|---|
| [22] | Green tea | – | Comet assay on intestinal cells | Rats + As | 10 mg/mL in water for 28 days | Claim protection |
| [23] | Spinach | Total polyphenols | Comet assay on leukocytes | Hyperlipidemic rats | 5% (powder) in diet, for 6 weeks | $H_2O_2$-induced DNA SBs in leukocytes ↓ |
| | | | | **In Vitro** | | |
| [24] | Green tea | – | Comet assay with Fpg | Human PBMN cells | 7–71 µM catechins | DNA damage ↓ at lower concentrations but ↑ at highest concentration |
| [25] | Herbal preparation | Total phenolics | Comet assay | YAC-1 (mouse lymphoma) cells | 1–13 mg/mL | DNA SBs ↑ at 8.7 mg/mL |
| | | | | Rat fibroblasts | 1–13 mg/mL | DNA SBs ↑ at 2.2 mg/mL |
| [26] | Various honeys | – | Comet assay | HepG2 (human liver carcinoma) cells treated with B(a)P, PhIP, nitrosamines | 0.1–100 mg/mL | Slight decreases in DNA SBs in most cases, not dose-dependent |

PBMN: peripheral blood mononuclear; SB: strand break; Fpg: formamidopyrimidine DNA glycosylase; UV: ultraviolet; VIS: visible; MN: micronucleus/micronuclei; Dox: doxorubicin; EndoIII: endonuclease III (Nth); 8-OH-G: 8-oxo-7,8-dihydroguanine; B(a)P: benzo(a)pyrene; PhIP: 2-amino-1-methyl-6-phenylimidazo[4,5-b]pyridine.

**Table 2.** Effects of plant extracts on various genetic damage endpoints, in humans, in animals ('in vivo'), and in cultured cells ('in vitro').

| Reference | Material Tested | Analysis | Assays | System | Concentration/Dose | Result |
|---|---|---|---|---|---|---|
| | | | | **In Humans** | | |
| [27] | Green tea polyphenols | | Urinary 8-OH-G by HPLC | Postmenopausal women with osteoporosis | 500 mg/day (capsules, 6 months) | 8-OH-G ↓ over 6 months |
| | | | | **In Vivo** | | |
| | | | | **Tea-Related** | | |
| [28] | Green tea polyphenols | | 8-OH-G in brain by Ab assay | Rats | 400 mg/day (gastric intubation, 4 weeks) | 8-OH-G ↓ |
| [29] | Green tea polyphenols | Epicatechin derivatives | CPD on skin and lymph nodes by Ab assay | Mice (NER+ and-) + UV | 0.2% in drinking water (7 days before UV irradiation) | Enhanced removal of CPDs in NER-proficient mice |
| [30] | Green tea extract | | MN in polychromatic erythrocytes | Mice + Cr(VI) | 30 mg/kg (one dose—gavage) | MN ↓ |
| [31] | Green tea polyphenols | | Comet assay with Fpg on blood; 8-OH-G in brain by HPLC | Rats + acrylonitrile | 0.4% in diet (1 week before acrylonitrile and then throughout acrylonitrile treatment for 28 days) | ↓ Fpg-sensitive sites and 8-OH-G ↓ |
| [32] | *Calluna vulgaris* polyphenol extract | | CPDs in skin by Ab assay | Mice + UV(B) | 4 mg. cm² (30 min before exposure to UV, repeated on 10 days) | CPDs ↓ |
| [33] | *Podophyllum hexandrum* extract | Total phenolics | Alkaline halo assay; DNA repair (SB rejoining—PCR assay) | Thymocytes from γ-irradiated mice | 15 mg/kg (one dose, i.p.) | Protection against γ-ray-induced DNA SBs and accelerated rejoining |
| [34] | *Cotinus coggyria* extract | | Comet assay on liver | Rats + pyrogallol | 0.5–2 g/kg (single dose, i.p.) | SBs at highest dose of extract alone: protection against pyrogallol-induced SBs at 0.5 g/kg |
| | | | | **In Vitro** | | |
| | | | | **Tea-Related** | | |
| [35] | Green tea polyphenols | | Comet assay | Melanoma cell lines | 20–60 μg/mL (time) | 40, 60 μg/mL; DNA SBs ↑ |
| [36] | Green tea extract | | Comet assay | Human laryngeal carcinoma cell line (HEp2) + drug-resistant cell line CK2 | IC = 2 g/200 mL H₂O₂ Concentration tested = 0.1× | SBs ↑ at 72 h, not 48 h |
| | | | | **Lamiaceae** | | |
| [37] | Citrus and rosemary bioflavonoid extract | Total polyphenols | Comet assay | HaCaT (human keratinocytes) + UV(B) | 100 μg/mL | Pre-treatment: UV(B)-induced DNA SBs ↓ |
| | | | MN | Human lymphocytes + X-ray | 1 mg/mL | X-ray induced MN ↓ |

**Table 2.** *Cont.*

| Reference | Material Tested | Analysis | Assays | System | Concentration/Dose | Result |
|---|---|---|---|---|---|---|
| [38] | *Thymus vulgaris* extract | | Comet assay and γ-H2AX by Ab | Human skin model exposed to UV(B) | 1.8 µg/mL | Protection against DNA damage |
| [39] | *Thymus vulgaris* extract | | Comet assay 24 h after UV | NCTC (human keratinocytes) + UV(A) or UV(B) | 1.82 µg/mL | DNA SBs ↓ |
| | | | MN | | | No effect seen |
| | | | γ-H2AX by Ab | | | No effect seen |
| [40] | Lemon balm extract | Polyphenols | Comet assay and γ-H2AX by Ab assay | Human keratinocytes + UV(B) | 15–100 µg/mL | DNA SBs ↓ (100 µg/mL); γH2AX ↓ (15 µg/mL) |
| [41] | *Ocimum sanctum* extract ("Holy basil") | Total phenolics | Comet assay | SH-SY5Y (human neuroblastoma) cells | 75 µg/mL | $H_2O_2$-induced DNA SBs ↓ |
| [42] | Various *Lamiaceae* leaf extracts | Total polyphenols, flavonoids | Comet assay | HepG2 (human liver carcinoma) cells + $CdCl_2$ | 50–350 µg/mL for 4 h | Dose-dependent decrease in Cd-induced DNA SBs |
| | **Fruits and Berries** | | | | | |
| [43] | Strawberry extract | Anthocyanins | Comet assay | Human dermal fibroblasts exposed to UV(A) | 0.05–0.5 mg/mL | Protection against DNA SBs at 0.25, 0.5 mg/mL |
| [44] | Strawberry extract | Total phenolics, flavonoids, anthocyanins, vitamin C, β-carotene | Comet assay | Human dermal fibroblasts exposed to $H_2O_2$ | 0.5 mg/mL | DNA SBs ↓ |
| [45] | *Vaccinium* berries extract | Total polyphenols and anthocyanins | Comet assay | A549 (human lung adenocarcinoma) cells | 21–167 µg/mL | Dose-dependent protection against DNA SBs induced by t-BOOH |
| [46] | Blackcurrant extract | | Comet assay ($H_2O_2$ resistance) | TK6 (human lymphoblastoid) cells | 0.5–3 mg/mL | $H_2O_2$-induced DNA SBs ↓ |
| | | | MN ± $H_2O_2$ | | 1 mg/mL | $H_2O_2$-induced MN ↓ |
| [47] | Various apple polyphenol s extract | Monomeric polyphenols oligosaccharides and oligomeric procyanidins. | Comet assay with Fpg | Caco2 (colon carcinoma) cells | 1–100 µg/mL | Menadione-induced DNA SBs and Fpg-sensitive sites ↓ Greatest protection at low concentrations; with some extracts, damage ↑ at high doses |
| [48] | Polyphenol extracts of Australian fruits | Phenolic acids and anthocyanins | MN | HT29 (human colon adenocarcinoma) cells | 0.5–1 mg/mL | MN ↑ with one extract |

**Table 2.** *Cont.*

| Reference | Material Tested | Analysis | Assays | System | Concentration/Dose | Result |
|---|---|---|---|---|---|---|
| [49] | Red wine extract | | Comet assay | HUVECs (human umbilical vein endothelial) cells + *t*-BOOH | 25 μg/mL | DNA SBs ↓ |
| **Honey-Related** | | | | | | |
| [16] | Honey extract | Phenolic compounds | Comet assay with EndoIII, Fpg | Bronchial epithelial and neuronal cells | 5 μg/mL | Pesticide (glyphosate, chlorpyrifos)-induced damage (SBs, EndoIII and Fpg sites) ↓ |
| | | | Cellular DNA repair | | | Protection against inhibition of repair of DNA SBs by pesticides |
| [50] | Propolis extr | | Comet assay | Fibroblasts | 0.1–0.3 μg/mL | γ-Ray-induced DNA SBs ↓ |
| [51] | Propolis | | Comet assay + Fpg, EndoIII | Human gastric cancer cell line AGS | 0.3 μg/mL | High DNA damage, suppressed by antioxidants or catalase |

Ab: antibody; CPD: cyclobutane pyrimidine dimer; NER: nucleotide excision repair; i.p.: intraperitoneal; *t*-BOOH: *tert*-butyl hydroperoxide; HUVEC: human umbilical vein endothelial cell.

**Table 3.** Effects of individual polyphenolic compounds on various genetic damage endpoints, in humans, in animals ('in vivo'), and in cultured cells ('in vitro').

| Reference | Material Tested | Assays | System | Concentration/Dose | Result |
|---|---|---|---|---|---|
| **In Humans** | | | | | |
| [52] | Epigallocatechin gallate | 8-OH-G in leukocyte DNA (HPLC/UV/MS) | Prostate cancer patients | 800 mg/day (3 to 6 weeks before surgery) | Decrease in 8-OH-G not significant |
| [53] | Xanthohumol (drink) | Comet assay and urinary 8-OH-G (UPLC) | Cross over intervention trial, healthy subjects | 12 mg/day for 14 days | FPG-sites ↓; H$_2$O$_2$-induced SBs ↓; 8-OH-G ↓ |
| | Xanthohumol (pills) | Comet assay | Parallel intervention trial, healthy subjects | | FPG-sites ↓; H$_2$O$_2$-induced SBs ↓ |
| **In Vivo** | | | | | |
| [54] | Luteolin | Comet assay and MN on blood and bone marrow | Mice + ochratoxin A | 2.5 mg/kg (one dose i.p.) | No effect |
| | Chlorogenic acid | | | 10 mg/kg (one dose i.p.) | DNA SBs ↓; also MN ↓ |
| | Caffeic acid | | | 10 mg/kg (one dose i.p.) | DNA SBs ↓ |
| | Curcumin | | | 100 or 200 mg/kg/day (7 days, gavage) | Pretreatment → etoposide-induced DNA damage ↓ |
| [55] | Epicatechin | Comet assay with FPG on bone marrow | Rats + etoposide | 20 or 40 mg/kg/day (7 days, gavage) | Pretreatment → etoposide-induced oxidative DNA damage ↓ (less than with Curcumin) but not DNA SBs. |
| [56] | Ellagic acid | MN in polychromatic erythrocytes; alkaline unwinding | Swiss albino mice + cyclophosphamide | 50/100 mg/kg/day (orally, 7 days) | Protection against MN formation and DNA SBs |
| [57] | Epigallocatechin gallate and theaflavin | Alkaline unwinding assay | Mouse skin + dimethylbenzanthracene | 100 µg/mouse (topical application, 1 h) | Topical pretreatment → DNA SBs ↓ |
| | Epigallocatechin gallate and theaflavin as NPs (PLGA) | | | 5–20 µg/mouse (topical application, 1 h) | NP form has ~30-fold dose-advantage |
| [58] | Epigallocatechin gallate | γ-H2AX by Western blot and Ab and 8-OH-G by Ab assay | H1299 (human lung cancer cells) xenografts in mice | 0.1%–0.5% in diet, 30 mg/kg/day injection | Dose-dependent ↑ in γ-H2AX and 8-OH-G |
| [59] | Silibinin | 8-OH-G in various brain regions by ELISA | Diabetic mice | 20 mg/kg/day i.p. (4 weeks) | 8-OH-G ↓ in different regions of brain |
| [60] | Quercetin | MN in bone marrow and blood | Rats + PCBs | 50 mg/kg/day for 25 days | PCB-induced MN ↓ |
| [61] | Quercetin | Chrom abs and MN in bone marrow; Comet assay on blood | Mice + γ-irradiation | 20 mg/kg/day for 5 days | Radiation-induced Chrom abs, SBs, MN ↓ |
| | Rutin | | | 10 mg/kg/day for 5 days | |
| [62] | Chrysin | Comet assay (hepatocytes and leukocytes) | Rats + methyl mercury | 0.1, 1, 10 mg/kg/day for 45 days | MeHg-induced SBs ↓ at higher doses |

**Table 3.** *Cont.*

| Reference | Material Tested | Assays | System | Concentration/Dose | Result |
|---|---|---|---|---|---|
| [63] | Puerarin | 8-OH-G in kidney by HPLC | Mice + CCl4 | 0.2 or 0.4 g/kg/day for 4 weeks | 8-OH-G ↓ |
| [64] | Quercetin | 8-OH-G in kidney by HPLC | Rats + lead | 10 mg/kg/day for 10 week | 8-OH-G ↓ |
| [65] | Myricitrin, Myricetin | MN (reticulocytes); Comet assay (liver, duodenum, stomach) | Mice | 1, 1.5, 2 g/kg/day for 3 days | No increase in MN, SBs only in liver + myricetin |
| [66] | Quercetin | Comet assay on liver | Rats + DEN | 10, 30, 100 mg/kg/day for 3 days | DEN-induced SBs ↓ |
| [34] | Myricetin | Comet assay on liver | Rats + pyrogallol | 255.5 µg/kg 2 h and 12 h b-fore pyrogallol | SBs ↓ in liver |
| [67] | Quercetin | Comet assay on liver | Rats + acrylamide | 10 mg/kg/day for 5 days | No effect of quercetin alone. Acrylamide-induced SBs ↓ |
| | | 8-OH-G in liver by ELISA | | | No effect of quercetin alone. Acrylamide-induced 8-OH-G ↓ |
| [68] | Naringin | Comet assay | Mice (hepatocytes and cardiocytes) | 50, 250 or 500 mg/kg oral (one dose) | No effect |
| | | | | 50, 250 or 500 mg/kg oral (one dose) + Dau i.p. | DNA SBs induced by Dau ↓ |
| [69] | Apigenin | Chrom abs and MN in bone marrow; comet assay on skin; DNA repair (removal of CPDs by Ab) | Mice + UV(B) | 1.5-3 mg/cm² (24 h; during UV irradiation) | Chrom abs and MN ↓; tail length ↓. Removal of dimers apparently stimulated by apigenin |

**In Vitro**

**Tea-Related**

| Reference | Material Tested | Assays | System | Concentration/Dose | Result |
|---|---|---|---|---|---|
| [70] | Chlorogenic acid | Comet assay | HaCaT (human keratinocytes) cells + UV(B) | Not stated. Probably 5-50 µM | DNA SBs ↓ |
| [71] | Chlorogenic acid | Comet assay | K562 (human leukaemia) cells | 0.5-5 mM | DNA SBs ↑ |
| | | γ-H2AX by Ab | Chinese hamster AA8 cell line and K562 | 0.5 mM | γ-H2AX foci ↑ |
| [73] | Ellagic acid | Comet assay | Prostate cancer cell lines LNCaP, DU145, BPH-1 | 4.5-300 µM | DNA SBs ↑ at 9 µM in BPH-1, 37 µM in DU 145, 150 µM in LnCap |
| [74] | Epicatechin gallate | Comet assay; MN | C6 astroglial cells | 0.1-1 µM | H2O2-induced DNA SBs and MN formation ↓ |
| [58] | Epigallocatechin gallate | γ-H2AX and 8-OH-G by Ab assay | H1299 (human lung adenocarcinoma) cells | 50 µM | γ-H2AX and 8-OH-G ↑ |
| [75] | Metabolites of quercetin, chlorogenic acid | Comet assay | L197 (human colorectal adenoma) cells + cumene hydroperoxide | 2.5 µM/5 µM | Decrease in DNA SBs |

**Table 3.** *Cont.*

| Reference | Material Tested | Assays | System | Concentration/Dose | Result |
|---|---|---|---|---|---|
| [76] | Epigallocatechin gallate | Comet assay | HeLa (human cervical cancer) cells, p53R (cells with p53 reporter) | 10, 20 µg/mL | DNA SBs ↑ |
| [77] | Ethyl gallate | Comet assay | Human carcinoma cell line KB | 20–50 µg/mL | DNA SBs ↑ |
| [78] | Tannic acid | Comet assay with Fpg | Human neutrophils | 10–150 µM | DNA SBs ↑ (dose-dependent); weak effect (↑) in TPA-stimulated cells. Fpg sites also ↑, but ↓ in TPA-stimulated cells |
| | Resveratrol | | | | DNA damage (SBs) ↑ (dose-dependent); but ↓ (dose-dependent) in TPA-stimulated cells. Same pattern with FPG sites |
| [72] | Chafuroside B (tea polyphenol) | CPDs by Ab | Human keratinocytes + UV(B) | 1 µM | CPDs ↓ after 24 h |
| [36] | Epigallocatechin gallate; Epicatechin gallate | Comet assay | HEp2 (human laryngeal carcinoma cell line) | 50 µM | With either ECG or EGCG, SBs ↓ at 48 h (from background); no effect at 72 h |
| | | | CK2 (drug resistant, from HEp2) | | No effect at 48 or 72 h |
| **Curcumin** | | | | | |
| [79] | Curcumin; Ellagic acid | Comet assay | HeLa (human cervical cancer) cells | 25 µM | DNA SBs ↑ (with both together; not significant alone) |
| [80]; | Curcumin | Chrom abs and PCC | Human lymphocytes, with/without stimulation | 0.14–7 µM | Radioprotective effects seen for both reagents in PCC assay (non-cycling cells) |
| | Resveratrol | | | 2.2–220 µM | Radiosensitisation of cycling cells (chrom abs) by both reagents |
| [81] | Curcumin | 8-OH-G by Ab assay | Smooth muscle cells | up to 10 µM | 8-OH-G ↑ |
| [82] | Quercetin; Curcumin | γ-H2AX by Ab assay | HT1080 human fibrosarcoma cell line | 30 and 80 µM Quercetin; 10 and 15 µM Curcumin, | Significant increases in γ H2AX |
| | | MN | | 30 µM Quercetin; 10 µM Curcumin | Significant increases in MN. (Quercetin less effective.) |
| [83] | Soy isoflavones | γ-H2AX by Ab assay | LNCaP (human prostate cancer) cells | 10 µg/mL | No effect on H2AX |
| | Curcumin | | | 25 µg/mL | γ-H2AX ↑ |
| [84] | Polyphenols | Comet assay | Lymphocytes + B(a)P | 5 µg/mL | DNA SBs ↓ |
| | Curcumin | | | 5 and 10 µg/mL | DNA SBs ↓ |
| [85] | Curcumin | Comet assay | HCT-116 (human colon cancer) cells | 50 µM | DNA SBs ↑ |
| [86] | Curcumin | Comet assay | K562 (human leukaemia) cells | 12.5–200 µM | DNA SBs ↑ |
| **Resveratrol** | | | | | |

**Table 3.** *Cont.*

| Reference | Material Tested | Assays | System | Concentration/Dose | Result |
|---|---|---|---|---|---|
| [87] | Resveratrol | Chrom abs | Human lymphocytes + aflatoxin | 10–100 µM | No effect of resveratrol alone. Dose-dependent decrease in aflatoxin-induced chrom abs |
| [88] | Resveratrol | MN; Comet assay | Human bronchial epithelial cell line HBE + Na arsenite | 5 µM | ↓ DNA SBs and MN induced by arsenite |
| [89] | Resveratrol | γ-H2AX by Ab assay | HCT-116 (human colon cancer) cells | 25 µM | γ-H2AX foci ↑; DNA damage due to toposiomerase II poisoning |
| [90] | Resveratrol | γ-H2AX by Ab assay | Prostate epithelial cells | 5 µM | Ionising radiation-induced damage enhanced |
| [91] | Resveratrol | Comet assay | Rat astrocytes + ethanol | 1–10 µM | ↓ DNA SBs induced by ethanol |
| **Lamiaceae** | | | | | |
| [39] | Thymol | Comet assay 24 h after UV | NCTC (human keratinocytes) + UV(A) or UV(B) | 1 µg/mL | DNA SBs ↓ |
| | | MN | | | No effect seen |
| | | γ-H2AX by Ab assay | | | No effect seen |
| **Flavonoids** | | | | | |
| [92] | Naringin | Chromosome aberrations | Human lymphocytes treated with Cd | 1, 2 µg/mL | Cd-induced chrom abs ↓ |
| | | SCE | | | No significant effect on SCE |
| [93] | Rutin | Comet assay | Rat hepatic cell line HTC | 10–810 µg/mL (24 h) | SBs at highest concentration |
| | | MN | | | No significant increase in MN—but protection against MN induced by B(a)P |
| [94] | Quercetin; Rutin | à-H2AX by Ab assay | V79 lung fibroblast hamster cells | 100 µg/mL for 12 h | Massive foci, results of lethality |
| [95] | Kaempferol | Comet assay | HL-60 human leukemia cells | 75 µM, 6–48 h | SBs induced |
| [96] | Quercetin | Comet assay | Lymphocytes from healthy subjects and colon cancer patients, + food mutagens PhIP and IQ | 100, 250, 500 µM | SBs induced by PhIP or IQ ↓ |
| | Rutin | | | 50, 250, 500 µM | |
| [97] | Fisetin, Kaempferol; Galangin; Quercetin; Luteolin; Chrysin; 7-hydroxyflavone; 7,8-dihydroxyflavone; Baicalein; Rutin | Comet assay; MN | HepG2 (human liver carcinoma) cells + B(a)P | 2.5–25 µM | SBs induced by B(a)P ↓ (all except rutin); MN induced by B(a)P ↓ (all except rutin); Fi>Qu>Ga>Ka>Lu (more effective group); Ch, 7Fl, 7,8Fl, Ba (less effective group) |
| [98] | Fisetin | Comet assay | Human hepatic Huth-7 cells | 60 µM | SBs ↑ |
| [99] | Kaempferol | Comet assay | Human osteosarcoma cells U2-OS | 50, 100, 150 µM | SBs ↑ (not quantitated) |
| [65] | Myricitrin | MN | TK6 (human lymphoblastoid) cells | 20–500 µg/mL for 24 h | MN ↑ (Dose-dependent) |
| | Myricetin | | | 2.5–75 µg/mL for 24 h | MN ↑ (significant?) |

**Table 3.** *Cont.*

| Reference | Material Tested | Assays | System | Concentration/Dose | Result |
|---|---|---|---|---|---|
| [100] | Quercetin and rutin | Comet assay | Human hepatoma cell line HepG2 | 0.1, 1 and 5 µg/mL (2 h of treatment) | No induction of SBs (quercetin and rutin alone) |
| | | | HepG2 + Aflatoxin B, MMS, Dox | Pre-, co- and post-treatment | DNA damage induced by AFB1, MMS, Dox ↓ in all treatment conditions |
| [101] | Quercetin | Comet assay; 8-OH-G (HPLC) | Human hepatoma cell line HepG2 cells | 0.1, 1 and 5 µg/mL (24 h of treatment) | No effect |
| | | | HepG2 cells + HgCl$_2$ and MeHg | Pre-, co- and post-treatment | DNA damage induced by HgCl$_2$ and MeHg ↓ in pre- and co-treatment |
| [102] | Quercitrin | Comet assay | Mouse epidermal cell line JB6 + UV(B) | 10, 20 and 80 µM, 30 min | No effect |
| | | | | 10, 20 and 80 µM, 30 min + UV(B) | UV(B)-induced SBs ↓ |
| [51] | Galangin, chrysin | Comet assay + FPG, EndoIII | AGS human gastric adenocarcinoma cells | 20 µM (1 h) | Base oxidation ↑ |
| [69] | Apigenin | Comet assay: Chrom abs; MN | HaCaT human keratinocytes + UV(B) | 15–25 µg/mL | DNA damage ↓, Chrom abs ↓, MN ↓ |

PCB: polychlorinated biphenyls; chrom ab: chromosome aberration; DEN: diethylnitrosamine; Dau: Daunorubicin; TPA: tetradecanoyl phorbol acetate; ECG: epicatechin gallate; EGCG: epigallocatechin gallate; PCC: premature chromosome condensation; SCE: sister chromatid exchange; IQ: 2-amino-3-methylimidazo[4,5-f]quinolone; MMS: methylmethanesulphonate; AFB1: aflatoxin B1.

## 3. Results

### 3.1. Whole Foods and Drinks

Relatively few investigations of effects of whole foods on genetic damage endpoints have been published. A variety of fruit-derived drinks as well as tea (though this could be considered an extract), and dark chocolate, were tested in human supplementation trials. A decrease in urinary 8-OH–G was seen in overweight or obese adults supplemented with orange juice [10] but levels of plasma 8-OH–G in triathletes were too low to see any effect of Aronia-citrus juice [11]. De-alcoholised wine given daily for one month was without effect on DNA SBs or Fpg-sites in peripheral blood mononuclear (PBMN) cells of post-menopausal women [13]. However, a daily blueberry drink taken for 6 weeks protected PBMN cells from $H_2O_2$-induced damage, but had no effect on SBs or DNA repair capacity [14]. Malhomme de la Roche et al. [15] found that ingestion of green tea protected PBMN cells challenged ex vivo with UV(A)/VIS (ultraviolet(A)/visible) radiation, but only in some subjects, described as responders. Alleva et al. [16] gave a honey supplement to humans exposed to pesticides, and found, after two weeks' supplementation, lower levels of EndoIII- and Fpg-sensitive sites in lymphocytes as well as an enhanced capacity for DNA repair. Dark chocolate induced a transient protection against $H_2O_2$-induced DNA damage in PBMN cells ex vivo [12].

Most of the animal studies have looked at the possible protection afforded by polyphenol-rich foods or drinks against DNA damage induced by treating the animals (rats or mice) with known carcinogens such as doxorubicin (Dox), n-nitrosodiethylamine, or sodium arsenite. Protection was claimed with *Chrysobalanus icaco* fruit [17], Piquia pulp [19], Açai pulp [20], and tea [18,22]; but cloudy apple juice actually increased SBs and had no effect on nitrosamine-induced damage [21]. Treatment of hyperlipidemic rats with spinach increased the resistance of blood cells ex vivo to $H_2O_2$-induced damage [23].

Experiments with cultured cells and whole foods/drinks are understandably rarely performed. Incubation of PBMN cells with green tea decreased DNA damage at low concentrations but increased it at the highest concentration tested (representing 71 mM catechins) [24]. Various honeys afforded slight protection of HepG2 cells against SBs produced by treatment with certain organic carcinogens [26]. A Chinese herbal preparation caused SBs in mouse lymphoma cells and rat fibroblasts, but at extreme concentrations (1–13 mg/mL) [25].

### 3.2. Extracts of Plants

#### 3.2.1. Tea-Related Extracts

One human trial and several animal experiments have been reported with tea-related extracts. Post-menopausal women with osteoporosis were supplemented with green tea polyphenols for 6 months; the level of urinary 8-OH–G decreased [27]. Xu et al. [28] found a decrease in 8-OH–G in rats given a very high dose of green tea polyphenols. Protective effects of green tea extracts against genetic damage were reported by Garcia-Rodriguez et al. [30] in mice treated with Cr(IV); and by Pu et al. [31] in rats treated with acrylonitrile. Katiyar et al. [29] found that green tea polyphenols promoted the repair of UV-induced DNA lesions in mice proficient in nucleotide excision repair (NER), but not in NER- mice. Two studies with cultured cells have found increases in DNA SBs induced by green tea extract; Prasad et al. [35] in melanoma cell lines (though at rather high concentrations), and Durgo et al. [36] in a human laryngeal carcinoma cell line.

#### 3.2.2. Lamiaceae Family Plants

The *Lamiaceae* family includes many plants used as culinary herbs, and so they have been grouped together here. All publications in our search deal with effects in cell culture.

Calo et al. [39] tested an extract of *Thymus vulgaris* (and thymol in parallel) on keratinocytes irradiated with UV(A) or UV(B); they found a decrease in SBs, though no effect on MN or γ-H2AX foci. A similar protective effect was reported by Cornaghi et al. [38] in a human skin model exposed to UV(B). A citrus and rosemary extract (but at high concentrations) decreased the frequency of MN induced by X-rays in human lymphocytes, and decreased UV(B)-induced SBs in keratinocytes [37]. This last group also tested lemon balm extract on UV(B)-irradiated keratinocytes and found a decrease in SBs (at a high concentration) and in γ-H2AX foci at a more moderate concentration [40]. Thirugnanasampandan et al. [42] studied three *Lamiaceae* species; HepG2 cells were incubated for 4 h with an extract before treating with CdCl$_2$. Dose-dependent decreases in SBs were seen with all three (though even the lowest concentration tested was high). An extract of *Ocimum sanctum* (a form of basil) was tested by Venuprasad et al. [41] on human neuroblastoma cells; it protected against H$_2$O$_2$-induced SBs (at a high concentration).

### 3.2.3. Honey-Related Extracts

In parallel experiments to their human honey trial, Alleva et al. [16] showed that pre-treatment of cells with honey extract protected against pesticide-induced DNA damage and inhibition of DNA repair. Propolis extract (at high concentration) decreased the frequency of γ-ray-induced SBs in fibroblasts [50], and yet—at a much lower concentration—it caused oxidative damage (SBs measured with Fpg and EndoIII together in the comet assay) in a human cancer cell line, which was suppressed by antioxidants or catalase and so was imputed to the production of H$_2$O$_2$ [51].

### 3.2.4. Fruits and Berries

All papers on extracts of fruits and berries reviewed here describe cell culture experiments and with one exception they have made use of high to extremely high extract concentrations. The extract of one Australian fruit (among several studied) caused an increase in MN [48]. Other reports are of protection against oxidation damage caused by H$_2$O$_2$ [43,44,46]; or tert-butyl-hydroperoxide (t-BOOH) [45,49]. The exception to usage of high doses is a report by Bellion et al. [47] with apple polyphenol extracts; they found that 24 h pre-incubation of Caco2 cells decreased the DNA damage induced by menadione (low concentrations actually giving the greatest protection).

### 3.2.5. Miscellaneous Plant Extracts

Animal experiments with various plant extracts have shown protection against SB production in liver cells of pyrogallol-treated rats (at very high doses of extract) [34]; accelerated rejoining of γ-ray-induced DNA SBs [33]; and a decrease in pyrimidine dimers in the skin of UV(B)-irradiated mice [32].

## 4. Isolated Phytochemicals

### 4.1. Compounds Related to Tea and Coffee

Compounds tested—caffeic acid, chafuroside B, chlorogenic acid, ellagic acid, epicatechin, epicatechin gallate, epigallocatechin gallate, theaflavin.

One human trial with epigallocatechin gallate in prostate cancer patients showed no significant effect on 8-OH–G in leukocytes [52]. Animal studies with single polyphenols have generally involved treating mice or rats with a known DNA-damaging agent and looking for protection against DNA breaks, MN and chrom abs. Generally, protection is seen [54,57] though in some cases at rather high doses [56,63]. Pretreatment of rats with epicatechin reduced the level of DNA breaks induced in bone marrow cells by the topoisomerase poison etoposide [55]. High concentrations have also been used in in vitro experiments with cultured cells, and have given increases in SBs and γ-H2AX foci [71] and in γ-H2AX and 8-OH–G [58]. Kumar et al. [79] found that a combination of ellagic acid with curcumin (25 µM each) caused SBs while the separate compounds had no significant effect. A decrease in (background) SBs with epigallocatechin gallate or epicatechin gallate was reported by Durgo et al. [36] at 48 but not 72 h. At more reasonable concentrations, the results are mixed: decreases in UV(B)-induced SBs [70] and cyclobutane pyrimidine dimers [72]; decreases in $H_2O_2$-induced SBs and MN [74]; a decrease in SBs induced by cumene hydroperoxide [75]; but SBs and Fpg-sites increased in tetradecanoyl phorbol acetate (TPA)-stimulated neutrophils [78] and an increase in SBs with ellagic acid in prostate cancer cells was reported by Vanella et al. [73] at concentrations of 9 µM in one of the cell lines but higher concentrations in two other lines.

## 4.2. Curcumin

Curcumin was examined alongside epicatechin by Papiez [55]; at high concentration (up to 0.2 g/kg/day), it decreased DNA damage in the bone marrow of rats treated with etoposide. In cultured cells, curcumin at rather high concentrations caused SBs [85,86] and γ-H2AX foci [83]. The production of SBs in combination with ellagic acid was noted above [79]. Lewinska et al. [81] reported a pro-oxidant effect of curcumin at concentrations of 10 µM (and below), indicated by an increase in 8-oxo–G in smooth muscle cells. Sebastia et al. [80] compared effects of curcumin on human lymphocytes, both stimulated by TPA and unstimulated, and γ-irradiated. In non-cycling cells, the phytochemical was radioprotective (decreasing the level of premature chromosome condensation), whereas in cycling cells it acted as a radiosensitiser, increasing the frequency of chrom abs.

## 4.3. Resveratrol

At high concentration, in human lymphocytes, resveratrol decreased the frequency of chromosome aberrations caused by aflatoxin [87]. At a lower concentration, it protected human epithelial cells against SBs and MN induced by sodium arsenite [88], and rat astrocytes against SBs caused by ethanol [91]. However, a low dose enhanced the frequency of γ-H2AX foci after ionising irradiation of prostate epithelial cells [90]. A moderately high concentration applied to colon cancer cells caused γ-H2AX foci, apparently as a result of topoisomerase II poisoning [89]. SBs as well as Fpg-sites were increased in non-cycling cells but decreased in TPA-stimulated, cycling cells [78]. In contrast, Sebastia et al. [80] found that, as with curcumin, effects of resveratrol on irradiated lymphocytes differed depending on whether the cells were non-cycling (showing a decrease in premature chromosome condensation), or cycling (in which it had the opposite effect, acting as a radiosensitiser, increasing chromosome aberrations).

## 4.4. Flavonoids

Kozics et al. [97] performed a useful comparative study of 10 flavonoids, concluding that their effectiveness at protecting against B(a)P-induced SBs and MN depended on their chemical structure. Tested over a relatively low concentration range, fisetin, quercetin, galangin, kaempferol and luteolin (in order of decreasing effectiveness) were more effective than chrysin,7-hydroxyflavone, 7,8-dihydroxyflavone or baicalein, while rutin was without effect.

Among the flavonoids, quercetin appears most often in this survey. At low concentrations, SBs induced by aflatoxin B1 (AFB1), methyl methanesulphonate (MMS), Dox, $HgCl_2$ or methyl mercury in HepG2 cells were decreased [100,101]. At high concentrations, quercetin and also rutin (glycoside of quercetin with rutinose) caused massive γ-H2AX foci, probably reflecting lethality [94], and yet they decreased DNA damage (SBs) induced by food mutagens PhIP and IQ [96].

Quercitrin, the rhamnose glycoside of quercetin, protected mouse epidermal cells against UV(B)-induced SBs [102]. Rutin at low concentrations showed the same protective effect as quercetin on HepG2 cells treated with AFB1, MMS or Dox [100]; at much higher concentrations, it caused SBs, but still protected against MN induced by B(a)P [93].

The myricetin rhamnoside, myricitrin, at high concentrations, induced MN in TK6 cells; the aglycone myricetin, being more cytotoxic, was tested at lower concentrations, and gave equivocal results [65]. Kaempferol at high concentrations induced SBs [95,99], as did fisetin [98]. Galangin and chrysin caused base oxidation at the moderate concentration of 20 µM [51], while a low concentration of naringin was protective against cadmium-induced chromosome aberrations [92]. Apigenin at a high concentration decreased SBs, chrom abs and MN [69].

## 5. Discussion and Conclusions

Many of the papers that we have reviewed report experiments with high or very high concentrations of phytochemicals. When investigating the role of phytochemicals in normal human nutrition, the aim should always be to study concentrations close to those likely to be present in humans as a result of dietary intake. As a rule of thumb, we have assumed this concentration to be in the low micromolar range. Many papers quote concentrations in µg/mL. To convert these concentrations to micromolar, again as a rule of thumb, we have assumed a molecular weight of 500; then 1 µg/mL = 2 µM. We would regard a concentration of over 20 µM or 10 µg/mL as high, and over 50 µM or 25 µg/mL as very high. Clearly, in functional foods or phytochemical supplements, the concentration is likely to be higher than in natural foods, and experiments showing genotoxicity of phytochemicals at high doses should at least serve as a warning to designers of functional foods.

It is always instructive to carry out experiments over a range of concentrations. Often, in the case of micronutrients in general, the dose–response curve is U-shaped, i.e., a beneficial effect at low concentrations changes to a detrimental effect at higher concentrations, and this tendency is clear in many of the reports described here.

Of course, if genotoxicity is specifically directed to cancer cells while healthy cells are unaffected, it is regarded as beneficial, and it is evidently the aim of some of the papers that we have reviewed to identify plant extracts or particular polyphenols that have such targeted action and so might have potential value as therapeutic agents. The differential response of cycling vs non-cycling cells to certain polyphenols might be exploited therapeutically in targeting dividing cancer cells.

With such a wide-ranging set of phytochemicals, not to mention the variety of test systems, experimental designs and assays applied in their study, it is difficult to generalise. However, high concentrations are likely to show DNA-damaging effects, while also in many cases protecting cells against damaging effects of other agents, apparently acting as pro-oxidants when present alone, but as anti-oxidants in combination. This is not a novel observation: many years ago, Duthie et al. reported DNA-damaging effects of quercetin at 50 µM [103] alongside an ability to protect cells against $H_2O_2$-induced DNA damage at concentrations of 10–50 µM [104]. Low concentrations are generally protective, in some cases even decreasing the already low background level of cellular DNA damage.

To summarise, results reported in the recent literature, on the whole, lend support to the hypothesis that dietary polyphenols protect the body against the effects of reactive oxygen species on DNA integrity, but do so reliably only when present at low concentrations. We recommend that greater attention be paid to the concentrations used, particularly in in vitro experiments, if the results are to be extrapolated to issues of human health. An important consideration when extrapolating is that plant foods contain a variety of micronutrients which might be expected to act in concert, whereas most experiments are carried out with single compounds. In this respect, there are clear advantages in using plant extracts or whole foods, though this approach does present practical difficulties. We also recommend that, since oxidative damage to DNA, and its prevention, are of major concern, the modified comet assay incorporating Fpg or EndoIII should be employed, since it provides increased sensitivity and specificity.

**Acknowledgments:** A.A. thanks the Ministerio de Economía y Competitividad ('Ramón y Cajal' programme, RYC-2013-14370) of the Spanish Government for personal support. This work was also supported by the BIOGENSA project (AGL2015-70640-R) of the 'Ministerio de Economía y Competitividad' of the Spanish Government.

**Conflicts of Interest:** The authors declare no conflict of interest.

## Abbreviations

| | |
|---|---|
| SB | strand break |
| Fpg | formamidopyrimidine DNA glycosylase |
| EndoIII | endonuclease III (Nth) |
| 8-OH–Gua (8-OH–G) | 8-oxo–7,8-dihydroguanine |
| PBMN | peripheral blood mononuclear |
| NER | nucleotide excision repair |
| Ab | antibody |
| NP | nanoparticle |
| Dox | doxorubicin |
| B(a)P | benzo(a)phenol |
| CPD | cyclobutane pyrimidine dimer |
| *t*-BOOH | *tert*-butyl hydroperoxide |
| PCB | polychlorinated biphenyls |
| DEN | diethylnitrosamine |
| TPA | tetradecanoyl-phorbol acetate |

## References

1. Bjelakovic, G.; Nikolova, D.; Gluud, L.L.; Simonetti, R.G.; Gluud, C. Mortality in randomized trials of antioxidant supplements for primary and secondary prevention: Systematic review and meta-analysis. *J. Am. Med. Assoc.* **2007**, *297*, 842–857. [CrossRef] [PubMed]
2. Azqueta, A.; Collins, A.R. The essential comet assay: A comprehensive guide to measuring DNA damage and repair. *Arch. Toxicol.* **2013**, *87*, 949–968. [CrossRef] [PubMed]
3. Kasai, H. Analysis of a form of oxidative DNA damage, 8-hydroxy-2'-deoxyguanosine, as a marker of cellular oxidative stress during carcinogenesis. *Mutat. Res./Rev. Mutat. Res.* **1997**, *387*, 147–163. [CrossRef]
4. Kasai, H.; Kawai, K. 8-hydroxyguanine, an oxidative DNA and RNA modification. In *Modified Nucleic Acids in Biology and Medicine*; Jurga, S.E., Erdmann, V.A., Barciszewski, J., Eds.; Springer: Basel, Switzerland, 2016; pp. 147–185.
5. Sedelnikova, O.A.; Rogakou, E.P.; Panyutin, I.G.; Bonner, W.M. Quantitative detection of (125)idu-induced DNA double-strand breaks with gamma-h2ax antibody. *Radiat. Res.* **2002**, *158*, 486–492. [CrossRef]
6. Huang, X.; Darzynkiewicz, Z. Cytometric assessment of histone h2ax phosphorylation: A reporter of DNA damage. *Methods Mol. Biol.* **2006**, *314*, 73–80. [PubMed]
7. Fenech, M. Cytokinesis-block micronucleus cytome assay. *Nat. Protoc.* **2007**, *2*, 1084–1104. [CrossRef] [PubMed]
8. Bonassi, S.; Norppa, H.; Ceppi, M.; Stromberg, U.; Vermeulen, R.; Znaor, A.; Cebulska-Wasilewska, A.; Fabianova, E.; Fucic, A.; Gundy, S.; et al. Chromosomal aberration frequency in lymphocytes predicts the risk of cancer: Results from a pooled cohort study of 22,358 subjects in 11 countries. *Carcinogenesis* **2008**, *29*, 1178–1183. [CrossRef] [PubMed]
9. Bonassi, S.; El-Zein, R.; Bolognesi, C.; Fenech, M. Micronuclei frequency in peripheral blood lymphocytes and cancer risk: Evidence from human studies. *Mutagenesis* **2011**, *26*, 93–100. [CrossRef] [PubMed]
10. Rangel-Huerta, O.D.; Aguilera, C.M.; Martin, M.V.; Soto, M.J.; Rico, M.C.; Vallejo, F.; Tomas-Barberan, F.; Perez-de-la-Cruz, A.J.; Gil, A.; Mesa, M.D. Normal or high polyphenol concentration in orange juice affects antioxidant activity, blood pressure, and body weight in obese or overweight adults. *J. Nutr.* **2015**, *145*, 1808–1816. [CrossRef] [PubMed]
11. Garcia-Flores, L.A.; Medina, S.; Cejuela-Anta, R.; Martinez-Sanz, J.M.; Abellan, A.; Genieser, H.G.; Ferreres, F.; Gil-Izquierdo, A. DNA catabolites in triathletes: Effects of supplementation with an aronia-citrus juice (polyphenols-rich juice). *Food Funct.* **2016**, *7*, 2084–2093. [CrossRef] [PubMed]
12. Spadafranca, A.; Martinez Conesa, C.; Sirini, S.; Testolin, G. Effect of dark chocolate on plasma epicatechin levels, DNA resistance to oxidative stress and total antioxidant activity in healthy subjects. *Br. J. Nutr.* **2010**, *103*, 1008–1014. [CrossRef] [PubMed]
13. Giovannelli, L.; Pitozzi, V.; Luceri, C.; Giannini, L.; Toti, S.; Salvini, S.; Sera, F.; Souquet, J.M.; Cheynier, V.; Sofi, F.; et al. Effects of de-alcoholised wines with different polyphenol content on DNA oxidative damage,

gene expression of peripheral lymphocytes, and haemorheology: An intervention study in post-menopausal women. *Eur. J. Nutr.* **2011**, *50*, 19–29. [CrossRef] [PubMed]

14. Riso, P.; Klimis-Zacas, D.; Del Bo, C.; Martini, D.; Campolo, J.; Vendrame, S.; Moller, P.; Loft, S.; De Maria, R.; Porrini, M. Effect of a wild blueberry (vaccinium angustifolium) drink intervention on markers of oxidative stress, inflammation and endothelial function in humans with cardiovascular risk factors. *Eur. J. Nutr.* **2013**, *52*, 949–961. [CrossRef] [PubMed]

15. Malhomme de la Roche, H.; Seagrove, S.; Mehta, A.; Divekar, P.; Campbell, S.; Curnow, A. Using natural dietary sources of antioxidants to protect against ultraviolet and visible radiation-induced DNA damage: An investigation of human green tea ingestion. *J. Photochem. Photobiol. B Biol.* **2010**, *101*, 169–173. [CrossRef] [PubMed]

16. Alleva, R.; Manzella, N.; Gaetani, S.; Ciarapica, V.; Bracci, M.; Caboni, M.F.; Pasini, F.; Monaco, F.; Amati, M.; Borghi, B.; et al. Organic honey supplementation reverses pesticide-induced genotoxicity by modulating dna damage response. *Mol. Nutr. Food Res.* **2016**, *60*, 2243–2255. [CrossRef] [PubMed]

17. Venancio, V.P.; Marques, M.C.; Almeida, M.R.; Mariutti, L.R.; Souza, V.C.; Barbosa, F., Jr.; Pires Bianchi, M.L.; Marzocchi-Machado, C.M.; Mercadante, A.Z.; Antunes, L.M. Chrysobalanus icaco l. Fruits inhibit nadph oxidase complex and protect DNA against doxorubicin-induced damage in wistar male rats. *J. Toxicol. Environ. Health Part A* **2016**, *79*, 885–893. [CrossRef] [PubMed]

18. Sinha, D.; Roy, M. Antagonistic role of tea against sodium arsenite-induced oxidative DNA damage and inhibition of DNA repair in swiss albino mice. *J. Environ. Pathol. Toxicol. Oncol.* **2011**, *30*, 311–322. [CrossRef] [PubMed]

19. Almeida, M.R.; Darin, J.D.; Hernandes, L.C.; Aissa, A.F.; Chiste, R.C.; Mercadante, A.Z.; Antunes, L.M.; Bianchi, M.L. Antigenotoxic effects of piquia (caryocar villosum) in multiple rat organs. *Plant Foods Hum. Nutr.* **2012**, *67*, 171–177. [CrossRef] [PubMed]

20. Ribeiro, J.C.; Antunes, L.M.; Aissa, A.F.; Darin, J.D.; De Rosso, V.V.; Mercadante, A.Z.; Bianchi Mde, L. Evaluation of the genotoxic and antigenotoxic effects after acute and subacute treatments with acai pulp (euterpe oleracea mart.) on mice using the erythrocytes micronucleus test and the comet assay. *Mutat. Res.* **2010**, *695*, 22–28. [CrossRef] [PubMed]

21. Krajka-Kuzniak, V.; Szaefer, H.; Ignatowicz, E.; Adamska, T.; Markowski, J.; Baer-Dubowska, W. Influence of cloudy apple juice on n-nitrosodiethylamine- induced liver injury and phases i and ii biotransformation enzymes in rat liver. *Acta Pol. Pharm.* **2015**, *72*, 267–276. [PubMed]

22. Acharyya, N.; Sajed Ali, S.; Deb, B.; Chattopadhyay, S.; Maiti, S. Green tea (camellia sinensis) alleviates arsenic-induced damages to DNA and intestinal tissues in rat and in situ intestinal loop by reinforcing antioxidant system. *Environ. Toxicol.* **2015**, *30*, 1033–1044. [CrossRef] [PubMed]

23. Ko, S.H.; Park, J.H.; Kim, S.Y.; Lee, S.W.; Chun, S.S.; Park, E. Antioxidant effects of spinach (*Spinacia oleracea* L.) supplementation in hyperlipidemic rats. *Prev. Nutr. Food Sci.* **2014**, *19*, 19–26. [CrossRef] [PubMed]

24. Ho, C.K.; Siu-wai, C.; Siu, P.M.; Benzie, I.F. Genoprotection and genotoxicity of green tea (camellia sinensis): Are they two sides of the same redox coin? *Redox Rep. Commun. Free Radic. Res.* **2013**, *18*, 150–154. [CrossRef] [PubMed]

25. Kuhnel, H.; Adilijiang, A.; Dadak, A.; Wieser, M.; Upur, H.; Stolze, K.; Grillari, J.; Strasser, A. Investigations into cytotoxic effects of the herbal preparation abnormal savda munziq. *Chin. J. Integr. Med.* **2015**, *53*, 1–9. [CrossRef] [PubMed]

26. Haza, A.I.; Morales, P. Spanish honeys protect against food mutagen-induced DNA damage. *J. Sci. Food Agric.* **2013**, *93*, 2995–3000. [CrossRef] [PubMed]

27. Qian, G.; Xue, K.; Tang, L.; Wang, F.; Song, X.; Chyu, M.C.; Pence, B.C.; Shen, C.L.; Wang, J.S. Mitigation of oxidative damage by green tea polyphenols and tai chi exercise in postmenopausal women with osteopenia. *PLoS ONE* **2012**, *7*, e48090. [CrossRef] [PubMed]

28. Xu, Y.; Zhang, J.J.; Xiong, L.; Zhang, L.; Sun, D.; Liu, H. Green tea polyphenols inhibit cognitive impairment induced by chronic cerebral hypoperfusion via modulating oxidative stress. *J. Nutr. Biochem.* **2010**, *21*, 741–748. [PubMed]

29. Katiyar, S.K.; Vaid, M.; van Steeg, H.; Meeran, S.M. Green tea polyphenols prevent uv-induced immunosuppression by rapid repair of DNA damage and enhancement of nucleotide excision repair genes. *Cancer Prev. Res.* **2010**, *3*, 179–189. [CrossRef] [PubMed]

30. Garcia-Rodriguez Mdel, C.; Carvente-Juarez, M.M.; Altamirano-Lozano, M.A. Antigenotoxic and apoptotic activity of green tea polyphenol extracts on hexavalent chromium-induced DNA damage in peripheral blood of cd-1 mice: Analysis with differential acridine orange/ethidium bromide staining. *Oxidative Med. Cell. Longev.* **2013**, *2013*, 486419. [CrossRef] [PubMed]

31. Pu, X.; Wang, Z.; Zhou, S.; Klaunig, J.E. Protective effects of antioxidants on acrylonitrile-induced oxidative stress in female f344 rats. *Environ. Toxicol.* **2015**. [CrossRef] [PubMed]

32. Olteanu, E.D.; Filip, A.; Clichici, S.; Daicoviciu, D.; Achim, M.; Postescu, I.D.; Bolfa, P.; Bolojan, L.; Vlase, L.; Muresan, A. Photochemoprotective effect of calluna vulgaris extract on skin exposed to multiple doses of ultraviolet b in skh-1 hairless mice. *J. Environ. Pathol. Toxicol. Oncol.* **2012**, *31*, 233–243. [CrossRef] [PubMed]

33. Chaudhary, P.; Shukla, S.K.; Sharma, R.K. Rec-2006-a fractionated extract of podophyllum hexandrum protects cellular DNA from radiation-induced damage by reducing the initial damage and enhancing its repair in vivo. *Evid.-Based Complement. Altern. Med.* **2011**, *2011*, 473953. [CrossRef] [PubMed]

34. Matic, S.; Stanic, S.; Bogojevic, D.; Vidakovic, M.; Grdovic, N.; Dinic, S.; Solujic, S.; Mladenovic, M.; Stankovic, N.; Mihailovic, M. Methanol extract from the stem of cotinus coggygria scop., and its major bioactive phytochemical constituent myricetin modulate pyrogallol-induced DNA damage and liver injury. *Mutat. Res.* **2013**, *755*, 81–89. [CrossRef] [PubMed]

35. Prasad, R.; Katiyar, S.K. Polyphenols from green tea inhibit the growth of melanoma cells through inhibition of class i histone deacetylases and induction of DNA damage. *Genes Cancer* **2015**, *6*, 49–61. [PubMed]

36. Durgo, K.; Kostic, S.; Gradiski, K.; Komes, D.; Osmak, M.; Franekic, J. Genotoxic effects of green tea extract on human laryngeal carcinoma cells in vitro. *Arch. Hig. Rada Toksikol.* **2011**, *62*, 139–146. [CrossRef] [PubMed]

37. Perez-Sanchez, A.; Barrajon-Catalan, E.; Caturla, N.; Castillo, J.; Benavente-Garcia, O.; Alcaraz, M.; Micol, V. Protective effects of citrus and rosemary extracts on uv-induced damage in skin cell model and human volunteers. *J. Photochem. Photobiol. B Biol.* **2014**, *136*, 12–18. [CrossRef] [PubMed]

38. Cornaghi, L.; Arnaboldi, F.; Calo, R.; Landoni, F.; Baruffaldi Preis, W.F.; Marabini, L.; Donetti, E. Effects of uv rays and thymol/thymus vulgaris l. Extract in an ex vivo human skin model: Morphological and genotoxicological assessment. *Cells Tissues Organs* **2016**, *201*, 180–192. [CrossRef] [PubMed]

39. Calo, R.; Visone, C.M.; Marabini, L. Thymol and thymus vulgaris L. Activity against uva- and uvb-induced damage in nctc 2544 cell line. *Mutat. Res. Genet. Toxicol. Environ. Mutagen.* **2015**, *791*, 30–37. [CrossRef] [PubMed]

40. Perez-Sanchez, A.; Barrajon-Catalan, E.; Herranz-Lopez, M.; Castillo, J.; Micol, V. Lemon balm extract (*Melissa officinalis* L.) promotes melanogenesis and prevents uvb-induced oxidative stress and DNA damage in a skin cell model. *J. Dermatol. Sci.* **2016**, *84*, 169–177. [CrossRef] [PubMed]

41. Venuprasad, M.P.; Hemanth Kumar, K.; Khanum, F. Neuroprotective effects of hydroalcoholic extract of ocimum sanctum against h2o2 induced neuronal cell damage in sh-sy5y cells via its antioxidative defence mechanism. *Neurochem. Res.* **2013**, *38*, 2190–2200. [CrossRef] [PubMed]

42. Thirugnanasampandan, R.; Jayakumar, R. Protection of cadmium chloride induced DNA damage by lamiaceae plants. *Asian Pac. J. Trop. Biomed.* **2011**, *1*, 391–394. [CrossRef]

43. Giampieri, F.; Alvarez-Suarez, J.M.; Tulipani, S.; Gonzales-Paramas, A.M.; Santos-Buelga, C.; Bompadre, S.; Quiles, J.L.; Mezzetti, B.; Battino, M. Photoprotective potential of strawberry (fragaria x ananassa) extract against uv-a irradiation damage on human fibroblasts. *J. Agric. Food Chem.* **2012**, *60*, 2322–2327. [CrossRef] [PubMed]

44. Giampieri, F.; Alvarez-Suarez, J.M.; Mazzoni, L.; Forbes-Hernandez, T.Y.; Gasparrini, M.; Gonzalez-Paramas, A.M.; Santos-Buelga, C.; Quiles, J.L.; Bompadre, S.; Mezzetti, B.; et al. Polyphenol-rich strawberry extract protects human dermal fibroblasts against hydrogen peroxide oxidative damage and improves mitochondrial functionality. *Molecules* **2014**, *19*, 7798–7816. [CrossRef] [PubMed]

45. Braga, P.C.; Antonacci, R.; Wang, Y.Y.; Lattuada, N.; Dal Sasso, M.; Marabini, L.; Fibiani, M.; Lo Scalzo, R. Comparative antioxidant activity of cultivated and wild vaccinium species investigated by epr, human neutrophil burst and comet assay. *Eur. Rev. Med. Pharmacol. Sci.* **2013**, *17*, 1987–1999. [PubMed]

46. Yamamoto, A.; Nakashima, K.; Kawamorita, S.; Sugiyama, A.; Miura, M.; Kamitai, Y.; Kato, Y. Protective effects of raw and cooked blackcurrant extract on DNA damage induced by hydrogen peroxide in human lymphoblastoid cells. *Pharm. Biol.* **2014**, *52*, 782–788. [CrossRef] [PubMed]

47. Bellion, P.; Digles, J.; Will, F.; Dietrich, H.; Baum, M.; Eisenbrand, G.; Janzowski, C. Polyphenolic apple extracts: Effects of raw material and production method on antioxidant effectiveness and reduction of DNA damage in caco-2 cells. *J. Agric. Food Chem.* **2010**, *58*, 6636–6642. [CrossRef] [PubMed]

48. Tan, A.C.; Konczak, I.; Ramzan, I.; Sze, D.M. Native australian fruit polyphenols inhibit cell viability and induce apoptosis in human cancer cell lines. *Nutr. Cancer* **2011**, *63*, 444–455. [CrossRef] [PubMed]

49. Botden, I.P.; Oeseburg, H.; Durik, M.; Leijten, F.P.; Van Vark-Van Der Zee, L.C.; Musterd-Bhaggoe, U.M.; Garrelds, I.M.; Seynhaeve, A.L.; Langendonk, J.G.; Sijbrands, E.J.; et al. Red wine extract protects against oxidative-stress-induced endothelial senescence. *Clin. Sci.* **2012**, *123*, 499–507. [CrossRef] [PubMed]

50. Yalcin, C.O.; Aliyazicioglu, Y.; Demir, S.; Turan, I.; Bahat, Z.; Misir, S.; Deger, O. Evaluation of the radioprotective effect of turkish propolis on foreskin fibroblast cells. *J. Cancer Res. Ther.* **2016**, *12*, 990–994. [PubMed]

51. Tsai, Y.C.; Wang, Y.H.; Liou, C.C.; Lin, Y.C.; Huang, H.; Liu, Y.C. Induction of oxidative DNA damage by flavonoids of propolis: Its mechanism and implication about antioxidant capacity. *Chem. Res. Toxicol.* **2012**, *25*, 191–196. [CrossRef] [PubMed]

52. Nguyen, M.M.; Ahmann, F.R.; Nagle, R.B.; Hsu, C.H.; Tangrea, J.A.; Parnes, H.L.; Sokoloff, M.H.; Gretzer, M.B.; Chow, H.H. Randomized, double-blind, placebo-controlled trial of polyphenon e in prostate cancer patients before prostatectomy: Evaluation of potential chemopreventive activities. *Cancer Prev. Res.* **2012**, *5*, 290–298. [CrossRef] [PubMed]

53. Ferk, F.; Misik, M.; Nersesyan, A.; Pichler, C.; Jager, W.; Szekeres, T.; Marculescu, R.; Poulsen, H.E.; Henriksen, T.; Bono, R.; et al. Impact of xanthohumol (a prenylated flavonoid from hops) on DNA stability and other health-related biochemical parameters: Results of human intervention trials. *Mol. Nutr. Food Res.* **2016**, *60*, 773–786. [CrossRef] [PubMed]

54. Cariddi, L.N.; Sabini, M.C.; Escobar, F.M.; Montironi, I.; Manas, F.; Iglesias, D.; Comini, L.R.; Sabini, L.I.; Dalcero, A.M. Polyphenols as possible bioprotectors against cytotoxicity and DNA damage induced by ochratoxin A. *Environ. Toxicol. Pharmacol.* **2015**, *39*, 1008–1018. [CrossRef] [PubMed]

55. Papiez, M.A. The influence of curcumin and (−)-epicatechin on the genotoxicity and myelosuppression induced by etoposide in bone marrow cells of male rats. *Drug Chem. Toxicol.* **2013**, *36*, 93–101. [CrossRef] [PubMed]

56. Rehman, M.U.; Tahir, M.; Ali, F.; Qamar, W.; Lateef, A.; Khan, R.; Quaiyoom, A.; Oday, O.H.; Sultana, S. Cyclophosphamide-induced nephrotoxicity, genotoxicity, and damage in kidney genomic DNA of swiss albino mice: The protective effect of ellagic acid. *Mol. Cell. Biochem.* **2012**, *365*, 119–127. [CrossRef] [PubMed]

57. Srivastava, A.K.; Bhatnagar, P.; Singh, M.; Mishra, S.; Kumar, P.; Shukla, Y.; Gupta, K.C. Synthesis of plga nanoparticles of tea polyphenols and their strong in vivo protective effect against chemically induced DNA damage. *Int. J. Nanomed.* **2013**, *8*, 1451–1462.

58. Li, G.X.; Chen, Y.K.; Hou, Z.; Xiao, H.; Jin, H.; Lu, G.; Lee, M.J.; Liu, B.; Guan, F.; Yang, Z.; et al. Pro-oxidative activities and dose-response relationship of (−)-epigallocatechin-3-gallate in the inhibition of lung cancer cell growth: A comparative study in vivo and in vitro. *Carcinogenesis* **2010**, *31*, 902–910. [CrossRef] [PubMed]

59. Marrazzo, G.; Bosco, P.; La Delia, F.; Scapagnini, G.; Di Giacomo, C.; Malaguarnera, M.; Galvano, F.; Nicolosi, A.; Li Volti, G. Neuroprotective effect of silibinin in diabetic mice. *Neurosci. Lett.* **2011**, *504*, 252–256. [CrossRef] [PubMed]

60. Rocha de Oliveira, C.; Ceolin, J.; Rocha de Oliveira, R.; Goncalves Schemitt, E.; Raskopf Colares, J.; De Freitas Bauermann, L.; Hilda Costabeber, I.; Morgan-Martins, M.I.; Mauriz, J.L.; Da Silva, J.; et al. Effects of quercetin on polychlorinated biphenyls-induced liver injury in rats. *Nutr. Hosp.* **2014**, *29*, 1141–1148. [PubMed]

61. Patil, S.L.; Rao, N.B.; Somashekarappa, H.M.; Rajashekhar, K.P. Antigenotoxic potential of rutin and quercetin in swiss mice exposed to gamma radiation. *Biomed. J.* **2014**, *37*, 305–313. [CrossRef] [PubMed]

62. Manzolli, E.S.; Serpeloni, J.M.; Grotto, D. Protective effects of the flavonoid chrysin against methylmercury-induced genotoxicity and alterations of antioxidant status, in vivo. *Oxidative Med. Cell. Longev.* **2015**, *2015*, 602360. [CrossRef] [PubMed]

63. Ma, J.Q.; Ding, J.; Xiao, Z.H.; Liu, C.M. Puerarin ameliorates carbon tetrachloride-induced oxidative DNA damage and inflammation in mouse kidney through erk/nrf2/are pathway. *Food Chem. Toxicol.* **2014**, *71*, 264–271. [CrossRef] [PubMed]

64. Liu, C.M.; Ma, J.Q.; Sun, Y.Z. Quercetin protects the rat kidney against oxidative stress-mediated DNA damage and apoptosis induced by lead. *Environ. Toxicol. Pharmacol.* **2010**, *30*, 264–271. [CrossRef] [PubMed]

65. Hobbs, C.A.; Swartz, C.; Maronpot, R.; Davis, J.; Recio, L.; Koyanagi, M.; Hayashi, S.M. Genotoxicity evaluation of the flavonoid, myricitrin, and its aglycone, myricetin. *Food Chem. Toxicol.* **2015**, *83*, 283–292. [CrossRef] [PubMed]

66. Gupta, C.; Vikram, A.; Tripathi, D.N.; Ramarao, P.; Jena, G.B. Antioxidant and antimutagenic effect of quercetin against den induced hepatotoxicity in rat. *Phytother. Res.* **2010**, *24*, 119–128. [CrossRef] [PubMed]

67. Ansar, S.; Siddiqi, N.J.; Zargar, S.; Ganaie, M.A.; Abudawood, M. Hepatoprotective effect of quercetin supplementation against acrylamide-induced DNA damage in wistar rats. *BMC Complement. Altern. Med.* **2016**, *16*, 327. [CrossRef] [PubMed]

68. Carino-Cortes, R.; Alvarez-Gonzalez, I.; Martino-Roaro, L.; Madrigal-Bujaidar, E. Effect of naringin on the DNA damage induced by daunorubicin in mouse hepatocytes and cardiocytes. *Biol. Pharm. Bull.* **2010**, *33*, 697–701. [CrossRef] [PubMed]

69. Das, S.; Das, J.; Paul, A.; Samadder, A.; Khuda-Bukhsh, A.R. Apigenin, a bioactive flavonoid from lycopodium clavatum, stimulates nucleotide excision repair genes to protect skin keratinocytes from ultraviolet b-induced reactive oxygen species and DNA damage. *J. Acupunct. Meridian Stud.* **2013**, *6*, 252–262. [CrossRef] [PubMed]

70. Cha, J.W.; Piao, M.J.; Kim, K.C.; Yao, C.W.; Zheng, J.; Kim, S.M.; Hyun, C.L.; Ahn, Y.S.; Hyun, J.W. The polyphenol chlorogenic acid attenuates uvb-mediated oxidative stress in human hacat keratinocytes. *Biomol. Ther.* **2014**, *22*, 136–142. [CrossRef] [PubMed]

71. Burgos-Moron, E.; Calderon-Montano, J.M.; Orta, M.L.; Pastor, N.; Perez-Guerrero, C.; Austin, C.; Mateos, S.; Lopez-Lazaro, M. The coffee constituent chlorogenic acid induces cellular DNA damage and formation of topoisomerase I- and II- DNA complexes in cells. *J. Agric. Food Chem.* **2012**, *60*, 7384–7391. [CrossRef] [PubMed]

72. Hasegawa, T.; Shimada, S.; Ishida, H.; Nakashima, M. Chafuroside b, an oolong tea polyphenol, ameliorates uvb-induced DNA damage and generation of photo-immunosuppression related mediators in human keratinocytes. *PLoS ONE* **2013**, *8*, e77308. [CrossRef] [PubMed]

73. Vanella, L.; Barbagallo, I.; Acquaviva, R.; Di Giacomo, C.; Cardile, V.; Abraham, N.G.; Sorrenti, V. Ellagic acid: Cytodifferentiating and antiproliferative effects in human prostatic cancer cell lines. *Curr. Pharm. Des.* **2013**, *19*, 2728–2736. [CrossRef] [PubMed]

74. Abib, R.T.; Quincozes-Santos, A.; Zanotto, C.; Zeidan-Chulia, F.; Lunardi, P.S.; Goncalves, C.A.; Gottfried, C. Genoprotective effects of the green tea-derived polyphenol/epicatechin gallate in c6 astroglial cells. *J. Med. Food* **2010**, *13*, 1111–1115. [CrossRef] [PubMed]

75. Miene, C.; Weise, A.; Glei, M. Impact of polyphenol metabolites produced by colonic microbiota on expression of cox-2 and gstt2 in human colon cells (lt97). *Nutr. Cancer* **2011**, *63*, 653–662. [CrossRef] [PubMed]

76. Hossain, M.Z.; Patel, K.; Kern, S.E. Salivary alpha-amylase, serum albumin, and myoglobin protect against DNA-damaging activities of ingested dietary agents in vitro. *Food Chem. Toxicol.* **2014**, *70*, 114–119. [CrossRef] [PubMed]

77. Mohan, S.; Thiagarajan, K.; Chandrasekaran, R. In vitro evaluation of antiproliferative effect of ethyl gallate against human oral squamous carcinoma cell line kb. *Nat. Prod. Res.* **2015**, *29*, 366–369. [CrossRef] [PubMed]

78. Zielinska-Przyjemska, M.; Ignatowicz, E.; Krajka-Kuzniak, V.; Baer-Dubowska, W. Effect of tannic acid, resveratrol and its derivatives, on oxidative damage and apoptosis in human neutrophils. *Food Chem. Toxicol.* **2015**, *84*, 37–46. [CrossRef] [PubMed]

79. Kumar, D.; Basu, S.; Parija, L.; Rout, D.; Manna, S.; Dandapat, J.; Debata, P.R. Curcumin and ellagic acid synergistically induce ros generation, DNA damage, p53 accumulation and apoptosis in hela cervical carcinoma cells. *Biomed. Pharmacother.* **2016**, *81*, 31–37. [CrossRef] [PubMed]

80. Sebastia, N.; Montoro, A.; Hervas, D.; Pantelias, G.; Hatzi, V.I.; Soriano, J.M.; Villaescusa, J.I.; Terzoudi, G.I. Curcumin and trans-resveratrol exert cell cycle-dependent radioprotective or radiosensitizing effects as elucidated by the pcc and g2-assay. *Mutat. Res.* **2014**, *766–767*, 49–55. [CrossRef] [PubMed]

81. Lewinska, A.; Wnuk, M.; Grabowska, W.; Zabek, T.; Semik, E.; Sikora, E.; Bielak-Zmijewska, A. Curcumin induces oxidation-dependent cell cycle arrest mediated by sirt7 inhibition of rdna transcription in human aortic smooth muscle cells. *Toxicol. Lett.* **2015**, *233*, 227–238. [CrossRef] [PubMed]

82. Sun, B.; Ross, S.M.; Trask, O.J.; Carmichael, P.L.; Dent, M.; White, A.; Andersen, M.E.; Clewell, R.A. Assessing dose-dependent differences in DNA-damage, p53 response and genotoxicity for quercetin and curcumin. *Toxicol. In Vitro* **2013**, *27*, 1877–1887. [CrossRef] [PubMed]

83. Ide, H.; Yu, J.; Lu, Y.; China, T.; Kumamoto, T.; Koseki, T.; Muto, S.; Horie, S. Testosterone augments polyphenol-induced DNA damage response in prostate cancer cell line, LNCaP. *Cancer Sci.* **2011**, *102*, 468–471. [CrossRef] [PubMed]

84. Seo, Y.N.; Lee, M.Y. Inhibitory effect of antioxidants on the benz[a]anthracene-induced oxidative DNA damage in lymphocyte. *J. Environ. Biol./Acad. Environ. Biol. India* **2011**, *32*, 7–10.

85. Lu, J.J.; Cai, Y.J.; Ding, J. Curcumin induces DNA damage and caffeine-insensitive cell cycle arrest in colorectal carcinoma hct116 cells. *Mol. Cell. Biochem.* **2011**, *354*, 247–252. [CrossRef] [PubMed]

86. Lu, J.J.; Cai, Y.J.; Ding, J. The short-time treatment with curcumin sufficiently decreases cell viability, induces apoptosis and copper enhances these effects in multidrug-resistant k562/a02 cells. *Mol. Cell. Biochem.* **2012**, *360*, 253–260. [CrossRef] [PubMed]

87. Turkez, H.; Sisman, T. The genoprotective activity of resveratrol on aflatoxin b(1)-induced DNA damage in human lymphocytes in vitro. *Toxicol. Ind. Health* **2012**, *28*, 474–480. [CrossRef] [PubMed]

88. Chen, C.; Jiang, X.; Hu, Y.; Zhang, Z. The protective role of resveratrol in the sodium arsenite-induced oxidative damage via modulation of intracellular gsh homeostasis. *Biol. Trace Element Res.* **2013**, *155*, 119–131. [CrossRef] [PubMed]

89. Demoulin, B.; Hermant, M.; Castrogiovanni, C.; Staudt, C.; Dumont, P. Resveratrol induces DNA damage in colon cancer cells by poisoning topoisomerase ii and activates the atm kinase to trigger p53-dependent apoptosis. *Toxicol. In Vitro* **2015**, *29*, 1156–1165. [CrossRef] [PubMed]

90. Rashid, A.; Liu, C.; Sanli, T.; Tsiani, E.; Singh, G.; Bristow, R.G.; Dayes, I.; Lukka, H.; Wright, J.; Tsakiridis, T. Resveratrol enhances prostate cancer cell response to ionizing radiation. Modulation of the ampk, akt and mtor pathways. *Radiat. Oncol.* **2011**, *6*, 669–672. [CrossRef] [PubMed]

91. Gonthier, B.; Allibe, N.; Cottet-Rousselle, C.; Lamarche, F.; Nuiry, L.; Barret, L. Specific conditions for resveratrol neuroprotection against ethanol-induced toxicity. *J. Toxicol.* **2012**, *2012*, 973134. [CrossRef] [PubMed]

92. Yilmaz, D.; Aydemir, N.C.; Vatan, O.; Tuzun, E.; Bilaloglu, R. Influence of naringin on cadmium-induced genomic damage in human lymphocytes in vitro. *Toxicol. Ind. Health* **2012**, *28*, 114–121. [CrossRef] [PubMed]

93. Cristina Marcarini, J.; Ferreira Tsuboy, M.S.; Cabral Luiz, R.; Regina Ribeiro, L.; Beatriz Hoffmann-Campo, C.; Segio Mantovani, M. Investigation of cytotoxic, apoptosis-inducing, genotoxic and protective effects of the flavonoid rutin in htc hepatic cells. *Exp. Toxicol. Pathol.* **2011**, *63*, 459–465. [CrossRef] [PubMed]

94. Maeda, J.; Roybal, E.J.; Brents, C.A.; Uesaka, M.; Aizawa, Y.; Kato, T.A. Natural and glucosyl flavonoids inhibit poly(adp-ribose) polymerase activity and induce synthetic lethality in brca mutant cells. *Oncol. Rep.* **2014**, *31*, 551–556. [PubMed]

95. Wu, L.Y.; Lu, H.F.; Chou, Y.C.; Shih, Y.L.; Bau, D.T.; Chen, J.C.; Hsu, S.C.; Chung, J.G. Kaempferol induces DNA damage and inhibits DNA repair associated protein expressions in human promyelocytic leukemia hl-60 cells. *Am. J. Chin. Med.* **2015**, *43*, 365–382. [CrossRef] [PubMed]

96. Kurzawa-Zegota, M.; Najafzadeh, M.; Baumgartner, A.; Anderson, D. The protective effect of the flavonoids on food-mutagen-induced DNA damage in peripheral blood lymphocytes from colon cancer patients. *Food Chem. Toxicol.* **2012**, *50*, 124–129. [CrossRef] [PubMed]

97. Kozics, K.; Valovicova, Z.; Slamenova, D. Structure of flavonoids influences the degree inhibition of benzo(a)pyrene—Induced DNA damage and micronuclei in hepg2 cells. *Neoplasma* **2011**, *58*, 516–524. [CrossRef] [PubMed]

98. Kim, J.Y.; Jeon, Y.K.; Jeon, W.; Nam, M.J. Fisetin induces apoptosis in huh-7 cells via downregulation of birc8 and bcl2l2. *Food Chem. Toxicol.* **2010**, *48*, 2259–2264. [CrossRef] [PubMed]

99. Huang, W.W.; Chiu, Y.J.; Fan, M.J.; Lu, H.F.; Yeh, H.F.; Li, K.H.; Chen, P.Y.; Chung, J.G.; Yang, J.S. Kaempferol induced apoptosis via endoplasmic reticulum stress and mitochondria-dependent pathway in human osteosarcoma u-2 os cells. *Mol. Nutr. Food Res.* **2010**, *54*, 1585–1595. [CrossRef] [PubMed]

100. Barcelos, G.R.; Grotto, D.; Angeli, J.P.; Serpeloni, J.M.; Rocha, B.A.; Bastos, J.K.; Barbosa, F., Jr. Evaluation of antigenotoxic effects of plant flavonoids quercetin and rutin on hepg2 cells. *Phytother. Res.* **2011**, *25*, 1381–1388. [CrossRef] [PubMed]

101. Barcelos, G.R.; Angeli, J.P.; Serpeloni, J.M.; Grotto, D.; Rocha, B.A.; Bastos, J.K.; Knasmuller, S.; Junior, F.B. Quercetin protects human-derived liver cells against mercury-induced DNA-damage and alterations of the redox status. *Mutat. Res.* **2011**, *726*, 109–115. [CrossRef] [PubMed]

102. Ding, M.; Zhao, J.; Bowman, L.; Lu, Y.; Shi, X. Inhibition of ap-1 and mapk signaling and activation of nrf2/are pathway by quercitrin. *Int. J. Oncol.* **2010**, *36*, 59–67. [CrossRef] [PubMed]
103. Duthie, S.J.; Johnson, W.; Dobson, V.L. The effect of dietary flavonoids on DNA damage (strand breaks and oxidised pyrimdines) and growth in human cells. *Mutat. Res.* **1997**, *390*, 141–151. [CrossRef]
104. Duthie, S.J.; Collins, A.R.; Duthie, G.G.; Dobson, V.L. Quercetin and myricetin protect against hydrogen peroxide-induced DNA damage (strand breaks and oxidised pyrimidines) in human lymphocytes. *Mutat. Res.* **1997**, *393*, 223–231. [CrossRef]

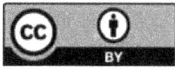

*nutrients*

MDPI

*Review*

# Anticancer Effects of Rosemary (*Rosmarinus officinalis* L.) Extract and Rosemary Extract Polyphenols

**Jessy Moore [1], Michael Yousef [1] and Evangelia Tsiani [1,2,***

[1] Department of Health Sciences, Brock University, St. Catharines, ON L2S 3A1, Canada;
jessy.moore@brocku.ca (J.M.); my11dq@brocku.ca (M.Y.)

[2] Centre for Bone and Muscle Health, Brock University, St. Catharines, ON L2S 3A1, Canada

* Correspondence: ltsiani@brocku.ca; Tel.: +1-905-688-5550 (ext. 3881)

Received: 23 August 2016; Accepted: 8 November 2016; Published: 17 November 2016

**Abstract:** Cancer cells display enhanced growth rates and a resistance to apoptosis. The ability of cancer cells to evade homeostasis and proliferate uncontrollably while avoiding programmed cell death/apoptosis is acquired through mutations to key signaling molecules, which regulate pathways involved in cell proliferation and survival. Compounds of plant origin, including food components, have attracted scientific attention for use as agents for cancer prevention and treatment. The exploration into natural products offers great opportunity to evaluate new anticancer agents as well as understand novel and potentially relevant mechanisms of action. Rosemary extract has been reported to have antioxidant, anti-inflammatory, antidiabetic and anticancer properties. Rosemary extract contains many polyphenols with carnosic acid and rosmarinic acid found in highest concentrations. The present review summarizes the existing in vitro and in vivo studies focusing on the anticancer effects of rosemary extract and the rosemary extract polyphenols carnosic acid and rosmarinic acid, and their effects on key signaling molecules.

**Keywords:** rosemary extract; carnosic acid; rosmarinic acid; cancer; proliferation; survival; cell signaling

## 1. Introduction

Arguably the most fundamental traits of cancer cells are their enhanced proliferative and decreased apoptotic capacities [1]. Normal cells tightly control the production and release of growth factors, which regulate cell growth/proliferation, thereby ensuring cellular homeostasis and maintenance of normal tissue architecture. In cancer cells, these signals are deregulated and thus, homeostasis within the cell is disrupted. Proliferation of cancer cells may be enhanced in a number of ways. Cancer cells may produce growth factors to which they can respond via the expression of cognate receptors. The level of receptor proteins displayed on the surface of cancer cells can also be elevated, rendering these cells hyperresponsive to growth factors; the same outcome can result from alterations to the receptor molecules that facilitate activation of downstream signaling pathways independent of growth factor binding [1]. Alternatively, cancer cells can signal normal neighbouring cells resulting in mutations/alterations in signaling pathways. These alterations stimulate the release of growth factors which are supplied back to the cancer cells, enhancing their proliferation [2,3]. Growth factor receptors (GFR), such as epidermal GFR (EGFR) are plasma membrane proteins with intrinsic tyrosine kinase (TK) activity. Growth factor binding enhances the tyrosine kinase activity of the receptor causing receptor autophosphorylation. The phosphorylated tyrosine residues of the receptor act as docking sites for intracellular proteins containing Src-homology 2 (SH2) domains, leading to stimulation of intracellular signaling cascades such as the phosphatidylinositol 3-kinase

(PI3K-Akt) and the Ras-mitogen activated protein kinase (Ras-MAPK) cascades, that result in enhanced proliferation and inhibition of apoptosis/enhanced survival.

The development of cancer is divided into three stages: initiation, promotion and progression. Initiation involves a change to the genetic makeup of a cell which primes the cell to become cancerous. During the stage of promotion various factors permit a single mutated cell to survive (resist apoptosis) and replicate, promoting growth of a tumor. Finally, as the cancerous cell replicates and develops into a tumor, the disease state progresses. As normal, healthy cells progress to a neoplastic state they acquire a series of hallmark capabilities which enable them to become malignant. The 6 hallmarks of cancer proposed by Hanahan and Weinberg include sustaining proliferative signaling, evading growth suppressors, resisting cell death, enabling replicative immortality, inducing angiogenesis, and activating invasion and metastasis [1]. As tumors progress and become more aggressive they will begin to exhibit more of these hallmarks. Current anticancer agents may be classified as chemopreventive or chemotherapeutic depending on which stage of carcinogenesis they target. To explore the chemopreventive potential of anticancer agents, cells in culture or animal models can be exposed to an anticancer agent before being exposed to a carcinogen. This provides evidence of the effect of an anticancer agent on the initiation and promotion stages of cancer. Alternatively, cells in culture or animal models may be exposed to a carcinogen to establish a neoplastic state prior to being treated with an anticancer agent and this provides evidence of the effect of an anticancer agent on the progression of cancer.

Many pharmaceutical agents have been discovered by screening natural products from plants. Some of these drugs such as the chemotherapeutics etoposide, isolated from the mandrake plant and Queen Anne's lace, and paclitaxel and docetaxel, isolated from the wood and bark of the Nyssaceae tree, are currently successfully employed in cancer treatment [4]. The exploration into natural products offers great opportunity to evaluate new chemical classes of anticancer agents as well as study novel and potentially relevant mechanisms of action. Many labs, including ours have shown metformin, a drug derived from the lilac, has anticancer properties [5]. In addition, the polyphenol resveratrol, found in high concentrations in wine, has been shown to have anticancer effects in vitro and in vivo [6–10]. Importantly, metformin and resveratrol exhibit both chemopreventive and chemotherapeutic effects.

The plant *Rosmarinus Officinalis* L. a member of the mint family *Lamiaceae*, is native to the Mediterranean region and has many culinary and medicinal uses. The main polyphenols found in rosemary extract (RE) include the diterpenes carnosic acid (CA) and rosmarinic acid (RA) [11]. Rosemary extract and its polyphenols CA and RA have recently been explored and found to exert potent anticancer effects (reviewed recently in [12–14]). To establish a systematic literature review we used the online search engine Pubmed. We searched the key phrases: rosemary extract and cancer, carnosic acid and cancer, rosmarinic acid and cancer. We also included subtypes of cancer such as breast cancer, colon cancer, etc., as keywords in our search. All studies pertaining to our topic and published after the year 2000 were included in the current review. In the following sections, in vitro and in vivo studies on the effects of RE and its main polyphenols have been summarized and sorted by cancer cell type, in chronological order from earliest to most recent. Chronology was chosen as the sorting method to highlight how the literature has progressed and what knowledge is currently available. Initially we focused on the studies examining the anticancer effects of RE, we then highlighted studies in which mechanisms of action have been investigated and separately summarized the studies using the polyphenols CA and RA. The studies presented in the text are also summarized, organized and presented in a table format to allow the reader to extract the information easily.

This is a comprehensive systematic review and adds to the existing literature by summarizing all relevant studies using RE, CA and RA in each cancer subtype. The review is organized by experimental treatment (RE, CA, RA), type of cancer (histology) and the study model (in vitro or in vivo) resulting in a clear, detailed and inclusive summary of the existing literature. This review also focuses on the mechanistic data provided by these studies, which will be beneficial for future research to help focus efforts on identifying the main mechanisms involved in the anticancer action of RE, CA and RA.

## 2. Anticancer Effects of Rosemary Extract (RE): In Vitro Studies

Several in vitro studies using colon cancer cell lines have shown RE to exhibit anticancer properties (Table 1). Exposure of CaCo-2 colon cancer cells to RE drastically decreased colony formation at 30 µg/mL (24 h) [15]. Yi, et al. (2011) examined the anti-tumorigenic effect of several culinary and medicinal herbs on SW480 colon cancer cells and found RE to significantly decrease cell growth at a concentration of 31.25 µg/mL (48 h), with an IC50 of approximately 71.8 µg/mL [16]. Cell proliferation was dramatically decreased and cell cycle arrest was induced in HT-29 and SW480 cells using extracts that were standardized to CA (25%–43%) or to total polyphenol content (10 µM) [17–19]. Cell growth of SW620 and DLD-1 colon cancer cells was significantly inhibited by RE at 30 µg/mL (48 h), with an IC50 as low as 34.6 µg/mL. Furthermore, RE enhanced the inhibitory effects of the chemotherapeutic drug 5-fluorouracil (5-FU) on proliferation and sensitized 5-FU resistant cells [20].

In SW620 and DLD-1 colon cancer cells RE inhibited cell viability dose-dependently resulting in significant inhibition at concentrations as low as 20 µg/mL, and an IC50 around 25 µg/mL (48 h). This study used 5 different RE's, containing increasing levels of carnosol (CN: 1%–3.8% $w/w$) and CA (10%–30% $w/w$). Inhibition of cell viability was correlated with increasing CA content. Furthermore, CA alone (at doses found in RE) decreased cell viability and this effect was potentiated by the addition of CN (at doses found in RE). However, the inhibition seen using RE was greater than the response seen with CA or CN alone or in combination suggesting that chemicals other than CA and CN present in RE, also contribute to its anticancer effects [21]. Similarly, RE inhibited cell viability in HT29, SW480 and HGUE-C-1 colon cells at comparable doses (1.5–100 µg/mL; 48 h) and the authors reported that individual fractions of RE containing CA and other polyphenols, while potent, were not as potent as the complete extract [22]. Using HCT116 and SW480 cells, 10–100 µg/mL RE standardized to 23% CA (24–72 h) inhibited cell viability and induced apoptosis [23]. Valdes, et al. have shown, using HT-29 colon cells, that 30–60 µg/mL RE (24–72 h) inhibits cell proliferation (IC50 16.2 µg/mL). Moreover, RE induced cell cycle arrest, necrosis, cholesterol accumulation and ROS accumulation [24–26]. These studies provide evidence for the role of RE as an anticancer agent in colon cancer cells, capable of consistently inhibiting cell growth and viability at relatively low concentrations in the 20–100 µg/mL range.

**Table 1.** Anticancer effects of Rosemary Extract (RE). In vitro studies: colon cancer.

| Cancer Cell | Dose/Duration | Findings | Mechanism | Reference |
|---|---|---|---|---|
| CaCo-2 (Colorectal adenocarcinoma) | 0.1–30 µg/mL (3–24 h) | ↓ cell colony formation. Long and short term antioxidant effects | ↓ H$_2$O$_2$-induced DNA strand breaks and oxidative damage. ↓ visible light-induced oxidative damage | [15] |
| SW480 (Colorectal adenocarcinoma) | 31.25–500 µg/mL (48 h) | ↓ cell proliferation. Cytotoxic above 250 µg/mL. IC50~71.8 µg/mL | | [16] |
| HT-29 (Colorectal adenocarcinoma) | RE containing 10 µM total polyphenols (72 h) | ↓ cell proliferation ↑ cell cycle arrest ↑ apoptosis | | [17] |
| HT29 (Colorectal adenocarcinoma) | 1.95–62.5 µg/mL (48 h) 3 RE's standardized to 25.9%, 36.2%, 42.4% CA | ↓ cell proliferation IC50 > 62.5 µg/mL | | [18] |
| SW480 (Colorectal adenocarcinoma), HT29 (Colorectal adenocarcinoma) | RE containing 10 µM total polyphenols (48 h) | ↓ cell proliferation SW480 more sensitive ↑ cell cycle arrest | ↑ antioxidant and xenobiotic effects Modulates: Nrf2, ER stress genes, cell cycle, proliferation genes | [19] |
| SW620 (Colorectal adenocarcinoma), DLD-1 (Colorectal adenocarcinoma) | 20–110 µg/mL (24–48 h) | ↓ cell proliferation IC50 36.4 and 34.6 µg/mL Effect on 5-FU sensitive and resistant cells ↑ apoptosis ↓ cell transformation | Modulates TYMS and TK1. ↑ PARP cleavage | [20] |

**Table 1.** *Cont.*

| Cancer Cell | Dose/Duration | Findings | Mechanism | Reference |
|---|---|---|---|---|
| SW620 (Colorectal adenocarcinoma), DLD-1 (Colorectal adenocarcinoma) | 20–120 µg/mL (48 h) | ↓ cell viability IC50 25 µg/mL | ↑ PARP cleavage. ↑ GCNT3. ↓ miR-15b gene expression | [21] |
| HT-29 (Colorectal adenocarcinoma), W480 (Colorectal adenocarcinoma), HGUE-C-1 (Colorectal carcinoma) | 1.5–100 µg/mL (24–48 h) | ↓ cell viability | | [22] |
| HCT116 (Colorectal carcinoma), SW480 (Colorectal adenocarcinoma) | 10–100 µg/mL (24 h, 48 h, 72 h) Standardized to 23% CA | ↓ cell viability ↑ apoptosis | ↑ Nrf2 ↑ PERK ↑ sestrin-2 ↑ HO-1 ↑ cleaved-casp 3 | [23] |
| HT-29 (Colorectal adenocarcinoma) | 30 µg/mL (2–72 h) | ↓ cell proliferation ↑ cell cycle arrest ↑ cholesterol accumulation ↑ ROS accumulation | ↑ UPR ↑ ER-stress ↓ cell cycle genes Altered cholesterol-modulating genes | [24] |
| HT-29 (Colorectal adenocarcinoma) | 30–70 µg/mL (24 h, 48 h) | ↓ cell proliferation IC50 16.2 µg/mL ↑ necrosis | ↓ Nrf2 pathway ↑ UPR ↑ autophagy | [25] |
| HT-29 (Colorectal adenocarcinoma) | 30–60 µg/mL (6 h, 24 h) | ↓ cell proliferation ↑ cell cycle arrest | ↑ H2O2 in media ↑ ROS levels ↑ HO-1 and CHOP expression | [26] |

$H_2O_2$ (hydrogen peroxide), 5-FU (fluorouracil), TYMS (thymidylate synthase), TK1 (thymidine kinase 1), PARP (poly ADP ribose polymerase), GCNT3 (glucosaminyl (*N*-acetyl) transferase 3), miR-15b (microRNA-15b). GI50 (50% growth inhibition), TGI (total growth inhibition), Nrf2 (nuclear factor erythroid 2-related factor 2), casp (caspase), UPR (unfolded protein response), ER (endoplasmic reticulum), HO-1 (heme oxygenase protein-1), CHOP (C/EBP homologous protein).

In rat RINm5F insulinoma cells, RE significantly inhibited cell proliferation at 25 µg/mL (24 h), viability at 12 µg/mL (24 h) and increased apoptosis at 25 µg/mL (24 h) [27] (Table 2). Exposure of pancreatic cancer cells PANC-1 and MIA-PaCa-2 to RE containing increasing concentrations of CN (1%–3.8% *w/w*) and CA (10%–30% *w/w*) resulted in significant inhibition of cell viability with an IC50 of 50 µg/mL (48 h) and 30 µg/mL (48 h) respectively. The RE containing 25.66% *w/w* CA (sub-max) caused maximal inhibition compared to other RE's in PANC-1 cells, significantly inhibiting cell viability to approximately 60% at 40 µg/mL (48 h) [21].

Breast cancer can be classified under three subtypes based on the sensitivity of the tumors to chemotherapeutic agents. The subtypes are (i) estrogen receptor positive (ER+), which express ERα and therefore respond to estrogens; (ii) human epidermal growth factor receptor 2 positive (HER2+) which overexpress HER2 and can be either ER+ or ER−; (iii) triple negative (TN) which lack expression of ERα, progesterone receptor and HER2. One study used MCF-7 (ER+) breast cancer cells and a cigarette smoke solution (in PBS) collected from a cigarette with or without 40 mg RE added to the filter. The control used in this experiment was cells stimulated with 2.5 µM benzopyrene for 12–18 h and exposed to 1:19 *v/v* cigarette smoke solution for 2 h without an RE filter. The presence of RE in the filter lead to considerably reduced benzopyrene levels and associated DNA adduct formation [28] (Table 2).

RE inhibited cell proliferation in breast cancer cells with an IC50 of 90 µg/mL and 26.8 µg/mL in MCF-7 (ER+) and MDA-MB-468 (TN) cell lines respectively [29] (Table 2). In a similar study, dose-dependent inhibition of cell viability by 6.25–50 µg/mL (48 h) RE was seen in MDA-MB-231 (TN) and MCF-7 (ER+) breast cancer cells and MCF-7 cells had an IC50 of ~24.02 µg/mL. There is a discrepancy seen in the reported IC50 values which may be attributed to the different extraction methods used for the preparation of rosemary extract; supercritical $CO_2$ [30] and ethanol extraction [29].

Furthermore, MCF-7 cells were used in 2 additional studies and while both were found to inhibit cell proliferation, the IC50 values varied greatly from 187 µg/mL [31] to 9.95–13.89 µg/mL (RE standardized to 25%–43% CA) [18]. In agreement with the aforementioned studies, the RE resulting in a higher IC50 value was obtained from an alcohol based, methanol extraction [31].

The effects of RE at 1–120 µg/mL (48 h) were explored in all three breast cancer subtypes, ER+, HER2+ and TN. RE caused dose-dependent inhibition of cell viability in all subtypes of breast cancer cells. Furthermore RE enhanced the effectiveness of the monoclonal antibody (mAb) trastusumab and the chemotherapeutic drugs tamoxifen and paclitaxel, used in the treatment of breast cancer [32]. Taken together, these studies suggest a role for RE to inhibit pancreatic and breast cancer cell viability and proliferation, and induce apoptosis at concentrations in the 10–100 µg/mL range.

**Table 2.** Anticancer effects of Rosemary Extract (RE). In vitro studies: pancreatic and breast cancer.

| Cancer Cell | Dose/Duration | Findings | Mechanism | Reference |
|---|---|---|---|---|
| RINm5F (Insulinoma) | 12–100 µg/mL (24–48 h) | ↓ cell proliferation ↓ cell viability ↑ apoptosis | ↑ nitrate accumulation. ↑ TNFα production. | [27] |
| MIA-PaCa-2 (Pancreatic carcinoma), PANC-1 (Pancreatic carcinoma) | 20–120 µg/mL (48 h) | ↓ cell viability | ↑ PARP-cleavage | [21] |
| MCF-7 (*ER+*) (Breast adenocarcinoma) | 40 mg RE powder filter (inserted into cigarette) (2 h) | | ↓ BP levels and associated DNA adduct formation. | [28] |
| MCF-7 (*ER+*) (Breast adenocarcinoma), MDA-MB-468 (Breast adenocarcinoma) | 0.1%–20% (5–120 h) | IC50 ~90 µg/mL and 26.8 µg/mL | | [29] |
| MCF-7 (*ER+*) (Breast adenocarcinoma), MDA-MB-231 (Breast adenocarcinoma) | 6.25–50 µg/mL (48 h) | ↓ cell viability IC50 ~20.42 µg/mL | | [30] |
| MCF-7 (Breast adenocarcinoma) | 1–250 µg/mL (48 h) | ↓ cell proliferation IC50 187 µg/mL | | [31] |
| MCF-7 (Breast adenocarcinoma) | 1.95–62.5 µg/mL (48 h) 3 REs standardized to 25.9%, 36.2%, 42.4% CA | ↓ cell proliferation IC50 9.95–13.89 µg/mL | | [18] |
| SK-BR-3 (*HER2+*) (Breast adenocarcinoma), UACC-812 (*HER2+*) (Breast ductal carcinoma), T-47D (*ER+*) (Breast ductal carcinoma), MCF-7 (*ER+*) (Breast adenocarcinoma), MDA-MB-231 (Breast adenocarcinoma) | 10–120 µg/mL (48 h) | ↓ cell viability Enhanced effect of chemotherapeutics ↑ apoptosis ↓ cell transformation | ↑ FOS levels ↑ PARP cleavage ↓ HER2 ↓ ERBB2 ↓ ERα receptor. | [32] |

TNFα (tumor necrosis factor), PARP (poly ADP ribose polymerase), BP (benzopyrene), Fos (FBJ murine osteogenic sarcoma virus), HER2 (human epidermal growth factor receptor 2), ERBB2 (HER2/neu gene), ERα (estrogen receptor α).

Rosemary extract (6.25–50 µg/mL; 48 h) inhibited viability of DU145 and PC3 prostate cancer cells [30] (Table 3). In agreement with these data, significant inhibition of LNCaP and 22RV1 prostate cancer cell proliferation and viability, and an induction of apoptosis were seen with RE (50 µg/mL standardized to 40% CA; 24–48 h) [33]. RE was able to combat the enhanced prostate specific antigen (PSA) levels measured in cell culture media, indicative of prostate cancer, inhibiting levels to less than a fifth of what was seen in the control group. Correspondingly, levels of the androgen receptor, to which PSA binds, were significantly decreased by 50 µg/mL RE [33]. The inhibitory effects on both androgen sensitive and insensitive cell lines are important and suggest potential chemotherapeutic effects in different prostate cancer subtypes.

Using 5637 bladder cancer cells Mothana, et al. (2011) showed that RE inhibited cell proliferation with an IC50 of 48.3 µg/mL (48 h) [31] (Table 3). Exposure of A2780 ovarian cancer cells to 0.08% (0.8 mg/mL; 48 h) RE containing media resulted in significant inhibition of proliferation and induction of apoptosis and cell cycle arrest. Cisplatin is a chemotherapeutic agent used often in cancer treatment however, as with many chemotherapeutics, patients often develop resistance to treatment. At 0.08% RE enhanced the sensitivity of A2780 and cisplatin-resistant A2780CP70 cell lines to growth inhibition by cisplatin treatment, suggesting that RE may be of use in combination with cisplatin or potentially other chemotherapeutic drugs in patients who have developed an acquired resistance [34]. In HeLa cervical cancer cells, RE inhibited cell proliferation with an IC50 of 23.31 µg/mL (72 h) [35] and RE standardized to CA (25%–43%) inhibited cell proliferation with an IC50 of ~10 µg/mL (48 h) [18], suggesting that standardized extracts containing higher concentrations of CA may have greater anticancer effects. Furthermore, in human ovarian cancer cells SK-OV3 and HO-8910 rosemary essential oil (0.0625%–1%) inhibited cell viability with an IC50 of 0.025% and 0.076% in each cell line respectively (48 h) (Table 3) [36]. This study noted that the rosemary essential oil was more potent than its individual components (α-pinene, β-pinene, 1,8-cineole) when tested alone at the same concentrations.

**Table 3.** Anticancer effects of Rosemary Extract (RE). In vitro studies: prostate, ovarian, cervical and bladder cancer.

| Cancer Cell | Dose/Duration | Findings | Mechanism | Reference |
|---|---|---|---|---|
| DU145 (Prostate adenocarcinoma), PC3 (Prostate adenocarcinoma) | 6.25–50 µg/mL (48 h) | ↓ cell viability IC50 ~8.82 µg/mL | | [30] |
| LNCaP (Prostate adenocarcinoma), 22RV1 (Prostate carcinoma) | 10–50 µg/mL (24–48 h) RE standardized to 40% CA | ↓ cell proliferation ↑ cell cycle arrest ↑ apoptosis modulates endoplasmic reticulum stress proteins. | ↑ CHOP ↓ PSA production ↑ Bax ↑ cleaved-casp 3 ↓ androgen receptor expression | [33] |
| 5637 (Bladder carcinoma) | 0–250 µg/mL (48 h) | ↓ cell proliferation IC50 48.3 µg/mL | | [31] |
| A2780 (Ovarian carcinoma), A2780CP70 (cisplatin-resistant) (Ovarian carcinoma) | 0.05%–0.25% (24–48 h) | ↓ cell proliferation Enhanced sensitivity of cisplatin -resistant cell lines. ↑apoptosis ↑ cell cycle arrest Modulates expression of apoptotic genes. | ↓ P-glyco protein ↑ cytochrome c gene ↑ hsp70 gene | [34] |
| HeLa (Cervical adenocarcinoma) | 1.56–400 µg/mL (72 h) | ↓ cell proliferation IC50 23.31µg/mL | | [35] |
| HeLa (Cervical adenocarcinoma) | 1.95–62.5 µg/mL (48 h) 3 REs standardized to 25.9%, 36.2%, 42.4% CA | ↓ cell proliferation IC50 10.02–11.32 µg/mL | | [18] |
| SK-OV3 (Ovarian adenocarcinoma), HO-8910 (Ovarian carcinoma) | 0.0625%–1% rosemary essential oil (48 h) | ↓ cell viability IC50 0.025% (SK-OV3) IC50 0.076% (HO-8910) | | [36] |

CHOP (C/EBP homologous protein), PSA (prostate specific antigen), Bax (Bcl-2 associated X protein), casp (caspase), hsp70 (heat shock protein 70).

In human liver Hep-3B cells, RE at 0–50 µg/mL (24–48 h) dose-dependently decreased cell viability [30,37] with an IC50 of 22.88 µg/mL [30] (Table 4). Cell viability was inhibited in Bel-7402 liver cells by rosemary essential oil with an IC50 of 0.13% (1.3 mg/mL; 48 h) [36] and in HepG2 liver cells by RE with an IC50 of 42 µg/mL (48 h) [38]. The latter study also found that of the 4 different extracts tested, those with higher concentrations of CA resulted in more potent inhibition of cell proliferation [38]. In lung cancer cells, RE decreased viability of NCI-H82 small cell carcinoma cells (6.25–50 µg/mL; 48 h) [30] and decreased proliferation of A549 non-small cell carcinoma cells (2.5–200 µg/mL) [39] with an IC50 or 24.08 µg/mL and 15.9 µg/mL in each cell line respectively

(Table 4). In a V79 normal hamster lung fibroblast cell line RE was cytotoxic at 30 µg/mL (24 h) [15]. The cytotoxicity of RE in normal fibroblasts raises questions about its potential as a successful treatment option however, further research is required to fully examine the cytotoxicity issue in normal tissues.

**Table 4.** Anticancer effects of Rosemary Extract (RE). In vitro studies: liver and lung cancer.

| Cancer Cell | Dose/Duration | Findings | Mechanism | Reference |
|---|---|---|---|---|
| Hep-3B (Hepatocellular carcinoma) | 0.5–5 µg/mL (24 h) | ↓ cell viability | ↑ TNFα | [37] |
| Hep-3B (Hepatocellular carcinoma) | 6.25–50 µg/mL (48 h) | ↓ cell viability IC50 ~22.88 µg/mL | | [30] |
| Bel-7402 (Hepatocellular carcinoma) | 0.0625%–1% rosemary essential oil (48 h) | ↓ cell viability IC50 0.13% | | [36] |
| HepG2 (Hepatocellular carcinoma) | 10–120 µg/mL (48 h) | ↓ cell viability IC50 42 µg/mL GI50 20 µg/mL | | [38] |
| NCI-H82 (Lung carcinoma; SCLC) | 6.25–50 µg/mL (48 h) | ↓ cell viability IC50 ~24.08 | | [30] |
| V79 (Normal hamster lung) | 0.1–30 µg/mL (3–24 h) | Cytotoxic to cells at 30 µg/mL (24 h) Long and short term antioxidant effects | ↓ $H_2O_2$-induced DNA strand breaks and oxidative damage. ↓ visible-light induced oxidative damage | [15] |
| A549 (Lung adenocarcinoma) | 2.5–200 µg/mL (48–72 h) | ↓ cell proliferation ↓ cell survival ↑ apoptosis IC50 ~15.9 | ↓ p-Akt ↓ p-mTOR ↓ p-P70S6K ↑ PARP cleavage | [39] |

mTOR (mammalian target of rapamycin), PARP (poly(ADP-ribose) polymerase).

Vitamin D analogues (VDA) are commonly used in clinical differentiation therapy of acute myeloid leukemia (AML) to attempt to restore a defect in the capacity of myeloid progenitor cells to mature into non-replicating adult cells. However, pharmacologically relevant doses have been found to result in many adverse events such as hypercalcemia and attempts to circumvent these adverse events have been unsuccessful. RE containing 10 µM equivalent of CA, or 10 µM CA alone (96 h) potentiated the ability of vitamin D derivatives to inhibit cell viability and proliferation, induce apoptosis and cell cycle arrest and increase differentiation of WEHI-3BD murine leukemic and human HL-60 leukemic cells [40,41] (Table 5). A study examining the human leukemia HL-60 and K-562 cell lines and the murine RAW264.7 macrophage/monocyte cell line found significant inhibition of proliferation with an IC50 of 0.14% (1.4 mg/mL) and 0.25% (2.5 mg/mL) for the HL-60 and K-562 cells, respectively. In addition 0.1% (1 mg/mL; 72 h) RE significantly increased differentiation of HL-60 cells [29]. RE inhibited viability at 50 µg/mL (48 h) in K-562 leukemia cells [30]. Similar effects of RE (50 µg/mL; 24 h) were reported by others that lead to decreased proliferation of K-562 cells [42].

**Table 5.** Anticancer effects of Rosemary Extract (RE). In vitro studies: leukemia.

| Cancer Cell | Dose/Duration | Findings | Mechanism | Reference |
|---|---|---|---|---|
| WEHI-3B D (Murine myeloid leukemia), HL-60 (Myeloid leukemia), U937 (Myeloid leukemia) | RE (10 µM equivalent of CA) (48–96 h) | Potentiated following effects of VDA: ↓ cell proliferation ↑ cell cycle arrest ↑ cell differentiation ↑ apoptosis | ↑ G1 phase | [41] |

**Table 5.** *Cont.*

| Cancer Cell | Dose/Duration | Findings | Mechanism | Reference |
|---|---|---|---|---|
| RAW 264.7 (Murine leukemia; macrophage), HL-60 (Myeloid leukemia), K-562 (Human leukemia) | 0.1%–20% (5–120 h) (1–200 mg/mL) | ↓ cell proliferation IC50 ~18.76 µg/mL and 33.5 µg/mL ↑ cell differentiation ↓ LPS-stimulated (LS) antioxidant activity | ↓ (LS) NO ↑ antioxid-ant activity ↔ basal TNFα, IL-1β, iNOS or COX2 ↓ (LS) IL-1β and COX2 | [29] |
| WEHI-3B D (Murine myeloid leukemia) | RE (10 µM equivalent of CA) (48–96 h) | Potentiated following effects of VDA: ↑ cell differentiation ↓ cell viability ↓ cell proliferation | ↓ ROS ↑ antioxid-ant activity ↑ NADP(H)-quinone reductase | [40] |
| K-562 (Human leukemia) | 6.25–50 µg/mL (48 h) | ↓ cell viability IC50 ~12.50 µg/mL | | [30] |
| K-562 (Human leukemia), U937 (Myeloid leukemia) | 50 µg/mL (0–96 h) | ↓ cell proliferation | ↓ AKT1 ↑ Rb2 ↔ ERK2 | [42] |

VDA (vitamin D analogue), LPS (lipopolysaccharide), NO (nitric oxide), TNFα (tumor necrosis factor α), IL-1β (interleukin 1β), iNOS (inducible nitric oxide synthase), COX2 (cyclooxygenase 2), ROS (reactive oxygen species), NADP (nicotinamide adenine dinucleotide phosphate), Rb2 (retinoblastoma-related gene 2).

## 0. Anticancer Effects of Rosemary Extract (RE): In Vivo Animal Studies

A limited number of studies have examined the effects of RE administration on tumor growth in animals in vivo (Table 6). Administration of RE (1 mg/mL) in the drinking water ad libitum for 32–35 days resulted in a significant decrease in tumor size in nude mice xenografted with SW620 colon cancer cells [21]. A similar study using HCT116 colon cancer xenografted athymic nude mice fed 100 mg/kg/day RE dissolved in olive oil (4 weeks) significantly decreased tumor size in treated animals compared to control [23]. Biochemical analysis of serum samples collected from Sprague Dawley rats with N-methylnitrosourea-induced colon cancer showed significant anticancer effects by both high (3333.3 mg/kg/day) and low (1666.6 mg/kg/day) dose RE after 4 months of treatment with significant alteration of gene and protein signaling and aggregation of lymphoid cells [43]. A significant reduction in tumor volume was seen in mice xenografted with 22RV1 prostate cancer cells by RE (100 mg/kg/day) which was administered, dissolved in olive oil for 22 days [33].

In a diethylnitrosamine (DEN)-induced liver cancer model in F344 rats, RE at 100 mg/kg/day (5 days) was administered intragastrically with an intraperitoneal (i.p) injection of DEN on day 4. From this point, rats were fed a normal diet for 3 weeks until undergoing partial hepatectomy. Examination of liver tissue suggested RE may exert some protective antioxidant effects [44]. In accordance with this, use of Swiss mice exposed to 6 Grays (Gy) ionizing radiation (IR) in their liver once, followed by treatment with 1000 mg/kg RE fed orally, daily for 5 days suggested protective, antioxidant activity by RE. A delayed onset of IR-induced mortality and attenuated increases in glycogen and protein levels were seen in livers of mice exposed to IR and fed RE, compared to IR-exposed mice not fed RE [45]. Caution should be taken however, due to the high concentration (1000 mg/kg) used [45] which is at least 10 times greater than what has been found to exert potent anticancer effects in other studies. Taken together, these studies suggest a role for RE inhibiting chemical- or IR-induced carcinogenesis by exerting protective, antioxidant effects on healthy tissues. Thus, RE may display radio-protective effects, which would benefit healthy tissue during radiation treatment.

In WEHI-3BD myeloid leukemia xenografted mice fed 1% *w/w* RE in their food ad libitum (29 days), investigators noted a significant decrease in both tumor volume and incidence. Furthermore, RE showed an additive effect when combined with Vitamin D analogues (VDA) [41]. In WEHI-3BD xenografted mice administered RE (4% *w/w* in food) for up to 15 weeks combined with VDAs, median survival time was significantly increased and white blood cell count decreased to levels comparable to those seen in the control group of healthy mice [40].

Using a 7,12-dimethylbenz(a)anthracene (DMBA)-induced skin cancer nude mouse model, RE (500 or 1000 mg/kg/day; 15 weeks) administered orally in water resulted in a significant decrease in tumor number, diameter, weight and decrease in tumor incidence and burden, and an increase in latency period compared to control mice treated with DMBA only [46,47]. One group of mice, which were administered RE for 7 days prior to the first application of DMBA, showed a 50% reduction in tumor growth compared to the DMBA-only treated mice, suggesting potent chemo protective effects [47].

**Table 6.** Anticancer effects of Rosemary Extract (RE). In vivo studies.

| Animal Model | Dose/Duration | Findings | Mechanism | Reference |
|---|---|---|---|---|
| SW620 colon xenograft (nude mice) | 1 mg/mL in drinking water (32–35 days) ad libitum | ↓ tumor size | ↓ miR-15b in plasma | [21] |
| HCT116 colon xenograft (athymic nude mice) | 100 mg/kg/day in 100 μL olive oil by oral gavage (4 weeks) | ↓ tumor size | ↑ Nrf2 expression ↑ sestrin-2 expression | [23] |
| NMN-induced colon cancer (Sprague-Dawley rats) | 1666.6 mg/kg/day (low dose) RE or 3333.3 mg/kg/day (high dose) RE orally (4 months) | Both RE showed comparable effects. Lead to lymphoid cell aggregation in submucosa | ↑ cyt C ↑ PCDP4 ↓CEA ↓ CCSA-4 ↓ β-catenin, K-ras, c-myc gene expression | [43] |
| 22RV1 prostate xenograft (athymic nude mice) | 100 mg/kg/day in olive oil, orally (22 days) | ↓ tumor volume (induces apoptosis) | ↓ androgen receptor expression ↓ PSA ↑ CHOP | [33] |
| DEN-induced liver cancer (F344 rats) | 100 mg/kg/day RE intragastrically (5 days) Injected i.p with 20 mg/kg DEN on day 4. Fed normal diet until week 3 (underwent partial hepatectomy) | ↑ antioxidant activity | ↓ GST positive foci | [44] |
| Swiss mice exposed to γ-IR (liver) | 6Gy γ-IR (once) followed by 1000 mg/kg/day RE orally (5 days) | Delayed onset of IR-induced mortality Attenuated negative IR effects Protective effect on liver and blood | ↓ LPx levels ↑ GSH levels | [45] |
| Myeloid leukemia inoculated mice | 1% RE *w/w* in food ad libitum (29 days) | ↓ tumor volume ↓ tumor incidence Potentiated VDA ability to ↓ tumor volume | | [41] |
| Myeloid leukemia inoculated mice | 4% *w/w* in food ad libitum (15 weeks) | RE alone ↔ median survival time RE+VDA ↑ median survival time | ↓ WBC | [40] |
| DMBA-induced skin cancer (nude mice) | 1000 mg/kg/day RE orally in water or by gavage (15 weeks) | ↓ tumor number ↓ tumor incidence ↓ tumor burden ↓ tumor yield ↑ latency period | ↓ LPx levels ↑ GSH levels | [46] |
| DMBA-induced skin cancer (nude mice) | 500 mg/kg/day RE orally in water or by gavage (15 weeks) | ↓ tumor number ↓ tumor diameter ↓ tumor weight | ↓ LPx levels ↑ GSH levels | [47] |

miR-15b (microRNA 15b), PSA (prostate specific antigen), CHOP (C/EBP homologous protein), VDA (vitamin D analogue), WBC (white blood cell), GST (glutathione *S* transferase), IR (ionizing radiation), LPx (lipid peroxidase), GSH (glutathione), DEN (diethylnitrosamine), DMBA (7,12-dimethylbenz(a)anthracene), NMN (*N*-methylnitrosourea), cyt C (cytochrome C), PCDP4 (programmed cell death protein 4), CEA (carcinoembryonic antigen), CCSA-4 (colon cancer specific antigen 4), LPx (lipid peroxidase), GSH (glutathione).

## 4. Mechanisms of Anticancer Effects of Rosemary Extract (RE): In Vitro Studies

Many studies have examined the anti-proliferative and colony forming abilities of RE in vitro in colon [15–20,24–26], pancreas [27], breast [18,29,31,32], prostate [33], cervical [18,35], bladder [31], ovarian [34], lung [39] and leukemia [29,40–42] cell lines however, little is known concerning the underlying mechanism. RE was shown to have an inhibitory effect on AKT1 mRNA and protein expression, a protein involved in the PI3K/Akt survival signaling pathway, in a leukemic cell line [42] however, no measure of Akt activity was mentioned. No effect on ERK2 protein levels, involved in cell proliferation and differentiation, were seen in these cells. Cell cycle arrest prevents further division by proliferating cells and RE was shown to induce cell cycle arrest in a number of cancer cell lines [17,19,24,25,33,34,41] and increase retinoblastoma-related gene 2 (Rb2) [42] which regulates entry into cell division. Recently, Moore, et al. (2016) found RE inhibited activation of the Akt/mTOR/p70S6K signaling pathway which was associated with a significant decrease in cell proliferation and survival [39].

The viability of various cancer cell lines was shown to be significantly inhibited by treatment with RE which many studies attributed to enhanced apoptosis and cell death. Increased poly ADP ribose polymerase (PARP) cleavage, which is an established indicator of enhanced apoptosis, was seen in colon [20,21], pancreas [21], breast [32] and lung [39] cancer cell lines following treatments with RE. Alternatively, RE enhanced nitrate accumulation (i.e., increased nitric oxide production) and TNFα production in pancreatic [27] and liver [37] cancer cells, indicative of enhanced cell death capabilities and nitric oxide-induced apoptosis. In ovarian cancer cells [34] enhanced apoptosis was associated with increased gene expression of mitochondrial-regulated apoptosis proteins cytochrome c, involved in the electron transport chain, and heat shock protein 70 (hsp70) which is involved in protein folding and protecting the cell from heat stress and toxic chemicals. Other mechanisms of apoptosis by RE include enhanced protein expression of pro-apoptotic Bax and cleaved-caspase 3 [23,33], increased expression of binding immunoglobulin protein (BiP) and CCAAT/-enhancer-binding protein homologous protein (CHOP) proteins which induce endoplasmic reticular stress [25,33], and the unfolded protein response [24–26,33] in prostate and colon cancer cells. Interestingly, in normal prostate epithelial cells RE treatment resulted in a decrease in endoplasmic reticular stress related protein PRKR-like endoplasmic reticulum kinase (PERK), suggesting RE selectively induces endoplasmic reticular stress in prostate cancer cells but spares normal prostate cells [33]. Similarly, in breast cancer cells [32] RE decreased expression of estrogen receptor α (ERα) in the ER+ subtype and human epidermal growth factor receptor 2 (HER2) in the HER2+ subtype, and it was suggested the decreased receptor expression was correlated with enhanced apoptosis in these cell subtypes. Correspondingly, increased levels of Fos, an oncogenic transcription factor, were detected in ER+ and HER2+ cell lines, and this event is thought to precede apoptosis and correspond to the PARP-cleavage seen in these cells. Although RE was also capable of inducing anticancer effects in triple negative (TN) breast cancer cells, its mechanism has yet to be elucidated [32].

Induction of apoptosis by endoplasmic reticular stress has been found by several studies in colon cancer cells [19,23,24,26] and has been shown to involve translocation of nuclear factor erythroid 2-related factor 2 (Nrf2) into the nucleus and induction of p38 MAPK and PERK activity. The Nrf2/antioxidant response element (ARE) signaling pathway has been considered to protect cells against carcinogenesis and attenuate cancer development by neutralizing ROS and carcinogens and members of this pathway, including sestrin-2 and heme oxygenase-1 (HO-1), are upregulated by RE in colon cancer cells [23,25]. Overall, the majority of existing studies indicate that the anticancer effects of RE may be due largely to induction of apoptosis.

Antioxidants are molecules, which scavenge harmful free radicals, protecting cells from oxidative DNA damage and potentially death. RE has been shown to exert antioxidant effects in colon [15], breast [28], and leukemia [29,40] cell lines. Colon cancer cells pretreated with RE followed by treatment with hydrogen peroxide, often used in cell culture to induce oxidative DNA damage, showed reduced DNA double-strand breaks and oxidative damage compared to control cells treated with hydrogen peroxide only. Similarly, RE reduced oxidative damage induced by methylene blue (oxidizes purines) in these cells [15]. RE treatment resulted in increased levels of antioxidants and NAPD(H)-quinone reductase (oxidoreductase involved in the transfer of electrons from a reduced molecule to an oxidized molecule) which decreased reactive oxygen species (ROS) levels, and inhibited lipopolysaccharide (LPS)-stimulated production of the free radical nitric oxide (NO) in leukemia cell lines [29,40]. In an in vitro model of cigarette smoking, the use of an RE containing cigarette filter considerably reduced benzopyrene (carcinogen) levels and associated DNA adduct formation in breast cancer cells [28]. An effect of RE treatment, to inhibit ROS levels in cancer cells, may be viewed as a beneficial and not an anticancer effect for cancer cells. Traditionally treatments for cancer should result in apoptosis/killing of cancer cells. The antioxidant properties exerted by RE treatment indicate a potential for RE as a preventative strategy which may target the initiation and promotion stages of cancer. Antioxidants work to restore damaged DNA back to normal and protect the cell from further damage thus, preventing the potential mutation into a cancer cell and subsequent tumor formation.

In addition to the antiproliferative, apoptotic and antioxidant mechanisms noted above, some evidence indicates that RE may (i) exert anti-inflammatory effects [29] through inhibition of interleukin-1 (IL-1) and cyclooxygenase 2 (COX2) molecules; (ii) aid in the reversal of acquired drug resistance [34] by inhibiting P-glycoprotein levels (involved in drug resistance); and (iii) alter metabolic-related genes [21] such as glycosyltransferase (GCNT3) which forms glycosidic linkages in a variety of macromolecules and its potential epigenetic regulator microRNA-15b. Induction of autophagy [26] and alterations to cholesterol metabolism [24] may also be mechanisms of RE in colon cancer cells.

## 5. Mechanisms of Anticancer Effects of Rosemary Extract (RE): In Vivo Animal Studies

Limited evidence exists regarding RE's mechanism in vivo however, few studies list potential antioxidant effects and serum biomarkers for RE's anticancer effects. Increases in glutathione (GSH), an antioxidant, and reductions in lipid peroxidase (LPx), an oxidizing agent resulting in free radical production and cell damage, have been recorded in IR-induced mouse liver [45] and DMBA-induced mouse skin cancer [46,47] models treated with RE. Similarly, RE decreased glutathione-S transferase (GST) positive foci, which are associated with oxidative damage from the reduction of GSH [40], in a rat DEN-induced liver cancer model however, results were not significant and should be taken with caution [44].

Serum samples from mice xenografted with prostate cancer cells and fed RE in their diet showed a decrease in prostate-specific antigen (PSA) levels (high levels would be suggestive of prostate cancer) and examination of tissue samples showed decreased androgen receptor and CHOP expression, indicative of an induction of apoptosis associated with endoplasmic reticular stress [33]. Similarly, HCT116 colon cancer xenografted mice showed increased Nrf2 and Sestrin-2 expression which are indicative of endoplasmic reticular stress and can lead to enhanced apoptosis [23]. A significant decrease in microRNA-15b (miR-15b) plasma levels after administration of RE in colon cancer xenografted mice suggested circulating miR-15b levels may act as a minimally invasive method to monitor the antitumor effects of RE in vivo [21]. Furthermore, rats with *N*-methylnitrosourea (NMN)-induced colon cancer fed RE, showed significant alterations in cell death modulating proteins including cytochrome c, programmed cell death protein 4 (PCDP4), carcinoembryonic antigen (CEA) and colon-cancer specific antigen-4 (CCSA-4) [43]. Sufficient evidence exists to support the potential use of RE in chemotherapeutics however, it is still not well understood whether the anticancer effects seen by RE are attributable to individual polyphenols within the extract or rely on the combination of all the components within the extract combined. The next section of this review explores the role of two of RE's main polyphenols, CA and RA, and their potential contribution to RE's anticancer effects.

## 6. Anticancer Effects of Carnosic Acid (CA): In Vitro Studies

Treatment of different colon cancer cells with CA resulted in significant inhibition of cell viability using concentrations ranging from 1 to 400 µM, and having IC50 values in the 20–90 µM range (Table 7). In addition, CA induced apoptosis and cell cycle arrest in Caco-2 cells [48,49] and inhibited cell adhesion and migration in Caco-2, HT-29 and LoVo cells [49] by inhibiting activity of the cell cycle regulator cyclin A [48] and by inhibiting MMP-9, uPA and COX-2 activity, associated with cell adhesion and migration properties [49]. Similarly, in SW480 colorectal cancer cells with hyperactive β-catenin which is oncogenic, CA targeted β-catenin for proteasomal degradation and this suggests a potential for CA to be used as a small molecule oncogenic β-catenin inhibitor [50]. In SLW620 and DLD-1 cells CA inhibited cell viability and this was associated with downregulation of miR-15b and enhanced GCNT3 activity which are associated with regulation of metabolic related genes [21]. Furthermore, in HT-29 colon cells CA inhibited cell proliferation and enhanced cell cycle arrest, which was correlated with altered expression of an array of transport and biosynthesis genes and altered activity of detoxifying enzymes and metabolites. Of note, levels of GSH, an important antioxidant, were enhanced and levels of *N*-acetylputrescine, which are toxic in high doses, were decreased [51]. In HT-29 cells co-cultured with 3T3-L1 adipocytes, CA attenuated the negative effects of the adipocytes on the colon cancer cells by inhibiting triglyceride accumulation and downregulating expression of the Ob-R receptor [52]. In these cells CA also inhibited cell viability by decreasing phosphorylation of the cell survival regulators Akt and Bcl-xL and enhancing Bax expression. Furthermore, cell cycle arrest was induced by inhibition of cyclin D1 and CDK4 [52]. Similarly, a fraction of rosemary extract which was found to consist mainly of CA (98.7% pure) was tested on HT-29, SW480 and HGUE-C-1 colon cancer cells and significantly inhibited cell viability. Among several different fractions of the RE that were tested, the fraction containing CA was found to be among the most active and it was suggested that synergism between many components of the extract plays a role in rosemary's anticancer effects [22]. Inhibition of cell proliferation and increased cell cycle arrest by CA in HT-29 cells was found to be orchestrated by the unfolded protein response and triggered by endoplasmic reticular stress [24] which can lead to apoptosis and thus destruction of cancerous cells. Enhanced cholesterol and ROS accumulation in CA treated cancer cells was also shown to contribute to the inhibition of proliferation seen [24]. Similarly, activity of pro-apoptotic markers including p53, Bax, caspases and PARP were enhanced and anti-apoptotic markers MDM2, Bcl-2 and Bcl-xL were decreased in HT-29, HCT116 and SW480 colon cells [53]. Levels of ROS and $H_2O_2$ were increased in vitro in the cell medium [25,53] by CA which can trigger cellular stress and thus cancer cell death. The signaling molecules STAT3 and survivin play a key role in regulating cell survival and CA inhibited activity of these molecules in colon cancer cells [53]. These studies provide strong evidence that CA at relatively low doses (1–100 µM) is capable of inhibiting colon cancer cell growth and survival by modulating expression of key signaling molecules and altering cell metabolism.

In breast cancer cells, including MCF-7, MDA-MB-231 and MDA-MB-468, CA inhibited cell proliferation and enhanced apoptosis at concentrations of 1.5–150 µM [30,54–56] (Table 8). The inhibitory effects of CA were found to be dependent on increasing levels of the antioxidant glutathione in breast cancer cells and accordingly, expression of genes involved in glutathione biosynthesis (CYP4F3, GCLC) and transport (SLC7A11) were significantly increased as well [54]. Importantly, the sensitivity of CA was found to be associated with HER2 expression and thus the MCF-7 cells were more sensitive to the CA treatment, compared to the triple-negative MDA-MB-468 cell line which does not express HER2 [54]. In the triple negative MDA-MB-361 cell line CA induced TRAIL-mediated apoptosis through down-regulation of c-FLIP and Bcl-2 expression and through CHOP-dependent upregulation of DR5, Bim and PUMA expression (ER stress associated proteins) [56] suggesting that CA is capable of inhibiting breast cancer cell survival through different mechanisms depending on the mutations that are present.

**Table 7.** Anticancer effects of Carnosic Acid (CA). In vitro studies: colon cancer.

| Cell Type | Dose/Duration | Findings | Mechanism | Reference |
|---|---|---|---|---|
| Caco-2 (Colorectal adenocarcinoma) | 1–50 μM CA (48 h) | ↓ cell proliferation ↑ cell cycle arrest ↑ cell doubling time IC50 23 μM | ↓ cyclin A | [48] |
| Caco-2 (Colorectal adenocarcinoma), HT-29 (Colorectal adenocarcinoma), LoVo (Colorectal adenocarcinoma) | 1–388 μM CA (48 h) | ↑ apoptosis ↓ cell adhesion and migration IC50 26.4–92.1 μM (high in Caco2) | ↓ MMP-9 and uPA activity, COX-2 expression | [49] |
| SW480 (Colorectal adenocarcinoma) | 25–100 μM CA (6 h) | targets activated β-catenin for proteasomal degradation and destabilizes oncogenic β-catenin | ↓ BCL9-β-catenin interaction | [50] |
| SW620 (Colorectal adenocarcinoma), DLD-1 (Colorectal adenocarcinoma) | 2–18 μg/mL (6.02–54.15 μM) CA (48 h) | ↓ cell viability | ↑ GCNT3. ↓ miR-15b gene expression. | [21] |
| HT-29 (Colorectal adenocarcinoma) | 5–35 μg/mL (15–105 μM) CA (24–72 h) | ↓ cell proliferation ↑ cell cycle arrest Alters activity of detoxifying enzymes and metabolites | ↑ GSH levels Altered expression of transport and biosynthesis genes ↓ N-acetylputrescine | [51] |
| HT-29 (Colorectal adenocarcinoma) | 1–10 μM CA (24–48 h) | ↓ cell viability ↑ cell cycle arrest ↓ triglyceride accumulation of 3T3-L1 adipocytes | ↓ p-Akt, cyclin D1, CDK4, Bcl-xL ↑ Bax expression, Ob-R expression | [52] |
| HT-29 (Colorectal adenocarcinoma), SW480 (Colorectal adenocarcinoma), HGUE-C-1 (Colorectal carcinoma) | 30–60 μg/mL (24–48 h) CA fraction of RE (98.7% purity) | ↓ cell viability | | [22] |
| HT-29 (Colorectal adenocarcinoma) | 12.5 μg/mL (37.6 μM) CA (2–72 h) | ↓ cell proliferation ↑ cell cycle arrest ↑ cholesterol accumulation ↑ ROS accumulation | ↑ UPR ↑ ER-stress ↓ cell cycle genes Altered cholesterol-modulating genes | [24] |
| HT-29 (Colorectal adenocarcinoma), HCT116 (Colorectal carcinoma), SW480 (Colorectal adenocarcinoma) | 20–100 μM CA (24 h) | ↓ cell viability ↑ apoptosis | ↑ p53, Bax, casp 3, casp 9, PARP cleavage ↑ ROS generation ↓ MDM2, Bcl-2, Bcl-xL ↓ survivin, cyclins STAT3 | [53] |
| HT-29 (Colorectal adenocarcinoma) | 8.3–16.6 μg/mL (25–50 μM) CA (24 h) | ↓ cell proliferation | ↑ H₂O₂ ↑ ROS | [25] |

MMP-9 (matrix metallopeptidase 9), uPA (urokinase plasminogen activator), COX-2 (cyclooxygenase 2), BCL9-β (B-cell CLL/lymphoma 9), GCNT3 (glucosaminyl (*N*-Acetyl) transferase 3), GSH (glutathione), CDK4 (cyclin-dependent kinase 4), Bcl-xL (B-cell lymphoma-extra large), Bax (Bcl-2-like protein 4), Ob-R (leptin receptor), ROS (reactive oxygen species), UPR (unfolded protein response), ER (endoplasmic reticulum), casp (caspase), p53 (tumor protein p53), PARP (poly(ADP-ribose) polymerase), MDM2 (mouse double minute 2 homolog), Bcl-2 (B-cell CLL/lymphoma 2), STAT3 (signal transducer and activator of transcription 3), $H_2O_2$ (hydrogen peroxide).

Inhibition of cell viability by CA was shown in rat insulinoma (RINm5F) and human (MIA-PaCa-2, PANC-1) pancreatic cancer cells at doses of 6–300 μM [21,27]. In prostate cancer cells, lower doses of CA (<100 μM) inhibited cell viability and enhanced apoptosis [30,57,58]. Induction of apoptosis in PC-3 prostate cells was associated with activation of both intrinsic and extrinsic apoptotic pathways. Inhibition of caspase 8 and 9, Bcl-2, Bid, IAP, p-Akt, p-GSK3 and NF-κB and activation of caspase 3 and 7, PARP, Bax, cytochrome c and PP2A all contribute to enhanced apoptosis within these cells [58]. The use of a pan-caspase inhibitor attenuated the apoptotic effects of CA and provides strong evidence for the involvement of caspases in the apoptotic mechanism of CA in prostate cancer cells [58]. Low doses of CA both alone and in combination with other phytonutrients such as curcumin showed potent anticancer effects in LNCaP, PC3 and DU145 prostate cells and inhibited androgen receptor activity. The inhibition of proliferation of these cells was associated with an inhibition of the EpRE/ARE antioxidant transcription system and inhibition of PSA secretion [57]. Furthermore, CA inhibited proliferation of A2780 ovarian cancer cells and enhanced the sensitivity of a resistant A2780CP70 cell line to cisplatin, a potent chemotherapeutic agent [34]. Carnosic acid has potent anticancer effects on its own but also acts synergistically with other compounds including phytonutrients and chemotherapeutics and this represents a promising route for future cancer therapies using combinations of anticancer agents at lower doses.

**Table 8.** Anticancer effects of Carnosic Acid (CA). In vitro studies: breast, pancreatic, prostate and ovarian cancer.

| Cell Type | Dose/Duration | Findings | Mechanism | Reference |
|---|---|---|---|---|
| MCF-7 *(ER+)* (Breast adenocarcinoma), MDA-MB-231 (Breast adenocarcinoma) | 6.25–50 μg/mL (18.8–150 μM) CA (48 h) | ↓ cell viability | | [30] |
| MCF-7 (Breast adenocarcinoma), MDA-MB-468 (Breast adenocarcinoma) | 0.5–40 μg/mL (1.5–120 μM) CA (6–96 h) | ↓ proliferation ↑ apoptosis ↑ cell cycle arrest IC50: 3μg/mL (9 μM) (88 h) | ↑ CYP4F3, GCLC, SLC7A11, CDKN1A expression | [54] |
| MDA-MB-468 (Breast adenocarcinoma) | 10–30 μM CA (?4 h) | ↑ apoptosis | | [55] |
| MDA-MB-361 (Breast adenocarcinoma) | 20 μM CA (24 h) | ↓ proliferation ↑ apoptosis | ↑ TRAIL-mediated apoptosis ↓ c-FLIP, Bcl-2 ↑ DR5, Bim, PUMA, CHOP | [56] |
| RINm5F (Insulinoma) | 12–100 μg/mL (36.1–300 μM) CA (24–48 h) | ↓ cell viability | | [27] |
| MIA-PaCa-2 (Pancreatic carcinoma), PANC-1 (Pancreatic carcinoma) | 2–18 μg/mL (6.02–54.15 μM) CA (48 h) | ↓ cell viability | | [21] |
| DU145 (Prostate carcinoma), PC3 (Prostate adenocarcinoma) | 6.25–50 μg/mL (18.8–150 μM) CA (48h) | ↓ cell viability | | [30] |
| PC3 (Prostate adenocarcinoma) | 20–100 μM CA (0–72 h) | ↓ proliferation ↑ apoptosis | ↓ casp 8, casp 9, Bcl-2, Bid, IAP, p-Akt, p-GSK3, NF-κB ↑ casp 3, casp 7, PARP cleavage, Bax, cyt c, PP2A | [58] |
| LNCaP (Prostate carcinoma), PC3 (Prostate adenocarcinoma), DU-145 (Prostate carcinoma) | 10 μM CA (72 h) | ↓ proliferation | ↓ EpRE/ARE transcription system ↓ PSA secretion | [57] |
| A2780 (Ovarian carcinoma), A2780CP70 (cisplatin-resistant) (Ovarian carcinoma) | 2.5–10 μg/mL (7.2–30 μM) CA (48 h) | ↓ cell proliferation Enhanced sensitivity of cisplatin-resistant cells | | [34] |

CYP4F3 (leukotriene-B(4)omega-hydroxylase 2), GCLC (glutamate-cysteine ligase catalytic subunit), SLC7A11 (solute carrier family 7 member 11), CDKN1A (cyclin-dependent kinase inhibitor 1A), TRAIL (TNF-related apoptosis-inducing ligand), c-FLIP (cellular FLICE (FADD-like-IL-1β-converting enzyme)-inhibiting protein), DR5 (death receptor 5), Bim (Bcl-2-like protein 11), PUMA (p53 upregulated modulator of apoptosis), CHOP (C/EBP homologous protein), casp (caspase), Bcl-2 (B-cell CLL/lymphoma 2), Bid (BH3 interacting-domain), IAP (inhibitor of apoptosis), p-Akt (phosphorylated protein kinase B), p-GSK3 (phosphorylated glycogen synthase kinase 3), NF-κB (nuclear factor kappa B), PARP (poly (ADP-ribose) polymerase), Bax (Bcl-2-like protein 4), cyt c (cytochrome c), PP2A (protein phosphatase 2A), EpRE (electrophile responsive element), ARE (antioxidant response element), PSA (prostate specific antigen).

In Hep-3B, HepG2 and SK-HEP1 human liver cancer cells, CA inhibited cell viability and enhanced apoptosis [30,55,56,59] (Table 9). In Hep-G2 cells the formation of autophagic vacuoles and autolysosomes contributed to enhanced cell death by CA and this was induced through inhibition of the Akt/mTOR cell survival pathway [59]. Furthermore, in SK-HEP1 cells CA induced TRAIL-mediated apoptosis by altering apoptotic markers such as c-FLIP, Bcl-2, DR5, Bim, PUMA and CHOP [56]. Rat liver clone 9 cells are often used as a model for screening hepatotoxicity and CA was found to enhance activity of enhancer element GPEI which regulates the pi class of glutathione *S*-transferase and modulates antioxidant and detoxification systems within the cell [60]. CA was found to exert a protective effect in these non-cancerous liver cells which was modulated by the Nrf2/p38 MAPK signaling pathway [60,61]. Furthermore, CA inhibited viability of small-cell lung cancer NCI-H82 cells [30].

**Table 9.** Anticancer effects of Carnosic Acid (CA). In vitro studies: liver, lung, skin and kidney cancer.

| Cell Type | Dose/Duration | Findings | Mechanism | Reference |
|---|---|---|---|---|
| Hep-3B (Hepatocellular carcinoma) | 6.25–50 µg/mL (18.8–150 µM) CA (48 h) | ↓ cell viability | | [30] |
| HepG2 (Hepatocellular carcinoma) | 20–100 µM for (12–48 h) | ↓ proliferation ↑ apoptosis ↑ autophagic vacuoles and autolysosomes | ↑ LC-3 ↓ p-Akt, p-mTOR | [59] |
| SK-HEP1 (Hepatocellular carcinoma) | 20–60 µM CA (24 h) | ↑ apoptosis | | [55] |
| SK-HEP1 (Hepatocellular carcinoma) | 20 µM CA (24 h) | ↓ proliferation ↑ apoptosis | ↑ TRAIL-mediated apoptosis ↓ c-FLIP, Bcl-2 ↑ DR5, Bim, PUMA, CHOP | [56] |
| Rat clone 9 (Normal rat liver) | 1–20 µM CA (24 h) | ↑ reporter activity of enhancer element GPEI ↑ detoxification systems | ↑ GSTP expression ↑ Nrf2 translocation ↑ p38 | [60] |
| Rat clone 9 (Normal rat liver) | 1–20 µM CA (0–24 h) | ↓ cell survival | ↑ NQO1 ↑ Nrf2 ↑ p-p38 ↑ p-ERK | [61] |
| NCI-H82 (Lung carcinoma; SCLC) | 6.25–50 µg/mL (18.8–150 µM) CA (48 h) | ↓ cell viability | | [30] |
| HT-1080 (Fibrosarcoma) | 25–100 µM CA (4–72 h) | ↑ apoptosis ↑ cell cycle arrest ↑ chromatin condensation and DNA fragmentation IC50 9 µM | | [62] |
| BAEC Aortic endothelial cells), HUVEC (Umbilical vein endothelial cells) | 25–100 µM CA (4–72 h) | ↓ cell survival ↑ apoptosis ↑ cell cycle arrest ↓ migration IC50 36µM | ↓ MMP-2 ↓ endothelial cell tubulogenesis. | [62] |
| B16F10 (Skin melanoma) | 2.5–10 µM CA (12 h) | ↓ cell migration and adhesion Suppressed mesenchymal markers Induced epithelial markers | ↓ MMP-9, TIMP-1, uPA, VCAM-1 ↓ p-Src, p-FAK, p-Akt | [63] |
| Caki (Kidney clear cell carcinoma) | 20–60 µM CA (24 h) | ↑ apoptosis Promotes ROS production | ↑ PARP cleavage, casp 3, ATF4, CHOP | [55] |
| Caki (Kidney clear cell carcinoma), AHCN (Kidney renal cell adenocarcinoma), A498 (Kidney carcinoma) | 20 µM CA (24 h) | ↓ proliferation ↑ apoptosis | ↑ TRAIL-mediated apoptosis ↓ c-FLIP, Bcl-2 ↑ DR5, Bim, PUMA, CHOP | [56] |

LC3 (light chain 3), p-mTOR (phosphorylated mammalian target of rapamycin), TRAIL (TNF-regulated apoptosis-inducing ligand), c-FLIP (cellular FLICE (FADD-like-IL-1β-converting enzyme)-inhibiting protein), Bcl-2 (B-cell CLL/lymphoma 2), DR5 (death receptor 5), Bim (Bcl-2-like protein 11), PUMA (p53 upregulated modulator of apoptosis), CHOP (C/EBP homologous protein), GSTP (Glutathione *S*-transferase P), Nrf2 (nuclear factor E2-related factor-2), NQO1 (NAD(P)H-quinone oxidoreductase 1), p-ERK (phosphorylated extracellular signal-regulated kinases), MMP-2 (matrix metalloproteinase-2), MMP-9 (matrix metallopeptidase-9), TIMP-1 (TIMP metallopeptidase inhibitor 1), uPA (urokinase plasminogen activator), VCAM-1 (vascular cell adhesion protein 1), p-Src (proto-oncogene tyrosine-protein kinase Src), p-FAK (phosphorylated focal adhesion kinase), PARP (poly(ADP-ribose)polymerase), casp (caspase).

In several models of skin cancer, including HT-1080, BEAC, HUVEC and B16F10 cells, CA inhibited cell survival, cell migration and cell adhesion, enhanced apoptosis and induced cell cycle arrest [62,63] (Table 9). Chromatin condensation and DNA fragmentation were seen in HT-1080 cells which lead to apoptosis [62]. In human umbilical and bovine aortic endothelial cell lines, CA inhibited tubulogenesis and MMP-2 expression suggesting anti-angiogenic properties of CA which would be beneficial in anticancer therapies [62]. Inhibition of the epithelial-mesenchymal transition in B16F10 melanoma cells suggests a possible mechanism for the inhibition of cell migration by CA. Inhibition of cell migration markers MMP-9, TIMP-1, uPA and VCAM-1 was seen in this cell line using low doses of CA (10 μM). Inhibition of phosphorylation of signaling molecules Akt, FAK and Src were also associated with inhibition of the epithelial-mesenchymal transition and cell migration in B16F10 cells [63]. In Caki, kidney cancer cells, CA induced apoptosis through ROS-mediated endoplasmic reticular stress. Activity of apoptotic markers PARP, caspase 3, ATF4 and CHOP was increased in these cells [55]. Similarly, TRAIL-mediated apoptosis was induced in Caki, AHCN and A498 kidney cells through modulation of endoplasmic reticular stress related proteins c-FLIP, Bcl-2, DR5, Bim, PUMA and CHOP [56].

In T98G glioblastoma cells CA promotes production of nerve growth factor and this was found to be regulated by the Nrf2 signaling pathway [64,65] (Table 10). Nerve growth factor is involved in the regulation of growth and the maintenance and survival of certain target neurons, and thus can act to protect neural cells from toxic agents that may cause cancer. In IMR-32 neuroblastoma cells CA induced apoptosis by activation of caspases, PARP and the p38 MAPK pathway and inhibited cell viability, which was associated with decreased ERK activation [66]. Interestingly however, in SH-SY5Y neuroblastoma cells CA attenuated apoptosis induced by the neurotoxic compounds methylglyoxal and amyloid β, exerting a cytoprotective effect [67,68]. This protective effect was associated with increased activation of PI3K/Akt signaling, inhibition of cytochrome c release and inhibition of caspase cascades which results in a pro-survival effect on the cell [36,67]. Similarly, in U373MG astrocytoma cells CA inhibited amyloid β peptide production and release and this was associated, at least partially, with activation of the α-secretase TACE/ADAM17 [69]. The use of CA may have potential in the prevention of amyloid β-mediated diseases. Furthermore, in GBM glioblastoma cells, CA promoted apoptosis by inducing cell cycle arrest and degradation of cyclin B1, RB, SOx2 and GFAP, molecules involved in cell survival and maturation processes [70].

**Table 10.** Anticancer effects of Carnosic Acid (CA). In vitro studies: brain and neural cancer.

| Cell Type | Dose/Duration | Findings | Mechanism | Reference |
|---|---|---|---|---|
| T98G (Glioblastoma) | 5–100 μM CA (0–48 h) | | ↑ NGF synthesis | [64] |
| T98G (Glioblastoma) | 2–50 μM CA (24 h) | | ↑ NGF synthesis<br>↑ Nrf2, HO-1, TXNRD1 | [65] |
| IMR-32 (Neuroblastoma) | 5–40 μM CA (0–48 h) | ↓ cell viability<br>↑ apoptosis<br>↑ ROS generation | ↑ casp 3, casp 9, PARP, p-p38<br>↓ p-ERK | [66] |
| U373MG (Glioblastoma) | 50 μM CA (8 h) | ↓ amyloid beta peptide release | ↑ α-secretase<br>TACE/ADAM17 | [69] |
| SH-SY5Y (Neuroblastoma) | 1 μM CA (12 h) | ↑ antioxidant defense<br>↑ detoxification systems<br>Blocked activation of apoptosis | ↑ PI3K/Akt<br>↓ cytochrome c release<br>↓ caspase cascade | [67] |
| SH-SY5Y (Neuroblastoma) | 10 μM CA (1 h) | ↓ apoptosis | ↓ caspase cascade | [68] |
| GBM (Glioblastoma) | 17.5–40 μM CA (48 h) | ↓ cell survival<br>↑ cell cycle arrest<br>↑ apoptosis | ↓ CDK activity<br>↓ cyclin B1<br>↓ RB<br>↓ SOX2<br>↓ GFAP | [70] |

NGF (nerve growth factor), Nrf2 (nuclear factor E2-related factor 2), HO-1 (heme oxygenase-1), TXNRD1 (thioredoxin reductase 1), casp (caspase), PARP (poly(ADP-ribose)polymerase), p-ERK (phosphorylated extracellular signal-regulated kinases), TACE (TNF-α converting enzyme), ADAM17 (ADAM metallopeptidase domain 17), PI3K (phosphatidylinositol-4,5-bisphosphate 3-kinase), Akt (protein kinase B), cyt c (cytochrome c), CDK (cyclin dependent kinase), RB (retinoblastoma), SOX2 (sex determining region Y-box 2), GFAP (glial fibrillary acidic protein).

Leukemia is a cancer that usually develops in the bone marrow and results in a high number of white blood cells that are not fully developed being released into the bloodstream. Most treatment options for leukemia involve agents that promote the differentiation of these immature white blood cells into mature, differentiated cells. Unfortunately, there are many side effects associated with higher doses of these differentiating agents and strategies are required to lower the dose necessary to see anticancer effects. One such agent which is used is 1α25-dihydroxyviatmin D (1,25D). Many studies have found that low doses of CA (5–10 µM) are able to potentiate the pro-differentiation effects of 1,25D and help sensitize leukemia cells including human HL-60, U937, MOLM-13 and mouse WEHI-3B cells [40,41,71–78] to its anticancer effects (Table 11). Furthermore, CA inhibited cell viability and induced apoptosis and cell cycle arrest in these cells using a multitude of different strategies. In HL-60 cells, CA enhanced expression of the vitamin D and retinoic acid receptors thus, enhancing the sensitivity of cells to 1,25D [71], and enhanced expression of cell cycle regulators p21$^{Waf1}$, p27$^{Kip1}$ which may have tumor suppressor functions [72]. Carnosic acid also increased levels of the antioxidant GSH and phase II enzyme NADP(H)-quinone reductase which help protect cells from chemically-induced carcinogenesis, and enhanced signaling through MAPK pathways including ERK and JNK which are involved in the proliferation and differentiation of cells [40,73–75,79]. In K562 leukemia cells CA inhibited cell viability and sensitized resistant cells to adriamycin, a chemotherapeutic agent [30,80]. Similarly, CA enhanced the activity of doxercaliferol, an agent which helps prevent the common problem of calcification associated with administration of vitamin D derivatives such as 1,25D, and decreased levels of microRNA181a which are linked to cell proliferation [81]. Antioxidant effects were also produced by CA in U937, HL-60 and NB4 leukemic cells which exhibited increased GSH and NADPH levels and CA ameliorated arsenic trioxide-induced cytotoxic effects [79]. Activation of the Nrf2/ARE signalling pathway which can alter cell survival was also seen [77,79]. The authors suggest that the Nrf2/ARE pathway likely plays an important role in the cooperative induction of leukemia cell differentiation by 1,25D and CA [77]. Importantly, in HL-60 cells CA increased PTEN expression and caspase cleavage and inhibited phosphorylation of Bad and Akt which are associated with enhanced apoptosis [62,82]. The strong inhibitory effects of CA on the PTEN/Akt survival pathway make it a good candidate to be combined with other therapies for leukemia treatment.

**Table 11.** Anticancer effects of Carnosic Acid (CA). In vitro studies: leukemia.

| Cell Type | Dose/Duration | Findings | Mechanism | Reference |
|---|---|---|---|---|
| HL-60 (Myeloid leukemia) | 10 µM CA (0–48 h) | CA potentiated effects of 1,25D ↑ differentiation ↓ proliferation ↑ cell cycle arrest | ↑ vitamin D receptor, retinoic acid receptor | [71] |
| HL-60 (Myeloid leukemia), U937 (Myeloid leukemia) | 2.5–10 µM CA (0–48 h) | CA potentiated effects of 1,25D ↑ differentiation ↓ proliferation ↑ cell cycle arrest IC50 6–7µM | ↑ p21$^{Waf1}$, p27$^{Kip1}$ | [72] |
| HL-60-G (Myeloid leukemia) | 10 µM CA (0–48 h) | CA potentiated effects of 1,25D ↑ differentiation ↓ ROS | ↑ GSH ↑ Raf/MAPK/ERK, AP-1 | [73] |
| HL-60 (Myeloid leukemia) | 10 µM CA (0–72 h) | CA potentiated effects of 1,25D ↑ differentiation | ↑ JNK pathway | [74] |
| WEHI-3B (Murine myeloid leukemia), HL-60 (Myeloid leukemia), U937 (Myeloid leukemia) | 10 µM CA (0–96 h) | CA potentiated effects of 1,25D ↑ differentiation ↓ proliferation ↑ cell cycle arrest | | [41] |
| WEHI-3B D (Murine myeloid leukemia) | 10 µM CA (48–96 h) | CA potentiated effects of 1,25D ↑ cell differentiation ↓ cell viability ↓ cell proliferation | ↓ ROS ↑ NADP(H)-quinone reductase | [40] |
| K562 (Myeloid leukemia) | 2.5–50 µM CA (24–72 h) | ↓ cell viability CA sensitized resistant cells to Adriamycin | | [80] |

Table 11. *Cont.*

| Cell Type | Dose/Duration | Findings | Mechanism | Reference |
|---|---|---|---|---|
| HL-60G (Myeloid leukemia), HL-60-40AF (Myeloid leukemia) | 10 μM CA (0–48 h) | CA potentiated effects of 1,25-D ↑ differentiation | ↑ JNK1, c-jun-ATF2, C/EBP | [75] |
| K-562 (Myeloid leukemia) | 6.25–50 μg/mL (18.8– μM) CA (48 h) | ↓ cell viability | | [30] |
| U937 (Myeloid leukemia) | 10 μM CA (96 h) | CA potentiated effects of 1,25-D ↑ differentiation | ↑ Nrf2, ARE, NADPH, | [77] |
| HL-60 (Myeloid leukemia), U937 (Myeloid leukemia) | 10 μM CA (48 h) | Enhances activity of 1,25D ↑ cell cycle arrest Induces differentiation Sensitizes 1,25D resistant cells | ↑ HPK1 | [76] |
| HL-60 (Myeloid leukemia), U937 | 10 μM CA (48 h) | Enhances activity of doxercalciferol ↑ cell cycle arrest Induces differentiation | ↓ microRNA181a | [81] |
| HL-60 (Myeloid leukemia) | 5–25 μM CA (24–72 h) | ↓ viability ↑ apoptosis ↑ cell cycle arrest | ↑ p27, cleaved casp 9, PTEN expression ↓ p-BAD, p-Akt | [82] |
| HL-60 (Myeloid leukemia) | 25–100 μM CA (4–72 h) | ↓ cell survival ↑ apoptosis ↑ cell cycle arrest IC50 5.9 μM | ↑ casp 3 | [62] |
| HL-60 (Myeloid leukemia), U937 (Myeloid leukemia), MOLM-13 (Acute monocytic leukemia) | 10 μM CA (96 h) | CA potentiated effects of 1,25-D ↑ differentiation | | [78] |
| NB4 (Human promyelocytic leukemia) | 5 μM CA (24 h) | Ameliorates arsenic trioxide-induced cytotoxic effects | ↑ GSH levels Activation of Nrf2 | [79] |

1,25-D (1α25-dihydroxyviatminD), GSH (glutathione), Raf (rapidly accelerated fibrosarcoma), MAPK (mitogen-activated protein kinase), ERK (extracellular signal-regulated kinases), AP-1 (activator protein 1), JNK (c-jun N-terminal kinases), ROS (reactive oxygen species), c-jun (v-jun sarcoma virus 17 oncogene), ATF2 (activating transcription factor 2), Nrf2 (nuclear factor E2-regulated factor-2), ARE (antioxidant response element), HPK1 (hematopoietic progenitor kinase 1), casp (caspase), PTEN (phosphatase and tensin homolog).

## 7. Anticancer Effects of Carnosic Acid (CA): In Vivo Animal Studies

The above studies in vitro provide strong evidence for the anticancer effects if CA in various cancer cell lines. Several studies using animal models have also explored the effects of CA in vivo and found significant anticancer effects which supports future research exploring the anticancer mechanisms of CA in both animal and human models (Table 12). In DMBA-induced models of oral cancer using hamsters, it was shown that using 10 mg/kg/day CA administered orally for 14 weeks, caused the number of tumors on the animals to significantly decrease. Furthermore, expression of detoxification enzymes was enhanced [83], markers of apoptosis including p53, Bax, Bcl-2 and caspases were increased [84], and regulators of cell growth including COX-2, c-fos, KF-κB and cyclin D1 were decreased [84]. Using the same hamster model, 750 μg CA dissolved in 0.1mL saline (20 μM) administered daily for 11 weeks significantly slowed the progression of lesions and oral cancer development [85]. In mice xenografted with prostate samples from human biopsies, 100 mg CA dissolved in 100 μL of cottonseed oil administered daily for 25 days decreased tumor growth [86]. Azoxymethane was used to induce colon cancer in mice and 0.01%–0.02% CA fed with a high fat (45%) diet for 11 weeks decreased both tumor size and number of tumors, and modulated signaling molecules involved in cell metabolism and cell growth [52]. Serum samples taken from the mice after treatment showed decreased levels of insulin, leptin and IGF-1 and analysis of tissue samples showed a decrease in the associated insulin and leptin receptors, as well as decreased activity of ERK and expression of cyclin D1 and Bcl-xL which regulate cell survival [52]. In K562 leukemia inoculated mice fed 1% CA with standard powder diet, there was a decrease in the number of leukemic cells which was partially attributed to enhanced apoptosis [87]. Furthermore, survival time of the animals increased significantly [87]. Overall, CA shows significant anticancer effects in mouse and hamster models of several types of cancer and this evidence provide support of its potential to be used against cancer in humans.

**Table 12.** Anticancer effects of Carnosic Acid (CA). In vivo studies.

| Animal Model | Dose/Duration | Findings | Mechanism | Reference |
|---|---|---|---|---|
| DMBA-induced oral cancer-hamster | 10 mg/kg/day CA (14 weeks) | ↓ # of tumors Anti-lipid peroxidative function ↑ detoxification enzymes | | [83] |
| DMBA-induced oral cancer-hamster | 10 mg/kg/day CA orally for (14 weeks) | ↓ # of tumors | ↑ p53, Bax, Bcl-2, casp 3, casp 9 ↓ COX-2, c-fos, NF-κB, cyclin D1 | [84] |
| Human prostate biopsies xenografted into mice | 100 mg/mouse dissolved in 100 μL cottonseed oil daily (25 days) | ↓ tumor growth | | [86] |
| DMBA-induced oral cancer-hamster | 750 μg CA dissolved in 0.1 mL saline (20 μM) daily for (11 weeks) | ↓ progression of cancer and development of lesions | | [85] |
| AOM-induced colon cancer-mice | 0.01%–0.02% CA fed with a high fat (45%) diet for (11 weeks) | ↓ # of tumors ↓ tumor size | ↓ insulin, leptin and IGF-1 serum levels compared to mice fed HFD alone ↓ insulin receptor, leptin receptor, p-ERK, cyclin D1, Bcl-xL expression | [52] |
| K562 leukemia inoculated mouse | 1% (*v/v*) CA with standard powdered rodent diet *Ad libitum* | ↓ # of leukemia cells ↑ apoptotic cells ↑ survival time | | [87] |

Bax (Bcl-2-like protein 4), Bcl-2 (B-cell CLL/lymphoma 2), casp (caspase), COX2 (cyclooxygenase 2), NF-κB (nuclear factor kappa B), IGF-1 (insulin-like growth factor 1), HFD (high fat diet), p-ERK (phosphorylated extracellular signal-regulated kinase), Bcl-xL (B-cell lymphoma-extra large), # (number).

## 8. Anticancer Effects of Rosmarinic Acid (RA): In Vitro Studies

Treatment of HT29 colon cancer cells with RA (5–20 μM) lead to a reduction in COX2 promoter activity and COX2 protein levels [88] (Table 13). In HCT15 and CO115 colon cancer cells, RA (10–100 μM) induced apoptosis and decreased levels of phosphorylated-ERK which regulates cell proliferation [89]. Rosmarinic acid (55–832.6 μM) decreased ROS levels which was associated with decreased migration and adhesion rates in Ls174-T colon cells [90]. Furthermore, treatment of CO115 cells with RA (50 μM) protected against BCNU-induced DNA damage, suggesting potential chemopreventive effects [91]. Treatment of MCF-7 and MDA-MB-231 breast cancer cells with RA (0–300 μM) decreased cell viability [30,92–94] (Table 13). Rosmarinic acid decreased methyltransferase activity, which inhibits hyper-methylation of DNA, associated with disease [93], and sensitized a resistant cell line (MCF-7/Adr) to the chemotherapeutic agent Adriamycin [94].

In DU145 and PC3 prostate cancer cells RA (17.3–138.8 μM) decreased cell viability [30] and in A2780 and A2790CP70 ovarian cancer cells RA (6.9–27.8 μM) lead to a reduction in cell proliferation and increased the sensitivity of cisplatin-resistant cells [34] (Table 13). In SGC7901/Adr gastric cancer cells, RA (0.096–60 μM) was found to decrease cell viability, drug resistance, expression and activity of p-glycoprotein [95]. Furthermore, treatment of MKN45 gastric cancer cells with RA (200–300 μM) lead to a decrease in cell viability, the Warburg effect/glucose uptake and pro-inflammatory cytokines [96]. In B16 melanoma cells, RA (1–100 μM) was found to increase melanin content, tyrosinase expression and CREB phosphorylation [97].

**Table 13.** Anticancer effects of Rosmarinic Acid (RA). In vitro studies: colon, breast, prostate, ovarian, gastric and skin cancer.

| Cell Type | Dose and Duration | Findings | Mechanisms | Reference |
|---|---|---|---|---|
| HT-29 (Colorectal adenocarcinoma) | 5–20 μM RA (1 h) | ↓ TPA induced COX2 promoter activity | ↓ COX2 protein levels | [88] |
| HCT15 (Colorectal adenocarcinoma), CO115 (Colorectal carcinoma) | 10–100 μM RA (48 h) | ↑ apoptosis of HCT15 (50 μM) and CO115 (100 μM) | ↓ p-ERK levels in HCT15 cells | [89] |
| Ls174-T (Colorectal adenocarcinoma) | 20–300 μg/mL (55.5–832.6 μM) RA (24 h) | ↓ migration rate ↓ adhesion IC50 70 μg/mL | ↓ ROS | [90] |
| CO115 (Colorectal carcinoma) | 50 μM RA (24 h) | ↓ BCNU-induced DNA damage | | [91] |
| MCF-7 (Breast adenocarcinoma) | 60 μM RA (24 h) | ↓ cell viability | | [92] |
| MCF7 (Breast adenocarcinoma) | 2–200 μM RA (72 h) | ↓ DNA methyltransferase activity | | [93] |
| MCF-7 (ER+) (Breast adenocarcinoma), MDA-MB-231 (Breast adenocarcinoma) | 6.25–50 μg/mL (17.3–138.8 μM) RA (48 h) | ↓ cell viability | | [30] |
| MCF-7/Adr (Breast adenocarcinoma), MCF-7/wt (Breast adenocarcinoma) | 0.08–10 mM RA EC values 0.74 mM (in wt) and 0.81 mM (in Adr resistant) | 0.08–0.32 mM RA effective ↑ cytotoxicity to MCF-7 cells | | [94] |
| DU145 (Prostate carcinoma), PC3 (Prostate adenocarcinoma) | 6.25–50 μg/mL (17.3–138.8 μM) RA (48h) | ↓ cell viability | | [30] |
| A2780 (Ovarian carcinoma), A2780CP70 (Ovarian carcinoma) | 2.5–10 μg/mL (6.9–27.8 μM) RA (48 h) | ↓ cell proliferation Enhanced sensitivity of cisplatin-resistant cells | | [34] |
| SGC7901/Adr (Gastric carcinoma) | 0.096–60 μM RA (48 h) | ↓ cell viability Reversed drug resistance | ↓ expression of p-glycoprotein ↓ activity of p-glycoprotein | [95] |
| MKN45 (Gastric carcinoma) | 200–300 μM RA | ↓ cell viability ↓ Warburg effect | ↓ glucose uptake ↓ pro-inflammatory cytokines (IL-6 and STAT3) | [96] |
| B16 (Skin melanoma) | 1–100 μM RA (48 h) | ↑ melanin content ↑ tyrosinase expression | ↑ phosphorylation of CREB | [97] |

TPA (12-*O*-tetradecanoylphorbol-13-acetate), COX2 (cyclooxygenase 2), ERK (extracellular signal-regulated kinases), ROS (reactive oxygen species), BCNU (1,3-*bis*-(2-chloroethyl)-1-nitosourea), IL-6 (interleukin-6), STAT3 (signal transducer and activator of transcription 3) CREB (cAMP response element-binding protein) wt (wild type), Adr (Adriamycin).

Treatment of HepG2 liver cancer cells with RA (25–250 μM) decreased ochratoxin and aflatoxin-mediated cell damage, apoptosis, ROS levels and caspase 3 activation [98] (Table 14), suggesting that RA can exert protective effects and prevent cytotoxicity induced by toxic agents. Alternatively, in HepG2 cells without the presence of cytotoxic agents, RA (13.9 and 27.8 μM) lead to an increase in apoptosis, which was associated with an increase in caspase 8, NFBIA, TNFSF9 and Jun mRNA and a decrease in Bcl-2 mRNA levels [99]. Thus, RA has several potential anticancer mechanisms in liver cells. In Hep-3B liver cancer cells, RA (17.3–138.8 μM) was found to decrease cell viability [30], while treatment of HepG2 liver cancer cells with RA (20–80 μM) showed no significant changes to cell viability but an increase in Nrf2 nuclear translocation, ARE-luciferin activity, MRP2 levels, intracellular ATP levels and efflux of p-glycoprotein was seen [100]. In NCI-H82 and A549 lung cancer cells RA (10–500 μM) decreased cell growth [30,101] which was associated with decreased hCOX2 activity, suggesting an anti-inflammatory role of RA [101].

**Table 14.** Anticancer effects of Rosmarinic Acid (RA). In vitro studies: liver and lung cancer.

| Cell Type | Dose and Duration | Findings | Mechanisms | Reference |
|---|---|---|---|---|
| HepG2 (Hepatocellular carcinoma) | 25–250 µM RA (24 h) | ↓ OTA- and AFB-induced cell damage and apoptosis ↓ DNA and protein synthesis inhibition induced by OTA- and AFB- | ↓ ROS production ↓ capase-3 activation | [98] |
| HepG2 (Hepatocellular carcinoma) | 5–10 µg/mL (13.9–27.8 µM) RA (72 h) | ↑ apoptosis | ↑ casp 8, NFBIA, TNFSF9 and Jun mRNA ↓ Bcl-2 mRNA expression | [99] |
| HepG2 (Hepatocellular carcinoma) | 60 µM RA (24 h) | ↓ cell viability | | [92] |
| Hep-3B (Hepatocellular carcinoma) | 6.25–50 µg/mL (17.3–138.8 µM) RA (48 h) | ↓ cell viability | | [30] |
| HepG2 (Hepatocellular carcinoma) | 20–80 µM RA (24 h or 4 days) | ↔ cell viability | ↑ translocation of Nrf2 ↑ ARE-luciferin activity ↑ efflux of p-glycoprotein ↑ MRP2 ↑ intracellular ATP | [100] |
| NCI-H82 (Lung carcinoma; SCLC) | 6.25–50 µg/mL (17.3–138.8 µM) RA (48 h) | ↓ cell viability | | [30] |
| A549 (Lung adenocarcinoma) | 10–500 µM RA (48 h) IC50 198.12 | ↓ cell proliferation | ↓ hCOX2 activity | [101] |

OTA (ochratoxin), AFB (Aflatoxin), ROS (reactive oxygen species), casp (caspase), NFBIA (nuclear factor of kappa light polypeptide gene enhancer in B-cells inhibitor-alpha), TNFSF9 (tumor necrosis factor ligand superfamily-member 9), Jun (v-jun sarcoma virus 17 oncogene), Bcl-2 (B-cell CLL/lymphoma 2), Nrf2 (nuclear factor E2-related factor-2), ARE (antioxidant response element), MRP2 (multidrug resistance-associated protein 2), ATP (adenosine triphosphate), hCOX2 (human cyclooxygenase 2).

Treatment of K562 leukemia cells with RA inhibited cell viability [30] and reversed the induction of hyperosmosis-induced apoptosis and associated ROS/RNS production [102] (Table 15). In U937 leukemia cells, RA (60 µM) enhanced TNF-α induced apoptosis and decreased TNF-α induced-NF-κB activation and ROS production [92]. Surprisingly AKT1 and ERK2 levels, which regulate cell survival, were not affected by RA treatment in U937 or K562 cells [42]. Rosmarinic acid (40 µM) increased macrophage differentiation induced by ATRA which was mediated by an increase in CD11b expression on the cell surface [103]. In HL-60 leukemia cells, RA (50–150 µM) inhibited cell growth and induced apoptosis, which was associated with decreased dNTP levels [104]. CCRF-CEM, CEM/ADR5000 leukemia cells treated with RA (3–100 µM) developed increased cytotoxicity, apoptosis, necrosis, cell cycle arrest and caspase-independent apoptosis which was mediated by increased PARP cleavage and blockage of p65 nuclear translocation [105]. In agreement with other studies, RA (0.07–2.2 mM) exerted DNA protective and anti-carcinogenic effects in HL-60 leukemia cells [106].

**Table 15.** Anticancer effects of Rosmarinic Acid (RA). In vitro studies: leukemia.

| Cell Type | Dose and Duration | Findings | Mechanisms | Reference |
|---|---|---|---|---|
| K562 (Myeloid leukemia) | 25 µM RA (1 h) | ↓ hyperosmotic-mediated ROS/RNS production and apoptosis | | [102] |
| U937 (Myeloid leukemia) | 60 µM RA (24 h) | ↑ TNF-α induced apoptosis | ↓ NF-κB activation ↓ ROS production ↑ caspases | [92] |
| K562 (Myeloid leukemia) | 6.25–50 µg/mL (17.3–138.8 µM) (48 h) | ↓ cell viability | | [30] |
| K562 (Myeloid leukemia), U937 (Myeloid leukemia) | 0.2 mM RA (48 h) | Not tested on proliferation | ↔ AKT1 ↔ ERK2 | [42] |
| NB4 (Human promyelocytic leukemia) | 40 µM RA (72 h) | ↑ ATRA-induced macrophage differentiation | ↑ expression of CD11b | [103] |

**Table 15.** *Cont.*

| Cell Type | Dose and Duration | Findings | Mechanisms | Reference |
|---|---|---|---|---|
| HL-60 (Myeloid leukemia) | 50–150 μM RA (24–72 h) | ↓ cell growth<br>↑ apoptosis<br>IC50 147 μM (24 h), 74 μM (48 h), 69 μM (72 h) | ↓ dNTP levels | [104] |
| CCRF-CEM (Lymphoblastic leukemia), CEM/ADR5000 (Lymphoblastic leukemia) | 3–100 μM RA (72 h) | ↑ cytotoxicity<br>↑ apoptosis and necrosis<br>↑ cell cycle arrest<br>↑ caspase-independent apoptosis | ↑ PARP-cleavage Blocked p65 nuclear translocation from the cytosol | [105] |
| HL-60 (Myeloid leukemia) | 0.07–2.2 mM RA (72 h) | DNA protection and anticarcinogenic effects | | [106] |

ROS (reactive oxygen species), RNS (reactive nitrogen species), TNF-α (tumor necrosis factor-alpha), NF-κB (nuclear factor kappa-light-chain-enhancer of activated B cells), Akt (protein kinase B), ERK (extracellular signal-regulated kinases), ATRA (all-*trans* retinoic acid), dNTP (deoxy-nucleoside triphosphate), PARP (poly(ADP-ribose) polymerase).

## 9. Anticancer Effects of Rosmarinic Acid (RA): In Vivo Animal Studies

Apart from the in vitro studies using different cancer cell lines, several studies using RA in animal cancer models have been performed. Administration of 0.25–1.35 mg of RA (30 min) prior to TPA treatment was found to decrease myeloperoxidase activity and COX2 induction in mice [107] (Table 16). Using 1–4 mg/kg RA (20 days) in Lewis lung carcinoma xenografted mice lead to decreased tumor growth [90] and 100 mg/kg RA (14 weeks) reduced DMBA-induced tumor formation in the buccal pouches of hamsters [108]. Administration of 360 mg/kg RA from weeks 4 to 12 of the animal's life decreased the frequency of large adenomas in mice [109]. Rats given 2.5–10 mg/kg RA for 16 weeks, showed a decrease in development of DMH-induced aberrant crypt foci by decreasing DMH-induced elevation of bacterial enzymes [110]. Administration of 100 mg/kg RA 1 week before DMBA treatment in mice decreased skin tumors by increasing the levels of phase I (cyt p450) and phase II (GST, GR, GSH) detoxification agents and restoring levels of caspase 3, caspase 9, p53 and Bcl-2 [111]. Venkatachalam, et al. found that 2.5, 5 and 10 mg/kg RA given to rats for 4 weeks, decreased DMH-induced colon tumor formation, number of polyps, antioxidant status, CYP450 content, PNPH activity and reversed the markers of oxidative stress [112]. Hamsters given 1.3 mg/mL RA for 2 weeks were found to have a decreased incidence of tumors induced by DMBA, decreased tumor grade scoring and increased tumor differentiation [113]. Rosmarinic acid administered at 2 mg/kg for 14 days to mice had an anti-Warburg effect, mediated through decreased glucose uptake [96]. Furthermore, administration of 5 mg/kg RA for 30 weeks was found to decrease DMH-induced colon tumor formation in rats through decreased TNF-α, IL-6 and COX2 levels [110]. Taken together, these studies provide evidence for RA's anticancer effects in animal models and suggest several mechanisms which may be responsible for the inhibition of tumor growth and progression.

**Table 16.** Anticancer effects of Rosmarinic Acid (RA). In vivo studies.

| Animal Model | Dose and Duration | Findings | Mechanisms | Reference |
|---|---|---|---|---|
| Seven-Nine week old male Balb/c mice | 0.25, 0.5, 1.0 and 1.35 mg/mouse (30 months) before TPA treatment | ↓ myeloperoxidase activity | ↓ COX2 induction | [107] |
| C57BL/6 mice implanted with Lewis lung carcinoma | 1, 2 and 4 mg/kg RA (20 days) | ↓ tumor growth | | [90] |
| Golden Syrian hamsters | 100 mg/kg RA (14 weeks) | Completely prevented tumor formation in DMBA-treated hamsters | ↓ p53<br>↓ Bcl-2 | [108] |
| C57BL/6J Min/+ (Apc$^{Min}$) mice | 360 mg/kg RA (8 weeks) | ↓ the frequency of large adenomas | ↑ levels of parent compound in plasma | [109] |

**Table 16.** *Cont.*

| Animal Model | Dose and Duration | Findings | Mechanisms | Reference |
|---|---|---|---|---|
| DMH induced colon cancer (Albino Wistar male rats) | 2.5–10 mg/kg RA (16 weeks) through intragastric intubation | ↓ DMH induced aberrant crypt foci | ↓ DMH induced increase in bacterial enzymes | [110] |
| DMBA induced skin cancer (Swiss albino mice) | 100 mg/kg RA administered (1 weeks) before DMBA treatment | ↓ skin tumors | ↑ status of phase I (cyt p450) detoxification agents ↑ status of phase II (GST, GR, GSH) detoxification agents. Restored activity levels of casp 3, casp 9, p53 and Bcl-2. | [111] |
| DMH induced colon cancer (Male Wistar rats) | 2.5, 5 and 10 mg/kg RA (4 weeks) | ↓ DMH induced aberrant crypt foci, number of polyps, reversed the markers of oxidative stress, antioxidant status, CYP450 content and PNPH activity | | [112] |
| Five month old Syrian hamsters | 1.3 mg/mL RA (2 weeks) pretreatment | ↓ incidence of tumors ↑ differentiation ↓ scores in the tumor invasion front grading system. | | [113] |
| 5 week old male nude Balb/c mice incubated sub-cutaneously with MKN45 cells into their flanks. | 2 mg/kg RA via celiac injection daily (14 days) | ↓ Warburg effect | ↓ glucose uptake | [114] |
| DMH induced colon cancer (Male Wistar rats) | 5 mg/kg RA orally (30 weeks) | ↓ DMH induced colon tumor formation | ↓ TNF-α ↓ IL-6 ↓ COX2 | [96] |

TPA (12-*O*-tetradecanoylpheorbol-13-acetate), COX2 (cyclooxygenase 2), DMBA (7,12-dimethylbenz(a)anthracene), DMH (1,2-dimethylhydrazine), p53 (tumor protein p53), casp (caspase), Bcl-2 (B-cell CLL/lymphoma 2), CYP450 (cytochrome p450), GST (Glutathione *S*-transferase), GR (glucocorticoid receptor), GSH (glutathione), PNPH (p-nitrophenol hydroxylase), TNF-α (tumor necrosis factor alpha), IL-6 (interleukin-6).

## 10. Dosage and Bioavailability

The effects of RE have been studied in many cancer cell lines and although the concentrations used in the in vitro studies are variable (0.1–500 μg/mL) it appears that the concentrations in the range of 0.1–100 μg/mL are most effective. Similar to in vitro studies, the reported doses of RE used in vivo are within a wide range (1 mg/mL drinking water −3333.3 mg/kg/day). This high variability suggests the need for more systematic studies to identify effective RE doses in vivo. One study has examined the levels of RE components in the plasma and tissue samples of animals administered with RE. Administration of a single dose of RE (100 mg/mL water) enriched in CA (40% *w/w*) by intragastric gavage in rats was followed by measurements of RE compounds and metabolites in plasma, liver, small intestine content and brain. The researchers tentatively identified 26 compounds and the main metabolites detected in plasma, liver and gut were glucuronide conjugates of CA, carnosol and rosmanol [115]. Metabolites were detected as early as 25 min after oral administration and most of the compounds remained present at substantial concentrations (micromolar range) for several hours [115]. Doolaege, et al. reported that 64.3 mg/kg (193.43 mM) CA orally administered to rats resulted in a plasma concentration of 0.015 mg/mL (45.12 μM) [116]. Another study reported that ingestion of 360 mg/kg/day RA after 8 weeks resulted in a plasma concentration of 1.1 μM [117]. The reported plasma concentrations of CA, carnosol and their metabolites were in the micromolar range indicating that absorption and bioavailability are likely not barriers for these components of RE [114,115,118].

Another important issue that must be systematically examined in well-designed studies are the potential toxicity of chronic administration of RE and RE polyphenols. Rosemary extract has already been approved as a safe food additive by the European Food and Safety Authority (EFSA) [119] and is considered to be generally recognized as safe by the United States Food and Drug Administration (FDA) (21CFR182.10). In a study reviewed by the EFSA, rosemary was found to have low acute and sub-chronic toxicity in rats and the only effect at high doses was a slight increase in relative liver weight, which has been shown to be reversible. Overall, 90 day RE administration (180–400 mg/kg/day, equivalent to 20–60 mg/kg/day of carnosol plus CA) in rats revealed no observed adverse effect levels (NOAEL) (reviewed in [119]). Furthermore, an acute single dose of 24 and 28.5 g/kg RE to female and male mice respectively or the daily administration of 11.8 and 14.1 g/kg to female and male mice respectively for 5 days resulted in no gross macroscopic lesions observed on autopsy besides fatty liver in mice subjected to repeat administration of the extract indicating low acute toxicity (reviewed in [119]). In another study, it was reported that an LD50 of 169.9 mg/kg/day RA was found in mice implanted with Lewis lung carcinoma cells [90]. One study performed in humans used a powdered RE mixed with citrus extract (1:1 ratio) (Nutroxsun™) which was consumed daily (250 mg) for 3 months. Results showed a protective effect against UV-induced skin damage. Significant results were seen after 8 weeks and continued to increase after 85 days of treatment [120]. Overall, the limited in vivo studies report doses of RE or RE components that are relatively high and showed minimal to no adverse effects, indicating low toxicity. Nonetheless, further research should be performed to confirm maximum recommended doses of RE and RE components.

In humans, to achieve RE polyphenol levels that will provide health benefits high intake of rosemary would be required, which is not practical. A more reasonable direction for the potential future use of RE and its polyphenols as anticancer agents would be to develop easily ingestible and soluble pills containing RE or RE components. Overall, the studies available currently suggest that RE and its polyphenols CA and RA are good candidates for drug development and further research examining the effective doses in animals is required before any clinical studies in humans are initiated. In addition, systematic studies in animals to examine if chronic administration results in any toxicity are required before clinical human studies.

It should be noted that in recent years, scientists have recognized that the gut microbiota plays an important role in overall health and disease prevention. Although certain plant bioactive compounds may be poorly bioavailable, the gut bacteria may generate metabolites that are more potent than the parent compounds. A recent study found that administration of RE rich in CA (40% *w/w*) in rats had a selective effect on caecum microbiota (increased the Blautia coccoides and Bacteroides/Prevotella groups and reduced the Lactobacillus/Leuconostoc/Pediococccus group), decreased β-glucosidase activity and increased fiber fecal elimination [121]. These data are associated with the decreased body weight and the improvement of the metabolic and inflammatory status seen with RE [121]. Although the above study suggests a potential prebiotic effect of RE administration against metabolic disorders and obesity, there are no studies specifically examining the effect of gut microbiota on RE metabolites.

## 11. Conclusions

It should be noted that the levels of polyphenols and bioactive compounds present in RE may be affected by many factors such as the plant growing conditions (soil, climate, exposure to stressors). Additionally, the extraction method and storage of RE may affect its potency. Water, methanol, ethanol and supercritical carbon dioxide extraction are methods which have been used in different studies and evidence suggests that methanol (alcoholic-solvent) extraction may lead to RE with higher potency (lower IC50) [31]. Since the source and extraction method of RE may affect its potency/biological activity, this issue should be taken into consideration when future studies are planned.

In recent years, focus has shifted towards establishing new targeted cancer treatments that can modulate specific pathways often mutated in cancer. RE and its polyphenols CA and RA may be used as chemicals to target specific pathways leading to induction of apoptosis and decreased cell survival. In addition, RE, CA and RA may be used as neutraceuticals to enhance the anticancer effects of current chemotherapeutics. This could allow for lower doses to be used and less toxicity induced in healthy surrounding tissue. Although studies examining signalling molecules and pathways targeted by RE, CA and RA are limited, the existing studies provide supporting evidence for the use of these compounds both on their own and in combination with other cancer therapies.

Overall, RE, CA and RA have been shown to have various potent and effective anticancer properties. However, more systematic studies are required in animals before human studies are initiated. The in vivo animal studies should find (1) the doses to be administered; (2) the best route of administration; (3) the plasma levels of CA, RA and other RE bioactive ingredients; (4) the signaling molecules/pathways affected; and (5) any possible toxic effects associated with chronic administration.

**Acknowledgments:** This work was supported in part by a Brock University Advancement Fund (BUAF) grant to E.T.

**Author Contributions:** J.M. and E.T. formulated the review topic, wrote the manuscript and reviewed the manuscript. M.Y. contributed to writing and reviewing the manuscript. All authors read and approved the final manuscript.

**Conflicts of Interest:** The authors declare no conflict of interest.

## References

1. Hanahan, D.; Weinberg, R.A. Hallmarks of Cancer: The Next Generation. *Cell* **2011**, *144*, 646–674. [CrossRef] [PubMed]
2. Bhowmick, N.A.; Neilson, E.G.; Moses, H.L. Stromal fibroblasts in cancer initiation and progression. *Nature* **2004**, *432*, 332–337. [CrossRef] [PubMed]
3. Cheng, N.; Chytil, A.; Shyr, Y.; Joly, A.; Moses, H.L. Transforming Growth Factor-β Signaling-Deficient Fibroblasts Enhance Hepatocyte Growth Factor Signaling in Mammary Carcinoma Cells to Promote Scattering and Invasion. *Mol. Cancer Res.* **2008**, *6*, 1521–1533. [CrossRef] [PubMed]
4. Da Rocha, A.B.; Lopes, R.M.; Schwartsmann, G. Natural products in anticancer therapy. *Curr. Opin. Pharmacol.* **2001**, *1*, 364–369. [CrossRef]
5. Storozhuk, Y.; Hopmans, S.N.; Sanli, T.; Barron, C.; Tsiani, E.; Cutz, J.-C.; Pond, G.; Wright, J.; Singh, G.; Tsakiridis, T. Metformin inhibits growth and enhances radiation response of non-small cell lung cancer (NSCLC) through ATM and AMPK. *Br. J. Cancer* **2013**, *108*, 2021–2032. [CrossRef] [PubMed]
6. Bai, Y.; Mao, Q.-Q.; Qin, J.; Zheng, X.-Y.; Wang, Y.-B.; Yang, K.; Shen, H.-F.; Xie, L.-P. Resveratrol induces apoptosis and cell cycle arrest of human T24 bladder cancer cells in vitro and inhibits tumor growth in vivo. *Cancer Sci.* **2010**, *101*, 488–493. [CrossRef] [PubMed]
7. Rashid, A.; Liu, C.; Sanli, T.; Tsiani, E.; Singh, G.; Bristow, R.G.; Dayes, I.; Lukka, H.; Wright, J.; Tsakiridis, T. Resveratrol enhances prostate cancer cell response to ionizing radiation. Modulation of the AMPK, Akt and mTOR pathways. *Radiat. Oncol.* **2011**, *6*, 144. [CrossRef] [PubMed]
8. Varoni, E.M.; Lo Faro, A.F.; Sharifi-Rad, J.; Iriti, M. Anticancer Molecular Mechanisms of Resveratrol. *Front. Nutr.* **2016**, *3*. [CrossRef] [PubMed]
9. Aggarwal, B.B.; Bhardwaj, A.; Aggarwal, R.S.; Seeram, N.P.; Shishodia, S.; Takada, Y. Role of Resveratrol in Prevention and Therapy of Cancer: Preclinical and Clinical Studies. *Anticancer Res.* **2004**, *24*, 2783–2840. [PubMed]
10. Barron, C.C.; Moore, J.; Tsakiridis, T.; Pickering, G.; Tsiani, E. Inhibition of human lung cancer cell proliferation and survival by wine. *Cancer Cell Int.* **2014**, *14*, 6. [CrossRef] [PubMed]
11. Cuvelier, M.E.; Berset, C.; Richard, H. Antioxidant Constituents in Sage (*Salvia officinalis*). *J. Agric. Food Chem.* **1994**, *42*, 665–669. [CrossRef]
12. González-Vallinas, M.; Reglero, G.; Ramírez de Molina, A. Rosemary (*Rosmarinus officinalis* L.) Extract as a Potential Complementary Agent in Anticancer Therapy. *Nutr. Cancer* **2015**, *67*, 1221–1229. [CrossRef] [PubMed]
13. Petiwala, S.M.; Puthenveetil, A.G.; Johnson, J.J. Polyphenols from the Mediterranean herb rosemary (*Rosmarinus officinalis*) for prostate cancer. *Front. Pharmacol.* **2013**, *4*, e1–e4. [CrossRef] [PubMed]
14. Petiwala, S.M.; Johnson, J.J. Diterpenes from rosemary (*Rosmarinus officinalis*): Defining their potential for anti-cancer activity. *Cancer Lett.* **2015**, *367*, 93–102. [CrossRef] [PubMed]

15. Slamenova, D.; Kuboskova, K.; Horvathova, E.; Robichova, S. Rosemary-stimulated reduction of DNA strand breaks and FPG-sensitive sites in mammalian cells treated with $H_2O_2$ or visible light-excited Methylene Blue. *Cancer Lett.* **2002**, *177*, 145–153. [CrossRef]

16. Yi, W.; Wetzstein, H.Y. Anti-tumorigenic activity of five culinary and medicinal herbs grown under greenhouse conditions and their combination effects. *J. Sci. Food Agric.* **2011**, *91*, 1849–1854. [CrossRef] [PubMed]

17. Ibáñez, C.; Simó, C.; García-Cañas, V.; Gómez-Martínez, Á.; Ferragut, J.A.; Cifuentes, A. CE/LC-MS multiplatform for broad metabolomic analysis of dietary polyphenols effect on colon cancer cells proliferation. *Electrophoresis* **2012**, *33*, 2328–2336. [CrossRef] [PubMed]

18. Đilas, S.; Knez, Ž.; Četojević-Simin, D.; Tumbas, V.; Škerget, M.; Čanadanović-Brunet, J.; Ćetković, G. In vitro antioxidant and antiproliferative activity of three rosemary (*Rosmarinus officinalis* L.) extract formulations. *Int. J. Food Sci. Technol.* **2012**, *47*, 2052–2062. [CrossRef]

19. Valdés, A.; Garcia-Canas, V.; Rocamora-Reverte, L.; Gomez-Martinez, A.; Ferragut, J.A.; Cifuentes, A. Effect of rosemary polyphenols on human colon cancer cells: Transcriptomic profiling and functional enrichment analysis. *Genes Nutr.* **2013**, *8*, 43–60. [CrossRef] [PubMed]

20. González-Vallinas, M.; Molina, S.; Vicente, G.; de la Cueva, A.; Vargas, T.; Santoyo, S.; García-Risco, M.R.; Fornari, T.; Reglero, G.; Ramírez de Molina, A. Antitumor effect of 5-fluorouracil is enhanced by rosemary extract in both drug sensitive and resistant colon cancer cells. *Pharmacol. Res.* **2013**, *72*, 61–68. [CrossRef] [PubMed]

21. González-Vallinas, M.; Molina, S.; Vicente, G.; Zarza, V.; Martín-Hernández, R.; García-Risco, M.R.; Fornari, T.; Reglero, G.; de Molina, A.R. Expression of MicroRNA-15b and the Glycosyltransferase GCNT3 Correlates with Antitumor Efficacy of Rosemary Diterpenes in Colon and Pancreatic Cancer. *PLoS ONE* **2014**, *9*, e98556. [CrossRef] [PubMed]

22. Borrás-Linares, I.; Pérez-Sánchez, A.; Lozano-Sánchez, J.; Barrajón-Catalán, E.; Arráez-Román, D.; Cifuentes, A.; Micol, V.; Carretero, A.S. A bioguided identification of the active compounds that contribute to the antiproliferative/cytotoxic effects of rosemary extract on colon cancer cells. *Food Chem. Toxicol. Int. J. Publ. Br. Ind. Biol. Res. Assoc.* **2015**, *80*, 215–222. [CrossRef] [PubMed]

23. Yan, M.; Li, G.; Petiwala, S.M.; Householter, E.; Johnson, J.J. Standardized rosemary (*Rosmarinus officinalis*) extract induces Nrf2/sestrin-2 pathway in colon cancer cells. *J. Funct. Foods* **2015**, *13*, 137–147. [CrossRef]

24. Valdés, A.; Sullini, G.; Ibáñez, E.; Cifuentes, A.; García-Cañas, V. Rosemary polyphenols induce unfolded protein response and changes in cholesterol metabolism in colon cancer cells. *J. Funct. Foods* **2015**, *15*, 429–439. [CrossRef]

25. Valdés, A.; García-Cañas, V.; Koçak, E.; Simó, C.; Cifuentes, A. Foodomics study on the effects of extracellular production of hydrogen peroxide by rosemary polyphenols on the anti-proliferative activity of rosemary polyphenols against HT-29 cells. *Electrophoresis* **2016**, *37*, 1795–1804. [CrossRef] [PubMed]

26. Valdés, A.; Artemenko, K.A.; Bergquist, J.; García-Cañas, V.; Cifuentes, A. Comprehensive Proteomic Study of the Antiproliferative Activity of a Polyphenol-Enriched Rosemary Extract on Colon Cancer Cells Using Nanoliquid Chromatography-Orbitrap MS/MS. *J. Proteome Res.* **2016**, *15*, 1971–1985. [CrossRef] [PubMed]

27. Kontogianni, V.G.; Tomic, G.; Nikolic, I.; Nerantzaki, A.A.; Sayyad, N.; Stosic-Grujicic, S.; Stojanovic, I.; Gerothanassis, I.P.; Tzakos, A.G. Phytochemical profile of *Rosmarinus officinalis* and *Salvia officinalis* extracts and correlation to their antioxidant and anti-proliferative activity. *Food Chem.* **2013**, *136*, 120–129. [CrossRef] [PubMed]

28. Alexandrov, K.; Rojas, M.; Rolando, C. DNA damage by benzo(a)pyrene in human cells is increased by cigarette smoke and decreased by a filter containing rosemary extract, which lowers free radicals. *Cancer Res.* **2006**, *66*, 11938–11945. [CrossRef] [PubMed]

29. Cheung, S.; Tai, J. Anti-proliferative and antioxidant properties of rosemary *Rosmarinus officinalis*. *Oncol. Rep.* **2007**, *17*, 1525–1531. [CrossRef] [PubMed]

30. Yesil-Celiktas, O.; Sevimli, C.; Bedir, E.; Vardar-Sukan, F. Inhibitory Effects of Rosemary Extracts, Carnosic Acid and Rosmarinic Acid on the Growth of Various Human Cancer Cell Lines. *Plant Foods Hum. Nutr.* **2010**, *65*, 158–163. [CrossRef] [PubMed]

31. Mothana, R.A.A.; Kriegisch, S.; Harms, M.; Wende, K.; Lindequist, U. Assessment of selected Yemeni medicinal plants for their in vitro antimicrobial, anticancer, and antioxidant activities. *Pharm. Biol.* **2011**, *49*, 200–210. [CrossRef] [PubMed]

32. González-Vallinas, M.; Molina, S.; Vicente, G.; Sánchez-Martínez, R.; Vargas, T.; García-Risco, M.R.; Fornari, T.; Reglero, G.; Ramírez de Molina, A. Modulation of estrogen and epidermal growth factor receptors by rosemary extract in breast cancer cells. *Electrophoresis* **2014**, *35*, 1719–1727. [CrossRef] [PubMed]

33. Petiwala, S.M.; Berhe, S.; Li, G.; Puthenveetil, A.G.; Rahman, O.; Nonn, L.; Johnson, J.J. Rosemary (*Rosmarinus officinalis*) Extract Modulates CHOP/GADD153 to Promote Androgen Receptor Degradation and Decreases Xenograft Tumor Growth. *PLoS ONE* **2014**, *9*, e89772. [CrossRef] [PubMed]

34. Tai, J.; Cheung, S.; Wu, M.; Hasman, D. Antiproliferation effect of Rosemary (*Rosmarinus officinalis*) on human ovarian cancer cells in vitro. *Phytomedicine* **2012**, *19*, 436–443. [CrossRef] [PubMed]

35. Berrington, D.; Lall, N. Anticancer Activity of Certain Herbs and Spices on the Cervical Epithelial Carcinoma (HeLa) Cell Line. *Evid. Based Complement. Alternat. Med.* **2012**, *2012*, e564927. [CrossRef] [PubMed]

36. Wang, W.; Li, N.; Luo, M.; Zu, Y.; Efferth, T. Antibacterial Activity and Anticancer Activity of *Rosmarinus officinalis* L. Essential Oil Compared to That of Its Main Components. *Molecules* **2012**, *17*, 2704–2713. [CrossRef] [PubMed]

37. Peng, C.-H.; Su, J.-D.; Chyau, C.-C.; Sung, T.-Y.; Ho, S.-S.; Peng, C.-C.; Peng, R.Y. Supercritical Fluid Extracts of Rosemary Leaves Exhibit Potent Anti-Inflammation and Anti-Tumor Effects. *Biosci. Biotechnol. Biochem.* **2007**, *71*, 2223–2232. [CrossRef] [PubMed]

38. Vicente, G.; Molina, S.; González-Vallinas, M.; García-Risco, M.R.; Fornari, T.; Reglero, G.; de Molina, A.R. Supercritical rosemary extracts, their antioxidant activity and effect on hepatic tumor progression. *J. Supercrit. Fluids* **2013**, *79*, 101–108. [CrossRef]

39. Moore, J.; Megaly, M.; MacNeil, A.J.; Klentrou, P.; Tsiani, E. Rosemary extract reduces Akt/mTOR/p70S6K activation and inhibits proliferation and survival of A549 human lung cancer cells. *Biomed. Pharmacother.* **2016**, *83*, 725–732. [CrossRef] [PubMed]

40. Shabtay, A.; Sharabani, H.; Barvish, Z.; Kafka, M.; Amichay, D.; Levy, J.; Sharoni, Y.; Uskokovic, M.R.; Studzinski, G.P.; Danilenko, M. Synergistic Antileukemic Activity of Carnosic Acid-Rich Rosemary Extract and the 19-nor Gemini Vitamin D Analogue in a Mouse Model of Systemic Acute Myeloid Leukemia. *Oncology* **2008**, *75*, 203–214. [CrossRef] [PubMed]

41. Sharabani, H.; Izumchenko, E.; Wang, Q.; Kreinin, R.; Steiner, M.; Barvish, Z.; Kafka, M.; Sharoni, Y.; Levy, J.; Uskokovic, M.; et al. Cooperative antitumor effects of vitamin D3 derivatives and rosemary preparations in a mouse model of myeloid leukemia. *Int. J. Cancer* **2006**, *118*, 3012–3021. [CrossRef] [PubMed]

42. Okumura, N.; Yoshida, H.; Nishimura, Y.; Kitagishi, Y.; Matsuda, S. Terpinolene, a component of herbal sage, downregulates AKT1 expression in K562 cells. *Oncol. Lett.* **2012**, *3*, 321–324. [PubMed]

43. Ahmad, H.H.; Hamza, A.H.; Hassan, A.Z.; Sayed, A.H. Promising therapeutic role of *Rosmarinus officinalis* successive methanolic fraction against colorectal cancer. *Int. J. Pharm. Pharm. Sci.* **2013**, *5*, 164–170.

44. Kitano, M.; Wanibuchi, H.; Kikuzaki, H.; Nakatani, N.; Imaoka, S.; Funae, Y.; Hayashi, S.; Fukushima, S. Chemopreventive effects of coumaperine from pepper on the initiation stage of chemical hepatocarcinogenesis in the rat. *Jpn. J. Cancer Res. Gann* **2000**, *91*, 674–680. [CrossRef] [PubMed]

45. Soyal, D.; Jindal, A.; Singh, I.; Goyal, P.K. Modulation of radiation-induced biochemical alterations in mice by rosemary (*Rosmarinus officinalis*) extract. *Phytomed. Int. J. Phytother. Phytopharm.* **2007**, *14*, 701–705. [CrossRef] [PubMed]

46. Sancheti, G.; Goyal, P. Modulatory influence of *Rosemarinus officinalis* on DMBA-induced mouse skin tumorigenesis. *Asian Pac. J. Cancer Prev.* **2006**, *7*, 331–335. [PubMed]

47. Sancheti, G.; Goyal, P.K. Effect of *Rosmarinus officinalis* in modulating 7,12-dimethylbenz(a)anthracene induced skin tumorigenesis in mice. *Phytother. Res.* **2006**, *20*, 981–986. [CrossRef] [PubMed]

48. Visanji, J.M.; Thompson, D.G.; Padfield, P.J. Induction of G2/M phase cell cycle arrest by carnosol and carnosic acid is associated with alteration of cyclin A and cyclin B1 levels. *Cancer Lett.* **2006**, *237*, 130–136. [CrossRef] [PubMed]

49. Barni, M.V.; Carlini, M.J.; Cafferata, E.G.; Puricelli, L.; Moreno, S. Carnosic acid inhibits the proliferation and migration capacity of human colorectal cancer cells. *Oncol. Rep.* **2012**, *27*, 1041–1048. [PubMed]

50. De la Roche, M.; Rutherford, T.J.; Gupta, D.; Veprintsev, D.B.; Saxty, B.; Freund, S.M.; Bienz, M. An intrinsically labile α-helix abutting the BCL9-binding site of β-catenin is required for its inhibition by carnosic acid. *Nat. Commun.* **2012**, *3*, 680. [CrossRef] [PubMed]

51. Valdés, A.; García-Cañas, V.; Simó, C.; Ibáñez, C.; Micol, V.; Ferragut, J.A.; Cifuentes, A. Comprehensive Foodomics Study on the Mechanisms Operating at Various Molecular Levels in Cancer Cells in Response to Individual Rosemary Polyphenols. *Anal. Chem.* **2014**, *86*, 9807–9815. [CrossRef] [PubMed]

52. Kim, Y.-J.; Kim, J.-S.; Seo, Y.-R.; Park, J.-H.Y.; Choi, M.-S.; Sung, M.-K. Carnosic acid suppresses colon tumor formation in association with anti-adipogenic activity. *Mol. Nutr. Food Res.* **2014**, *58*, 2274–2285. [CrossRef] [PubMed]

53. Kim, D.-H.; Park, K.-W.; Chae, I.G.; Kundu, J.; Kim, E.-H.; Kundu, J.K.; Chun, K.-S. Carnosic acid inhibits STAT3 signaling and induces apoptosis through generation of ROS in human colon cancer HCT116 cells. *Mol. Carcinog.* **2016**, *55*, 1096–1110. [CrossRef] [PubMed]

54. Einbond, L.S.; Wu, H.; Kashiwazaki, R.; He, K.; Roller, M.; Su, T.; Wang, X.; Goldsberry, S. Carnosic acid inhibits the growth of ER-negative human breast cancer cells and synergizes with curcumin. *Fitoterapia* **2012**, *83*, 1160–1168. [CrossRef] [PubMed]

55. Min, K.-J.; Jung, K.-J.; Kwon, T.K. Carnosic Acid Induces Apoptosis Through Reactive Oxygen Species-mediated Endoplasmic Reticulum Stress Induction in Human Renal Carcinoma Caki Cells. *J. Cancer Prev.* **2014**, *19*, 170–178. [CrossRef] [PubMed]

56. Jung, K.-J.; Min, K.; Bae, J.H.; Kwon, T.K. Carnosic acid sensitized TRAIL-mediated apoptosis through down-regulation of c FLIP and Bcl-2 expression at the post translational levels and CHOP-dependent up-regulation of DR5, Bim, and PUMA expression in human carcinoma caki cells. *Oncotarget* **2015**, *6*, 1556–1568. [CrossRef] [PubMed]

57. Linnewiel-Hermoni, K.; Khanin, M.; Danilenko, M.; Zango, G.; Amosi, Y.; Levy, J.; Sharoni, Y. The anti-cancer effects of carotenoids and other phytonutrients resides in their combined activity. *Arch. Biochem. Biophys.* **2015**, *572*, 28–35. [CrossRef] [PubMed]

58. Kar, S.; Palit, S.; Ball, W.B.; Das, P.K. Carnosic acid modulates Akt/IKK/NF-κB signaling by PP2A and induces intrinsic and extrinsic pathway mediated apoptosis in human prostate carcinoma PC-3 cells. *Apoptosis Int. J. Program. Cell Death* **2012**, *17*, 735–747. [CrossRef] [PubMed]

59. Gao, Q.; Liu, H.; Yao, Y.; Geng, L.; Zhang, X.; Jiang, L.; Shi, B.; Yang, F. Carnosic acid induces autophagic cell death through inhibition of the Akt/mTOR pathway in human hepatoma cells. *J. Appl. Toxicol.* **2014**, 485–492. [CrossRef] [PubMed]

60. Lin, C.-Y.; Wu, C.-R.; Chang, S.-W.; Wang, Y.-J.; Wu, J.-J.; Tsai, C.-W. Induction of the pi class of glutathione S-transferase by carnosic acid in rat Clone 9 cells via the p38/Nrf2 pathway. *Food Funct.* **2015**, *6*, 1936–1943. [CrossRef] [PubMed]

61. Tsai, C.-W.; Lin, C.-Y.; Wang, Y.-J. Carnosic acid induces the NAD(P)H: Quinone oxidoreductase 1 expression in rat clone 9 cells through the p38/nuclear factor erythroid-2 related factor 2 pathway. *J. Nutr.* **2011**, *141*, 2119–2125. [CrossRef] [PubMed]

62. López-Jiménez, A.; García-Caballero, M.; Medina, M.Á.; Quesada, A.R. Anti-angiogenic properties of carnosol and carnosic acid, two major dietary compounds from rosemary. *Eur. J. Nutr.* **2013**, *52*, 85–95. [CrossRef] [PubMed]

63. Park, S.Y.; Song, H.; Sung, M.-K.; Kang, Y.-H.; Lee, K.W.; Park, J.H.Y. Carnosic Acid Inhibits the Epithelial-Mesenchymal Transition in B16F10 Melanoma Cells: A Possible Mechanism for the Inhibition of Cell Migration. *Int. J. Mol. Sci.* **2014**, *15*, 12698–12713. [CrossRef] [PubMed]

64. Kosaka, K.; Yokoi, T. Carnosic acid, a component of rosemary (*Rosmarinus officinalis* L.), promotes synthesis of nerve growth factor in T98G human glioblastoma cells. *Biol. Pharm. Bull.* **2003**, *26*, 1620–1622. [CrossRef] [PubMed]

65. Mimura, J.; Kosaka, K.; Maruyama, A.; Satoh, T.; Harada, N.; Yoshida, H.; Satoh, K.; Yamamoto, M.; Itoh, K. Nrf2 regulates NGF mRNA induction by carnosic acid in T98G glioblastoma cells and normal human astrocytes. *J. Biochem.* **2011**, *150*, 209–217. [CrossRef] [PubMed]

66. Tsai, C.-W.; Lin, C.-Y.; Lin, H.-H.; Chen, J.-H. Carnosic acid, a rosemary phenolic compound, induces apoptosis through reactive oxygen species-mediated p38 activation in human neuroblastoma IMR-32 cells. *Neurochem. Res.* **2011**, *36*, 2442–2451. [CrossRef] [PubMed]

67. De Oliveira, M.R.; Ferreira, G.C.; Schuck, P.F.; dal Bosco, S.M. Role for the PI3K/Akt/Nrf2 signaling pathway in the protective effects of carnosic acid against methylglyoxal-induced neurotoxicity in SH-SY5Y neuroblastoma cells. *Chem. Biol. Interact.* **2015**, *242*, 396–406. [CrossRef] [PubMed]

68. Meng, P.; Yoshida, H.; Tanji, K.; Matsumiya, T.; Xing, F.; Hayakari, R.; Wang, L.; Tsuruga, K.; Tanaka, H.; Mimura, J.; et al. Carnosic acid attenuates apoptosis induced by amyloid-β 1–42 or 1–43 in SH-SY5Y human neuroblastoma cells. *Neurosci. Res.* **2015**, *94*, 1–9. [CrossRef] [PubMed]

69. Yoshida, H.; Meng, P.; Matsumiya, T.; Tanji, K.; Hayakari, R.; Xing, F.; Wang, L.; Tsuruga, K.; Tanaka, H.; Mimura, J.; et al. Carnosic acid suppresses the production of amyloid-β 1–42 and 1–43 by inducing an α-secretase TACE/ADAM17 in U373MG human astrocytoma cells. *Neurosci. Res.* **2014**, *79*, 83–93. [CrossRef] [PubMed]

70. Cortese, K.; Daga, A.; Monticone, M.; Tavella, S.; Stefanelli, A.; Aiello, C.; Bisio, A.; Bellese, G.; Castagnola, P. Carnosic acid induces proteasomal degradation of Cyclin B1, RB and SOX2 along with cell growth arrest and apoptosis in GBM cells. *Phytomed. Int. J. Phytother. Phytopharm.* **2016**, *23*, 679–685. [CrossRef] [PubMed]

71. Danilenko, M.; Wang, X.; Studzinski, G.P. Carnosic acid and promotion of monocytic differentiation of HL60-G cells initiated by other agents. *J. Natl. Cancer Inst.* **2001**, *93*, 1224–1233. [CrossRef] [PubMed]

72. Steiner, M. Carnosic Acid Inhibits Proliferation and Augments Differentiation of Human Leukemic Cells Induced by 1,25-Dihydroxyvitamin Dsub3 and Retinoic Acid. *Nutr. Cancer* **2001**, *41*, 135–144. [CrossRef] [PubMed]

73. Danilenko, M.; Wang, Q.; Wang, X.; Levy, J.; Sharoni, Y.; Studzinski, G.P. Carnosic acid potentiates the antioxidant and prodifferentiation effects of 1alpha,25-dihydroxyvitamin D3 in leukemia cells but does not promote elevation of basal levels of intracellular calcium. *Cancer Res.* **2003**, *63*, 1325–1332. [PubMed]

74. Wang, Q.; Harrison, J.S.; Uskokovic, M.; Kutner, A.; Studzinski, G.P. Translational study of vitamin D differentiation therapy of myeloid leukemia: Effects of the combination with a p38 MAPK inhibitor and an antioxidant. *Leukemia* **2005**, *19*, 1812–1817. [CrossRef] [PubMed]

75. Chen-Deutsch, X.; Garay, E.; Zhang, J.; Harrison, J.S.; Studzinski, G.P. c-Jun *N*-terminal kinase 2 (JNK2) antagonizes the signaling of differentiation by JNK1 in human myeloid leukemia cells resistant to vitamin D. *Leuk. Res.* **2009**, *33*, 1372–1378. [CrossRef] [PubMed]

76. Chen-Deutsch, X.; Studzinski, G.P. Dual role of hematopoietic progenitor kinase 1 (HPK1) as a positive regulator of 1α,25-dihydroxyvitamin D-induced differentiation and cell cycle arrest of AML cells and as a mediator of vitamin D resistance. *Cell. Cycle Georget. Tex* **2012**, *11*, 1364–1373. [CrossRef] [PubMed]

77. Bobilev, I.; Novik, V.; Levi, I.; Shpilberg, O.; Levy, J.; Sharoni, Y.; Studzinski, G.P.; Danilenko, M. The Nrf2 transcription factor is a positive regulator of myeloid differentiation of acute myeloid leukemia cells. *Cancer Biol. Ther.* **2011**, *11*, 317–329. [CrossRef] [PubMed]

78. Nachliely, M.; Sharony, E.; Kutner, A.; Danilenko, M. Novel analogs of 1,25-dihydroxyvitamin D2 combined with a plant polyphenol as highly efficient inducers of differentiation in human acute myeloid leukemia cells. *J. Steroid Biochem. Mol. Biol.* **2016**, *164*, 59–65. [CrossRef] [PubMed]

79. Nishimoto, S.; Suzuki, T.; Koike, S.; Yuan, B.; Takagi, N.; Ogasawara, Y. Nrf2 activation ameliorates cytotoxic effects of arsenic trioxide in acute promyelocytic leukemia cells through increased glutathione levels and arsenic efflux from cells. *Toxicol. Appl. Pharmacol.* **2016**, *305*, 161–168. [CrossRef] [PubMed]

80. Yu, X.-N.; Chen, X.-L.; Li, H.; Li, X.-X.; Li, H.-Q.; Jin, W.-R. Reversion of P-glycoprotein-mediated multidrug resistance in human leukemic cell line by carnosic acid. *Chin. J. Physiol.* **2008**, *51*, 348–356. [PubMed]

81. Duggal, J.; Harrison, J.S.; Studzinski, G.P.; Wang, X. Involvement of microRNA181a in differentiation and cell cycle arrest induced by a plant-derived antioxidant carnosic acid and vitamin D analog doxercalciferol in human leukemia cells. *MicroRNA Shāriqah. United Arab Emir.* **2012**, *1*, 26–33. [CrossRef]

82. Wang, R.; Cong, W.; Guo, G.; Li, X.; Chen, X.; Yu, X.; Li, H. Synergism between carnosic acid and arsenic trioxide on induction of acute myeloid leukemia cell apoptosis is associated with modulation of PTEN/Akt signaling pathway. *Chin. J. Integr. Med.* **2012**, *18*, 934–941. [CrossRef] [PubMed]

83. Manoharan, S.; Vasanthaselvan, M.; Silvan, S.; Baskaran, N.; Kumar Singh, A.; Vinoth Kumar, V. Carnosic acid: A potent chemopreventive agent against oral carcinogenesis. *Chem. Biol. Interact.* **2010**, *188*, 616–622. [CrossRef] [PubMed]

84. Rajasekaran, D.; Manoharan, S.; Silvan, S.; Vasudevan, K.; Baskaran, N.; Palanimuthu, D. Proapoptotic, anti-cell proliferative, anti-inflammatory and anti-angiogenic potential of carnosic acid during 7,12

dimethylbenz[a]anthracene-induced hamster buccal pouch carcinogenesis. *Afr. J. Tradit. Complement. Altern. Med. AJTCAM Afr. Netw. Ethnomed.* **2012**, *10*, 102–112.

85. Gómez-García, F.; López-Jornet, M.; Álvarez-Sánchez, N.; Castillo-Sánchez, J.; Benavente-García, O.; Vicente Ortega, V. Effect of the phenolic compounds apigenin and carnosic acid on oral carcinogenesis in hamster induced by DMBA. *Oral Dis.* **2013**, *19*, 279–286. [CrossRef] [PubMed]

86. Petiwala, S.M.; Li, G.; Bosland, M.C.; Lantvit, D.D.; Petukhov, P.A.; Johnson, J.J. Carnosic acid promotes degradation of the androgen receptor and is regulated by the unfolded protein response pathway in vitro and in vivo. *Carcinogenesis* **2016**, *37*, 827–838. [CrossRef] [PubMed]

87. Wang, L.-Q.; Wang, R.; Li, X.-X.; Yu, X.-N.; Chen, X.-L.; Li, H. The anti-leukemic effect of carnosic acid combined with Adriamycin in a K562/A02/SCID leukemia mouse model. *Int. J. Clin. Exp. Med.* **2015**, *8*, 11708–11717. [PubMed]

88. Scheckel, K.A.; Degner, S.C.; Romagnolo, D.F. Rosmarinic acid antagonizes activator protein-1-dependent activation of cyclooxygenase-2 expression in human cancer and nonmalignant cell lines. *J. Nutr.* **2008**, *138*, 2098–2105. [CrossRef] [PubMed]

89. Xavier, C.P.R.; Lima, C.F.; Fernandes-Ferreira, M.; Pereira-Wilson, C. *Salvia fruticosa, Salvia officinalis*, and rosmarinic acid induce apoptosis and inhibit proliferation of human colorectal cell lines: The role in MAPK/ERK pathway. *Nutr. Cancer* **2009**, *61*, 564–571. [CrossRef] [PubMed]

90. Xu, Y.; Xu, G.; Liu, L.; Xu, D.; Liu, J. Anti-invasion effect of rosmarinic acid via the extracellular signal-regulated kinase and oxidation-reduction pathway in Ls174-T cells. *J. Cell. Biochem.* **2010**, *111*, 370–379. [CrossRef] [PubMed]

91. Ramos, A.A.; Pedro, D.; Collins, A.R.; Pereira-Wilson, C. Protection by Salvia extracts against oxidative and alkylation damage to DNA in human HCT15 and CO115 cells. *J. Toxicol. Environ. Health A* **2012**, *75*, 765–775. [CrossRef] [PubMed]

92. Moon, D.-O.; Kim, M.-O.; Lee, J.-D.; Choi, Y.H.; Kim, G.-Y. Rosmarinic acid sensitizes cell death through suppression of TNF-α-induced NF-κB activation and ROS generation in human leukemia U937 cells. *Cancer Lett.* **2010**, *288*, 183–191. [CrossRef] [PubMed]

93. Paluszczak, J.; Krajka-Kuźniak, V.; Baer-Dubowska, W. The effect of dietary polyphenols on the epigenetic regulation of gene expression in MCF7 breast cancer cells. *Toxicol. Lett.* **2010**, *192*, 119–125. [CrossRef] [PubMed]

94. Berdowska, I.; Zieliński, B.; Fecka, I.; Kulbacka, J.; Saczko, J.; Gamian, A. Cytotoxic impact of phenolics from Lamiaceae species on human breast cancer cells. *Food Chem.* **2013**, *141*, 1313–1321. [CrossRef] [PubMed]

95. Li, F.-R.; Fu, Y.-Y.; Jiang, D.-H.; Wu, Z.; Zhou, Y.-J.; Guo, L.; Dong, Z.-M.; Wang, Z.-Z. Reversal effect of rosmarinic acid on multidrug resistance in SGC7901/Adr cell. *J. Asian Nat. Prod. Res.* **2013**, *15*, 276–285. [CrossRef] [PubMed]

96. Han, S.; Yang, S.; Cai, Z.; Pan, D.; Li, Z.; Huang, Z.; Zhang, P.; Zhu, H.; Lei, L.; Wang, W. Anti-Warburg effect of rosmarinic acid via miR-155 in gastric cancer cells. *Drug Des. Dev. Ther.* **2015**, *9*, 2695–2703.

97. Lee, J.; Kim, Y.S.; Park, D. Rosmarinic acid induces melanogenesis through protein kinase A activation signaling. *Biochem. Pharmacol.* **2007**, *74*, 960–968. [CrossRef] [PubMed]

98. Renzulli, C.; Galvano, F.; Pierdomenico, L.; Speroni, E.; Guerra, M.C. Effects of rosmarinic acid against aflatoxin B1 and ochratoxin-A-induced cell damage in a human hepatoma cell line (HepG2). *J. Appl. Toxicol.* **2004**, *24*, 289–296. [CrossRef] [PubMed]

99. Lin, C.-S.; Kuo, C.-L.; Wang, J.-P.; Cheng, J.-S.; Huang, Z.-W.; Chen, C.-F. Growth inhibitory and apoptosis inducing effect of *Perilla frutescens* extract on human hepatoma HepG2 cells. *J. Ethnopharmacol.* **2007**, *112*, 557–567. [CrossRef] [PubMed]

100. Wu, J.; Zhu, Y.; Li, F.; Zhang, G.; Shi, J.; Ou, R.; Tong, Y.; Liu, Y.; Liu, L.; Lu, L.; et al. Spica prunellae and its marker compound rosmarinic acid induced the expression of efflux transporters through activation of Nrf2-mediated signaling pathway in HepG2 cells. *J. Ethnopharmacol.* **2016**, *193*, 1–11. [CrossRef] [PubMed]

101. Tao, L.; Wang, S.; Zhao, Y.; Sheng, X.; Wang, A.; Zheng, S.; Lu, Y. Phenolcarboxylic acids from medicinal herbs exert anticancer effects through disruption of COX-2 activity. *Phytomed. Int. J. Phytother. Phytopharm.* **2014**, *21*, 1473–1482. [CrossRef] [PubMed]

102. Aquilano, K.; Filomeni, G.; Di Renzo, L.; Vito, M.D.; Stefano, C.D.; Salimei, P.S.; Ciriolo, M.R.; Marfè, G. Reactive oxygen and nitrogen species are involved in sorbitol-induced apoptosis of human erithroleukaemia cells K562. *Free Radic. Res.* **2007**, *41*, 452–460. [CrossRef] [PubMed]

103. Heo, S.-K.; Noh, E.-K.; Yoon, D.-J.; Jo, J.-C.; Koh, S.; Baek, J.H.; Park, J.-H.; Min, Y.J.; Kim, H. Rosmarinic acid potentiates ATRA-induced macrophage differentiation in acute promyelocytic leukemia NB4 cells. *Eur. J. Pharmacol.* **2015**, *747*, 36–44. [CrossRef] [PubMed]

104. Saiko, P.; Steinmann, M.-T.; Schuster, H.; Graser, G.; Bressler, S.; Giessrigl, B.; Lackner, A.; Grusch, M.; Krupitza, G.; Bago-Horvath, Z.; et al. Epigallocatechin gallate, ellagic acid, and rosmarinic acid perturb dNTP pools and inhibit de novo DNA synthesis and proliferation of human HL-60 promyelocytic leukemia cells: Synergism with arabinofuranosylcytosine. *Phytomedicine* **2015**, *22*, 213–222. [CrossRef] [PubMed]

105. Wu, C.-F.; Hong, C.; Klauck, S.M.; Lin, Y.-L.; Efferth, T. Molecular mechanisms of rosmarinic acid from *Salvia miltiorrhiza* in acute lymphoblastic leukemia cells. *J. Ethnopharmacol.* **2015**, *176*, 55–68. [CrossRef] [PubMed]

106. Lozano-Baena, M.-D.; Tasset, I.; Muñoz-Serrano, A.; Alonso-Moraga, Á.; de Haro-Bailón, A. Cancer Prevention and Health Benefices of Traditionally Consumed *Borago officinalis* Plants. *Nutrients* **2016**, *8*, 48. [CrossRef] [PubMed]

107. Osakabe, N.; Yasuda, A.; Natsume, M.; Yoshikawa, T. Rosmarinic acid inhibits epidermal inflammatory responses: Anticarcinogenic effect of *Perilla frutescens* extract in the murine two-stage skin model. *Carcinogenesis* **2004**, *25*, 549–557. [CrossRef] [PubMed]

108. Anusuya, C.; Manoharan, S. Antitumor initiating potential of rosmarinic acid in 7,12-dimethylbenz(a)anthracene-induced hamster buccal pouch carcinogenesis. *J. Environ. Pathol. Toxicol. Oncol. Off. Organ Int. Soc. Environ. Toxicol. Cancer* **2011**, *30*, 199–211. [CrossRef]

109. Karmokar, A.; Marczylo, T.H.; Cai, H.; Steward, W.P.; Gescher, A.J.; Brown, K. Dietary intake of rosmarinic acid by Apc(Min) mice, a model of colorectal carcinogenesis: Levels of parent agent in the target tissue and effect on adenoma development. *Mol. Nutr. Food Res.* **2012**, *56*, 775–783. [CrossRef] [PubMed]

110. Karthikkumar, V.; Sivagami, G.; Vinothkumar, R.; Rajkumar, D.; Nalini, N. Modulatory efficacy of rosmarinic acid on premalignant lesions and antioxidant status in 1,2-dimethylhydrazine induced rat colon carcinogenesis. *Environ. Toxicol. Pharmacol.* **2012**, *34*, 949–958. [CrossRef] [PubMed]

111. Sharmila, R.; Manoharan, S. Anti-tumor activity of rosmarinic acid in 7,12-dimethylbenz(a)anthracene (DMBA) induced skin carcinogenesis in Swiss albino mice. *Indian J. Exp. Biol.* **2012**, *50*, 187–194. [PubMed]

112. Venkatachalam, K.; Gunasekaran, S.; Jesudoss, V.A.S.; Namasivayam, N. The effect of rosmarinic acid on 1,2-dimethylhydrazine induced colon carcinogenesis. *Exp. Toxicol. Pathol.* **2013**, *65*, 409–418. [CrossRef] [PubMed]

113. Baldasquin-Caceres, B.; Gomez-Garcia, F.J.; López-Jornet, P.; Castillo-Sanchez, J.; Vicente-Ortega, V. Chemopreventive potential of phenolic compounds in oral carcinogenesis. *Arch. Oral Biol.* **2014**, *59*, 1101–1107. [CrossRef] [PubMed]

114. Furtado, R.A.; Oliveira, B.R.; Silva, L.R.; Cleto, S.S.; Munari, C.C.; Cunha, W.R.; Tavares, D.C. Chemopreventive effects of rosmarinic acid on rat colon carcinogenesis. *Eur. J. Cancer Prev. Off. J. Eur. Cancer Prev. Organ. ECP* **2015**, *24*, 106–112. [CrossRef] [PubMed]

115. Romo Vaquero, M.; García Villalba, R.; Larrosa, M.; Yáñez-Gascón, M.J.; Fromentin, E.; Flanagan, J.; Roller, M.; Tomás-Barberán, F.A.; Espín, J.C.; García-Conesa, M.-T. Bioavailability of the major bioactive diterpenoids in a rosemary extract: Metabolic profile in the intestine, liver, plasma, and brain of Zucker rats. *Mol. Nutr. Food Res.* **2013**, *57*, 1834–1846. [CrossRef] [PubMed]

116. Doolaege, E.H.A.; Raes, K.; Vos, F.D.; Verhé, R.; Smet, S.D. Absorption, Distribution and Elimination of Carnosic Acid, A Natural Antioxidant from *Rosmarinus officinalis*, in Rats. *Plant Foods Hum. Nutr.* **2011**, *66*, 196–202. [CrossRef] [PubMed]

117. Karthikkumar, V.; Sivagami, G.; Viswanathan, P.; Nalini, N. Rosmarinic acid inhibits DMH-induced cell proliferation in experimental rats. *J. Basic Clin. Physiol. Pharmacol.* **2015**, *26*, 185–200. [CrossRef] [PubMed]

118. Romo-Vaquero, M.; Larrosa, M.; Yáñez-Gascón, M.J.; Issaly, N.; Flanagan, J.; Roller, M.; Tomás-Barberán, F.A.; Espín, J.C.; García-Conesa, M.-T. A rosemary extract enriched in carnosic acid improves circulating adipocytokines and modulates key metabolic sensors in lean Zucker rats: Critical and contrasting differences in the obese genotype. *Mol. Nutr. Food Res.* **2014**, *58*, 942–953. [CrossRef] [PubMed]

119. European Food Safety Authority (EFSA). Use of rosemary extracts as a food additive—Scientific Opinion of the Panel on Food Additives, Flavourings, Processing Aids and Materials in Contact with Food. *EFSA J.* **2008**, *6*, 1–29.

120. Pérez-Sánchez, A.; Barrajón-Catalán, E.; Caturla, N.; Castillo, J.; Benavente-García, O.; Alcaraz, M.; Micol, V. Protective effects of citrus and rosemary extracts on UV-induced damage in skin cell model and human volunteers. *J. Photochem. Photobiol. B* **2014**, *136*, 12–18. [CrossRef] [PubMed]

121. Romo-Vaquero, M.; Selma, M.-V.; Larrosa, M.; Obiol, M.; García-Villalba, R.; González-Barrio, R.; Issaly, N.; Flanagan, J.; Roller, M.; Tomás-Barberán, F.A.; et al. A Rosemary Extract Rich in Carnosic Acid Selectively Modulates Caecum Microbiota and Inhibits β-Glucosidase Activity, Altering Fiber and Short Chain Fatty Acids Fecal Excretion in Lean and Obese Female Rats. *PLoS ONE* **2014**, *9*, e94687. [CrossRef] [PubMed]

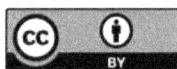

*nutrients*

MDPI

*Article*

# Unraveling the Anticancer Effect of Curcumin and Resveratrol

Aline Renata Pavan [†], Gabriel Dalio Bernardes da Silva [†], Daniela Hartmann Jornada [†], Diego Eidy Chiba [†], Guilherme Felipe dos Santos Fernandes [†], Chung Man Chin [†] and Jean Leandro dos Santos *,[†]

School of Pharmaceutical Sciences, UNESP–University Estadual Paulista, Araraquara 14800903, Brazil; alinerenatapavan2004@yahoo.com.br (A.R.P.); gabriel.dalio@hotmail.com (G.D.B.d.S.); daniela.hj@hotmail.com (D.H.J.); chiba.diego@outlook.com (D.E.C.); guilhermefelipe@outlook.com (G.F.d.S.F.); chungmc@fcfar.unesp.br (C.M.C.)
* Correspondence: santosjl@fcfar.unesp.br; Tel.: +55-16-3301-6972; Fax: +55-16-3301-6960
† All authors contributed equally to this work.

Received: 4 September 2016; Accepted: 27 September 2016; Published: 10 November 2016

**Abstract:** Resveratrol and curcumin are natural products with important therapeutic properties useful to treat several human diseases, including cancer. In the last years, the number of studies describing the effect of both polyphenols against cancer has increased; however, the mechanism of action in all of those cases is not completely comprehended. The unspecific effect and the ability to interfere in assays by both polyphenols make this challenge even more difficult. Herein, we analyzed the anticancer activity of resveratrol and curcumin reported in the literature in the last 11 years, in order to unravel the molecular mechanism of action of both compounds. Molecular targets and cellular pathways will be described. Furthermore, we also discussed the ability of these natural products act as chemopreventive and its use in association with other anticancer drugs.

**Keywords:** cancer; resveratrol; curcumin; polyphenols; anticancer

---

## 1. Introduction

Over the last years, the number of searchers involving polyphenols has increased meaningly. The major reason for that includes the presence of these compounds in our diet contributing to prevention of several diseases. In addition, potent antioxidant properties of polyphenols reduce oxidative stress-associated with some diseases, including cancer. It has been described that polyphenols inhibit carcinogenesis and induce tumor cell death [1].

Among the polyphenols, the interest in two of them has increased in the last years. Papers describing curcumin and/or resveratrol are present in almost fifteen thousand of publications in the last ten years. Both polyphenols have been described as promising anticancer compounds; however, the mode of action for them are still unclear and not fully comprehended [2].

Curcumin (diferuloylmethane) is an active ingredient of the perennial herb *Curcuma longa*, also known as turmeric. The yellow color of this polyphenol is chemically related to its major fraction, which contains curcuminoids [3]. Curcumin has been used for a long time in countries such as China and India as traditional medicines. This ancient remedy has brought the attention of scientific community for a wide range of beneficial properties including anti-inflammatory, antioxidant and chemopreventive [4,5].

By the other hand, resveratrol (*trans*-3,5,4′-trihydroxystilbene) is a stilbene phytoalexin synthetized by a variety of plants, specially vine in response to fungi infections and ultraviolet radiation [6]. This compound is found at high concentration in grapes and red wine, which antioxidant effect is well established in several different assays. Resveratrol has been investigated as potential compound for the treatment of several diseases, regulation of immune system and chemoprevention [7,8].

In clinical studies, the common issue regarding both compounds is the reduced aqueous solubility and low bioavailability [3,9–11]. In order to overcome these limitations, studies have been conducted using several strategies. For curcumin, for example, these strategies include: (a) complexation with metal ions, such as $Zn^{2+}$, $Cu^{2+}$, $Se^{2+}$ and $Mg^{2+}$ [12]; (b) co-administration with piperine, which inhibits the phase II metabolism of curcumin and increases its bioavailability [13,14]; (c) Pharmaceutical technologies such as micelles formation and nanoencapsulation were used to increase the bioavailability of curcumin [15–23]. Resveratrol has been extensively studied aiming to enhance its aqueous solubility and bioavailability and a number of techniques were used to achieve this goal [24], including: (a) nanoencapsulation [25–28]; (b) prodrug approach [29]; and (c) co-administration with piperine [30]. These polyphenols have exhibited very low or not-observed toxic effects at daily intake of 0–3 mg·kg$^{-1}$ body weight for curcumin [3] and 0.073 mg–5 g for resveratrol [31]. However, in humans at high doses either curcumin and resveratrol can cause side effects such as diarrhea, skin rash, and headaches [3,31–34].

Another concern about these both polyphenols is the ability to perturb membranes and alter protein function, that leads to false-results in a series of assays described in the literature [35–37]. Therefore, this review article proposes to investigate the real mechanisms involved in the anticancer effect of resveratrol and curcumin in order to clarify the mode of action of both compounds as anticancer drugs useful for prevention and treatment.

## 2. Cell Proliferation

The antiproliferative effects of curcumin and resveratrol are associated with the modulation of transcription factors, protein kinases, cell cycle regulatory proteins, and inhibition of angiogenesis [9,10]. Some targets related to its effect are presented as following (Figure 1).

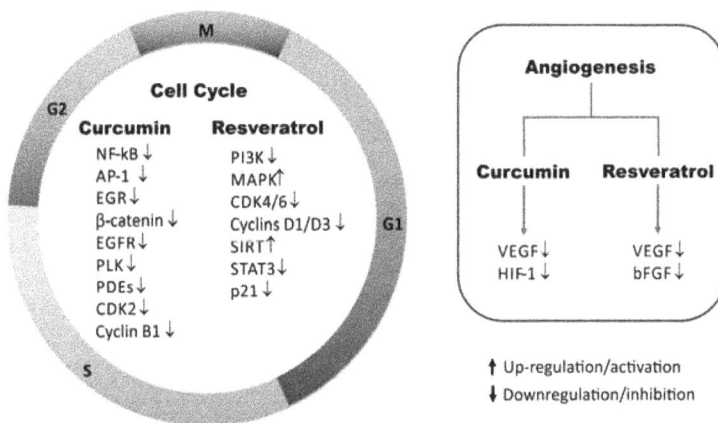

**Figure 1.** Effects of curcumin and resveratrol in cellular proliferation and angiogenesis.

### 2.1. Transcription Factors

#### 2.1.1. NF-κB

Nuclear Factor-kappa B (NF-κB) is a pro-inflammatory transcription factor that regulates the expression of more than 200 genes, which are involved in innate and adaptive immunity, cellular transformation, proliferation, antiapoptosis, angiogenesis, invasion and metastasis [38]. Moreover, NF-κB regulates several pro-inflammatory cytokines including, IL-1, IL-2, IL-6, TNF-α and monocyte chemotactic protein 1 (MCP-1). These cytokines are released in chronic inflammation states associated to various cancers [39–42].

NF-κB is found in an inactive state in the cytoplasm and its activation occurs through the action of a variety of stimuli, such as, carcinogens, mitogens, chemotherapeutic agents, radiation, hypoxia, protein kinases, and degradation of the NF-κB cytoplasmic inhibitor (I-κB) [43–45]. Subsequently its activation, NF-κB translocate to the cell nucleus and binds to the target DNA gene promoter region [46].

Luciferase assay was performed transfecting series of plasmids into PC-3 cells with luciferase reporter gene. The data showed down regulation of NF-κB blocking the development and progression of prostate cancer cells (PC-3) [47].

Curcumin showed a potent antiproliferative effect on melanoma cell lines by NF-κB inhibition. Three melanoma cell lines were treated with curcumin and it has shown a decreasing of NF-κB binding activity through electrophoretic mobility shift assay (EMSA), and an inhibition of cell viability in a dose-dependent manner with $IC_{50}$ ranging from 6.1 μM to 7.7 μM [48].

### 2.1.2. AP-1

The activating protein-1 (AP-1) transcription factor is related to control an extensive range of cellular processes, including cell proliferation. Dysfunctions in the AP-1 transcription factor levels are associated to the growth and progression of many types of cancer [49]. AP-1 showed to be required for binding in the involucrin (hINV), which is a marker of keratinocyte differentiation [50].

Using a High-Throughput Cell-Based Assay, it was identified potentials AP-1 inhibitors. In this assay, curcumin has shown inhibiting AP-1 in the dose-dependent manner with $IC_{50}$ values of 100 μM [51].

In a different study, using fluorescent cell-staining assay it was shown that curcumin also suppress the in vitro growth of PC-3 cells. By a luciferase assay, it was determined the intracellular signal pathway via inhibition of androgen-induced AP-1 activity in prostate cancer cells (PC-3). Flow cytometry data indicated that curcumin arrested 57.29% of PC-3 cells in G2/M phase, and reduced to 23.89% of cells in the S phase [47].

### 2.1.3. EGR—Early Growth Response

The Early Growth Response gene (EGR-1) is activated by stress, injury, mitogens and differentiation [52]. This gene regulates the expression of other genes, which are involved in the control of growth and apoptosis such as: p21, p53, PTEN, Gadd45 [53].

Curcumin suppressed proliferation in human high-metastatic NSCLC cells 95D by EGR-1 in a dose-dependent manner. NSCLC cells transfected with EGR-1 siRNA notably inhibited EGR-1 expression, specifically siRNA3 [52]. Also, it has been found that curcumin inhibits human colon cancer cell growth via suppressing EGR-1 [54].

### 2.1.4. β-Catenin

The β-catenin is located in three cellular pools (cell membrane, cytoplasm and nucleus), mainly in the cell membrane [55]. The main event of the activation of Wnt/β-catenin pathway is the nuclear translocation of beta-catenin, which binds to T-cell factor (TCF) in the nucleus [56]. The intracellular levels of beta-catenin are regulated by the phosphorylation of GSK-3β. Curcumin showed suppressing this phosphorylation in LNCaP prostate cancer cells, inducing the degradation of beta-catenin affecting the cell proliferation [56].

Curcumin suppressed cell growth by inhibiting the activation of Wnt/β-catenin pathway in desmoplastic cerebellar medulloblastoma (DAOY) cells. In this study, the expression of nuclear beta-catenin was significantly decreased; however, there was no effect on the expression of cytoplasmic beta-catenin levels. In addition, curcumin promote the activation of GSK-3β and its downstream target cyclin D1. The authors concluded that curcumin could be useful in the medulloblastoma treatment [57].

*2.2. Protein Kinases*

Protein kinases are a group of tyrosine or serine/threonine kinase enzymes whose function is to modify others proteins by attaching phosphate groups through the phosphorylation process. Tyrosine phosphorylation has a vital role in several important cellular pathways of eukaryote physiology, as well as in human diseases [58,59].

Protein kinases mediate most of the intracellular signal-transduction pathways in eukaryotic cells, control metabolism, transcription, mRNA processing, cell division, apoptosis and differentiation. Moreover, tyrosine phosphorylation mediated by protein kinases also regulate communication between neighboring cells, motility of cells and transport of molecules to within the cell [60,61]. Deregulation in tyrosine phosphorylation has been associated to a variety of cellular disorders and human diseases, such as cancer, diabetes, cardiovascular disorders, inflammatory diseases and immune deficiencies [62–65]. Specifically related to cancer, several studies have shown that deregulation of several protein kinases, including MAPK, Raf kinase, Akt, mTOR, MLK3, Src kinase, AMPK and protein kinase D are associated to a variety of cancers, such breast, gastric, thyroid, prostate, lung, liver and colorectal cancer [66–74].

2.2.1. EGFR—Epidermal Growth Factor Receptor

Also known as ErbB1 or HER1, EGFR is a member of the ErbB family of receptors. The structure of EGF receptor is represented by an extracellular ligand-binding domain, a single transmembrane region with hydrophobic characteristics, and an intracellular module including the tyrosine kinase domain [75].

The EGFR pathway contributes in many ways to cancer proliferation and angiogenesis to many types of cancer. Curcumin decreased expression of EGFR, and also EGFR mRNA levels in bladder cancer cells [76].

An autophosphorylation activity of the EGFR tyrosine kinase have been observed after a short-term treatment of curcumin in dose and time dependent manner in human epithelial cancer cells (A431). Curcumin was able to inhibit EGFR tyrosine kinase in a concentration of 1 µM after 4 h of cell exposure. The exact molecular mechanism of this short-term inhibition remains unknown [75].

2.2.2. Polo-Like Kinase (PLK)

Polo-like kinases are important proteins on regulation of the cell cycle. It is related to spindle assembly, which has been found in high levels in colorectal cancer than normal colon tissues [77]. Curcumin downregulates PLK resulting in inhibition of the cell growth. It was characterized that curcumin promote cell cycle arrest in the G2/M phase and decrease the expression of some genes including tubulin genes and p53 related to colon cancer [78]. In some cancer cell lines, inhibition of PLK leads to cellular senescence correlating to the number of cells arrested in mitosis [79].

2.2.3. Phosphatidylinositol 3-Kinase (PI3K) Pathway

PI3K is a protein that acts in the mechanism of cell survival. Its expression or activation is upregulated in diseases, such as diabetes and cancer. Akt is a mediator of PI3K signaling and affects directly the apoptosis process, targeting related proteins [80].

The influence of PI3K/Akt pathway and the effect of RES on cell growth were evaluated in different cancers cells. PI3K and MAPK are associated with HIF-$1\alpha$ accumulation and increase of VEGF expression, leading to angiogenesis [81]. In a study conducted to evaluate the influence of the RES in the accumulation of HIF-$1\alpha$ and VEGF expression in human tongue squamous cell carcinoma and hepatoma cells induced by hypoxia condition, it was observed that resveratrol was able to reduce the accumulation of HIF-$1\alpha$ and the expression of VEGF through inhibition of Akt and p42 and p44 MAPK phosphorylation [82].

In another study using human diffuse large B-cell lymphoma, it was observed that the resveratrol inhibited Akt phosphorylation following downstream targets, such as p70 S6K, S6 ribosomal and FOXO-3a. More specifically, it provides an improved comprehension of one possible mechanism of action, which involves the inhibition of PI3K pathway. This inhibitory effect exhibited a direct relationship with a decreased activity in the glycolysis pathway and may be the cause of cell cycle arrest in G0/G1 phase according authors observations [83].

The exposure of prostate cancer cells to resveratrol demonstrated that inhibition of the PI3K pathway reduces the phosphorylation of GSK-3 protein, which is related with the modulation of expression of cyclin D1, and decreases the activation NF-κβ [84,85].

### 2.2.4. MAPK (p38 e ERK)

Resveratrol effects on MAPK are described in the literature. Using breast cancer cells, it was demonstrated that this polyphenol causes cycle cell arrest in S/G2M phase and upregulates the levels of phosphorylated p38 e ERK and increase p21 and p53R2 levels [86]. Another study using the same type of cancer cells also demonstrated the activity of resveratrol in the activation of p38. Resveratrol caused cycle cell arrest in G0/G1 phase. It also increased the activation of p38, p21 and p53 levels and decreased pRb hyperphosphorylated. Additionally, it was observed inhibition of ER expression, related to p53 activity. ER is described to play an important role in breast cancer cell proliferation [87].

### 2.3. Phosphodiesterases (PDEs)

Phosphodiesterases consist of a family containing 11 isoenzymes, which are responsible for hydrolyze two important second messengers that regulate cellular responses to external stimuli: the cyclic adenosine-3′,5′-monophosphate (cAMP) and the cyclic guanosine-3′,5′-monophosphate (cGMP).

These isoenzymes play an important role in cancer, and were found to be upregulated in angiogenesis and various types of tumors. For curcumin, it was found modifications in the pattern of PDE1A expression at transcriptional level. After curcumin treatment, the expression of PDE1A was dramatically reduced in B16F10 melanoma cancer cells. These findings indicate that PDE1A has an important role in the anti-proliferative effects of curcumin, and its inhibition may recover normal intracellular signaling contributing to the treatment [88]. Other isoforms (PDE2 and PDE4) were described to be upregulated in human umbilical vein endothelial cells (HUVECs). In these cells, the inhibition of PDE2 and PDE4 activities decrease the angiogenesis and cell proliferation [89].

### 2.4. Angiogenesis

Angiogenesis is involved in several biological processes. Nonetheless, its involvement in pathological processes, notably in tumor growth and metastasis still have been extensively investigated [90]. Some important pro-angiogenic and anti-angiogenic factors include: VEGF, MMPs, FGF (fibroblast growth factor) and HGF (hepatocyte growth factor). However, among these factors, VEGF and its receptors were described to be key regulators of both physiological and pathological vasculogenesis and angiogenesis [91,92].

VEGF is an important and multifunctional signaling glycoprotein that comprises a family of structurally related mitogens: VEGF-A, VEGF-B, VEGF-C, VEGF-D and placental growth factor (PlGF). These growth factors regulate a family VEGF receptors tyrosine kinases (VEGFR-1, VEGFR-2 and VEGFR-3) and promote endothelium regeneration, blood vessel regeneration and increase vascular permeability. However, VEGF-A (commonly known as VEGF) is the central member of the VEGF family and the majority of angiogenic effects related to these growth factor family are attributed to the interaction of VEGF-A with VEGFR-2 [93,94].

HIF-1/VEGF/bFGF

Cancer tumors activate hypoxia-inducible factor (HIF) under hypoxic conditions as a survival mechanism that ultimately leads to angiogenesis progression. It has been reported the effect of curcumin on vascular endothelial cells under hypoxic conditions using human umbilical vein endothelial cells (HUVECs). Specifically, curcumin downregulates HIF-1$\alpha$ protein and VEGF expression by blocking hypoxia-stimulated angiogenesis [95] and demonstrates anti-proliferative and anti-angiogenic properties [96].

During the tumor development, VEGF is a critical pro-angiogenic stimulator for neovascularization. The VEGF-VEGFR-2 complex is required to maintain a subset of vasculatures in healthy tissues and organs. Curcumin can block the VEGF-VEGFR-2 signaling pathways in HUVECs by suppressing the phosphorylation of VEGFR-2 induced by VEGF [97].

The effects of resveratrol against VEGF alter cell proliferation in endometrial cancer [98], myeloma [99], osteosarcoma [100], renal cancer [101] and melanoma [102]. High levels of VEGF were observed in endometrial carcinoma cells cultured in vitro under hypoxia conditions. However, after resveratrol treatment it was observed a reduced level of VEGF in a dose dependent manner, suggesting an anti-angiogenic activity when angiogenesis is induced under hypoxia [98].

The cellular viability of osteosarcoma cells and human renal cancer cells was evaluated in the presence of resveratrol. It was observed a dose dependent inhibition of growth in both cells, with no detectable VEGF and VEGF mRNA even at high doses of resveratrol (up to 40 $\mu$mol/L) [100,101].

Resveratrol also inhibited in a dose dependent manner the proliferation, migration and tube formation of HUVEC induced by co-culture with myeloma cell. In order to comprehend the mechanism that resveratrol acts in angiogenesis, it was determinate the levels of VEGF, basic fibroblast growth factor (bFGF) and metalloproteinases 2 and 9 (MMP-2 and MMP-9) [99]. Interestingly, it was found that resveratrol inhibited the expression of VEGF and bFGF, besides to suppress the expression of MMPs, which may explain its effect in the angiogenesis [99].

Additionally, studies to characterize the antiangiogenic effect of RES were evaluated in a chick chorioallantoic membrane (CAM) model. Resveratrol reduced the angiogenesis in the membrane induced by fibroblast growth factor-2 (FGF-2). Moreover, the tumor growth in the CAM model was inhibited, as well as, the angiogenesis. The level of p53 was quantified and a significant reduction was determinated after treatment using resveratrol. This results suggest an apoptotic effect induced by resveratrol, which might be responsible to stop tumor growth and angiogenesis [103].

*2.5. Cell Cycle Regulators*

The cell cycle is divided into four main phases: G1-S-G2-M. The G1 phase, also known as GAP 1, is the first growth stage of the cell cycle. During the S (synthesis) stage, the chromosomes of somatic cells are replicating. The G2 phase (GAP 2) is the final sub-phase of interphase in the cell cycle, prior to mitosis (M phase) [104].

Cyclin B1 is overexpressed in many tumors and is needed to forward cells from G2 phase to M phase during the cellular cycle. It was demonstrated that after 24 h of curcumin treatment, protein and mRNA levels of cyclin B1 were downregulated. In addition, flow cytometry data have shown arrested effect on cell cycle involving G2/M phase in small cell lung cancer (SCLC) cells [105].

Curcumin inhibits cyclin-dependent kinase 2 (CDK2) activity in vitro and decrease the proliferation of colon cancer cells, indicating G1 cell cycle arrest in a dose-dependent manner. The percentage of sh-CKD2-transfected HCT116 colon cancer cells in G1 phase was higher after curcumin treatment that those of control groups. Computational molecular docking studies have demonstrated a very good binding affinity between CDK2 and curcumin with a score of $-12.69$ kcal/mol, validating previous in vitro data [106].

Resveratrol has been described to cause cell cycle arrest in different types of cancers, mainly at low concentrations. Cycle cell arrest between the G1 and S phases were observed in prostate cancer cells [107], pituitary prolactinoma [108], human epidermoid carcinoma [109] and lung cancer cells [110].

Similar results were found in these studies, showing that resveratrol decreased the levels of cyclins (D1 and D3) and of CDK (4 and 6). In addition, resveratrol increased the expression of p21 and p27.

Furthermore, the inhibition of cell proliferation of pituitary prolactinoma cells, an estrogen-dependent tumor, caused by resveratrol persists after the end of the exposure of this compound, which indicates an irreversible suppressive effect [108]. The phosphorylation of pRb was inhibited in two different type of cells exposed to resveratrol [108,109]. Resveratrol was described to inhibit kinases, therefore, authors assumed that a reduction of cyclin D1 levels could be associated with this effect [109].

The exposition of hepatocarcinoma cells to resveratrol induces cell accumulation in S phase, by a reversible process. Regarding cell cycle regulators, it was observed reduction in the levels of cyclin D1 and p21. However, the levels of phosphorylated CDK2 and Chk2 have been increased. PI3K pathway may be related, in part, with cell cycle arrest in S phase [111].

In addition, it was observed that resveratrol treatment of oral squamous carcinoma cells resulted in cell cycle arrest in G2/M phase. It was also observed an increase in cyclin A and B levels, possibly related to the high expression of protein kinase Myt-1 [112].

## 2.6. SIRT

Sirtuin family is composed by seven sirtuins types, defined as $NAD^+$-dependent histone deacetylases. SIRT-1 is responsible for deacetylation of transcriptional factors, DNA repair proteins and signaling factors. It regulates important biological activity, including cell survival, gene expression, metabolism and senescence [113].

Resveratrol has been described as a potential SIRT activator, since this compound inhibited cell proliferation in a SIRT-1 dependent way. In this study, the anti-proliferative effect of this compound was studied only in gastric cancer cells that could express SIRT-1. It was observed that resveratrol treatment caused a G1 phase arrest, decrease the levels of cyclin D1, CDK4 and CDK6 and increase the levels of p21. In knockout cells that can express SIRT-1, resveratrol was not capable to inhibit cell proliferation [114].

Similary, in a study using breast cancer cells, resveratrol inhibited cell proliferation by stimulating SIRT-1. Activation of AMPK pathway leads to mTOR activation, which stimulates the cell proliferation. It was observed that resveratrol can block AMPK phosphorylation by SIRT-1 activity overexpressed in tumor cells [115].

The effects of resveratrol on cell proliferation of hepatocarcinoma cell under high concentration of glucose were evaluated in another study. The results showed that high glucose concentration upregulated activated STAT-3 and enhanced cellular viability. Resveratrol was able to suppress proliferation and activation of STAT-3 and Akt [116].

## 2.7. Others Targets

Others proteins, enzymes, and transcription factors involved in cell proliferation and described as target for curcumin and resveratrol are described in Tables 1 and 2.

**Table 1.** Antiproliferative targets for curcumin.

| Target | Effect | Cancer Type | Reference |
| --- | --- | --- | --- |
| GRP78 | downregulation | Colon | [117] |
| EphA2 | downregulation | Melanoma | [118] |
| SOCS1 & 3 | upregulation | Leukemia | [119] |
| Nrf2 | downregulation | Breast | [120] |
| miR-15a/16-1 | downregulation | Leukemia | [121] |
| DLEC1 | upregulation | Colon | [122] |
| Skp2 | downregulation | Glioma | [123] |

Table 2. Antiproliferative targets for resveratrol.

| Target | Effect | Cancer Type | Reference |
|--------|--------|-------------|-----------|
| PKC | downregulation | gastric | [124] |
| eEF1A2 | downregulation | ovarian | [125] |
| pro-IGFII | upregulation | breast | [126] |
| PTEN | upregulation | breast | [127] |
| MIC-1 | upregulation | pancreas | [128] |
| 6-PF1K | inhibition | breast | [129] |
| RNF20 | activation | breast | [130] |
| Nox5 | upregulation | lung | [131] |
| uH2B | downregulation | glioma | [132] |

## 3. Metastasis

Although several advances have been achieved in the last years against cancer, the mortality rate related to metastasis is still about 90% [133–135]. Therefore, cellular pathways involved in metastasis have been extensively described as promising therapeutic target for a variety of cancers [136–138]. Metastasis is the spread and growth process of solid cancers cells from the original neoplasm to distant organs through several cellular mechanisms, such as angiogenesis, invasion and proliferation [139,140]. The process involved in metastasis is fairly complex and begins when primary cancer cells break away from their original tumor environmental and invade through the basement membrane reaching the circulation. Subsequently, these metastasizing cells will reach and settle microenvironment in distant organs [141]. This metastatic progression depends on several biochemical, genetic and epigenetic factors in the original tumor cells and association to the new microenvironment [142].

Curcumin and resveratrol modulate many of these cellular pathways, including transcription factors, proteins, enzymes and growth factors (Figure 2) [143]. Although the precise mechanism of action of polyphenols remains unclear, several studies have highlighted the inhibitory effect of these compounds in a number of molecular targets and signaling pathways involved in cancer metastasis [144–147]. In this section, we highlighted the major cellular targets involved in metastasis that curcumin and resveratrol have the ability to modulate.

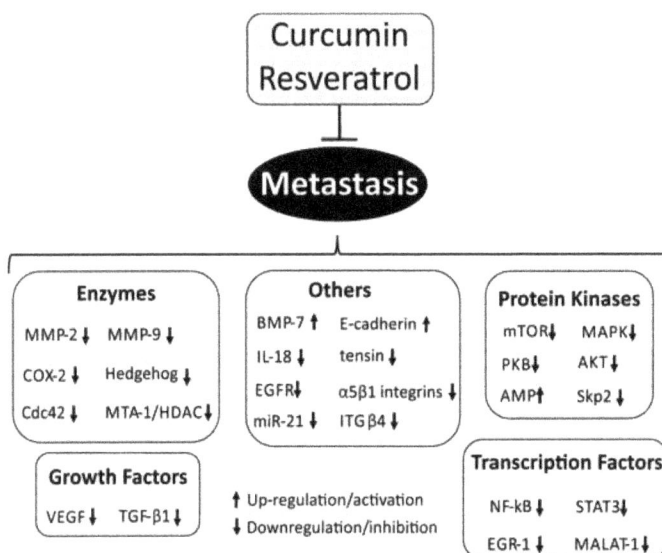

Figure 2. The control of metastasis by curcumin and resveratrol.

### 3.1. NF-κB Signaling Pathway

Curcumin is able to modulate NF-κB signaling pathway directly and indirectly by downregulation or upregulation some key factors. Aggarwal and coworkers demonstrated that curcumin inhibited tumor cell invasion through inhibition of I-κB kinase complex (IKK) and protein kinase B (Akt) in human myeloid leukemia and human embryonic kidney cells. The inhibition of IKK and Akt blocks the phosphorylation of p65, which led to a suppression of cellular events required for NF-κB gene expression. As a result, the inhibition of NF-κB by curcumin resulted in downregulating of several NF-κB-regulated gene products involved in cellular proliferation and metastasis including COX-2, cyclin D1, c-myc, MMP-9, VEGF and intercellular adhesion molecule-1 [148].

Similarly, it was also demonstrated that curcumin inhibits translocation of NF-κB from the cell nucleus by inhibition of the I-κB kinase complex in both, breast and prostate cancer cells [149,150]. The authors have demonstrated that inhibition of NF-κB activity reduces the expression of inflammatory cytokines, such as, CXCL1 and CXCL2. Some cancer cells with potential to metastasize to lung overexpress these inflammatory cytokines and promotes infiltration of inflammatory cells, which lead to angiogenesis and metastasis process [151]. Moreover, in vivo experiments using mice demonstrated that curcumin was able to reduce the number of lung metastases formed from circulating prostate cancer cells after 35 days of treatment [150].

In fact, several studies have demonstrated the narrow relationship between curcumin and NF-κB signaling pathway in cancer metastasis. Narasimhan and Ammanamanchi have shown that curcumin was able to block the invasion of breast carcinoma cells using a matrigel invasion experiment. They have concluded that curcumin reduced the expression and transcriptional activity of NF-κB p65 protein and decreased the levels of the Recepteur d'Origine Nantais tyrosine kinase (RON) [152]. RON plays an important role in cell proliferation, differentiation and metastasis. Its overexpression in patients with breast cancer is associated to a poor prognostic [153].

Zong and colleagues also demonstrated the potential therapeutic application of curcumin to inhibit metastatic progression of breast cancer cells. They investigated the urokinase-type plasminogen activator (uPA), a serine protease protein that plays an important role in tumor growth and metastasis. The authors found that curcumin was able to reduce uPA expression through downregulating NF-κB activity [154].

In a different work, the inhibition of the human astroglioma cells invasion and metastasis was reported for curcumin. The authors proposed that mechanism of action involves the downregulation of NF-κB, which resulted in an inhibition of matrix metalloproteinase-9 [155]. Interestingly, an in vivo study using human prostate adenocarcinoma LNCaP xenograft cells demonstrated that curcumin was able to reduce metastatic process in mice though inhibition of NF-κB activity leading to a reduction in the expression of its related genes, including VEGF, Bcl-2, Bcl-XL, uPA, cyclin D1, MMP-2, MMP-9, COX-2 and IL-8 [156].

By the other hand, the activity of resveratrol against NF-κB during metastasis is also described by several groups. Chen and colleagues have reported that resveratrol successfully inhibited epithelial-mesenchymal transition in mouse melanoma model and reduced cancer migration and metastasis. The authors concluded that resveratrol downregulated NF-κB activity and influenced in epithelial-mesenchymal transition [157]. In another study, it was demonstrated that resveratrol was able to block the migration and invasion of human metastatic lung and cervical cancer cells. Resveratrol inhibited the activity of NF-κB and AP-1 leading to reduction in MMP-9 expression [158]. Liu and coworkers also demonstrated the effect of resveratrol on NF-κB inhibition and its downstream events in human lung adenocarcinoma cell metastasis [159].

Heme oxygenase 1 (HO-1) is an important enzyme involved in angiogenesis and tumor metastasis and its activity have been associated to matrix metalloproteinases expression [160]. Resveratrol suppressed NF-κB activity leading to inhibition of HO-1 and subsequently downregulating the expression of MMP-2 and MMP-9 in lung cancer cells [159]. Resveratrol was also reported acting as an inhibitor of cancer invasion and metastasis of human hepatocellular carcinoma cells.

The authors have demonstrated that resveratrol suppressed TNF-α-mediated MMP-9 expression through downregulation of NF-κB signaling pathway activity [161].

Ryu and coworkers have reported the antimetastatic activity of resveratrol in human glioma cancer cells induced by TNF-α overexpression. Resveratrol suppressed NF-κB activation and downregulated the expression of urokinase plasminogen activator (uPA), thereby leading to a reduction of TNF-α-induced cell invasion [162]. Adhesion molecules, such as intracellular adhesion molecule-1 (ICAM-1), vascular cell adhesion molecule-1 (VCAM-1), E-cadherin and E-selectin plays a central role in endothelial adhesion of a number of cancer cells and are closely related to cancer invasion and metastasis [163,164]. Therefore, the inhibition of cellular pathways related to adhesion molecules have been considering as a promising anti-metastasis target [165]. Park and colleagues have demonstrated the anti-metastatic activity of resveratrol in human fibrosarcoma cells. Resveratrol blocked cancer cell adhesion to endothelial cells through inhibition of ICAM-1 expression; however, they observed that this downregulation of ICAM-1 expression was due to suppression of NF-κB activation. Therefore, indirectly the inhibition of NF-κB pathway has an important role in ICAM-1 expression [166].

### 3.2. Matrix Metalloproteinase (MMP)

Matrix metalloproteinases (MMPs), collectively called matrixins, represents a group of enzymes with proteolytic activity that exist in the extracellular matrix (ECM) and are involved in most of the physiological conditions, including embryogenesis, reproduction, organ development, wound healing, angiogenesis and apoptosis [167,168]. These zinc-dependent endopeptidases also plays a vital role in the spread and dissemination of cancer and are closely related to tumor metastasis process [169]. The proteolytic activity of MMPs involves the ECM degradation and evidences have shown that the expression of specific MMPs, such as MMP-2 (Gelatinase A) and MMP-9 (Gelatinase B), are associated with a wide range of human cancers [170–173].

Several studies have shown the potential use of curcumin in cancer metastasis by reducing the expression and activity of matrix metalloproteinases. Chen and colleagues have demonstrated that curcumin suppressed migration and invasion of human endometrial carcinoma cells. Curcumin successfully reduced the expression of MMP-2 and MMP-9 through downregulation of the extracellular signal regulated kinase (ERK) signaling pathway [174]. This protein kinase is involved in the biosynthesis of MMP and plays a vital role to regulate the proliferation and invasion of endometrial carcinoma cells [175]. Another study demonstrated that curcumin also suppress the tumor growth and metastasis in prostate cancer cells by inhibition of MMP-9. Furthermore, curcumin also inhibited the expression of cellular matriptase, a membrane-anchored serine protease that is associated to a number of tumors with poor prognosis [176].

Indeed, MMP-2 and MMP-9 are the main enzymes associated with metastasis whose activities are inhibited by curcumin. This inhibitory activity may occur through different pathways. For instance, it was demonstrated that curcumin inhibited lung cancer cells invasion by modulating the PKCα/Nox-2/ROS/ATF-2 signaling pathway leading to downregulation of MMP-9 expression. During the metastasis process, the activation of MMP-9 gene promoter enhances MMP-9 transcription [177]. Another study pointed out that Rac1/PAK1 pathway is a promising target in MMPs activation pathway. The authors have demonstrated that curcumin reduces lung cancer cell metastasis through inhibition of MMP-2 and MMP-9 expression mainly by downregulation of Rac1/PAK1 [178]. Banerji and coworkers demonstrated the effect of curcumin on MMP-2 activity in murine melanoma cells. They observed a reduction in membrane type-1 matrix metalloproteinase (MT1-MMP) and focal adhesion kinase (FAK) production, leading to a reduction of MMP-2 expression after 15 days of curcumin treatment [179]. FAK and MT1-MMP plays a vital role in intracellular signaling pathway and studies have associated its activity to MMP expression [180,181]. Further, the same research group has demonstrated that curcumin was able to reduce tumor cell invasion and metastasis in human laryngeal squamous carcinoma cells. The authors suggested that curcumin inhibited MMP-2 expression through modulation of FAK and MT1-MMP signaling pathway [182]. Liao and colleagues also demonstrated the inhibitory effect of curcumin in MMP-2 expression on lung cancer cells due to downregulation of the expression of glucose transporter 1 (GLUT-1) and MT1-MMP [183].

For resveratrol, studies have demonstrated its anti-metastatic effect against several types of cancers by downregulation of MMP expression and its enzymatic activities, mainly MMP-2 and MMP-9. Among the types of cancer that resveratrol was active, we included glioblastoma [184], breast [185,186], multiple myeloma [99,187] and hepatocellular carcinoma [188].

### 3.3. E-Cadherin

The epithelial cell–cell adhesion molecule cadherin 1, also known as epithelial cadherin (E-cadherin) is a transmembrane glycoprotein that mediates cell-cell adhesion through calcium-dependent binding between two E-cadherin molecules at surface of adjacent cells [189,190]. E-cadherin is essential for the epithelial cell behavior and evidence have shown that loss of its function is associated with the proliferation of a number of cancers, including lung [191], pancreatic [192], oral [193], liver [194], gastric [195], prostate [196] and ovarian [197]. The cellular function of E-cadherin depends on the interaction with the catenin protein family, such as $\alpha$-, $\beta$- and p120 catenins [198]. $\beta$-catenin is a key cytoplasmic protein that acts in association with $\alpha$-catenin and creates a link between E-cadherin and the actin cytoskeleton [189,199].

Chen and colleagues described the cell invasion and metastasis inhibitory activity of curcumin in a mice lung cancer [200]. Specifically, curcumin up-regulated the expression of E-cadherin through activation of the tumor suppressor DnaJ-like heat shock protein 40 (HLJ1), which has been associated with cell proliferation, invasion and metastasis against a variety of human cancers [201]. The authors also suggested that curcumin modulates HLJ1 by enhancing the JNK/JunD expression [200]. Further, the same research group demonstrated the anti-metastatic effect of curcumin against colorectal cancer cells using in vivo assays [202]. Curcumin played its activity by upregulation of E-cadherin expression leading to an inhibition of mesenchymal transition (EMT). EMT-related genes has been associated with cancer progression and metastasis [203]. Likewise, not only E-cadherin overexpression was observed for curcumin activity, but also the suppression of Sp-1 transcriptional activity and the inhibition of focal adhesion kinase (FAK) phosphorylation [202]. Curcumin was able to block papillary thyroid cancer cells migration and invasion in a dual pathway, by increasing E-cadherin expression and inhibition of MMP-9 activity [204–206]. Zhang and coworkers have shown the potential application of curcumin in reducing progression and metastasis of colon cancer cells through the overexpression of E-cadherin. Moreover, the authors demonstrated that others signaling pathways were involved, including downregulation of vimentin, inhibition of Wnt signaling pathway and downregulation of CXCR4 [207].

### 3.4. Protein Kinases

Du and colleagues have reported the effect of curcumin in the inhibition of cancer invasion and metastasis in human prostate-associated fibroblasts. Curcumin suppressed the MAOA/mTOR/HIF-1$\alpha$ signaling pathway thereby leading to a downregulation of reactive oxygen species (ROS), CXC chemokine receptor 4 (CXCR4) and interleukin-6 (IL-6) receptor, which has been associated to migration of prostate carcinoma cells [208]. The inhibition of the Akt/mTOR/P70S6K kinase-signaling pathway by curcumin was also reported in human melanoma cells. Curcumin reduced the phosphorylation of this kinase-signaling pathway leading to an inhibition of cell invasion. The authors have demonstrated that curcumin was able to reduce melanoma growth against an in vivo melanoma model [209].

Guan and coworkers have reported the antiproliferative and antimetastatic activity of curcumin in breast cancer cells. They concluded that for these cells, curcumin increased AMP-kinase phosphorylation leading to a reduction of Akt protein expression and subsequently cell migration suppression [210].

Another study has demonstrated that curcumin inhibited cell growth and invasion through downregulation of S-phase kinase associated protein 2 (Skp2)-pathway in glioma cancer cells. The authors concluded that the suppression of Skp2 activity promotes an upregulation of p57 [123], which acts as an regulator of apoptosis, differentiation and migration in tumorigenesis and its inhibition is related to tumor growth [211].

Mitogen-activated protein kinase (MAPK) pathway comprises a family of protein kinases, including extracellular-signal regulated kinases (ERK), c-Jun *N*-terminal Kinase (JNK) and p38 MAPK. These protein kinases plays an important role in the regulation of genes involved in cell migration and invasion [212]. Several in vitro and in vivo studies have reported the anti-metastatic activity of resveratrol through downregulation of MAPK pathways against cancers, such as ovarian [213,214], oral [215], breast [216,217], fibrosarcoma [218], hepatocellular carcinoma [219] and osteosarcoma [220].

Akt/protein kinase B (PKB) is another important serine/threonine kinase that plays a central role in many signaling pathways involved in cell growth, proliferation and tumorigenesis, such as PI3K, PTEN, NF1, LKB1, TSC2, FOXO and eIF4E [221,222]. Resveratrol have been described as an inhibitor of the Akt signaling pathway in a number of human cancer, including cutaneous melanoma [223], glioblastoma [224], pancreatic [225], and breast [226]. In most cases, the inhibition of this pathway leads to a reduction in MMP expression, and consequently inhibition of cancer invasion and metastasis.

### 3.5. Vascular Endothelial Growth Factor (VEGF)

Kalinski and colleagues have reported the angiogenesis and anti-metastatic activity of curcumin in human chondrosarcoma cells. Curcumin inhibited interleukin-1 (IL-1) signaling by blocking the recruitment of IL-1 receptor associated kinase (IRAK) to the IL-1 receptor. IL-1 plays a central role in inflammatory, immune and malignant processes and its downstream events are associated with activation of NF-κB and metastasis-related genes, such as, VEGF-A [227]. Curcumin was also described with anti-metastatic activity through mice gastric cancer model. The authors reported that curcumin downregulated the expression of vascular endothelial growth factor receptor 3 (VEGFR-3) and its mRNA, prospero homeobox 1 (Prox-1) and podoplanin. This compound leads to a suppression of lymphatic vessel density, which is associated with poor prognosis in gastric cancer [228].

### 3.6. Hedgehog Signaling Pathway

The Hedgehog signaling pathway is an important family of proteins recognized for its importance in a number of cellular events including, proliferation, survival and differentiation [229]. Cumulative evidence strongly suggests its regulatory effect in the development of cancer angiogenesis and metastasis by modulating the expression of central proteins and transcription factors involved in cancer invasion, such as Snail protein, E-cadherin, angiogenic factors, cyclins, anti-apoptotic and apoptotic genes [230,231].

It was demonstrated the effect of resveratrol on metastatic prostate cancer cells by modulating the Hedgehog pathway. The authors have demonstrated that resveratrol-treated cells resulted in inhibition of epithelial-mesenchymal transition, exhibited an enhancement of E-cadherin expression and reduction of vimentin expression. In addition, resveratrol inhibited the expression of the transcription factor glioma-associated oncogene homolog 1 (Gli-1) [232], which plays an important role in the downstream events upon Hedgehog activation [233]. Gao and colleagues also demonstrated the anti-metastatic activity of resveratrol against gastric cancer cells by modulation of the Hedgehog signaling pathway through downregulation of Gli-1 expression. Moreover, resveratrol upregulated the expression of E-cadherin gene, decrease Snail protein and N-cadherin expression [234].

In different study, the role of Hedgehog pathway was once again described. Authors have found that the beneficial effect of resveratrol in the inhibition pancreatic cancer cells migration and invasion by suppression of this signaling pathway. Resveratrol was able to reduce Gli-1 expression and hypoxia-induced reactive oxygen species production leading to a downregulation of Hedgehog activity and thereby inhibiting the cell invasion. Furthermore, resveratrol also inhibited HIF-1$\alpha$, uPA and MMP-2 expression [235].

*3.7. STAT-3 Signaling Pathway*

Signal transducer and activator of transcription-3 (STAT-3) is a transcription factor that belongs to the STAT protein family [236]. This signaling pathway is present in cytoplasm in their inactive state and upon activation-dependent tyrosine phosphorylation; this transcription factor translocates into the cell nucleus and binds to specific enhancer elements for transcription process initiation. A number of stimuli are known to activate STAT-3 pathway, including cytokines, growth factors and oncogenic proteins. Currently, there is cumulative evidence that point out its important role in metastasis process of a variety of human cancers, such as leukemias, lymphomas, head and neck, breast, lung, gastric, hepatocellular, colorectal and prostate cancers [237]. STAT-3 target genes are involved in several cellular events related to cancer metastasis, such as invasion, cell survival, angiogenesis and tumor-cell immune evasion [238].

Lee-Chang and coworkers have reported the in vivo anti-metastatic activity of resveratrol against metastatic lung cancer. The authors described that resveratrol downregulates STAT-3 activity and reduces the tumor-evoked regulatory B cells (tBregs) production and activity [239]. tBregs is thought to be an important mediator in the protection of metastatic cancer cells by modulation of CD4+ T cells to inactivate antitumor NK cells and the effector CD8+ T cells conversion [240].

Resveratrol was also reported as an inhibitor of tumor growth and metastasis against tumor-associated macrophages. The mechanism seems to be through inhibition of lymphangiogenesis and M2 macrophage activation and differentiation [241]. M2 macrophage activation has been associated to tumor growth and metastasis in tumor-associated macrophages [242]. The authors demonstrated the inhibitory effect of resveratrol on STAT-3 phosphorylation during M2 macrophage differentiation. This effect blocks the differentiation process, decreases VEGF-C-induced migration/invasion, and capillary-like tube formation in lymphatic endothelial cells by modulation of IL-10, MCP-1 and TGF-$\beta$1 [241]. Wang and colleagues also reported the inhibitory effect of resveratrol in the STAT-3 phosphorylation in human glioblastoma cells leading to a reduction of hypoxia-induced migration and invasion [243]. Mechanistically, resveratrol inhibited cancer metastasis through upregulation of microRNA-34a activity, which act as an important tumor suppressor and is downregulated by STAT-3 [243,244].

*3.8. Others*

For resveratrol and curcumin, not only those mechanisms described above are responsible to inhibit the metastasis process, but different biochemical signaling pathways has shown an important contribution to modulate this process as well. For instance, Chen and colleagues reported the effect of curcumin to prevent cancer progression and metastasis using an in vivo lung cancer model. In this work, it was demonstrated that curcumin downregulated the expression of Cdc42 and Rho GTPase protein that plays an important role in proliferation, invasion and metastasis [245]. In fact, several studies have associated the overexpression of Cdc42 and the progression of a variety of human cancers [246]. The same research group has demonstrated the anti-metastatic activity of curcumin in non-small cell lung cancer by decreasing the expression of early growth response protein 1 (EGR-1), and thereby reducing the adherens junctions and Wnt signaling pathway activity. This signaling pathway is essential for cancer cells detach from the epithelium and achieve metastasis to distant tissues [52].

Integrin $\beta$4 (ITG $\beta$4) is a heterodimeric transmembrane receptor that act as structural link between cells or cells to the extracellular matrix. Cumulative evidences reveal that ITG $\beta$4 is associated in several signaling pathways leading to a variety of cellular events, including cell apoptosis, differentiation, cancer invasion and metastasis [247]. It was demonstrated that curcumin successfully inhibited the palmitoylation process of ITG β4 in breast cancer cells. This process is a post-translational modification and it is essential for ITG β4 signaling activity that promote a reduction in cancer invasion [248].

Dorai and coworkers have reported the anti-metastatic activity of curcumin in bone cancer. Curcumin was able to inhibit metastasis process from bone cancer to prostate using an in vivo model. The authors suggested that curcumin upregulated the bone morphogenic protein-7 (BMP-7), which act as a metastasis inhibitory protein and its upregulation promoted a modulation of transforming growth factor-β (TGF-β) function [249]. TGF-β plays a vital role in the cycle of bone metastasis. Studies have shown that its binding with BMP-7 leads to increased expression of E-cadherin and therefore, the inhibition of bone cancer metastasis [250].

Curcumin also inhibited in vivo tumor progression and metastasis in colorectal cancer. The study concluded that curcumin reduced miR-21 transcriptional regulation and expression through inhibition of activator protein-1 (AP-1) [251]. miR-21 is a microRNA that plays an important role in cellular proliferation, differentiation and apoptosis and studies have associated its overexpression in a variety of human cancer, including glioblastoma, ovarian carcinoma, hepatocellular carcinomas, head and neck cancer and chronic lymphocytic leukaemia [252]. In another study, curcumin suppressed migration of cancer glioma cells by decreasing miR-21 expression [253].

Phosphatase of regenerating liver-3 (PRL-3) is a tyrosine phosphatase and cumulative evidence have associated its overexpression with a number of human cancer metastasis [254,255]. Wang and collaborators have demonstrated that curcumin inhibits in vivo metastasis through downregulation of PRL-3 expression in melanoma cells. Specifically, the inhibition of PRL-3 cause a reduction of Src and STAT-3 phosphorylation [256].

Several others proteins, enzymes, and transcription factors have been described as a target for resveratrol leading to inhibition of cancer metastasis. Some examples reported in the literature are presented in Table 3.

**Table 3.** Antimetastatic targets for resveratrol.

| Target | Effect | Cancer Type | Reference |
|---|---|---|---|
| MTA-1/HDAC | downregulation | prostate | [257] |
| EGFR | downregulation | ovarian | [258] |
| MALAT-1 | downregulation | colorectal | [259] |
| TGF-β1/Smads | downregulation | colorectal | [260] |
| α5β1 integrins/hyaluronic acid | downregulation/upregulation | ovarian | [261] |
| tensin | upregulation | erythroleukemia | [262] |
| TGF-β1 | downregulation | lung | [263] |
| COX-2 | downregulation | colon adenocarcinoma | [264] |
| interleukin-18 | downregulation | hepatic melanoma | [265] |

## 4. Cellular Death

### 4.1. Apoptosis

An important event in the intrinsic apoptotic pathway, or mitochondrial pathway, is the change in mitochondrial membrane potential that leads to an increase in permeabilization of the outer mitochondrial membrane and the release of the proteins found in the space between the inner and outer mitochondrial membranes. The regulation of this permeabilization is coordinated by proteins of the Bcl-2 family and others components [266]. Bcl-2 is an antiapoptotic protein inserted in the outer of mitochondrial membrane. It has your antiapoptotic properties by regulating the activity of Bax and Bak, for example. These two proteins are able to move to the mitochondria, disrupt the function of Bcl-2, allow the permeabilization of the outer mitochondrial membrane and release the content of the intermembrane space [267].

Cytochrome c is an example of the released content of the mitochondrial intermembrane space. Once in the cytosol, cytochrome c binds to the C-terminal region of Apaf-1 (apoptotic protease activating factor-1), a cytosolic protein with an N-terminal caspase-recruitment domain (CARD), a nucleotide-binding domain and a C-terminal domain [268]. The association of dATP with Apaf-1 is facilitated by this binding and exposes its N-terminal CARD, which now is able to oligomerize and become a platform on which the initiator caspase-9 is activated through a CARD-CARD interaction [269]. This complex is called apoptosome and it is the responsible for caspase-3, that it is able to induce apoptosis [270,271].

Smac/DIABLO and Omi/HtrA2 are two others examples of the released mitochondrial proteins. They facilitate caspase activation by inhibiting the IAPs (inhibitor of apoptosis proteins), an endogenous inhibitor of caspases [272]. XIAP, cIAP1, cIAP2, survivin and livin (ML-IAP) are examples of IAPs. AIF (apoptosis inducing factor) is another protein of the mitochondrial intermembrane space that induces apoptosis caspase-independent. After an apoptotic insult, AIF translocate to the nucleus and induces chromatin condensation and DNA fragmentation. On the other hand, an overexpression of Bcl-2 blocks the AIF redistribution, inhibiting this apoptotic pathway [273]. A general scheme about apoptosis is presented in Figure 3.

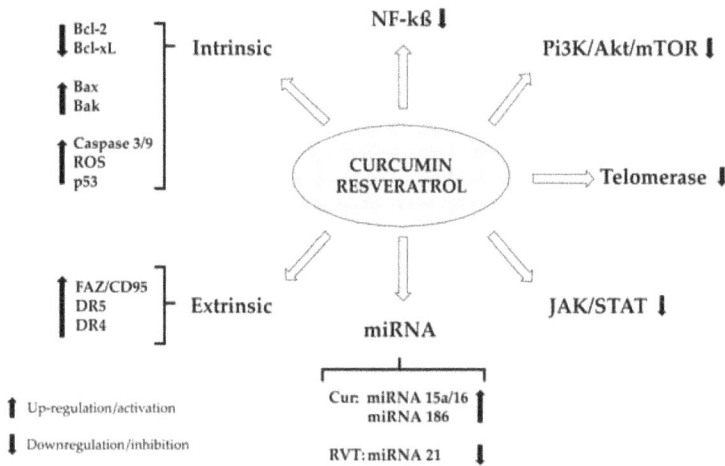

**Figure 3.** General scheme about curcumin and resveratrol effects in apoptosis.

The ability of resveratrol to direct target mitochondria was shown in bladder cancer cells and neuroblastoma cell lines. Experiments with intact cancer cell and isolated mitochondria were run and both of them resulted in a loss of mitochondrial membrane potential. Thus, it was shown that resveratrol was able to induce the release of cytochrome c and Smac/diablo in the intact cancer cell. An interesting result came from the neuroblastoma cell lines, which demonstrated that isolated mitochondria cytochrome c was not able to be released, indicating that the cytoplasmic content is important for this process [274,275].

In breast cancer cells [276] and glioma cells [277], resveratrol has demonstrated potential to activate caspase-3 and increase its activity. In breast cancer cell study, the cleavage of caspase-3 into its active form was observed. In addition, the role of caspase-3 in apoptosis was tested using a caspase-3 inhibitor, resulting in a decrease of cell death. Beyond that, in glioma cells study was also demonstrated the induction in the caspase-3 mRNA expression.

In human lung adenocarcinoma, has been demonstrated that the resveratrol-induced apoptosis is predominantly via intrinsic pathway and caspase-independent. It was demonstrated that in these cells AIF is the protein released from mitochondria. Also, resveratrol was able to induce Bak, but not

Bax, activation and, when the first one is silenced, the release of AIF is prevented and the apoptosis is inhibited, indicating that Bak has an essential role in this caspase-independent AIF signaling pathway [278,279].

### 4.1.1. ROS

Curcumin is capable to activate antioxidant enzymes, such as, glutathione-*S*-transferase (GST), quinine reductase and hemeoxygenase-1 [280]. There are a lot of works demonstrating that apoptotic induced effect by curcumin is due to reactive oxygen species (ROS) formation. It was reported that both papillary thyroid cancer cell line and cutaneous T cell lymphoma cells have a previous increased levels of ROS that is responsible to promote loss of mitochondrial membrane potential (MMP). These deregulations culminated in Bcl-2 reduction, cleavage of poly ADP-ribose polymerase (PARP) and apoptosis induction [281,282].

Curcumin has increased the levels of ROS and superoxide radicals (SOR) against human lung adenocarcinoma epithelial cells, leading to high levels of lipid peroxidation. They described that the antioxidant agent—*N*-acetyl cysteine—has prevented curcumin-induced ROS formation and apoptosis. They suggested that ROS formation induced by curcumin was able to activate the apoptosis in these cells [283].

In diffuse large B cell lymphoma cells lines (DLBCL) was demonstrated that resveratrol-induced apoptosis is related to release of ROS (reactive oxygen species). In a sequence of events, the ROS released is able to inactive Akt and FOXO1, GSK3 and Bad. Inactivated Bad allows a change in Bax protein conformation, which leads to variations in mitochondrial membrane potential, release of cytochrome c and apoptosis via intrinsic pathway. Moreover, ROS release also results in up-regulation of DR5, a death receptor, which increased the apoptosis in DLBCL, demonstrating, in this cell, that resveratrol is able to induce apoptosis via intrinsic and extrinsic pathway [284].

In SGC7901 cells, resveratrol was able to induce apoptosis and developed a pro-oxidant role, inducing the generation of reactive oxygen species. A treatment of this cells with a scavenger eliminated the pro-apoptotic effect of resveratrol, indicating that the pro-oxidant role of this polyphenol is essential for the apoptosis [285].

### 4.1.2. Calcium Homeostasis

Calcium also appears to be an important role in apoptosis induces for curcumin. This polyphenol promoted apoptosis in color cancer cells through the increase in $[Ca^{2+}]$ and ROS formation. These effects promote a reduction in MMP and generate caspase-3 activation. The use of an intracellular calcium chelator promote a reversion in apoptosis [286]. A similar result was observed in human leukemia cells and was also verified that the caspase-3 inhibitor (z-VAD-fmk) was capable to block curcumin-induced apoptosis [287].

In a different study, the levels of ROS and intracellular $[Ca^{2+}]$ increased by curcumin have shown an important contribution to cause apoptosis. The use of the mitochondrial uniporter inhibitor (RU-360) partially suppressed curcumin-induced apoptosis. Moreover, the use of SKF-96365, a store-operated $Ca^{2+}$ channel blocker, blocked the elevation of mitochondrial calcium, promoting a potentiation in curcumin-induced apoptosis [288].

Using human hepatocellular carcinoma J5 cells, it was also demonstrated for curcumin the ability to induce apoptosis through $Ca^{2+}$-regulated mitochondria-dependent pathway. In vitro assays have demonstrated an increased level of cytoplasmatic cytochrome c, corroborating with reduced mitochondrial membrane potential hypothesis. Once again, for these cells it was observed an increase in ROS formation and cytoplasmic calcium accumulation. BAPTA, an intracellular calcium chelator, was capable to reduce curcumin-induced apoptosis, suggesting that this process is calcium dependent in these cells lines [289].

In mesothelioma cells (REN cells), resveratrol was able to induce a transient intracellular $[Ca^{2+}]$ elevation possibly by T-type $Ca^{2+}$ channels. Experiments were run toward to Cav 3.2 isoform of this channel because its shown to be highly expressed in REN cells. The results have demonstrated that it is the major responsible for $Ca^{2+}$ entry. Besides, Cav 3.2 siRNA inhibited the effect of resveratrol, which indicates the role of this channel. A comparison between normal cells and mesothelioma cells was studied and a difference in the peak levels of calcium have demonstrated a higher sensibility of cancer cells to resveratrol-induced changes. Furthermore, in cancer cells resveratrol was able to inhibit proliferation whereas in normal cells it was ineffective [290].

### 4.1.3. Bcl-2 Family

In follicular lymphoma cell lines, curcumin inhibited the cellular proliferation and induced apoptosis through the increase in bcl-2 family proteins. The authors demonstrated a reduction in Bcl-xL levels for all cell lines. In addition, they characterized cell line-dependent changes in the level of Mcl-1, bcl-w, Bak, and Bok. All these process promotes increased levels of ROS. Curcumin also increase the lysosomal membrane permeability [291].

Similar observations were made for other cancer cell lines, including glioblastoma, colorectal, lung and endometrial carcinoma [292,293]. In human prostate cancer cells, it was observed reduction of pro-apoptotic proteins and induction of caspase 3 and PARP cleavage [294]. Yu and Shah (2007) verified through transfected human endometrial adenocarcinoma HEC-1-A cells the possibility of proto-oncogene Ets-1 promote Bcl-2 regulation [295]. The authors observed that curcumin was capable to downregulate the Ets-1 gene and reduce Bcl-2 expression. For HEC-1-A cells, it was found DNA fragmentation induced by curcumin in a dose-dependent manner.

The in vivo effect of Curcumin on Bcl-2 and Bax expression was described using nude mice prostate cancer (PC3 cell line) [296]. Three groups were treated with different concentrations of this compound and showed an expressive reduction in tumor volume at all concentrations compared to control groups.

Huang and colleagues have shown the apoptotic effect of resveratrol in nasopharyngeal carcinoma cells. In their study, Bcl-2 was downregulated and Bax protein was upregulated. The expressive increase in the Bax/Bcl-2 ratio is responsible for the apoptosis due to the apoptotic properties of Bax. Besides that, it was also observed the release of cytochrome c due to the disruption of the mitochondrial membrane potential, and the activation of caspase-9 and -3. The last one responsible to cause DNA fragmentation and apoptosis [297].

Corroborating with previous results, Wang and co-workers have demonstrated in human leukemia cells the apoptotic effect of resveratrol and its ability to interfere in the regulation of proteins of Bcl-2 family. The ratio Bax/Bcl-2 increases, which induces the permeabilization of the outer mitochondrial membrane and the release of pro-apoptotic proteins. In their study, it was shown the decrease of cytochrome c level of the intermembrane space in the mitochondria and its increase in the cytosol. In addition, caspase-3 activity was increased as well [298].

Cholangiocarcinoma, human acute leukemia, liver and pancreatic cancer cell lines have demonstrated to be sensitive to resveratrol. In all four-cell lines, this polyphenol was able to induce apoptosis by reducing Bcl-2 levels and increase caspase-3 activity. Furthermore, in pancreatic cells was also demonstrated an up-regulation in Bax and downregulation in Bcx-xL and XIAP, and in liver cancer cells an increase in p53 expression protein was also detected [299–301].

### 4.1.4. p53 Family

The TP53 gene is responsible for p53 protein codification, which is a transcription factor involved in cellular regulation, as well as, tumor suppression. Its effect occurs due to activation of repair proteins or induction of apoptosis, when cellular damages are irreversible [302–304]. This factor are present in both intrinsic and extrinsic pathways, and acts on the changes of mitochondrial membrane potential as cell sensitization to apoptosis [304].

According to He and co-workers [57], curcumin can ameliorate the general health state of patients with colorectal cancer through the increase of p53 expression in tumor cells. This study conducted with 126 patients, revealed that curcumin promotes an increase in weight body of the individuals when compared to control group (vehicle). After surgery, immunoblotting assay revealed that anti-apoptotic protein Bcl-2 was reduced and Bax was elevated. TNF-α level was also lower than control group, probably for p53 modulation. Thus, the authors have suggested that curcumin can be used in the treatment to ameliorate cachexia in these patients.

In breast cancer, it was demonstrated that resveratrol was not able to induce p53 protein expression, but expressively increased the phosphorylation in Ser15, resulting in a higher level of phospho-p53. When phosphorylated, p53 protein reduce its interaction with MDM2, an oncoprotein that regulates it negatively, what results in cell cycle arrest or apoptosis [305].

Notch-1 is a transmembrane receptor that mediates intracellular signalling involved in cell differentiation and cell survival [306]. In glioblastoma cells were demonstrated that Notch-1 activation and p-53 restoration by resveratrol was correlated. Glioblastoma cells were treated with a Notch-1 inhibitor (MRK-003) and resulted in a decrease of p53 restoration and significantly inhibition of p53 translocation to the nucleus, which indicates that Notch-1 activated is able to augment p53 expression and restore its function. In these cells, the activation of Notch-1-p53 signaling pathway indicates to be an initiating factor of apoptosis induced by resveratrol, with increased Bax expression and decreased Bcl-2 expression [307].

p73 is another transcription factor, belonging to p53 family, related to apoptosis and cancer progression. The p73 presents several functions in nervous system. Structurally, it is more complex than p53 because the conserved region in DNA-binding domain is also more complex [303]. p73 is responsible to perform the transcription of two isoform of proteins: TAp73 (related with tumor suppression and chemotherapy induced-apoptosis); and DNp73 (present in tumor cells and associated with chemoresistance) [308,309]. A research with p73 transfected Hep3B (p53-deficient) showed apoptosis induction when treated with curcumin at concentrations ranging from 40 to 80 μM. Western blot data have revealed an increase of TAp73 and reduction of DNp73 protein in the same concentrations necessary to induce apoptosis. MMP (mitochondrial membrane potential) were reduced and it was accompanied for cytochrome c release, cleavage of pro-caspase-9, pro-caspase-3, and pro-PARP [310].

### 4.1.5. Extrinsic Pathway (Receptor-Mediated Pathway)

The extrinsic pathway is mediated by triggering cell surface death receptors of the tumor necrosis factor (TNF) receptor superfamily (TNF-R1, Fas/CD95, TRAIL-R1/DR4 and TRAIL-R2/DR5). After that, an adaptor, FADD (Fas-associated death domain protein), for example, binds to the receptor and a trimerized receptor-ligand complex (DISC—death-inducing signaling complex) is shaped. Thus, DISC recruits the initiator caspase-8, which is now activated [311]. In type I cells, caspase-8 activation is sufficient to apoptosis occurrence as a direct consequence, with activating downstream caspases such as caspase-3. In type II cells, the apoptosis is dependent on the amplification of death receptors via the mitochondrial pathway. The link between these two pathways occurs via Bid cleavage by caspase-8. The truncated bid interacts with Bax, promoting cytochrome c release and downstream events [312].

TRAIL (TNF-related apoptosis-inducing ligand) is the ligand of the death receptors DR4 and DR5. Some types of cells, like LNCaP (prostate cancer), are resistant to TRAIL-induced apoptosis. Shankar et al. have studied the resveratrol and curcumin ability to sensitize this prostate cancer cells to TRAIL. The results have demonstrated that these polyphenols were able to sensitize the cells to TRAIL, and they were also able to upregulate the TRAILs receptors, DR4 and DR5. Furthermore, the death receptor pathway was demonstrated to be involved in sensitization of TRAIL-resistant cells by resveratrol and curcumin [313,314].

An in vivo study with curcumin corroborates with the data above. LNCaP cells were xenografted in Balb nude mice and treatments with curcumin, TRAIL and curcumin + TRAIL was evaluated. Curcumin alone is able to induce apoptosis in tumor cells, while TRAIL is ineffective. When together, they are able to increase the cell death to values higher than curcumin alone, demonstrating that this natural product sensitize TRAIL-resistant cells [156].

In chondrosarcoma cells, curcumin was able to induce the cleavage of caspase-3, -7 and -8, but not -9, which indicates the activation of extrinsic pathway. Furthermore, it was also demonstrated an increase in Fas, FasL and DR5 expression by curcumin treatment, and transfection with siRNA of this components reduced apoptosis. p53 was also evaluated in this study, and it was shown to be able to participate of death receptor increased expression. Taken together, these results suggest that curcumin-induced cell death in chondrosarcoma cells occurs by extrinsic pathway [315].

In anaplastic large-cell lymphoma, resveratrol has induced apoptosis in a dose-dependent manner. In the same study, it was demonstrated that this phytoalexin was also able to induce the expression of the death receptor Fas/CD95 about twice folds when cells were treated with 25 μM of resveratrol for 48 h, indicating that extrinsic pathway may be a mechanism of this cellular apoptosis [316].

A link between intrinsic and extrinsic apoptotic pathway induced by resveratrol was demonstrated in multiple myeloma and T-cell leukemia cells. In the death receptor pathway, resveratrol induced the association of membrane rafts and Fas/CD95 and translocated DR4 and DR5 (TRAIL-receptors) to rafts. FADD, procaspase-8 and -10 were also translocated into rafts, as well as its actives forms. These data indicate that the constituents of DISC (FADD, Fas/CD95 and procaspase-8) are recruited into rafts, and this apoptotic complex in death receptor signaling is activated. Furthermore, Bid, which is a linker between Fas signaling and mitochondria was also translocated to raft. This data indicates a connection between intrinsic and extrinsic apoptotic pathway, which was demonstrated by blocking Fas/CD95 downstream signaling what prevented loss in membrane mitochondrial potential [317].

Endoplasmatic Reticulum (ER) Stress

Curcumin promotes apoptosis induction at a dose and time-dependent manner in human lung cancer cells. Besides the upregulation of the pro-apoptotic proteins Bax and Bad, an increased level of ROS accompanied for ER stress in these cells after treatment with curcumin was observed. These alterations conduce to MMP (mitochondrial membrane potential) modification and caspase-3 activation. The authors concluded that an activation of extrinsic pathway through increased FAS/CD95 expression promotes caspase-8 activation. This data was confirmed by using a caspase-8 inhibitor, which decreased the apoptosis in these cells [318].

4.1.6. NF-κβ

The levels of NF-κβ are increased in pancreatic carcinoma cells. It was demonstrated that curcumin reduces this levels, promotes apoptosis and inhibits cellular proliferation. Reduction in the levels of I-κB kinase (IKK), NF-κβ, as well as, cyclooxygenase-2 (COX-2), prostaglandin E2 (PGE-2), and interleukin-8 (IL-8) were observed after treatment using curcumin [319].

Similar results were obtained using melanoma cells, where curcumin inhibited NF-kβ and IKK independently from B-Raf mutations or PI3K/Akt pathway. The authors did not found a direct correlation between IL-8 and NF-κβ for melanoma cells, and they hypothesized that IL-8 regulation could occur through AP-1 transcription factor [48].

In a different study using glioblastoma cells, curcumin was selective against cancer cells and promoted a reduction in NF-κβ and IKK leading to apoptosis [320].

Sun et al. have investigated the role of the inhibition of NF-κB in resveratrol-induced apoptosis in human multiple myeloma cells. When activated, p65 subunit of NF-κB is translocated to the nucleus, which lead the researches to evaluate its presence in the cytoplasm. As result, they found the vast majority of NF-κB in this compartment, where it could not function as transcription factor. Furthermore, the targets genes of NF-κB were also evaluated, and as expected, they were down regulated. Bcl-2, Bcl-xL, XIAP, c-IAP and VEGF are proteins resultant from the target genes activated by NF-κB [321].

Another example of the role of NF-κB in resveratrol-induced apoptosis was demonstrated in human breast cancer cells. EMSA experiments have shown a decrease in the p65(RelA)/p50 binding to the DNA at resveratrol levels that induces apoptosis. This result may be attributed to the lower level of NF-κB activated in nucleus due to the increase of the protein I-κB in the cytosol. These data were confirmed through the dose-dependent increased level of p65/(RelA) immunoprecipitated by an anti I-κB antibody. In this case, Bcl-2 was down regulated [322].

A study with multiple myeloma cells has demonstrated the ability of resveratrol to suppress the constitutively active IKK, which is necessary for NF-κB activation. Furthermore, resveratrol also inhibited the appearance of subunit p65 in the nucleus [323].

### 4.1.7. PI3K, Akt/mTOR

Phosphotydilinositol-3 kinase (PI3K) is a lipid kinase family, which is activated by receptors with protein tyrosine kinase activity (RPTK). When RPTK is activated, PI3K associates with the receptor leading to the catalytic subunit activation and formation of the second messenger phosphatidylinositol-3,4,5-trisphosphate (PIP3). PIP3 recruits signaling proteins with pleckstrin homology (PH) domains to the membrane, including PDK1 and Akt. Akt activated has the ability to modulate the function of various substrates that are involved in cell survival, cell cycle progression and cellular growth [221].

Akt/PI3K is an important pathway for apoptosis regulation. In breast cancer cells, curcumin induced an Akt and glycogen synthase kinase 3b (GSK3B) phosphorylation. This kinase is involved in apoptosis process [324]. However, curiously in both cells: T-cell acute lymphoblastic leukemia (T-ALL) malignant cells and upper aero-digestive tract cancer cell; curcumin promotes the de-phosphorylation/inactivation of Akt, FOXO transcription factor and GSK3 [325,326].

FOXO transcription factors have been correlated with induction and cancer regulation. Pancreatic cancer cells treated with curcumin, presented an increased in FOXO1 (Forkhead box O1) expression, which is correlated with inhibition in phosphorylation/activation of PI3K and Akt [327].

mTOR, an Akt upstream modulator, was inhibited in vitro by curcumin using uterine leiomyosarcoma cells. Western Blot data revealed that curcumin has restrained p70S6 and S6 phosphorylations; both ribosomal proteins are downstream targets of mTOR. Interestingly, in the presence of a mTOR inhibitor (rapamycin), it was not observed apoptosis [328]. In vivo assay, using female nude mice, shows that curcumin decreases m-TOR and S6 phosphorylation leading to a reduction in tumor size [329].

In a time-dependent manner, resveratrol was able to reduce Akt phosphorylation, decrease the level of Akt protein and the phosphorylation of caspase-9, sequentially, in human breast cancer cells. Assuming that caspase-9 is a site for Akt and now it is activated, it indicates that this is one of the pathways for resveratrol-induced apoptosis [330].

Another pathway involving Akt activity and resveratrol-induced apoptosis was studied in human chronic myeloid leukemia cells. Hsp70, a heat shock protein, is responsible for helping the cell to maintain protein homeostasis and scape apoptosis and, in the cited cells, is overexpressed. The expression of Hsp genes is regulated by transcription factors of HSF (heat shock factor) family. In this study, resveratrol was able to decrease the phosphorylation of Akt, which is essential for its activity. GSK3B is a target of Akt and its phosphorylated form is inactive. Assuming that Akt is not able to phosphorylate GSK3B, then it is able to prevent HSF-1 to enter the nucleus and activate Hsp70 expression [331,332].

Studies have demonstrated that Akt is a direct regulator of miR21 expression [333]. PC-3M-MM2 cells exhibit a high level of phosphorylated Akt, which it is shown, in this study, to be decreased by resveratrol as well as miR-21 expression. To corroborate with this supposition, this androgen-independent human prostate carcinoma cells was treated with LY294002, a well-known inhibitor of Akt activity. The results demonstrated that the expression of miR-21 was also decreased, indicating that Akt may be a target for cancer treatment [334].

Dai et al. have studied in chondrosarcoma cells the ability of resveratrol to interfere in PI3K activity. By western blot analysis, it was demonstrated that the PI3K, Akt and AMPK levels decreased significantly in a concentration of resveratrol enough to cause apoptosis. This result suggest that the inhibition of PI3K pathway by resveratrol may be a molecular mechanism to suppress cancer cell proliferation [335].

### 4.1.8. Telomerase

Telomerase is a reverse transcriptase, responsible to regulation of telomeric length of chromosomes, doing addition of repetitive sequences with guanine. This enzyme is expressed in proliferations cells, as germinal cells and cancer [336].

High levels of telomerase are found in tumor cells, and studies suggest this target as potential for anticancer drug development. In human leukemia cells and acute myeloblastic leukemia cells curcumin has inhibited telomerase activity, at dose and time-dependent manner. This activity is probably due to suppression of translocation of the catalytic subunit of telomerase (TERT—telomerase reverse transcriptase) from nucleus to cytosol. Curcumin induced apoptosis by increasing Bax and reducing Bcl-2, which promotes activation of caspase-3 and release of cytochrome c. The authors have suggested that a relationship between curcumin-induced apoptosis parameters and telomerase inhibition can exist [337,338].

Similar results were obtained using brain tumor cells. Khaw and collaborators identified that curcumin binds to cell surface and hen seeps into the cytoplasm in order to initiate the apoptotic cascade. TRAP assay and PCR revealed that curcumin inhibited telomerase activity through the inhibition in hTERT mRNA expression. This effect provokes a reduction of a telomere size. Moreover, caspase-3 and caspase-7 levels are increased [339].

A study carried out with MCF-7 cells has demonstrated the effect of resveratrol in telomerase activity. In a dose dependent manner, resveratrol was able to decrease the cellular viability and induce apoptosis. These events were related to resveratrol ability to down regulated TLMA, reduce the level of hTERT (catalytic subunit of human telomerase reverse transcriptase) of the nuclear compartment, where it is able to elongate the telomere and increase its levels in the cytoplasm, indicating that this phitoalexin is able to interfere in the process of translocation of this subunit to the nucleus [340].

In A431 epidermoid carcinoma cells, resveratrol was able to inhibit telomerase activity in a dose independent manner. Moreover, resveratrol was also able to decrease the expression of hTERT by inhibition of RNA transcription [341].

### 4.1.9. JAK/STAT

STAT-3 (Signal transducer and activator of transcription 3) is a protein that has a dual role in normal cells, as cytoplasmic signaling proteins and as nuclear transcription factors that activates diverse genes. Among the genes regulated by STATs are the genes that control proliferation, apoptosis, angiogenesis and immune responses [342]. Simplistically, JAK2 is a tyrosine kinase responsible for the phosphorylation and activation of STAT-3, which is now able to enter into the nucleus and activate its target genes [343].

In human leukemia cells curcumin reduced the nuclear expression of STAT-3, 5a and 5b in dose and time-dependent manner. In addition, STAT-5a and 5b was followed by truncated isoforms formation, indicating that curcumin was able to induce the cleavage of STAT-5 into its dominant negative variants (lacking the STAT5 C-terminal region). However, it was not observed modifications in STAT-1 expression, only reduction in its transactivation. STAT-3, 5a and 5b phosphorylation was maintained and mRNA of Jak-2 was reduced as well as cyclin D1 and v-src gene expression [344].

Similar results were obtained in other researches with primary effusion lymphoma, Hodgkin's lymphoma, cutaneous T-cell lymphoma and melanoma cells. These studies have found that curcumin reduces phosphorylation in Jak-2 or Jak-1 and STAT-3. These regulations provoke an apoptosis induction, reduction in Bcl-2, activation in caspase-3 and PARP cleavage [345–348].

In head and neck tumor cells, STAT-3 is overexpressed in comparison to others tumor cells. It was shown that resveratrol has inhibited the constitutive activation of STAT-3 and JAK2, the tyrosine kinase of the Janus family responsible for the STAT-3 phosphorylation. Beyond that, resveratrol inhibited STAT-3-DNA binding, because of the decreased phosphorylation level, which inhibits STAT-3 to translocate to the nucleus. Furthermore, resveratrol was also able to induce the expression of SOCS-1 (suppressor of cytokine signaling 1) protein and mRNA. SOCS-1 is a negative regulator of STAT-3 by inhibiting JAK2. STAT-3 is also known for its expression regulation of various genes products involved in anti-apoptosis (Bcl-2, Bcl-xL, survivin and others), which was found to be downregulated in resveratrol treatment [349].

In NK leukemia cells, resveratrol, in a time and dose-dependent manner, inhibited constitutively phosphorylation of STAT-3 and JAK2, which resulted in a decrease of downstream anti-apoptotic proteins MCL1, surviving and Bcl-10 [350].

In bladder and ovarian cancer cells, beyond the inhibition of STAT-3 expression and phosphorylation, it was demonstrated the reduction of STAT-3 into the nucleus. In consequence of this event, STAT-3 downstream anti apoptotic products genes were suppressed [351,352].

### 4.1.10. miRNA

miRNAs are portions of RNA that can not be transcript in proteins, and lately several works have established its role in many diseases, including cancer. Despite of this importance, until now is not known its exact function in many human diseases [353].

According to the literature, Bcl-2 is a target of miRNA15a and miRNA16 [354]. In human breast adenocarcinoma (MCF-7 cells), it was observed a downregulation in Bcl-2 and upregulation of mi-R15a and mi-R16 when exposed to different concentration of curcumin. In breast carcinoma cell lines, it was also found that curcumin was capable to upregulate these miRNA and the use of anti-miRNA15a and anti-miRNA16 promoted a renovation of Bcl-2 expression. Thus, curcumin can induce miR-15a and miR-16 expression and it can probably serve as potential gene therapy targets for Bcl-2-overexpressing tumors [355].

Curcumin increased miRNA16 in A549 human lung adenocarcinoma cell line, but promoted a significantly downregulation in miRNA186*. Authors observed that the use of an inhibitor for mRNA186*, not only reduce cellular proliferation but also promote apoptosis, indicating that miR-186* may play an oncogenic role in the development of lung cancer. Moreover, it was observed that modifications in miR-186* levels cause changes in caspase-10 levels. This enzyme appears to be increased in cell treated with curcumin [356].

Another study showed the relationship between curcumin and miRNA186* in treatment of multidrug-resistant cells of lung carcinoma (A549/DDP cells). These cells are sensitive to curcumin treatment, which can modify miRNA186* expression. The authors concluded that mRNA-186* can be a target for lung cancer susceptible to curcumin treatment [357].

In human glioma cells, resveratrol was able to inhibit the expression of the microRNA 21 (miR-21) that is found to be overexpressed in this type of cancer. Furthermore, it was studied the involvement of miR-21 and the resveratrol-induced apoptosis in these cells. It was found that the downregulation of miR-21 expression decreases the phosphorylation of I-kB and nuclear p65 protein levels, which leads to an inactivation of NF-κB signaling and, consequently, apoptosis [358].

Bcl-2 is a key regulator of apoptosis and it has been reported to be positive regulated by miR-21. To analyze if this is the mechanism involved in resveratrol-induced apoptosis in pancreatic cancer cells, Liu et al. have studied this purpose. Real-time PCR has demonstrated the ability of resveratrol to decreased the expression of miR-21, and western blot has demonstrated that Bcl-2 is downregulated by resveratrol, but it is restored by overexpression of miR-21. These results indicate that in pancreatic cancer cells the apoptosis induced by resveratrol is due to inhibiting miR-21 regulation of Bcl-2 expression [359].

A study realized by Zhou et al. in bladder cancer cells, resulted in the same data that Liu et al. demonstrating the ability of resveratrol to reduce miR-21 and Bcl-2. Furthermore, this study was able to indicate that Akt also participates of this process. It was demonstrated that resveratrol inhibits miR-21 expression, and as a consequence decreases Akt phosphorylation and Bcl-2 expression. The inhibition of Bcl-2 was counteracted by an Akt stimulator, demonstrating that in these cells, resveratrol is able to induce apoptosis by the regulation of Akt/Bcl-2 signaling pathway by inhibiting miR-21 expression [360].

## 4.2. Autophagy

This kind of cellular death are characterized for the formation of vesicles with cellular organelles (autophagosome), that promote an auto phagocytic process [361,362]. An important difference when compared to apoptosis, is that autophagy do not promote chromatin condensation and it is accompanied by massive autophagic vacuolization of the cytoplasm [362]. At cellular level the autophagic death can be considered as reversible process, once the stimuli is removed the cellular death process is interrupted [362].

Curcumin can induce autophagy in glioma cell lines, regulated by simultaneous inhibition of the Akt/mTOR/p70S6K pathway and stimulation of the ERK1/2 pathway. The last one regulates extracellular signalization, and when are activated promote autophagy. In vivo models using nude mice have revealed that curcumin reduced the tumor size by inducing autophagy. The mechanism seems to be related to LC3, an autophagosome-specific protein, that was increased in tumor treated for this polyphenol [363].

AMP is a kinase involved in metabolism of eukaryotic cells and its deregulation seems to be related with cancer process [364]. Similarly, in human adenocarcinoma cell line curcumin has promoted an autophagy process that was not observed in human normal lung cells. In this study, the authors observed an increased phosphorylation of AMP (AMPK) and acetylCoA carboxylase. The use of a si-RNA knockdown of a catalytic subunit of AMP kinase (AMPK$\alpha$1) promotes a reduction in LC3-II, suggesting that this pathway is important to autophagy in these cell lines [365].

An in vitro and in vivo study with breast cancer stem-like cells has demonstrated the ability of resveratrol to decreased the cell viability in both systems. Thus, the cell death by autophagy was studied. It was demonstrated that resveratrol treatment increased the number of autophagossomes, upregulated the expression of LC3-II, Beclin1 and Atg 7, which are required for autophagossome formation, and GFP-LC3-II puncta formation assay demonstrated an increase in the percentage of cells with autophagossomes compared with control. It was also demonstrated that resveratrol induces autophagy, at least partially, via suppressing Wnt/$\beta$catenin signaling pathway [366].

In melanoma cells, resveratrol treatment has induced a dose and time-dependent accumulation of LC3-II, significantly upregulation of Beclin-1 and induction of the formation of LC3 puncta, suggesting that resveratrol induces autophagy in these cells, and this event is regulated by ceramides, which regulates Akt/mTOR pathway. Interestingly results appeared when the conversion of LC3-I in LC3-II and Beclin-1 formation were inhibited. The cytotoxic effect of resveratrol increased as well as the apoptosis. It indicates that, in this case, autophagy acts as a resistance mechanism against apoptotic cell death, and inhibition of this event could be a novel strategy of treatment [367].

Others apoptotic targets have been studied for curcumin (Table 4) and resveratrol (Table 5).

**Table 4.** Others apoptotic targets for curcumin.

| Target | Effect | Cancer Type | Reference |
|---|---|---|---|
| AP-2γ | inhibition | testicular | [368] |
| MST1 | activation | melanoma | [369] |
| Hexoquinase-2 | downregulation | colorectal | [370] |
| Skp2/Her2 | downregulation | breast | [371] |
| GADD45/153 | upregulation | lung | [372] |
| Proteasome | inhibition | colon | [373] |
| Aurora A | downregulation | bladder | [374] |
| AMPK | activation | colon | [375] |
| Cdc27/APC3 | inhibition | medulloblastoma | [376] |
| HDAC 4 | inhibition | medulloblastoma | [377] |
| PKC | downregulation | liver | [378] |
| Sp1 | inhibition | lung | [379] |
| Microtúbulo | inhibition | breast | [380] |
| Ras/ERK signaling | activation | gastric | [381] |
| Fatty acid synthase | inhibition | liver | [382] |

**Table 5.** Others examples of apoptotic targets for resveratrol.

| Target | Effect | Cancer Type | Reference |
|---|---|---|---|
| 5-LOX | downregulation | mammary | [383] |
| COX 2 | upregulation | ovarian | [384,385] |
| ΔNp63 | downregulation | nasopharyngeal | [386] |
| Hexoquinase 2 | downregulation | hepatocellular | [387] |
| MTA1 | downregulation | prostate | [388] |
| Specificity protein 1 | inhibition | mesothelioma | [389] |
| GADD45α/Annexin A1 | upregulation | leukemia | [390] |
| p21 | upregulation | breast | [391] |
| ASPP1 | upregulation | breast | [392] |
| TIGAR | downregulation | Lung/breast | [393] |
| Casein kinase (CK2) | downregulation | prostate | [394] |
| IRE1α/XBP1 | upregulation | Multiple myeloma | [395] |
| Androgen receptor | downregulation | prostate | [396] |
| Caspase-6 | upregulation | colon | [397] |
| CHOP | upregulation | colon | [398] |
| Cathepsin L/B | activation | Cervical/colorectal | [399,400] |
| ATF3 | upregulation | colorectal | [401] |
| Fatty acid synthase | downregulation | breast | [402] |
| Hedgehog signaling | downregulation | pancreas | [403] |
| Tristetraprolin | activation | glioma | [404] |
| SphK1/S1P | downregulation | leukemia | [405] |
| Proteasome | activation | leukemia | [406] |
| Pentose phosphate and talin-FAK pathway | downregulation | colon | [407] |

## 5. Perspectives

The antitumoral properties of resveratrol and curcumin have been described in a number of studies using different types of cancers, including lung, breast, colon, leukemia, lymphoma, melanoma, multiple myeloma, neuroblastoma, osteosarcoma, ovarian, pancreatic, and prostate [107,108,277,278]. The majority of these studies have evaluated the anticancer properties of resveratrol or curcumin by itself (no-association) through in vitro or in vivo assays [408,409]. These studies conducted to hypothesis about the mechanism of action, whereby these polyphenols acted in the cell through down- or upregulation of important proteins, transcription factors and cytokines. Nevertheless, these polyphenols present non-specific action, considering the wide range of molecular targets that they can act. These non-specific activities are in fact, very different from the traditional chemotherapeutics that hit only one (or very few targets) in most of the cases [410]. This plurality of molecular targets associated to polyphenols have been generating divergent opinions in literature about the real contribution that such phytochemicals may have in anticancer therapy [37,145,410–413]. Nonetheless, there are a number of reviews in literature that highlight the cancer chemoprevention effect exerted by these polyphenols [414–419]. This chemopreventive effect has been associated to the anti-inflammatory properties of these phytochemicals, especially through the antioxidant activity [420–423].

Not only those targets discussed in this review, but also ability to complex with the DNA was described for both polyphenols. Using infrared spectroscopy, it was demonstrated that curcumin is able to interact with guanine, adenine and thymine, and the backbone $PO_2$ in the DNA structure. It was also shown the ability of curcumin to complex the RNA molecule, which maintain its A-RNA conformation upon curcumin complexation [424,425].

Furthermore, there are a variety of studies involving these polyphenols in combination with approved anti-cancer drugs and its implication in anticancer combination therapy. These studies highlight the application of curcumin and resveratrol along with anticancer drugs aiming to improve the efficacy of the treatment. We highlighted in Table 6 some examples of polyphenols and anticancer drugs in combination regimens evaluated in vitro or in vivo.

**Table 6.** Combination therapy of polyphenols and approved anti-cancer drugs.

| Polyphenol | Drug | Cancer Type | Reference |
|------------|------|-------------|-----------|
| curcumin | cisplatin | lung | [426] |
| curcumin | cisplatin | head and neck | [427] |
| curcumin | valproic acid | leukemia | [428] |
| curcumin | gemcitabine | pancreatic | [429] |
| curcumin | 5-fluorouracil | breast | [430] |
| curcumin | 5-fluorouracil | gastric | [431] |
| curcumin | 5-fluorouracil + oxaliplatin | colon | [432] |
| curcumin | bevacizumab | liver | [433] |
| curcumin | imatinib | leukemia | [434] |
| curcumin | paclitaxel | brain | [435] |
| curcumin | oxaliplatin | colorectal | [436] |
| curcumin | temozolomide | glioblastoma | [437] |
| curcumin | gefitinib | lung | [438] |
| resveratrol | cisplatin | ovarian | [439] |
| resveratrol | cisplatin | colorectal | [440] |
| resveratrol | 5-fluorouracil | colorectal | [441] |
| resveratrol | 5-fluorouracil | melanoma | [442] |
| resveratrol | doxorubicin | breast | [443] |
| resveratrol | doxorubicin | leukemia | [444] |
| resveratrol | melphalan | breast | [445] |
| resveratrol | temozolomide | glioma | [446] |
| resveratrol | gemcitabine | pancreatic | [447] |
| resveratrol | paclitaxel | neuroblastoma | [448] |
| resveratrol | tamoxifen | breast | [449] |
| resveratrol | cyclophosphamide | breast | [450] |

The combinations of polyphenols (resveratrol and curcumin) within anticancer drugs have demonstrated in several cases a synergic effect and it seems to be a useful strategy to treat cancer.

Studies involving humans to test both polyphenols against cancer is being performed. Tables 7 and 8 describe the current studies registered in US at different stages. It is possible to observe a high number of studies recruiting volunteers, which reveals the interest in both polyphenols by scientific community. Not only treatment against cancer but also chemoprevention and palliative care is being investigated (Tables 7 and 8).

**Table 7.** Human studies using curcumin in cancer.

| Cancer Treatment | | | |
|---|---|---|---|
| **Intervention** | **Study** | **Status** | **NCT Number** |
| Curcumin and 5-fluoracil (5-FU) | Curcumin in combination with 5-FU for colon cancer | Recruiting | NCT02724202 (Phase 0) |
| Curcumin and capecitabine | Curcumin, capecitabine and radiation therapy followed by surgery for rectal cancer | Ongoing, but not recruiting | NCT00745134 (Phase II) |
| Curcumin | Trial of curcumin in advanced-pancreatic cancer | Completed | NCT00094445 (Phase II) |
| Curcumin | Phase II study of curcumin versus placebo for chemotherapy-treated breast cancer patients undergoing radiotherapy | Recruiting | NCT01740323 (Phase II) |
| Avastin and Curcumin | Avastin/folfiri in combination with curcumin in colorectal cancer patients with metastasis | Recruiting | NCT02439385 (Phase II) |
| Gemcitabine and curcumin | Gemcitabine With Curcumin for Pancreatic Cancer | Completed | NCT00192842 (Phase II) |
| Curcumin | Effect of Curcumin in Treatment of Squamous Cervical Intraepithelial Neoplasias (CINs) | Recruiting | NCT02554344 |
| Gemcitabine, curcumin and celecoxib | Phase III Trial of Gemcitabine, Curcumin and Celebrex in Patients with Metastatic Colon Cancer | Unknown | NCT00295035 |
| Curcumin and Docetaxel | Multicenter Study Comparing Taxotere Plus Curcumin Versus Taxotere Plus Placebo Combination in First-line Treatment of Prostate Cancer Metastatic Castration Resistant (CURTAXEL) (CURTAXEL) | Ongoing, but not recruiting | NCT02095717 (Phase II) |
| Curcumin and Docetaxel | Docetaxel With or Without a Phytochemical in Treating Patients with Breast Cancer | Recruiting | NCT00852332 (Phase II) |
| Gemcitabine, curcumin and celebrex | Phase III trial of gemcitabine, curcumin and celebrex in patients with advance or inoperable pancreatic cancer | Unknown | NCT00486460 (Phase III) |
| Curcumin and cholecalciferol | Curcumin and cholecalciferol in treating patients with previously untreated stage 0-II Chronic lymphocytic leukemia or small lymphocytic lymphoma | Recruiting | NCT0210042 (Phase II) |
| Curcumin and bioperine | Pilot study of curcumin (diferuloylmethane derivative) with or without bioperine in patients with multiple myeloma | Completed | NCT00113841 |
| Curcumin | Use of curcumin for treatment of intestinal adenomas in familial adenomatous polyposis (FAP) | Recruiting | NCT00927485 |
| Anthocyanins and curcumin | Randomized window of opportunity trial of anthocyanin extract and phospholipid curcumin in subjects with colorectal adenoma | Recruiting | NCT0194866 (Phase II) |
| Curcumin and Ashwagandha extract | Pilot study of curcumin formulation and Ashwagandha extract in advanced osteosarcoma | Unknown | NCT00689195 (Phase I/II) |
| Curcumin | Turmeric effect on reduction of serum prolactin and related hormonal change and adenoma size in prolactinoma patients | Unknown | NCT0134429 (Phase I) |
| **Adverse Effects Management Induced by Chemotherapy** | | | |
| **Intervention** | **Study** | **Status** | **NCT Number** |
| Curcumin | Curcumin for the Prevention of Radiation-induced Dermatitis in Breast Cancer Patients | Completed | NCT01042938 (Phase II) |
| Curcumin | Radiosensitizing and Radioprotectve Effects of Curcumin in Prostate Cancer | Completed | NCT01917890 |
| Curcumin and FOLFOX | Combining Curcumin With FOLFOX Chemotherapy in Patients with Inoperable Colorectal Cancer (CUFOX) | Ongoing, but no Recruiting | NCT01490996 (Phase I/II) |
| Curcumin | Nanocurcumin for Prostate Cancer Patients Undergoing Radiotherapy (RT) | Recruiting | NCT02724618 (Phase II) |

Table 7. *Cont.*

| Adverse Effects Management Induced by Chemotherapy | | | |
|---|---|---|---|
| Intervention | Study | Status | NCT Number |
| Curcumin and Tirosine kinase inhibitors | An Open-label Prospective Cohort Trial of Curcumin Plus Tyrosine Kinase Inhibitors (TKI) for EGFR -Mutant Advanced NSCLC (CURCUMIN) | Recruiting | NCT02321293 (Phase I) |
| Curcumin | Prophylactic Topical Agents in Reducing Radiation-Induced Dermatitis in Patients with Non-inflammatory Breast Cancer or Breast Cancer in Situ (Curcumin-II) | Ongoing, but no recruiting | NCT02556632 (Phase II) |
| Curcumin | Effect of curcumin addition to standard treatment on tumor-induced inflammation in endometrial carcinoma | Recruiting | NCT02017353 (Phase II) |
| Curcumin | Curcumin for prevention of oral mucositis in children using chemotherapy | Completed | NCT00475683 (Phase III) |
| Curcumin | Oral curcumin for radiation dermatitis in breast cancer patients | Completed | NCT01246973 (Phase II/III) |
| Chemoprevention | | | |
| Intervention | Study | Status | NCT Number |
| Curcumin | Curcumin in Treating Patients with Familial Adenomatous Polyposis | Ongoing, but not recruiting | NCT00641147 (Phase II) |
| Curcumin | Curcumin in Preventing Gastric Cancer in Patients with Chronic Atrophic Gastritis or Gastric Intestinal Metaplasia | Not yet recruiting | NCT02782949 (Phase II) |
| Curcumin | Sulindac and plant compounds in preventing colon cancer | Completed | NCT00003365 |
| Curcumin | Curcumin for the chemoprevention of colorectal cancer | Completed | NCT00118989 (Phase II) |
| Curcumin and sulindac | The effects of curcuminoids on aberrant crypt foci in the human colon | Unknown | NCT00176618 |
| Curcumin | Randomized trial of adjuvant curcumin after prostatectomy | Recruiting | NCT02064673 |

Table 8. Human studies using resveratrol in cancer.

| Cancer Treatment | | | |
|---|---|---|---|
| Intervention | Study | Status | NCT Number |
| Resveratrol | Resveratrol for patients with colon cancer | Completed | NCT00256334 (Phase I) |
| Resveratrol | Resveratrol in treating patients with colorectal cancer that can be removed by surgery | Completed | NCT00433576 (Phase I) |
| Resveratrol | A biological study of resveratrol's effects on notch-1 signaling in subjects with low grade gastrointestinal tumors | Ongoing, not recruiting | NCT01476592 |
| Resveratrol and others | Dietary intervention in follicular lymphoma (KLYMF) | Unknown | NCT00455416 (Phase II) |
| Adverse Effects Management Induced by Chemotherapy | | | |
| Intervention | Study | Status | NCT Number |
| SRT501 (new formulation of resveratrol) | A clinical study to assess the safety, pharmacokinetics, and pharmacodynamics of SRT501 in subjects with colorectal cancer and hepatic metastases | Completed | NCT00920803 (Phase I) |
| Chemoprevention | | | |
| Intervention | Study | Status | NCT Number |
| Resveratrol | UMCC 2003-064 Resveratrol in Preventing Cancer in Healthy Participants (IRB 2004-535) | Completed | NCT00098969 (Phase I) |

## 6. Conclusions

Curcumin and resveratrol are natural products with promising anticancer activity. Both compounds can act against proliferation, metastasis and cellular death through different mechanisms. Not only in vitro, but also in vivo data have demonstrated the potential of these polyphenols to treat and prevent cancer. In addition, the association of these polyphenols with current anticancer drugs has demonstrated synergic effect useful to improve the treatment. Different groups worldwide are conducting several clinical trials aiming to investigate the beneficial effects of curcumin and resveratrol in humans. Therefore, the use of resveratrol and curcumin seems to contribute to anticancer therapy.

**Acknowledgments:** The authors thank the Programa de Apoio ao Desenvolvimento Científico da Faculdade de Ciências Farmacêuticas da UNESP (PADC-FCF UNESP) and Fundação de Amparo à Pesquisa do Estado de São Paulo (FAPESP 2015/19531-1; 2016/08470-4; 2015/21252-3; 2014/14980-0; 2014/02240-1 and 2014/24811-0) for financial support.

**Author Contributions:** Authors A.R.P., G.D.B.d.S., D.H.J., D.E.C., G.F.d.S.F., C.M.C. and J.L.S. designed the study, analyzed and organized the literature papers. J.L.S. and C.M.C. revised the manuscript and approved it in its final form. All authors edited and contributed to drafts of the manuscript. All authors approved the final form of the manuscript.

**Conflicts of Interest:** The authors declare no conflict of interest.

## References

1. Cimino, S.; Sortino, G.; Favilla, V.; Castelli, T.; Madonia, M.; Sansalone, S.; Russo, G.I.; Morgia, G. Polyphenols. Key issues involved in chemoprevention of prostate cancer. *Oxid. Med. Cell. Longev.* **2012**, *2012*, 1–9. [CrossRef] [PubMed]
2. Rodríguez, M.L.; Estrela, J.M.; Ortega, Á.L. Carcinogenesis & mutagenesis natural polyphenols and apoptosis Induction in cancer therapy. *J. Carcinog. Mutagen.* **2013**, *6*, 1–10.
3. Esatbeyoglu, T.; Huebbe, P.; Ernst, I.M.A.; Chin, D.; Wagner, A.E.; Rimbach, G. Curcumin—From molecule to biological function. *Angew. Chem. Int. Ed.* **2012**, *51*, 5308–5332. [CrossRef] [PubMed]
4. Hatcher, H.; Planalp, R.; Cho, J.; Torti, F.M.; Torti, S.V. Curcumin: From ancient medicine to current clinical trials. *Cell. Mol. Life Sci.* **2008**, *65*, 1631–1652. [CrossRef] [PubMed]
5. Kunnumakkara, A.B.; Anand, P.; Aggarwal, B.B. Curcumin inhibits proliferation, invasion, angiogenesis and metastasis of different cancers through interaction with multiple cell signaling proteins. *Cancer Lett.* **2008**, *269*, 199–225. [CrossRef] [PubMed]
6. Leischner, C.; Burkard, M.; Pfeiffer, M.M.; Lauer, U.M.; Busch, C.; Venturelli, S. Nutritional immunology: Function of natural killer cells and their modulation by resveratrol for cancer prevention and treatment. *Nutr. J.* **2016**, *15*, 47. [CrossRef] [PubMed]
7. Chakraborty, S.; Kumar, A.; Butt, N.A.; Zhang, L.; Williams, R.; Rimando, A.M.; Biswas, P.K.; Levenson, A.S. Molecular insight into the differential anti-androgenic activity of resveratrol and its natural analogs: In silico approach to understand biological actions. *Mol. BioSyst.* **2016**, *12*, 1702–1709. [CrossRef] [PubMed]
8. Das, J.; Ramani, R.; Suraju, M.O. Polyphenol compounds and PKC signaling. *Biochim. Biophys. Acta Gen. Subj.* **2016**, *1860*, 2107–2121. [CrossRef] [PubMed]
9. Walle, T. Bioavailability of resveratrol. *Ann. N. Y. Acad. Sci.* **2011**, *1215*, 9–15. [CrossRef] [PubMed]
10. Anand, P.; Kunnumakkara, A.B.; Newman, R.A.; Aggarwal, B.B. Bioavailability of curcumin: Problems and promises. *Mol. Pharm.* **2007**, *4*, 807–818. [CrossRef] [PubMed]
11. Jäger, R.; Lowery, R.P.; Calvanese, A.V.; Joy, J.M.; Purpura, M.; Wilson, J.M. Comparative absorption of curcumin formulations. *Nutr. J.* **2014**, *13*, 1–8. [CrossRef] [PubMed]
12. Zebib, B.; Mouloungui, Z.; Noirot, V. Stabilization of curcumin by complexation with divalent cations in glycerol/water system. *Bioinorg. Chem. Appl.* **2010**, *2010*, 1–8. [CrossRef] [PubMed]
13. Shoba, G.; Joy, D.; Joseph, T.; Majeed, M.; Rajendran, R.; Srinivas, P.S. Influence of piperine on the pharmacokinetics of curcumin in animals and human volunteers. *Planta Med.* **1998**, *64*, 353–356. [CrossRef] [PubMed]
14. Suresh, D.; Srinivasan, K. Tissue distribution & elimination of capsaicin, piperine & curcumin following oral intake in rats. *Indian J. Med. Res.* **2010**, *131*, 682–691. [PubMed]

15. Xie, X.; Tao, Q.; Zou, Y.; Zhang, F.; Guo, M.; Wang, Y.; Wang, H.; Zhou, Q.; Yu, S. PLGA nanoparticles improve the oral bioavailability of curcumin in rats: Characterizations and mechanisms. *J. Agric. Food Chem.* **2011**, *59*, 9280–9289. [CrossRef] [PubMed]

16. Tsai, Y.-M.; Jan, W.-C.; Chien, C.-F.; Lee, W.-C.; Lin, L.-C.; Tsai, T.-H. Optimised nano-formulation on the bioavailability of hydrophobic polyphenol, curcumin, in freely-moving rats. *Food Chem.* **2011**, *127*, 918–925. [CrossRef] [PubMed]

17. Shaikh, J.; Ankola, D.D.; Beniwal, V.; Singh, D.; Kumar, M.N.V.R. Nanoparticle encapsulation improves oral bioavailability of curcumin by at least 9-fold when compared to curcumin administered with piperine as absorption enhancer. *Eur. J. Pharm. Sci.* **2009**, *37*, 223–230. [CrossRef] [PubMed]

18. Yallapu, M.M.; Jaggi, M.; Chauhan, S.C. Poly(β-cyclodextrin)/curcumin self-assembly: A novel approach to improve curcumin delivery and its therapeutic efficacy in prostate cancer cells. *Macromol. Biosci.* **2010**, *10*, 1141–1151. [CrossRef] [PubMed]

19. Sasaki, H.; Sunagawa, Y.; Takahashi, K.; Imaizumi, A.; Fukuda, H.; Hashimoto, T.; Wada, H.; Katanasaka, Y.; Kakeya, H.; Fujita, M.; et al. Innovative preparation of curcumin for improved oral bioavailability. *Biol. Pharm. Bull.* **2011**, *34*, 660–665. [CrossRef] [PubMed]

20. Prasad, S.; Tyagi, A.K.; Aggarwal, B.B. Recent developments in delivery, bioavailability, absorption and metabolism of curcumin: The golden pigment from golden spice. *Cancer Res. Treat.* **2014**, *46*, 2–18. [CrossRef] [PubMed]

21. Cuomo, J.; Appendino, G.; Dern, A.S.; Schneider, E.; Mckinnon, T.P.; Brown, M.J.; Togni, S.; Dixon, B.M. Comparative absorption of a standardized curcuminoid mixture and its lecithin formulation. *J. Nat. Prod.* **2011**, *74*, 664–669. [CrossRef] [PubMed]

22. Imaizumi, A. Highly bioavailable curcumin (Theracurmin): Its development and clinical application. *PharmaNutrition* **2015**, *3*, 123–130. [CrossRef]

23. Sunagawa, Y.; Katanasaka, Y.; Hasegawa, K.; Morimoto, T. Clinical applications of curcumin. *PharmaNutrition* **2015**, *3*, 131–135. [CrossRef]

24. Smoliga, J.M.; Blanchard, O. Enhancing the delivery of resveratrol in humans: If low bioavailability is the problem, what is the solution? *Molecules* **2014**, *19*, 17154–17172. [CrossRef] [PubMed]

25. Wang, S.; Su, R.; Nie, S.; Sun, M.; Zhang, J.; Wu, D.; Moustaid-Moussa, N. Application of nanotechnology in improving bioavailability and bioactivity of diet-derived phytochemicals. *J. Nutr. Biochem.* **2014**, *25*, 363–376. [CrossRef] [PubMed]

26. Pageni, R.; Sahni, J.K.; Ali, J.; Sharma, S.; Baboota, S. Resveratrol: Review on therapeutic potential and recent advances in drug delivery. *Expert Opin. Drug Deliv.* **2014**, *11*, 1285–1298. [CrossRef] [PubMed]

27. Sessa, M.; Tsao, R.; Liu, R.; Ferrari, G.; Donsì, F. Evaluation of the stability and antioxidant activity of nanoencapsulated resveratrol during in vitro digestion. *J. Agric. Food Chem.* **2011**, *59*, 12352–12360. [CrossRef] [PubMed]

28. Ansari, K.A.; Vavia, P.R.; Trotta, F.; Cavalli, R. Cyclodextrin-based nanosponges for delivery of resveratrol: In vitro characterisation, stability, cytotoxicity and permeation study. *AAPS Pharm. Sci. Tech.* **2011**, *12*, 279–286. [CrossRef] [PubMed]

29. Liang, L.; Liu, X.; Wang, Q.; Cheng, S.; Zhang, S.; Zhang, M. Pharmacokinetics, tissue distribution and excretion study of resveratrol and its prodrug 3,5,4′-tri-$O$-acetylresveratrol in rats. *Phytomedicine* **2013**, *20*, 558–563. [CrossRef] [PubMed]

30. Johnson, J.J.; Nihal, M.; Siddiqui, I.A.; Scarlett, C.O.; Bailey, H.H.; Mukhtar, H.; Ahmad, N. Enhancing the bioavailability of resveratrol by combining it with piperine. *Mol. Nutr. Food Res.* **2011**, *55*, 1169–1176. [CrossRef] [PubMed]

31. Cottart, C.-H.; Nivet-Antoine, V.; Beaudeux, J.-L. Review of recent data on the metabolism, biologicaleffects, and toxicity of resveratrol in humans. *Mol. Nutr. Food Res.* **2014**, *58*, 7–21. [CrossRef] [PubMed]

32. Cottart, C.-H.; Nivet-Antoine, V.; Laguillier-Morizot, C.; Beaudeux, J.-L. Resveratrol bioavailability and toxicity in humans. *Mol. Nutr. Food Res.* **2010**, *54*, 7–16. [CrossRef] [PubMed]

33. Mukherjee, S.; Dudley, J.I.; Das, D.K. Dose-dependency of resveratrol in providing health benefits. *Dose Response* **2010**, *8*, 478–500. [CrossRef] [PubMed]

34. Lao, C.D.; Ruffin, M.T.; Normolle, D.; Heath, D.D.; Murray, S.I.; Bailey, J.M.; Boggs, M.E.; Crowell, J.; Rock, C.L.; Brenner, D.E. Dose escalation of a curcuminoid formulation. *BMC Complement. Altern. Med.* **2006**, *6*, 10. [CrossRef] [PubMed]

35. Dutra, L.A.; de Melo, T.R.F. The paradigma of the interference in assays for natural products. *Biochem. Pharmacol.* **2016**, *5*, 1000e183. [CrossRef]

36. Dos Santos, J.L.; Chin, C.M. Pan-assay interference compounds (PAINS): Warning signs in biochemical-pharmacological evaluations. *Biochem. Pharmacol.* **2015**, *4*, 1000e173. [CrossRef]

37. Ingólfsson, H.I.; Thakur, P.; Herold, K.F.; Hobart, E.A.; Ramsey, N.B.; Periole, X.; de Jong, D.H.; Zwama, M.; Yilmaz, D.; Hall, K.; et al. Phytochemicals perturb membranes and promiscuously alter protein function. *ACS Chem. Biol.* **2014**, *9*, 1788–1798. [CrossRef] [PubMed]

38. Shishodia, S. Molecular mechanisms of curcumin action: Gene expression. *Biofactors* **2013**, *39*, 37–55. [CrossRef] [PubMed]

39. Coussens, L.M.; Werb, Z. Inflammation and cancer. *Nature* **2002**, *420*, 860–867. [CrossRef] [PubMed]

40. Mantovani, A.; Allavena, P.; Sica, A.; Balkwill, F. Cancer-related inflammation. *Nature* **2008**, *454*, 444. [CrossRef] [PubMed]

41. Karin, M. Nuclear factor-kappaB in cancer development and progression. *Nature* **2006**, *441*, 431–436. [CrossRef] [PubMed]

42. Balkwill, F.; Mantovani, A. Inflammation and cancer: Back to virchow? *Lancet* **2001**, *357*, 539–545. [CrossRef]

43. Jobin, C.; Bradham, C.A.; Russo, M.P.; Juma, B.; Narula, A.S.; Brenner, D.A.; Sartor, R.B. Curcumin blocks cytokine-mediated NF-κB activation and proinflammatory gene expression by inhibiting inhibitory factor I-κB kinase activity. *J. Immunol.* **1999**, *163*, 3474–3483. [PubMed]

44. Aggarwal, B.B. Nuclear factor-kappaB: The enemy within. *Cancer Cell* **2004**, *6*, 203–208. [CrossRef] [PubMed]

45. Pahl, H.L. Activators and target genes of Rel/NF-kappaB transcription factors. *Oncogene* **1999**, *18*, 6853–6866. [CrossRef] [PubMed]

46. Baldwin, A.S. Series introduction: The transcription factor NF-kappaB and human disease. *J. Clin. Investig.* **2001**, *107*, 3–6. [CrossRef] [PubMed]

47. Liu, S.; Wang, Z.; Hu, Z.; Zeng, X.; Li, Y.; Su, Y.; Zhang, C.; Ye, Z. Anti-tumor activity of curcumin against androgen-independent prostate cancer cells via inhibition of NF-κB and AP-1 pathway in vitro. *J. Huazhong Univ. Sci. Technol. Med. Sci.* **2011**, *31*, 530–534. [CrossRef] [PubMed]

48. Siwak, D.R.; Shishodia, S.; Aggarwal, B.B.; Kurzrock, R. Curcumin-induced antiproliferative and proapoptotic effects in melanoma cells are associated with suppression of IkappaB kinase and nuclear factor kappaB activity and are independent of the B-Raf/mitogen-activated/extracellular signal-regulated protein ki. *Cancer* **2005**, *104*, 879–890. [CrossRef] [PubMed]

49. Hu, L.; Xia, L.; Zhou, H.; Wu, B.; Mu, Y.; Wu, Y.; Yan, J. TF/FVIIa/PAR2 promotes cell proliferation and migration via PKCα and ERK-dependent c-Jun/AP-1 pathway in colon cancer cell line SW620. *Tumor Biol.* **2013**, *34*, 2573–2581. [CrossRef] [PubMed]

50. Balasubramanian, S.; Eckert, R.L. Curcumin suppresses AP1 transcription factor-dependent differentiation and activates apoptosis in human epidermal keratinocytes. *J. Biol. Chem.* **2007**, *282*, 6707–6715. [CrossRef] [PubMed]

51. Ruocco, K.M.; Goncharova, E.I.; Young, M.R.; Colburn, N.H.; McMahon, J.B.; Henrich, C.J. A high-throughput cell-based assay to identify specific inhibitors of transcription factor AP-1. *J. Biomol. Screen.* **2006**, *12*, 133–139. [CrossRef] [PubMed]

52. Chen, Q.; Jiao, D.; Wang, L.; Wang, L.; Hu, H.; Song, J.; Yan, J.; Wu, L.; Shi, J. Curcumin inhibits proliferation-migration of NSCLC by steering crosstalk between a Wnt signaling pathway and an adherens junction via EGR-1. *Mol. Biosyst.* **2015**, *11*, 859–868. [CrossRef] [PubMed]

53. Byeong, H.C.; Chang, G.K.; Bae, Y.S.; Lim, Y.; Young, H.L.; Soon, Y.S. p21Waf1/Cip1 expression by curcumin in U-87MG human glioma cells: Role of early growth response-1 expression. *Cancer Res.* **2008**, *68*, 1369–1377.

54. Chen, A.; Xu, J.; Johnson, A. Curcumin inhibits human colon cancer cell growth by suppressing gene expression of epidermal growth factor receptor through reducing the activity of the transcription factor Egr-1. *Oncogene* **2006**, *25*, 278–287. [CrossRef] [PubMed]

55. Hong, J.H.; Lee, G.; Choi, H.Y. Effect of curcumin on the interaction between androgen receptor and Wnt/β-catenin in LNCaP xenografts. *Korean J. Urol.* **2015**, *56*, 656–665. [CrossRef] [PubMed]

56. Choi, H.Y.; Lim, J.E.; Hong, J.H. Curcumin interrupts the interaction between the androgen receptor and Wnt/beta-catenin signaling pathway in LNCaP prostate cancer cells. *Prostate Cancer Prostatic Dis.* **2010**, *13*, 343–349. [CrossRef] [PubMed]

57. He, M.; Li, Y.; Zhang, L.; Li, L.; Shen, Y.; Lin, L.; Zheng, W.; Chen, L.; Bian, X.; Ng, H.K.; Tang, L. Curcumin suppresses cell proliferation through inhibition of the Wnt/β-catenin signaling pathway in medulloblastoma. *Oncol. Rep.* **2014**, *32*, 173–180. [CrossRef] [PubMed]

58. Alonso, A.; Sasin, J.; Bottini, N.; Friedberg, I.; Friedberg, I.; Osterman, A.; Godzik, A.; Hunter, T.; Dixon, J.; Mustelin, T. Protein tyrosine phosphatases in the human genome. *Cell* **2004**, *117*, 699–711. [CrossRef] [PubMed]

59. Hunter, T. A thousand and one protein kinases. *Cell* **1987**, *50*, 823–829. [CrossRef]

60. Manning, G.; Whyte, D.B.; Martinez, R.; Hunter, T.; Sudarsanam, S. The protein kinase complement of the human genome. *Science* **2002**, *298*, 1912–1934. [CrossRef] [PubMed]

61. Roskoski, R. A historical overview of protein kinases and their targeted small molecule inhibitors. *Pharmacol. Res.* **2015**, *100*, 1–23. [CrossRef] [PubMed]

62. Cohen, P. The role of protein phosphorylation in human health and disease. *Eur. J. Biochem.* **2001**, *268*, 5001–5010. [CrossRef] [PubMed]

63. Blume-Jensen, P.; Hunter, T. Oncogenic kinase signalling. *Nature* **2001**, *411*, 355–365. [CrossRef] [PubMed]

64. Lahiry, P.; Torkamani, A.; Schork, N.J.; Hegele, R. A kinase mutations in human disease: Interpreting genotype-phenotype relationships. *Nat. Rev. Genet.* **2010**, *11*, 60–74. [CrossRef] [PubMed]

65. Fabbro, D.; Cowan-Jacob, S.W.; Moebitz, H. Ten things you should know about protein kinases: IUPHAR Review 14. *Br. J. Pharmacol.* **2015**, *172*, 2675–2700. [CrossRef] [PubMed]

66. Yang, M.; Huang, C.-Z. Mitogen-activated protein kinase signaling pathway and invasion and metastasis of gastric cancer. *World J. Gastroenterol.* **2015**, *21*, 11673–11679. [CrossRef] [PubMed]

67. Yesilkanal, A.E.; Rosner, M.R. Raf kinase inhibitory protein (RKIP) as a metastasis suppressor: Regulation of signaling networks in cancer. *Crit. Rev. Oncog.* **2014**, *19*, 447–454. [CrossRef] [PubMed]

68. Almhanna, K.; Strosberg, J.; Malafa, M. Targeting AKT protein kinase in gastric cancer. *Anticancer Res.* **2011**, *31*, 4387–4392. [PubMed]

69. Zhou, H.; Huang, S. Role of mTOR signaling in tumor cell motility, invasion and metastasis. *Curr. Protein Pept. Sci.* **2011**, *12*, 30–42. [PubMed]

70. Rattanasinchai, C.; Gallo, K. MLK3 signaling in cancer invasion. *Cancers* **2016**, *8*, 51. [CrossRef] [PubMed]

71. Varkaris, A.; Katsiampoura, A.D.; Araujo, J.C.; Gallick, G.E.; Corn, P.G. Src signaling pathways in prostate cancer. *Cancer Metastasis Rev.* **2014**, *33*, 595–606. [CrossRef] [PubMed]

72. Durand, N.; Borges, S.; Storz, P. Functional and therapeutic significance of protein kinase D enzymes in invasive breast cancer. *Cell. Mol. Life Sci.* **2015**, *72*, 4369–4382. [CrossRef] [PubMed]

73. Igea, A.; Nebreda, A.R. The stress kinase p38α as a target for cancer therapy. *Cancer Res.* **2015**, *75*, 3997–4002. [CrossRef] [PubMed]

74. Li, N.; Huang, D.; Lu, N.; Luo, L. Role of the LKB1/AMPK pathway in tumor invasion and metastasis of cancer cells (Review). *Oncol. Rep.* **2015**, *34*, 2821–2826. [CrossRef] [PubMed]

75. Starok, M.; Preira, P.; Vayssade, M.; Haupt, K.; Salomé, L.; Rossi, C. EGFR inhibition by curcumin in cancer cells: A dual mode of action. *Biomacromolecules* **2015**, *16*, 1634–1642. [CrossRef] [PubMed]

76. Chadalapaka, G.; Jutooru, I.; Burghardt, R.; Safe, S. Drugs that target specificity proteins downregulate epidermal growth factor receptor in bladder cancer cells. *Mol. Cancer Res.* **2010**, *8*, 739–750. [CrossRef] [PubMed]

77. Amani, V.; Prince, E.W.; Alimova, I.; Balakrishnan, I.; Birks, D.; Donson, A.M.; Harris, P.; Levy, J.M.M.; Handler, M.; Foreman, N.K.; et al. Polo-like Kinase 1 as a potential therapeutic target in Diffuse Intrinsic Pontine Glioma. *BMC Cancer* **2016**, *16*, 647. [CrossRef] [PubMed]

78. Van Erk, M.J.; Teuling, E.; Staal, Y.C.; Huybers, S.; Van Bladeren, P.J.; Aarts, J.M.; Van Ommen, B. Time- and dose-dependent effects of curcumin on gene expression in human colon cancer cells. *J. Carcinog.* **2004**, *3*, 1–17. [CrossRef] [PubMed]

79. Mosieniak, G.; Sliwinska, M.A.; Przybylska, D.; Grabowska, W.; Sunderland, P.; Bielak-Zmijewska, A.; Sikora, E. Curcumin-treated cancer cells show mitotic disturbances leading to growth arrest and induction of senescence phenotype. *Int. J. Biochem. Cell Biol.* **2016**, *74*, 33–43. [CrossRef] [PubMed]

80. Downward, J. PI 3-kinase, Akt and cell survival. *Semin. Cell Dev. Biol.* **2004**, *15*, 177–182. [CrossRef] [PubMed]

81. Minet, E.; Michel, G.; Mottet, D.; Raes, M.; Michiels, C. Transduction pathways involved in hypoxia-inducible factor-1 phosphorylation and activation. *Free Radic. Biol. Med.* **2001**, *31*, 847–855. [CrossRef]

82. Zhang, Q.; Tang, X.; Lu, Q.Y.; Zhang, Z.F.; Brown, J.; Le, A.D. Resveratrol inhibits hypoxia-induced accumulation of hypoxia-inducible factor-1α and VEGF expression in human tongue squamous cell carcinoma and hepatoma cells. *Mol. Cancer Ther.* **2005**, *4*, 1465–1474. [CrossRef] [PubMed]

83. Faber, A.C.; Dufort, F.J.; Blair, D.; Wagner, D.; Roberts, M.F.; Chiles, T.C. Inhibition of phosphatidylinositol 3-kinase-mediated glucose metabolism coincides with resveratrol-induced cell cycle arrest in human diffuse large B-cell lymphomas. *Biochem. Pharmacol.* **2006**, *72*, 1246–1256. [CrossRef] [PubMed]

84. Benitez, D.A.; Pozo-Guisado, E.; Clementi, M.; Castellón, E.A.; Fernandez-Salguero, P.M. Non-genomic action of resveratrol on androgen and oestrogen receptors in prostate cancer: Modulation of the phosphoinositide 3-kinase pathway. *Br. J. Cancer* **2007**, *96*, 1595–1604. [CrossRef] [PubMed]

85. Benitez, D.A.; Hermoso, M.A.; Pozo-Guisado, E.; Fernández-Salguero, P.M.; Castellón, E.A. Regulation of cell survival by resveratrol involves inhibition of NFκβ-regulated gene expression in prostate cancer cells. *Prostate* **2009**, *69*, 1045–1054. [CrossRef] [PubMed]

86. Hsieh, T.C.; Wong, C.; Bennett, D.J.; Wu, J.M. Regulation of p53 and cell proliferation by resveratrol and its derivatives in breast cancer cells: An in silico and biochemical approach targeting integrin αvβ3. *Int. J. Cancer* **2011**, *129*, 2732–2743. [CrossRef] [PubMed]

87. De Amicis, F.; Giordano, F.; Vivacqua, A.; Pellegrino, M.; Panno, M.L.; Tramontano, D.; Fuqua, S.A.W.; Ando, S. Resveratrol, through NF-Y/p53/Sin3/HDAC1 complex phosphorylation, inhibits estrogen receptor gene expression via p38MAPK/CK2 signaling in human breast cancer cells. *FASEB J.* **2011**, *25*, 3695–3707. [CrossRef] [PubMed]

88. Abusnina, A.; Keravis, T.; Himheur, D.; Bronner, C.; Lugnier, C. Anti-proliferative effect of curcumin on melanoma cells is mediated by PDE1A inhibition that regulates the epigenetic integrin UHRF1. *Mol. Nutr. Food Res.* **2011**, *55*, 1677–1689. [CrossRef] [PubMed]

89. Abusnina, A.; Keravis, T.; Zhou, Q.; Justiniano, H.; Lobstein, A.; Lugnier, C. Tumour growth inhibition and anti-angiogenic effects using curcumin correspond to combined PDE2 and PDE4 inhibition. *Thromb. Haemost.* **2015**, *113*, 319–328. [CrossRef] [PubMed]

90. Weis, S.M.; Cheresh, D.A. Tumor angiogenesis: Molecular pathways and therapeutic targets. *Nat. Med.* **2011**, *17*, 1359–1370. [CrossRef] [PubMed]

91. Zhao, Y.; Adjei, A.A. Targeting angiogenesis in cancer therapy: Moving beyond vascular endothelial growth factor. *Oncologist* **2015**, *20*, 660–673. [CrossRef] [PubMed]

92. Shojaei, F. Anti-angiogenesis therapy in cancer: Current challenges and future perspectives. *Cancer Lett.* **2012**, *320*, 130–137. [CrossRef] [PubMed]

93. Ellis, L.M.; Hicklin, D.J. VEGF-targeted therapy: Mechanisms of anti-tumour activity. *Nat. Rev. Cancer* **2008**, *8*, 579–591. [CrossRef] [PubMed]

94. Ferrara, N.; Gerber, H.P.; LeCouter, J. The biology of VEGF and its receptors. *Nat. Med.* **2003**, *9*, 669–676. [CrossRef] [PubMed]

95. Bae, M.K.; Kim, S.H.; Jeong, J.W.; Lee, Y.M.; Kim, H.S.; Kim, S.R.; Yun, I.; Bae, S.K.; Kim, K.W. Curcumin inhibits hypoxia-induced angiogenesis via down-regulation of HIF-1. *Oncol. Rep.* **2006**, *15*, 1557–1562. [CrossRef] [PubMed]

96. Shan, B.; Schaaf, C.; Schmidt, A.; Lucia, K.; Buchfelder, M.; Losa, M.; Kuhlen, D.; Kreutzer, J.; Perone, M.J.; Arzt, E.; et al. Curcumin suppresses HIF1A synthesis and VEGFA release in pituitary adenomas. *J. Endocrinol.* **2012**, *214*, 389–398. [CrossRef] [PubMed]

97. Fu, Z.; Chen, X.; Guan, S.; Yan, Y.; Lin, H.; Hua, Z.-C. Curcumin inhibits angiogenesis and improves defective hematopoiesis induced by tumor-derived VEGF in tumor model through modulating VEGF-VEGFR2 signaling pathway. *Oncotarget* **2015**, *6*, 19469–19482. [CrossRef] [PubMed]

98. Dann, J.M.; Sykes, P.H.; Mason, D.R.; Evans, J.J. Regulation of vascular endothelial growth factor in endometrial tumour cells by resveratrol and EGCG. *Gynecol. Oncol.* **2009**, *113*, 374–378. [CrossRef] [PubMed]

99. Hu, Y.; Sun, C.; Huang, J.; Hong, L.; Zhang, L.; Chu, Z. Antimyeloma effects of resveratrol through inhibition of angiogenesis. *Chin. Med. J.* **2007**, *120*, 1672–1677. [PubMed]

100. Liu, Z.; Li, Y.; Yang, R. Effects of resveratrol on vascular endothelial growth factor expression in osteosarcoma cells and cell proliferation. *Oncol. Lett.* **2012**, *4*, 837–839. [PubMed]

101. Yang, R.; Zhang, H.; Zhu, L. Inhibitory effect of resveratrol on the expression of the VEGF gene and proliferation in renal cancer cells. *Mol. Med. Rep.* **2011**, *4*, 981–983. [PubMed]

102. Trapp, V.; Parmakhtiar, B.; Papazian, V.; Willmott, L.; Fruehauf, J.P. Anti-angiogenic effects of resveratrol mediated by decreased VEGF and increased TSP1 expression in melanoma-endothelial cell co-culture. *Angiogenesis* **2010**, *13*, 305–315. [CrossRef] [PubMed]

103. Mousa, S.S.; Mousa, S.S.; Mousa, S.A. Effect of resveratrol on angiogenesis and platelet/fibrin-accelerated tumor growth in the chick chorioallantoic membrane model. *Nutr. Cancer* **2005**, *52*, 59–65. [CrossRef] [PubMed]

104. Ravindran, J.; Prasad, S.; Aggarwal, B.B. Curcumin and cancer cells: How many ways can curry kill tumor cells selectively? *AAPS J.* **2009**, *11*, 495–510. [CrossRef] [PubMed]

105. Yang, C.L.; Liu, Y.Y.; Ma, Y.G.; Xue, Y.X.; Liu, D.G.; Ren, Y.; Liu, X.B.; Li, Y.; Li, Z. Curcumin blocks small cell lung cancer cells migration, invasion, angiogenesis, cell cycle and neoplasia through janus kinase-STAT3 signalling pathway. *PLoS ONE* **2012**, *7*, e37960. [CrossRef] [PubMed]

106. Lim, T.-G.; Lee, S.-Y.; Huang, Z.; Lim, D.Y.; Chen, H.; Jung, S.K.; Bode, A.M.; Lee, K.W.; Dong, Z. Curcumin suppresses proliferation of colon cancer cells by targeting CDK2. *Cancer Prev. Res.* **2014**, *7*, 466–474. [CrossRef] [PubMed]

107. Hudson, T.S.; Hartle, D.K.; Hursting, S.D.; Nunez, N.P.; Wang, T.T.Y.; Young, H.A.; Arany, P.; Green, J.E. Inhibition of prostate cancer growth by muscadine grape skin extract and resveratrol through distinct mechanisms. *Cancer Res.* **2007**, *67*, 8396–8405. [CrossRef] [PubMed]

108. Wang, C.; Hu, Z.; Chu, M.; Wang, Z.; Zhang, W.; Wang, L.; Li, C.; Wang, J. Resveratrol inhibited GH3 cell growth and decreased prolactin level via estrogen receptors. *Clin. Neurol. Neurosurg.* **2012**, *114*, 241–248. [CrossRef] [PubMed]

109. Kim, A.L.; Zhu, Y.; Zhu, H.; Han, L.; Kopelovich, L.; Bickers, D.R.; Athar, M. Resveratrol inhibits proliferation of human epidermoid carcinoma A431 cells by modulating MEK1 and AP-1 signalling pathways. *Exp. Dermatol.* **2006**, *15*, 538–546. [CrossRef] [PubMed]

110. Yuan, L.; Zhang, Y.; Xia, J.; Liu, B.; Zhang, Q.; Liu, J.; Luo, L.; Peng, Z.; Song, Z.; Zhu, R. Resveratrol induces cell cycle arrest via a p53-independent pathway in A549 cells. *Mol. Med. Rep.* **2015**, *11*, 2459–2464. [CrossRef] [PubMed]

111. Zhou, R.; Fukui, M.; Choi, H.J.; Zhu, B.T. Induction of a reversible, non-cytotoxic S-phase delay by resveratrol: Implications for a mechanism of lifespan prolongation and cancer protection. *Br. J. Pharmacol.* **2009**, *158*, 462–474. [CrossRef] [PubMed]

112. Yu, X.-D.; Yang, J.; Zhang, W.-L.; Liu, D.-X. Resveratrol inhibits oral squamous cell carcinoma through induction of apoptosis and G2/M phase cell cycle arrest. *Tumor Biol.* **2016**, *37*, 2871–2877. [CrossRef] [PubMed]

113. Carafa, V.; Nebbioso, A.; Altucci, L. Sirtuins and disease: The road ahead. *Front. Pharmacol.* **2012**, *3*, 1–6. [CrossRef] [PubMed]

114. Yang, Q.; Wang, B.; Zang, W.; Wang, X.; Liu, Z.; Li, W.; Jia, J. Resveratrol inhibits the growth of gastric cancer by inducing G1 phase arrest and senescence in a Sirt1-dependent manner. *PLoS ONE* **2013**, *8*, e70627. [CrossRef] [PubMed]

115. Lin, J.-N.; Lin, V.C.-H.; Rau, K.-M.; Shieh, P.-C.; Kuo, D.-H.; Shieh, J.-C.; Chen, W.-J.; Tsai, S.-C.; Way, T.-D. Resveratrol modulates tumor cell proliferation and protein translation via SIRT1-dependent AMPK activation. *J. Agric. Food Chem.* **2010**, *58*, 1584–1592. [CrossRef] [PubMed]

116. Li, Y.; Zhu, W.; Li, J.; Liu, M.; Wei, M. Resveratrol suppresses the STAT3 signaling pathway and inhibits proliferation of high glucose-exposed HepG2 cells partly through SIRT1. *Oncol. Rep.* **2013**, *30*, 2820–2828. [PubMed]

117. Chang, Y.J.; Huang, C.Y.; Hung, C.S.; Chen, W.Y.; Wei, P.L. GRP78 mediates the therapeutic efficacy of curcumin on colon cancer. *Tumor Biol.* **2015**, *36*, 633–641. [CrossRef] [PubMed]

118. Chen, L.X.; He, Y.J.; Zhao, S.Z.; Wu, J.G.; Wang, J.T.; Zhu, L.M.; Lin, T.T.; Sun, B.C.; Li, X.R. Inhibition of tumor growth and vasculogenic mimicry by cucumin through downregulation of the EphA2/PI3K/MMP pathway in a murine choroidal melanoma model. *Cancer Biol. Ther.* **2011**, *11*, 229–235. [CrossRef] [PubMed]

119. Chen, C.Q.; Yu, K.; Yan, Q.X.; Xing, C.Y.; Chen, Y.; Yan, Z.; Shi, Y.F.; Zhao, K.W.; Gao, S.M. Pure curcumin increases the expression of SOCS$_1$ and SOCS$_3$ in myeloproliferative neoplasms through suppressing class I histone deacetylases. *Carcinogenesis* **2013**, *34*, 1442–1449. [CrossRef] [PubMed]

120. Chen, B.; Zhang, Y.; Wang, Y.; Rao, J.; Jiang, X.; Xu, Z. Curcumin inhibits proliferation of breast cancer cells through Nrf2-mediated down-regulation of Fen1 expression. *J. Steroid Biochem. Mol. Biol.* **2014**, *143*, 11–18. [CrossRef] [PubMed]

121. Gao, S.; Yang, J.; Chen, C.; Chen, J.; Ye, L.; Wang, L.; Wu, J.; Xing, C.; Yu, K. Pure curcumin decreases the expression of WT1 by upregulation of miR-15a and miR-16-1 in leukemic cells. *J. Exp. Clin. Cancer Res.* **2012**, *31*, 27. [CrossRef] [PubMed]

122. Guo, Y.; Shu, L.; Zhang, C.; Su, Z.-Y.; Kong, A.-N.T. Curcumin inhibits anchorage-independent growth of HT29 human colon cancer cells by targeting epigenetic restoration of the tumor suppressor gene DLEC1. *Biochem. Pharmacol.* **2015**, *94*, 69–78. [CrossRef] [PubMed]

123. Wang, L.; Ye, X.; Cai, X.; Su, J.; Ma, R.; Yin, X.; Zhou, X.; Li, H.; Wang, Z. Curcumin suppresses cell growth and invasion and induces apoptosis by down-regulation of Skp2 pathway in glioma cells. *Oncotarget* **2015**, *6*, 18027–18037. [CrossRef] [PubMed]

124. Atten, M.J.; Godoy-romero, E.; Attar, B.M.; Milson, T.; Zopel, M.; Holian, O. Resveratrol regulates cellular PKC $\alpha$ and $\delta$ to inhibit growth and induce apoptosis in gastric cancer cells. *Investig. New Drugs* **2005**, *23*, 111–119. [CrossRef] [PubMed]

125. Lee, M.-H.; Choi, B.Y.; Kundu, J.K.; Shin, Y.K.; Na, H.-K.; Surh, Y.-J. Resveratrol suppresses growth of human ovarian cancer cells in culture and in a murine xenograft model: Eukaryotic elongation factor 1A2 as a potential target. *Cancer Res.* **2009**, *69*, 7449–7458. [CrossRef] [PubMed]

126. Vyas, S.; Asmerom, Y.; De León, D.D. Resveratrol regulates insulin-like growth factor-II in breast cancer cells. *Endocrinology* **2005**, *146*, 4224–4233. [CrossRef] [PubMed]

127. Waite, K.A.; Sinden, M.R.; Eng, C. Phytoestrogen exposure elevates PTEN levels. *Hum. Mol. Genet.* **2005**, *14*, 1457–1463. [CrossRef] [PubMed]

128. Golkar, L.; Ding, X.Z.; Ujiki, M.B.; Salabat, M.R.; Kelly, D.L.; Scholtens, D.; Fought, A.J.; Bentrem, D.J.; Talamonti, M.S.; Bell, R.H.; Adrian, T.E. Resveratrol inhibits pancreatic cancer cell proliferation through transcriptional induction of Macrophage Inhibitory Cytokine-1. *J. Surg. Res.* **2007**, *138*, 163–169. [CrossRef] [PubMed]

129. Gomez, L.S.; Zancan, P.; Marcondes, M.C.; Ramos-Santos, L.; Meyer-Fernandes, J.R.; Sola-Penna, M.; Da Silva, D. Resveratrol decreases breast cancer cell viability and glucose metabolism by inhibiting 6-phosphofructo-1-kinase. *Biochimie* **2013**, *95*, 1336–1343. [CrossRef] [PubMed]

130. Lin, C.Y.; Hsiao, W.C.; Wright, D.E.; Hsu, C.L.; Lo, Y.C.; Wang Hsu, G.S.; Kao, C.F. Resveratrol activates the histone H2B ubiquitin ligase, RNF20, in MDA-MB-231 breast cancer cells. *J. Funct. Foods* **2013**, *5*, 790–800. [CrossRef]

131. Luo, H.; Yang, A.; Schulte, B.A.; Wargovich, M.J.; Wang, G.Y. Resveratrol induces premature senescence in lung cancer cells via ROS-mediated DNA damage. *PLoS ONE* **2013**, *8*, e60065. [CrossRef] [PubMed]

132. Gao, Z.; Xu, M.S.; Barnett, T.L.; Xu, C.W. Resveratrol induces cellular senescence with attenuated mono-ubiquitination of histone H2B in glioma cells. *Biochem. Biophys. Res. Commun.* **2011**, *407*, 271–276. [CrossRef] [PubMed]

133. Chaffer, C.L.; Weinberg, R. A perspective on cancer cell metastasis. *Science* **2011**, *331*, 1559–1564. [CrossRef] [PubMed]

134. Eccles, S.A.; Welch, D.R. Metastasis: Recent discoveries and novel treatment strategies. *Lancet* **2007**, *369*, 1742–1757. [CrossRef]

135. Wan, L.; Pantel, K.; Kang, Y. Tumor metastasis: Moving new biological insights into the clinic. *Nat. Med.* **2013**, *19*, 1450–1464. [CrossRef] [PubMed]

136. Steeg, P.; Theodorescu, D. Metastasis: A therapeutic target for cancer. *Nat. Clin. Pract. Oncol.* **2008**, *5*, 206–219. [CrossRef] [PubMed]

137. Steeg, P.S. Targeting metastasis. *Nat. Rev. Cancer* **2016**, *16*, 201–218. [CrossRef] [PubMed]

138. Sleeman, J.; Steeg, P.S. Metastasis: A therapeutic target for cancer. *Eur. J. Cancer* **2010**, *46*, 1177–1180. [CrossRef] [PubMed]

139. Fidler, I.J. The pathogenesis of cancer metastasis: The "seed and soil" hypothesis revisited. *Nat. Rev. Cancer* **2003**, *3*, 453–458. [CrossRef] [PubMed]

140. Yang, W.; Zou, L.; Huang, C.; Lei, Y. Redox regulation of cancer metastasis: Molecular signaling and therapeutic opportunities. *Drug Dev. Res.* **2014**, *75*, 331–341. [CrossRef] [PubMed]

141. Sun, Y.; Ma, L. The emerging molecular machinery and therapeutic targets of metastasis. *Trends Pharmacol. Sci.* **2015**, *36*, 349–359. [CrossRef] [PubMed]

142. Weiss, L. The molecular genetics of progression and metastasis. *Cancer Metastasis Rev.* **2000**, *19*, 327–344. [CrossRef]

143. Shehzad, A.; Wahid, F.; Lee, Y.S. Curcumin in cancer chemoprevention: Molecular targets, pharmacokinetics, bioavailability, and clinical trials. *Arch. Pharm.* **2010**, *343*, 489–499. [CrossRef] [PubMed]

144. Pulido-Moran, M.; Moreno-Fernandez, J.; Ramirez-Tortosa, C.; Ramirez-Tortosa, M.C. Curcumin and health. *Molecules* **2016**, *21*, 264. [CrossRef] [PubMed]

145. Shanmugam, M.K.; Rane, G.; Kanchi, M.M.; Arfuso, F.; Chinnathambi, A.; Zayed, M.E.; Alharbi, S.A.; Tan, B.K.H.; Kumar, A.P.; Sethi, G. The Multifaceted Role of Curcumin in Cancer Prevention and Treatment. *Molecules* **2015**, *20*, 2728–2769. [CrossRef] [PubMed]

146. Shehzad, A.; Lee, J.; Lee, Y.S. Curcumin in various cancers. *BioFactors* **2013**, *39*, 56–68. [CrossRef] [PubMed]

147. Gupta, S.C.; Prasad, S.; Kim, J.H.; Patchva, S.; Webb, L.J.; Priyadarsini, I.K.; Aggarwal, B.B. Multitargeting by curcumin as revealed by molecular interaction studies. *Nat. Prod. Rep.* **2011**, *28*, 1937–1955. [CrossRef] [PubMed]

148. Aggarwal, S.; Ichikawa, H.; Takada, Y.; Sandur, S.K.; Shishodia, S.; Aggarwal, B.B. Curcumin (Diferuloylmethane) down-regulates expression of cell proliferation and antiapoptotic and metastatic gene products through suppression of IκBα Kinase and Akt activation. *Mol. Pharmacol.* **2006**, *69*, 195–206. [PubMed]

149. Bachmeier, B.E.; Mohrenz, I.V.; Mirisola, V.; Schleicher, E.; Romeo, F.; Höhneke, C.; Jochum, M.; Nerlich, A.G.; Pfeffer, U. Curcumin downregulates the inflammatory cytokines CXCL1 and -2 in breast cancer cells via NFκB. *Carcinogenesis* **2008**, *29*, 779–789. [CrossRef] [PubMed]

150. Killian, P.H.; Kronski, E.; Michalik, K.M.; Barbieri, O.; Astigiano, S.; Sommerhoff, C.P.; Pfeffer, U.; Nerlich, A.G.; Bachmeier, B.E. Curcumin inhibits prostate cancer metastasis in vivo by targeting the inflammatory cytokines CXCL1 and -2. *Carcinogenesis* **2012**, *33*, 2507–2519. [CrossRef] [PubMed]

151. Minn, A.J.; Gupta, G.P.; Siegel, P.M.; Bos, P.D.; Shu, W.; Giri, D.D.; Viale, A.; Olshen, A.B.; Gerald, W.L.; Massague, J. Genes that mediate breast cancer metastasis to lung. *Nature* **2005**, *436*, 518–524. [CrossRef] [PubMed]

152. Narasimhan, M.; Ammanamanchi, S. Curcumin blocks RON tyrosine kinase-mediated invasion of breast carcinoma cells. *Cancer Res.* **2008**, *68*, 5185–5192. [CrossRef] [PubMed]

153. Thangasamy, A.; Rogge, J.; Ammanamanchi, S. Recepteur d'Origine nantais tyrosine kinase is a direct target of hypoxia-inducible factor-1α-mediated invasion of breast carcinoma cells. *J. Biol. Chem.* **2009**, *284*, 14001–14010. [CrossRef] [PubMed]

154. Zong, H.; Wang, F.; Fan, Q.-X.; Wang, L.-X. Curcumin inhibits metastatic progression of breast cancer cell through suppression of urokinase-type plasminogen activator by NF-kappa B signaling pathways. *Mol. Biol. Rep.* **2012**, *39*, 4803–4808. [CrossRef] [PubMed]

155. Woo, M.S.; Jung, S.H.; Kim, S.Y.; Hyun, J.W.; Ko, K.H.; Kim, W.K.; Kim, H.S. Curcumin suppresses phorbol ester-induced matrix metalloproteinase-9 expression by inhibiting the PKC to MAPK signaling pathways in human astroglioma cells. *Biochem. Biophys. Res. Commun.* **2005**, *335*, 1017–1025. [CrossRef] [PubMed]

156. Shankar, S.; Ganapathy, S.; Chen, Q.; Srivastava, R.K. Curcumin sensitizes TRAIL-resistant xenografts: Molecular mechanisms of apoptosis, metastasis and angiogenesis. *Mol. Cancer* **2008**, *7*, 16. [CrossRef] [PubMed]

157. Chen, M.-C.; Chang, W.-W.; Kuan, Y.-D.; Lin, S.-T.; Hsu, H.-C.; Lee, C.-H. Resveratrol inhibits LPS-induced epithelial-mesenchymal transition in mouse melanoma model. *Innate Immun.* **2012**, *18*, 685–693. [CrossRef] [PubMed]

158. Kim, Y.S.; Sull, J.W.; Sung, H.J. Suppressing effect of resveratrol on the migration and invasion of human metastatic lung and cervical cancer cells. *Mol. Biol. Rep.* **2012**, *39*, 8709–8716. [CrossRef] [PubMed]

159. Liu, P.L.; Tsai, J.R.; Charles, A.L.; Hwang, J.J.; Chou, S.H.; Ping, Y.H.; Lin, F.Y.; Chen, Y.L.; Hung, C.Y.; Chen, W.C.; et al. Resveratrol inhibits human lung adenocarcinoma cell metastasis by suppressing heme oxygenase 1-mediated nuclear factor-κB pathway and subsequently downregulating expression of matrix metalloproteinases. *Mol. Nutr. Food Res.* **2010**, *54*, 196–204. [CrossRef] [PubMed]

160. Dulak, J.; Łoboda, A.; Zagórska, A.; Józkowicz, A. Complex role of heme oxygenase-1 in angiogenesis. *Antioxid. Redox Signal.* **2004**, *6*, 858–866. [CrossRef] [PubMed]

161. Yu, H.; Pan, C.; Zhao, S.; Wang, Z.; Zhang, H.; Wu, W. Resveratrol inhibits tumor necrosis factor-alpha-mediated matrix metalloproteinase-9 expression and invasion of human hepatocellular carcinoma cells. *Biomed. Pharmacother.* **2008**, *62*, 366–372. [CrossRef] [PubMed]

162. Ryu, J.; Ku, B.M.; Lee, Y.K.; Jeong, J.Y.; Kang, S.; Choi, J.; Yang, Y.; Lee, D.H.; Roh, G.S.; Kim, H.J.; et al. Resveratrol reduces TNF-alpha-induced U373MG human glioma cell invasion through regulating NF-kappaB activation and uPA/uPAR expression. *Anticancer Res.* **2011**, *31*, 4223–4230. [PubMed]

163. Behrens, J. The role of cell adhesion molecules in cancer invasion and metastasis. *Breast Cancer Res. Treat.* **1993**, *24*, 175–184. [CrossRef] [PubMed]

164. Reymond, N.; D'Água, B.B.; Ridley, A.J. Crossing the endothelial barrier during metastasis. *Nat. Rev. Cancer* **2013**, *13*, 858–870. [CrossRef] [PubMed]

165. Okegawa, T.; Pong, R.-C.; Li, Y.; Hsieh, J.-T. The role of cell adhesion molecule in cancer progression and its application in cancer therapy. *Acta Biochim. Pol.* **2004**, *51*, 445–457. [PubMed]

166. Park, J.S.; Kim, K.M.; Kim, M.H.; Chang, H.J.; Baek, M.K.; Kim, S.M.; Jung, Y. Do resveratrol inhibits tumor cell adhesion to endothelial cells by blocking ICAM-1 expression. *Anticancer Res.* **2009**, *29*, 355–362. [PubMed]

167. Visse, R.; Nagase, H. Matrix metalloproteinases and tissue inhibitors of metalloproteinases: Structure, function, and biochemistry. *Circ. Res.* **2003**, *92*, 827–839. [CrossRef] [PubMed]

168. Kumar, D.; Kumar, M.; Saravanan, C.; Singh, S.K. Curcumin: A potential candidate for matrix metalloproteinase inhibitors. *Expert Opin. Ther. Targets* **2012**, *16*, 959–972. [CrossRef] [PubMed]

169. Brown, G.T.; Murray, G.I. Current mechanistic insights into the roles of matrix metalloproteinases in tumour invasion and metastasis. *J. Pathol.* **2015**, *237*, 273–281. [CrossRef] [PubMed]

170. Choe, G.; Park, J.K.; Jouben-Steele, L.; Kremen, T.J.; Liau, L.M.; Vinters, H.V.; Cloughesy, T.F.; Mischel, P.S. Active matrix metalloproteinase 9 expression is associated with primary glioblastoma subtype. *Clin. Cancer Res.* **2002**, *8*, 2894–2901. [PubMed]

171. Roomi, M.W.; Monterrey, J.C.; Kalinovsky, T.; Rath, M.; Niedzwiecki, A. Patterns of MMP-2 and MMP-9 expression in human cancer cell lines. *Oncol. Rep.* **2009**, *21*, 1323–1333. [PubMed]

172. Jezierska, A.; Motyl, T. Matrix metalloproteinase-2 involvement in breast cancer progression: A mini-review. *Med. Sci. Monit.* **2009**, *15*, 32–40.

173. Xu, X.; Wang, Y.; Chen, Z.; Sternlicht, M.D.; Hidalgo, M.; Steffensen, B. Matrix metalloproteinase-2 contributes to cancer cell migration on collagen. *Cancer Res.* **2005**, *65*, 130–136. [PubMed]

174. Chen, Q.; Gao, Q.; Chen, K.; Wang, Y.; Chen, L.; Li, X. Curcumin suppresses migration and invasion of human endometrial carcinoma cells. *Oncol. Lett.* **2015**, 1297–1302. [CrossRef] [PubMed]

175. Lakka, S.S.; Jasti, S.L.; Gondi, C.; Boyd, D.; Chandrasekar, N.; Dinh, D.H.; Olivero, W.C.; Gujrati, M.; Rao, J.S. Downregulation of MMP-9 in ERK-mutated stable transfectants inhibits glioma invasion in vitro. *Oncogene* **2002**, *21*, 5601–5608. [CrossRef] [PubMed]

176. Cheng, T.S.; Chen, W.C.; Lin, Y.Y.; Tsai, C.H.; Liao, C.I.; Shyu, H.Y.; Ko, C.J.; Tzeng, S.F.; Huang, C.Y.; Yang, P.C.; et al. Curcumin-targeting pericellular serine protease matriptase role in suppression of prostate cancer cell invasion, tumor growth, and metastasis. *Cancer Prev. Res.* **2013**, *6*, 495–505. [CrossRef] [PubMed]

177. Fan, Z.; Duan, X.; Cai, H.; Wang, L.; Li, M.; Qu, J.; Li, W.; Wang, Y.; Wang, J. Curcumin inhibits the invasion of lung cancer cells by modulating the PKCα/Nox-2/ROS/ATF-2/MMP-9 signaling pathway. *Oncol. Rep.* **2015**, *34*, 691–698. [CrossRef] [PubMed]

178. Chen, Q.-Y.; Zheng, Y.; Jiao, D.-M.; Chen, F.-Y.; Hu, H.-Z.; Wu, Y.-Q.; Song, J.; Yan, J.; Wu, L.-J.; Lv, G.-Y. Curcumin inhibits lung cancer cell migration and invasion through Rac1-dependent signaling pathway. *J. Nutr. Biochem.* **2014**, *25*, 177–185. [CrossRef] [PubMed]

179. Banerji, A.; Chakrabarti, J.; Mitra, A.; Chatterjee, A. Effect of curcumin on gelatinase a (MMP-2) activity in B16F10 melanoma cells. *Cancer Lett.* **2004**, *211*, 235–242. [CrossRef] [PubMed]

180. Kurschat, P.; Zigrino, P.; Nischt, R.; Breitkopf, K.; Steurer, P.; Klein, C.E.; Krieg, T.; Mauch, C. Tissue inhibitor of matrix metalloproteinase-2 regulates matrix metalloproteinase-2 activation by modulation of membrane-type 1 matrix metalloproteinase activity in high and low invasive melanoma cell lines. *J. Biol. Chem.* **1999**, *274*, 21056–21062. [CrossRef] [PubMed]

181. Sieg, D.J.; Hauck, C.R.; Ilic, D.; Klingbeil, C.K.; Schaefer, E.; Damsky, C.H.; Schlaepfer, D.D. FAK integrates growth-factor and integrin signals to promote cell migration. *Nat. Cell Biol.* **2000**, *2*, 249–256. [PubMed]

182. Mitra, A.; Chakrabarti, J.; Banerji, A.; Chatterjee, A.; Das, B.R. Curcumin, a potential inhibitor of MMP-2 in human laryngeal squamous carcinoma cells HEp2. *J. Environ. Pathol. Toxicol. Oncol.* **2006**, *25*, 679–690. [CrossRef] [PubMed]

183. Liao, H.; Wang, Z.; Deng, Z.; Ren, H.; Li, X. Curcumin inhibits lung cancer invasion and metastasis by attenuating GLUT1/MT1-MMP/MMP2 pathway. *Int. J. Clin. Exp. Med.* **2015**, *8*, 8948–8957. [PubMed]

184. Gagliano, N.; Moscheni, C.; Torri, C.; Magnani, I.; Bertelli, A.A.; Gioia, M. Effect of resveratrol on matrix metalloproteinase-2 (MMP-2) and Secreted Protein Acidic and Rich in Cysteine (SPARC) on human cultured glioblastoma cells. *Biomed. Pharmacother.* **2005**, *59*, 359–364. [CrossRef] [PubMed]

185. Gunther, S.; Ruhe, C.; Derikito, M.G.; Bose, G.; Sauer, H.; Wartenberg, M. Polyphenols prevent cell shedding from mouse mammary cancer spheroids and inhibit cancer cell invasion in confrontation cultures derived from embryonic stem cells. *Cancer Lett.* **2007**, *250*, 25–35. [CrossRef] [PubMed]

186. Lee, H.S.; Ha, A.W.; Kim, W.K. Effect of resveratrol on the metastasis of 4T1 mouse breast cancer cells in vitro and in vivo. *Nutr. Res. Pract.* **2012**, *6*, 294–300. [CrossRef] [PubMed]

187. Sun, C.; Hu, Y.; Guo, T.; Wang, H.; Zhang, X.; He, W.; Tan, H. Resveratrol as a novel agent for treatment of multiple myeloma with matrix metalloproteinase inhibitory activity. *Acta Pharmacol. Sin.* **2006**, *27*, 1447–1452. [CrossRef] [PubMed]

188. Weng, C.J.; Wu, C.F.; Huang, H.W.; Wu, C.H.; Ho, C.T.; Yen, G.C. Evaluation of anti-invasion effect of resveratrol and related methoxy analogues on human hepatocarcinoma cells. *J. Agric. Food Chem.* **2010**, *58*, 2886–2894. [CrossRef] [PubMed]

189. Cavallaro, U.; Christofori, G. Cell adhesion and signalling by cadherins and Ig-CAMs in cancer. *Nat. Rev. Cancer* **2004**, *4*, 118–132. [CrossRef] [PubMed]

190. Larue, L.; Antos, C.; Butz, S.; Huber, O.; Delmas, V.; Dominis, M.; Kemler, R. A role for cadherins in tissue formation. *Development* **1996**, *122*, 3185–3194. [PubMed]

191. Zhang, B.; Zhang, H.; Shen, G. Metastasis-associated protein 2 (MTA2) promotes the metastasis of non-small-cell lung cancer through the inhibition of the cell adhesion molecule Ep-CAM and E-cadherin. *Jpn. J. Clin. Oncol.* **2015**, *45*, 755–766. [CrossRef] [PubMed]

192. Galván, J.A.; Zlobec, I.; Wartenberg, M.; Lugli, A.; Gloor, B.; Perren, A.; Karamitopoulou, E. Expression of E-cadherin repressors SNAIL, ZEB1 and ZEB2 by tumour and stromal cells influences tumour-budding phenotype and suggests heterogeneity of stromal cells in pancreatic cancer. *Br. J. Cancer* **2015**, *112*, 1944–1950. [CrossRef] [PubMed]

193. Luo, S.-L.; Xie, Y.-G.; Li, Z.; Ma, J.-H.; Xu, X. E-cadherin expression and prognosis of oral cancer: A meta-analysis. *Tumour Biol.* **2014**, *35*, 5533–5537. [CrossRef] [PubMed]

194. Schneider, M.R.; Hiltwein, F.; Grill, J.; Blum, H.; Krebs, S.; Klanner, A.; Bauersachs, S.; Bruns, C.; Longerich, T.; Horst, D.; et al. Evidence for a role of E-cadherin in suppressing liver carcinogenesis in mice and men. *Carcinogenesis* **2014**, *35*, 1855–1862. [CrossRef] [PubMed]

195. Liu, X.; Chu, K.-M.; Liu, X.; Chu, K.-M. E-cadherin and gastric cancer: Cause, consequence, and applications. *Biomed. Res. Int.* **2014**, *2014*, 637308. [CrossRef] [PubMed]

196. Barber, A.G.; Castillo-Martin, M.; Bonal, D.M.; Jia, A.J.; Rybicki, B.A.; Christiano, A.M.; Cordon-Cardo, C. PI3K/AKT pathway regulates E-cadherin and Desmoglein 2 in aggressive prostate cancer. *Cancer Med.* **2015**, *4*, 1258–1271. [CrossRef] [PubMed]

197. Trillsch, F.; Kuerti, S.; Eulenburg, C.; Burandt, E.; Woelber, L.; Prieske, K.; Eylmann, K.; Oliveira-Ferrer, L.; Milde-Langosch, K.; Mahner, S. E-Cadherin fragments as potential mediators for peritoneal metastasis in advanced epithelial ovarian cancer. *Br. J. Cancer* **2016**, *114*, 207–212. [CrossRef] [PubMed]

198. Vergara, D.; Simeone, P.; Latorre, D.; Cascione, F.; Leporatti, S.; Trerotola, M.; Giudetti, A.M.; Capobianco, L.; Lunetti, P.; Rizzello, A.; et al. Proteomics analysis of E-cadherin knockdown in epithelial breast cancer cells. *J. Biotechnol.* **2015**, *202*, 3–11. [CrossRef] [PubMed]

199. Xu, W.; Kimelman, D. Mechanistic insights from structural studies of beta-catenin and its binding partners. *J. Cell Sci.* **2007**, *120*, 3337–3344. [CrossRef] [PubMed]

200. Chen, H.-W.; Lee, J.-Y.; Huang, J.-Y.; Wang, C.-C.; Chen, W.-J.; Su, S.-F.; Huang, C.-W.; Ho, C.-C.; Chen, J.J.W.; Tsai, M.-F.; et al. Curcumin inhibits lung cancer cell invasion and metastasis through the tumor suppressor HLJ1. *Cancer Res.* **2008**, *68*, 7428–7438. [CrossRef] [PubMed]

201. Calderwood, S.K.; Khaleque, M.A.; Sawyer, D.B.; Ciocca, D.R. Heat shock proteins in cancer: Chaperones of tumorigenesis. *Trends Biochem. Sci.* **2006**, *31*, 164–172. [CrossRef] [PubMed]

202. Chen, C.C.; Sureshbabul, M.; Chen, H.W.; Lin, Y.S.; Lee, J.Y.; Hong, Q.S.; Yang, Y.C.; Yu, S.L. Curcumin suppresses metastasis via Sp-1, FAK inhibition, and E-cadherin upregulation in colorectal cancer. *Evid. Based Complement. Altern. Med.* **2013**, *2013*, 1–17. [CrossRef] [PubMed]

203. Kalluri, R.; Weinberg, R.A. The basics of epithelial-mesenchymal transition. *J. Clin. Investig.* **2009**, *119*, 1420–1428. [CrossRef] [PubMed]

204. Tan, C.; Zhang, L.; Cheng, X.; Lin, X.-F.F.; Lu, R.-R.R.; Bao, J.-D.D.; Yu, H.-X.X. Curcumin inhibits hypoxia-induced migration in K1 papillary thyroid cancer cells. *Exp. Biol. Med.* **2015**, *240*, 925–935. [CrossRef] [PubMed]

205. Zhang, C.-Y.; Zhang, L.; Yu, H.-X.; Bao, J.-D.; Lu, R.-R. Curcumin inhibits the metastasis of K1 papillary thyroid cancer cells via modulating E-cadherin and matrix metalloproteinase-9 expression. *Biotechnol. Lett.* **2013**, *35*, 995–1000. [CrossRef] [PubMed]

206. Zhang, L.; Cheng, X.; Gao, Y.; Zhang, C.; Bao, J.; Guan, H.; Yu, H.; Lu, R.; Xu, Q.; Sun, Y. Curcumin inhibits metastasis in human papillary thyroid carcinoma BCPAP cells via down-regulation of the TGF-β/Smad2/3 signaling pathway. *Exp. Cell Res.* **2016**, *341*, 157–165. [CrossRef] [PubMed]

207. Zhang, Z.; Chen, H.; Xu, C.; Song, L.; Huang, L.; Lai, Y.; Wang, Y.; Chen, H.; Gu, D.; Ren, L.; Yao, Q. Curcumin inhibits tumor epithelial-mesenchymal transition by downregulating the Wnt signaling pathway and upregulating NKD2 expression in colon cancer cells. *Oncol. Rep.* **2016**, *35*, 2615–2623. [CrossRef] [PubMed]

208. Du, Y.; Long, Q.; Zhang, L.; Shi, Y.; Liu, X.; Li, X.; Guan, B.; Tian, Y.; Wang, X.; Li, L.; He, D. Curcumin inhibits cancer-associated fibroblast-driven prostate cancer invasion through MAOA/mTOR/HIF-1α signaling. *Int. J. Oncol.* **2015**, *47*, 2064–2072. [CrossRef] [PubMed]

209. Zhao, G.; Han, X.; Zheng, S.; Li, Z.; Sha, Y.; Ni, J.; Sun, Z.; Qiao, S.; Song, Z. Curcumin induces autophagy, inhibits proliferation and invasion by downregulating AKT/mTOR signaling pathway in human melanoma cells. *Oncol. Rep.* **2016**, *35*, 1065–1074. [CrossRef] [PubMed]

210. Guan, F.; Ding, Y.; Zhang, Y.; Zhou, Y.; Li, M.; Wang, C. Curcumin suppresses proliferation and migration of MDA-MB-231 breast cancer cells through autophagy-dependent Akt degradation. *PLoS ONE* **2016**, *11*, e0146553. [CrossRef] [PubMed]

211. Guo, H.; Tian, T.; Nan, K.; Wang, W. p57: A multifunctional protein in cancer (Review). *Int. J. Oncol.* **2010**, *36*, 1321–1329. [PubMed]

212. Dhillon, A.S.; Hagan, S.; Rath, O.; Kolch, W. MAP kinase signalling pathways in cancer. *Oncogene* **2007**, *26*, 3279–3290. [CrossRef] [PubMed]

213. Park, S.Y.; Jeong, K.J.; Lee, J.; Yoon, D.S.; Choi, W.S.; Kim, Y.K.; Han, J.W.; Kim, Y.M.; Kim, B.K.; Lee, H.Y. Hypoxia enhances LPA-induced HIF-1α and VEGF expression: Their inhibition by resveratrol. *Cancer Lett.* **2007**, *258*, 63–69. [CrossRef] [PubMed]

214. Baribeau, S.; Chaudhry, P.; Parent, S.; Asselin, E. Resveratrol inhibits cisplatin-induced epithelial-to-mesenchymal transition in ovarian cancer cell lines. *PLoS ONE* **2014**, *9*, e86987. [CrossRef] [PubMed]

215. Lin, F.; Hsieh, Y.; Yang, S.; Chen, C.; Tang, C.; Chuang, Y.; Lin, C.; Chen, M. Resveratrol suppresses TPA-induced matrix metalloproteinase-9 expression through the inhibition of MAPK pathways in oral cancer cells. *J. Oral Pathol. Med.* **2015**, *44*, 699–706. [CrossRef] [PubMed]

216. Sun, T.; Chen, Q.Y.; Wu, L.J.; Yao, X.M.; Sun, X.J. Antitumor and antimetastatic activities of grape skin polyphenols in a murine model of breast cancer. *Food Chem. Toxicol.* **2012**, *50*, 3462–3467. [CrossRef] [PubMed]

217. Tang, F.; Chiang, E.I.; Sun, Y. Resveratrol inhibits heregulin-β 1-mediated matrix metalloproteinase-9 expression and cell invasion in human breast cancer cells. *J. Nutr. Biochem.* **2008**, *19*, 287–294. [CrossRef] [PubMed]

218. Gweon, E.J.; Kim, S.J. Resveratrol induces MMP-9 and cell migration via the p38 kinase and PI-3K pathways in HT1080 human fbrosarcoma cells. *Oncol. Rep.* **2013**, *29*, 826–834. [PubMed]

219. Yeh, C.B.; Hsieh, M.J.; Lin, C.W.; Chiou, H.L.; Lin, P.Y.; Chen, T.Y.; Yang, S.F. The antimetastatic effects of resveratrol on hepatocellular carcinoma through the downregulation of a metastasis-associated protease by SP-1 modulation. *PLoS ONE* **2013**, *8*, e56661. [CrossRef] [PubMed]

220. Yang, S.; Lee, W.; Tan, P.; Tang, C.; Hsiao, M.; Hsieh, F.; Chien, M. Upregulation of miR-328 and inhibition of CREB-DNA-binding activity are critical for resveratrol-mediated suppression of matrix metalloproteinase-2 and subsequent metastatic ability in human osteosarcomas. *Oncotarget* **2015**, *6*, 2736–2753. [CrossRef] [PubMed]

221. Vara, J.Á.F.; Casado, E.; de Castro, J.; Cejas, P.; Belda-Iniesta, C.; González-Barón, M. PI3K/Akt signalling pathway and cancer. *Cancer Treat. Rev.* **2004**, *30*, 193–204. [CrossRef] [PubMed]

222. Altomare, D.A.; Testa, J.R. Perturbations of the AKT signaling pathway in human cancer. *Oncogene* **2005**, *24*, 7455–7464. [CrossRef] [PubMed]

223. Bhattacharya, S.; Darjatmoko, S.R.; Polans, A.S. Resveratrol modulates the malignant properties of cutaneous melanoma through changes in the activation and attenuation of the antiapoptotic protooncogenic protein Akt/PKB. *Melanoma Res.* **2011**, *21*, 180–187. [CrossRef] [PubMed]

224. Jiao, Y.; Li, H.; Liu, Y.; Guo, A.; Xu, X.; Qu, X.; Wang, S.; Zhao, J.; Li, Y.; Cao, Y. Resveratrol inhibits the invasion of glioblastoma-initiating cells via down-regulation of the PI3K/Akt/NF-κB signaling pathway. *Nutrients* **2015**, *7*, 4383–4402. [CrossRef] [PubMed]

225. Li, W.; Ma, J.; Ma, Q.; Li, B.; Han, L.; Liu, J.; Xu, Q.; Duan, W.; Yu, S.; Wang, F.; Wu, E. Resveratrol inhibits the epithelial-mesenchymal transition of pancreatic cancer cells via suppression of the PI-3K/Akt/NF-κB pathway. *Curr. Med. Chem.* **2013**, *20*, 4185–4194. [CrossRef] [PubMed]

226. Tang, F.Y.; Su, Y.C.; Chen, N.C.; Hsieh, H.S.; Chen, K.S. Resveratrol inhibits migration and invasion of human breast-cancer cells. *Mol. Nutr. Food Res.* **2008**, *52*, 683–691. [CrossRef] [PubMed]

227. Kalinski, T.; Sel, S.; Hutten, H.; Ropke, M.; Roessner, A.; Nass, N. Curcumin blocks interleukin-1 signaling in chondrosarcoma cells. *PLoS ONE* **2014**, *9*, e99296. [CrossRef] [PubMed]

228. Da, W.; Zhu, J.; Wang, L.; Sun, Q. Curcumin suppresses lymphatic vessel density in an in vivo human gastric cancer model. *Tumour Biol.* **2015**, *36*, 5215–5223. [CrossRef] [PubMed]

229. Rubin, L.L.; de Sauvage, F.J. Targeting the Hedgehog pathway in cancer. *Nat. Rev. Drug Discov.* **2006**, *5*, 1026–1033. [CrossRef] [PubMed]

230. Amakye, D.; Jagani, Z.; Dorsch, M. Unraveling the therapeutic potential of the Hedgehog pathway in cancer. *Nat. Med.* **2013**, *19*, 1410–1422. [CrossRef] [PubMed]

231. Gupta, S.; Takebe, N.; LoRusso, P. Targeting the Hedgehog pathway in cancer. *Ther. Adv. Med. Oncol.* **2010**, *2*, 237–250. [CrossRef] [PubMed]

232. Li, J.; Chong, T.; Wang, Z.; Chen, H.; Li, H.; Cao, J.; Zhang, P.; Li, H. A novel anti-cancer effect of resveratrol: Reversal of epithelial-mesenchymal transition in prostate cancer cells. *Mol. Med. Rep.* **2014**, *10*, 1717–1724. [CrossRef] [PubMed]

233. Matise, M.P.; Joyner, A.L. Gli genes in development and cancer. *Oncogene* **1999**, *18*, 7852–7859. [CrossRef] [PubMed]

234. Gao, Q.; Yuan, Y.; Gan, H.; Peng, Q. Resveratrol inhibits the hedgehog signaling pathway and epithelial-mesenchymal transition and suppresses gastric cancer invasion and metastasis. *Oncol. Lett.* **2015**, *9*, 2381–2387. [CrossRef] [PubMed]

235. Li, W.; Cao, L.; Chen, X.; Lei, J.; Ma, Q. Resveratrol inhibits hypoxia-driven ROS-induced invasive and migratory ability of pancreatic cancer cells via suppression of the Hedgehog signaling pathway. *Oncol. Rep.* **2016**, *35*, 1718–1726. [CrossRef] [PubMed]

236. Yu, H.; Lee, H.; Herrmann, A.; Buettner, R.; Jove, R. Revisiting STAT3 signalling in cancer: New and unexpected biological functions. *Nat. Rev. Cancer* **2014**, *17*, 736–746. [CrossRef] [PubMed]

237. Siveen, K.S.; Sikka, S.; Surana, R.; Daia, X.; Zhang, J.; Kumar, A.P.; Tan, B.K.H.; Sethi, G.; Bishayee, A. Targeting the STAT-3 signaling pathway in cancer: Role of synthetic and natural inhibitors. *Biochim. Biophys. Acta* **2014**, *1845*, 136–154. [PubMed]

238. Eswaran, D.; Huang, S. STAT-3 as a central regulator of tumor metastases. *Curr. Mol. Med.* **2009**, *9*, 626–633.

239. Lee-Chang, C.; Bodogai, M.; Martin-Montalvo, A.; Wejksza, K.; Sanghvi, M.; Moaddel, R.; de Cabo, R.; Biragyn, A. Inhibition of breast cancer metastasis by resveratrol-mediated inactivation of tumor-evoked regulatory B cells. *J. Immunol.* **2013**, *191*, 4141–4151. [CrossRef] [PubMed]

240. Olkhanud, P.B.; Damdinsuren, B.; Bodogai, M.; Gress, R.E.; Sen, R.; Wejksza, K.; Malchinkhuu, E.; Wersto, R.P.; Biragyn, A. Tumor-evoked regulatory B cells promote breast cancer metastasis by converting resting CD4+ T cells to T-regulatory cells. *Cancer Res.* **2011**, *71*, 3505–3515. [CrossRef] [PubMed]

241. Kimura, Y.; Sumiyoshi, M. Resveratrol prevents tumor growth and metastasis by inhibiting lymphangiogenesis and M2 macrophage activation and differentiation in tumor-associated macrophages. *Nutr. Cancer* **2016**, *68*, 667–678. [CrossRef] [PubMed]

242. Schmieder, A.; Michel, J.; Schönhaar, K.; Goerdt, S.; Schledzewski, K. Differentiation and gene expression profile of tumor-associated macrophages. *Semin. Cancer Biol.* **2012**, *22*, 289–297. [CrossRef] [PubMed]

243. Wang, H.; Feng, H.; Zhang, Y. Resveratrol inhibits hypoxia-induced glioma cell migration and invasion by the p-STAT-3/miR-34a axis. *Neoplasma* **2016**, *63*, 532–539. [CrossRef] [PubMed]

244. Misso, G.; Di Martino, M.T.; De Rosa, G.; Farooqi, A.A.; Lombardi, A.; Campani, V.; Zarone, M.R.; Gullà, A.; Tagliaferri, P.; Tassone, P.; et al. Mir-34: A New Weapon Against Cancer? *Mol. Ther. Nucleic Acids* **2014**, *3*, e194. [CrossRef] [PubMed]

245. Chen, Q.Y.; Jiao, D.E.M.; Yao, Q.H.; Yan, J.; Song, J.; Chen, F.Y.; Lu, G.H.; Zhou, J.Y. Expression analysis of Cdc42 in lung cancer and modulation of its expression by curcumin in lung cancer cell lines. *Int. J. Oncol.* **2012**, *40*, 1561–1568. [CrossRef] [PubMed]

246. Sahai, E.; Marshall, C.J. RHO-GTPases and cancer. *Nat. Rev. Cancer* **2002**, *2*, 133–142. [CrossRef] [PubMed]

247. Wang, L.; Dong, Z.; Zhang, Y.; Miao, J. The roles of integrin β4 in vascular endothelial cells. *J. Cell. Physiol.* **2012**, *227*, 474–478. [CrossRef] [PubMed]

248. Coleman, D.T.; Soung, Y.H.; Surh, Y.J.; Cardelli, J.A.; Chung, J. Curcumin prevents palmitoylation of integrin β4 in breast cancer cells. *PLoS ONE* **2015**, *10*, e0125399. [CrossRef] [PubMed]

249. Dorai, T.; Diouri, J.; O'Shea, O.; Doty, S.B. Curcumin inhibits prostate cancer bone metastasis by up-regulating bone morphogenic protein-7 in vivo. *J. Cancer Ther.* **2014**, *5*, 369–386. [CrossRef] [PubMed]

250. Buijs, J.T.; Rentsch, C.A.; van der Horst, G.; van Overveld, P.G.M.; Wetterwald, A.; Schwaninger, R.; Henriquez, N.V.; Ten Dijke, P.; Borovecki, F.; Markwalder, R.; et al. BMP7, a putative regulator of epithelial homeostasis in the human prostate, is a potent inhibitor of prostate cancer bone metastasis in vivo. *Am. J. Pathol.* **2007**, *171*, 1047–1057. [CrossRef] [PubMed]

251. Mudduluru, G.; George-William, J.N.; Muppala, S.; Asangani, I.A.; Kumarswamy, R.; Nelson, L.D.; Allgayer, H. Curcumin regulates miR-21 expression and inhibits invasion and metastasis in colorectal cancer. *Biosci. Rep.* **2011**, *31*, 185–197. [CrossRef] [PubMed]

252. Selcuklu, S.D.; Donoghue, M.T.; Spillane, C. miR-21 as a key regulator of oncogenic processes. *Biochem. Soc. Trans.* **2009**, *37*, 918–925. [CrossRef] [PubMed]

253. Yeh, W.; Lin, H.; Huang, C.; Huang, B. Migration-prone glioma cells show curcumin resistance associated with enhanced expression of miR-21 and invasion/anti-apoptosis-related proteins. *Oncotarget* **2015**, *6*, 37770–37781. [PubMed]

254. Bessette, D.C.; Wong, P.C.W.; Pallen, C.J. PRL-3: A metastasis-associated phosphatase in search of a function. *Cells Tissues Organs* **2007**, *185*, 232–236. [CrossRef] [PubMed]

255. Rouleau, C.; Roy, A.; St. Martin, T.; Dufault, M.R.; Boutin, P.; Liu, D.; Zhang, M.; Puorro-Radzwill, K.; Rulli, L.; Reczek, D.; et al. Protein tyrosine phosphatase PRL-3 in malignant cells and endothelial cells: Expression and function. *Mol. Cancer Ther.* **2006**, *5*, 219–229. [CrossRef] [PubMed]

256. Wang, L.; Shen, Y.; Song, R.; Sun, Y.; Xu, J.; Xu, Q. An anticancer effect of curcumin mediated by down-regulating phosphatase of regenerating liver-3 expression on highly metastatic melanoma cells. *Mol. Pharmacol.* **2009**, *76*, 1238–1245. [CrossRef] [PubMed]

257. Dhar, S.; Kumar, A.; Li, K.; Tzivion, G.; Levenson, A.S. Resveratrol regulates PTEN/Akt pathway through inhibition of MTA1/HDAC unit of the NuRD complex in prostate cancer. *Biochim. Biophys. Acta Mol. Cell Res.* **2015**, *1853*, 265–275. [CrossRef] [PubMed]

258. Jeong, K.J.; Cho, K.H.; Panupinthu, N.; Kim, H.; Kang, J.; Park, C.G.; Mills, G.B.; Lee, H.Y. EGFR mediates LPA-induced proteolytic enzyme expression and ovarian cancer invasion: Inhibition by resveratrol. *Mol. Oncol.* **2013**, *7*, 121–129. [CrossRef] [PubMed]

259. Ji, Q.; Liu, X.; Fu, X.; Zhang, L.; Sui, H.; Zhou, L.; Sun, J.; Cai, J.; Qin, J.; Ren, J.; Li, Q. Resveratrol inhibits invasion and metastasis of colorectal cancer cells via MALAT1 mediated Wnt/β-catenin signal pathway. *PLoS ONE* **2013**, *8*, e78700. [CrossRef] [PubMed]

260. Ji, Q.; Liu, X.; Han, Z.; Zhou, L.; Sui, H.; Yan, L.; Jiang, H.; Ren, J.; Cai, J.; Li, Q. Resveratrol suppresses epithelial-to-mesenchymal transition in colorectal cancer through TGF-β1/Smads signaling pathway mediated Snail/E-cadherin expression. *BMC Cancer* **2015**, *15*, 97. [CrossRef] [PubMed]

261. Mikula-Pietrasik, J.; Sosinska, P.; Ksiazek, K. Resveratrol inhibits ovarian cancer cell adhesion to peritoneal mesothelium in vitro by modulating the production of α5β1 integrins and hyaluronic acid. *Gynecol. Oncol.* **2014**, *134*, 624–630. [CrossRef] [PubMed]

262. Rodrigue, C.M.; Porteu, F.; Navarro, N.; Bruyneel, E.; Bracke, M.; Romeo, P.-H.; Gespach, C.; Garel, M.-C. The cancer chemopreventive agent resveratrol induces tensin, a cell–matrix adhesion protein with signaling and antitumor activities. *Oncogene* **2005**, *24*, 3274–3284. [CrossRef] [PubMed]

263. Wang, H.; Zhang, H.; Tang, L.; Chen, H.; Wu, C.; Zhao, M.; Yang, Y.; Chen, X.; Liu, G. Resveratrol inhibits TGF-β1-induced epithelial-to-mesenchymal transition and suppresses lung cancer invasion and metastasis. *Toxicology* **2013**, *303*, 139–146. [CrossRef] [PubMed]

264. Zykova, T.A.; Zhu, F.; Zhai, X.; Ma, W.Y.; Ermakova, S.P.; Ki, W.L.; Bode, A.M.; Dong, Z. Resveratrol directly targets COX-2 to inhibit carcinogenesis. *Mol. Carcinog.* **2008**, *47*, 797–805. [CrossRef] [PubMed]

265. Salado, C.; Olaso, E.; Gallot, N.; Valcarcel, M.; Egilegor, E.; Mendoza, L.; Vidal-Vanaclocha, F. Resveratrol prevents inflammation-dependent hepatic melanoma metastasis by inhibiting the secretion and effects of interleukin-18. *J. Transl. Med.* **2011**, *9*, 59. [CrossRef] [PubMed]

266. Green, D.R.; Kroemer, G. The pathophysiology of mitochondrial cell death. *Science* **2004**, *305*, 626–629. [CrossRef] [PubMed]

267. Henry-Mowatt, J.; Dive, C.; Martinou, J.; James, D. Role of mitochondrial membrane permeabilization in apoptosis and cancer. *Oncogene* **2004**, *23*, 2850–2860. [CrossRef] [PubMed]

268. Zou, H.; Henzel, W.J.; Liu, X.; Lutschg, A.; Wang, X. Apaf-1, a human protein homologous to *C. elegans* CED-4, participates in cytochrome c dependent activation of caspace 3. *Cell* **1997**, *90*, 405–413. [CrossRef]

269. Adrain, C.; Slee, E.A.; Harte, M.T.; Martin, S.J. Regulation of apoptotic protease activating factor-1 oligomerization and apoptosis by the WD-40 repeat region. *J. Biol. Chem.* **1999**, *274*, 20855–20860. [CrossRef] [PubMed]

270. Kroemer, G.; Galluzzi, L.; Brenner, C. Mitochondrial membrane permeabilization in cell death. *Physiol. Rev.* **2007**, *87*, 99–163. [CrossRef] [PubMed]

271. Bratton, S.B.; Walker, G.; Srinivasula, S.M.; Sun, X.M.; Butterworth, M.; Alnemri, E.S.; Cohen, G.M. Recruitment, activation and retention of caspases-9 and-3 by Apaf-1 apoptosome and associated XIAP complexes. *EMBO J.* **2001**, *20*, 998–1009. [CrossRef] [PubMed]

272. Fulda, S.; Debatin, K.-M. Extrinsic versus intrinsic apoptosis pathways in anticancer chemotherapy. *Oncogene* **2006**, *25*, 4798–4811. [CrossRef] [PubMed]

273. Susin, S.A.; Zamzami, N.; Castedo, M.; Hirsch, T.; Marchetti, P.; Macho, A.; Daugas, E.; Geuskens, M.; Kroemer, G. Bcl-2 inhibits the mitochondrial release of an apoptogenic protease. *J. Exp. Med.* **1996**, *184*, 1331–1341. [CrossRef] [PubMed]

274. Lin, X.; Wu, G.; Huo, W.Q.; Zhang, Y.; Jin, F.S. Resveratrol induces apoptosis associated with mitochondrial dysfunction in bladder carcinoma cells. *Int. J. Urol.* **2012**, *19*, 757–764. [CrossRef] [PubMed]

275. Van Ginkel, P.R.; Sareen, D.; Subramanian, L.; Walker, Q.; Darjatmoko, S.R.; Lindstrom, M.J.; Kulkarni, A.; Albert, D.M.; Polans, A.S. Resveratrol inhibits tumor growth of human neuroblastoma and mediates apoptosis by directly targeting mitochondria. *Clin. Cancer Res.* **2007**, *13*, 5162–5169. [CrossRef] [PubMed]

276. Alkhalaf, M.; El-Mowafy, A.; Renno, W.; Rachid, O.; Ali, A.; Al-Attyiah, R. Resveratrol-induced apoptosis in human breast cancer cells is mediated primarily through the caspase-3-dependent pathway. *Arch. Med. Res.* **2008**, *39*, 162–168. [CrossRef] [PubMed]

277. Zhang, W.; Fei, Z.; Zhen, H.-N.; Zhang, J.-N.; Zhang, X. Resveratrol inhibits cell growth and induces apoptosis of rat C6 glioma cells. *J. Neurooncol.* **2007**, *81*, 231–240. [CrossRef] [PubMed]

278. Zhang, W.; Wang, X.; Chen, T. Resveratrol induces mitochondria-mediated AIF and to a lesser extent caspase-9-dependent apoptosis in human lung adenocarcinoma ASTC-a-1 cells. *Mol. Cell. Biochem.* **2011**, *354*, 29–37. [CrossRef] [PubMed]

279. Zhang, W.; Wang, X.; Chen, T. Resveratrol induces apoptosis via a Bak-mediated intrinsic pathway in human lung adenocarcinoma cells. *Cell. Signal.* **2012**, *24*, 1037–1046. [CrossRef] [PubMed]

280. Qadir, M.I.; Naqvi, S.T.Q.; Muhammad, S.A. Curcumin: A polyphenol with molecular targets for cancer control. *Asian Pac. J. Cancer Prev.* **2016**, *17*, 2735–2739. [PubMed]

281. Song, F.; Zhang, L.; Yu, H.-X.; Lu, R.-R.; Bao, J.-D.; Tan, C.; Sun, Z. The mechanism underlying proliferation-inhibitory and apoptosis-inducing effects of curcumin on papillary thyroid cancer cells. *Food Chem.* **2012**, *132*, 43–50. [CrossRef] [PubMed]

282. Khan, M.A.; Gahlot, S.; Majumdar, S. Oxidative stress induced by curcumin promotes the death of cutaneous T-cell lymphoma (HuT-78) by disrupting the function of several molecular targets. *Mol. Cancer Ther.* **2012**, *11*, 1873–1883. [CrossRef] [PubMed]

283. Kaushik, G.; Kaushik, T.; Yadav, S.K.; Sharma, S.K.; Ranawat, P.; Khanduja, K.L.; Pathak, C.M. Curcumin sensitizes lung adenocarcinoma cells to apoptosis via intracellular redox status mediated pathway. *Indian J. Exp. Biol.* **2012**, *50*, 853–861. [PubMed]

284. Hussain, A.R.; Uddin, S.; Bu, R.; Khan, O.S.; Ahmed, S.O.; Ahmed, M.; Al-Kuraya, K.S. Resveratrol suppresses constitutive activation of AKT via generation of ROS and induces apoptosis in diffuse large B cell lymphoma cell lines. *PLoS ONE* **2011**, *6*, e24703. [CrossRef] [PubMed]

285. Wang, Z.; Li, W.; Meng, X.; Jia, B. Resveratrol induces gastric cancer cell apoptosis via reactive oxygen species, but independent of sirtuin1. *Clin. Exp. Pharmacol. Physiol.* **2012**, *39*, 227–232. [CrossRef] [PubMed]

286. Su, C.C.; Lin, J.G.; Li, T.M.; Chung, J.G.; Yang, J.S.; Ip, S.W.; Lin, W.C.; Chen, G.W. Curcumin-induced apoptosis of human colon cancer colo 205 cells through the production of ROS, $Ca^{2+}$ and the activation of caspase-3. *Anticancer Res.* **2006**, *26*, 4379–4389. [PubMed]

287. Tan, T.-W.; Tsai, H.-R.; Lu, H.-F.; Lin, H.-L.; Tsou, M.-F.; Lin, Y.-T.; Tsai, H.-Y.; Chen, Y.-F.; Chung, J.-G. Curcumin-induced cell cycle arrest and apoptosis in human acute promyelocytic leukemia HL-60 cells via MMP changes and caspase-3 activation. *Anticancer Res.* **2006**, *26*, 4361–4371. [PubMed]

288. Ibrahim, A.; El-Meligy, A.; Lungu, G.; Fetaih, H.; Dessouki, A.; Stoica, G.; Barhoumi, R. Curcumin induces apoptosis in a murine mammary gland adenocarcinoma cell line through the mitochondrial pathway. *Eur. J. Pharmacol.* **2011**, *668*, 127–132. [CrossRef] [PubMed]

289. Wang, W.; Chiang, I.; Ding, K.; Chung, J.-G.; Lin, W.-J.; Lin, S. L.; Hwang, J.-J. Curcumin-induced apoptosis in human hepatocellular carcinoma J5 cells: Critical role of $Ca^{+2}$-dependent pathway. *Evid. Based Complement. Altern. Med.* **2012**, *2012*, 1–7. [CrossRef] [PubMed]

290. Marchetti, C.; Ribulla, S.; Magnelli, V.; Patrone, M.; Burlando, B. Resveratrol induces intracellular $Ca^{2+}$ rise via T-type $Ca^{2+}$ channels in a mesothelioma cell line. *Life Sci.* **2016**, *148*, 125–131. [CrossRef] [PubMed]

291. Skommer, J.; Wlodkowic, D.; Pelkonen, J. Cellular foundation of curcumin-induced apoptosis in follicular lymphoma cell lines. *Exp. Hematol.* **2006**, *34*, 463–474. [CrossRef] [PubMed]

292. Guo, L.; Chen, X.; Hu, Y.; Yu, Z.; Wang, D.; Liu, J. Curcumin inhibits proliferation and induces apoptosis of human colorectal cancer cells by activating the mitochondria apoptotic pathway. *Phyther. Res.* **2013**, *27*, 422–430. [CrossRef] [PubMed]

293. Huang, T.Y.; Tsai, T.H.; Hsu, C.W.; Hsu, Y.C. Curcuminoids suppress the growth and induce apoptosis through caspase-3-dependent pathways in glioblastoma multiforme (GBM) 8401 cells. *J. Agric. Food Chem.* **2010**, *58*, 10639–10645. [CrossRef] [PubMed]

294. Shankar, S.; Srivastava, R.K. Involvement of Bcl-2 family members, phosphatidylinositol 3′-kinase/AKT and mitochondrial p53 in curcumin (diferulolylmethane)-induced apoptosis in prostate cancer. *Int. J. Oncol.* **2007**, *30*, 905–918. [CrossRef] [PubMed]

295. Yu, Z.; Shah, D.M. Curcumin down-regulates Ets-1 and Bcl-2 expression in human endometrial carcinoma HEC-1-A cells. *Gynecol. Oncol.* **2007**, *106*, 541–548. [CrossRef] [PubMed]

296. Yang, J.; Ning, J.; Peng, L.; He, D. Effect of curcumin on Bcl-2 and Bax expression in nude mice prostate cancer. *Int. J. Clin. Exp. Pathol.* **2015**, *8*, 9272–9278. [PubMed]

297. Huang, T.; Lin, H.; Chen, C.; Lu, C.; Wei, C.; Wu, T.; Liu, F.; Lai, H. Resveratrol induces apoptosis of human nasopharyngeal carcinoma cells via activation of multiple apoptotic pathways. *J. Cell. Physiol.* **2010**, *226*, 720–728. [CrossRef] [PubMed]

298. Wang, B.; Liu, J.; Gong, Z. Resveratrol induces apoptosis in K562 cells via the regulation of mitochondrial signaling pathways. *Int. J. Clin. Exp. Med.* **2015**, *8*, 16926–16933. [PubMed]

299. Cui, J.; Sun, R.; Yu, Y.; Gou, S.; Zhao, G.; Wang, C. Antiproliferative effect of resveratrol in pancreatic cancer cells. *Phyther. Res.* **2010**, *24*, 1637–1644. [CrossRef] [PubMed]

300. Fernández-Pérez, F.; Belchí-Navarro, S.; Almagro, L.; Bru, R.; Pedreño, M.A.; Gómez-Ros, L.V. Cytotoxic effect of natural trans-resveratrol obtained from elicited vitis vinifera cell cultures on three cancer cell lines. *Plant Foods Hum. Nutr.* **2012**, *67*, 422–429. [CrossRef] [PubMed]

301. Ou, X.; Chen, Y.; Cheng, X.; Zhang, X.; He, Q. Potentiation of resveratrol-induced apoptosis by matrine in human hepatoma HepG2 cells. *Oncol. Rep.* **2014**, *32*, 2803–2809. [CrossRef] [PubMed]

302. Benchimol, S. P53-dependent pathways of apoptosis. *Cell Death Differ.* **2001**, *8*, 1049–1051. [CrossRef] [PubMed]

303. Fridman, J.S.; Lowe, S.W. Control of apoptosis by p53. *Oncogene* **2003**, *22*, 9030–9040. [CrossRef] [PubMed]

304. Reuter, S.; Eifes, S.; Dicato, M.; Aggarwal, B.B.; Diederich, M. Modulation of anti-apoptotic and survival pathways by curcumin as a strategy to induce apoptosis in cancer cells. *Biochem. Pharmacol.* **2008**, *76*, 1340–1351. [CrossRef] [PubMed]

305. Alkhalaf, M. Resveratrol-induced apoptosis is associated with activation of p53 and inhibition of protein translation in T47D human breast cancer cells. *Pharmacology* **2007**, *80*, 134–143. [CrossRef] [PubMed]

306. Ellisen, L.W.; Bird, J.; West, D.C.; Soreng, A.L.; Reynolds, T.C.; Smith, S.D.; Sklar, J. TAN-l, the human homolog of the drosophila notch gene, is broken by chromosomal translocations in T lymphoblastic neoplasms. *Cell* **1991**, *66*, 649–661. [CrossRef]

307. Lin, H.; Xiong, W.; Zhang, X.; Liu, B.; Zhang, W.; Zhang, Y.; Cheng, J.; Huang, H. Notch-1 activation-dependent p53 restoration contributes to resveratrol-induced apoptosis in glioblastoma cells. *Oncol. Rep.* **2011**, *26*, 925–930. [PubMed]

308. Ozaki, T.; Nakagawara, A. P73, a sophisticated P53 family member in the cancer world. *Cancer Sci.* **2005**, *96*, 729–737. [CrossRef] [PubMed]

309. Moll, U.M.; Slade, N. P63 and P73: Roles in development and tumor formation. *Mol. Cancer Res.* **2004**, *2*, 371–386. [PubMed]

310. Wang, J.; Xie, H.; Gao, F.; Zhao, T.; Yang, H.; Kang, B. Curcumin induces apoptosis in p53-null Hep3B cells through a TAp73/DNp73-dependent pathway. *Tumor Biol.* **2016**, *37*, 4203–4212. [CrossRef] [PubMed]

311. Harper, N.; Hughes, M.; MacFarlane, M.; Cohen, G.M. Fas-associated death domain protein and caspase-8 are not recruited to the tumor necrosis factor receptor 1 signaling complex during tumor necrosis factor-induced apoptosis. *J. Biol. Chem.* **2003**, *278*, 25534–25541. [CrossRef] [PubMed]

312. Wang, S.; El-Deiry, W.S. TRAIL and apoptosis induction by TNF-family death receptors. *Oncogene* **2003**, *22*, 8628–8633. [CrossRef] [PubMed]

313. Shankar, S.; Chen, Q.; Siddiqui, I.; Sarva, K.; Srivastava, R.K. Sensitization of TRAIL-resistant LNCaP cells by resveratrol (3,4′,5 tri-hydroxystilbene): Molecular mechanisms and therapeutic potential. *J. Mol. Signal.* **2007**, *2*, 7. [CrossRef] [PubMed]

314. Shankar, S.; Chen, Q.; Sarva, K.; Siddiqui, I.; Srivastava, R.K. Curcumin enhances the apoptosis-inducing potential of TRAIL in prostate cancer cells: Molecular mechanisms of apoptosis, migration and angiogenesis. *J. Mol. Signal.* **2007**, *2*, 10. [CrossRef] [PubMed]

315. Lee, H.; Li, T.; Tsao, J.; Fong, Y.; Tang, C. Curcumin induces cell apoptosis in human chondrosarcoma through extrinsic death receptor pathway. *Int. Immunopharmacol.* **2012**, *13*, 163–169. [CrossRef] [PubMed]

316. Ko, Y.; Chang, C.; Chien, H.; Wu, C.; Lin, L. Resveratrol enhances the expression of death receptor Fas/CD95 and induces differentiation and apoptosis in anaplastic large-cell lymphoma cells. *Cancer Lett.* **2011**, *309*, 46–53. [CrossRef] [PubMed]

317. Reis-Sobreiro, M.; Gajate, C.; Mollinedo, F. Involvement of mitochondria and recruitment of Fas/CD95 signaling in lipid rafts in resveratrol-mediated antimyeloma and antileukemia actions. *Oncogene* **2009**, *28*, 3221–3234. [CrossRef] [PubMed]

318. Wu, S.H.; Hang, L.W.; Yang, J.S.; Chen, H.Y.; Lin, H.Y.; Chiang, J.H.; Lu, C.C.; Yang, J.L.; Lai, T.Y.; Ko, Y.C.; et al. Curcumin induces apoptosis in human non-small cell lung cancer NCI-H460 cells through ER stress and caspase cascade- and mitochondria-dependent pathways. *Anticancer Res.* **2010**, *30*, 2125–2133. [PubMed]

319. Li, L.; Aggarwal, B.B.; Shishodia, S.; Abbruzzese, J.; Kurzrock, R. Nuclear factor-kappaB and IkappaB kinase are constitutively active in human pancreatic cells, and their down-regulation by curcumin (diferuloylmethane) is associated with the suppression of proliferation and the induction of apoptosis. *Cancer* **2004**, *101*, 2351–2362. [CrossRef] [PubMed]

320. Zanotto-Filho, A.; Braganhol, E.; Schroder, R.; De Souza, L.H.T.; Dalmolin, R.J.S.; Pasquali, M.A.B.; Gelain, D.P.; Battastini, A.M.O.; Moreira, J.C.F. NFκB inhibitors induce cell death in glioblastomas. *Biochem. Pharmacol.* **2011**, *81*, 412–424. [CrossRef] [PubMed]

321. Sun, C.; Hu, Y.; Liu, X.; Wu, T.; Wang, Y.; He, W.; Wei, W. Resveratrol downregulates the constitutional activation of nuclear factor-κB in multiple myeloma cells, leading to suppression of proliferation and invasion, arrest of cell cycle, and induction of apoptosis. *Cancer Genet. Cytogenet.* **2006**, *165*, 9–19. [CrossRef] [PubMed]

322. Pozo-guisado, E.; Merino, J.M.; Mulero-navarro, S.; Jesús, M.; Centeno, F.; Alvarez-barrientos, A.; Salguero, P.M.F. Resveratrol-induced apoptosis in MCF-7 human breast cancer cells involves a caspase-independent mechanism with downregulation of Bcl-2 and NF-κB. *Int. J. Cancer* **2005**, *115*, 74–84. [CrossRef] [PubMed]

323. Hardwaj, A.; Sethi, G.; Vadhan-Raj, S.; Bueso-Ramos, C.; Takada, Y.; Gaur, U.; Nair, A.S.; Shishodia, S.; Aggarwal, B.B. Resveratrol inhibits proliferation, induces apoptosis, and overcomes chemoresistance through down-regulation of STAT-3 and nuclear factor-kappaB-regulated antiapoptotic and cell survival gene products in human multiple myeloma cells. *Blood* **2007**, *109*, 2293–2302. [CrossRef] [PubMed]

324. Kizhakkayil, J.; Thayyullathil, F.; Chathoth, S.; Hago, A.; Patel, M.; Galadari, S. Modulation of curcumin-induced Akt phosphorylation and apoptosis by PI3K inhibitor in MCF-7 cells. *Biochem. Biophys. Res. Commun.* **2010**, *394*, 476–481. [CrossRef] [PubMed]

325. Amin, A.R.M.R.; Haque, A.; Rahman, M.A.; Chen, Z.G.; Khuri, F.R.; Shin, D.M. Curcumin induces apoptosis of upper aerodigestive tract cancer cells by targeting multiple pathways. *PLoS ONE* **2015**, *10*, e0124218. [CrossRef] [PubMed]

326. Hussain, A.R.; Al-Rasheed, M.; Manogaran, P.S.; Al-Hussein, K.A.; Platanias, L.C.; Al Kuraya, K.; Uddin, S. Curcumin induces apoptosis via inhibition of PI3 kinase/AKT pathway in acute T cell leukemias. *Apoptosis* **2006**, *11*, 245–254. [CrossRef] [PubMed]

327. Zhao, Z.; Li, C.; Xi, H.; Gao, Y.; Xu, D. Curcumin induces apoptosis in pancreatic cancer cells through the induction of forkhead box O1 and inhibition of the PI3K/Akt pathway. *Mol. Med. Rep.* **2015**, *12*, 5415–5422. [PubMed]

328. Wong, T.F.; Takeda, T.; Li, B.; Tsuiji, K.; Kitamura, M.; Kondo, A.; Yaegashi, N. Curcumin disrupts uterine leiomyosarcoma cells through AKT-mTOR pathway inhibition. *Gynecol. Oncol.* **2011**, *122*, 141–148. [CrossRef] [PubMed]

329. Wong, T.F.; Takeda, T.; Li, B.; Tsuiji, K.; Kondo, A.; Tadakawa, M.; Nagase, S.; Yaegashi, N. Curcumin targets the AKT-mTOR pathway for uterine leiomyosarcoma tumor growth suppression. *Int. J. Clin. Oncol.* **2014**, *19*, 354–363. [CrossRef] [PubMed]

330. Li, Y.; Liu, J.; Liu, X.; Xing, K.; Wang, Y.; Li, F.; Yao, L. Resveratrol-induced cell inhibition of growth and apoptosis in MCF7 human breast cancer cells are associated with modulation of phosphorylated akt and caspase-9. *Appl. Biochem. Biotechnol.* **2006**, *135*, 181–192. [CrossRef]

331. Chakraborty, P.K.; Mustafi, S.B.; Ganguly, S.; Chatterjee, M.; Raha, S. Resveratrol induces apoptosis in K562 (chronic myelogenous leukemia) cells by targeting a key survival protein, heat shock protein 70. *Cancer Sci.* **2008**, *99*, 1109–1116. [CrossRef] [PubMed]

332. Mustafi, S.B.; Chakraborty, P.K.; Raha, S. Modulation of AKT and ERK1/2 pathways by resveratrol in chronic myelogenous leukemia (CML) cells results in the downregulation of Hsp70. *PLoS ONE* **2010**, *5*, e8719.

333. Sayed, D.; He, M.; Hong, C.; Gao, S.; Rane, S.; Yang, Z.; Abdellatif, M. MicroRNA-21 is a downstream effector of AKT that mediates its antiapoptotic effects via suppression of fas ligand. *J. Biol. Chem.* **2010**, *285*, 20281–20290. [CrossRef] [PubMed]

334. Sheth, S.; Jajoo, S.; Kaur, T.; Mukherjea, D.; Sheehan, K.; Rybak, L.P.; Ramkumar, V. Resveratrol reduces prostate cancer growth and metastasis by inhibiting the Akt/MicroRNA-21 pathway. *PLoS ONE* **2012**, *7*, e51655. [CrossRef] [PubMed]

335. Dai, Z.; Lei, P.; Xie, J.; Hu, Y. Antitumor effect of resveratrol on chondrosarcoma cells via phosphoinositide 3-kinase/AKT and p38 mitogen-activated protein kinase pathways. *Mol. Med. Rep.* **2015**, *12*, 3151–3155. [CrossRef] [PubMed]

336. Gomez, D.E.; Armando, R.G.; Farina, H.G.; Menna, P.L.; Cerrudo, C.S.; Ghiringhelli, P.D.; Alonso, D.F. Telomere structure and telomerase in health and disease (Review). *Int. J. Oncol.* **2012**, *41*, 1561–1569. [CrossRef] [PubMed]

337. Chakraborty, S.; Ghosh, U.; Bhattacharyya, N.P.; Bhattacharya, R.K.; Roy, M. Inhibition of telomerase activity and induction of apoptosis by curcumin in K-562 cells. *Mutat. Res.* **2006**, *596*, 81–90. [CrossRef] [PubMed]

338. Chakraborty, S.M.; Ghosh, U.; Bhattacharyya, N.P.; Bhattacharya, R.K.; Dey, S.; Roy, M. Curcumin-induced apoptosis in human leukemia cell HL-60 is associated with inhibition of telomerase activity. *Mol. Cell. Biochem.* **2007**, *297*, 31–39. [CrossRef] [PubMed]

339. Khaw, A.K.; Hande, M.P.; Kalthur, G.; Hande, M.P. Curcumin inhibits telomerase and induces telomere shortening and apoptosis in brain tumour cells. *J. Cell. Biochem.* **2013**, *114*, 1257–1270. [CrossRef] [PubMed]

340. Lanzilli, G.; Fuggetta, M.P.; Tricarico, M.; Cottarelli, A.; Serafino, A.; Falchetti, R.; Ravagnan, G.; Turriziani, M.; Adamo, R.; Franzese, O.; et al. Resveratrol down-regulates the growth and telomerase activity of breast cancer cells in vitro. *Int. J. Oncol.* **2006**, *28*, 641–648. [CrossRef] [PubMed]

341. Zhai, X.-X.; Ding, J.-C.; Tang, Z.-M.; Li, J.-G.; Li, Y.-C.; Yan, Y.-H.; Sun, J.-C.; Zhang, C.-X. Effects of resveratrol on the proliferation, apoptosis and telomerase ability of human A431 epidermoid carcinoma cells. *Oncol. Lett.* **2016**, *11*, 3015–3018. [CrossRef] [PubMed]

342. Yu, H.; Jove, R. The STATs of cancer—New molecular targets come of age. *Nat. Rev. Cancer* **2004**, *4*, 97–105. [CrossRef] [PubMed]

343. Ihle, J.N. STATs: Signal transducers and activators of transcription. *Cell* **1996**, *84*, 331–334. [CrossRef]

344. Blasius, R.; Reuter, S.; Henry, E.; Dicato, M.; Diederich, M. Curcumin regulates signal transducer and activator of transcription (STAT) expression in K562 cells. *Biochem. Pharmacol.* **2006**, *72*, 1547–1554. [CrossRef] [PubMed]

345. Zhang, Y.P.; Li, Y.Q.; Lv, Y.T.; Wang, J.M. Effect of curcumin on the proliferation, apoptosis, migration, and invasion of human melanoma A375 cells. *Genet. Mol. Res.* **2015**, *14*, 1056–1067. [CrossRef] [PubMed]

346. Zhang, C.; Li, B.; Zhang, X.; Hazarika, P.; Aggarwal, B.B.; Duvic, M. Curcumin selectively induces apoptosis in cutaneous T-cell lymphoma cell lines and patients' PBMCs: Potential role for STAT-3 and NF-kappaB signaling. *J. Investig. Dermatol.* **2010**, *130*, 2110–2119. [CrossRef] [PubMed]

347. Uddin, S.; Hussain, A.R.; Manogaran, P.S.; Al-Hussein, K.; Platanias, L.C.; Gutierrez, M.I.; Bhatia, K.G. Curcumin suppresses growth and induces apoptosis in primary effusion lymphoma. *Oncogene* **2005**, *24*, 7022–7030. [CrossRef] [PubMed]

348. Mackenzie, G.G.; Queisser, N.; Wolfson, M.L.; Fraga, C.G.; Adamo, A.M.; Oteiza, P.I. Curcumin induces cell-arrest and apoptosis in association with the inhibition of constitutively active NF-kappaB and STAT3 pathways in Hodgkin's lymphoma cells. *Int. J. Cancer* **2008**, *123*, 56–65. [CrossRef] [PubMed]

349. Baek, S.H.; Ko, J.; Lee, H.; Jung, J.; Kong, M.; Lee, J.; Lee, J.; Chinnathambi, A.; Zayed, M.E.; Alharbi, S.A.; et al. Resveratrol inhibits STAT-3 signaling pathway through the induction of SOCS-1: Role in apoptosis induction and radiosensitization in head and neck tumor cells. *Phytomedicine* **2016**, *23*, 566–577. [CrossRef] [PubMed]

350. Trung, L.Q.; Espinoza, J.L.; Takami, A.; Nakao, S. Resveratrol induces cell cycle arrest and apoptosis in malignant NK cells via JAK2/STAT-3 pathway inhibition. *PLoS ONE* **2013**, *8*, e55183.

351. Wu, M.-L. Short-term resveratrol exposure causes in vitro and in vivo growth inhibition and apoptosis of bladder cancer. *PLoS ONE* **2014**, *9*, e89806. [CrossRef] [PubMed]

352. Zhong, L.-X.; Li, H.; Wu, M.; Liu, X.-Y.; Zhong, M.; Chen, X.; Liu, J.; Zhang, Y. Inhibition of STAT3 signaling as critical molecular event in resveratrol-suppressed ovarian cancer cells. *J. Ovarian Res.* **2015**, *8*, 25. [CrossRef] [PubMed]

353. Ha, M.; Kim, V.N. Regulation of microRNA biogenesis. *Nat. Rev. Mol. Cell Biol.* **2014**, *15*, 509–524. [CrossRef] [PubMed]

354. Cimmino, A.; Calin, G.A.; Fabbri, M.; Iorio, M.V.; Ferracin, M.; Shimizu, M.; Wojcik, S.E.; Aqeilan, R.I.; Zupo, S.; Dono, M.; et al. miR-15 and miR-16 induce apoptosis by targeting BCL2. *Proc. Natl. Acad. Sci. USA* **2005**, *102*, 13944–13949. [CrossRef] [PubMed]

355. Yang, J.; Cao, Y.; Sun, J.; Zhang, Y. Curcumin reduces the expression of Bcl-2 by upregulating miR-15a and miR-16 in MCF-7 cells. *Med. Oncol.* **2010**, *27*, 1114–1118. [CrossRef] [PubMed]

356. Zhang, J.; Du, Y.; Wu, C.; Ren, X.; Ti, X.; Shi, J.; Zhao, F.; Yin, H. Curcumin promotes apoptosis in human lung adenocarcinoma cells through miR-186 signaling pathway. *Oncol. Rep.* **2010**, *24*, 1217–1223. [CrossRef] [PubMed]

357. Zhang, J.; Zhang, T.; Ti, X.; Shi, J.; Wu, C.; Ren, X.; Yin, H. Curcumin promotes apoptosis in A549/DDP multidrug-resistant human lung adenocarcinoma cells through an miRNA signaling pathway. *Biochem. Biophys. Res. Commun.* **2010**, *399*, 1–6. [CrossRef] [PubMed]

358. Li, H.; Jia, Z.; Li, A. Resveratrol repressed viability of U251 cells by miR-21 inhibiting of NF-κB pathway. *Mol. Cell. Biochem.* **2013**, *382*, 137–143. [CrossRef] [PubMed]

359. Liu, P.; Liang, H.; Xia, Q.; Li, P.; Kong, H.; Lei, P.; Wang, S.; Tu, Z. Resveratrol induces apoptosis of pancreatic cancers cells by inhibiting miR-21 regulation of BCL-2 expression. *Clin. Transl. Oncol.* **2013**, *15*, 741–746. [CrossRef] [PubMed]

360. Zhou, C.; Ding, J.U.N.; Wu, Y. Resveratrol induces apoptosis of bladder cancer cells via miR-21 regulation of the Akt/Bcl-2 signaling pathway. *Mol. Med. Rep.* **2014**, *9*, 1467–1473. [CrossRef] [PubMed]

361. Elmore, S. Apoptosis: A review of programmed cell death. *Toxicol. Pathol.* **2007**, *35*, 495–516. [CrossRef] [PubMed]

362. Kroemer, G.; Galluzzi, L.; Vandenabeele, P.; Abrams, J.; Alnemri, E.; Baehrecke, E.; Blagosklonny, M.; El-Deiry, W.; Golstein, P.; Green, D.; et al. Classification of cell death. *Cell Death Differ.* **2009**, *16*, 3–11. [CrossRef] [PubMed]

363. Aoki, H.; Takada, Y.; Kondo, S.; Sawaya, R.; Aggarwal, B.B.; Kondo, Y. Evidence that curcumin suppresses the growth of malignant gliomas in vitro and in vivo through induction of autophagy: Role of Akt and extracellular signal-regulated kinase signaling pathways. *Mol. Pharmacol.* **2007**, *72*, 29–39. [CrossRef] [PubMed]

364. Mihaylova, M.M.; Shaw, R.J. The AMPK signalling pathway coordinates cell growth, autophagy and metabolism. *Nat. Cell. Biol.* **2012**, *13*, 1016–1023. [CrossRef] [PubMed]

365. Xiao, K.; Jiang, J.; Guan, C.; Dong, C.; Wang, G.; Bai, L.; Sun, J.; Hu, C.; Bai, C. Curcumin induces autophagy via activating the AMPK signaling pathway in lung adenocarcinoma cells. *J. Pharmacol. Sci.* **2013**, *123*, 102–109. [CrossRef] [PubMed]

366. Fu, Y.; Chang, H.; Peng, X.; Bai, Q.; Yi, L.; Zhou, Y.; Zhu, J.; Mi, M. Resveratrol Inhibits Breast Cancer Stem-Like Cells and Induces Autophagy via Suppressing Wnt/b Catenin Signaling Pathway. *PLoS ONE* **2014**, *9*, e102535. [CrossRef] [PubMed]

367. Wang, M.; Yu, T.; Zhu, C.; Sun, H.; Qiu, Y.; Zhu, X.; Li, J. Resveratrol triggers protective autophagy through the Ceramide/Akt/mTOR pathway in melanoma B16 cells the ceramide/Akt/mTOR pathway in melanoma B16 cells. *Nutr. Cancer* **2014**, *66*, 435–440. [CrossRef] [PubMed]

368. Zhou, C.; Zhao, X.; Li, X.; Wang, C.; Zhang, X.; Liu, X.; Ding, X. Curcumin inhibits AP-2γ-induced apoptosis in the human malignant testicular germ cells in vitro. *Acta Pharmacol. Sin.* **2013**, *34*, 1192–1200. [CrossRef] [PubMed]

369. Yu, T.; Ji, J.; Guo, Y. Biochemical and Biophysical Research Communications MST1 activation by curcumin mediates JNK activation, Foxo3a nuclear translocation and apoptosis in melanoma cells. *Biochem. Biophys. Res. Commun.* **2013**, *441*, 53–58. [CrossRef] [PubMed]

370. Wang, K.; Fan, H.; Chen, Q.; Ma, G.; Zhu, M.; Zhang, X.; Zhang, Y.; Yu, J. Curcumin inhibits aerobic glycolysis and induces mitochondrial-mediated apoptosis through hexokinase II in human colorectal cancer cells in vitro. *Anticancer Drugs* **2015**, *26*, 15–24. [CrossRef] [PubMed]

371. Sun, S.; Huang, H.; Huang, C.; Lin, J. Cycle arrest and apoptosis in MDA-MB-231/Her2 cells induced by curcumin. *Eur. J. Pharmacol.* **2012**, *690*, 22–30. [CrossRef] [PubMed]

372. Saha, A.; Kuzuhara, T.; Echigo, N.; Fujii, A.; Suganuma, M.; Fujiki, H. Apoptosis of human lung cancer cells by curcumin mediated through up-regulation of "Growth arrest and DNA damage inducible genes 45 and 153". *Biol. Pharm. Bull.* **2010**, *33*, 1291–1299. [CrossRef] [PubMed]

373. Milacic, V.; Banerjee, S.; Landis-piwowar, K.R.; Sarkar, F.H.; Majumdar, A.P.N.; Dou, Q.P. Curcumin inhibits the proteasome activity in human colon cancer cells in vitro and in vivo. *Cancer Res.* **2008**, *68*, 7283–7292. [CrossRef] [PubMed]

374. Liu, H.; Ke, C.; Cheng, H.; Huang, C.F.; Su, C. Curcumin-induced mitotic spindle defect and cell cycle arrest in human bladder cancer cells occurs partly through inhibition of aurora A. *Mol. Pharmacol.* **2011**, *80*, 638–646. [CrossRef] [PubMed]

375. Lee, Y.; Park, S.Y.; Kim, Y.; Park, J.O. Regulatory effect of the AMPK-COX-2 signaling pathway in curcumin-induced apoptosis in HT-29 colon cancer cells. *Ann. N. Y. Acad. Sci.* **2009**, *1171*, 489–494. [CrossRef] [PubMed]

376. Lee, S.J.; Langhans, S.A. Anaphase-promoting complex/cyclosome protein Cdc27 is a target for curcumin-induced cell cycle arrest and apoptosis. *BMC Cancer* **2012**, *12*, 44. [CrossRef] [PubMed]

377. Lee, S.J.; Krauthauser, C.; Maduskuie, V.; Fawcett, P.T.; Olson, J.M.; Rajasekaran, S.A. Curcumin-induced HDAC inhibition and attenuation of medulloblastoma growth in vitro and in vivo. *BMC Cancer* **2011**, *11*, 144. [CrossRef] [PubMed]

378. Kao, H.; Wu, C.; Won, S.; Shin, J.-W.; Liu, H.-S.; Su, C.-L. Kinase gene expression and subcellular protein expression pattern of protein kinase c isoforms in curcumin-treated human hepatocellular carcinoma hep 3B cells. *Plant Foods Hum. Nutr.* **2011**, *66*, 136–142. [CrossRef] [PubMed]

379. Cui, J.; Meng, X.; Gao, X.; Tan, G. Curcumin decreases the expression of Pokemon by suppressing the binding activity of the Sp1 protein in human lung cancer cells. *Mol. Biol. Rep.* **2010**, *37*, 1627–1632. [CrossRef] [PubMed]

380. Banerjee, M.; Singh, P.; Panda, D. Curcumin suppresses the dynamic instability of microtubules, activates the mitotic checkpoint and induces apoptosis in MCF-7 cells. *FEBS J.* **2010**, *277*, 3437–3448. [CrossRef] [PubMed]

381. Cao, A.; Tang, Q.; Zhou, W.; Qiu, Y. Ras/ERK signaling pathway is involved in curcumin-induced cell cycle arrest and apoptosis in human gastric carcinoma AGS cells. *J. Asian Nat. Prod.* **2014**, 37–41. [CrossRef] [PubMed]

382. Fan, H.; Tian, W.; Ma, X. Curcumin induces apoptosis of HepG2 cells via inhibiting fatty acid synthase. *Target. Oncol.* **2014**, *9*, 279–286. [CrossRef] [PubMed]

383. Chatterjee, M.; Das, S.; Janarthan, M.; Ramachandran, H.K.; Chatterjee, M. Role of 5-lipoxygenase in resveratrol mediated suppression of 7,12-dimethylbenz (α) anthracene-induced mammary carcinogenesis in rats. *Eur. J. Pharmacol.* **2011**, *668*, 99–106. [CrossRef] [PubMed]

384. Lin, C.; Crawford, D.R.; Lin, S.; Sebuyira, A.; Meng, R.; Westfall, E.; Tang, H.; Lin, S.; Yu, P.; Davis, P.J.; et al. Inducible COX-2-dependent apoptosis in human ovarian cancer cells. *Carcinogenesis* **2011**, *32*, 19–26. [CrossRef] [PubMed]

385. Zhong, L.X.; Zhan, ZX.; Hunag, Z.H.; Feng, M.; Xiong, J.P. Resveratrol treatment inhibits proliferation of and induces apoptosis in human colon cancer. *Med. Sci. Monit.* **2016**, *22*, 1101–1108.

386. Chow, S.; Wang, J.; Chuang, S.; Chang, Y.; Chu, W.; Chen, W.; Chen, Y. Resveratrol-induced p53-independent apoptosis of human nasopharyngeal carcinoma cells is correlated with the downregulation of ΔNp63. *Cancer Gene Ther.* **2010**, *17*, 872–882. [CrossRef] [PubMed]

387. Dai, W.; Wang, F.; Lu, J.; Xia, Y.; He, L.; Chen, K.; Li, J.; Li, S.; Liu, T.; Zheng, Y.; et al. By reducing hexokinase 2, resveratrol induces apoptosis in HCC cells addicted to aerobic glycolysis and inhibits tumor growth in mice. *Oncotarget* **2015**, *6*, 13703–13717. [CrossRef] [PubMed]

388. Kai, L.; Samuel, S.K.; Levenson, A.S. Resveratrol enhances p53 acetylation and apoptosis in prostate cancer by inhibiting MTA1/NuRD complex. *Int. J. Cancer* **2010**, *126*, 1538–1548. [CrossRef] [PubMed]

389. Lee, K.-A.; Lee, Y.-J.; Ban, J.O.; Lee, Y.-J.; Lee, S.; Cho, M.; Nam, H.; Hong, J.T.; Shim, J. The flavonoid resveratrol suppresses growth of human malignant pleural mesothelioma cells through direct inhibition of specificity protein 1. *Int. J. Mol. Med.* **2012**, *30*, 21–27. [PubMed]

390. Li, G.; He, S.; Chang, L.; Lu, H.; Zhang, H.; Zhang, H.; Chiu, J. GADD45α and annexin A1 are involved in the apoptosis of HL-60 induced by resveratrol. *Phytomedicine* **2011**, *18*, 704–709. [CrossRef] [PubMed]

391. Mohapatra, P.; Ranjan, S.; Das, D.; Siddharth, S. Resveratrol mediated cell death in cigarette smoke transformed breast epithelial cells is through induction of p21Waf1 / Cip1 and inhibition of long patch base excision repair pathway. *Toxicol. Appl. Pharmacol.* **2014**, *275*, 221–231. [CrossRef] [PubMed]

392. Shi, Y.; Yang, S.; Troup, S.; Lu, X.; Callaghan, S.; Park, D.S.; Xing, Y.; Yang, X. Resveratrol induces apoptosis in breast cancer cells by E2F1-mediated up-regulation of ASPP1. *Oncol. Rep.* **2011**, *25*, 1713–1719. [PubMed]

393. Kumar, B.; Iqbal, M.A.; Singh, R.K.; Bamezai, R.N.K. Biochimie resveratrol inhibits TIGAR to promote ROS induced apoptosis and autophagy. *Biochimie* **2015**, *118*, 26–35. [CrossRef] [PubMed]

394. Ahmad, K.A.; Harris, N.H.; Johnson, A.D.; Lindvall, H.C.N.; Wang, G.; Ahmed, K. Protein kinase CK2 modulates apoptosis induced by resveratrol and epigallocatechin-3-gallate in prostate cancer cells. *Mol. Cancer Ther.* **2007**, *6*, 1006–1012. [CrossRef] [PubMed]

395. Wang, F.; Galson, D.L.; Roodman, G.D.; Ouyang, H. Resveratrol triggers the pro-apoptotic endoplasmic reticulum stress response and represses pro-survival XBP1 signaling in human multiple myeloma cells. *Exp. Hematol.* **2011**, *39*, 999–1006. [CrossRef] [PubMed]

396. Seeni, A.; Takahashi, S.; Takeshita, K.; Tang, M.; Sugiura, S.; Sato, S.; Shirai, T. Suppression of prostate cancer growth by resveratrol in the transgenic rat for adenocarcinoma of prostate (TRAP) model. *Asian Pac. J. Cancer Prev.* **2008**, *9*, 7–14. [PubMed]

397. Lee, S.C.; Chan, J.; Clement, M.V.; Pervaiz, S. Functional proteomics of resveratrol-induced colon cancer cell apoptosis: Caspase-6-mediated cleavage of lamin A is a major signaling loop. *Proteomics* **2006**, *6*, 2386–2394. [CrossRef] [PubMed]

398. Woo, K.J.; Lee, T.J.; Lee, S.H.; Seo, J.H.; Jeong, Y.J.; Park, J.W.; Kwon, T.K. Elevated gadd153/chop expression during resveratrol-induced apoptosis in human colon cancer cells. *Biochem. Pharmacol.* **2007**, *73*, 68–76. [CrossRef] [PubMed]

399. Hsu, K.; Wu, C.; Huang, S.; Wu, C.; Yo, Y.; Chen, Y.; Shiau, A.; Chou, C. Cathepsin L mediates resveratrol-induced autophagy and apoptotic cell death in cervical cancer cells. *Autophagy* **2009**, *5*, 451–460. [CrossRef] [PubMed]

400. Trincheri, N.F.; Nicotra, G.; Follo, C.; Castino, R.; Isidoro, C. Resveratrol induces cell death in colorectal cancer cells by a novel pathway involving lysosomal cathepsin D. *Carcinogenesis* **2007**, *28*, 922–931. [CrossRef] [PubMed]

401. Whitlock, N.; Bahn, J.H.; Lee, S.H.; Eling, T.E.; Baek, S.J. Resveratrol-induced apoptosis is mediated by early growth response-1, Krüppel-like factor 4, and activating transcription factor 3. *Cancer Prev. Res.* **2011**, *4*, 116–127. [CrossRef] [PubMed]

402. Pandey, P.R.; Okuda, H.; Watabe, M.; Pai, S.K. Resveratrol suppresses growth of cancer stem-like cells by inhibiting fatty acid synthase. *Breast Cancer Res. Treat.* **2011**, *130*, 387–398. [CrossRef] [PubMed]

403. Qin, Y.; Ma, Z.; Dang, X.; Li, W.E.I.; Ma, Q. Effect of resveratrol on proliferation and apoptosis of human pancreatic cancer MIA PaCa-2 cells may involve inhibition of the Hedgehog signaling pathway. *Mol. Med. Rep.* **2014**, *10*, 2563–2567. [PubMed]

404. Ryu, J.; Yoon, N.A.; Seong, H.; Jeong, J.Y.; Kang, S.; Park, N.; Choi, J.; Lee, D.H.; Roh, G.S.; Kim, H.J.; et al. Resveratrol induces glioma cell apoptosis through activation of tristetraprolin. *Mol. Cells* **2015**, *38*, 991–997. [PubMed]

405. Tian, H.; Yu, Z. Resveratrol induces apoptosis of leukemia cell line K562 by modulation of sphingosine kinase-1 pathway. *Int. J. Clin. Exp. Pathol.* **2015**, *8*, 2755–2762. [PubMed]

406. Tomic, J.; Mccaw, L.; Li, Y.; Hough, M.R.; Ben-david, Y. Resveratrol has anti-leukemic activity associated with decreased *O*-GlcNAcylated proteins. *Exp. Hematol.* **2013**, *41*, 675–686. [CrossRef] [PubMed]

407. Vanamala, J.; Radhakrishnan, S.; Reddivari, L.; Bhat, V.B.; Ptitsyn, A.B. Resveratrol suppresses human colon cancer cell proliferation and induces apoptosis via targeting the pentose phosphate and the talin-FAK signaling pathways—A proteomic approach. *Proteome Sci.* **2011**, *9*, 49. [CrossRef] [PubMed]

408. Varoni, E.M.; Faro, A.F.L.; Sharifi-Rad, J.; Iriti, M. Anticancer molecular mechanisms of resveratrol. *Front. Nutr.* **2016**, *3*, 8. [CrossRef] [PubMed]

409. Carter, L.G.; D'Orazio, J.A.; Pearson, K.J. Resveratrol and cancer: Focus on in vivo evidence. *Endocr. Relat. Cancer* **2014**, *21*, R209–R225. [CrossRef] [PubMed]

410. D'Incalci, M.; Steward, W.P.; Gescher, A.J. Use of cancer chemopreventive phytochemicals as antineoplastic agents. *Lancet Oncol.* **2005**, *6*, 899–904. [CrossRef]

411. López-Lázaro, M. Anticancer and carcinogenic properties of curcumin: Considerations for its clinical development as a cancer chemopreventive and chemotherapeutic agent. *Mol. Nutr. Food Res.* **2008**, *52*, 103–127. [CrossRef] [PubMed]

412. Burgos-Morón, E.; Calderón-Montaño, J.M.; Salvador, J.; Robles, A.; López-Lázaro, M. The dark side of curcumin. *Int. J. Cancer* **2010**, *126*, 1771–1775. [CrossRef] [PubMed]

413. Kurien, B.T.; Dillon, S.P.; Dorri, Y.; D'Souza, A.; Scofield, R.H. Curcumin does not bind or intercalate into DNA and a note on the gray side of curcumin. *Int. J. Cancer* **2011**, *128*, 239–249. [CrossRef] [PubMed]

414. Maru, G.B. Understanding the molecular mechanisms of cancer prevention by dietary phytochemicals: From experimental models to clinical trials. *World J. Biol. Chem.* **2016**, *7*, 88. [CrossRef] [PubMed]

415. Zheng, Y.Y.; Viswanathan, B.; Kesarwani, P.; Mehrotra, S. Dietary agents in cancer prevention: An immunological perspective. *Photochem. Photobiol.* **2012**, *88*, 1083–1098. [CrossRef] [PubMed]

416. Shukla, Y.; Singh, R. Resveratrol and cellular mechanisms of cancer prevention. *Ann. N. Y. Acad. Sci.* **2011**, *1215*, 1–8. [CrossRef] [PubMed]

417. Duvoix, A.; Blasius, R.; Delhalle, S.; Schnekenburger, M.; Morceau, F.; Henry, E.; Dicato, M.; Diederich, M. Chemopreventive and therapeutic effects of curcumin. *Cancer Lett.* **2005**, *223*, 181–190. [CrossRef] [PubMed]

418. Nishino, H.; Tokuda, H.; Satomi, Y.; Masuda, M.; Osaka, Y.; Yogosawa, S.; Wada, S.; Mou, X.Y.; Takayasu, J.; Murakoshi, M.; et al. Cancer prevention by antioxidants. *BioFactors* **2004**, *22*, 57–61. [CrossRef] [PubMed]

419. Singh, S.; Khar, A. Biological effects of curcumin and its role in cancer chemoprevention and therapy. *Anticancer Agents Med. Chem.* **2006**, *6*, 259–270. [CrossRef] [PubMed]

420. Bhat, K.P.L.; Pezzuto, J.M. Cancer chemopreventive activity of resveratrol. *Ann. N. Y. Acad. Sci.* **2002**, *957*, 210–229. [CrossRef] [PubMed]

421. Aziz, M.H.; Kumar, R.A.J.; Ahmad, N. Cancer chemoprevention by resveratrol: In vitro and in vivo studies and the underlying mechanisms (Review). *Int. J. Oncol.* **2003**, *23*, 17–28. [CrossRef] [PubMed]

422. Stepanic, V.; Gasparovic, A.C.; Troselj, K.G.; Amic, D.; Zarkovic, N. Selected attributes of polyphenols in targeting oxidative stress in cancer. *Curr. Top. Med. Chem.* **2016**, *15*, 496–509. [CrossRef]

423. Mileo, A.M.; Miccadei, S. Polyphenols as modulator of oxidative stress in cancer disease: New therapeutic strategies. *Oxid. Med. Cell. Longev.* **2016**, *2016*, 1–17. [CrossRef] [PubMed]

424. Nafisi, S.; Adelzadeh, M.; Norouzi, Z.; Sarbolouki, M.N. Curcumin binding to DNA and RNA. *DNA Cell Biol.* **2009**, *28*, 201–208. [CrossRef] [PubMed]

425. N'soukpoé-Kossi, C.N.; Bourassa, P.; Mandeville, J.S.; Bekale, L.; Tajmir-Riahi, H.A. Structural modeling for DNA binding to antioxidants resveratrol, genistein and curcumin. *J. Photochem. Photobiol. B Biol.* **2015**, *151*, 69–75. [CrossRef] [PubMed]

426. Baharuddin, P.; Satar, N.; Fakiruddin, K.S.; Zakaria, N.; Lim, M.N.; Yusoff, N.M.; Zakaria, Z.; Yahaya, B.H. Curcumin improves the efficacy of cisplatin by targeting cancer stem-like cells through p21 and cyclin D1-mediated tumour cell inhibition in non-small cell lung cancer cell lines. *Oncol. Rep.* **2016**, *35*, 13–25. [CrossRef] [PubMed]

427. Duarte, V.M.; Han, E.; Veena, M.S.; Salvado, A.; Jeffrey, D.; Liang, L.; Faull, K.F.; Srivatsan, E.S.; Wang, M.B. Curcumin enhances the effect of cisplatin in suppression of head and neck squamous cell carcinoma via inhibition of IKKβ protein of the nuclear factor kB pathway. *Mol. Cancer Ther.* **2010**, *9*, 2665–2675. [CrossRef] [PubMed]

428. Chen, J.; Wang, G.; Wang, L.; Kang, J.; Wang, J. Curcumin p38-dependently enhances the anticancer activity of valproic acid in human leukemia cells. *Eur. J. Pharm. Sci.* **2010**, *41*, 210–218. [CrossRef] [PubMed]

429. Epelbaum, R.; Schaffer, M.; Vizel, B.; Badmaev, V.; Bar-Sela, G. Curcumin and gemcitabine in patients with advanced pancreatic cancer. *Nutr. Cancer* **2010**, *62*, 1137–1141. [CrossRef] [PubMed]

430. Ferguson, J.E.; Orlando, R.A. Curcumin reduces cytotoxicity of 5-Fluorouracil treatment in human breast cancer cells. *J. Med. Food* **2015**, *18*, 497–502. [CrossRef] [PubMed]

431. Pandey, A.; Vishnoi, K.; Mahata, S.; Tripathi, S.C.; Misra, S.P.; Misra, V.; Mehrotra, R.; Dwivedi, M.; Bharti, A.C. Berberine and curcumin target survivin and STAT-3 in gastric cancer cells and synergize actions of standard chemotherapeutic 5-fluorouracil. *Nutr. Cancer* **2015**, *67*, 1293–1304. [CrossRef] [PubMed]

432. Yu, Y.; Kanwar, S.S.; Patel, B.B.; Nautiyal, J.; Sarkar, F.H.; Majumdar, A.P. Elimination of colon cancer stem-like cells by the combination of curcumin and FOLFOX. *Transl. Oncol.* **2009**, *2*, 321–328. [CrossRef] [PubMed]

433. Gao, J.-Z.; Du, J.-L.; Wang, Y.-L.; Li, J.; Wei, L.-X.; Guo, M.-Z. Synergistic effects of curcumin and bevacizumab on cell signaling pathways in hepatocellular carcinoma. *Oncol. Lett.* **2015**, *9*, 295–299. [CrossRef] [PubMed]

434. Guo, Y.; Li, Y.; Shan, Q.; He, G.; Lin, J.; Gong, Y. Curcumin potentiates the anti-leukemia effects of imatinib by downregulation of the AKT/mTOR pathway and BCR/ABL gene expression in Ph+ acute lymphoblastic leukemia. *Int. J. Biochem. Cell Biol.* **2015**, *65*, 1–11. [CrossRef] [PubMed]

435. Hossain, M.M.; Banik, N.L.; Ray, S.K. Synergistic anti-cancer mechanisms of curcumin and paclitaxel for growth inhibition of human brain tumor stem cells and LN18 and U138MG cells. *Neurochem. Int.* **2012**, *61*, 1102–1113. [CrossRef] [PubMed]

436. De Ruiz Porras, V.; Bystrup, S.; Martínez-Cardús, A.; Pluvinet, R.; Sumoy, L.; Howells, L.; James, M.I.; Iwuji, C.; Manzano, J.L.; Layos, L.; et al. Curcumin mediates oxaliplatin-acquired resistance reversion in colorectal cancer cell lines through modulation of CXC-Chemokine/NF-κB signalling pathway. *Sci. Rep.* **2016**, *6*, 24675. [CrossRef] [PubMed]

437. Zanotto-Filho, A.; Braganhol, E.; Klafke, K.; Figueiró, F.; Terra, S.R.; Paludo, F.J.; Morrone, M.; Bristot, I.J.; Battastini, A.M.; Forcelini, C.M.; et al. Autophagy inhibition improves the efficacy of curcumin/ temozolomide combination therapy in glioblastomas. *Cancer Lett.* **2015**, *358*, 220–231. [CrossRef] [PubMed]

438. Lee, J.Y.; Lee, Y.M.; Chang, G.C.; Yu, S.L.; Hsieh, W.Y.; Chen, J.J.W.; Chen, H.W.; Yang, P.C. Curcumin induces EGFR degradation in lung adenocarcinoma and modulates p38 activation in intestine: The versatile adjuvant for gefitinib therapy. *PLoS ONE* **2011**, *6*, e23756. [CrossRef] [PubMed]

439. Björklund, M.; Roos, J.; Gogvadze, V.; Shoshan, M. Resveratrol induces SIRT-1- and energy-stress-independent inhibition of tumor cell regrowth after low-dose platinum treatment. *Cancer Chemother. Pharmacol.* **2011**, *68*, 1459–1467. [CrossRef] [PubMed]

440. Osman, A.M.M.; Al-Malki, H.S.; Al-Harthi, S.E.; El-Hanafy, A.A.; Elashmaoui, H.M.; Elshal, M.F. Modulatory role of resveratrol on cytotoxic activity of cisplatin, sensitization and modification of cisplatin resistance in colorectal cancer cells. *Mol. Med. Rep.* **2015**, *12*, 1368–1374. [CrossRef] [PubMed]

441. Buhrmann, C.; Shayan, P.; Kraehe, P.; Popper, B.; Goel, A.; Shakibaei, M. Resveratrol induces chemosensitization to 5-fluorouracil through up-regulation of intercellular junctions, Epithelial-to-mesenchymal transition and apoptosis in colorectal cancer. *Biochem. Pharmacol.* **2015**, *98*, 51–58. [CrossRef] [PubMed]

442. Lee, S.H.; Koo, B.S.; Park, S.Y.; Kim, Y.M. Anti-angiogenic effects of resveratrol in combination with 5-fluorouracil on B16 murine melanoma cells. *Mol. Med. Rep.* **2015**, *12*, 2777–2783. [CrossRef] [PubMed]

443. Díaz-Chavez, J.; Fonseca-Sanchez, M.A.; Arechaga-Ocampo, E.; Flores-Perez, A.; Palacios-Rodreguez, Y.; Domínguez-Góme, G.; Marchat, L.A.; Fuentes-Mera, L.; Mendoza-Hernandez, G.; Gariglio, P.; et al. Proteomic profiling reveals that resveratrol inhibits HSP27 expression and sensitizes breast cancer cells to doxorubicin therapy. *PLoS ONE* **2013**, *8*, e64378. [CrossRef] [PubMed]

444. Kweon, S.H.; Song, J.H.; Kim, T.S. Resveratrol-mediated reversal of doxorubicin resistance in acute myeloid leukemia cells via downregulation of MRP1 expression. *Biochem. Biophys. Res. Commun.* **2010**, *395*, 104–110. [CrossRef] [PubMed]

445. Casanova, F.; Quarti, J.; Ferraz Da Costa, D.C.; Ramos, C.A.; Da Silva, J.L.; Fialho, E. Resveratrol chemosensitizes breast cancer cells to melphalan by cell cycle arrest. *J. Cell. Biochem.* **2012**, *113*, 2586–2596. [CrossRef] [PubMed]

446. Filippi-Chiela, E.C.; Thomé, M.P.; Bueno e Silva, M.M.; Pelegrini, A.L.; Ledur, P.F.; Garicochea, B.; Zamin, L.L.; Lenz, G. Resveratrol abrogates the temozolomide-induced G2 arrest leading to mitotic catastrophe and reinforces the temozolomide-induced senescence in glioma cells. *BMC Cancer* **2013**, *13*, 147. [CrossRef] [PubMed]

447. Harikumar, K.B.; Kunnumakkara, A.B.; Sethi, G.; Diagaradjane, P.; Anand, P.; Pandey, M.K.; Gelovani, J.; Krishnan, S.; Guha, S.; Aggarwal, B.B. Resveratrol, a multitargeted agent, can enhance antitumor activity of gemcitabine in vitro and in orthotopic mouse model of human pancreatic cancer. *Int. J. Cancer* **2010**, *127*, 257–268. [PubMed]

448. Rigolio, R.; Miloso, M.; Nicolini, G.; Villa, D.; Scuteri, A.; Simone, M.; Tredici, G. Resveratrol interference with the cell cycle protects human neuroblastoma SH-SY5Y cell from paclitaxel-induced apoptosis. *Neurochem. Int.* **2005**, *46*, 205–211. [CrossRef] [PubMed]

449. Shi, X.P.; Miao, S.; Wu, Y.; Zhang, W.; Zhang, X.F.; Ma, H.Z.; Xin, H.L.; Feng, J.; Wen, A.D.; Li, Y. Resveratrol sensitizes tamoxifen in antiestrogen-resistant breast cancer cells with epithelial-mesenchymal transition features. *Int. J. Mol. Sci.* **2013**, *14*, 15655–15668. [CrossRef] [PubMed]

450. Singh, N.; Nigam, M.; Ranjan, V.; Zaidi, D.; Garg, V.K.; Sharma, S.; Chaturvedi, R.; Shankar, R.; Kumar, S.; Sharma, R.; et al. Resveratrol as an adjunct therapy in cyclophosphamide-treated MCF-7 cells and breast tumor explants. *Cancer Sci.* **2011**, *102*, 1059–1067. [CrossRef] [PubMed]

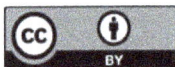

![nutrients logo] *nutrients*

MDPI

*Review*

# Chemopreventive Agents and Inhibitors of Cancer Hallmarks: May *Citrus* Offer New Perspectives?

Santa Cirmi [1,†], Nadia Ferlazzo [1,†], Giovanni E. Lombardo [2], Alessandro Maugeri [1], Gioacchino Calapai [3], Sebastiano Gangemi [4,5] and Michele Navarra [1,*]

[1]  Department of Chemical, Biological, Pharmaceutical and Environmental Sciences, University of Messina, Messina I-98168, Italy; scirmi@unime.it (S.C.); nadiaferlazzo@email.it (N.F.); maugeri.alessandro@gmail.com (A.M.)

[2]  Department of Health Sciences, University "Magna Graecia" of Catanzaro, Catanzaro I-88100, Italy; gelombardo@unicz.it

[3]  Department of Biomedical and Dental Sciences and Morphofunctional Imaging, University of Messina, Messina I-98125, Italy; gcalapai@unime.it

[4]  Department of Clinical and Experimental Medicine, University of Messina, Messina I-98125, Italy; gangemis@unime.it

[5]  Institute of Applied Sciences and Intelligent Systems (ISASI), National Research Council (CNR), Pozzuoli I-80078, Italy

*  Correspondence: mnavarra@unime.it; Tel.: +39-090-676-6431

†  These authors contributed equally to this work.

Received: 5 August 2016; Accepted: 13 October 2016; Published: 4 November 2016

**Abstract:** Fruits and vegetables have long been recognized as potentially important in the prevention of cancer risk. Thus, scientific interest in nutrition and cancer has grown over time, as shown by increasing number of experimental studies about the relationship between diet and cancer development. This review attempts to provide an insight into the anti-cancer effects of *Citrus* fruits, with a focus on their bioactive compounds, elucidating the main cellular and molecular mechanisms through which they may protect against cancer. Scientific literature was selected for this review with the aim of collecting the relevant experimental evidence for the anti-cancer effects of *Citrus* fruits and their flavonoids. The findings discussed in this review strongly support their potential as anti-cancer agents, and may represent a scientific basis to develop nutraceuticals, food supplements, or complementary and alternative drugs in a context of a multi-target pharmacological strategy in the oncology.

**Keywords:** *Citrus*; cancer; flavonoids; nutraceuticals; functional foods; natural product; complementary and alternative medicines

---

## 1. Introduction

Cancer and heart disease are two of the main pathologies worldwide, and the most common causes of death in old age. The decline in death rates over the last century has resulted in a large proportion of people beginning to live up to eighty years old or more, and an increased incidence of chronic diseases. Thus, cancer represents a crisis for public health, with an estimated 14 million cases globally with a total of 8.2 million deaths for cancer in 2012 [1]. The two most important ways to reduce cancer risk are the avoidance of cancer-causing agents and finding preventive strategies to stop cancer onset. Obviously, death to cancer can be reduced by the discovery of new drugs or novel therapeutic approaches, designed to stop the development of clinical cancer in the first instance.

Despite the ongoing development of synthetic drugs that represent the mainstay of pharmaceutical care, the plant kingdom still remains an attractive source of novel anti-cancer drugs. It provides biologically active molecules for use in pharmaceuticals applications, and it has been estimated that about 70% of anti-cancer drugs originate to some extent from natural sources [2]. Moreover, both observational and experimental studies suggest that regular consumption of fruits and vegetables may play an important role in reducing degenerative diseases such as cancer [3–5]. Recently, it has been suggested that, among tissues, a third of the variation in cancer risk is attributable to environmental factors or hereditary predisposition, and that changes in lifestyle can play a very important role in the development of certain types of cancer [6]. About 30%–40% of cancer incidence could be prevented by an healthy diet, doing regular physical activity, and maintaining correct body weight [7]. Overall, a high dietary intake vegetables and fruits (>400 g/day) could prevent at least 20% of all cancer cases [7,8].

The cancer protective effects of vegetables and fruits may be due to the presence of bioactive molecules acting through different mechanisms including the following: inhibition of carcinogen activation, stimulation of carcinogen detoxification, scavenging of free radical species, control of cell-cycle progression, inhibition of cell proliferation, induction of apoptosis, inhibition of oncogene activity of, inhibition of angiogenesis and metastasis, and inhibition of hormone or growth-factor activity [4,9–12].

*Citrus* fruits (CF), i.e., oranges, lemons, limes, bergamot, grapefruits, and tangerines, are popular all over the world. CF are the main winter fruits consumed in the Mediterranean diet, meaning they are the main source of dietary flavonoids. They are rich in vitamins and flavonoids, and have long been hypothesized to possess a protective effect against cancer

This review is an attempt to provide an insight into the anti-cancer effects of CF, with a focus on their bioactive compounds, elucidating the main cellular and molecular mechanisms by which they may protect against cancer.

## 2. The *Citrus* Flavonoids

Flavonoids are pigments commonly present in the genus *Citrus* that are responsible for flower and fruit color. They are low molecular weight polyphenolic compounds, widely found in the plant kingdom as secondary metabolites. They are characterized by a common C6-C3-C6 structure consisting of two benzene rings (A and B) linked through a heterocyclic pyran ring (C) (Figure 1).

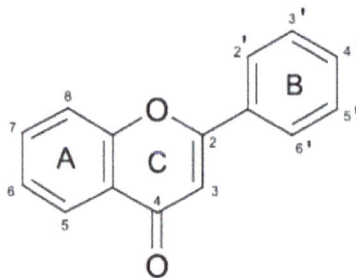

**Figure 1.** Basic chemical structure of *Citrus* flavonoids.

Flavonoids containing an hydroxyl group in position C-3 of the C ring are classified as 3-hydroxyflavonoids (flavonols, anthocyanidins, leucoanthocyanidins, and catechins), and those lacking it as 3-desoxyflavonoids (flavanones and flavones). At present, more than 9000 flavonoids have been characterized, some of which are clinically used. The large number of compounds arises from various combinations of multiple hydroxyl and methoxyl groups substituting the basic flavonoids skeleton. Flavonoids are divided into six classes on the basis of their chemical structures: flavones, flavanones, flavonols, isoflavones, anthocyanidins, and flavans. Flavonoids are mainly present in plants as glycosides, while aglycones (the forms lacking sugar moieties) occur less frequently. Therefore, a large number of flavonoids result from many different combinations of aglycones and sugars, among which mainly D-glucose and L-rhamnose bound to the hydroxyl group at the C-3 or C-7 position.

More than sixty types of flavonoids have been identified in CF: flavanones are the flavonoids most widely present, followed by flavones, flavonols, and anthocyanins (the latter only in blood oranges). Some flavonoids, such as hesperidin, naringin, and polymethoxylated flavones (PMFs) are characteristic compounds contained in *Citrus* while others like rutin and quercetin are common throughout the plant kingdom [13]. Figure 2 shows the main structural formula of some flavonoids isolated from CF, and their chemical substituents.

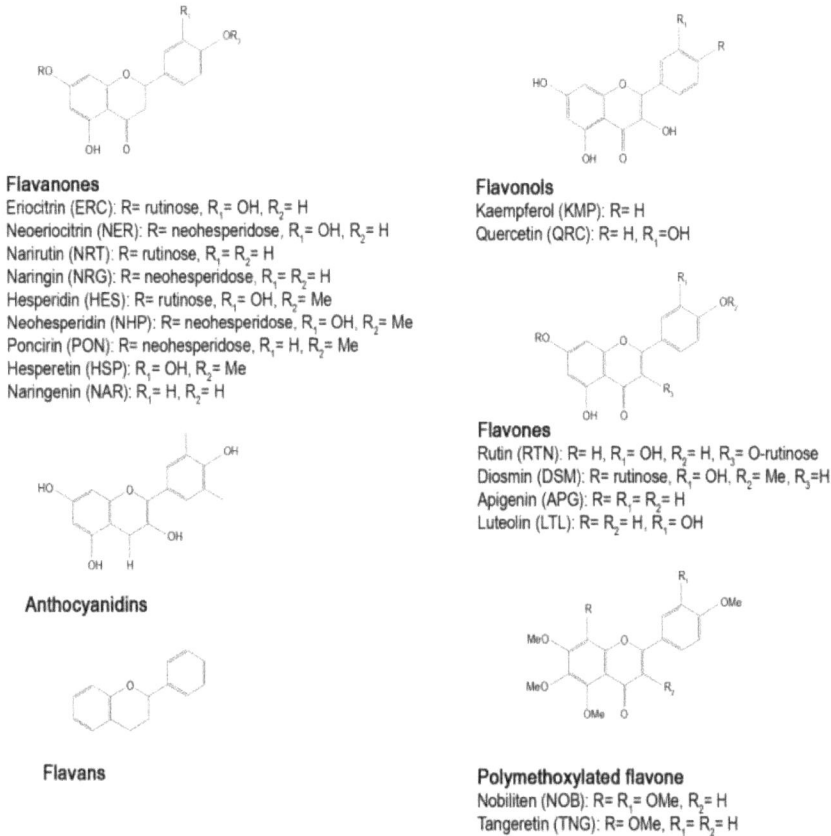

**Flavanones**
Eriocitrin (ERC): R= rutinose, $R_1$= OH, $R_2$= H
Neoeriocitrin (NER): R= neohesperidose, $R_1$= OH, $R_2$= H
Narirutin (NRT): R= rutinose, $R_1$= $R_2$= H
Naringin (NRG): R= neohesperidose, $R_1$= $R_2$= H
Hesperidin (HES): R= rutinose, $R_1$= OH, $R_2$= Me
Neohesperidin (NHP): R= neohesperidose, $R_1$= OH, $R_2$= Me
Poncirin (PON): R= neohesperidose, $R_1$= H, $R_2$= Me
Hesperetin (HSP): $R_1$= OH, $R_2$= Me
Naringenin (NAR): $R_1$= H, $R_2$= H

**Flavonols**
Kaempferol (KMP): R= H
Quercetin (QRC): R= H, $R_1$=OH

**Flavones**
Rutin (RTN): R= H, $R_1$= OH, $R_2$= H, $R_3$= O-rutinose
Diosmin (DSM): R= rutinose, $R_1$= OH, $R_2$= Me, $R_3$=H
Apigenin (APG): R= $R_1$= $R_2$= H
Luteolin (LTL): R= $R_2$= H, $R_1$= OH

**Anthocyanidins**

**Flavans**

**Polymethoxylated flavone**
Nobiliten (NOB): R= $R_1$= OMe, $R_2$= H
Tangeretin (TNG): R= OMe, $R_1$= $R_2$= H

**Figure 2.** Structural formula of some flavonoids isolated from *Citrus* fruits and their chemical substituents.

Flavanones (2,3-dihydro-2-phenylchromen-4-one) occur almost exclusively in CF and are present in both the glycoside or aglycone forms (Figure 3). Naringenin and hesperetin are the most important flavanones present in aglycone forms, while the glycosidic forms are grouped into two types: neohesperidosides and rutinosides. Glycosylation occurs at position 7, either by rutinose or neohesperidose, disaccharides formed by a glucose and a rhamnose molecule differing only in the type of linkage (1 → 6 or 1 → 2). Naringin, neoeriocitrin, neohesperedin, and poncirin consist of a flavanone with neohesperidose (rhamnosyl-α-1,2 glucose), and they have a bitter taste; while hesperidin, narirutin, eriocitrin, and didymin consist of a flavanone with rutinose (rhamnosyl-α-1,6 glucose), and have no taste. Flavanones, usually present in diglycoside form, give CF their characteristic taste.

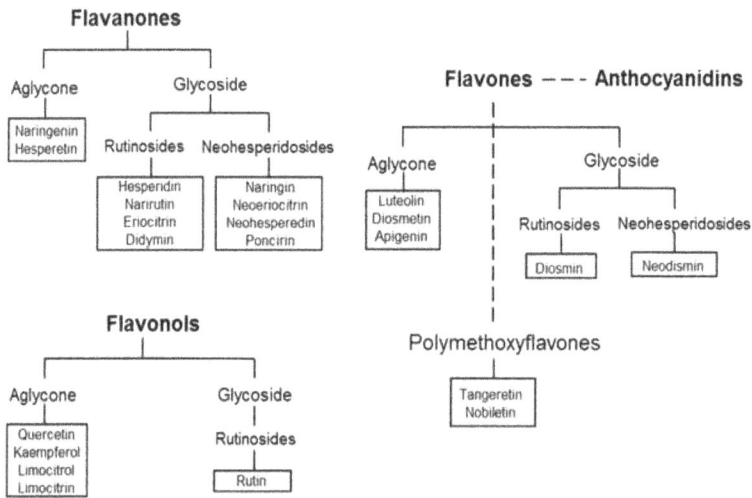

**Figure 3.** Classification of *Citrus* flavonoids.

Flavonols (3-hydroxy-2-phenylchromen-4-one) may be considered to be the 3-hydroxy derivatives of flavones. Glycosylation occurs preferentially at the 3-hydroxyl group of the central ring, and the predominant types are 3-*O*-monoglycosides. The most common flavonol aglycones are quercetin and kaempferol, while rutin and rutinosides are the main glycosidic forms.

The most abundant flavones (2-phenylchromen-4-one) present in the aglycone form are luteolin, diosmetin, and apigenin, while diosmin and neodismin represent the principal flavones present in the rutinoside and neohesperidoside forms, respectively. The PMFs tangeretin and nobiletin are present in smaller quantities.

Anthocyanins (2-phenylchromenylium), are metabolites of flavones structurally derived from pyran or flavan. In CF, they are present only in blood oranges. Anthocyanidins are anthocyanins with a sugar group, in which glycosylation with glucose, arabinose, or galactose almost always occurs at the 3-position.

The most abundant *Citrus* flavonoids are flavanones, e.g., hesperidin, naringin, or neohesperidin. However, there are flavones, e.g., diosmin, apigenin, or luteolin, that generally display higher biological activity, despite occuring in much lower concentrations. Of note are apigenin, which has shown particularly good anti-inflammatory activity, and diosmin and rutin that are important venotonic agents present in several pharmaceutical products. The beneficial effects of flavonoids are mainly due to their anti-oxidant properties which can play a key role in fighting several degenerative diseases. However, there is recent increasing evidence linking the pharmacological activity of *Citrus* flavonoids to their ability to inhibit the activity of intracellular signaling molecules, such as phosphodiesterases, kinases, topoisomerases, and other regulatory enzymes [14]. Blocking protein kinases and lipid-dependent signaling cascades results in alterations in the phosphorylation state of target molecules, with the consequent modulation of gene expression implicated in many degenerative diseases including cancer. Many studies designed to uncover a structure–activity relationship have demonstrated that anti-oxidant, enzyme-inhibitory, or anti-proliferative activities of some flavonoids are dependent upon particular structural factors. The structure oxidation state (flavanone, flavone, etc.), substituents (position, number, and nature of groups in both the A and B rings of the flavonoid structure), and the presence of glycosylation may be important determinant features of flavonoid activity [15,16]. More specifically, studies on melanoma cell lines using several flavonoids of *Citrus* origin have shown the presence of the C2–C3 double bond on the C ring, conjugated with the 4-oxo function, to be critical for this biological activity [17]. Moreover, the presence of three or more hydroxyls in any of the rings of the flavonoid skeleton significantly increased the anti-proliferative activity observed in melanoma B16-F10 cell cultures [18].

## 3. Preclinical Studies

Carcinogenesis is a multi-step process of genetic and epigenetic alterations leading to the progressive transformation of normal cells towards malignancy. The process of carcinogenesis can be divided into three main stages: (i) initiation, a phase in which cellular exposition to a carcinogenic agent leads to irreversible alterations, usually at the DNA level. In this phase cells react to carcinogens by the activation of enzymes involved in the metabolism of xenobiotics that, while aiming to inactivate, may generate a mutagenic compound responsible for DNA damage and mutations, thereby initiating cancer development; (ii) the tumor promotion stage is characterized by the proliferation of abnormal cells that may initiate a pre-neoplastic focus. In this phase over-activation and/or over-expression of enzymes involved in the synthesis of nucleotides and DNA (e.g., ornithine decarboxylase), as well as in the regulation of the differentiation process (DNA polymerase or topoisomerases) occur. Moreover, oxidative stress caused by the overproduction of reactive oxygen species (ROS) induces further cell damage and genome instability; (iii) progression is the final stage of carcinogenesis. It is characterized by an uncontrolled proliferation of tumor cells which also acquire the ability to invade neighboring tissues and to form metastasis at distant sites, coupled with a loss of capacity for apoptosis or senescence. Hence, metastasis is the spread of cancer cells from a primary tumor to distant sites in the cancer patient's body. Angiogenesis is the first step of the metastatic process that leads to the formation of new blood capillaries by outgrowth or sprouting of pre-existing blood vessels. It allows the tumor to be fed and facilitates the access of tumor cells to the bloodstream. Indeed, tumor vessels are more permeable than normal ones, since tumor-associated endothelial cells are enlarged and loosely connected. Therefore, the metastatic process is the end result of a complex series of events depending on the ability of tumor cells to detach from the primary tumor, migrate, and invade connective tissues, entering the vascular or lymphatic system, through which vital organs are reached where they proliferate to form a distant metastasis. The tendency of a primary tumor to form metastasis is the hallmark of malignant cancer, and has important diagnostic, prognostic, and therapeutic implications.

Interest in nutrition and cancer has grown considerably, as evidenced by the rapid proliferation of studies examining nutritional exposure in relation to cancer risk [19]. A large body of in vitro and in vivo studies have shown that fruits and vegetables may have an important role in the maintenance of a healthy lifestyle and the reduction of cancer risk. Their potential health benefits are probably due to the presence of secondary metabolites ubiquitous in the plant kingdom that are considered non-nutritional but which are essential for the maintenance of health. Thus, in the last decade, bioactive compounds including flavonoids, carotenoids, ascorbic acid, and limonoids have been intensively investigated for their potential antioxidant, anti-inflammatory, and anti-cancer activities. Several compounds are responsible for *Citrus* antitumoral effects; of these, vitamin C is considered an important micronutrient through which CF exert their antioxidant effects by trapping free radicals and reactive oxygen molecules, thus protecting against oxidative damage, inhibiting the formation of carcinogens and protecting DNA from damage [20]. Flavonoids also exhibit antioxidant and free radical scavenging properties, interfering with the oxidative/anti-oxidative potential of the cell [21]. Furthermore, there are numerous reports showing flavonoids to be able to act at various stages of carcinogenesis, and specifically to interact with proteins involved in cancer development.

Growing experimental evidence supports the view that *Citrus* flavonoids exert their anti-cancer effects through a number of different mechanisms. They may act as suppressing agents, preventing the formation of new cancers from pro-carcinogens or as blocking agents, disenabling carcinogens from achieving initiation, as well as preventing the onset of the tumor promotion stage. Moreover, *Citrus* flavonoids may function as transformation agents, facilitating the biotransformation of carcinogens into inactive metabolites. Finally, they behave as both anti-angiogenic and anti-metastatic agents, preventing the formation of new vessels and metastasis [14,22]. Table 1 shows the principal cancer-related processes modulated by *Citrus* flavonoids.

**Table 1.** Main mechanisms through which *Citrus* flavonoids may act as anti-cancer drugs.

| Mechanism by Which Citrus Flavonoids May Fight against Cancer |
|---|
| Antioxidant activity, thus counteract oxidative stress |
| Anti-inflammatory effect |
| Phase II enzyme induction, hence enhancing detoxification |
| Phase I enzyme inhibition, thus stopping activation of carcinogens |
| Inhibition of cell proliferation |
| Inhibition of oncogene and/or induction of tumor suppressor gene |
| Induction of cell-cycle arrest |
| Induction of apoptosis |
| Inhibition of signal transduction pathways |
| Anti-angiogenic effect |
| Inhibition of cell adhesion, migration and invasion |

*3.1. Initiation Phase Inhibition by* Citrus *Flavonoids*

In the last twenty years, there has been an increasing awareness that flavonoids and other naturally-occurring substances in plants have protective effects against environmental mutagens/ carcinogens and endogenous mutagens [23]. In support of this, there are numerous experimental findings suggesting that certain *Citrus* flavonoids may exert preventive effects against DNA damage induced by a variety of carcinogens [24]. Naringenin and rutin prevent the accumulation of ultraviolet radiation-B (UV-B)-induced DNA damage [25] by a mechanism that may involve the ability of flavonoids to neutralize free radicals generated near DNA, promoting mutations. The radical scavenging property of flavonoids is also responsible for quercetin protective effect against mercury-induced DNA damage and oxidative stress in a human-derived liver cell line (HepG2), that seems to be due to the maintenance of redox status [26]. Moreover, it has been observed that naringenin at low doses (10–80 µM) can stimulate DNA repair following oxidative damage in a human lymph node prostate cancer cell line (LNCaP), leading to a significant increase in the levels of several major enzymes in the DNA base excision repair pathway [27]. In in vivo experiments, naringenin has demonstrated its capability to inhibit N-diethylnitrosamine (NDEA)-induced hepatocarcinogenesis [28,29]. Naringin has been found to reduce the rate of micronuclei formed by ifosfamide in mouse blood cells [30] and to exert protective action against DNA deterioration induced by daunorubicin in mouse hepatocytes and cardiocytes, suggesting that this flavonoid may be useful in reducing the adverse effects found in anthracycline treatments [31]. Moreover, it accelerated the regression of pre-neoplastic lesions in rats exposed to 1,2-dimethylhydrazine (DMH) [32]. Experiments performed using in vivo models of genotoxicity induced by cyclophosphamide show that the antioxidative activity of hesperidin (100, 200, and 400 mg/kg body weight (BW) administered by gavages for five consecutive days) may reduce the frequency of micronucleated polychromatic erythrocytes (MnPCEs) induced by chemotherapy drugs [33]. Furthermore, in the presence of a mammalian metabolic activation system, naringin, apigenin, hesperetin, and other flavonoids (300 µg/plate) have been shown to produce antimutagenic effects against aflatoxin B1 (1 µg/plate), with an inhibition rate of more than a 70% in *Salmonella typhimurium*. In this study, the structure–activity relationship analysis suggests the flavonoid configuration containing the free 5-, 7-hydroxyl group to be essential [34].

Flavonoids may also inhibit the first phase of carcinogenesis through an increase in detoxification processes by modulating enzyme activity resulting in the decreased carcinogenicity of xenobiotics. For example, naringenin inhibits the activity of aromatase (CYP19) in Chinese hamster ovary (CHO) cells, thereby decreasing estrogen biosynthesis and inducing antiestrogenic effects, which are important in breast and prostate cancers [35]. Quercetin has instead proven to be a potent non-competitive inhibitor of sulfotransferase 1A1, suggesting a role for potential chemopreventive agents in sulfation-induced carcinogenesis [36]. The chemopreventive potential of diosmin, naringenin, naringin, and rutin against CYP1A2-mediated mutagenesis of heterocyclic amines produced by high temperature cooking of meat was hinted by Bear and Teel [37]. Several reports have described the potential anti-mutagenic properties of apigenin. For instance, exposure to apigenin prior to a carcinogenic insult has been shown to offer a protective effect in both murine skin and colon cancer models [38], as well as to prevent the genotoxic effects of benzo(α)pyrene (BP) in vivo. Indeed, Khan et al. [39] demonstrated that apigenin (2.5 and 5 mg/kg orally) reverts BP-induced depletion in the levels of glutathione (GSH), quinone reductase (QR), and glutathione-*S*-transferase (GST), while also reducing DNA strand breaks and damage. Increased GSH by apigenin also enhances endogenous defense against oxidative stress [40]. Moreover, topical application of apigenin has been proven to reduce dimethyl benzanthracene-induced skin tumors by strongly inhibiting epidermal ornithine decarboxylase, an enzyme that plays a key role in tumor promotion [41]. In addition, apigenin administration has been reported diminish the incidence of UV light-induced cancers and to increase tumor-free survival in vivo [42]. Moreover, apigenin as well naringenin, suppress colon carcinogenesis in azoxymethane (AOM)-treated rats [43].

The antigenotoxic activity of hesperidin was investigated by Nandakumar et al., [44]. They reported that daily administration of hesperidin at a concentration of 30 mg/kg BW for 45 days prevented 7,12-dimethylbenz(α)anthracene (DMBA)-induced experimental breast cancer formation, presumably by the regulation of both phase I and phase II metabolizing enzymes, and through its strong antioxidant activity. The results also revealed that the flavanone may act both by modulating the energy reservoir of the cell and by maintaining oxidative phosphorylation. Also, the aglycone hesperetin has been reported to modulate xenobiotic-metabolizing enzymes during DMH-induced colon carcinogenesis [45]. Tangeretin, a pentamethoxy flavone present in significant amounts in CF peel, was found to suppress DMBA-induced breast cancer in rats [46].

Chronic inflammation is closely connected to the carcinogenic process. Indeed, nobiletin has been shown to inhibit DMBA/tetradecanoyl-13-phorbol acetate (TPA)-induced skin tumor formation by reducing the number of tumors per mouse, manifesting its potential in inflammation-associated tumorigenesis [47]. The studies discussed above are summarized in Table 2.

**Table 2.** Studies investigating the ability of *Citrus* flavonoids to inhibit the initiation phase of carcinogenesis.

| | Initiation Phase | | |
|---|---|---|---|
| **Flavonoid** | **Concentration/Dose** | **Experimental Model** | **Reference** |
| Quercetin | 0.1–5.0 µM | $HgCl_2$/MeHg-treated HepG2 cells | [26] |
| Naringenin | 10–80 µM | Ferrous sulfate-exposed LNCaP cells | [27] |
| Naringenin | 200 mg/kg | NDEA-treated rats | [28] |
| Naringenin | 200 mg/kg | NDEA-treated rats | [29] |
| Naringin | 50–500 mg/kg | Ifos-treated mice | [30] |
| Naringin | 50–500 mg/kg | Dau-treated mice | [31] |
| Naringin | 10–200 mg/kg | DMH-injected rats | [32] |
| Hesperidin | 50–400 mg/kg | Cyclophosphamide-treated mice | [33] |
| Naringin, apigenin, hesperetin | 300 µg/plate | Aflatoxin B1-exposed *Salmonella typhimurium* TA100 | [34] |
| Diosmin, naringenin, naringin, rutin | 0.25–1.0 µM | Heterocyclic amines-exposed *Salmonella typhimurium* TA98 | [37] |
| Apigenin | 10–100 µM | 308 and HCT116 cells | [38] |
| Apigenin | 2.5 and 5 mg/kg | BP-treated mice | [39] |
| Quercetin, kaempferol, myricetin, apigenin | 5–25 µM | COS-1 cells | [40] |
| Apigenin | 1–50 µM | DMBA/TPA-exposed mice | [41] |
| Apigenin | 5 and 10 µmoles in 200 µL | UV-A/B-exposed SKH-1 mice | [42] |
| Apigenin, naringenin | 0.1% and 0.02% | AOM-treated rats | [43] |
| Hesperidin | 30 mg/kg | DMBA-treated rats | [44] |
| Hesperetin | 20 mg/kg | DMH-treated rats | [45] |
| Tangeretin | 50 mg/kg | DMBA-treated rats | [46] |
| Nobiletin | 160 and 320 nM | DMBA/TPA-exposed mice | [47] |

AOM: azoxymethane; BP: benzo(α)pyrene; Dau: daunorubicin; DMBA: 7,12-dimethylbenz(α)anthracene; DMH: 1,2-dimethylhydrazine; Ifos: ifosfamide; NDEA: *N*-diethylnitrosamine; TPA: tetradecanoyl-13-phorbol acetate.

*3.2. Inhibition of Tumor Development*

A great number of in vitro studies have demonstrated that *Citrus* flavonoids reduce the growth of several types of tumor cells in cultures. Tangeretin, nobiletin, quercetin and taxifolin have anti-proliferative effects on squamous cell carcinoma HTB43 [48], as well as on many other tumoral cell lines. Tangeretin, a PMF present mainly in the peel of tangerine and other CF, induced apoptosis in human myeloid leukaemia HL-60 cells, without causing cytotoxicity in human peripheral blood mononuclear cells [49,50]. Tangeretin and nobiletin (another PMF widely found in the mandarin epicarp) also inhibited the proliferation of both human breast cancer cell lines (MDA-MB-435 and MCF-7) and a human colon cancer cell line (HT-29) in a concentration- and time-dependent manner, by blocking cell cycle progression at the G1 phase without inducing cell death [51]. This study showed tangeretin $IC_{50}$ values of 30–40 µM for breast and colon cell lines, and slightly higher values for nobiletin, while in other reports tangeretin exhibited much greater potency [49,50]. However, this discrepancy could be caused by differences related to both cell type and experimental procedures. The inhibition of the activity of cyclin-dependent kinases 2 (Cdk2) and 4 (Cdk4), accompanied by an increase in Cdk inhibitors p21 and p27 seems to be the mechanism through which tangeretin arrests cell cycle progression at the G1 phase in colon adenocarcinoma COLO 205 cells [52]. Yoshimizu et al. [53] documented the growth-inhibitory action of nobiletin, both alone and in combination with cisplatin, in various human gastric cancer cell lines (TMK-1, MKN-45, MKN-74, and KATO-III), through the induction of apoptosis and cell cycle deregulation. Interestingly, orange peel extract (OPE) containing 30% polymethoxyflavones, such as tangeretin (19.0%), heptamethoxyflavone (15.24%), tetramethoxyflavone (13.6%), nobiletin (12.49%), hexamethoxyflavone (11.06%) and sinensitin (9.16%), inhibited tumorigenesis in Apc[(Min/+)] mice by increasing apoptosis [54]. OPE also decreased the development of hyperplastic lesions in mouse mammary glands [55]. The reduction of mammary cancer cell growth caused by tangeretin may be related to the inhibition of mitogen-activated protein kinase (MAPK)/extracellular-signal-regulated kinase (ERK) phosphorylation and of other proteins like adducin α and γ, protein kinase Cδ, signal transducer and activator of transcription (STAT) 1 and 3, and stress-activated protein kinase (JNK) [56]. Tangeretin and nobiletin also inhibited the proliferation of both SH-SY5Y neuroblastoma cells [57] and brain tumor cells [58], reducing also invasion, migration, and adhesive properties. Moreover, it has been reported that tangeretin sensitizes cisplatin-resistant human ovarian cancer cells through the downregulation of the phosphoinositide 3-kinase (PI3K)/protein kinase B (also known as Akt) signaling pathway, suggesting a potential approach for the treatment of drug-resistant cancers [59]. Tangeretin also induced apoptosis in gastric cancer AGS cells through the activation of both extrinsic and intrinsic signaling pathways [60]. Nobiletin and the coumarin auraptene have been reported to counteract prostate carcinogenesis both in vitro and in vivo. In particular, nobiletin inhibited the growth of several prostate cancer cell lines with $IC_{50}$ values of around 100 µM, by a mechanism involving apoptosis and cell cycle arrest at the $G_0/G_1$ phase, as well as inhibited development of prostate adenocarcinomas in a transgenic rat model [61]. The preventive effects of nobiletin on prostate cancer have recently been confirmed in a study that also reported the ability of this flavonoid to reduce the risk of colon cancer [62]. Furthermore, nobiletin reduces AOM-induced rat colon carcinogenesis [63] and, like quercetin (100 ppm), is able to decrease preneoplastic lesions and serum levels of both leptin and insulin in an in vivo model of colon carcinogenesis, suggesting a promising role in preventing tumors associated with obesity [64,65]. Experiments performed using both in vitro and in vivo models showed the anti-proliferative property of nobiletin on lung cancer cells. The mechanism involves the activation of the apoptotic process and cell cycle arrest at the G2/M phase due to decreased Bcl-2 and increased Bax protein expression, both of which positively correlated with elevated expression of p53 [66]. As reported by Ohnishi et al. [67], nobiletin treatment suppressed HepG2 and MH1C1 hepatocarcinoma cell growth by inducing cell cycle inhibition and apoptosis, but without apparent effects in the early stages of in vivo hepatocarcinogenesis. In glioma cells, it suppresses proliferation by inhibiting Ras activity and mitogen-activated protein/extracellular signal-regulated kinase (MEK/ERK) signaling cascade, probably via a $Ca^{2+}$-sensitive protein kinase C (PKC)-dependent mechanism [68]. There are more recent results that demonstrate the ability of nobiletin to inhibit cell growth and migration via cell-cycle arrest and suppression of the MAPK and Akt pathways [69]. In human gastric p53-mutated SNU-16 cells, nobiletin was found to be effective in inhibiting cell proliferation, inducing apoptosis, and enhancing the efficacy of 5-Fluorouracil (FU) [70]. Its anti-cancer effects have also been demonstrated in acute myeloid leukemia cells [71], where it was responsible for the induction of cell-cycle arrest and apoptosis. Moreover, orally administrated nobiletin inhibited colitis-associated colon carcinogenesis in AOM/dextran sulfate sodium-treated mice [72].

Apigenin is a flavone present mainly in fruits and vegetables, and among *Citrus* species it is abundant in grapefruit. It possesses anti-inflammatory and free radical scavenging activity, and as a candidate anti-cancer agent, is capable of reducing cancer cell proliferation of without affecting normal cells. It has been reported that apigenin possesses growth inhibitory properties in breast cancer, inducing apoptosis by: (i) the involvement of the caspase cascade [73]; (ii) inhibiting STAT3 and nuclear factor kappa B (NF-κB) signaling in HER2-overexpressing breast cancer cells [74]; (iii) reducing the activity of both PI3K and Akt kinase [75] and regulating the p14ARF-Mdm2-p53 pathway [76]. Apigenin is reported to exert growth inhibitory effects by increasing the stability of p53, leading to cell cycle arrest in many cancer cell lines, including rat neural and liver epithelial cells, as well as human breast, ovarian, cervical, prostate, colon, and thyroid cancers [77]. In epidermal cells and fibroblasts reversible G2/M and G0/G1 arrest is also mediated by the inhibition of p34 (Cdc2) kinase activity [78,79], while in breast carcinoma the G2/M phase cell cycle arrest after apigenin treatment led to a significant decrease in cyclins (B1, D1, and A) and cyclin-dependent kinase (Cdk1 and 4) protein levels [80]. In pancreatic cancer cell lines, apigenin caused both time- and concentration-dependent inhibition of DNA synthesis and cell proliferation through G2/M phase cell cycle arrest caused by the suppression of cyclin B-associated Cdc2 activity [81,82]. Moreover, in the same cell lines, it inhibited the glycogen synthase kinase-3β/NF-kB signaling pathway and upregulated the expression of cytokine genes, which potentially contributed to its anti-cancer properties [83]. In addition, apigenin has been shown to induce WAF1/p21 levels, resulting in G1 phase cell cycle arrest in androgen-responsive (LNCaP) and androgen-refractory (DU145) human prostate cancer cells [84,85]. Indeed, the apoptosis observed in these cell lines appeared to be correlated with: (i) the alteration in Bax/Bcl-2 ratio; (ii) the down- regulation of the constitutive expression of NF-kB/p65; (iii) the release of cytochrome c; (iv) the induction of apoptotic protease activating factor-1 (Apaf-1), which leads to caspase activation and PARP-cleavage [84,85]. Apigenin-induced growth inhibition by different mechanisms has also been reported in colon [86,87], prostate [88], and neuroblastoma [89,90] cancer cells. In endothelial cells, the anti-proliferative effect exerted by the flavanone is due to the blocking of cells in the G2/M phase, as a result of the accumulation of the hyperphosphorylated form of retinoblastoma protein [91]. Diosmin, another important *Citrus* flavone (mostly due to its venotonic activity), occurs naturally as a glycoside, and after ingestion is rapidly transformed by intestinal flora to its aglycone form, diosmetin. Diosmin has been shown to inhibit Caco-2 and HT-29 colon cancer cell growth [92]. In the hepatocellular carcinoma HA22T cells, it inhibited cell viability, reduced cellular proliferative proteins, and induced cell cycle arrest in the G2/M phase through p53 activation and inhibition of the PI3K-Akt-mouse double minute 2 homolog (MDM2) signaling pathway. In addition, it suppressed tumor growth through protein phosphatase 2 (PP2A) activation in HA22T-implanted xeno-graft nude activation [93]. The effectiveness of diosmin as an anti-cancer agent has also been demonstrated in DU145 prostate cancer cells, where it promotes genotoxic events and apoptotic cell death [94]. Moreover, it has been shown that diosmin may reduce the development of esophageal cancer induced by *N*-methyl-*N*-amylnitrosamine (MNAN) when given during the initiation phase [95], decreases oral carcinogenesis initiated by 4-nitroquinoline 1-oxide (4-NQO) [96], counteracts *N*-butyl-*N*-(4-hydroxybutyl)nitrosamine (OH-BBN)-induced urinary-bladder carcinogenesis [97], and prevents AOM-induced rat colon carcinogenesis, either alone or in combination with hesperidin [98]. In these cases [95–98], rats were fed a diet containing diosmin (1000 ppm), hesperidin (1000 ppm), or diosmin + hesperidin (900 ppm and 100 ppm, respectively), and the cancer inhibition found could be related to the suppression of the increased cell proliferation caused by the carcinogens in the affected mucous membranes.

Quercetin is a water-soluble flavonol, widely distributed in nature and the most common dietary flavonol. It represents the aglycone form of a number of other flavonoid glycosides, such as rutin and quercitin. In CF it is present mainly in lemon peel. Experimental data have shown quercetin to be a potential anti-carcinogenic agent against several human tumor cell lines, including HL-60 (promyelocytic leukemia cells), A431 (epithelial carcinoma cell line), SK-OV-3 (ovary adenocarcinoma), HeLa (cervical carcinoma) and HOS (osteosarcoma) [99]. The inhibitory effect of quercetin on HL-60 growth may be due to the induction of apoptosis mediated by an up-regulation of pro-apoptotic Bax and post-translational modification (phosphorylation) of anti-apoptotic Bcl2 [100]. This flavonol also demonstrated concentration-dependent anti-proliferative activity against both meningioma [101] and colon cancer cells (CRC) [102]. Growth inhibition of several CRC cells has been reported and numerous mechanisms explaining the in vitro anti-proliferative effect of quercetin have been proposed [103]. Interestingly the combination of quercetin and low-frequency ultrasound selectively induced cytotoxicity in skin and prostate cancer cells, while having minimal effect on corresponding normal cell lines [104]. Quercetin has been reported to induce cell growth inhibition in MDA-MB-231 breast cancer cells by inhibition of the F-box protein S-phase kinase-associated protein 2 (Skp2) and induction of p27 expression, thereby blocking cell cycle progression [105]. Moreover, several reports have shown that if quercetin is associated with antineoplastic drugs it may then play a relevant role in development of chemotherapeutic combinations. For example, in human breast cancer cells, quercetin inhibits lapatinib-sensitive and -resistant breast cancer cell growth by modifying levels of factors that regulate cell cycle G2/M progression and apoptosis, such as cyclin B1, p-Cdc25c (Ser216), Chk1, caspase 3, caspase 7, and PARP [106]. In breast cancer cells, it potentiated the antitumor effects of doxorubicin, attenuating unwanted cytotoxicity to non-tumoral cells [107], and markedly increased the effect of adriamycin in a multidrug-resistant MCF-7 human breast cancer cell line [108] and in MCT-15 human colon carcinoma cells [109].

Naringin and naringenin are two of the most abundant flavanones in CF, although the amounts differ. Naringenin is the aglycone and is a metabolite of naringin (naringenin-7-neohesperoside), the main flavonoid of grapefruit. Diverse biological and pharmacological properties, including anti-carcinogenic activity, have been reported for both of these flavanones. Kanno et al. [110] showed the anti-proliferative effect of naringenin in a range of human cancer cell lines (breast, stomach, liver, cervix, pancreas, and colon) as well as its ability to inhibit tumor growth in sarcoma S-180-implanted mice. The same authors reported that the exposure of human promyeloleukemia HL-60 cells to naringenin at concentrations up to 0.5 mM induced apoptosis via the activation of NF-κB, while a higher concentration (1 mM) reduced intracellular ATP levels, causing mitochondrial dysfunctions leading to necrosis [111]. Naringenin-induced inhibition of colon cancer cell proliferation has also been reported by Frydoonfar et al. [112]. A mechanism through which naringenin might cause a reduction of breast cancer growth seems to be the impairment of glucose uptake. Indeed, in MCF-7 cells, the flavanone impaired the insulin-stimulated glucose uptake, thus decreasing the availability of glucose concentration in the culture medium and inhibiting proliferation [113]. In human leukemia THP-1 cells, naringenin exerts an anti-proliferative effect in a concentration-dependent manner, inducing apoptosis through the modulation of the Bcl-2 family, mitochondrial dysfunction, activation of caspases, and PARP degradation that correlate with inactivation of the PI3K/Akt pathway [114]. Using the same cell line, Shi et al. [115] have demonstrated naringenin may enhance curcumin-induced apoptosis through inhibition of the Akt and ERK pathways, and by activating the JNK and p53 pathways. In human epidermoid carcinoma A431 cells, the ability of naringenin to induce apoptotic cascade and cell cycle arrest in the G0/G1 phase has been demonstrated [116]. Several in vitro studies have demonstrated the naringenin-induced intrinsic apoptotic pathway initiated by the caspase cascade [111,114,117]. It has also been reported activation of the apoptosis extrinsic pathway, triggered by ligands binding plasma membrane death receptors. Indeed, it has been observed that naringenin enhances tumor necrosis factor-related apoptosis-inducing ligand

(TRAIL)-induced apoptosis in TRAIL-resistant A549 human lung cancer cells by the upregulation of TRAIL receptor 5 (death receptor 5, DR5, also named TRAIL-R2)) without inhibition of cell growth in human normal lung fibroblast WI-38 cells [118]. Moreover, naringenin (50 μM) and other flavonoids, among which hesperetin and apigenin, produced a more than three-fold increase in mitoxantrone accumulation by inhibition of breast cancer resistance protein (BCRP; an ATP-binding cassette transporter conferring multidrug resistance to a number of important anti-cancer agents) in BCRP-overexpressing MCF-7 (breast cancer) and NCI-H460 (lung cancer) cells, whereas the glycoside form (naringin) had no significant effects [119]. The presence of the 2,3-double bond in the C ring of flavonoids, as well as ring B being attached at position 2, hydroxylation at position 5, lack of hydroxylation at position 3, and hydrophobic substitution at positions 6, 7, 8, or 40, are structural properties important for potent flavonoid–BCRP interaction, and critical for potent BCRP inhibition [120]. Some studies have suggested that naringenin also inhibits the P-glycoprotein (P-gp), thus improving antitumor activity both in vitro [121] and in vivo [122,123]. Conversely, other experimental studies indicate that naringenin modulates drug efflux pathways by inhibiting the activity of multidrug resistance-associated proteins (MRPs) but not P-gp [124]. Similarly, Zhang and collaborators [124] have claimed that doxorubicin in combination with naringenin enhanced antitumor activity in vivo, while others have asserted that the pharmacokinetics of intravenously administered doxorubicin (the plasma concentration, biliary, and urinary clearance and tissue distribution) is not altered by pre-treatment with naringin, naringenin, and quercetin [125]. A number of in vivo studies on the antitumor effects of naringenin have also been performed. These found that it suppresses colon carcinogenesis through the aberrant crypt stage in AOM-treated rats [43], reduces tumor size and weight loss in *N*-methyl-*N'*-nitro-*N*-nitrosoguanidine-induced gastric carcinogenesis [126,127], promotes apoptosis in cerebrally-implanted C6 glioma cells rat model [128] and, like naringin, inhibits oral carcinogenesis [129].

Several findings have identified naringin to be a promising chemotherapeutic agent for diverse types of cancers. Naringin (750 μM) showed an anti-proliferative effect on SiHa human cervical cancer cells through cell cycle arrest in the G2/M phase and apoptosis induction via disruption of mitochondrial transmembrane potential, and the activation of both the intrinsic and extrinsic pathways [130]. By contrast, naringin (1 mM) induced growth inhibition and apoptosis by suppressing the NF-κB/COX-2-caspase-1 pathway on HeLa cells [131]. Recently, the role of glycoconjugates in cancer cells has been a focus because of their regulatory effects on malignant phenotypes. A study by Yoshinaga [132] reported naringin to suppress HeLa and A549 cell growth through the alteration of glycolipids. This effect may largely be due to the attenuation of epidermal growth factor receptor (EGFR) signaling through GM3 ganglioside accumulation. Triple-negative (ER-/PR-/HER2-) breast cancer is an aggressive cancer with poor prognosis and a lack of targeted therapies. In this kind of tumor, Li et al. [133] demonstrated that naringin inhibited cell proliferation and promoted cell apoptosis and G1 cycle arrest. These effects were accompanied by increased p21 levels and decreased survival by modulation of the β-catenin pathway.

Moreover, 100 μM naringin resulted in a significant concentration-dependent growth inhibition of 5637 bladder cancer cells together with of cell-cycle blocking [134]. In this cell line, the naringin-induced anti-proliferative effect seems to be linked to the activation of Ras/Raf/ERK-mediated p21WAF1 induction, which in turn leads to a decrease in the levels of cyclin D1/CDK4 and cyclin E-CDK2 complexes, causing G1-phase cell-cycle arrest [134]. Recently, naringin has been investigated regarding its ability to induce autophagy. Several studies have reported that autophagy promotes cancer cell death in response to various anti-cancer agents on apoptosis-defective cells [135,136]. Accordingly, over-activation of autophagy in cancer cells has been proposed to be an important death mechanism occurring in the tumor progression phase, where apoptosis is limited [136]. In AGS gastric adenocarcinoma cells, naringin showed autophagy-mediated growth inhibition by suppressing the PI3K/Akt/mTOR cascade through MAPKs activation [137]. Naringin has been demonstrated to reduce glioblastoma cell proliferation by inhibiting the FAK/cyclin D1 pathway, and promoting cell apoptosis by influencing the FAK/bads pathway [138].

Furthermore, an in vivo study documented that grapefruit pulp powder (13.7 g/kg) or isolated naringin (200 mg/kg) or limonin (200 mg/kg) protect against AOM-induced aberrant crypt foci (ACF) by suppressing proliferation and elevating apoptosis through anti-inflammatory activities, suggesting that the consumption of grapefruit or its flavonoids may help to suppress colon cancer development [139]. Camargo et al. [140] showed that the treatment of rats bearing Walker 256 carcinosarcoma (W256) with 25 mg/kg of naringin reduced tumor necrosis factor-$\alpha$ (TNF-$\alpha$) and interleukin-6 (IL-6) levels and tumor growth by ~75%. Very recently, it has been proven that naringin prevent intestinal tumorigenesis in a adenomatous polyposis coli multiple intestinal neoplasia (Apc$^{(Min/+)}$) mouse model [141].

Another important *Citrus* flavanone is hesperidin (hesperetin-7-rutinoside), the principal flavonoid in sweet orange and lemon, being the glycosides form of hesperetin (free state). It is water-soluble as a glycoside conjugate due to the presence of the sugar in its structure, which on ingestion releases its aglycone hesperetin. Along with other flavonoid compounds, hesperidin has been widely reported to possess venotonic and vasculo-protective pharmacological properties, and it is effectively used as a supplement in patients suffering from blood vessel disorders including capillary fragility and excessive permeability [142]. Both hesperidin and hesperetin have shown anti-cancer activities, although the latter exhibited higher anti-proliferative activity in vitro. Chen et al. [143] showed hesperetin to exert stronger cytotoxic activity than hesperidin in the HL-60 human leukemia cell line. Moreover, at the higher concentrations (40 and 80 µM), hesperetin induced apoptosis, while hesperidin did not. The Authors suggest that the rutinoside group at C-7 attenuate the reduction of apoptotic induction on HL-60 cells by hesperidin. This hypothesis is strengthened by evidence that the aglycone naringenin also induces anti-proliferative and pro-apoptotic effects, but not the glycone naringin. Furthermore, hesperetin inhibits the expression of CDK2, CDK4, and cyclin D, thus inducing cell cycle arrest in the G1 phase, which in turn reduces MCF-7 cell proliferation in a concentration-dependent manner [144]. Moreover, hesperetin (5 to 100 µM) inhibits human colon adenocarcinoma HT-29 cellular growth and induces apoptosis via the Bax-dependent mitochondrial pathway, involving oxidant/antioxidant imbalance [145]. It also enhances Notch1 levels, that in turn decreases the expression of the neuroendocrine tumor markers ASCL1 and CgA, causing inhibition of human gastrointestinal carcinoid (BON) cell growth [146]. Furthermore, hesperetin exerts anti-proliferative and pro-apoptotic effects in human cervical cancer SiHa cells, via both death receptor- and mitochondria-related mechanisms [147], while it induces ROS-mediated cell death in hepatocarcinoma cells [148]. In the same study, the Authors showed that hesperetin significantly inhibited the growth of xenograft tumors [148]. Hesperidin (20 mg/kg BW) suppressed cell proliferation markers, angiogenic growth factors, COX-2 mRNA expression, enhanced apoptosis, and reduced aberrant crypt foci in DMH-induced colon carcinogenesis in rats [149,150].

Anti-proliferative activity has also been described for the glycone hesperidin: Patil et al. [151] found that it inhibits cell cycle progression in Panc-28 human pancreatic carcinoma cells, while Park et al. [152] described its cytotoxic and pro-apoptotic effects on SNU-C4 human colon cancer cells. In HepG2 hepatocarcinoma cells, its ability to induce apoptosis via both mitochondrial and death receptor pathways has been demonstrated [153], as well as the non-apoptotic programmed cell death namely paraptosis [154]. Hesperidin also inhibits proliferation of Ramos Burkitt's lymphoma cells and sensitizes them to doxorubicin-induced apoptosis through the inhibition of both constitutive and doxorubicin-mediated NF-κB activation in a PPARγ-independent manner [155]. In hematopoietic malignancies, hesperidin promoted p53 accumulation and downregulated constitutive NF-κB activity in both PPARγ-dependent and -independent pathways [156]. Induction of apoptosis by hesperidin has also been reported in human mammary carcinoma MCF-7 [157,158] and human cervical cancer HeLa cells [159].

Other reports have shown that hesperidin and neohesperidin increase the sensitivity of Caco-2 cells to doxorubicin, which is consistent with decreased Pgp activity demonstrated in drug-resistant human leukaemia cells (CEM/ADR5000) at non-toxic concentrations (0.32–32 µM) [160]. Inhibition of Pgp has also been described for hesperetin and quercetin in breast cancer resistance protein (BCRP/ABCG2)-overexpressing cell lines [161]. Moreover, hesperidin has been reported suppress proliferation of both human breast cancer and androgen-dependent prostate cancer cells through mechanisms other than antimitotic ones, suggesting a possible interaction with androgenic receptors [162].

Encouraging results in vivo of carcinogenesis inhibition by hesperidin have also been observed. The compound (500 ppm/kg BW) was found to inhibit 4-NQO-induced oral carcinogenesis and to decrease the number of lesions, polyamine levels in tongue tissue, and cell proliferation activity [163]. Later, the same group reported the inhibition of 4-NQO, AOM, MNAN, and OH-BBN-initiated tumorigenesis by hesperidin alone or in combination with diosmin, as described above [95,97]. Moreover, when administered subcutaneously to CD-1 mice, hesperidin inhibited TPA-induced tumor promotion, although it did not inhibit DMBA-induced tumor initiation [164]. Later, they documented the protective effect of hesperidin against the TPA-stimulated infiltration of neutrophils, suggesting its potential as a chemopreventive agent against tumor promoter-induced inflammation and hyperplasia [165]. Daily administration of hesperetin (20 mg/kg BW) *per os* for 15 weeks inhibited rat colon carcinogenesis during and after DMH initiation [166]. Further, in rats with DMBA-induced mammary gland tumors, pretreatment with hesperetin (50 mg/kg BW/day) significantly reduced the tumor burden and the overexpression of the proliferating cell nuclear antigen (PCNA), as well as restoring the decreased Bcl-2 and increased Bax expression. By contrast, in the liver of mice treated with DMBA, at a dosage of 10 mg/kg BW, it prevented DNA fragmentation and decreased Bax expression and cleaved caspase-3, caspase-9 and PARP [167]. This study suggests that hesperetin may act as either pro-apoptotic or anti-apoptotic agent depending on the circumstance [167]. Attenuation of BP-induced lung cancer afforded by hesperidin supplementation (25 mg/kg BW) has also been reported [168]. Finally, dietary administration of hesperetin at 1000 ppm and 5000 ppm significantly deterred xenograft growth in athymic mice ovariectomized and transplanted with aromatase-overexpressing MCF-7 cells, while no such effect was observed in mice treated with apigenin or naringenin. Western blot analysis indicated that cyclin D1, CDK4, and Bcl-XL were reduced in the tumors of hesperetin-treated mice, and there are also results suggesting that the flavonone reduces plasma estrogen [169].

Didymin and poncirin are two flavanones that have been investigated less. However, studies have shown their ability to induce the extrinsic apoptosis pathway in human non-small cell lung cancer cells [170] and gastric cancer cells [171], respectively.

Anthocyanidins and anthocyanins occur ubiquitously in the plant kingdom and confer the bright red, blue, and purple colors to fruits and vegetables. In CF, they are found most commonly in oranges, predominantly as mixture of them. Several investigations have shown the antiproliferative effects of anthocyanidins and anthocyanins both in vitro (towards multiple cancer cell types) and in vivo [172]. The main characteristics of the studies presented in this section are reported in Table 3.

**Table 3.** Studies on the ability of *Citrus* flavonoids to inhibit tumor development.

| | Promotion Phase | | |
| --- | --- | --- | --- |
| Flavonoid | Concentration/Dose | Experimental Model | Reference |
| Quercetin, taxifolin, nobiletin, tangeretin | 2–8 µg/mL | HTB43 cells | [48] |
| Tangeretin | 50–100 µM | HL-60 cells | [49] |
| Tangeretin | 2.7–27 µM | HL-60 cells | [50] |
| Tangeretin, nobiletin | 54 µM (tangeretin) 100–200 µM for MDA-MB-435 60 µM for MCF-7 200 µM for HT-29 (nobiletin) | MDA-MB-435, MCF-7, and HT-29 cells | [51] |
| Tangeretin | 10–50 µM | COLO 205 cells | [52] |
| Nobiletin | 20–200 µM | TMK-1, MKN-45, MKN-74, and KATO-III cells | [53] |
| Tangeretin | $10^{-7}$–$10^{-4}$ M | T47D cells | [56] |
| Nobiletin | 20–30 µM | $H_2O_2$-treated SH-SY5Y cells | [57] |
| Tangeretin, nobiletin | $IC_{50}$ 4 mg/mL | Brain tumor cells | [58] |
| Tangeretin | 150 µM | A2780/CP70 and 2008/C13 cells | [59] |

**Table 3.** *Cont.*

| Promotion Phase | | | |
|---|---|---|---|
| Flavonoid | Concentration/Dose | Experimental Model | Reference |
| Tangeretin | 5–240 µM | AGS cells | [60] |
| Nobiletin | $1 \times 10^{-7}$–$5 \times 10^{-4}$ mol/L | TRAP rats | [61] |
| Nobiletin | 0.05% | PhIP-treated rats | [62] |
| Nobiletin | 0.01%–0.05% | AOM-treated rats | [63] |
| Chrysin, quercetin, nobiletin | 100 ppm | AOM-treated mice | [64] |
| Nobiletin | 100 ppm | AOM/DSS-treated mice | [65] |
| Nobiletin | 1.25–80 µM | A549 cells | [66] |
| Nobiletin | $10^{-3}$ M | MH1C1 and HepG2 cells | [67] |
| Nobiletin | 10–100 µM | C6 cells | [68] |
| Nobiletin | 20–100 µM | U87 and Hs683 cells | [69] |
| Nobiletin | 0–200 µM | AGS, MKN-45, SNU-1, and SNU-16 cells | [70] |
| Nobiletin | 0–160 µM | HL-60, U937, THP-1, OCI-AML3, and MV4-11 cells | [71] |
| Nobiletin | 0.05 wt% | AOM/DSS-treated CD-1 mice | [72] |
| Apigenin | 1–100 µM | MDA-MB-453 cells | [73] |
| Apigenin | 0–40 µM | MCF-7, MCF-7 HER2, SK-BR-3 cells | [74] |
| Apigenin | 10–70 µM | MDA-MB-453, BT-474, SKBr-3, MCF-7, and HBL-100 cells | [75] |
| Apigenin | 0–60 µM | HT-29 and MG63 cells | [77] |
| Apigenin | 10–50 µM | HDF cells | [79] |
| Apigenin | IC$_{50}$: 7.8 µg/mL for MCF-7 and 8.9 µg/mL for MDA-MB-468 cells | MCF-7 and MDA-MB-468 cells | [80] |
| Apigenin | 1–100 µM | BxPC-3 and MiaPaCa-2 cells | [81] |
| Apigenin | 6.25–100 µM | AsPC-1, CD18, MIA PaCa2, and S2-013 cells | [82] |
| Apigenin | 10–100 µM | BxPC-3 and PANC-1 cells | [83] |
| Apigenin | 10–80 µM | LNCaP cells | [84] |
| Apigenin | 1–20 µM | DU145 cells | [85] |
| Apigenin | 0–80 µM | SW480, HT-29, and Caco-2 cells | [86] |
| Apigenin | 10–10 µM | HCT-116, SW480, HT-29, and LoVo cells | [87] |
| Apigenin | 20–50 µg/mouse | 22Rv1 and PC-3 cells-implanted mice | [88] |
| Apigenin | 50 µM | SH-SY5Y cells | [89] |
| Apigenin | 15–60 µM and 25 mg/kg | NUB-7, LAN-5, and SK-N-BE cells and NUB-7 inoculated xenograft mice | [90] |
| Flavonids | 25–250 µM | HT-29, Caco-2, LLC-PK1, and MCF-7 cells | [92] |
| Diosmin | 0–120 µM and 15 mg/kg | HA22T cells and HA22T xenograft mice | [93] |
| Diosmin | 50–250 µM | DU145 cells | [94] |
| Diosmin, hesperidin | 1000 ppm | MNAN-injected rats | [95] |
| Diosmin, hesperidin | 1000 ppm | 4-NQO-exposed rats | [96] |
| Diosmin, hesperidin | 500–1000 ppm | OH-BBN-exposed rats | [97] |
| Diosmin, hesperidin | 1000 ppm | AOM-injected rats | [98] |
| 22 flavonoids | 0–10 µM | HL-60, A431, SK-OV-3, HeLa, HOS cells | [99] |
| Quercetin | 0–100 µM | Caco-2 and HT-29 and IEC-6 cells | [102] |
| Quercetin | 0–50 µM | Prostate and skin cells | [104] |
| Quercetin | 0–50 µM | MDA-MB-231, MDA-MB-453, AU565, BT483, BT474, and MCF-7 cells | [105] |
| Quercetin | 0–10 µM | SK-Br-3 and SK-Br-3-Lap R cells | [106] |
| Quercetin | 2.5–40 µM | MDA-MB-231, MCF-7, and MCF-10A cells | [107] |
| Quercetin | 1–10 µM | MCF-7ADR-resistant cells | [108] |
| Naringenin | 0–1 mM | HL-60 cells | [110] |
| Naringenin | 0.02–2.85 mmol | HT-29 cells | [112] |
| Naringenin | 10 µM | MCF-7 cells | [113] |
| Naringenin | 0–400 µM | THP-1 cells | [114] |
| Naringenin | 50–750 µM | HaCaT and A431 cells | [116] |
| Naringenin | 0.1–0.5 mM | HL-60 cells | [117] |
| Naringenin | 100 µM | A549, H460, and WI-38 cells | [118] |
| Naringenin, hesperetin, apigenin | 50 µM | MCF-7 and NCI-H460 cells | [119] |

**Table 3.** *Cont.*

| Promotion Phase | | | |
|---|---|---|---|
| Flavonoid | Concentration/Dose | Experimental Model | Reference |
| Naringenin, kaempferol | 25–100 μM | HK-2 cells | [121] |
| Naringenin | 10 mg/kg | Rats | [122] |
| Naringenin, naringin | 0.7 mg/kg (naringenin) and 2.4–9.4 mg/kg (naringin) | Rats | [123] |
| Naringenin | 100 μM | A549, MCF-7, HepG2, and MCF-7/DOX cells | [124] |
| Naringin, naringenin, quercetin | 50 mg/kg (naringin or naringenin) and 100 mg/kg (quercetin) | Rats | [125] |
| Naringenin | 200 mg/kg | MNNG-treated rats | [126] |
| Naringenin | 200 mg/kg | MNNG-treated rats | [127] |
| Naringenin | 50 mg/kg | C6 cells-injected rats | [128] |
| Naringin, naringenin | 2.5% | Hamsters | [129] |
| Naringin | 250–2000 μM | SiHa cells | [130] |
| Naringin | 1000 μmol/L | HeLa cells | [131] |
| Naringin | 0–3200 μM | HeLa and A549 cells | [132] |
| Naringin | 50–200 μM and 100 mg/kg | MDA-MB-231, MDA-MB-468, and BT-549 cells/MDA-MB-231 xenograft mice | [133] |
| Naringin | 0–150 μM | 5637 and T24 cells | [134] |
| Naringin | 1.2–3 mM | AGS cells | [137] |
| Naringin | 50–200 μM | MDA-MB-231, MDA-MB-468, and BT-549 cells | [138] |
| Naringin | 200 mg/kg | AOM-injected rats | [139] |
| Naringin | 10.25–35 mg/kg | W256 rats | [140] |
| Naringin | 150 mg/kg | Apc(Min/+) mice | [141] |
| Hesperetin, hesperidin, naringenin, naringin | 40–80 μM | HL-60, THP-1, and PMN cells | [143] |
| Hesperetin | 0–200 μM | MCF-7 cells | [144] |
| Hesperetin | 5–100 μM | HT-29 cells | [145] |
| Hesperetin | 0–125 μmol/L | BON cells | [146] |
| Hesperetin | 125–1000 μM | SiHa cells | [147] |
| Hesperetin | 0–600 μM and 10–40 mg/kg | HepG-2, SMMC-7721, and Huh-7/hepatocellular carcinoma xenograft mice | [148] |
| Hesperetin | 20 mg/kg | DMH-injected rats | [149] |
| Hesperidin, hesperitin, rutin, neohesperidin | 25–100 μg/mL | Panc-28 cells | [151] |
| Hesperidin | 1–100 μM | SNU-C4 cells | [152] |
| Hesperidin | 0–200 μM | HepG2 cells | [153] |
| Hesperidin | 0.1–2 mM | HepG2 cells | [154] |
| Hesperidin | 0–100 μM | Ramos cells | [155] |
| Hesperidin | 10–100 μM | NALM-6 cells | [156] |
| Hesperidin | 0–200 μM | MCF-7, MCF-10A, HMEC and MDA-MB-231 cells | [157] |
| Hesperidin | 20–100 μM | MCF-7 cells | [158] |
| Hesperidin | 0–100 μM | HeLa cells | [159] |
| Hesperidin | 0.32–32 μM | Caco-2, CCRF-CEM and CEM/ADR5000 cells | [160] |
| Hesperetin, quercetin | 30 μM | K562, K562/BCRP, MCF7/WT, and MCF7/MR cells | [161] |
| Hesperidin | 0–100 μM | MCF-7, LNCaP, PC-3 and DU-145 cells | [162] |
| Hesperidin | 500 ppm | 4-NQO-treated rats | [163] |
| Hesperidin | 1% | DMBA/TPA-treated mice | [164] |
| Hesperetin | 20 mg/kg | DMH-treated rats | [166] |
| Hesperetin | 10–50 mg/kg | DMBA-treated rats | [167] |
| Hesperidin | 25 mg/kg | BP-exposed mice | [168] |
| Hesperetin | 1000–5000 ppm | MCF-7 xenograft mice | [169] |
| Didymin | 0–20 μM | A549 and H460 cells | [170] |
| Poncirin | 50–200 μM | AGS cells | [171] |

4-NQO: 4-nitroquinoline 1-oxide; AOM: azoxymethane; DMH: 1,2-dimethylhydrazine; DSS: dextran sulfate sodium; MNAN: *N*-methyl-*N*-amylnitrosamine; MNNG: *N*-methyl-*N'*-nitro-*N*-nitrosoguanidine OH-BBN: *N*-butyl-*N*-(4-hydroxybutyl)nitrosamine; PhIP: 2-amino-1-methyl-6-phenylimidazo[4,5-b]pyridine.

*3.3. Inhibition of Tumor Progression: Focus on Angiogenesis and Metastatization*

Both development and progression of solid neoplasms requires rapid and persistent growth of new blood vessels (neo-angiogenesis) around the cancer tissue to supply the growing tumor with nutrients and oxygen. Cancer cells can stimulate angiogenesis by secreting angiogenesis-promoting growth factors, such as the vascular endothelial growth factor (VEGF), the most important endothelial cell-selective mitogen in vitro. VEGF also produces a substantial increase in vascular permeability that allows tumor cells access to the bloodstream, thereby linking angiogenesis and metastases with a poor prognosis [91].

It has been reported that some flavonoids, including naringin, apigenin, and rutin, are able to inhibit VEGF release in MDA human breast cancer cells [173], and VEGF and transforming growth factor-β1 (TGF-β1) in the GL-15 glioblastoma cell lines [174]. Several findings suggest that apigenin can be considered a natural anti-angiogenic compound. Indeed, it reduces VEGF transcriptional activation via hypoxia-inducible factor 1 (HIF-1) pathway in A549 lung cancer cells, and inhibits angiogenesis in the tumor tissues of nude mice [175]. The inhibition of HIF-1 and VEGF expression has been described in different cancer cells in normoxic or hypoxic conditions [176]. The Authors described the inhibition of tumor angiogenesis using both chicken chorioallantoic membrane and Matrigel plug assays [176]. Apigenin-induced reduction of neo-angiogenesis in the human umbilical vein endothelial cell (HUVEC) seems to be mediated by inhibition of matrix-degrading proteases [177]. Recently, it has been shown that apigenin may act by modulating the inflammatory cytokine IL-6/activators of transcription 3 (STAT3) (IL-6/STAT3) signaling pathways in HUVEC cells. Angiogenesis inhibition resulted in modulation of the activation of extracellular signal-regulated kinase 1/2 (ERK 1/2) signaling triggered by IL-6, as well as in a marked reduction in the proliferation, migration, and morphogenic differentiation of endothelial cells. These effects were coupled with reduced expression of the IL-6 signal transducing receptor-alpha (IL-6Rα) and suppression of cytokine signaling (SOCS3) protein, as well as the secretion of extracellular matrix metalloproteinase (MMP)-2 [178].

Other *Citrus* flavonoids have been evaluated for their potential anti-angiogenic capability. Lam et al. [179] demonstrated the anti-angiogenic activity of some polymethoxylated flavonoids, including hesperetin and nobiletin, both in vitro (HUVEC cells) and in vivo (the zebrafish embryo model). The structure–activity relationship (SAR) analysis indicated that a flavonoid with a methoxylated group at the C3$'$ position offers stronger anti-angiogenic activity, whereas the absence of a methoxylated group at the C8 position causes lower lethal toxicity in addition to enhancing anti-angiogenic activity. Anti-angiogenic activity of nobiletin in vitro and in vivo previously reported by Kunimasa et al. [180], gave an in-depth description of the mechanisms underlying its inhibitory action on multiple functions of the proliferation, migration, and tube formation of HUVEC cells. Wang et al. [181] reported nobiletin to inhibit tumor growth and angiogenesis by reducing VEGF expression of K562 cells xenograft in nude mice. Moreover, quercetin inhibited tube formation in HUVEC cells and suppressed the angiogenic process in a chick chorioallantoic membrane assay [182]. Interestingly, the flavonoid quercetin possessed strong inhibitory effects on vessel formation and on endothelial cell proliferation, and concomitantly showed strong antioxidant activity [183].

Many studies have reported that flavonoids, many of which are abundant in the *Citrus* genus, are an effective natural inhibitor of cancer invasion and metastasis [184]. In particular, tangeretin and nobiletin appear to be able to inhibit the progression phase of carcinogenesis.

In MCF-7/6 breast cancer cells, tangeretin was found to upregulate the function of the E-cadherin/catenin complex, which consequently led to firm cell–cell adhesions and inhibited cell invasion [185]. In brain tumor cells, nobiletin, and to a lesser extent, tangeretin, exhibited inhibitory activity on the adhesion, migration, invasion, and secretion of MMP-2/MMP-9. In glioblastoma, nobiletin inhibited human U87 and Hs683 glioma cell growth and migration by arresting cell cycle and suppressing the MAPK and Akt pathways [69]. Naringin inhibited the invasion and migration of glioblastoma U87 MG cells by increasing the expression of tissue inhibitors of metalloproteinases (TIMP-1 and TIMP-2), thereby decreasing the expression and proteinase activity of MMP-2 and MMP-9 and enhancing the focal adhesion kinase (FAK)/MMPs pathway [138]. Moreover, naringin inhibited cell migration and invasion of chondrosarcoma cells via vascular cell adhesion molecule 1 (VCAM-1) down-regulation by increasing miR-126 [186], while in bladder cancer cells it downregulated the Akt and MMP-2 pathways [187]. In an experimental model of pulmonary metastasis generated by inoculating albino Swiss mice with highly metastatic murine melanoma cells B16F10, diosmin reduced the number of metastatic nodules in the lung more effectively than tangeretin and rutin [188]. Furthermore, oral administration of naringenin or hesperitin reduced the number of lung metastases in C57BL6/N mice inoculated with B16F10 cells, and increased survival time after tumor cell inoculation [189]. In addition, in a breast cancer resection model that mimics clinical situations after surgery, orally administered naringenin significantly decreased the number of metastatic tumor cells in the lung and extended the life span of tumor resected mice. Both in vitro and in vivo experimental results have further demonstrated that relief of immunosuppression caused by regulatory T cells might be the fundamental mechanism underlying metastasis inhibition by naringenin [190]. Some reports have illustrated the mechanisms by which nobiletin may reduce tumor invasion and metastasis in vitro. In human fibrosarcoma HT-1080 cells stimulated with TPA, it directly inhibited the phosphorylation of mitogen-activated protein/extracellular signal-regulated kinase (MEK), thereby suppressing either the sequential phosphorylation of extracellular regulated kinases (ERK) and the expression of MMP [191]. MMP-1 and -9 expression were suppressed by nobiletin in fibrosarcoma cells with an associated increase in tissue inhibitors of MMPs [192]. Additionally, MMP-7 was down-regulated in colorectal cells [193], while MMP-2 in human nasopharyngeal carcinoma cells [194]. Nobiletin exerts antimetastatic effects on human breast cancer cells [195] through the down-regulation of both CXC chemokine receptor type 4 (CXCR4) and MMP-9 via a mechanism involving NF-κB inhibition and MAPKs activation. Minagawa et al. [196] showed that pro-MMP-9 activity was inhibited by nobiletin in gastric cell lines, and reported a significant reduction in the peritoneal dissemination of stomach cancer nodules when the polymethoxylated flavone was administered subcutaneously to severe combined immune deficient (SCID) mice. Moreover, nobiletin has been shown to reduce adhesion, invasion, and migration of highly metastatic human gastric adenocarcinoma AGS cells by inhibiting the activation of FAK and PI3K/Akt signals, which in turn downregulates MMP-2 and -9 expression and activity [197]. Finally, nobiletin inhibited the epithelial–mesenchymal transition of human non-small cell lung cancer cells by antagonizing the TGF-β1/Smad3 signaling pathway, thus prohibiting the growth of metastatic nodules in the lungs of nude mice [198].

Treatment of MDA-MB-231 breast tumor cells with apigenin (ranging from 2.5 to 10 μg/mL) led to a partial decrease in urokinase-plasminogen activator (uPA) expression and completely inhibited phorbol 12-myristate 13-acetate (PMA)-induced MMP-9 secretion [199]. Apigenin also inhibited hepatocyte growth factor (HGF)-induced migration and invasion and decreased HGF-stimulated integrin β4 and Akt phosphorylation in MDA-MB-231 cells. It also inhibited HGF-promoted metastasis in nude mice and in chick embryos [200]. In prostate cancer, the motility and invasion of PC3-M cells were inhibited by apigenin through a FAK/Src signaling mechanism [201]. In ovarian cancer, it inhibited FAK-mediated migration and invasion of A2780 cells, and repressed spontaneous metastasis formation on the ovaries of nude mice following inoculation with A2780 cells [202]. In cervical cancer, apigenin inhibited the motility and invasiveness of HeLa cells [203]. Moreover, its administration significantly decreased the incidence of cancer metastasis in AOM-induced intestinal adenocarcinoma in rats [204]. Noh et al. [205] further reported that this flavone inhibited PMA-induced migration and invasion of human cervical carcinoma Caski cell line via the suppression of p38 MAPK-dependent MMP-9 expression. Finally, intraperitoneal administration of apigenin and quercetin into syngeneic mice injected with B16-BL6 melanoma cells resulted in a significant delay in tumor growth and lungs metastases, with flavonoids being more effective than tamoxifen [206].

Over the last decade, there has been extensive researches into the potential anti-invasive role of quercetin. In breast cancer, the invasive activity of PMA-induced MCF-7 cells was blocked by the flavonol by reducing MMP-9 expression and by blocking activation of the protein kinase C (PKC)/ERK/AP-1 signaling cascade [207]. In MDA-MB-231 cells the anti-invasive effect was mediated by inhibiting MMP-3 activity [208]. In PC-3 prostate cancer cells, quercetin (50 and 100 μM for 24 h) decreased MMP-2/MMP-9 expression [209] and downregulated the mRNA of uPA, uPA receptor (uPA-R), EGF, and EGF receptor (EGF-R), thereby inhibiting invasion and migration [210]. In human glioblastoma U87 cells, quercetin blocked PMA-induced migration and invasion by inhibiting ERK-dependent COX-2 activation and MMP-9 activity [211], while in the DAOY medulloblastoma cell line, it reduced both Met-induced cell migration and HGF-mediated Akt activation [212]. Moreover, quercetin decreased the invasiveness of A431 epidermal cancer cells by increasing EGF-depressed E-cadherin, by down-regulating both epithelial–mesenchymal transition (EMT) markers and MMP-9, leading to the restoration of cell–cell junctions [213]. In addition, it inhibited cell–matrix adhesion, migration, and invasion of HeLa cells [214] and inhibited the motility and invasion of murine melanoma B16-BL6 cells by decreasing pro-MMP-9 via the PKC pathway [215]. The administration of quercetin to DMBA-induced mammary carcinoma rats has been reported to significantly decrease both tissue type plasminogen activator (t-PA) and u-PA [216]. Lastly, didymin was observed to suppress phthalate-mediated breast cancer cell proliferation, migration, and invasion, suggesting that it is capable of preventing phthalate ester-associated cancer aggravation [217]. Table 4 summarizes the essential features of the studies on the anti-angiogenic and anti-metastatic activity of *Citrus* flavonoids.

**Table 4.** Studies on the ability of *Citrus* flavonoids to inhibit angiogenesis and metastasis and their characteristics.

| Flavonoid | Concentration/Dose | Experimental Model | Reference |
|---|---|---|---|
| | | **Progression Phase** | |
| Flavonoids | 0.1–100 μmol/L | MDA, U343, and U118 cells | [173] |
| Rutin | 50–100 μM | GL-15 cells | [174] |
| Apigenin | 0–20 μM | A549 cells | [175] |
| Apigenin | 0–30 μM | PC-3, DU145, LNCaP, OVCAR-3, HCT-8, MCF-7 cells | [176] |
| Apigenin | 5 mg/L | HUVEC cells | [177] |
| Apigenin | 25 μM | HUVEC, HMVECs-d-Ad cells | [178] |
| Hesperetin and nobiletin | 0–100 μM and 30 μM | HUVECs cells and zebrafish | [179] |
| Nobiletin | 0–128 μM and 100 μg/egg | HUVEC and HDMEC cells and CAM | [180] |
| Nobiletin | 12.5–50 mg/kg | K562 cells xenograft mice | [181] |
| Quercetin | 0–100 μM and 50–100 nmol/10 μL/egg | HUVEC cells and CAM | [182] |
| Quercetin | 3.13–50 μg/mL | HUVEC cells | [183] |
| Naringin | 0–30 μM | JJ012 and SW1353 cells | [186] |
| Neringenin | 0–300 μM | TSGH-8301 cells | [187] |
| Tangeretin, rutin, and diosmin | 20 mg/animal | B16F10-inoculated mice | [188] |
| Naringenin and hesperitin | 10 μM/20 mg/g of pellets | B16-F10 cells/B16-F10-inoculated C57BL6/N mice | [189] |
| Naringenin | 0–200 μM and 100 mg/kg | 4T1 cells/4T1-injected BALB/c and C57BL/6 mice | [190] |
| Nobiletin | 64 μM | TPA-stimulated HT-1080 cells | [191] |
| Nobiletin | 0–64 μM | TPA-stimulated HT-1080 cells | [192] |
| Nobiletin | 0–100 μM | Caco-2, HT-29, Colo205, Colo320DM, LS174T, and LS180 cells | [193] |
| Nobiletin | 0–200 μM | MDA MB-231 cells | [195] |
| Nobiletin | 0–256 μM/16–64 μM | TMK-1, MKN-45, and St-4 cell/TMK-1-injected mice | [196] |
| Nobiletin | 0–4.5 μM | HepG2, Caco-2, and AGS cells | [197] |
| Apigenin | 2.5–10 μg/mL | MDA-MB231 cells | [199] |
| Apigenin | 0–320 μM | MDA-MB-231, A549, SK-Hep1 cells | [200] |
| Apigenin | 0–50 μM | PC3-M, C4-2B, and DU145 cells | [201] |
| Apigenin | 20/40 μM | A2780 cells | [202] |
| Apigenin | 10–50 μM | HeLa cells | [203] |
| Apigenin | 0.75–1.5 mg/kg | AOM-treated rats | [204] |
| Apigenin | 5–20 μM | PMA-exposed SK-Hep1 and MDA-231 cells | [205] |
| Apigenin and quercetin | 1–10,000 nM/25–50 mg/kg | B16-BL6-injected mice | [206] |
| Quercetin | 80 μM | TPA-treated MCF-7 cells | [207] |
| Quercetin | 0–100 μmol/L | MDA-MB-231 cells | [208] |
| Quercetin | 50–100 μM | PC-3 cells | [209] |
| Quercetin | 25–125 mM | PC-3 cells | [210] |
| Quercetin | 50 μM | TPA-exposed U87 cells | [211] |
| Quercetin | 1–20 μM | HGF-exposed DAOY cells | [212] |
| Quercetin and luteolin | 10–20 μM | A431 cells | [213] |
| Quercetin | 20 to 80 μM/L | HeLa cells | [214] |
| Quercetin | $3.3 \times 10^{-1}$ mM | B16-BL6 cells | [215] |
| Quercetin | 25 mg/kg | DMBA-treated rats | [216] |

DMBA: 7,12-dimethylbenz(α)anthracene; HGF: hepatocyte growth factor; TPA: tetradecanoyl-13-phorbol acetate.

## 4. Anti-Cancer Properties of *Citrus* Juices and Extracts

As described above, a number of studies have investigated the anti-cancer effect of single *Citrus* flavonoids as pure compounds. However, few studies have focused on the biological activity of *Citrus* juices and extracts. A very interesting paper [218] explains why a single bioactive compound may not replicate the same effect as the phytocomplex in which it is contained. Indeed, often, even at high concentrations, no single active principle can replace the combination of natural phytochemicals present in an extract in achieving the same magnitude of pharmacological effect. Liu [218] suggests that the additive and synergistic effects of phytochemicals in fruits and vegetables are responsible for these potent antioxidant and anti-cancer activities, and that the benefits of a diet rich in fruits and vegetables is attributable to the complex mixture of phytochemicals present in whole foods. This concept has been supported through data obtained employing several nutraceuticals by Surh [10].

In line with this, some preclinical studies have indicated that *Citrus* juices and extracts may reduce cancer formation and progression. To the best of our knowledge, So et al. [219] were the first to show that concentrated *Citrus sinensis* (orange) juice inhibits the development of mammary tumors induced by 5 mg of DMBA in rats, also suggesting the anti-cancer properties of naringin and quercetin. Two years later, the same Authors [220] showed that a double-strength orange juice administration inhibited DMBA-induced mammary tumorigenesis in rats more effectively than double-strength grapefruit juice. Moreover, Miyagi and coworkers [221] showed that orange juice inhibits AOM-induced colon cancer in male rats, suggesting that flavonoids and limonoid glucosides might be responsible for this anti-cancer activity. *Citrus reticulata* (mandarin) juice has also long been investigated regarding its antitumoral activity. In particular, studies have demonstrated the capability of mandarin juice to suppress the chemically-induced carcinogenesis in colon, tongue, and lung cancers, especially when it is supplemented with added amounts of flavonoids, such as beta-cryptoxanthin and hesperidin [222–225]. Recently, we have investigated the effects of a flavonoid-rich extract from mandarin juice (MJe) on three human anaplastic thyroid carcinoma cell lines (CAL-62, C-643, and 8505C cells), showing that MJe reduced cell proliferation through a block of the cell cycle in the G2/M phase, accompanied by low cell death due to autophagy. Moreover, MJe reduced activity of MMP-2, thus decreasing cell migration [226]. In another study, Vanamala and coworkers [139] showed that grapefruit juice and limonin produce suppressive effects on AOM-induced colon carcinogenesis by lowering inducible nitric oxide synthases iNOS and cyclooxygenase-2 COX-2 levels and upregulating apoptosis, thereby reducing the formation of aberrant crypt foci. Furthermore, methanolic extract of lemon fruit triggered apoptosis of MCF-7 human breast cancer cells [227]. An analogous effect was achieved on the same cell line using lemon seed extract [228].

In recent years, *Citrus bergamia* (bergamot) fruit has attracted attention due to its potential anti-cancer effects. In particular, we have shown that bergamot juice (BJ) to reduce the growth rate of different cancer cell lines by different molecular mechanisms, depending on cancer type. In SH-SY5Y human neuroblastoma cells, BJ stimulated the cell cycle arrest in the G1 phase without inducing apoptosis, and caused a modification in cellular morphology associated with a marked increase in detached cells. The inhibition of adhesive ability onto different physiologic substrates and onto endothelial cell monolayer was correlated with BJ-induced impairment of actin filaments and with the reduction in the expression of the active form of FAK, in turn causing inhibition of cell migration [229]. Contrariwise, in human hepatocellular carcinoma HepG2 cells, we demonstrated that BJ reduces the growth rate through the involvement of p53, p21, and NF-κB pathways, as well as the activation of both intrinsic and extrinsic apoptotic pathways [230]. Moreover, we documented that the BJ-induced reduction of both cell adhesiveness and motility could be responsible for the slight inhibitory effects on lung metastasis colonization observed in an animal model of spontaneous neuroblastoma metastasis formation in SCID mouse [231]. In order to assess which bioactive component of BJ was responsible for its antitumor activity, we focused on the flavonoid-rich fraction from bergamot juice (BJe). Our results suggested that BJe inhibits HT-29 human colorectal carcinoma cell growth and induces apoptosis through multiple mechanisms. Molecular assays revealed that higher concentrations of BJe increase

ROS production, which causes a loss of mitochondrial membrane potential and oxidative DNA damage. Lower concentrations of BJe inhibited MAPK pathways and modified apoptosis-related proteins, which in turn induced cell cycle arrest and apoptosis [232].

It is well known that chronic inflammation might lead to carcinogenesis, and that both inflammatory cells and cytokines contribute to tumor growth, progression, and immunosuppression [233]. Moreover, there is evidence to support the hypothesis that dysregulation of both inflammatory and redox pathways in tumor cells and in their stromal environment play an essential role in tumorigenesis, invasion, and systemic spread [234]. Furthermore, inflammatory pathways are constitutively active in most cancers. Therefore, the use of medicines with antioxidant and anti-inflammatory activities is desirable in oncological applications. In addition, although natural remedies are not risk free, they are generally safer than both synthetic and biological drugs. In this context, we have recently shown that BJe has antioxidant properties [235,236] and is able to suppress pro-inflammatory responses in both in vitro [237,238] and in vivo models [239,240]. Interestingly, evidence showing that BJ did not significantly affect the viability of normal human diploid fibroblast WI-38 cells [229], as well as not provoking any apparent sign of systemic toxicity [231], together with its antimicrobial activity [241,242] and favorable safety/efficacy balance [243], reveals the potential of BJe as an anti-cancer remedy, highlighting that it could represent a novel strategic approach in oncology field.

Other studies have been performed using extracts of *Citrus* derivatives. For examples, Mak and collaborators [244] reported that an extract from the pericarpium of *Citrus reticulata* inhibited the proliferation of murine myeloid leukemia WEHI 3B cells and induced their differentiation into macrophages and granulocytes, identifying nobiletin and tangeretin as the active components. Kim and coworkers [245] reported the anti-proliferative and pro-apoptotic effects of a *Citrus reticulata* Blanco peel extract on the human gastric cancer cell line SNU-668. Park et al. [246] used a flavonoid extract from the peel of Korean *Citrus aurantium* L. and found it was able to induce cell cycle arrest and apoptosis in A549 lung cancer cells, while Han and collaborators [247] suggested that a crude methanol extract of *Citrus aurantium* L. peel should induce caspase-dependent apoptosis through the inhibition of Akt in U937 human leukemia cells. Two animal studies using an orange peel extract abundant in polymethoxyflavones, showed its ability to reduce the development of hyperplastic lesions and to increase apoptosis in ductal epithelial cells of mouse mammary glands [55], and to inhibit intestinal tumorigenesis in Apc$^{(Min/+)}$ mice [54]. Moreover, the ethanolic extract of peel from *Citrus aurantifolia* increased the sensitivity of MCF-7 cells to doxorubicin, enhancing both cell cycle arrest and apoptosis [248]. Similarly, total flavonoids from *Citrus paradisi* Macfadyen peel, when combined with arsenic trioxide, produced a synergistic effect in reducing the proliferation of leukemia cells and triggering apoptosis [249], suggesting that *Citrus* extracts could be used as co-adjuvants in cancer therapy. Finally, we have shown that the bergamot essential oil (BEO) obtained by rasping the peel of *Citrus bergamia* fruits decreased the growth rate of SH-SY5Y neuroblastoma cells [250] by a mechanism correlated to both apoptotic and necrotic cell death [251]. Table 5 summarizes the main characteristics of the above investigations into the anti-cancer properties of *Citrus* juices and extracts.

**Table 5.** Essential features of the studies evaluating the anti-cancer properties of *Citrus* juices and extracts.

| *Citrus* Juices and Extracts | Experimental Model | Reference |
|---|---|---|
| *Citrus sinensis* juice | DMBA-injected rats | [219] |
| *Citrus sinensis* juice | DMBA-injected rats | [220] |
| *Citrus sinensis* juice | AOM-injected rats | [221] |
| *Citrus reticulata* juice | AOM-injected rats | [222] |
| *Citrus reticulata* juice | NNK-injected mice | [223] |
| *Citrus reticulata* juice | AOM-injected rats | [225] |
| *Citrus reticulata* juice | CAL-62, C-643, 8505C cells | [226] |
| Lemon fruit extract | MCF-7 cells | [227] |

Table 5. *Cont.*

| *Citrus* Juices and Extracts | Experimental Model | Reference |
|---|---|---|
| Lemon seed extracts | MCF-7 cells | [228] |
| *Citrus bergamia* juice | SH-SY5Y cells | [229] |
| *Citrus bergamia* juice | HepG2 cells | [230] |
| *Citrus bergamia* juice | SK-*N*-SH/LAN-1 xenograft mice | [231] |
| Flavonoid-rich extract of bergamot juice | HT-29 cells | [232] |
| *Citrus reticulata* pericarpium extract | WEHI 3B cells | [244] |
| *Citrus reticulata* Blanco peel extract | SNU-668 cells | [245] |
| *Citrus aurantium* peel extract | A549 cells | [246] |
| *Citrus aurantium* peel extract | U937 cells | [247] |
| Orange peel extract | C57Bl/6 mice | [55] |
| Orange peel extract | Apc$^{(Min/+)}$ mice | [54] |
| *Citrus aurantifolia* peel extract | MCF-7 cells | [248] |
| *Citrus paradis* peel extract | Kasumi-1 cells | [249] |
| *Citrus bergamia* essential oil | SH-SY5Y cells | [250] |
| *Citrus bergamia* essential oil | SH-SY5Y cells | [251] |

AOM: azoxymethane; DMBA: 7,12-dimethylbenz(α)anthracene; NNK: 4-(methyl-nitrosoamino)-1-(3-pyridyl)-1-butanone.

## 5. Epidemiological Studies

Over the last few decades, epidemiological and clinical studies have suggested that regular intake of CF may protect against cancer development. The majority of the clinical evidence supporting the potential anti-cancer effects of *Citrus* is derived from case–control studies. One of the first population-based case-control studies evaluating whether *Citrus* intake is associated with a reduced cancer risk was carried out in Shanghai at the end of the 1990s. The aim of this study was to investigate the association between dietary factors and risk of nasopharyngeal carcinoma (NPC), Yuan et al. [252] found that high intake of oranges and tangerines was associated with a statistically significant reduction in the risk of NPC. The study included 935 NPC patients aged 15 to 74 years interviewed by a questionnaire. Authors concluded that oranges and tangerines are a rich source of vitamin C that can block nitrosamine formation, thereby offering a biological rationale for the anti-NPC effect. In the 1990s, Bosetti et al. [253] conducted a hospital-based case–control study in three areas of northern Italy on 304 patients affected by a squamous cell carcinoma of the esophagus and 743 controls who were asked to complete a questionnaire. The results of this observational study provide further evidence to support the theory that consumption of CF is inversely related to esophageal cancer risk. Steevens et al. [254] reached the same conclusions when studying a Netherlands cohort. High intake of CF has also been associated with reduced risk of cancer of the oral cavity and pharynx [255]. Some years later, the same research group, performed a population-based case control study recruiting subjects in Northern Italy and Swiss Canton of Vaud in the 1990s showed that intake of CF may also reduce laryngeal cancer [256]. In line with these findings, a prospective study on 42,311 US men in the Health Professionals Follow-up Study [257] reported that histologically-diagnosed oral premalignant lesions were suppressed by consumption of CF and CF juices (30% to 40% lower risk), thus upholding results previously obtained in Europe on smaller subject groups. Interestingly, a meta-analysis showed that the CF consumption exerts the strongest protective effect against oral cancer compared to all other kinds of fruits [258]. Pourfarzi et al. [259] reported that regular intake of fruits could reduce the risk of gastric cancer by more than half. In particular, consumption of CF was more protective than all other fruits, and subjects eating them more than three times per week had about a 70% lower risk than those who never or infrequently ate CF. The beneficial effects of CF with respect to stomach cancer prevention were confirmed by a more recent cohort study performed in Netherlands [254]. Epidemiological data from a network of case–control studies strengthen the hypothesis that increasing consumption of CF may reduce the risk of cancers of the digestive and upper respiratory tract [260]. Gonzalez and co-workers [261] also observed a significant inverse correlation between total CF ingestion and gastric cancer risk.

However, the possibility that intake of CF can prevent the development of colon cancer is quite controversial [262,263]. A large population-based case–control study was conducted on Chinese women in Shanghai by interview. Tangerines, oranges, and grapefruits were found to be inversely associated with breast cancer risk among pre-menopausal women, but the same data was not found to be statistically significant in post-menopausal women [264]. However, a more recent study revealed a significant protective effect against breast cancer by oranges, orange juice, and other CF [265]. Intake of either CF [266] or orange, grapefruit, and their juice [267] also reduced the risk of developing pancreatic cancer. Moreover, CF intake also seems to be inversely associated with prostate cancer risk [268], and high consumption of both tangerines and oranges was found to be protective against melanoma [269]. Recently, a prospective study showed that *Citrus* consumption, especially if eaten daily, was correlated with reduced incidence of all cancers, although significant results were only obtained for prostate and pancreatic cancer [270]. About 40,000 Japanese patients of Ohsaki were followed for up to 9 years to assess the *Citrus* consumption by a self-administered questionnaire. This study overcomes the bias of other studies described above due to their retrospective nature, confirming the ability of CF to reduce risk of first and second primary tumors [270]. Interestingly, one prospective study indicated that high intake of CF may confer protection against the development of second pulmonary cancers, particularly in the lung [271].

Furthermore, meta-analyses have confirmed the relationship between CF intake and decreased risk of cancers. In particular, Bae et al. [272] have provided evidence for the protective effects of high CF ingestion against stomach cancer risk. Another quantitative systematic review [273] has reported an inverse association between CF consumption and pancreatic cancer risk, although the effect was limited due to the weakness of study design. More recently, different meta-analyses have highlighted an inverse association between CF intake and the risk of various types of cancers, such as breast cancer [274], bladder cancers [275–277], and esophageal cancer [278]. A very recent systematic literature review of prospective studies on CF intake and risk of esophageal and gastric cancers revealed only a marginally significant decreased risk of esophageal cancer and reported no significant inverse association for gastric cardia cancer, but data are still limited [279].

However, some researchers have reported the ineffectiveness of CF in cancer prevention. For instance, the results from a large European prospective cohort suggested that higher consumption of fruits and vegetables is not associated with decreased risk of pancreatic cancer [280]. Moreover, Bae and coworkers [273] found no association between CF intake and risk of prostate cancer.

The reasons for this variability are multi-factorial, but probably reflect the ability of *Citrus* flavonoids to interact with their molecular targets, and are due to their poor bioavailability and issues linked to the study design. The latter include: fluctuations in CF intake, the qualitative/quantitative composition of CF, the relative concentration of bioactive molecules, the eventual standardization (in the case of natural remedies), the patient's compliance with the instructions provided by the investigator, and other numerous possible confounding elements. Nevertheless, although evidence linking CF intake and cancer prevention are conflicting, epidemiological data seem to support the hypothesis of some protection against certain types of cancer by CF. Table 6 collects the studies presented in this paragraph.

**Table 6.** The main epidemiological and clinical studies, systematic review, and meta-analysis on the anti-cancer effects of *Citrus* fruits.

| Study Design | Subjects | Reference |
|---|---|---|
| Case–control study | 935 nasopharyngeal carcinoma (NPC) patients aged 15 to 74 years and 1032 community controls | [252] |
| Case–control study | 304 esophagus squamous cell carcinoma patients and 743 hospital controls | [253] |
| Cohort study | 120,852 Dutch men and women aged 55–69 | [254] |
| Case–control study | 512 men and 86 women with cancer of the oral cavity and pharynx and 1008 men and 483 women controls | [255] |
| Case–control study | 527 incident, histologically confirmed cases and 1297 frequency-matched controls | [256] |
| Prospective study | 42,311 US men | [257] |
| Case–control study | 217 people with gastric cancer and 394 controls | [259] |
| Population-based case–control study | 1459 incident breast cancer cases and 1556 frequency-matched controls | [264] |
| Clinic-based case–control study | 384 cases of pancreatic cancer and 983 controls | [266] |
| Population-based case–control study | 532 cases of pancreatic cancer and 1701 controls | [267] |
| Case–control study | 130 incident patients with adenocarcinoma of the prostate and 274 controls | [268] |
| Hospital-based case–control study | 304 incident cases of cutaneous melanoma and 305 controls | [269] |
| Cohort Study | 42,470 Japanese adults with age ranging fron 40 to 79 years | [270] |
| Population-based case–control study | 876 male patients with laryngeal/hypopharyngeal carcinoma | [271] |
| Systematic review | Stomach cancer | [272] |
| Systematic review | Pancreatic cancer | [273] |
| Systematic review | Breast cancer | [274] |
| Meta-analysis | Bladder cancer | [275] |
| Systematic review and meta-analysis | Bladder cancer | [276] |
| Meta-analysis | Bladder cancer | [277] |
| Meta-analysis | Esophageal cancer | [278] |
| Systematic review | Esophageal and gastric cancers | [279] |

## 6. Concluding Remarks

Overall, knowledge about the effects of flavonoids on cancer development has progressively grown over recent years, as well as people's desire to maintain good health through increasing use of nutraceuticals, functional foods, and natural remedies. Numerous in vitro and in vivo studies have shown the ability of flavonoids to exert anti-cancer effect, and some epidemiological studies support this hypothesis. Moreover, evidence showing that flavonoids act not only as free radical scavengers but also as modulators of several key molecular events implicated in cell survival and death, has heightened scientific interest in these plant secondary metabolites. The main sources of dietary flavonoids for humans are fruits, especially *Citrus* fruits and their juices, along with vegetables, wine, and tea. Over the last few decades, experimental research and epidemiological studies indicate that CF and their flavonoids could have anti-tumor properties. The experimental results discussed in this review have clearly shown that *Citrus* flavonoids may act as chemopreventive and chemotherapeutic agents, either as single agents or as co-adjuvants for other drugs. However, the majority of studies on the anti-cancer potential of *Citrus* extracts and their single components have been carried out in in vitro and in vivo models, and the extrapolation of preclinical results for human use is difficult to achieve, particularly, but not solely, due to problems linked to pharmacokinetics. Indeed, the modest bioavailability of flavonoids and their limited duration of action are the main obstacles restricting their clinical use. Some flavonoids, such as quercetin and anthocyanins, can be absorbed at the gastric level, while others—resistant to acid hydrolysis in the stomach— intact reach the intestine where are absorbed. However, most of the flavonoids present in food are esters, glycosides, or polymers, which are not absorbed in their native form because of their extensive modification by intestinal enzymes such as β-glucosidases and lactase-phlorizin hydrolase present in the resident bacterial flora. Moreover, flavonoids may be subjected to intestinal and hepatic first-pass extraction that can further affect their bioavailability. However, some metabolic reactions lead to the formation of biologically active metabolites. While some flavonoids undergo an extensive pre-systemic elimination, others are less vulnerable, depending on their chemical structure. Inter-individual variations have also been observed, probably due to the different composition of the colonic microflora which can affect their metabolism in different ways. Nevertheless, despite bioavailability problems, numerous experimental and clinical data have demonstrated the ability of *Citrus* flavonoids to exert important systemic pharmacological effects [14,281,282]. In addition, *Citrus* flavonoids also display neuroprotective effects [283,284], suggesting that they are able to cross the blood–brain barrier. One explanation for the apparent discrepancy between the poor bioavailability of flavonoids and their biological activity in humans would be to assume that a significant part of the biological actions exhibited by *Citrus* flavonoids are due to their active metabolites. Another hypothesis is the underestimation of plasma concentration and half-life due to their large volume of distribution values, to their relatively rapid post-systemic metabolization, and to the limits of assay sensitivity. In addition, to the best of our knowledge, there are few appropriately designed clinical trials to assess both pharmacological efficacy and pharmacokinetic profile of the bioactive molecules contained in CF. However, clinical studies evaluating the effectiveness of CF extracts or flavonoids mixtures in which one or more was from CF are a little more numerous. This evidence, together with the findings of other Authors [10,218,285], strengthens our thesis that given the multi-factorial pathogenesis of cancer, the complex mixture of phytochemicals present in a whole extract acts better than a single constituent. This is because all molecules present in a phytocomplex can simultaneously modulate different targets of action in both human cells and microorganisms, leading to a pool of pharmacological effects contributing together to improve the patient's health. On the bases of several preclinical and epidemiological studies summarized in this review, we believe that regular intake of CF and their derivatives, linked to a healthy life style, might be an important way to reduce cancer risk.

**Acknowledgments:** This review has been written within the framework of the "MEPRA" (PO FESR Sicilia 2007/2013, Linea d'Intervento 4.1.1.1, CUP G73F11000050004) and "ABSIB" (PSR Calabria 2007/2013 misura 124) projects to MN.

**Author Contributions:** Santa Cirmi assisted in both collecting the literature and writing the paper; Nadia Ferlazzo assisted in writing the paper; Giovanni Enrico Lombardo and Alessandro Maugeri assisted in collecting the literature; Gioacchino Calapai and Sebastiano Gangemi revised the paper. Michele Navarra conceived and designed the study, collected the literature and wrote the paper. All authors read and approved the final manuscript.

**Conflicts of Interest:** The authors declare no conflict of interests.

## References

1. International Agency for Research on Cancer (IARC). World Cancer Report 2014. Available online: http://publications.iarc.fr/Non-Series-Publications/World-Cancer-Reports/World-Cancer-Report-2014 (accessed on 5 August 2016).

2. Newman, D.J.; Cragg, G.M. Natural products as sources of new drugs over the last 25 years. *J. Nat. Prod.* **2007**, *70*, 461–477. [CrossRef] [PubMed]

3. Gerber, M. The comprehensive approach to diet: A critical review. *J. Nutr.* **2001**, *131*, 3051S–3055S. [PubMed]

4. Manson, M.M. Cancer prevention—The potential for diet to modulate molecular signalling. *Trends Mol. Med.* **2003**, *9*, 11–18. [CrossRef]

5.	Middleton, E.; Kandaswami, C.; Theoharides, T.C. The effects of plant flavonoids on mammalian cells: Implications for inflammation, heart disease, and cancer. *Pharmacol. Rev.* **2000**, *52*, 673–751. [PubMed]

6.	Tomasetti, C.; Vogelstein, B. Variation in cancer risk among tissues can be explained by the number of stem cell divisions. *Science* **2015**, *347*, 78–81. [CrossRef] [PubMed]

7.	Amin, A.R.M.R.; Kucuk, O.; Khuri, F.R.; Shin, D.M. Perspectives for cancer prevention with natural compounds. *J. Clin. Oncol.* **2009**, *27*, 2712–2725. [CrossRef] [PubMed]

8.	Gullett, N.P.; Ruhul Amin, A.R.; Bayraktar, S.; Pezzuto, J.M.; Shin, D.M.; Khuri, F.R.; Aggarwal, B.B.; Surh, Y.J.; Kucuk, O. Cancer prevention with natural compounds. *Semin. Oncol.* **2010**, *37*, 258–281. [CrossRef] [PubMed]

9.	Milner, J.A.; McDonald, S.S.; Anderson, D.E.; Greenwald, P. Molecular targets for nutrients involved with cancer prevention. *Nutr. Cancer Int. J.* **2001**, *41*, 1–16.

10.	Surh, Y.J. Cancer chemoprevention with dietary phytochemicals. *Nat. Rev. Cancer* **2003**, *3*, 768–780.

11.	Micali, S.; Isgro, G.; Bianchi, G.; Miceli, N.; Calapai, G.; Navarra, M. Cranberry and recurrent cystitis: More than marketing? *Crit. Rev. Food Sci. Nutr.* **2014**, *54*, 1063–1075.

12.	Paterniti, I.; Cordaro, M.; Campolo, M.; Siracusa, R.; Cornelius, C.; Navarra, M.; Cuzzocrea, S.; Esposito, E. Neuroprotection by association of palmitoylethanolamide with luteolin in experimental alzheimer's disease models: The control of neuroinflammation. *CNS Neurol. Disord. Drug Targets* **2014**, *13*, 1530–1541.

13.	Nogata, Y.; Sakamoto, K.; Shiratsuchi, H.; Ishii, T.; Yano, M.; Ohta, H. Flavonoid composition of fruit tissues of citrus species. *Biosci. Biotechnol. Biochem.* **2006**, *70*, 178–192.

14.	Benavente-Garcia, O.; Castillo, J. Update on uses and properties of citrus flavonoids: New findings in anticancer, cardiovascular, and anti-inflammatory activity. *J. Agric. Food Chem.* **2008**, *56*, 6185–6205.

15.	Pouget, C.; Lauthier, F.; Simon, A.; Fagnere, C.; Basly, J.P.; Delage, C.; Chulia, A.J. Flavonoids: Structural requirements for antiproliferative activity on breast cancer cells. *Bioorg. Med. Chem. Lett.* **2001**, *11*, 3095–3097.

16.	Yanez, J.; Vicente, V.; Alcaraz, M.; Castillo, J.; Benavente-Garcia, O.; Canteras, M.; Teruel, J.A.L. Cytotoxicity and antiproliferative activities of several phenolic compounds against three melanocytes cell lines: Relationship between structure and activity. *Nutr. Cancer Int. J.* **2004**, *49*, 191–199.

17.	Rodriguez, J.; Yanez, J.; Vicente, V.; Alcaraz, M.; Benavente-Garcia, O.; Castillo, J.; Lorente, J.; Lozano, J.A. Effects of several flavonoids on the growth of B16F10 and SK-MEL-1 melanoma cell lines: Relationship between structure and activity. *Melanoma Res.* **2002**, *12*, 99–107.

18.	Martinez, C.; Yanez, J.; Vicente, V.; Alcaraz, M.; Benavente-Garcia, O.; Castillo, J.; Lorente, J.; Lozano, J.A. Effects of several polyhydroxylated flavonoids on the growth of B16F10 melanoma and melan-a melanocyte cell lines: Influence of the sequential oxidation state of the flavonoid skeleton. *Melanoma Res.* **2003**, *13*, 3–9.

19.	Hursting, S.D.; Cantwell, M.M.; Sansbury, L.B.; Forman, M.R. Nutrition and cancer prevention: Targets, strategies, and the importance of early life interventions. In Proceedings of the 57th Nestlé Nutrition Workshop, Pediatric Program, Half Moon Bay, San Francisco, CA, USA, 24–28 May 2005; Lucas, A., Sampson, H.A., Eds.; Nestec Ltd.: Basel, Switzerland, 2006; pp. 153–202.

20.	Mandl, J.; Szarka, A.; Banhegyi, G. Vitamin C: Update on physiology and pharmacology. *Br. J. Pharmacol.* **2009**, *157*, 1097–1110.

21.	Williams, R.J.; Spencer, J.P.; Rice-Evans, C. Flavonoids: Antioxidants or signalling molecules? *Free Radic. Biol. Med.* **2004**, *36*, 838–849.

22.	Manthey, J.A.; Grohmann, K.; Guthrie, N. Biological properties of citrus flavonoids pertaining to cancer and inflammation. *Curr. Med. Chem.* **2001**, *8*, 135–153.

23.	Nyberg, F.; Hou, S.M.; Pershagen, G.; Lambert, B. Dietary fruit and vegetables protect against somatic mutation in vivo, but low or high intake of carotenoids does not. *Carcinogenesis* **2003**, *24*, 689–696.

24.	Calomme, M.; Pieters, L.; Vlietinck, A.; Vanden Berghe, D. Inhibition of bacterial mutagenesis by citrus flavonoids. *Planta Med.* **1996**, *62*, 222–226.

25.	Kootstra, A. Protection from UV-B-induced DNA damage by flavonoids. *Plant Mol. Biol.* **1994**, *26*, 771–774.

26.	Barcelos, G.R.; Angeli, J.P.; Serpeloni, J.M.; Grotto, D.; Rocha, B.A.; Bastos, J.K.; Knasmuller, S.; Junior, F.B. Quercetin protects human-derived liver cells against mercury-induced DNA-damage and alterations of the redox status. *Mutat. Res.* **2011**, *726*, 109–115.

27.	Gao, K.; Henning, S.M.; Niu, Y.T.; Youssefian, A.A.; Seeram, N.P.; Xu, A.L.; Heber, D. The citrus flavonoid naringenin stimulates DNA repair in prostate cancer cells. *J. Nutr. Biochem.* **2006**, *17*, 89–95.

28.	Arul, D.; Subramanian, P. Inhibitory effect of naringenin (*Citrus* flavonone) on *N*-nitrosodiethylamine induced hepatocarcinogenesis in rats. *Biochem. Biophys. Res. Commun.* **2013**, *434*, 203–209.

29. Subramanian, P.; Arul, D. Attenuation of ndea-induced hepatocarcinogenesis by naringenin in rats. *Cell Biochem. Funct.* **2013**, *31*, 511–517.

30. Alvarez-Gonzalez, I.; Madrigal-Bujaidar, E.; Dorado, V.; Espinosa-Aguirre, J.J. Inhibitory effect of naringin on the micronuclei induced by ifosfamide in mouse, and evaluation of its modulatory effect on the CYP3A subfamily. *Mutat. Res.* **2001**, *480*, 171–178.

31. Carino-Cortes, R.; Alvarez-Gonzalez, I.; Martino-Roaro, L.; Madrigal-Bujaidar, E. Effect of naringin on the DNA damage induced by daunorubicin in mouse hepatocytes and cardiocytes. *Biol. Pharm. Bull.* **2010**, *33*, 697–701.

32. Sequetto, P.L.; Oliveira, T.T.; Maldonado, I.R.; Augusto, L.E.; Mello, V.J.; Pizziolo, V.R.; Almeida, M.R.; Silva, M.E.; Novaes, R.D. Naringin accelerates the regression of pre-neoplastic lesions and the colorectal structural reorganization in a murine model of chemical carcinogenesis. *Food Chem. Toxicol.* **2014**, *64*, 200–209.

33. Ahmadi, A.; Hosseinimehr, S.J.; Naghshvar, F.; Hajir, E.; Ghahremani, M. Chemoprotective effects of hesperidin against genotoxicity induced by cyclophosphamide in mice bone marrow cells. *Arch. Pharm. Res.* **2008**, *31*, 794–797.

34. Choi, J.S.; Park, K.Y.; Moon, S.H.; Rhee, S.H.; Young, H.S. Antimutagenic effect of plant flavonoids in the salmonella assay system. *Arch. Pharm. Res.* **1994**, *17*, 71–75.

35. Kao, Y.C.; Zhou, C.; Sherman, M.; Laughton, C.A.; Chen, S. Molecular basis of the inhibition of human aromatase (estrogen synthetase) by flavone and isoflavone phytoestrogens: A site-directed mutagenesis study. *Environ. Health Perspect.* **1998**, *106*, 85–92.

36. Harris, R.M.; Wood, D.M.; Bottomley, L.; Blagg, S.; Owen, K.; Hughes, P.J.; Waring, R.H.; Kirk, C.J. Phytoestrogens are potent inhibitors of estrogen sulfation: Implications for breast cancer risk and treatment. *J. Clin. Endocrinol. Metab.* **2004**, *89*, 1779–1787.

37. Bear, W.L.; Teel, R.W. Effects of *Citrus* flavonoids on the mutagenicity of heterocyclic amines and on cytochrome P450 1A2 activity. *Anticancer Res.* **2000**, *20*, 3609–3614.

38. Van Dross, R.; Xue, Y.; Knudson, A.; Pelling, J.C. The chemopreventive bioflavonoid apigenin modulates signal transduction pathways in keratinocyte and colon carcinoma cell lines. *J. Nutr.* **2003**, *133*, 3800S–3804S.

39. Khan, T.H.; Jahangir, T.; Prasad, L.; Sultana, S. Inhibitory effect of apigenin on benzo(a)pyrene-mediated genotoxicity in swiss albino mice. *J. Pharm. Pharmacol.* **2006**, *58*, 1655–1660.

40. Myhrstad, M.C.; Carlsen, H.; Nordstrom, O.; Blomhoff, R.; Moskaug, J.O. Flavonoids increase the intracellular glutathione level by transactivation of the gamma-glutamylcysteine synthetase catalytical subunit promoter. *Free Radic. Biol. Med.* **2002**, *32*, 386–393.

41. Wei, H.; Tye, L.; Bresnick, E.; Birt, D.F. Inhibitory effect of apigenin, a plant flavonoid, on epidermal ornithine decarboxylase and skin tumor promotion in mice. *Cancer Res.* **1990**, *50*, 499–502.

42. Birt, D.F.; Mitchell, D.; Gold, B.; Pour, P.; Pinch, H.C. Inhibition of ultraviolet light induced skin carcinogenesis in SKH-1 mice by apigenin, a plant flavonoid. *Anticancer Res.* **1997**, *17*, 85–91.

43. Leonardi, T.; Vanamala, J.; Taddeo, S.S.; Davidson, L.A.; Murphy, M.E.; Patil, B.S.; Wang, N.; Carroll, R.J.; Chapkin, R.S.; Lupton, J.R.; et al. Apigenin and naringenin suppress colon carcinogenesis through the aberrant crypt stage in azoxymethane-treated rats. *Exp. Biol. Med. (Maywood)* **2010**, *235*, 710–717.

44. Nandakumar, N.; Balasubramanian, M.P. Hesperidin protects renal and hepatic tissues against free radical-mediated oxidative stress during DMBA-induced experimental breast cancer. *J. Environ. Pathol. Toxicol. Oncol.* **2011**, *30*, 283–300.

45. Aranganathan, S.; Selvam, J.P.; Sangeetha, N.; Nalini, N. Modulatory efficacy of hesperetin (*Citrus* flavanone) on xenobiotic-metabolizing enzymes during 1,2-dimethylhydrazine-induced colon carcinogenesis. *Chem. Biol. Interact.* **2009**, *180*, 254–261.

46. Lakshmi, A.; Subramanian, S. Chemotherapeutic effect of tangeretin, a polymethoxylated flavone studied in 7,12-dimethylbenz(a)anthracene induced mammary carcinoma in experimental rats. *Biochimie* **2014**, *99*, 96–109.

47. Murakami, A.; Nakamura, Y.; Torikai, K.; Tanaka, T.; Koshiba, T.; Koshimizu, K.; Kuwahara, S.; Takahashi, Y.; Ogawa, K.; Yano, M.; et al. Inhibitory effect of *Citrus* nobiletin on phorbol ester-induced skin inflammation, oxidative stress, and tumor promotion in mice. *Cancer Res.* **2000**, *60*, 5059–5066.

48. Kandaswami, C.; Perkins, E.; Soloniuk, D.S.; Drzewiecki, G.; Middleton, E., Jr. Antiproliferative effects of citrus flavonoids on a human squamous cell carcinoma in vitro. *Cancer Lett.* **1991**, *56*, 147–152.

49. Sugiyama, S.; Umehara, K.; Kuroyanagi, M.; Ueno, A.; Taki, T. Studies on the differentiation inducers of myeloid leukemic cells from *Citrus* species. *Chem. Pharm. Bull. (Tokyo)* **1993**, *41*, 714–719.

50. Hirano, T.; Abe, K.; Gotoh, M.; Oka, K. Citrus flavone tangeretin inhibits leukaemic HL-60 cell growth partially through induction of apoptosis with less cytotoxicity on normal lymphocytes. *Br. J. Cancer* **1995**, *72*, 1380–1388.

51. Morley, K.L.; Ferguson, P.J.; Koropatnick, J. Tangeretin and nobiletin induce G1 cell cycle arrest but not apoptosis in human breast and colon cancer cells. *Cancer Lett.* **2007**, *251*, 168–178.

52. Pan, M.H.; Chen, W.J.; Lin-Shiau, S.Y.; Ho, C.T.; Lin, J.K. Tangeretin induces cell-cycle G1 arrest through inhibiting cyclin-dependent kinases 2 and 4 activities as well as elevating cdk inhibitors p21 and p27 in human colorectal carcinoma cells. *Carcinogenesis* **2002**, *23*, 1677–1684.

53. Yoshimizu, N.; Otani, Y.; Saikawa, Y.; Kubota, T.; Yoshida, M.; Furukawa, T.; Kumai, K.; Kameyama, K.; Fujii, M.; Yano, M.; et al. Anti-tumour effects of nobiletin, a *Citrus* flavonoid, on gastric cancer include: Antiproliferative effects, induction of apoptosis and cell cycle deregulation. *Aliment. Pharmacol. Ther.* **2004**, *20* (Suppl. 1), 95–101.

54. Fan, K.; Kurihara, N.; Abe, S.; Ho, C.T.; Ghai, G.; Yang, K. Chemopreventive effects of orange peel extract (OPE) I: Ope inhibits intestinal tumor growth in Apc$^{(min/+)}$ mice. *J. Med. Food* **2007**, *10*, 11–17.

55. Abe, S.; Fan, K.; Ho, C.T.; Ghai, G.; Yang, K. Chemopreventive effects of orange peel extract (OPE) II: OPE inhibits atypical hyperplastic lesions in rodent mammary gland. *J. Med. Food* **2007**, *10*, 18–24.

56. Van Slambrouck, S.; Parmar, V.S.; Sharma, S.K.; de Bondt, B.; Fore, F.; Coopman, P.; Vanhoecke, B.W.; Boterberg, T.; Depypere, H.T.; Leclercq, G.; et al. Tangeretin inhibits extracellular-signal-regulated kinase (ERK) phosphorylation. *FEBS Lett.* **2005**, *579*, 1665–1669.

57. Akao, Y.; Itoh, T.; Ohguchi, K.; Iinuma, M.; Nozawa, Y. Interactive effects of polymethoxy flavones from *Citrus* on cell growth inhibition in human neuroblastoma SH-SY5Y cells. *Bioorg. Med. Chem.* **2008**, *16*, 2803–2810.

58. Rooprai, H.K.; Kandanearatchi, A.; Maidment, S.L.; Christidou, M.; Trillo-Pazos, G.; Dexter, D.T.; Rucklidge, G.J.; Widmer, W.; Pilkington, G.J. Evaluation of the effects of swainsonine, captopril, tangeretin and nobiletin on the biological behaviour of brain tumour cells in vitro. *Neuropathol. Appl. Neurobiol.* **2001**, *27*, 29–39.

59. Arafa el, S.A.; Zhu, Q.; Barakat, B.M.; Wani, G.; Zhao, Q.; El-Mahdy, M.A.; Wani, A.A. Tangeretin sensitizes cisplatin-resistant human ovarian cancer cells through downregulation of phosphoinositide 3-kinase/Akt signaling pathway. *Cancer Res.* **2009**, *69*, 8910–8917.

60. Dong, Y.; Cao, A.L.; Shi, J.R.; Yin, P.H.; Wang, L.; Ji, G.; Xie, J.Q.; Wu, D.Z. Tangeretin, a citrus polymethoxyflavonoid, induces apoptosis of human gastric cancer AGS cells through extrinsic and intrinsic signaling pathways. *Oncol. Rep.* **2014**, *31*, 1788–1794.

61. Tang, M.; Ogawa, K.; Asamoto, M.; Hokaiwado, N.; Seeni, A.; Suzuki, S.; Takahashi, S.; Tanaka, T.; Ichikawa, K.; Shirai, T. Protective effects of *Citrus* nobiletin and auraptene in transgenic rats developing adenocarcinoma of the prostate (TRAP) and human prostate carcinoma cells. *Cancer Sci.* **2007**, *98*, 471–477.

62. Tang, M.X.; Ogawa, K.; Asamoto, M.; Chewonarin, T.; Suzuki, S.; Tanaka, T.; Shirai, T. Effects of nobiletin on PhIP-induced prostate and colon carcinogenesis in F344 rats. *Nutr. Cancer* **2011**, *63*, 227–233.

63. Suzuki, R.; Kohno, H.; Murakami, A.; Koshimizu, K.; Ohigashi, H.; Yano, M.; Tokuda, H.; Nishino, H.; Tanaka, T. *Citrus* nobiletin inhibits azoxymethane-induced large bowel carcinogenesis in rats. *Biofactors* **2004**, *22*, 111–114.

64. Miyamoto, S.; Yasui, Y.; Ohigashi, H.; Tanaka, T.; Murakami, A. Dietary flavonoids suppress azoxymethane-induced colonic preneoplastic lesions in male C57BL/KSJ-DB/DB mice. *Chem. Biol. Interact.* **2010**, *183*, 276–283.

65. Miyamoto, S.; Yasui, Y.; Tanaka, T.; Ohigashi, H.; Murakami, A. Suppressive effects of nobiletin on hyperleptinemia and colitis-related colon carcinogenesis in male ICR mice. *Carcinogenesis* **2008**, *29*, 1057–1063.

66. Luo, G.; Guan, X.; Zhou, L. Apoptotic effect of *Citrus* fruit extract nobiletin on lung cancer cell line a549 in vitro and in vivo. *Cancer Biol. Ther.* **2008**, *7*, 966–973.

67. Ohnishi, H.; Asamoto, M.; Tujimura, K.; Hokaiwado, N.; Takahashi, S.; Ogawa, K.; Kuribayashi, M.; Ogiso, T.; Okuyama, H.; Shirai, T. Inhibition of cell proliferation by nobiletin, a dietary phytochemical, associated with apoptosis and characteristic gene expression, but lack of effect on early rat hepatocarcinogenesis in vivo. *Cancer Sci.* **2004**, *95*, 936–942.

68. Aoki, K.; Yokosuka, A.; Mimaki, Y.; Fukunaga, K.; Yamakuni, T. Nobiletin induces inhibitions of RAS activity and mitogen-activated protein kinase kinase/extracellular signal-regulated kinase signaling to suppress cell proliferation in C6 rat glioma cells. *Biol. Pharm. Bull.* **2013**, *36*, 540–547.

69. Lien, L.M.; Wang, M.J.; Chen, R.J.; Chiu, H.C.; Wu, J.L.; Shen, M.Y.; Chou, D.S.; Sheu, J.R.; Lin, K.H.; Lu, W.J. Nobiletin, a polymethoxylated flavone, inhibits glioma cell growth and migration via arresting cell cycle and suppressing MAPK and Akt pathways. *Phytother. Res.* **2016**, *30*, 214–221.

70. Moon, J.Y.; Cho, M.; Ahn, K.S.; Cho, S.K. Nobiletin induces apoptosis and potentiates the effects of the anticancer drug 5-fluorouracil in p53-mutated SNU-16 human gastric cancer cells. *Nutr. Cancer Int. J.* **2013**, *65*, 286–295.

71. Hsiao, P.C.; Lee, W.J.; Yang, S.F.; Tan, P.; Chen, H.Y.; Lee, L.M.; Chang, J.L.; Lai, G.M.; Chow, J.M.; Chien, M.H. Nobiletin suppresses the proliferation and induces apoptosis involving MAPKs and caspase-8/-9/-3 signals in human acute myeloid leukemia cells. *Tumor Biol.* **2014**, *35*, 11903–11911.

72. Wu, X.; Song, M.Y.; Wang, M.Q.; Zheng, J.K.; Gao, Z.L.; Xu, F.; Zhang, G.D.; Xiao, H. Chemopreventive effects of nobiletin and its colonic metabolites on colon carcinogenesis. *Mol. Nutr. Food Res.* **2015**, *59*, 2383–2394.

73. Choi, E.J.; Kim, G.H. Apigenin induces apoptosis through a mitochondria/caspase-pathway in human breast cancer MDA-MB-453 cells. *J. Clin. Biochem. Nutr.* **2009**, *44*, 260–265.

74. Seo, H.S.; Choi, H.S.; Kim, S.R.; Choi, Y.K.; Woo, S.M.; Shin, I.; Woo, J.K.; Park, S.Y.; Shin, Y.C.; Ko, S.K. Apigenin induces apoptosis via extrinsic pathway, inducing p53 and inhibiting STAT3 and NFκB signaling in HER2-overexpressing breast cancer cells. *Mol. Cell. Biochem.* **2012**, *366*, 319–334.

75. Way, T.D.; Kao, M.C.; Lin, J.K. Apigenin induces apoptosis through proteasomal degradation of HER2/NEU in HER2/NEU-overexpressing breast cancer cells via the phosphatidylinositol 3-kinase/Akt-dependent pathway. *J. Biol. Chem.* **2004**, *279*, 4479–4489.

76. Agrawal, A.; Yang, J.; Murphy, R.F.; Agrawal, D.K. Regulation of the p14ARF-MDM2-p53 pathway: An overview in breast cancer. *Exp. Mol. Pathol.* **2006**, *81*, 115–122.

77. Takagaki, N.; Sowa, Y.; Oki, T.; Nakanishi, R.; Yogosawa, S.; Sakai, T. Apigenin induces cell cycle arrest and p21/WAF1 expression in a p53-independent pathway. *Int. J. Oncol.* **2005**, *26*, 185–189.

78. Lepley, D.M.; Pelling, J.C. Induction of p21/WAF1 and G1 cell-cycle arrest by the chemopreventive agent apigenin. *Mol. Carcinog.* **1997**, *19*, 74–82.

79. Plaumann, B.; Fritsche, M.; Rimpler, H.; Brandner, G.; Hess, R.D. Flavonoids activate wild-type p53. *Oncogene* **1996**, *13*, 1605–1614.

80. Yin, F.; Giuliano, A.E.; Law, R.E.; Van Herle, A.J. Apigenin inhibits growth and induces G2/M arrest by modulating cyclin-CDK regulators and ERK MAP Kinase activation in breast carcinoma cells. *Anticancer Res.* **2001**, *21*, 413–420.

81. King, J.C.; Lu, Q.Y.; Li, G.; Moro, A.; Takahashi, H.; Chen, M.; Go, V.L.; Reber, H.A.; Eibl, G.; Hines, O.J. Evidence for activation of mutated p53 by apigenin in human pancreatic cancer. *Biochim. Biophys. Acta* **2012**, *1823*, 593–604.

82. Ujiki, M.B.; Ding, X.Z.; Salabat, M.R.; Bentrem, D.J.; Golkar, L.; Milam, B.; Talamonti, M.S.; Bell, R.H., Jr.; Iwamura, T.; Adrian, T.E. Apigenin inhibits pancreatic cancer cell proliferation through G2/M cell cycle arrest. *Mol. Cancer* **2006**, *5*, 76. [CrossRef]

83. Johnson, J.L.; de Mejia, E.G. Flavonoid apigenin modified gene expression associated with inflammation and cancer and induced apoptosis in human pancreatic cancer cells through inhibition of GSK-3 beta/NFκB signaling cascade. *Mol. Nutr. Food Res.* **2013**, *57*, 2112–2127.

84. Gupta, S.; Afaq, F.; Mukhtar, H. Involvement of nuclear factor-kappa B, BAX and BCL-2 in induction of cell cycle arrest and apoptosis by apigenin in human prostate carcinoma cells. *Oncogene* **2002**, *21*, 3727–3738.

85. Shukla, S.; Gupta, S. Molecular mechanisms for apigenin-induced cell-cycle arrest and apoptosis of hormone refractory human prostate carcinoma DU145 cells. *Mol. Carcinog.* **2004**, *39*, 114–126.

86. Wang, W.; Heideman, L.; Chung, C.S.; Pelling, J.C.; Koehler, K.J.; Birt, D.F. Cell-cycle arrest at G2/M and growth inhibition by apigenin in human colon carcinoma cell lines. *Mol. Carcinog.* **2000**, *28*, 102–110.

87. Zhong, Y.; Krisanapun, C.; Lee, S.H.; Nualsanit, T.; Sams, C.; Peungvicha, P.; Baek, S.J. Molecular targets of apigenin in colorectal cancer cells: Involvement of p21, NAG-1 and p53. *Eur. J. Cancer* **2010**, *46*, 3365–3374.

88. Shukla, S.; Gupta, S. Molecular targets for apigenin-induced cell cycle arrest and apoptosis in prostate cancer cell xenograft. *Mol. Cancer Ther.* **2006**, *5*, 843–852.

89.  Das, A.; Banik, N.L.; Ray, S.K. Mechanism of apoptosis with the involvement of calpain and caspase cascades in human malignant neuroblastoma SH-SY5Y cells exposed to flavonoids. *Int. J. Cancer* **2006**, *119*, 2575–2585.
90.  Torkin, R.; Lavoie, J.F.; Kaplan, D.R.; Yeger, H. Induction of caspase-dependent, p53-mediated apoptosis by apigenin in human neuroblastoma. *Mol. Cancer Ther.* **2005**, *4*, 1–11.
91.  Hanahan, D.; Weinberg, R.A. Hallmarks of cancer: The next generation. *Cell* **2011**, *144*, 646–674.
92.  Kuntz, S.; Wenzel, U.; Daniel, H. Comparative analysis of the effects of flavonoids on proliferation, cytotoxicity, and apoptosis in human colon cancer cell lines. *Eur. J. Nutr.* **1999**, *38*, 133–142.
93.  Dung, T.D.; Day, C.H.; Binh, T.V.; Lin, C.H.; Hsu, H.H.; Su, C.C.; Lin, Y.M.; Tsai, F.J.; Kuo, W.W.; Chen, L.M.; et al. PP2A mediates diosmin p53 activation to block HA22T cell proliferation and tumor growth in xenografted nude mice through PI3K-Akt-MDM2 signaling suppression. *Food Chem. Toxicol.* **2012**, *50*, 1802–1810.
94.  Lewinska, A.; Siwak, J.; Rzeszutek, I.; Wnuk, M. Diosmin induces genotoxicity and apoptosis in DU145 prostate cancer cell line. *Toxicol. Vitr.* **2015**, *29*, 417–425.
95.  Tanaka, T.; Makita, H.; Kawabata, K.; Mori, H.; Kakumoto, M.; Satoh, K.; Hara, A.; Sumida, T.; Fukutani, K.; Tanaka, T.; et al. Modulation of *N*-methyl-*N*-amylnitrosamine-induced rat oesophageal tumourigenesis by dietary feeding of diosmin and hesperidin, both alone and in combination. *Carcinogenesis* **1997**, *18*, 761–769.
96.  Tanaka, T.; Makita, H.; Ohnishi, M.; Mori, H.; Satoh, K.; Hara, A.; Sumida, T.; Fukutani, K.; Tanaka, T.; Ogawa, H. Chemoprevention of 4-nitroquinoline 1-oxide-induced oral carcinogenesis in rats by flavonoids diosmin and hesperidin, each alone and in combination. *Cancer Res.* **1997**, *57*, 246–252.
97.  Yang, M.; Tanaka, T.; Hirose, Y.; Deguchi, T.; Mori, H.; Kawada, Y. Chemopreventive effects of diosmin and hesperidin on *N*-butyl-*N*-(4-hydroxybutyl)nitrosamine-induced urinary-bladder carcinogenesis in male ICR mice. *Int. J. Cancer* **1997**, *73*, 719–724.
98.  Tanaka, T.; Makita, H.; Kawabata, K.; Mori, H.; Kakumoto, M.; Satoh, K.; Hara, A.; Sumida, T.; Tanaka, T.; Ogawa, H. Chemoprevention of azoxymethane-induced rat colon carcinogenesis by the naturally occurring flavonoids, diosmin and hesperidin. *Carcinogenesis* **1997**, *18*, 957–965.
99.  Rubio, S.; Quintana, J.; Lopez, M.; Eiroa, J.L.; Triana, J.; Estevez, F. Phenylbenzopyrones structure-activity studies identify betuletol derivatives as potential antitumoral agents. *Eur. J. Pharmacol.* **2006**, *548*, 9–20.
100. Duraj, J.; Zazrivcova, K.; Bodo, J.; Sulikova, M.; Sedlak, J. Flavonoid quercetin, but not apigenin or luteolin, induced apoptosis in human myeloid leukemia cells and their resistant variants. *Neoplasma* **2005**, *52*, 273–279.
101. Piantelli, M.; Rinelli, A.; Macri, E.; Maggiano, N.; Larocca, L.M.; Scerrati, M.; Roselli, R.; Iacoangeli, M.; Scambia, G.; Capelli, A.; et al. Type II estrogen binding sites and antiproliferative activity of quercetin in human meningiomas. *Cancer* **1993**, *71*, 193–198.
102. Kuo, S.M. Antiproliferative potency of structurally distinct dietary flavonoids on human colon cancer cells. *Cancer Lett.* **1996**, *110*, 41–48.
103. Araujo, J.R.; Goncalves, P.; Martel, F. Chemopreventive effect of dietary polyphenols in colorectal cancer cell lines. *Nutr. Res.* **2011**, *31*, 77–87.
104. Paliwal, S.; Sundaram, J.; Mitragotri, S. Induction of cancer-specific cytotoxicity towards human prostate and skin cells using quercetin and ultrasound. *Br. J. Cancer* **2005**, *92*, 499–502.
105. Huang, H.C.; Lin, C.L.; Lin, J.K. 1,2,3,4,6-penta-*O*-galloyl-beta-D-glucose, quercetin, curcumin and lycopene induce cell-cycle arrest in MDA-MB-231 and BT474 cells through downregulation of SKP2 protein. *J. Agric. Food Chem.* **2011**, *59*, 6765–6775.
106. Li, J.; Zhu, F.; Lubet, R.A.; De Luca, A.; Grubbs, C.; Ericson, M.E.; D'Alessio, A.; Normanno, N.; Dong, Z.; Bode, A.M. Quercetin-3-methyl ether inhibits lapatinib-sensitive and -resistant breast cancer cell growth by inducing G(2)/M arrest and apoptosis. *Mol. Carcinog.* **2011**, *52*, 134–143.
107. Staedler, D.; Idrizi, E.; Kenzaoui, B.H.; Juillerat-Jeanneret, L. Drug combinations with quercetin: Doxorubicin plus quercetin in human breast cancer cells. *Cancer Chemother. Pharmacol.* **2011**, *68*, 1161–1172.
108. Scambia, G.; Ranelletti, F.O.; Panici, P.B.; De Vincenzo, R.; Bonanno, G.; Ferrandina, G.; Piantelli, M.; Bussa, S.; Rumi, C.; Cianfriglia, M.; et al. Quercetin potentiates the effect of adriamycin in a multidrug-resistant MCF-7 human breast-cancer cell line: P-glycoprotein as a possible target. *Cancer Chemother. Pharmacol.* **1994**, *34*, 459–464.
109. Critchfield, J.W.; Welsh, C.J.; Phang, J.M.; Yeh, G.C. Modulation of adriamycin accumulation and efflux by flavonoids in HCT-15 colon cells. Activation of p-glycoprotein as a putative mechanism. *Biochem. Pharmacol.* **1994**, *48*, 1437–1445.

110. Kanno, S.; Tomizawa, A.; Hiura, T.; Osanai, Y.; Shouji, A.; Ujibe, M.; Ohtake, T.; Kimura, K.; Ishikawa, M. Inhibitory effects of naringenin on tumor growth in human cancer cell lines and sarcoma S-180-implanted mice. *Biol. Pharm. Bull.* **2005**, *28*, 527–530.

111. Kanno, S.; Tomizawa, A.; Ohtake, T.; Koiwai, K.; Ujibe, M.; Ishikawa, M. Naringenin-induced apoptosis via activation of NF-κB and necrosis involving the loss of ATP in human promyeloleukemia HL-60 cells. *Toxicol. Lett.* **2006**, *166*, 131–139.

112. Frydoonfar, H.R.; McGrath, D.R.; Spigelman, A.D. The variable effect on proliferation of a colon cancer cell line by the *Citrus* fruit flavonoid naringenin. *Colorectal Dis.* **2003**, *5*, 149–152.

113. Harmon, A.W.; Patel, Y.M. Naringenin inhibits glucose uptake in MCF-7 breast cancer cells: A mechanism for impaired cellular proliferation. *Breast Cancer Res. Treat.* **2004**, *85*, 103–110.

114. Park, J.H.; Jin, C.Y.; Lee, B.K.; Kim, G.Y.; Choi, Y.H.; Jeong, Y.K. Naringenin induces apoptosis through downregulation of AKT and caspase-3 activation in human leukemia THP-1 cells. *Food Chem. Toxicol.* **2008**, *46*, 3684–3690.

115. Shi, D.; Xu, Y.; Du, X.; Chen, X.; Zhang, X.; Lou, J.; Li, M.; Zhuo, J. Co-treatment of THP-1 cells with naringenin and curcumin induces cell cycle arrest and apoptosis via numerous pathways. *Mol. Med. Rep.* **2015**, *12*, 8223–8228.

116. Ahamad, M.S.; Siddiqui, S.; Jafri, A.; Ahmad, S.; Afzal, M.; Arshad, M. Induction of apoptosis and antiproliferative activity of naringenin in human epidermoid carcinoma cell through ROS generation and cell cycle arrest. *PLoS ONE* **2014**, *9*, e110003.

117. Naoghare, P.K.; Ki, H.A.; Paek, S.M.; Tak, Y.K.; Suh, Y.G.; Kim, S.G.; Lee, I.C.H.; Dong, J.M. Simultaneous quantitative monitoring of drug-induced caspase cascade pathways in carcinoma cells. *Integr. Biol.* **2010**, *2*, 46–57.

118. Jin, C.Y.; Park, C.; Hwang, H.J.; Kim, G.Y.; Choi, B.T.; Kim, W.J.; Choi, Y.H. Naringenin up-regulates the expression of death receptor 5 and enhances TRAIL-induced apoptosis in human lung cancer A549 cells. *Mol. Nutr. Food Res.* **2011**, *55*, 300–309.

119. Zhang, S.Z.; Yang, X.N.; Morris, M.E. Flavonoids are inhibitors of breast cancer resistance protein (ABCG2)-mediated transport. *Mol. Pharmacol.* **2004**, *65*, 1208–1216.

120. Zhang, S.Z.; Yang, X.N.; Coburn, R.A.; Morris, M.E. Structure activity relationships and quantitative structure activity relationships for the flavonoid-mediated inhibition of breast cancer resistance protein. *Biochem. Pharmacol.* **2005**, *70*, 627–639.

121. Romiti, N.; Tramonti, G.; Donati, A.; Chieli, E. Effects of grapefruit juice on the multidrug transporter p-glycoprotein in the human proximal tubular cell line HK-2. *Life Sci.* **2004**, *76*, 293–302.

122. Tsai, T.H.; Lee, C.H.; Yeh, P.H. Effect of p-glycoprotein modulators on the pharmacokinetics of camptothecin using microdialysis. *Br. J. Pharmacol.* **2001**, *134*, 1245–1252.

123. De Castro, W.V.; Mertens-Talcott, S.; Derendorf, H.; Butterweck, V. Effect of grapefruit juice, naringin, naringenin, and bergamottin on the intestinal carrier-mediated transport of talinolol in rats. *J. Agric. Food Chem.* **2008**, *56*, 4840–4845.

124. Zhang, F.Y.; Du, G.J.; Zhang, L.; Zhang, C.L.; Lu, W.L.; Liang, W. Naringenin enhances the anti-tumor effect of doxorubicin through selectively inhibiting the activity of multidrug resistance-associated proteins but not p-glycoprotein. *Pharm. Res.* **2009**, *26*, 914–925.

125. Park, H.S.; Oh, J.H.; Lee, J.H.; Lee, Y.J. Minor effects of the citrus flavonoids naringin, naringenin and quercetin, on the pharmacokinetics of doxorubicin in rats. *Pharmazie* **2011**, *66*, 424–429.

126. Ekambaram, G.; Rajendran, P.; Magesh, V.; Sakthisekaran, D. Naringenin reduces tumor size and weight lost in *N*-methyl-*N'*-nitro-*N*-nitrosoguanidine-induced gastric carcinogenesis in rats. *Nutr. Res.* **2008**, *28*, 106–112.

127. Ganapathy, E.; Peramaiyan, R.; Rajasekaran, D.; Venkataraman, M.; Dhanapal, S. Modulatory effect of naringenin on *N*-methyl-*N'*-nitro-*N*-nitrosoguanidine-and saturated sodium chloride-induced gastric carcinogenesis in male wistar rats. *Clin. Exp. Pharmacol. Physiol.* **2008**, *35*, 1190–1196.

128. Sabarinathan, D.; Mahalakshmi, P.; Vanisree, A.J. Naringenin promote apoptosis in cerebrally implanted C6 glioma cells. *Mol. Cell. Biochem.* **2010**, *345*, 215–222.

129. Miller, E.G.; Peacock, J.J.; Bourland, T.C.; Taylor, S.E.; Wright, J.A.; Patil, B.S.; Miller, E.G. Inhibition of oral carcinogenesis by *Citrus* flavonoids. *Nutr. Cancer Int. J.* **2008**, *60*, 69–74.

130. Ramesh, E.; Alshatwi, A.A. Naringin induces death receptor and mitochondria-mediated apoptosis in human cervical cancer (SiHa) cells. *Food Chem. Toxicol.* **2013**, *51*, 97–105.

131. Zeng, L.; Zhen, Y.; Chen, Y.; Zou, L.; Zhang, Y.; Hu, F.; Feng, J.; Shen, J.; Wei, B. Naringin inhibits growth and induces apoptosis by a mechanism dependent on reduced activation of NFκB/COX2caspase-1 pathway in HeLa cervical cancer cells. *Int. J. Oncol.* **2014**, *45*, 1929–1936.

132. Yoshinaga, A.; Kajiya, N.; Oishi, K.; Kamada, Y.; Ikeda, A.; Chigwechokha, P.K.; Kibe, T.; Kishida, M.; Kishida, S.; Komatsu, M.; et al. Neu3 inhibitory effect of naringin suppresses cancer cell growth by attenuation of EGFR signaling through GM3 ganglioside accumulation. *Eur. J. Pharmacol.* **2016**, *782*, 21–29.

133. Li, H.; Yang, B.; Huang, J.; Xiang, T.; Yin, X.; Wan, J.; Luo, F.; Zhang, L.; Li, H.; Ren, G. Naringin inhibits growth potential of human triple-negative breast cancer cells by targeting beta-catenin signaling pathway. *Toxicol. Lett.* **2013**, *220*, 219–228.

134. Kim, D.I.; Lee, S.J.; Lee, S.B.; Park, K.; Kim, W.J.; Moon, S.K. Requirement for RAS/RAF/ERK pathway in naringin-induced G(1)-cell-cycle arrest via p21WAF1 expression. *Carcinogenesis* **2008**, *29*, 1701–1709.

135. Xie, C.M.; Chan, W.Y.; Yu, S.; Zhao, J.; Cheng, C.H. Bufalin induces autophagy-mediated cell death in human colon cancer cells through reactive oxygen species generation and JNK activation. *Free Radic. Biol. Med.* **2011**, *51*, 1365–1375.

136. Chen, Y.J.; Chi, C.W.; Su, W.C.; Huang, H.L. Lapatinib induces autophagic cell death and inhibits growth of human hepatocellular carcinoma. *Oncotarget* **2014**, *5*, 4845–4854.

137. Raha, S.; Yumnam, S.; Hong, G.E.; Lee, H.J.; Saralamma, V.V.; Park, H.S.; Heo, J.D.; Lee, S.J.; Kim, E.H.; Kim, J.A.; et al. Naringin induces autophagy-mediated growth inhibition by downregulating the PI3K/AKT/MTOR cascade via activation of MAPK pathways in AGS cancer cells. *Int. J. Oncol.* **2015**, *47*, 1061–1069.

138. Li, J.; Dong, Y.; Hao, G.; Wang, B.; Wang, J.; Liang, Y.; Liu, Y.; Zhen, E.; Feng, D.; Liang, G. Naringin suppresses the development of glioblastoma by inhibiting FAK activity. *J. Drug Target.* **2016**. [CrossRef]

139. Vanamala, J.; Leonardi, T.; Patil, B.S.; Taddeo, S.S.; Murphy, M.E.; Pike, L.M.; Chapkin, R.S.; Lupton, J.R.; Turner, N.D. Suppression of colon carcinogenesis by bioactive compounds in grapefruit. *Carcinogenesis* **2006**, *27*, 1257–1265.

140. Camargo, C.A.; Gomes-Marcondes, M.C.C.; Wutzki, N.C.; Aoyama, H. Naringin inhibits tumor growth and reduces interleukin-6 and tumor necrosis factor alpha levels in rats with Walker 256 carcinosarcoma. *Anticancer Res.* **2012**, *32*, 129–133.

141. Zhang, Y.S.; Li, Y.; Wang, Y.; Sun, S.Y.; Jiang, T.; Li, C.; Cui, S.X.; Qu, X.J. Naringin, a natural dietary compound, prevents intestinal tumorigenesis in Apc$^{(min/+)}$ mouse model. *J. Cancer Res. Clin. Oncol.* **2016**, *142*, 913–925.

142. Garg, A.; Garg, S.; Zaneveld, L.J.; Singla, A.K. Chemistry and pharmacology of the *Citrus* bioflavonoid hesperidin. *Phytother. Res.* **2001**, *15*, 655–669.

143. Chen, Y.C.; Shen, S.C.; Lin, H.Y. Rutinoside at C7 attenuates the apoptosis-inducing activity of flavonoids. *Biochem. Pharmacol.* **2003**, *66*, 1139–1150.

144. Choi, E.J. Hesperetin induced G1-phase cell cycle arrest in human breast cancer MCF-7 cells: Involvement of CDK4 and p21. *Nutr. Cancer Int. J.* **2007**, *59*, 115–119.

145. Sivagami, G.; Vinothkumar, R.; Preethy, C.P.; Riyasdeen, A.; Akbarsha, M.A.; Menon, V.P.; Nalini, N. Role of hesperetin (a natural flavonoid) and its analogue on apoptosis in HT-29 human colon adenocarcinoma cell line—A comparative study. *Food Chem. Toxicol.* **2012**, *50*, 660–671.

146. Zarebczan, B.; Pinchot, S.N.; Kunnimalaiyaan, M.; Chen, H. Hesperetin, a potential therapy for carcinoid cancer. *Am. J. Surg.* **2011**, *201*, 329–333.

147. Alshatwi, A.A.; Ramesh, E.; Periasamy, V.S.; Subash-Babu, P. The apoptotic effect of hesperetin on human cervical cancer cells is mediated through cell cycle arrest, death receptor, and mitochondrial pathways. *Fundam. Clin. Pharmacol.* **2013**, *27*, 581–592.

148. Zhang, J.; Song, J.; Wu, D.; Wang, J.; Dong, W. Hesperetin induces the apoptosis of hepatocellular carcinoma cells via mitochondrial pathway mediated by the increased intracellular reactive oxygen species, ATP and calcium. *Med. Oncol.* **2015**, *32*, 101. [CrossRef]

149. Aranganathan, S.; Nalini, N. Antiproliferative efficacy of hesperetin (*Citrus* flavonoid) in 1,2-dimethylhydrazine-induced colon cancer. *Phytother. Res.* **2013**, *27*, 999–1005.

150. Nalini, N.; Aranganathan, S.; Kabalimurthy, J. Chemopreventive efficacy of hesperetin (*Citrus* flavonone) against 1,2-dimethylhydrazine-induced rat colon carcinogenesis. *Toxicol. Mech. Methods* **2012**, *22*, 397–408.

151. Patil, J.R.; Murthy, K.N.C.; Jayaprakasha, G.K.; Chetti, M.B.; Patil, B.S. Bioactive compounds from mexican lime (*Citrus aurantifolia*) juice induce apoptosis in human pancreatic cells. *J. Agric. Food Chem.* **2009**, *57*, 10933–10942.

152. Park, H.J.; Kim, M.J.; Ha, E.; Chung, J.H. Apoptotic effect of hesperidin through caspase3 activation in human colon cancer cells, SNU-C4. *Phytomedicine* **2008**, *15*, 147–151.

153. Banjerdpongchai, R.; Wudtiwai, B.; Khaw-On, P.; Rachakhom, W.; Duangnil, N.; Kongtawelert, P. Hesperidin from *Citrus* seed induces human hepatocellular carcinoma HepG2 cell apoptosis via both mitochondrial and death receptor pathways. *Tumour Biol.* **2016**, *37*, 227–237.

154. Yumnam, S.; Park, H.S.; Kim, M.K.; Nagappan, A.; Hong, G.E.; Lee, H.J.; Lee, W.S.; Kim, E.H.; Cho, J.H.; Shin, S.C.; et al. Hesperidin induces paraptosis like cell death in hepatoblastoma, hepg2 cells: Involvement of ERK1/2 MAPK. *PLoS ONE* **2014**, *9*, e101321.

155. Nazari, M.; Ghorbani, A.; Hekmat-Doost, A.; Jeddi-Tehrani, M.; Zand, H. Inactivation of nuclear factor-κB by *Citrus* flavanone hesperidin contributes to apoptosis and chemo-sensitizing effect in ramos cells. *Eur. J. Pharmacol.* **2011**, *650*, 526–533.

156. Ghorbani, A.; Nazari, M.; Jeddi-Tehrani, M.; Zand, H. The *Citrus* flavonoid hesperidin induces p53 and inhibits NF-kB activation in order to trigger apoptosis in NALM-6 cells: Involvement of ppar gamma-dependent mechanism. *Eur. J. Nutr.* **2012**, *51*, 39–46.

157. Palit, S.; Kar, S.; Sharma, G.; Das, P.K. Hesperetin induced apoptosis in breast carcinoma by triggering accumulation of ROS and activation of ASK1/JNK pathway. *J. Cell. Physiol.* **2015**, *230*, 1729–1739.

158. Natarajan, N.; Thamaraiselvan, R.; Lingaiah, H.; Srinivasan, P.; Periyasamy, B.M. Effect of flavonone hesperidin on the apoptosis of human mammary carcinoma cell line MCF-7. *Biomed. Prev. Nutr.* **2011**, *1*, 207–215.

159. Wang, Y.X.; Yu, H.; Zhang, J.; Gao, J.; Ge, X.; Lou, G. Hesperidin inhibits HeLa cell proliferation through apoptosis mediated by endoplasmic reticulum stress pathways and cell cycle arrest. *BMC Cancer* **2015**, *15*. [CrossRef]

160. El-Readi, M.Z.; Hamdan, D.; Farrag, N.; El-Shazly, A.; Wink, M. Inhibition of p-glycoprotein activity by limonin and other secondary metabolites from *Citrus* species in human colon and leukaemia cell lines. *Eur. J. Pharmacol.* **2010**, *626*, 139–145. [PubMed]

161. Cooray, H.C.; Janvilisri, T.; van Veen, H.W.; Hladky, S.B.; Barrand, M.A. Interaction of the breast cancer resistance protein with plant polyphenols. *Biochem. Biophys. Res. Commun.* **2004**, *317*, 269–275.

162. Lee, C.J.; Wilson, L.; Jordan, M.A.; Nguyen, V.; Tang, J.; Smiyun, G. Hesperidin suppressed proliferations of both human breast cancer and androgen-dependent prostate cancer cells. *Phytother. Res.* **2010**, *24*, S15–S19.

163. Tanaka, T.; Makita, H.; Ohnishi, M.; Hirose, Y.; Wang, A.J.; Mori, H.; Satoh, K.; Hara, A.; Ogawa, H. Chemoprevention of 4-nitroquinoline 1-oxide-induced oral carcinogenesis by dietary curcumin and hesperidin—Comparison with the protective effect of beta-carotene. *Cancer Res.* **1994**, *54*, 4653–4659.

164. Berkarda, B.; Koyuncu, H.; Soybir, G.; Baykut, F. Inhibitory effect of hesperidin on tumour initiation and promotion in mouse skin. *Res. Exp. Med.* **1998**, *198*, 93–99.

165. Koyuncu, H.; Berkarda, B.; Baykut, F.; Soybir, G.; Alatli, C.; Gul, H.; Altun, M. Preventive effect of hesperidin against inflammation in CD-1 mouse skin caused by tumor promoter. *Anticancer Res.* **1999**, *19*, 3237–3241.

166. Aranganathan, S.; Nalini, N. Efficacy of the potential chemopreventive agent, hesperetin (*Citrus* flavonone), on 1,2-dimethylhydrazine induced colon carcinogenesis. *Food Chem. Toxicol.* **2009**, *47*, 2594–2600.

167. Choi, E.J.; Kim, G.H. Anti-/pro-apoptotic effects of hesperetin against 7,12-dimetylbenz(a)anthracene-induced alteration in animals. *Oncol. Rep.* **2011**, *25*, 545–550.

168. Kamaraj, S.; Ramakrishnan, G.; Anandakumar, P.; Jagan, S.; Devaki, T. Antioxidant and anticancer efficacy of hesperidin in benzo(a)pyrene induced lung carcinogenesis in mice. *Investig. New Drugs* **2009**, *27*, 214–222.

169. Ye, L.; Chan, F.L.; Chen, S.A.; Leung, L.K. The *Citrus* flavonone hesperetin inhibits growth of aromatase-expressing MCF-7 tumor in ovariectomized athymic mice. *J. Nutr. Biochem.* **2012**, *23*, 1230–1237.

170. Hung, J.Y.; Hsu, Y.L.; Ko, Y.C.; Tsai, Y.M.; Yang, C.J.; Huang, M.S.; Kuo, P.L. Didymin, a dietary flavonoid glycoside from *Citrus* fruits, induces FAS-mediated apoptotic pathway in human non-small-cell lung cancer cells in vitro and in vivo. *Lung Cancer* **2010**, *68*, 366–374.

171. Saralamma, V.V.G.; Nagappan, A.; Hong, G.E.; Lee, H.J.; Yumnam, S.; Raha, S.; Heo, J.D.; Lee, S.J.; Lee, W.S.; Kim, E.H.; et al. Poncirin induces apoptosis in AGS human gastric cancer cells through extrinsic apoptotic pathway by up-regulation of FAS ligand. *Int. J. Mol. Sci.* **2015**, *16*, 22676–22691.

172. Wang, L.S.; Stoner, G.D. Anthocyanins and their role in cancer prevention. *Cancer Lett.* **2008**, *269*, 281–290.

173. Schindler, R.; Mentlein, R. Flavonoids and vitamin E reduce the release of the angiogenic peptide vascular endothelial growth factor from human tumor cells. *J. Nutr.* **2006**, *136*, 1477–1482.

174. Freitas, S.; Costa, S.; Azevedo, C.; Carvalho, G.; Freire, S.; Barbosa, P.; Velozo, E.; Schaer, R.; Tardy, M.; Meyer, R.; et al. Flavonoids inhibit angiogenic cytokine production by human glioma cells. *Phytother. Res.* **2011**, *25*, 916–921.

175. Liu, L.Z.; Fang, J.; Zhou, Q.; Hu, X.W.; Shi, X.L.; Jiang, B.H. Apigenin inhibits expression of vascular endothelial growth factor and angiogenesis in human lung cancer cells: Implication of chemoprevention of lung cancer. *Mol. Pharmacol.* **2005**, *68*, 635–643.

176. Fang, J.; Zhou, Q.; Liu, L.Z.; Xia, C.; Hu, X.W.; Shi, X.L.; Jiang, B.H. Apigenin inhibits tumor angiogenesis through decreasing HIF-1 alpha and VEGF expression. *Carcinogenesis* **2007**, *28*, 858–864.

177. Kim, M.H. Flavonoids inhibit VEGF/BFGF-induced angiogenesis in vitro by inhibiting the matrix-degrading proteases. *J. Cell. Biochem.* **2003**, *89*, 529–538.

178. Lamy, S.; Akla, N.; Ouanouki, A.; Lord-Dufour, S.; Beliveau, R. Diet-derived polyphenols inhibit angiogenesis by modulating the interleukin-6/Stat3 pathway. *Exp. Cell Res.* **2012**, *318*, 1586–1596.

179. Lam, I.K.; Alex, D.; Wang, Y.H.; Liu, P.; Liu, A.L.; Du, G.H.; Lee, S.M. In vitro and in vivo structure and activity relationship analysis of polymethoxylated flavonoids: Identifying sinensetin as a novel antiangiogenesis agent. *Mol. Nutr. Food Res.* **2012**, *56*, 945–956.

180. Kunimasa, K.; Ikekita, M.; Sato, M.; Ohta, T.; Yamori, Y.; Ikeda, M.; Kuranuki, S.; Oikawa, T. Nobiletin, a *Citrus* polymethoxyflavonoid, suppresses multiple angiogenesis-related endothelial cell functions and angiogenesis in vivo. *Cancer Sci.* **2010**, *101*, 2462–2469.

181. Wang, Y.; Su, M.; Yin, J.; Zhang, H. Effect of nobiletin on K562 cells xenograft in nude mice. *Zhongguo Zhong Yao Za Zhi* **2009**, *34*, 1410–1414.

182. Tan, W.F.; Lin, L.P.; Li, M.H.; Zhang, Y.X.; Tong, Y.G.; Xiao, D.; Ding, J. Quercetin, a dietary-derived flavonoid, possesses antiangiogenic potential. *Eur. J. Pharmacol.* **2003**, *459*, 255–262.

183. Ahn, M.R.; Kunimasa, K.; Kumazawa, S.; Nakayama, T.; Kaji, K.; Uto, Y.; Hori, H.; Nagasawa, H.; Ohta, T. Correlation between antiangiogenic activity and antioxidant activity of various components from propolis. *Mol. Nutr. Food Res.* **2009**, *53*, 643–651.

184. Weng, C.J.; Yen, G.C. Flavonoids, a ubiquitous dietary phenolic subclass, exert extensive in vitro anti-invasive and in vivo anti-metastatic activities. *Cancer Metastas. Rev.* **2012**, *31*, 323–351.

185. Bracke, M.E.; Boterberg, T.; Depypere, H.T.; Stove, C.; Leclercq, G.; Mareel, M.M. The *Citrus* methoxyflavone tangeretin affects human cell-cell interactions. *Flavonoids Cell Funct.* **2002**, *505*, 135–139.

186. Tan, T.W.; Chou, Y.E.; Yang, W.H.; Hsu, C.J.; Fong, Y.C.; Tang, C.H. Naringin suppress chondrosarcoma migration through inhibition vascular adhesion molecule-1 expression by modulating mir-126. *Int. Immunopharmacol.* **2014**, *22*, 107–114.

187. Liao, A.C.H.; Kuo, C.C.; Huang, Y.C.; Yeh, C.W.; Hseu, Y.C.; Liu, J.Y.; Hsu, L.S. Naringenin inhibits migration of bladder cancer cells through downregulation of AKT and MMP-2. *Mol. Med. Rep.* **2014**, *10*, 1531–1536.

188. Martinez Conesa, C.; Vicente Ortega, V.; Yanez Gascon, M.J.; Alcaraz Banos, M.; Canteras Jordana, M.; Benavente-Garcia, O.; Castillo, J. Treatment of metastatic melanoma B16F10 by the flavonoids tangeretin, rutin, and diosmin. *J. Agric. Food Chem.* **2005**, *53*, 6791–6797.

189. Lentini, A.; Forni, C.; Provenzano, B.; Beninati, S. Enhancement of transglutaminase activity and polyamine depletion in B16-F10 melanoma cells by flavonoids naringenin and hesperitin correlate to reduction of the in vivo metastatic potential. *Amino Acids* **2007**, *32*, 95–100.

190. Qin, L.; Jin, L.T.; Lu, L.L.; Lu, X.Y.; Zhang, C.L.; Zhang, F.Y.; Liang, W. Naringenin reduces lung metastasis in a breast cancer resection model. *Protein Cell* **2011**, *2*, 507–516.

191. Miyata, Y.; Sato, T.; Imada, K.; Dobashi, A.; Yano, M.; Ito, A. A *Citrus* polymethoxyflavonoid, nobiletin, is a novel mek inhibitor that exhibits antitumor metastasis in human fibrosarcoma HT-1080 cells. *Biochem. Biophys. Res. Commun.* **2008**, *366*, 168–173.

271

192. Sato, T.; Koike, L.; Miyata, Y.; Hirata, M.; Mimaki, Y.; Sashida, Y.; Yano, M.; Ito, A. Inhibition of activator protein-1 binding activity and phosphatidylinositol 3-kinase pathway by nobiletin, a polymethoxy flavonoid, results in augmentation of tissue inhibitor of metalloproteinases-1 production and suppression of production of matrix metalloproteinases-1 and-9 in human fibrosarcoma HT-1080 cells. *Cancer Res.* **2002**, *62*, 1025–1029.

193. Kawabata, K.; Murakami, A.; Ohigashi, H. Nobiletin, a *Citrus* flavonoid, down-regulates matrix metalloproteinase-7 (matrilysin) expression in HT-29 human colorectal cancer cells. *Biosci. Biotechnol. Biochem.* **2005**, *69*, 307–314.

194. Chien, S.Y.; Hsieh, M.J.; Chen, C.J.; Yang, S.F.; Chen, M.K. Nobiletin inhibits invasion and migration of human nasopharyngeal carcinoma cell lines by involving ERK1/2 and transcriptional inhibition of MMP-2. *Expert Opin. Ther. Targets* **2015**, *19*, 307–320.

195. Baek, S.H.; Kim, S.M.; Nam, D.; Lee, J.H.; Ahn, K.S.; Choi, S.H.; Kim, S.H.; Shim, B.S.; Chang, I.M.; Ahn, K.S. Antimetastatic effect of nobiletin through the down-regulation of CXC chemokine receptor type 4 and matrix metallopeptidase-9. *Pharm. Biol.* **2012**, *50*, 1210–1218.

196. Minagawa, A.; Otani, Y.; Kubota, T.; Wada, N.; Furukawa, T.; Kumai, K.; Kameyama, K.; Okada, Y.; Fujii, M.; Yano, M.; et al. The *Citrus* flavonoid, nobiletin, inhibits peritoneal dissemination of human gastric carcinoma in SCID mice. *Jpn. J. Cancer Res.* **2001**, *92*, 1322–1328.

197. Lee, Y.C.; Cheng, T.H.; Lee, J.S.; Chen, J.H.; Liao, Y.C.; Fong, Y.; Wu, C.H.; Shih, Y.W. Nobiletin, a citrus flavonoid, suppresses invasion and migration involving FAK/PI3K/AKT and small GTPase signals in human gastric adenocarcinoma AGS cells. *Mol. Cell. Biochem.* **2011**, *347*, 103–115.

198. Da, C.; Liu, Y.; Zhan, Y.; Liu, K.; Wang, R. Nobiletin inhibits epithelial-mesenchymal transition of human non-small cell lung cancer cells by antagonizing the TGF-BETA1/SMAD3 signaling pathway. *Oncol. Rep.* **2016**, *35*, 2767–2774.

199. Lindenmeyer, F.; Li, H.; Menashi, S.; Soria, C.; Lu, H. Apigenin acts on the tumor cell invasion process and regulates protease production. *Nutr. Cancer Int. J.* **2001**, *39*, 139–147.

200. Lee, W.J.; Chen, W.K.; Wang, C.J.; Lin, W.L.; Tseng, T.H. Apigenin inhibits hgf-promoted invasive growth and metastasis involving blocking PI3K/AKT pathway and beta 4 integrin function in MDA-MB-231 breast cancer cells. *Toxicol. Appl. Pharmacol.* **2008**, *226*, 178–191.

201. Franzen, C.A.; Amargo, E.; Todorovic, V.; Desai, B.V.; Huda, S.; Mirzoeva, S.; Chiu, K.; Grzybowski, B.A.; Chew, T.L.; Green, K.J.; et al. The chemopreventive bioflavonoid apigenin inhibits prostate cancer cell motility through the focal adhesion kinase/Src signaling mechanism. *Cancer Prev. Res.* **2009**, *2*, 830–841.

202. Hu, X.W.; Meng, D.; Fang, J. Apigenin inhibited migration and invasion of human ovarian cancer A2780 cells through focal adhesion kinase. *Carcinogenesis* **2008**, *29*, 2369–2376.

203. Czyz, J.; Madeja, Z.; Irmer, U.; Korohoda, W.; Hulser, D.F. Flavonoid apigenin inhibits motility and invasiveness of carcinoma cells in vitro. *Int. J. Cancer* **2005**, *114*, 12–18.

204. Tatsuta, M.; Iishi, H.; Baba, M.; Yano, H.; Murata, K.; Mukai, M.; Akedo, H. Suppression by apigenin of peritoneal metastasis of intestinal adenocarcinomas induced by azoxymethane in wistar rats. *Clin. Exp. Metastas.* **2001**, *18*, 657–662.

205. Noh, H.J.; Sung, E.G.; Kim, J.Y.; Lee, T.J.; Song, I.H. Suppression of phorbol-12-myristate-13-acetate-induced tumor cell invasion by apigenin via the inhibition of p38 mitogen-activated protein kinase-dependent matrix metalloproteinase-9 expression. *Oncol. Rep.* **2010**, *24*, 277–283.

206. Caltagirone, S.; Rossi, C.; Poggi, A.; Ranelletti, F.O.; Natali, P.G.; Brunetti, M.; Aiello, F.B.; Piantelli, M. Flavonoids apigenin and quercetin inhibit melanoma growth and metastatic potential. *Int. J. Cancer* **2000**, *87*, 595–600.

207. Lin, C.W.; Hou, W.C.; Shen, S.C.; Juan, S.H.; Ko, C.H.; Wang, L.M.; Chen, Y.C. Quercetin inhibition of tumor invasion via suppressing PKC DELTA/ERK/AP-1-dependent matrix metalloproteinase-9 activation in breast carcinoma cells. *Carcinogenesis* **2008**, *29*, 1807–1815.

208. Phromnoi, K.; Yodkeeree, S.; Anuchapreeda, S.; Limtrakul, P. Inhibition of MMP-3 activity and invasion of the MDA-MB-231 human invasive breast carcinoma cell line by bioflavonoids. *Acta Pharmacol. Sin.* **2009**, *30*, 1169–1176.

209. Vijayababu, M.R.; Arunkumar, A.; Kanagaraj, P.; Venkataraman, P.; Krishnamoorthy, G.; Arunakaran, J. Quercetin downregulates matrix metalloproteinases 2 and 9 proteins expression in prostate cancer cells (PC-3). *Mol. Cell. Biochem.* **2006**, *287*, 109–116.

210. Senthilkumar, K.; Arunkumar, R.; Elumalai, P.; Sharmila, G.; Gunadharini, D.N.; Banudevi, S.; Krishnamoorthy, G.; Benson, C.S.; Arunakaran, J. Quercetin inhibits invasion, migration and signalling molecules involved in cell survival and proliferation of prostate cancer cell line (PC-3). *Cell Biochem. Funct.* **2011**, *29*, 87–95.

211. Chiu, W.T.; Shen, S.C.; Chow, J.M.; Lin, C.W.; Shia, L.T.; Chen, Y.C. Contribution of reactive oxygen species to migration/invasion of human glioblastoma cells U87 via ERK-dependent COX-2/PGE(2) activation. *Neurobiol. Dis.* **2010**, *37*, 118–129.

212. Labbe, D.; Provencal, M.; Lamy, S.; Boivin, D.; Gingras, D.; Beliveau, R. The flavonols quercetin, kaempferol, and myricetin inhibit hepatocyte growth factor-induced medulloblastoma cell migration. *J. Nutr.* **2009**, *139*, 646–652.

213. Lin, Y.S.; Tsai, P.H.; Kandaswami, C.C.; Cheng, C.H.; Ke, F.C.; Lee, P.P.; Hwang, J.J.; Lee, M.T. Effects of dietary flavonoids, luteolin, and quercetin on the reversal of epithelial-mesenchymal transition in A431 epidermal cancer cells. *Cancer Sci.* **2011**, *102*, 1829–1839.

214. Zhang, W.; Zhang, F. Effects of quercetin on proliferation, apoptosis, adhesion and migration, and invasion of HeLa cells. *Eur. J. Gynaecol. Oncol.* **2009**, *30*, 60–64.

215. Zhang, X.M.; Huang, S.P.; Xu, Q. Quercetin inhibits the invasion of murine melanoma B16-BL6 cells by decreasing pro-MMP-9 via the PKC pathway. *Cancer Chemother. Pharmacol.* **2004**, *53*, 82–88.

216. Devipriya, S.; Ganapathy, V.; Shyamaladevi, C.S. Suppression of tumor growth and invasion in 9,10 dimethyl benz(a) anthracene induced mammary carcinoma by the plant bioflavonoid quercetin. *Chem. Biol. Interact.* **2006**, *162*, 106–113.

217. Hsu, Y.L.; Hsieh, C.J.; Tsai, E.M.; Hung, J.Y.; Chang, W.A.; Hou, M.F.; Kuo, P.L. Didymin reverses phthalate ester-associated breast cancer aggravation in the breast cancer tumor microenvironment. *Oncol. Lett.* **2016**, *11*, 1035–1042.

218. Liu, R.H. Potential synergy of phytochemicals in cancer prevention: Mechanism of action. *J. Nutr.* **2004**, *134*, 3479S–3485S.

219. So, F.V.; Guthrie, N.; Chambers, A.F.; Moussa, M.; Carroll, K.K. Inhibition of human breast cancer cell proliferation and delay of mammary tumorigenesis by flavonoids and citrus juices. *Nutr. Cancer Int. J.* **1996**, *26*, 167–181.

220. Guthrie, N.; Carroll, K.K. Inhibition of mammary cancer by *Citrus* flavonoids. *Flavonoids Cell Funct.* **1998**, *439*, 227–236.

221. Miyagi, Y.; Om, A.S.; Chee, K.M.; Bennink, M.R. Inhibition of azoxymethane-induced colon cancer by orange juice. *Nutr. Cancer Int. J.* **2000**, *36*, 224–229.

222. Tanaka, T.; Kohno, H.; Murakami, M.; Shimada, R.; Kagami, S.; Sumida, T.; Azuma, Y.; Ogawa, H. Suppression of azoxymethane-induced colon carcinogenesis in male F344 rats by mandarin juices rich in beta-cryptoxanthin and hesperidin. *Int. J. Cancer* **2000**, *88*, 146–150.

223. Kohno, H.; Taima, M.; Sumida, T.; Azuma, Y.; Ogawa, H.; Tanaka, T. Inhibitory effect of mandarin juice rich in beta-cryptoxanthin and hesperidin on 4-(methylnitrosamino)-1-(3-pyridyl)-1-butanone-induced pulmonary tumorigenesis in mice. *Cancer Lett.* **2001**, *174*, 141–150.

224. Tanaka, T.; Tanaka, T.; Tanaka, M.; Kuno, T. Cancer chemoprevention by *Citrus* pulp and juices containing high amounts of beta-cryptoxanthin and hesperidin. *J. Biomed. Biotechnol.* **2012**, *2012*, 516981.

225. Kohno, H.; Maeda, M.; Honjo, S.; Murakami, M.; Shimada, R.; Masuda, S.; Sumida, T.; Azuma, Y.; Ogawa, H.; Tanaka, T. Prevention of colonic preneoplastic lesions by the β-cryptoxanthin and hesperidin rich powder prepared from *Citrus* unshiu marc. Juice in male f344 rats. *J. Toxicol. Pathol.* **1999**, *12*, 209–215.

226. Celano, M.; Maggisano, V.; De Rose, R.F.; Bulotta, S.; Maiuolo, J.; Navarra, M.; Russo, D. Flavonoid fraction of *Citrus* reticulata juice reduces proliferation and migration of anaplastic thyroid carcinoma cells. *Nutr. Cancer Int. J.* **2015**, *67*, 1183–1190.

227. Alshatwi, A.A.; Shafi, G.; Hasan, T.N.; Al-Hazzani, A.A.; Alsaif, M.A.; Alfawaz, M.A.; Lei, K.Y.; Munshi, A. Apoptosis-mediated inhibition of human breast cancer cell proliferation by lemon *Citrus* extract. *Asian Pac. J. Cancer Prev.* **2011**, *12*, 1555–1559.

228. Kim, J.; Jayaprakasha, G.K.; Uckoo, R.M.; Patil, B.S. Evaluation of chemopreventive and cytotoxic effect of lemon seed extracts on human breast cancer (MCF-7) cells. *Food Chem. Toxicol.* **2012**, *50*, 423–430.

229. Delle Monache, S.; Sanita, P.; Trapasso, E.; Ursino, M.R.; Dugo, P.; Russo, M.; Ferlazzo, N.; Calapai, G.; Angelucci, A.; Navarra, M. Mechanisms underlying the anti-tumoral effects of *Citrus* bergamia juice. *PLoS ONE* **2013**, *8*, e61484.

230. Ferlazzo, N.; Cirmi, S.; Russo, M.; Trapasso, E.; Ursino, M.R.; Lombardo, G.E.; Gangemi, S.; Calapai, G.; Navarra, M. NF-κB mediates the antiproliferative and proapoptotic effects of bergamot juice in HepG2 cells. *Life Sci.* **2016**, *146*, 81–91.

231. Navarra, M.; Ursino, M.R.; Ferlazzo, N.; Russo, M.; Schumacher, U.; Valentiner, U. Effect of *Citrus* bergamia juice on human neuroblastoma cells in vitro and in metastatic xenograft models. *Fitoterapia* **2014**, *95*, 83–92.

232. Visalli, G.; Ferlazzo, N.; Cirmi, S.; Campiglia, P.; Gangemi, S.; Di Pietro, A.; Calapai, G.; Navarra, M. Bergamot juice extract inhibits proliferation by inducing apoptosis in human colon cancer cells. *Anticancer Agents Med. Chem.* **2014**, *14*, 1402–1413.

233. Balkwill, F.; Mantovani, A. Inflammation and cancer: Back to virchow? *Lancet* **2001**, *357*, 539–545.

234. Crawford, S. Anti-inflammatory/antioxidant use in long-term maintenance cancer therapy: A new therapeutic approach to disease progression and recurrence. *Ther. Adv. Med. Oncol.* **2014**, *6*, 52–68.

235. Ferlazzo, N.; Visalli, G.; Smeriglio, A.; Cirmi, S.; Lombardo, G.E.; Campiglia, P.; di Pietro, A.; Navarra, M. Flavonoid fraction of orange and bergamot juices protect human lung epithelial cells from hydrogen peroxide-induced oxidative stress. *Evid. Based Complement. Altern. Med.* **2015**, *2015*, 957031.

236. Ferlazzo, N.; Visalli, G.; Cirmi, S.; Lombardo, G.E.; Lagana, P.; di Pietro, A.; Navarra, M. Natural iron chelators: Protective role in A549 cells of flavonoids-rich extracts of *Citrus* juices in Fe$^{3+}$-induced oxidative stress. *Environ. Toxicol. Pharmacol.* **2016**, *43*, 248–256.

237. Risitano, R.; Currò, M.; Cirmi, S.; Ferlazzo, N.; Campiglia, P.; Caccamo, D.; Ientile, R.; Navarra, M. Flavonoid fraction of bergamot juice reduces LPS-induced inflammatory response through SIRT1-mediated NF-kB inhibition in THP-1 monocytes. *PLoS ONE* **2014**, *9*, e107431.

238. Currò, M.; Risitano, R.; Ferlazzo, N.; Cirmi, S.; Gangemi, C.; Caccamo, D.; Ientile, R.; Navarra, M. *Citrus* bergamia juice extract attenuates beta-amyloid-induced pro-inflammatory activation of THP-1 cells through MAPK and AP-1 pathways. *Sci. Rep.* **2016**, *6*, 20809.

239. Impellizzeri, D.; Bruschetta, G.; di Paola, R.; Ahmad, A.; Campolo, M.; Cuzzocrea, S.; Esposito, E.; Navarra, M. The anti-inflammatory and antioxidant effects of bergamot juice extract (BJe) in an experimental model of inflammatory bowel disease. *Clin. Nutr.* **2015**, *34*, 1146–1154.

240. Impellizzeri, D.; Cordaro, M.; Campolo, M.; Gugliandolo, E.; Esposito, E.; Benedetto, F.; Cuzzocrea, S.; Navarra, M. Anti-inflammatory and antioxidant effects of flavonoid-rich fraction of bergamot juice (BJe) in a mouse model of intestinal ischemia/reperfusion injury. *FASEB J.* **2016**, *30* (Suppl. 1), 720–725.

241. Filocamo, A.; Bisignano, C.; Ferlazzo, N.; Cirmi, S.; Mandalari, G.; Navarra, M. In vitro effect of bergamot (*Citrus* bergamia) juice against cagA-positive and-negative clinical isolates of helicobacter pylori. *BMC Complement. Altern. Med.* **2015**, *15*. [CrossRef]

242. Cirmi, S.; Bisignano, C.; Mandalari, G.; Navarra, M. Anti-infective potential of *Citrus* bergamia risso et poiteau (bergamot) derivatives: A systematic review. *Phytother. Res.* **2016**. [CrossRef]

243. Marino, A.; Paterniti, I.; Cordaro, M.; Morabito, R.; Campolo, M.; Navarra, M.; Esposito, E.; Cuzzocrea, S. Role of natural antioxidants and potential use of bergamot in treating rheumatoid arthritis. *PharmaNutrition* **2015**, *3*, 53–59.

244. Mak, N.K.; WongLeung, Y.L.; Chan, S.C.; Wen, J.M.; Leung, K.N.; Fung, M.C. Isolation of anti-leukemia compounds from *Citrus* reticulata. *Life Sci.* **1996**, *58*, 1269–1276.

245. Kim, M.J.; Park, H.J.; Hong, M.S.; Park, H.J.; Kim, M.S.; Leem, K.H.; Kim, J.B.; Kim, Y.J.; Kim, H.K. *Citrus* reticulata blanco induces apoptosis in human gastric cancer cells SNU-668. *Nutr. Cancer* **2005**, *51*, 78–82.

246. Park, K.I.; Park, H.S.; Nagappan, A.; Hong, G.E.; Lee, D.H.; Kang, S.R.; Kim, J.A.; Zhang, J.; Kim, E.H.; Lee, W.S.; et al. Induction of the cell cycle arrest and apoptosis by flavonoids isolated from korean *Citrus aurantium* L. in non-small-cell lung cancer cells. *Food Chem.* **2012**, *135*, 2728–2735.

247. Han, M.H.; Lee, W.S.; Lu, J.N.; Kim, G.; Jung, J.M.; Ryu, C.H.; Kim, G.Y.; Hwang, H.J.; Kwon, T.K.; Choi, Y.H. *Citrus aurantium* L. exhibits apoptotic effects on U937 human leukemia cells partly through inhibition of AKT. *Int. J. Oncol.* **2012**, *40*, 2090–2096.

248. Adina, A.B.; Goenadi, F.A.; Handoko, F.F.; Nawangsari, D.A.; Hermawan, A.; Jenie, R.I.; Meiyanto, E. Combination of ethanolic extract of *Citrus* aurantifolia peels with doxorubicin modulate cell cycle and increase apoptosis induction on MCF-7 cells. *Iran. J. Pharm. Res.* **2014**, *13*, 919–926.

249. Wang, B.; Lin, S.Y.; Shen, Y.Y.; Wu, L.Q.; Chen, Z.Z.; Li, J.; Chen, Z.; Qian, W.B.; Jiang, J.P. Pure total flavonoids from *Citrus* paradisi Macfadyen act synergistically with arsenic trioxide in inducing apoptosis of kasumi-1 leukemia cells in vitro. *J. Zhejiang Univ. Sci. B* **2015**, *16*, 580–585.

250. Celia, C.; Trapasso, E.; Locatelli, M.; Navarra, M.; Ventura, C.A.; Wolfram, J.; Carafa, M.; Morittu, V.M.; Britti, D.; di Marzio, L.; et al. Anticancer activity of liposomal bergamot essential oil (BEO) on human neuroblastoma cells. *Colloids Surf. B Biointerfaces* **2013**, *112*, 548–553.

251. Navarra, M.; Ferlazzo, N.; Cirmi, S.; Trapasso, E.; Bramanti, P.; Lombardo, G.E.; Minciullo, P.L.; Calapai, G.; Gangemi, S. Effects of bergamot essential oil and its extractive fractions on SH-SY5Y human neuroblastoma cell growth. *J. Pharm. Pharmacol.* **2015**, *67*, 1042–1053.

252. Yuan, J.M.; Wang, X.L.; Xiang, Y.B.; Gao, Y.T.; Ross, R.K.; Yu, M.C. Preserved foods in relation to risk of nasopharyngeal carcinoma in Shanghai, China. *Int. J. Cancer* **2000**, *85*, 358–363.

253. Bosetti, C.; la Vecchia, C.; Talamini, R.; Simonato, L.; Zambon, P.; Negri, E.; Trichopoulos, D.; Lagiou, P.; Bardini, R.; Franceschi, S. Food groups and risk of squamous cell esophageal cancer in northern Italy. *Int. J. Cancer* **2000**, *87*, 289–294.

254. Steevens, J.; Schouten, L.J.; Goldbohm, R.A.; van den Brandt, P.A. Vegetables and fruits consumption and risk of esophageal and gastric cancer subtypes in the Netherlands cohort study. *Int. J. Cancer* **2011**, *129*, 2681–2693.

255. Franceschi, S.; Favero, A.; Conti, E.; Talamini, R.; Volpe, R.; Negri, E.; Barzan, L.; la Vecchia, C. Food groups, oils and butter, and cancer of the oral cavity and pharynx. *Br. J. Cancer* **1999**, *80*, 614–620.

256. Bosetti, C.; la Vecchia, C.; Talamini, R.; Negri, E.; Levi, F.; dal Maso, L.; Franceschi, S. Food groups and laryngeal cancer risk: A case-control study from Italy and Switzerland. *Int. J. Cancer* **2002**, *100*, 355–360.

257. Maserejian, N.N.; Giovannucci, E.; Rosner, B.; Zavras, A.; Joshipura, K. Prospective study of fruits and vegetables and risk of oral premalignant lesions in men. *Am. J. Epidemiol.* **2006**, *164*, 556–566.

258. Pavia, M.; Pileggi, C.; Nobile, C.G.A.; Angelillo, I.F. Association between fruit and vegetable consumption and oral cancer: A meta-analysis of observational studies. *Am. J. Clin. Nutr.* **2006**, *83*, 1126–1134.

259. Pourfarzi, F.; Whelan, A.; Kaldor, J.; Malekzadeh, R. The role of diet and other environmental factors in the causation of gastric cancer in Iran-a population based study. *Int. J. Cancer* **2009**, *125*, 1953–1960.

260. Foschi, R.; Pelucchi, C.; dal Maso, L.; Rossi, M.; Levi, F.; Talamini, R.; Bosetti, C.; Negri, E.; Serraino, D.; Giacosa, A.; et al. *Citrus* fruit and cancer risk in a network of case-control studies. *Cancer Causes Control* **2010**, *21*, 237–242.

261. Gonzalez, C.A.; Lujan-Barroso, L.; Bueno-de-Mesquita, H.B.; Jenab, M.; Duell, E.J.; Agudo, A.; Tjonneland, A.; Boutron-Ruault, M.C.; Clavel-Chapelon, F.; Touillaud, M.; et al. Fruit and vegetable intake and the risk of gastric adenocarcinoma: A reanalysis of the european prospective investigation into cancer and nutrition (epic-eurgast) study after a longer follow-up. *Int. J. Cancer* **2012**, *131*, 2910–2919.

262. Franceschi, S.; Favero, A.; la Vecchia, C.; Negri, E.; Conti, E.; Montella, M.; Giacosa, A.; Nanni, O.; Decarli, A. Food groups and risk of colorectal cancer in Italy. *Int. J. Cancer* **1997**, *72*, 56–61.

263. Levi, F.; Pasche, C.; la Vecchia, C.; Lucchini, F.; Franceschi, S. Food groups and colorectal cancer risk. *Br. J. Cancer* **1999**, *79*, 1283–1287.

264. Malin, A.S.; Qi, D.; Shu, X.O.; Gao, Y.T.; Friedmann, J.M.; Jin, F.; Zheng, W. Intake of fruits, vegetables and selected micronutrients in relation to the risk of breast cancer. *Int. J. Cancer* **2003**, *105*, 413–418.

265. Ronco, A.L.; de Stefani, E.; Stoll, M. Hormonal and metabolic modulation through nutrition: Towards a primary prevention of breast cancer. *Breast* **2010**, *19*, 322–332.

266. Jansen, R.J.; Robinson, D.P.; Stolzenberg-Solomon, R.Z.; Bamlet, W.R.; de Andrade, M.; Oberg, A.L.; Hammer, T.J.; Rabe, K.G.; Anderson, K.E.; Olson, J.E.; et al. Fruit and vegetable consumption is inversely associated with having pancreatic cancer. *Cancer Causes Control* **2011**, *22*, 1613–1625.

267. Chan, J.M.; Wang, F.; Holly, E.A. Vegetable and fruit intake and pancreatic cancer in a population-based case-control study in the San Francisco bay area. *Cancer Epidemiol. Biomark. Prev.* **2005**, *14*, 2093–2097.

268. Jian, L.; Du, C.J.; Lee, A.H.; Binns, C.W. Do dietary lycopene and other carotenoids protect against prostate cancer? *Int. J. Cancer* **2005**, *113*, 1010–1014.

269. Fortes, C.; Mastroeni, S.; Melchi, F.; Pilla, M.A.; Antonelli, G.; Camaioni, D.; Alotto, M.; Pasquini, P. A protective effect of the mediterranean diet for cutaneous melanoma. *Int. J. Epidemiol.* **2008**, *37*, 1018–1029.

270. Li, W.Q.; Kuriyama, S.; Li, Q.; Nagai, M.; Hozawa, A.; Nishino, Y.; Tsuji, I. *Citrus* consumption and cancer incidence: The Ohsaki cohort study. *Int. J. Cancer* **2010**, *127*, 1913–1922.

271. Dikshit, R.P.; Boffetta, P.; Bouchardy, C.; Merletti, F.; Crosignani, P.; Cuchi, T.; Ardanaz, E.; Brennan, P. Risk factors for the development of second primary tumors among men after laryngeal and hypopharyngeal carcinoma—A multicentric european study. *Cancer* **2005**, *103*, 2326–2333.

272. Bae, J.M.; Lee, E.J.; Guyatt, G. *Citrus* fruit intake and stomach cancer risk: A quantitative systematic review. *Gastric Cancer* **2008**, *11*, 23–32.

273. Bae, J.M.; Lee, E.J.; Guyatt, G. *Citrus* fruit intake and pancreatic cancer risk: A quantitative systematic review. *Pancreas* **2009**, *38*, 168–174.

274. Song, J.K.; Bae, J.M. *Citrus* fruit intake and breast cancer risk: A quantitative systematic review. *J. Breast Cancer* **2013**, *16*, 72–76.

275. Liang, S.; Lv, G.; Chen, W.; Jiang, J.; Wang, J. *Citrus* fruit intake and bladder cancer risk: A meta-analysis of observational studies. *Int. J. Food Sci. Nutr.* **2014**, *65*, 893–898.

276. Xu, C.; Zeng, X.T.; Liu, T.Z.; Zhang, C.; Yang, Z.H.; Li, S.; Chen, X.Y. Fruits and vegetables intake and risk of bladder cancer: A prisma-compliant systematic review and dose-response meta-analysis of prospective cohort studies. *Medicine* **2015**, *94*, e759.

277. Yao, B.; Yan, Y.; Ye, X.; Fang, H.; Xu, H.; Liu, Y.; Li, S.; Zhao, Y. Intake of fruit and vegetables and risk of bladder cancer: A dose-response meta-analysis of observational studies. *Cancer Causes Control* **2014**, *25*, 1645–1658.

278. Wang, A.; Zhu, C.; Fu, L.; Wan, X.; Yang, X.; Zhang, H.; Miao, R.; He, L.; Sang, X.; Zhao, H. *Citrus* fruit intake substantially reduces the risk of esophageal cancer: A meta-analysis of epidemiologic studies. *Medicine* **2015**, *94*, e1390.

279. Vingeliene, S.; Chan, D.S.; Aune, D.; Vieira, A.R.; Polemiti, E.; Stevens, C.; Abar, L.; Rosenblatt, D.N.; Greenwood, D.C.; Norat, T. An update of the WCRF/AICR systematic literature review on esophageal and gastric cancers and *Citrus* fruits intake. *Cancer Causes Control* **2016**, *27*, 837–851.

280. Vrieling, A.; Verhage, B.A.; van Duijnhoven, F.J.; Jenab, M.; Overvad, K.; Tjonneland, A.; Olsen, A.; Clavel-Chapelon, F.; Boutron-Ruault, M.C.; Kaaks, R.; et al. Fruit and vegetable consumption and pancreatic cancer risk in the european prospective investigation into cancer and nutrition. *Int. J. Cancer* **2009**, *124*, 1926–1934.

281. Ferlazzo, N.; Cirmi, S.; Calapai, G.; Ventura-Spagnolo, E.; Gangemi, S.; Navarra, M. Anti-inflammatory activity of *Citrus* bergamia derivatives: Where do we stand? *Molecules* **2016**, *21*, 1273. [CrossRef]

282. Mannucci, C.; Navarra, M.; Calapai, F.; Squeri, R.; Gangemi, S.; Calapai, G. Clinical Pharmacology of Citrus bergamia: A Systematic Review. *Phytother. Res.* **2016**. [CrossRef]

283. Cirmi, S.; Ferlazzo, N.; Lombardo, G.E.; Ventura-Spagnolo, E.; Gangemi, S.; Calapai, G.; Navarra, M. Neurodegenerative diseases: Might *Citrus* flavonoids play a protective role? *Molecules* **2016**, *21*, 1312. [CrossRef]

284. Citraro, R.; Navarra, M.; Leo, A.; Donato Di Paola, E.; Santangelo, E.; Lippiello, P.; Aiello, R.; Russo, E.; De Sarro, G. The anticonvulsant activity of a flavonoid rich extract from orange juice involves both NMDA and GABA-benzodiazepine receptor complexes. *Molecules* **2016**, *21*. [CrossRef]

285. Efferth, T.; Koch, E. Complex interactions between phytochemicals. The multi-target therapeutic concept of phytotherapy. *Curr. Drug Targets* **2011**, *12*, 122–132.

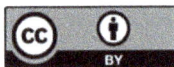

*nutrients*

MDPI

*Review*

# The Anti-Cancer Effect of Polyphenols against Breast Cancer and Cancer Stem Cells: Molecular Mechanisms

Ahmed Abdal Dayem, Hye Yeon Choi, Gwang-Mo Yang, Kyeongseok Kim, Subbroto Kumar Saha and Ssang-Goo Cho *

Department of Stem Cell & Regenerative Biotechnology, Incurable Disease Animal Model and Stem Cell Institute (IDASI), Konkuk University, Gwangjin-gu, Seoul 05029, Korea; ahmed_morsy86@yahoo.com (A.A.D.); hyeon.choi24@gmail.com (H.Y.C.); slayersgod@nate.com (G.-M.Y.); proproggs@naver.com (K.K.); subbroto@konkuk.ac.kr (S.K.S.)
*   Correspondence: ssangoo@konkuk.ac.kr; Tel.: +82-2-450-4207

Received: 8 July 2016; Accepted: 9 September 2016; Published: 21 September 2016

**Abstract:** The high incidence of breast cancer in developed and developing countries, and its correlation to cancer-related deaths, has prompted concerned scientists to discover novel alternatives to deal with this challenge. In this review, we will provide a brief overview of polyphenol structures and classifications, as well as on the carcinogenic process. The biology of breast cancer cells will also be discussed. The molecular mechanisms involved in the anti-cancer activities of numerous polyphenols, against a wide range of breast cancer cells, in vitro and in vivo, will be explained in detail. The interplay between autophagy and apoptosis in the anti-cancer activity of polyphenols will also be highlighted. In addition, the potential of polyphenols to target cancer stem cells (CSCs) via various mechanisms will be explained. Recently, the use of natural products as chemotherapeutics and chemopreventive drugs to overcome the side effects and resistance that arise from using chemical-based agents has garnered the attention of the scientific community. Polyphenol research is considered a promising field in the treatment and prevention of breast cancer.

**Keywords:** polyphenols; breast cancer; anti-cancer activity; autophagy; apoptosis; cancer stem cells

## 1. Introduction

Currently, cancer is one of the most common life-threatening diseases worldwide, and breast cancer has the highest rate of diagnosis amongst women. There are three main strategies to block and postpone the stages of carcinogenesis [1–3]. The primary strategy considered is a preventive approach, which blocks the toxic, as well as the mutagenic, effects, which consequently inhibits tumor initiation and promotion. The secondary strategy presents anti-cancer potential during the early stages of carcinogenesis via various mechanisms, such as control of signal transduction, blocking angiogenesis, antioxidant mechanisms, hormones, and modulation of immunity, which finally result in the blockage of cancer progression. The third strategy for cancer treatment and prevention involves blocking the invasiveness and metastatic properties of a tumor via regulation of cell-adhesion molecules, protection of the extracellular matrix (ECM) from degradation, and up-regulation of genes that block metastasis [1,2].

The link between a diet that is rich in fruits and vegetables, and the prevention, as well as the reduction, of the occurrence of health-daunting diseases has been evidenced, and is partially ascribed to polyphenols [4–6]. The term polyphenol was first given to natural compounds bearing multiple (poly) phenol rings, which are widespread in various fruits, vegetables, wine, nuts, tea, coffee, and in many foods that are consumed daily by humans [7]. Polyphenols possess a broad spectrum of structural variations, which lead to a wide range of biological functions; among them, anti-cancer functions. Polyphenols possess a broad spectrum of structural variations in the carbon backbone chains, as well as alterations to primary and secondary structures due to methylation, glycosylation, and hydroxylation [6,8]. These structural variations may be responsible for their various health benefits, including antioxidant [9,10], anti-inflammatory, anti-angiogenic [11,12], and anti-proliferative mechanisms, as well as regulation of key signaling protein and enzyme functions [13].

## 2. Carcinogenesis: Overview and Molecular Basis

The tumorigenic process is complicated and occurs through a multistep procedure, including initiation, promotion, and progression, as illustrated in Figure 1 [14,15]. Initiation includes the entrance and distribution of cancer-causing agents in the cell, in particular, the nucleus, and interaction with DNA that finally results in the mutagenesis and emergence of the toxic effect [16]. This stage is irreversible, but can be prevented by phase I and phase II metabolizing enzymes, which transform the carcinogens into less toxic and soluble products [17,18].

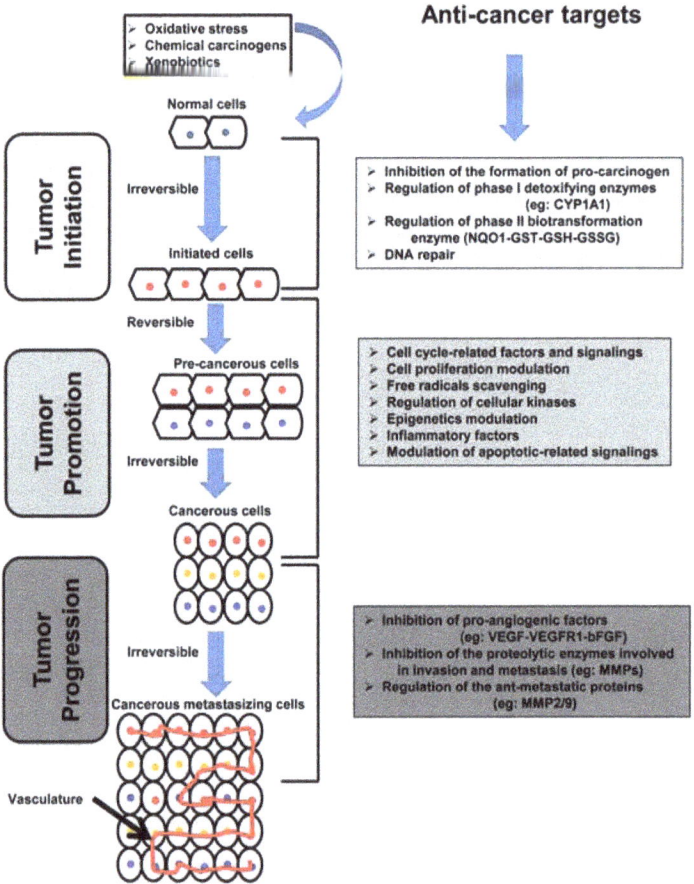

**Figure 1.** Schematic representation depicting the multistage process, including initiation, promotion, and progression, of carcinogenesis, and the biological targets of polyphenols at each step.

Polyphenols present preventive effects against tumor initiation via numerous mechanisms, such as prevention of the formation of genotoxic molecules and blocking the activity of the mutagens-transforming enzymes [19,20]; regulation of heme-containing phase I enzymes, such as cytochrome P450s (CYPs) [21,22]; regulation of carcinogen-detoxifying phase II enzymes, such as NADPH-quinone oxidoreductase-1 (NQO1), quinone reductase (QR), glutathione $S$-transferase (GST), and uridine diphospho (UDP) glucuronosyl transferase (UGT) [23,24]; and prevention of the formation of DNA adducts [25].

The promotion stage, which takes time, is related to the proliferation of tumor-initiating cells. It is considered a reversible stage of tumorigenesis, and gives rise to pre-cancerous cells. The main features of this stage are cell proliferation and apoptosis. The tumor progression stage is the stage in which cells gradually transform to the malignant state. Metastasis and invasiveness also emerge during this stage, via the angiogenesis process, with the growth of new blood capillaries in the tumor, which is enhanced by the secretion of specific growth factors and growth factor receptors, such as platelet-derived growth factor (PDGF), PDGF receptor (PDGFR), vascular endothelial growth factor (VEGF), and VEGF receptor (VEGFR), leading to overgrowth and spread of the tumor [26].

Cathepsins, which belong to the lysosomal proteases superfamily, are implicated in tumor progression [27]. Cathepsin D, an aspartic protease, is considered to be a candidate as a clinical marker for breast cancer, and is involved in the activation of the inactive form of cathepsin B (procathepsin B) [28]. Cathepsin B is essential for the growth of breast cancer [29] and its down-regulation leads to a reduction of tumor progression [30]. The up-regulation of cathepsin B is an indicator of cancer progression and is a poor prognosis [31].

The urokinase plasminogen activator (uPA) system consists of serine protease uPA and various serine protease inhibitors, such as plasminogen activator inhibitors 1 and 2 (PAI-1 and PAI-2). Upon binding of uPA to urokinase plasminogen activator anchored receptor (uPAR), the activation of plasminogen takes place and leads to the production of the broad spectrum protease, plasmin [32]. Plasmin directly degrades the ECM, or indirectly via the activation of the zymogens of metalloproteinases (MMPs) [33].

There are numerous polyphenols that show potent inhibitory effects on the invasiveness and metastatic properties of cancer, which will be explained in detail in the following sections.

## 3. Overview on Breast Cancer and Cancer Stem Cells (CSCs)

Breast cancer represents about 25.2% of cancer cases in women, and commonly occurs in US women at a rate of one in eight cases [34,35]. In 2012, approximately 522,000 deaths were due to breast cancer [36]. Despite the success of emergent breast cancer therapeutics in decreasing mortality cases, the prognosis, in particular for the stage IV cancer, remains poor and needs further improvement [37]. The presence of small populations of cells with unique tumor recurrence and metastases represents a serious challenge during cancer therapy, and may be ascribed to the presence of a small population of specialized malignant cells, which are believed to be cancer stem cells (CSCs) [38,39].

In 2003, Al-Hajj et al. discovered the presence of CSCs in breast cancer [40]. They carried out fluorescence-activated cell sorting (FACS) analyses of primary breast cancer cells for the expression of the following markers, cluster of differentiation 44 (CD44), cluster of differentiation 24 (CD24), and epithelial specific antigen (ESA). They confirmed that CD44$^+$ CD24$^{-/low}$ cells possess the same characteristic features of CSCs, including self-renewal, differentiation, and high tumor induction properties [40].

## 4. Therapeutic Approaches to Breast Cancer and Development of Resistance

The main approaches for the treatment of breast cancer are surgical intervention, hormonal therapy, immunotherapy, chemotherapy, and radiotherapy. However, the recovery rate after application of these conventional methods is about 60%–80% for primary cancers and about 50% for metastatic ones [41,42].

Previously, the heterogenic features of cancer were calibrated, based on the following parameters: histological analysis, tumor grading, condition of lymph nodes, and specific markers, such as estrogen receptor (ER), progesterone receptor (PR), and, recently, human epidermal growth factor receptor 2 (HER2) [43]. Furthermore, tumor heterogeneity was verified using gene expression analysis and cDNA microarrays analysis [44].

There are four fundamental groups of patients with metastatic breast cancer that are subjected to treatment, including hormone receptor (HR)-positive patients, who are classified into two classes: luminal A type, with the highest invasiveness and the best prognosis, which is characterized by ER+, PR+, HER2−, and low ki67, and luminal B, which is characterized by ER+, PR+, HER2+ or HER2−, and high ki67 [45,46]. HR+ breast cancers have the best prognosis and can be treated with tamoxifen, an ER antagonist, fulvestrant, which directly hampers ER synthesis, and aromatase inhibitors, namely, anastrozole, exemestane, and letrozole [47].

HER2+, another subtype of metastatic breast cancer, is an ER− breast cancer, and, therefore, is considered to be from the worst aggressive type of breast cancer [48,49]. To eliminate this type of cancer, various therapeutic strategies have been developed, such as a drug targeting HER2 receptor using humanized monoclonal antibodies, including trastuzumab (herceptin), pertuzumab, and lapatinib [49].

Triple-negative breast cancer (TNBC), voided of ER, PR, and HER2, is considered the worst type of metastatic breast cancer and has highly invasive proportion, a large tumor size, poor prognosis, a high chance to relapse, is not responsive to hormonal therapy, and has lymph node involvement. There are several approaches to counteract TNBC, such as neoadjuvant chemotherapy, anthracyclines, taxanes, poly (ADP-ribose) polymerase protein (PARP) inhibitors, epidermal growth factor receptor (EGFR) inhibitors, and platinum-containing chemotherapeutic agents [50–52].

Chemotherapy remains a crucial approach for cancer management in all patient groups. However, HER2-positive tumor patients, and patients with TNBC, need endocrine therapy in addition to chemotherapy [53]. Taken together, new, alternative therapeutics, in particular, natural products, need to be explored using mammosphere culture in order to overcome this problem.

## 5. Overview on Polyphenols

Polyphenols, a broad category of natural compounds and plant metabolites, possess one, or numerous, benzene rings that bear one, or several, hydroxyl groups. They are considered to be complicated antioxidants that are abundantly present in our daily diet, in particular, they can be found in fruits, legumes, spices, cocoa, vegetable, coffee, nuts, beer, wine, and olive oil [54]. Average daily consumption of polyphenols is estimated to be around one gram [55]. In nature, polyphenols generally exist conjugated with organic acids and sugars, and, accordingly, can be classified into two main categories; flavonoids and non-flavonoids, as shown in Figure 2.

The flavonoid category consists of two benzene rings, linked by a heterocyclic pyrone C-ring, and the non-flavonoid category contains more complicated molecules (benzoic acid, hydroxycinnamates, stilbenes, lignans, gallic acids tannins, and gallotannins) [56,57].

Polyphenols have been reported to possess special activities that are beneficial for human health, such as anti-oxidant [58], anti-infection [59–61], anti-cancer [62,63], neuroprotective [64], and anti-inflammatory [65] effects. Their broad activity could be attributed to several mechanisms, including interaction with, as well as modulation of, a wide range of proteins, enzymes, and membrane receptors, regulation of gene expression, apoptosis induction, vasodilatation, and modulation of cell signaling pathways [66–70].

There are similarities between some groups of flavonoids, such as isoflavones and lignans, and the estrogens, and, accordingly, they are considered as a phytoestrogen. Their anti-estrogenic activity has been exploited and applied in a wide range of studies [71]. Especially, the potent anti-cancer activity of polyphenols can be ascribed to their targeting of aromatase, antioxidant mechanisms, anti-inflammatory mechanisms, and anti-estrogenic mechanisms [72–76].

Flavonoids are considered to be the largest category of the polyphenols, and are characterized by their low molecular weight [77,78]. The structural characteristics of flavonoids can determine their functions and bioavailability, and can be used for classification into various groups.

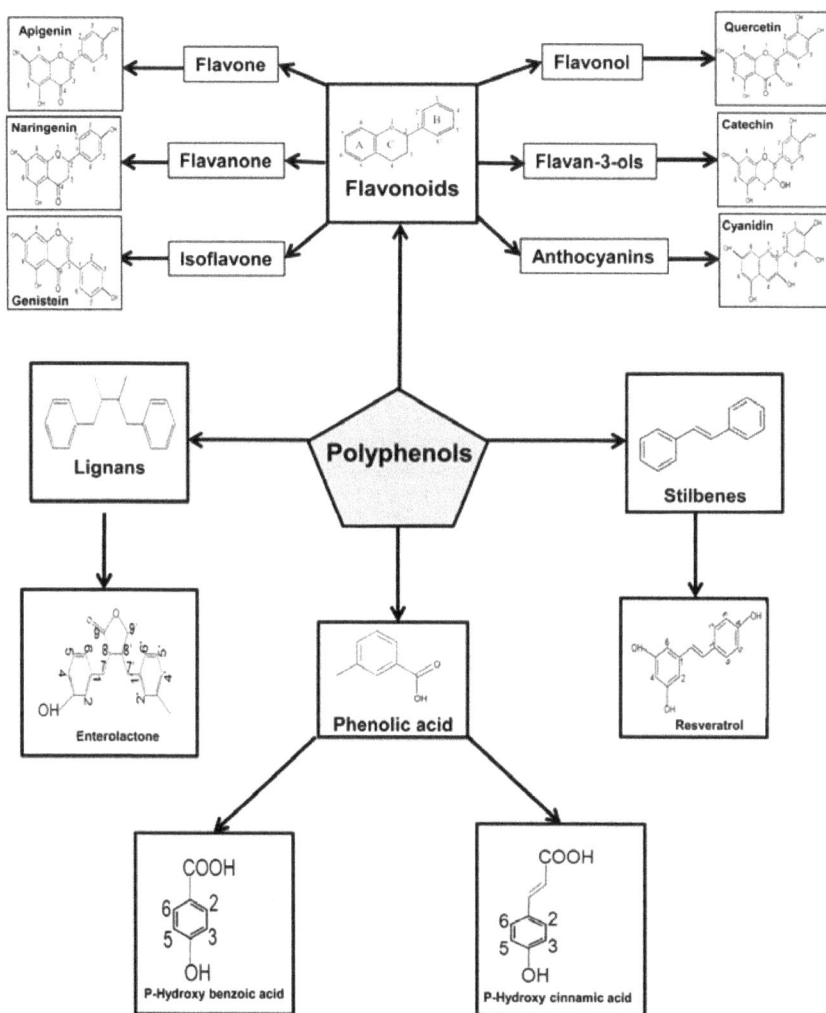

**Figure 2.** Diagram summarizing the classes of polyphenols and their basic chemical structures. Polyphenols can be separated into two main classes: flavonoids and non-flavonoids. The flavonoid class consists of two benzene rings, linked by a heterocyclic pyrone C-ring. The non-flavonoids class contains more intricate molecules, namely, benzoic acid, hydroxycinnamates, stilbenes, lignans, gallic acids tannins, and gallotannins.

The basic structure of flavonoids consists of a flavan nucleus (2-phenylchroman) containing 15 atoms that constitute three rings (A-ring (C6), B-ring (C6), and C-ring (C3)). The variation among flavonoids depends on the following: changes in the C-ring (presence of the 3-hydroxyl group, and double bond or 4-oxo group) and changes in the A- and B-rings, such as the difference in the number and the position of the hydroxyl and methoxyl groups. If one or more sugar group binds to the flavonoid structure, they are called "flavonoid glycosides", whereas flavonoids without a sugar group are described as "aglycones".

Dietary flavonoids are mainly "flavonoids glycosides", except for flavanols. Moreover, our research group revealed various aspects of the biological activities and health benefits of numerous flavonoids, such as antioxidant, antiviral, and anti-cancer properties, which were evidenced in vitro and in vivo [79–84].

Polyphenols are considered the main natural antioxidant component in fruits, vegetables, tea, oils, and cereals. The wide range of health benefits of dietary polyphenols is ascribed to their potential in reducing the risk, as well as preventing, serious diseases, such as cancer, metabolic diseases, neurodegenerative diseases, and heart diseases, which threaten human life and negatively affect quality of life, as summarized in Figure 3 [85].

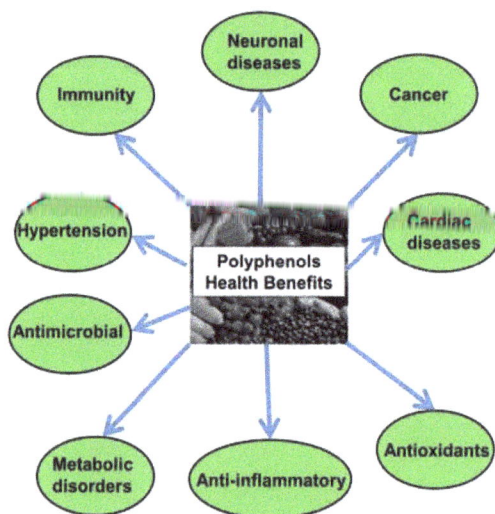

**Figure 3.** Overview summarizing the main health benefits of polyphenols. Polyphenols play key roles in the prevention of serious diseases that threaten human life and negatively affect quality of life, such as cancer, metabolic diseases, neurodegenerative diseases, hypertension, and cardiac diseases.

There is a large body of literature that describes the impact of polyphenols on human health and disease prevention [86,87]. Polyphenols are present in foods as intricate combinations of various chemical formulations of several polyphenol compounds, such as oligomers, chlorogenic acid, hydroxycinnamic acids, and epicatechin (in apples) [88]. Moreover, these dietary polyphenols are present in combination with sugar residues that conjugate with hydroxyl groups and aromatic carbons, can be combined with organic and carboxylic acids, and with amines [89]. In cereals, polyphenols are conjugated with polysaccharides of the cell wall [90], and in fruits, the amount of conjugated polyphenols is much higher than the amount of free polyphenols [91].

The absorption rate and site of polyphenols are modulated by their structures [92]. For instance, glycosides can be absorbed in the small intestine, except for glycosides that link to the rhamnose group metabolized by the enzyme, $\alpha$-rhamnosidase, which is secreted by microflora in the colon [93]. Glycosides can be metabolized by several enzymes, including cytosolic $\beta$-glucosidase and the membrane-located lactase phlorizin hydrolase [94,95].

On the other hand, the acylated polyphenol compounds, flavan-3-ols (epicatechin), are absorbed directly into the enterocyte without hydrolysis [96]. Hydroxycinnamic acids, which are esterified with organic acids, lipids, and sugar, are partially absorbed in the small intestine, and a major portion is metabolized by colonic microflora. The colon is considered a suitable site for the absorption of polymeric proanthocyanidins.

## 6. Correlation between Polyphenols' Anti-Cancer Activity and Autophagy

Autophagy is a cellular phenomenon that occurs as a response reaction against stress factors, such as starvation, oxidative stress, and toxicity [97]. During the autophagy process, catabolic lysosomal degradation takes place in order to maintain cellular homeostasis.

Autophagy-related genes (ATG) and their proteins are essential for the formation of the double-membrane vesicles needed for the engulfment of damaged cellular organelles in the cytosol. Beclin-1 (Atg6 in yeast), which is located on human chromosome 17q21, is considered one of the key components of ATG proteins. It exhibits haploinsufficiency, and its identification may have unveiled a crosslink between autophagy and human cancer. Its monoallelic deletion has been detected in breast, ovary, and prostate cancers [98,99].

The crosslink between diet and autophagy is well-known, and dietary restriction or starvation are related to autophagy induction and influence on health [100,101]. Autophagy induction is modulated by the level of cellular ATP and energy, which are detected by the cellular energy sensor, adenosine monophosphate kinase (AMPK). AMPK activation is enhanced as a response to the low ratio of ATP/AMP and nutrient deprivation via its upstream kinase, liver kinase BQ (LKB1 kinase). AMPK inhibits the activity of the mammalian target of rapamycin 1 (mTORC1) directly via phosphorylation of RAPTOR, or indirectly through activation of TSC1/2, which enhance the activity of GTP-Rheb [102,103]. Inactivated mTOR is involved in autophagy induction via activation of complexes, including ULK1, Atg13, and the FAK-family interacting protein of 200 kDa (FIP200) [104].

Below, we will discuss examples of polyphenols, and how autophagy signaling pathways and transcription factors are involved in their anti-cancer potentials, as summarized in Figure 4.

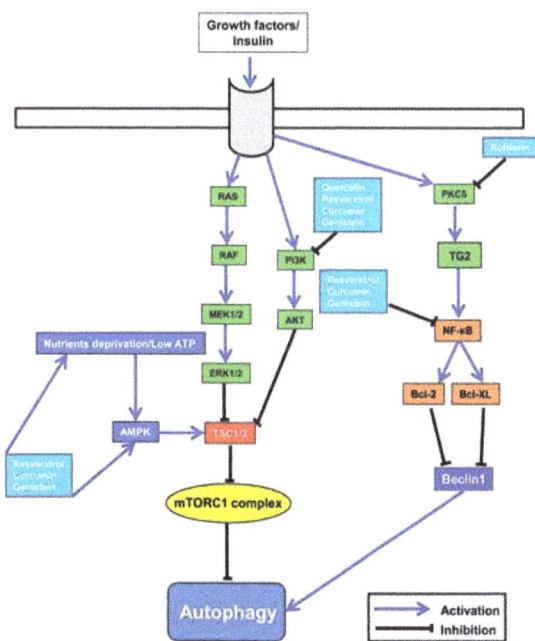

**Figure 4.** Role of polyphenols in the modulation of autophagy in breast cancer. Polyphenols modulate the autophagy process by regulating various signaling pathways, such as the PI3K/AKT, RAS/RAF/ERK, PKCδ, and AMPK signaling pathways.

## 6.1. Resveratrol

Resveratrol (3,4′,5-trihydroxy-trans-stilbene), the main polyphenol in grapes and peanuts, exists in red wine at a concentration of about 0.1–1.8 g per 100 mL. In mice, resveratrol potently mitigates the harmful consequences of a high-fat diet that influences longevity and lifespan [105]. This lifespan-increasing effect is attributed to the activation of sirtuin (SIRT1) via an autophagy-mediated mechanism [106]. The crosslink between SIRT1 and autophagy is attributed to the potency of SIRT1 to deacetylate the core elements, such as Atg5, Atg7, and Atg8, of autophagy induction [107]. Resveratrol is a well-known polyphenol modulating SIRT1 [108]. The anti-cancer activity of resveratrol has been proven in vitro and in vivo [109–111], and is mediated by numerous mechanisms, such as apoptosis, cell cycle arrest, kinase signaling pathways, and autophagy [109,112].

The implication of resveratrol in the induction of autophagy via the accumulation of autophagosomes has been proved in various cell lines [109,113,114]; however, resveratrol treatment induces non-canonical autophagy, which is independent of Beclin-1, vacuolar protein sorting 34 (Vps34), and Atg-dependent autophagy in breast cancer cells [115].

Apoptosis-resistant cell lines, such as breast cancer MCF-7 cells, which are deficient in caspase-3, showed sensitivity to resveratrol treatment, and, interestingly, activation of caspase-9, as well as chromatin condensation, were detected in resveratrol-treated MCF-7 cells [116].

Recently, FoxO transcription factors have been shown to play an important role in apoptosis and autophagy induced by resveratrol treatment [117]. In human colorectal cancer, resveratrol induced cell death was abolished upon genetic inhibition of the function of autophagy-related proteins, including PI3K, Lamp2b, and Beclin1 [113]. In human epidermoid carcinoma cells, exposure to resveratrol led to a decrease in the expression level of Rictor protein, and of mTORC2, and ultimately a reduction of RhoA-GTPase [118].

Reactive oxygen species (ROS) mediate the significant up-regulation of AMPK upon resveratrol treatment in etoposide-resistant HT-29 colon cancer cells, and, in turn, augment the potential of etoposide to induce apoptosis [119]. In addition, resveratrol exposure increased ROS generation and cleavage of caspase-8 and caspase-9, and ultimately induced autophagy via up-regulation of microtubule-associated protein 1 light chain 3-II (LC3-II) expression in colon cancer [120].

Resveratrol leads to autophagy induction via the up-regulation of p62/sequestome-1 (SQSTM1), and AMPK/mTOR-mediated, by JNK in imatinib-sensitive and imatinib-resistant chronic myelogenous leukemia cells (CML) K562 [121].

## 6.2. Silibinin

Silibinin, which is a flavonolignan extracted from milk thistle (*Silybum marianum*), possesses protective effects for the liver [122] and neurons [123,124]. Recently, the anti-cancer activity of silibinin has been demonstrated in vitro and in vivo [125–127]. In human colon cancer cells, silibinin treatment led to activation of the extrinsic (receptor-related) and intrinsic (mitochondria-related) apoptosis pathways, as well as activation of the autophagic process [128]. Pharmacological inhibition of autophagy with treatment of bafilomycin-A1 (Baf-A1) in silibinin-exposed human colon cancer cells resulted in autophagy inhibition, which is accompanied by activation of cell death. Accordingly, silibinin treatment of human cancer cells induced cytoprotective autophagy, and ROS was a mediator in silibinin-induced apoptosis and autophagy in tumor cells [129,130]. On the other hand, the ROS-scavenging activity of silibinin was also shown in vitro and in vivo [123,131].

An interesting study demonstrated the potential of silibinin to induce autophagic cell death in breast cancer cells. This effect was confirmed by high expression of LC3-II, increase of Beclin-1, high Atg-12-Atg-5, and down-regulation of Bcl-2 [132]. Upon treatment with pharmacological inhibitors of autophagy, 3-methyladenine (3-MA) and Baf-A1, silibinin-induced breast cancer cell death was mitigated. Silibinin treatment led to ROS generation, which was correlated with the disruption of mitochondrial membrane potential and ATP depletion, which were further blocked by treatment of *N*-acetyl cysteine (NAC) and ascorbic acid [132].

Of note, silibinin-exposed breast cancer cells showed up-regulation of Bcl-2 adenovirus E1B 19-kDa-interacting protein 3 (BNIP3). Small interfering RNA (siRNA) targeting BNIP3 abrogated silibinin-induced cell death, ROS generation, ATP depletion, and the disruption of mitochondrial membrane potential [132].

Silibinin-induced autophagy and apoptosis in MCF-7 cells are concomitant with the down-regulation of AKT, mTOR, and ERK [133]. Co-treatment of ERα antagonist, methyl-piperidinopyrazole (MPP) dihydrochloride, with silibinin led to the aggravation of the apoptosis and autophagy induced by silibinin treatment. These results indicate that ERα inhibition by silibinin mediates the down-regulation of AKT, mTOR, and ERK, and the final induction of apoptosis and autophagy in MCF-7 cells [133].

## 6.3. Quercetin

Quercetin (3,3′,4′,5,7-pentahydroxyflavanone), a flavonol, exists in a wide range of fruits and vegetables, such as onions, apples, and berries, and is considered one of the most common antioxidants in the human diet [134]. The application of quercetin to inhibit tyrosine kinase has been approved for clinical trials [135]. The anti-cancer potential of quercetin has been shown in various in vitro and in vivo studies [136–139]. Down-regulation of mTOR activity, and the subsequent formation of autophagosomes by quercetin treatment, have been evidenced [140].

In gastric cancer cells, quercetin induced cytoprotective autophagy that was abrogated upon treatment with the lysosomal inhibitor, chloroquine, or silencing of Atg5 or Beclin-1 using siRNA, and led to apoptotic cell death [141].

Hypoxia-induced factor 1α (HIF-1α) and Akt-mTOR signaling pathways are mediators of quercetin-induced cytoprotective autophagy. The components of the mTOR signaling pathway, in particular, mTORC1, play key roles in the maintenance of cellular homeostasis via modulation of protein synthesis through p70S6 kinase, which activates the ribosomal S6 subunit, and phosphorylation of 4E-BP1 (eIF4E binding protein 1) that inhibits the sequestration of the eukaryotic initiation factor of protein biosynthesis (eIF4). In various cancer cell lines, quercetin modulates the mTOR signaling pathway through down-regulation of the phosphorylation level of the ribosomal S6 subunit via p70S6 kinase, as well as via activation of 4E-BP1 [140].

## 6.4. Genistein

Genistein (4′,5,7-trihydroxyisoflavone), an isoflavone, is widely distributed in soybean and presents a broad spectrum of in vitro and in vivo anti-cancer potential in numerous cancer cells, through cell cycle arrest, induction of apoptosis, blocking of angiogenesis, inhibition of telomerase activity, and blocking inhibition of DNA topoisomerase II [142–145].

In ovarian cancer cells, genistein treatment led to cell death, which is independent of caspase signaling pathways and induced autophagy [146]. The autophagy induced by genistein treatment can be recovered upon treatment with methyl pyruvate, the substrate for oxidative phosphorylation and fatty acid synthesis.

Genistein-exposed ovarian cancer cells showed a marked reduction in glucose uptake that may be attributed to the inactivation of AKT signaling [146]. Inhibition of the aggregate that is formed by the interaction between cyclic AMP phosphodiesterase-4A4 (PDE4A4) and SQSTM1 protein (p62) is essential for the induction of autophagy. This can be explained by the role of SQSTM1 protein in interacting with LC3, which has a pivotal role in vesicle formation in autophagosomes [147]. Genistein-treated ovarian cancer cells showed marked autophagy due to inhibition of the formation of PDE4A4 and SQSTM1 aggregates, activated by ERK and PKC inhibitors [148].

## 6.5. Curcumin

Curcumin, diferuloylmethane extracted from *Curcuma longa*, is the key constituent of turmeric, and possesses various biological functions with minimal toxicity, such as antioxidant, anti-inflammatory, and anti-cancer functions [149,150]. In malignant glioma cells, curcumin exposure led to cell cycle arrest and autophagy induction through up-regulation of the ERK1/2 signaling pathways and down-regulation of the Akt/mTOR/p70S6K signaling pathways [151]. In bladder cancer cells, curcumin dephosphorylated AKT, and, in turn, activated LC3-II [152].

The autophagy-inducing capacity of curcumin was exploited in cellular protection against oxidative stress-induced cell death in human umbilical vein endothelial cells. This was mediated by modulation of the autophagy machinery, including activation of LC3-II, inhibition of PI3K/Akt/mTOR core signaling, and promotion of FOXO1 (autophagy mediator) [153]. In curcumin-exposed human colon cancer cells, there was a significant increase in the conversion of LC3-I to LC3-II, as well as degradation of SQSTM1 [154]. These effects were markedly abrogated after treatment with an ROS scavenging compound, NAC, indicating that ROS is a mediator of curcumin-induced autophagosome formation and cell death [154].

In malignant glioma cells, curcumin treatment induced autophagy that is attributed to the up-regulation of ERK signaling, which is concomitant with the down-regulation of the Akt/mTOR/p70 ribosomal protein S6 kinase (p70S6K) pathway [155]. Moreover, SIRT1 was modulated by curcumin in the regulation of autophagy and other cellular events [108].

Curcumin remarkably enhanced the expression of AMPK, accompanied by p38 signaling-mediated cell death in ovarian cancer cells [156]. Similarly, curcumin induced ROS generation at the beginning of apoptosis and autophagy in oral squamous cell carcinoma, and NAC treatment abolished curcumin modulated autophagosome formation [157]. In addition to the induction of autophagy, curcumin exposure led to apoptosis via inactivation of Bcl-2 protein and down regulation of NF-κB in cancer cells [158,159].

### 6.6. Rottlerin

Rottlerin, also called mallotoxin, is one of the active components of the Kamala tree (*Mallotus philippensis*), which grows widely in Southeast Asia. In 1994, the pharmacological effects of rottlerin were revealed, after its potential to specifically inhibit the activity of protein kinase C delta (PKCδ) was demonstrated [160]. Therefore, the potency of rottlerin to block PKCδ activity has been exploited in various biological functions related to PKCδ [161].

Recently, rottlerin was shown to exhibit various biological activities, including human T-cell response inhibition [162], potassium channel activation [163], in vitro and in vivo neuroprotection [164], antioxidant activity [165], antihistaminic activity [166], and anti-cancer activity [167]. The crosslink between tissue transglutaminase (TG2) and NF-κB was evidenced [168]. Moreover, implication of NF-κB in the autophagy process was proven [169].

In pancreatic cancer cells, rottlerin, as well as PKCδ siRNA treatment, led to a drastic decrease in cell proliferation, which was accompanied by a significant reduction in mRNA and protein levels of TG2, without showing any apoptotic changes [170]. However, rottlerin-treated pancreatic cancer cells showed significant autophagy, which was evidenced by cytoplasmic acidic vacuoles and the up-regulation of LC3-II, similar to that of TG2-specific siRNA-treated cells. Belin-1 knockdown abrogated the potential of rottlerin and TG2 siRNA to induce autophagy in pancreatic cancer cells.

In human pancreatic CSCs, rottlerin treatment led to early autophagy, evidenced by the formation of autophagosomes, LC3-II formation, up-regulation of Atg7 and Beclin-1, as well as down-regulation of the pro-apoptotic proteins, Bcl-2 and Bcl-$X_L$ [171]. Treatment of 3-MA or genetic inhibition of autophagy via silencing of the autophagy-specific genes, Atg7 and Beclin-1, blocked the potential of rottlerin to induce autophagy and enhanced rottlerin-induced apoptosis [171].

In human breast cancer cells, rottlerin treatment showed TSC2-dependent inhibition of the mTORC1 signaling pathway and the accumulation of autophagosomes as a consequence [172]. Taken together, we described the mechanisms of polyphenols in autophagy modulation in terms of their anti-cancer functions. However, these findings need to be scrutinized in depth with respect to breast cancer and in vivo using animal models that possess genetic modifications of autophagy-related genes.

## 7. Anti-Cancer Activity of Polyphenols against Breast Cancer: Molecular Mechanisms

The anti-cancer activities of polyphenols against a wide range of cancers, such as breast cancer [173], prostate cancer [174], colorectal cancer [175], pancreatic cancer, lung cancer, colorectal fibrosarcoma, and leukemia, have been proven [176]. The possible mechanisms underlying the anticancer activity of polyphenols against breast cancer are summarized in Figure 5, and the possible molecular mechanisms by which polyphenols kill breast cancer are described below.

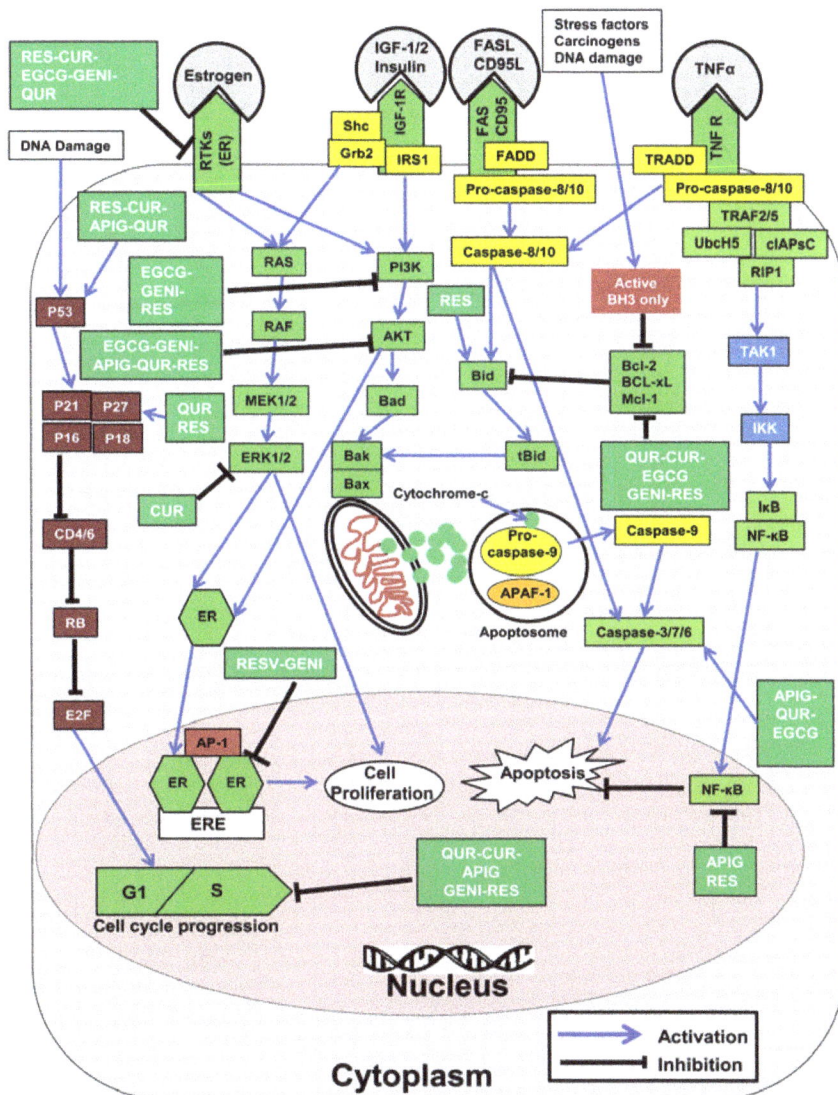

**Figure 5.** Comprehensive representation summarizing the possible mechanisms of action of polyphenols against breast cancer. The anti-cancer activity of polyphenols is mediated via the regulation of various signaling pathways, such as intrinsic and extrinsic apoptotic pathways, estrogen-related signaling pathways, cell cycle arrest, and inflammation-related signaling pathways. RES, resveratrol; CUR, curcumin; GENI, genistein; QUR, quercetin; APIG, apigenin.

### 7.1. Modulation of ROS

In fruits, polyphenols represent a major portion of the antioxidants compared to vitamin C [177]. Antioxidant activity is one of the key mechanisms that contribute to the protective effect of polyphenols against oxidative damage.

Cellular redox balance can be maintained by cellular antioxidant enzymes, including superoxide dismutase (SOD), peroxiredoxins (PRXs), catalase (CAT), glutathione peroxidase (GPx), and glutathione reductase (GR) [178]. However, mitigation of excessive generation of ROS by the cellular antioxidant enzymes is difficult [179].

Polyphenols are directly involved in the reduction of the Fenton reaction, via chelation of iron, thereby protecting cells from oxidation from highly reactive hydroxyl radicals [180–182]. The potent antioxidant activity of polyphenols is attributed to their ability to scavenge a broad spectrum of highly reactive species, such as ROS, reactive nitrogen species (NOS), chlorine species, peroxynitrous acid (ONOOH), and hypochlorous acid (HOCl) [183]; they also block the chain reactions of lipid peroxidation (chain breakers) as a consequence [180,184]. The antioxidant activity of flavonoid compounds is also mediated by targeting NFκB- and MAPK-related signaling pathways [185]. Polyphenols can work as co-antioxidants, as they show synergistic activity with other antioxidants, such as α-tocopherol (vitamin E), leading to the regeneration of vitamin E [186].

The polyphenols structures, such as the hydroxyl group's number and position, hydroxylation degree, and distance between the aromatic ring and the carbonyl group, play a pivotal role in its antioxidant activity and metal chelating property. For instance, within the flavonol group, quercetin showed the most potent antioxidant activity due to its 3-hydroxy group [187]. Additionally, polyphenol potential for metal chelation and scavenging of free radicals could be elevated with a B-ring bearing catechol moiety, C-ring bearing 4-oxo group, and the presence of a double bond [188].

Cinnamic acid and its derivatives showed relatively better antioxidant properties compared to benzoic acid, due to the longer distance between the aromatic ring and the carbonyl group. Additionally, the presence of the hydroxyl group at the para and/or ortho position on the benzoic ring enhances antioxidant potential compared to the presence of the hydroxyl group at other positions [189].

Biochanin A, an isoflavonoid purified from red clover (*Trifolium pratense*) showed preventive activity against the incidence of mammary gland cancer, after exposure to carcinogenic agents in prepubertal rat [190]. It potentially counteracted oxidative stress through a significant up-regulation of SOD, CAT, GPx, GST, and DT-diaphorase (DTD), as well as a remarkable reduction of lactate dehydrogenase (LDH) and lipid peroxidation (LPO) activities.

The protective action of resveratrol against 17β-estradiol (E2)-induced carcinogenesis was evidenced in vitro and in vivo, and was mediated by a significant increase in the expression of nuclear factor erythroid-related factor-2 (Nrf-2), which consequently up-regulated the expression of antioxidant genes, including NQO1, SOD3, and 8-oxoguanine DNA glycosylase 1 (OGG1) [191].

Green tea is composed of four main catechins, (−)-epicatechin (EC), (−)-epicatechin gallate (ECG), (−)-epigallocatechin (EGC), and (−)-epigallocatechin-3-gallate (EGCG). EGCG, the most abundant polyphenolic catechin, is considered the most active catechin, possessing various biological functions in vitro and in vivo [15,192]. Low concentrations of EGCG resulted in significant reduction in ROS generation, which was induced on exposure to environmental carcinogens [193]. However, it had no significant effect on the regulation of the antioxidant enzymes (SOD and CAT) in MCF-7 breast cancer cell lines, but showed up-regulated expression of NQO1, the main detoxification enzyme of phase II [193].

Genistein showed significant antioxidant action and better mitochondrial function in T47D with low ERα/ERβ ratios, whereas no significant antioxidant effect was shown in MCF-7 cells with high ERα/ERβ ratios [194]. Therefore, ERβ is essential for the antioxidant potential of genistein [194].

Curcumin-treated breast cancer cells showed a significant decrease in cell proliferation, mediated by Nrf-2 nuclear translocation, associated with the down-regulation of Flap endonuclease 1

(Fen1), which is a nuclease involved in DNA repair [195]. It also showed ROS scavenging actions in MCF-7 breast cancer cells exposed to nickel oxide nanoparticles [196].

On the other hand, polyphenols presented a pro-oxidant action that was determined by the application of high concentrations, or the presence of, metal ions that mediate the formation of chelates and the oxidation of polyphenols [197–199]. The pro-oxidant effects of polyphenols are involved in their anti-cancer activity. For example, the pro-oxidant activity of polyphenols was correlated with mitochondrial dysfunction and DNA damage mediated by high oxidative stress, and, in turn, resulted in apoptosis [200,201]. In breast cancer cells, 50 µM of soy isoflavone, genistein, showed a pro-oxidant action via mobilization of copper ions that led to DNA damage, an increase in ROS generation, and apoptosis [202]. The pro-oxidant effect of curcumin via ROS generation, in a time-dependent manner, in MCF-7 and MDA-MB-231 breast cancer cell lines, was demonstrated [203]. Additionally, high concentration of EGCG showed a marked increase in ROS generation in Hs578T breast cancer cells [204]. In vivo studies are needed to confirm, as well as explain, the contradictory findings of the antioxidant and the pro-oxidant effects of polyphenols.

## 7.2. Modulation of Inflammation-Related Factors

Cancer occurs at sites of chronic inflammation, and is proved by the presence of inflammatory cells in cancer [205]. For instance, inflammatory responses from microbial infection represent 15%–20% of cancer death cases worldwide [205], and, therefore, non-steroidal, anti-inflammatory drugs are one option to mitigate cancer deaths arising from inflammatory responses [206,207]. Chronic inflammation can give rise to an aggressive type of breast cancer, inflammatory breast cancer (IBC), which represents 5% of breast cancers and is associated with 8%–10% of breast cancer deaths [208,209].

Polyphenols from blueberry powder present potent in vitro and in vivo inhibitory properties against breast cancer proliferation and metastasis by regulation of interlukin-6 (IL-6) [210]. Polyphenol-enriched blueberry preparation (PEBP) potently inhibited breast cancer proliferation, cell movement, and migration, by targeting inflammatory signaling cascades, including the ERK, AKT, and STAT3 pathways [211]. In this regard, the anti-inflammatory activity of polyphenols may be important mechanisms underlying their anti-cancer and chemopreventive potentials. The anti-inflammatory activity of polyphenols is attributed to their ability to block properties against NF-κB [212], cyclooxygenase (COX-2) [213], and lipoxygenase (LOX) [214] activities.

NF-κB plays a pivotal role in the control of the expression level of inflammation-related cytokines, TNFα and IL-1 [215], as well as up-regulation of COX-2, which is an inducible prostaglandin G/H synthase that is highly expressed in numerous tumor cells [216]. The possible mechanisms by which dietary polyphenols block the up-regulation of NF-κB involve the inhibition of phosphorylation and/or proteasomal degradation of IκBs, inhibition of the liberation of NF-κB dimers from the cytoplasm into the nucleus, and hampering the interaction between NF-κB and target DNA [217,218]. Curcumin [219], green tea rich polyphenols [220], quercetin [221], and resveratrol [222] showed potent anti-cancer activities by blocking the expression level of NF-κB.

The potential of curcumin to inhibit cancer metastasis has been confirmed in vitro using breast cancer cells, as well as in vivo, using immunodeficient mice. In this study, the authors showed the crosslink between curcumin and the inhibition of the expression level of MMPs via down-regulation of the expression level of NF-κB and transcription factor AP-1, as well as inhibition of the phosphorylation of NF-κB, in turn, reducing the phosphorylation of IκB and p65 [223]. The anti-metastatic action of curcumin in breast cancer cells is explained by its inhibition of the nuclear translocation of NF-κB via dephosphorylation of IκB, resulting in the down-regulation of inflammation-related cytokines, such as CXCL1/2 [224].

Green tea catechin, EGCG, stimulated apoptosis in γ-radiation-exposed breast cancer cells, and was associated with the inactivation of NF-κB [225]. Combined treatment with EGCG and curcumin potently reduced the expression of the BCSC marker, CD44, via dephosphorylation of

STAT3, and, in turn, prevented its nuclear translocation and its interaction with NF-κB for activation of target transcription factors [226].

The activation of STAT3 is essential for the proliferation and metastasis of a wide range of cancer, and its high expression is indicative of a poor prognosis. Targeting the STAT3 pathway is considered one of the key therapeutic approaches to block cancer proliferation and metastasis [227,228]. The inhibitory activity of silibinin against the phosphorylation of STAT3 has been demonstrated in preclinical studies in various cancers [229]; however, further clinical trials are needed to fully characterize silibinin activity as a STAT3 inhibitor.

In nude mice inoculated with MCF-7 cells, oral administration of xanthohumol, a prenylated flavonoid that was purified from hops (*Humulus lupulus* L.), resulted in a significant reduction in infiltration of mononuclear and polymorphonuclear inflammatory cells, an increase in the percentage of apoptosis, a reduction in the density of microvessels, and a decrease in nuclear and cytoplasmic NF-κβ expression and cytoplasmic staining of Pi-Iκβα, compared to tumors in untreated control mice [230].

### 7.3. Modulation of the Estrogen Receptor

Estrogens are a commonly-listed human carcinogen, and high exposure to estrogen is highly related to the incidence of breast cancer via increased cell proliferation through interaction with ER [231]. Patients with breast cancer show a high level of estrogen in the circulating blood [232]. Simply, breast cancer could be treated by inhibition of this action, as well as the production of estrogens, or interference, in the binding to ER [233,234]. ER targeting can be performed using classical drugs, such as raloxifene and tamoxifen, which are collectively called selective estrogen receptor modulators (SERMs) and are effectively applied in pre-and post-menopausal women [235].

Two types of ER, ERα and ERβ, are differentially expressed in organs, and ERα is highly expressed in the uterus and is involved in the proliferation of the endometrium, whereas ERβ is abundant in mammary glands, ovary, and the hypothalamus [236]. ERβ was involved in the induction of various transcription factors that are related to the modulation of cell proliferation and death, the cell cycle, and differentiation [237,238].

Owing to the similarity in the structure of non-steroidal compounds or phytoestrogens and E2, several phytoestrogens were shown to bind to ERα and ERβ. The binding affinity of genistein to ERβ is about 7–48-fold higher than to ERα [239–241]. In contrast, a flavonoid, xanthohumol, showed potent anti-cancer activity against luminal-type breast cancer by inhibiting the interaction between the growth of luminal-type guanine nucleotide-exchange protein 3 (BIG3) and tumor suppressor prohibitin 2 (PHB2) [242]. The released PHB2 binds to the nuclear and cytoplasmic ERα, and blocks E2-associated signaling pathways, thereby inhibiting the proliferation of ERα-positive breast cancer cells in vitro and in vivo.

The flavonoid compound, ellagic acid, which is widely distributed in berries, grapes, and nuts, possesses phenolic rings and ortho-dihydroxyl groups involved in the recognition of ER receptors [243]. Ellagic acid significantly reduced cancer size and occurrence in ACI rats exposed to estrogen with decreased CYP1A1 activity [244].

Similar to most flavones, including fisetin, apigenin, and kaempferol, morin (3,5,7,2′,4′-pentahydroxyflavone), a flavonol compound that is found in copious amounts in onion, mill (*Prunus dulcis*), and fig (*Chlorophora tinctoria*), showed strong inhibitory effects against oxidative stress [245]. Morin possesses hydroxyl groups in the 7- and 4′-positions, parallel to the 3- and 4′-positions, on synthetic estrogen diethylstilbestrol (DES), and is therefore considered a phytoestrogen [246].

Luteolin (3′,4′,5,7-tetrahydroxyflavone) potentially decreased the expression of insulin-like growth factor-1 (IGF-1), which correlated with MCF-7 proliferation. This effect was attributed to the capacity of luteolin to down-regulate ERα expression [247]. Knockdown of ERα led to the abolishment of the potency of luteolin to inhibit MCF-7 cell proliferation.

The chemical structure (2 hydroxyl groups and phenolic ring) of quercetin is akin to the structure of estrogen and it is considered a phytoestrogen that potentially binds to ER and modulates cell cycle progression. It also presents anti-cancer actions via estrogen-related pathways [248,249].

Resveratrol inhibits the growth of various breast cancer cells (MCF-7 and MBA-MB-231) via modulation of the expression level of various transcription factors associated with cell cycle regulation, apoptosis, metastasis, and angiogenesis. These actions were more pronounced in ER$^+$ cells than in ER$^-$ cells, assuring the importance of the binding to ER in the enhancement of the anti-cancer activity of resveratrol against breast cancer [250].

In ER$\alpha$-positive MCF-7 cell lines, the physiological dose of EGCG induced a significant reduction in cell growth, which was correlated with the reduction in the protein levels of ER$\alpha$ and IGF-1 receptor (IGF-1R), as well as the up-regulation of p53 and p21 [251]. Whereas, in ER$\alpha$-positive T47D cell lines expressing mutated p53, EGCG treatment had no significant inhibitory effects on cell growth; however, EGCG treatment enhanced the expression of ER$\alpha$, and increased the sensitivity of cells to treatment with an ER$\alpha$ antagonist, tamoxifen. Moreover, EGCG-exposed ER$\alpha$-negative MDA-MB-231 cell lines, expressing mutated p53, showed a marked decrease in cell growth and up-regulation of ER$\alpha$ and IGF-1R, which resulted in an increased responsiveness of the cell to tamoxifen treatment [251].

There are paradoxical findings on the effect of genistein on the proliferation of ER$^+$ and ER$^-$ breast cancer cells that are associated with concentration of genistein [252,253]. For instance, ER$^+$ and ER$^-$ breast cancer cells treated with a high concentration of genistein showed a significant reduction in growth rate, while lower concentrations enhanced their growth rate. Similarly, tamoxifen and SERMs showed controversial effects, which correlated with the applied concentration and the type of tissue [254].

Taken together, the application of phytoestrogens is intricate, due to the controversial effects attributed to variations in doses [255]. Therefore, further comprehensive research is needed to characterize the side effects of using these phytoestrogens, which may be beneficial for endocrine disorder-related public health in the future.

*7.4. Modulation of the Aromatase Activity*

Aromatase, an estrogen synthase, belongs to the cytochrome P450 enzyme family [256,257]. It is highly expressed in breast cancer tissue compared to normal breast tissue [232]. Aromatase inhibitors showed a better capacity for the treatment of breast cancer when compared to tamoxifen [258]. Aromatase stimulation is correlated with ER-independent malignancy [259]. The efficiency of various synthetic aromatase inhibitors in the clinical application of breast cancer treatment, in ER$^+$ patients at the postmenopausal stage, was demonstrated [260].

Owing to the similarity between the A and C rings of flavonoids with D and C rings of androstenedione, which is the substrate of aromatase, as well as to the potential of the C4 position's oxo-group to interact with the heme group of the aromatase, flavonoid compounds potently inhibit aromatase activity [261]. Flavones and isoflavones were reported to bind to estrogen receptors and to the active sites of the aromatase [262]. The potential of flavonoids to influence the promoter activity of aromatase was demonstrated [263,264], additionally their role in the regulation of breast cancer's aromatase expression has been proven [265].

Aromatase activity is markedly inhibited by luteolin [266], but is up-regulated by hesperetin (3′,5,7-trihydroxy-4-methoxyflavanone) [265]. The imidazolyl quinoline derivative of flavonoids, XHN27, a potent aromatase inhibitor, significantly suppresses the proliferation of breast cancer T47D cells, determined after screening a library of 7000 compounds [267].

*7.5. Modulation of the Cell Cycle*

During carcinogenesis, there is an imbalance between the action of cell cycle progression proteins and cell cycle arrest proteins, resulting in marked cell division and proliferation. Cell cycle progression can be mediated by cyclins and cyclin-dependent kinases (CDK), and its arrest is mediated by CDK inhibitors (CDKi), such as p15, p16, p21, p27, p53, and retinoblastoma tumor suppressor protein (RB). Loss of function of RB, a tumor suppressor gene, is involved in resistance to chemotherapeutic drugs, such as tamoxifen.

Numerous polyphenol-treated cancer cells showed down-regulation of CDK, as well as modulation of CDKi, consequently leading to cell cycle arrest and apoptosis at the G2/M phase [268,269]. In breast cancer cells, the synergy between E2 and IGF-1 is essential for cell cycle progression via up-regulation of Cdk2, Cdk4, and cyclin D1 [270].

In breast and colon cancer cells, ginnalins A–C polyphenols isolated from *Acer saccharum* Marsh. sugar and red maple (*Acer rubrum* L.) species showed remarkable anti-cancer activities via induction of cell cycle arrest, in particular, in the S- and $G_2$/M-phases, as well as down-regulation of cyclins A and D1 proteins [268].

The potency of quercetin-3-methyl ether was exploited to induce cell cycle arrest in the G2/M phase, and up-regulation of the phosphorylation level of cyclin B1 (Ser 147) to potently block the growth of breast cancer cells that are resistant or sensitive to lapatinib, a reversible inhibitor of EGFR and HER2 [271]. Therefore, quercetin-3-methyl ether is considered a naturally occurring polyphenol that overcomes the resistance against the common anti-breast-cancer drug, lapatinib. In addition, quercetin-exposed MDA-MB-453 breast cancer cells showed a marked increase in the number of cells in the G2/M phase and a reduction in cell populations in the G1 phase [100].

Quercetin led to down-regulation of cyclin A and cyclin B, and a significant up-regulation of CDK inhibitors, including p53, p21CIP1/waf1, and p27Kip1 [272,273]. As a part of its anti-cancer activities, resveratrol also resulted in the modulation of cell cycle and apoptosis [274].

Curcumin possesses anti-cancer activities via the modulation of apoptosis and the cell cycle [275]. Curcumin-treated human MCF-7 breast cancer cells showed a drastic reduction in proliferation, mediated by cell-cycle arrest in the $G_2$/M phase [275]. Curcumin treatment led to apoptotic cell death, which was confirmed by the detection of a high fraction of cells accumulated in the $G_0$/$G_1$ phase, as well as by the up-regulation of Bax through a p53-dependent mechanism [276]. It was evidenced that curcumin can induce the monopolar spindle formation, accumulation of mitotic arrest deficient 2 (Mad2), and Mad3/BubR1, thereby activating the mitotic checkpoint [277].

Apigenin (4',5,7-trihydroxyflavone), a flavone, significantly inhibited the proliferation of SK-BR-3 breast cancer cells through inhibition of cell cycle progression at the G2M phase, with the up-regulation of p21$^{Cip1}$, as well as down-regulation of CDK1 and cyclin A and B [278].

EGCG inhibited the division and growth of cancer cells via dephosphorylation of the myosin II regulatory light chain (MRLC), which is essential for contractile ring formation [279]. Consequently, EGCG-treated cells showed high percentages of cell population in the G2/M phase and a decrease in cell growth and division. Of note, EGCG-induced dephosphorylation of MRLC was attributed to its interaction with metastasis-associated 67 kDa laminin receptor (67LR) [279].

*7.6. Modulation of Apoptosis*

Apoptosis is a type of programmed cell death, which is essential for various physiological processes, such as homeostasis and development. Intrinsic or mitochondrial type apoptosis is modulated by the B cell lymphoma (Bcl-2) family proteins [280]. The extrinsic apoptotic pathway is activated by binding of death receptors with their ligands, such as binding of tumor necrosis factor receptor 1 (TNFR1) and tumor necrosis factor (TNF), and the recruitment of receptor-interacting protein (RIP), TNFR1-associated death domain protein (TRADD), and TNFR-associated factor (TRAF), or binding of death-inducing signaling complexes [280].

Apoptosis plays important roles in the potential of quercetin to inhibit the proliferation of human MDA-MB-453 breast cancer cells that are mediated by up-regulation of BAX and down-regulation of Bcl-2 expression, as well as cleavage of caspase-3 and PARP proteins [138]. Quercetin-exposed MCF-7 breast cancer cells showed apoptotic cell death with a reduction in mitochondrial membrane potential, down-regulation of Bcl-2 protein, and activation of the initiator caspases, caspase-8 and caspase-9, and the effector caspase, caspase-6, which were attributed to the binding of quercetin to the Fas/CD95 receptor [273]. Moreover, quercetin significantly inhibited MD-MBA-231 breast cancer cells through the activation of caspase-3/-8/-9 [281].

Apigenin-treated SK-BR-3 breast cancer cells showed apoptotic cell death, evidenced by the up-regulation of p53 and its downstream effectors, BAX and cytochrome c [278]. A recent study detected a dramatic decrease in cell proliferation, as well as significant stimulation of apoptosis signaling pathways, such as PARP cleavage and caspase-8 and -9 cleavages in apigenin-treated SKBR3 breast cancer cells [282]. This study concluded that STAT3 inhibition mediated apigenin-enhanced apoptosis signaling pathways in SKBR3 cells.

On treatment with green tea polyphenols and EGCG, a significant reduction in cell growth associated with apoptotic changes, such as stimulation of BAX, cleavage of PARP, and down-regulation of Bcl-2, was observed in MD-MB-231 human breast cancer cells [283].

Resveratrol treatment led to apoptotic cell death in T47D breast cancer cells via activation of CD95L, which is involved in the extrinsic apoptotic pathway [284], as well as activation of p53 [285]. PARP cleavage was significantly induced in resveratrol-treated MDA-MB-231 cells, and was correlated with the activation of caspase-3 [286]. Moreover, resveratrol induced apoptosis in various malignant cells (including MDA-MB-231 and MDA-MB-468 cell lines), via inhibition of Src tyrosine kinase activity and blockage of STAT3 activation [287]. In estrogen-positive breast cancer cells, resveratrol markedly reduced growth rate by stimulating apoptosis through reduction of the ratio of Bcl2/BAX, which was independent of the presence of E2 [288]. Therefore, resveratrol is considered a potential and safe chemopreventive alternative to hormone replacement therapy (HRT), in particular, in postmenopausal women, and against hormone-dependent breast cancer.

Genistein-exposed MCF-7 cells showed up-regulation of BAX and reduction of Bcl-2 at the protein and mRNA levels, resulting in a reduction in the Bcl-2/BAX ratio [289]. This effect is mediated by blocking the activation of the IGF receptor (IGFR), as well as the phosphorylation of AKT.

Fisetin (3,3',4',7-tetrahydroxyflavone), a flavonoid, which is widely distributed in fruits and vegetables, induced an uncommon form of apoptosis in caspase-voided MCF-7 cells characterized by the activation of caspase-7/-8/-9, cleaved PARP, mitochondrial membrane depolarization, up-regulation of p53, and break in the plasma membrane, while no change was detected in DNA or phosphatidylserine (PS) [290]. These apoptotic changes were abolished upon treatment with a pan-caspase inhibitor, z-VAD-fmk.

### 7.7. Modulation of the Multidrug Resistance (MDR)

Despite the potency of anti-cancer drugs in decreasing cancer size, a few populations of CSCs potently resist chemotherapy and lead to tumor recurrence and MDR [291]. The crosslink between the virulence of CSCs and MDR is correlated with reduction of intracellular concentrations of anti-cancer drugs, continual growth, and cancer relapse [292].

The emergence of MDR is linked to over-expression of the ATP-binding cassette (ABC) transporters family, which is composed of energy-dependent transporter proteins, which act as pumps. ABC transporters are involved in drug efflux, thereby decreasing in intracellular concentrations [293]. Transporter proteins include various proteins, such as multidrug resistant-associated proteins (MRPs), mitoxantrone resistance protein (MXR or ABCG2), and P-glycoprotein (P-gp) or ABCB1.

EGCG treatment leads to the accumulation of rhodamine-123 dye in MDR cell lines and an increase in the intracellular concentration of anti-cancer drugs [294]. Moreover, a group of six common polyphenols (naringenin, silymarin, daidzein, quercetin, resveratrol, and hesperetin) potently inhibit the activity of MRP family proteins, thereby inhibiting efflux [295].

Curcumin treatment leads to down-regulation of MDR-1b expression by its interaction with PI3K/AKT/NF-κB signaling [296]. Moreover, it enhances the sensitivity of MDR cell lines to chemotherapeutic agents, such as cisplatin, vincristine, doxorubicin, tamoxifen, and mitoxantrone [297].

### 7.8. Modulation of Signaling Pathways Related to Self-Renewal Capacity and Transformation of CSCs

CD44$^+$/CD24$^{low}$ BCSCs showed a high degree of tumorigenicity with enhanced sphere formation and self-renewal capacities [298,299]. Embryonic development-related signaling pathways, such as Notch, Wnt/β-catenin, and Hedgehog, were significantly implicated in the self-renewal property of BCSCs [300]. We will discuss the potential of polyphenols to interfere with the stemness-related signaling pathways below.

### 7.8.1. Hedgehog (Hh) Signaling Pathway

Hh, encoding secreted proteins, modulates cellular differentiation, proliferation, and development processes via autocrine- and paracrine-mediated signaling pathways [301]. There are three main mammalian homologs of the Hh gene, namely Sonic hedgehog (Shh), Indian hedgehog, and Desert hedgehog [302]. The interaction of the Hh proteins with the transmembrane protein, patched (PTC), leads to activation or phosphorylation of another transmembrane protein, smoothened (SMO) [303]. The Hh pathway is correlated with the development and maintenance of CSCs in breast cancer, myeloid leukaemia, glioma, gastric cancer, and multiple myeloma [304–307]. Therefore, the discovery of new inhibitors targeting the Hh signaling pathway is a potent anti-cancer strategy and is under clinical trials (phases I and II) [308].

Cyclopamine, extracted from *Veratrum californicum* or corn lily, was the first discovered phytochemical that inhibits Hh signaling pathways by inactivation of SMO [306,309]. Cyclopamine inhibits breast CSC proliferation and mammosphere formation [304].

Genistein potently inhibits the growth of CD44$^+$/CD24$^-$ BCSCs by the notable down-regulation of mRNA levels and the protein levels of SMO and Gli1, which are key factors for modulation of Hedgehog-Gli1 signaling [310].

### 7.8.2. Notch Signaling Pathway

Notch proteins are composed of four transmembrane glycoproteins, namely, Notch1, Notch2, Notch3, and Notch4, and also have five ligands, Delta-like1, Delta-like3, Delta-like4, Jagged1, and Jagged2 [311]. The Notch signaling pathway is involved in cellular proliferation and differentiation [312]. Its activation is mediated by the interaction between the extracellular domains of receptors with ligands and the release of the Notch intracellular domain (NICD) into the nucleus through proteolytic cleavage.

Resveratrol leads to down-regulation of Notch proteins only at the post-translational level, a decrease in mRNA levels of pre-TCRα and HES1, an increase in p53, and a reduction of PI3K/AKT signaling in MOLT-4 acute lymphoblastic leukemia cells [313].

### 7.8.3. Wingless/Integration 1 (Wnt) and the β-Catenin Signaling Pathway

The Wnt/β-Catenin signaling pathway is considered one of the essential signaling pathways for the self-renewal of BCSCs [314]. β-Catenin is an integral effector of the Wnt signaling pathway in the nucleus. In response to Wnt activation, stabilized β-catenin moves to the nucleus and activates target genes by its interaction with the TC/LEF transcription factor [314,315]. Glycogen synthase kinase3β (GSK3β), axin, casein kinase1α, and adenomatous polyposis coli (APC) protein complex are linked to regulation of the intracellular level of β-Catenin.

EGCG significantly inhibits the formation and invasiveness of breast cancer by suppressing the Wnt signaling pathway and reducing c-myc expression [316]; additionally, it potently reduces nuclear β-Catenin [317]. Curcumin also targets β-Catenin in the caspase-mediated mechanism in colon cancer [318]. Sulforaphane, a product of the conversion of glucoraphanin, which is the main glucosinolate in broccoli and its sprouts, has potent chemoprevention activity against a wide range of cancers [319–321].

Sulforaphane-exposed human cervical carcinoma and hepatocarcinoma cell lines show a significant increase in apoptosis by degradation of the β-Catenin protein [322]. Sulforaphane potently eliminates BCSCs in vitro and in vivo by targeting the Wnt/β-Catenin-mediated self-renewal property of BCSCs [321].

Piperine, an alkaloid isolated from black pepper (*Piper nigrum*) and long pepper (*Piper longum*), shows potent in vivo reduction of lung metastasis [323]; in addition, it inhibits the self-renewal property of BCSCs through down-regulation of the Wnt signaling pathway [324].

Oxymatrine, an alkaloid isolated from *Sophora japonica*, markedly decreases the proliferation of breast cancer and its drastic reduction of the growth of the sorted side population (SP) of CSCs was demonstrated [325]. In addition, it significantly reduced the activity of the Wnt/β-catenin signaling pathway.

### 7.9. Modulation of Autophagy

Autophagy plays a pivotal role in maintaining stem cell characteristics. Conditional deletion of Atg7 leads to a loss in properties, and disturbance in hematopoietic stem cell function [326]. In BCSCs, a high basal level of autophagy was detected in ALDH1+ cell populations [327]. Autophagy is essential for the enhancement of the invasiveness and metastatic properties of glioblastoma stem cells, which are mediated by DRAM1 and p62 [328].

Rottlerin significantly inhibits the growth of human BCSCs and induces autophagy via up-regulation of Atg12 and Beclin-1, and conversion of LC3-I into LC3-II [329]. Up-regulation of BAX, reduction in phosphorylation of AKT, mTOR, and AMPK, and a significant decrease in the expression of anti-apoptotic factors, were demonstrated over a long period of time of rottlerin treatment. shRNAs targeting Atg7 and Beclin-1 abrogated the capacity of rottlerin to induce autophagy. Autophagy inhibitors, 3-MA, Baf-A1, and cycloheximide, alleviate rottlerin-induced apoptosis and phosphorylation of AMPK. Inactivation of AMPK was concomitant with the down-regulation of Beclin-1, Atg12, and LC3.

Resveratrol blocks the growth of BCSCs and number of mammospheres [330]. It showed significant up-regulation of LC3-II, Atg7, and Beclin1, which is concomitant with cell toxicity.

### 7.10. Modulation of the Epithelial Mesenchymal Transition (EMT)

EMT is an intricate developmental process, in which special differentiated polarized epithelial cells undergo morphogenesis via loss of their differentiation characteristics, such as cell–cell adhesion, cell polarity, immotile status, and the transformation into mesenchymal cells with invasive and migratory properties [331,332].

During EMT, there is a decrease in the expression of epithelial markers, such as γ-catenin and E-cadherin, and up-regulation of mesenchymal markers, including vimentin, N-cadherin, fibronectin, and MMP-2/9. In contrast, mesenchymal-epithelial transition (MET) takes place after the migration and invasion of cells to their designated sites [333]. E-cadherin, encoded by CDH1, plays a pivotal role in the inhibition of tumor invasiveness and malignancy, as well as suppression of EMT.

There are various transcription factors, the Snail superfamily of zinc-finger transcriptional repressors, such as Snail 1 and Snail 2 (also known as slug); the ZEB family, such as ZEB1 (also known as TCF8 and δEF1) and ZEB2 (also known as Smad-interacting protein 1 (SIP1)); and basic helix-loop-helix (bHLH), such as E47 (also known as TCF3), TCF4 (also known as E2-2), and TWIST1 [331], which represent transcription repressors of the CDH1 gene, and, thereby, inhibit tumor malignancy and invasiveness.

Up-regulation of the EMT transcription repressor is induced by a complicated signaling network that is enhanced by receptor tyrosine kinases (RTKs) and transforming growth factor β (TGFβ) [334]. The NF-κB signaling pathway is involved in the activation of Snail, Slug, ZEB-1/2, and Twist, as well as the up-regulation of mesenchymal markers, including MMPs, fibronectin, and vimentin [335].

Resveratrol treatment triggers apoptosis and recovers the expression of γ-catenin and E-cadherin in tamoxifen-resistant breast cancer cells (MCF-7/TR) via targeting of TGFβ and its downstream effector, Smad [336]. Moreover, resveratrol recovered epithelial characteristics in EGF-transformed breast cancer cell lines via repression of the ERK1/2 signaling pathways [337].

Baicalin and baicalein, the main flavones isolated from *Scutellaria baicalensis*, potently inhibit EMT by targeting TGF-β1, and the inactivation of NF-κB-induced activation of Slug [338]. Furthermore, Chrysin (5,7-dihydroxyflavone), a flavone isolated from passion flower (*Passiflora caerulea*) and honeycomb of *Apis mellifera*, significantly inhibits the metastatic and invasive characteristics of TNBC through down-regulation of Slug, Snail, and Vimentin, and inhibition of MMP-10 via blocking of the PI3K-AKT signaling pathway [339].

Honokiol, isolated from seed cones from *Magnolia grandiflora* led to inhibition of EMT, which was mediated by inactivation of STAT3 and, in turn, blocked off the repressive action of ZEB1 on E-cadherin [340].

To sum up, several interesting studies have showed the capacity of polyphenols to potently restore epithelial characteristics in transformed breast cancer cells, and prevented the emergence of CSC phenotype and drug resistance.

## 8. Conclusions and Perspectives

In this review, we provide detailed information on the broad spectrum of mechanistic actions of polyphenols against breast cancer and CSCs. Many studies revealed that apoptosis- and/or autophagy-related signaling pathways are modulated by polyphenol treatment. Pharmacological inhibition of autophagy plays a pivotal role in polyphenol-induced cell death. We also explained the potential of polyphenols to target breast cancer and CSCs via modulation of various stemness-related signaling pathways and transcription factors.

This review provides useful information that will guide future research, which will provide strategies for efficient, polyphenol-based prevention, or treatment, of breast cancer. Further efforts are needed to resolve several remaining hurdles, such as the variations in applied dose, the large discrepancy between the in vitro and in vivo doses, and exposure time. Moreover, a better understanding of the interconnection between apoptosis and autophagy in the polyphenol-mediated treatment of breast cancer is needed to characterize the key factors involved in the actions of polyphenols. However, the progress in technology continues to provide answers to unresolved questions. To determine the potential of polyphenols in curing breast cancer in clinical trials, discovered polyphenols need to be elucidated. Chemotherapy remains.

In fact, there is a paucity of information related to the application of polyphenols as chemopreventive compounds. What lies ahead is the application of previously-discovered polyphenols in the treatment of breast cancer in clinical trials. Collectively, the therapeutic applications of polyphenols in breast cancer are promising, as these compounds present various mechanistic actions and their clinical applications need to be tested.

**Acknowledgments:** This work was supported by grants from the National Research Foundation (NRF) funded by the Korean government (2013M3A9D3045880 and 2015R1A5A1009701), by a grant (No. 312062-05) from the Bio-industry Technology Development Program, Ministry of Agriculture, Food and Rural Affairs, Republic of Korea, and by the 2016 KU Brain Pool of Konkuk University.

**Author Contributions:** Ahmed Abdal Dayem designed this work, collected the data, and co-wrote the manuscript, Hye Yeon Choi, Gwang-Mo Yang, Kyeongseok Kim, and Subbroto Kumar Saha collected the data and helped edit the manuscript. Ssang-Goo Cho designed the work, collected and reorganized the data, and wrote and edited the manuscript.

**Conflicts of Interest:** The authors declare no conflicts of interest.

## References

1. De Flora, S.; Ferguson, L.R. Overview of mechanisms of cancer chemopreventive agents. *Mutat. Res. Fundam. Mol. Mech. Mutagen.* **2005**, *591*, 8–15. [CrossRef] [PubMed]

2. De Flora, S.; Izzotti, A.; D'Agostini, F.; Balansky, R.M.; Noonan, D.; Albini, A. Multiple points of intervention in the prevention of cancer and other mutation-related diseases. *Mutat. Res. Fundam. Mol. Mech. Mutagen.* **2001**, *480*, 9–22. [CrossRef]

3. Mocanu, M.M.; Nagy, P.; Szöllősi, J. Chemoprevention of breast cancer by dietary polyphenols. *Molecules* **2015**, *20*, 22578–22620. [CrossRef] [PubMed]

4. Ui, A.; Kuriyama, S.; Kakizaki, M.; Sone, T.; Nakaya, N.; Ohmori-Matsuda, K.; Hozawa, A.; Nishino, Y.; Tsuji, I. Green tea consumption and the risk of liver cancer in Japan: The Ohsaki Cohort study. *Cancer Causes Control* **2009**, *20*, 1939–1945. [CrossRef] [PubMed]

5. Wu, Y.; Zhang, L.; Na, R.; Xu, J.; Xiong, Z.; Zhang, N.; Dai, W.; Jiang, H.; Ding, Q. Plasma genistein and risk of prostate cancer in Chinese population. *Int. Urol. Nephrol.* **2015**, *47*, 965–970. [CrossRef] [PubMed]

6. Crozier, A.; Jaganath, I.B.; Clifford, M.N. Dietary phenolics: Chemistry, bioavailability and effects on health. *Natl. Prod. Rep.* **2009**, *26*, 1001–1043. [CrossRef] [PubMed]

7. Sharma, R. Polyphenols in health and disease: Practice and mechanisms of benefits. *Polyphen. Hum. Health Dis. Acad. San Diego* **2014**, 757–778.

8. Halbwirth, H. The creation and physiological relevance of divergent hydroxylation patterns in the flavonoid pathway. *Int. J. Mol. Sci.* **2010**, *11*, 595–621. [CrossRef] [PubMed]

9. Danesi, F.; Kroon, P.A.; Saha, S.; de Biase, D.; D'Antuono, L.F.; Bordoni, A. Mixed pro-and anti-oxidative effects of pomegranate polyphenols in cultured cells. *Int. J. Mol. Sci.* **2014**, *15*, 19458–19471. [CrossRef] [PubMed]

10. Hsieh, S.R.; Cheng, W.C.; Su, Y.M.; Chiu, C.H.; Liou, Y.M. Molecular targets for anti-oxidative protection of green tea polyphenols against myocardial ischemic injury. *BioMedicine* **2014**, *4*, 23. [CrossRef] [PubMed]

11. Lewandowska, U.; Szewczyk, K.; Owczarek, K.; Hrabec, Z.; Podsędek, A.; Sosnowska, D.; Hrabec, E. Procyanidins from evening primrose (oenothera paradoxa) defatted seeds inhibit invasiveness of breast cancer cells and modulate the expression of selected genes involved in angiogenesis, metastasis, and apoptosis. *Nutr. Cancer* **2013**, *65*, 1219–1231. [CrossRef] [PubMed]

12. Duluc, L.; Jacques, C.; Soleti, R.; Andriantsitohaina, R.; Simard, G. Delphinidin inhibits VEGF induced-mitochondrial biogenesis and Akt activation in endothelial cells. *Int. J. Biochem. Cell Biol.* **2014**, *53*, 9–14. [CrossRef] [PubMed]

13. Symonds, E.L.; Konczak, I.; Fenech, M. The Australian fruit Illawarra plum (*Podocarpus elatus* Endl., Podocarpaceae) inhibits telomerase, increases histone deacetylase activity and decreases proliferation of colon cancer cells. *Br. J. Nutr.* **2013**, *109*, 2117–2125. [CrossRef] [PubMed]

14. Steward, W.; Brown, K. Cancer chemoprevention: A rapidly evolving field. *Br. J. Cancer* **2013**, *109*, 1–7. [CrossRef] [PubMed]

15. Surh, Y.J. Cancer chemoprevention with dietary phytochemicals. *Nat. Rev. Cancer* **2003**, *3*, 768–780. [CrossRef] [PubMed]

16. Minamoto, T.; Mai, M.; Ronai, Z.E. Environmental factors as regulators and effectors of multistep carcinogenesis. *Carcinogenesis* **1999**, *20*, 519–527. [CrossRef] [PubMed]

17. Galati, G.; Teng, S.; Moridani, M.Y.; Chan, T.S.; O'Brien, P.J. Cancer chemoprevention and apoptosis mechanisms induced by dietary polyphenolics. *Drug Metab. Drug Interact.* **2000**, *17*, 311–350. [CrossRef]

18. Guengerich, F.P. Metabolism of chemical carcinogens. *Carcinogenesis* **2000**, *21*, 345–351. [CrossRef] [PubMed]

19. Frassinetti, S.; Della Croce, C.M.; Caltavuturo, L.; Longo, V. Antimutagenic and antioxidant activity of *Lisosan G* in *Saccharomyces cerevisiae*. *Food Chem.* **2012**, *135*, 2029–2034. [CrossRef] [PubMed]

20. Słoczyńska, K.; Powroźnik, B.; Pękala, E.; Waszkielewicz, A.M. Antimutagenic compounds and their possible mechanisms of action. *J. Appl. Genet.* **2014**, *55*, 273–285. [CrossRef] [PubMed]

21. Rodeiro, I.; Donato, M.T.; Jimenez, N.; Garrido, G.; Molina-Torres, J.; Menendez, R.; Castell, J.V.; Gómez-Lechón, M.J. Inhibition of human p450 enzymes by natural extracts used in traditional medicine. *Phytother. Res.* **2009**, *23*, 279–282. [CrossRef] [PubMed]

22. Basheer, L.; Kerem, Z. Interactions between cyp3a4 and dietary polyphenols. *Oxid. Med. Cell. Longev.* **2015**, *2015*, 854015. [CrossRef] [PubMed]

23. Munday, R.; Munday, C.M. Induction of phase ii detoxification enzymes in rats by plant-derived isothiocyanates: Comparison of allyl isothiocyanate with sulforaphane and related compounds. *J. Agric. Food Chem.* **2004**, *52*, 1867–1871. [CrossRef] [PubMed]

24. Kou, X.; Kirberger, M.; Yang, Y.; Chen, N. Natural products for cancer prevention associated with nrf2-ARE pathway. *Food Sci. Hum. Wellness* **2013**, *2*, 22–28. [CrossRef]

25. Lu, F.; Zahid, M.; Wang, C.; Saeed, M.; Cavalieri, E.L.; Rogan, E.G. Resveratrol prevents estrogen-DNA adduct formation and neoplastic transformation in MCF-10F cells. *Cancer Prev. Res.* **2008**, *1*, 135–145. [CrossRef] [PubMed]

26. Niu, G.; Chen, X. Vascular endothelial growth factor as an anti-angiogenic target for cancer therapy. *Curr. Drug Targets* **2010**, *11*, 1000–1017. [CrossRef] [PubMed]

27. Wu, S.; Huang, Y.; Yeh, C.; Tsai, M.; Liao, C.; Cheng, W.; Chen, W.; Lin, K. Cathepsin H regulated by the thyroid hormone receptors associate with tumor invasion in human hepatoma cells. *Oncogene* **2011**, *30*, 2057–2069. [CrossRef] [PubMed]

28. Van Der Stappen, J.W.; Williams, A.C.; Maciewicz, R.A.; Paraskeva, C. Activation of cathepsin B, secreted by a colorectal cancer cell line requires low pH and is mediated by cathepsin D. *Int. J. Cancer* **1996**, *67*, 547–554. [CrossRef]

29. Nouh, M.A.; Mohamed, M.M.; El-Shinawi, M.; Shaalan, M.A.; Cavallo-Medved, D.; Khaled, H.M.; Sloane, B.F. Cathepsin B: A potential prognostic marker for inflammatory breast cancer. *J. Transl. Med.* **2011**, *9*, 1. [CrossRef] [PubMed]

30. Zhang, C.; Sun, J.B.; Liu, D.C.; Cui, Y.Q.; Liu, S.; Sun, H.C. Preliminary research on the pathological role of cathepsin B in subcutaneous heteroplastic pancreatic carcinoma in nude mice. *Chin. Med. J.* **2009**, *122*, 2489. [PubMed]

31. Sevenich, L.; Werner, F.; Gajda, M.; Schurigt, U.; Sieber, C.; Müller, S.; Follo, M.; Peters, C.; Reinheckel, T. Transgenic expression of human cathepsin B promotes progression and metastasis of polyoma-middle-t-induced breast cancer in mice. *Oncogene* **2011**, *30*, 54–64. [CrossRef] [PubMed]

32. Ellis, V.; Behrendt, N.; Danø, K. Plasminogen activation by receptor-bound urokinase. A kinetic study with both cell-associated and isolated receptor. *J. Biol. Chem.* **1991**, *266*, 12752–12758. [PubMed]

33. Curran, S.; Murray, G.I. Matrix metalloproteinases in tumour invasion and metastasis. *J. Pathol.* **1999**, *189*, 300–308. [CrossRef]

34. Van Pham, P. *Breast Cancer Stem Cells & Therapy Resistance*; Springer: Berlin, Germany, 2015.

35. Stewart, B.; Wild, C. World Cancer Report 2014. In *International Agency for Research on Cancer*; World Health Organization: Geneva, Swizerland, 2014.

36. IARC; World Heath Organization. *Globocan: Estimated Cancer Incidence, Mortality, Prevalence Worldwide in 2012*; IARC: Lyon, France, 2014.

37. Torre, L.A.; Bray, F.; Siegel, R.L.; Ferlay, J.; Lortet-Tieulent, J.; Jemal, A. Global cancer statistics, 2012. *CA Cancer J. Clin.* **2015**, *65*, 87–108. [CrossRef] [PubMed]

38. Visvader, J.E.; Lindeman, G.J. Cancer stem cells in solid tumours: Accumulating evidence and unresolved questions. *Nat. Rev. Cancer* **2008**, *8*, 755–768. [CrossRef] [PubMed]

39. Eyler, C.E.; Rich, J.N. Survival of the fittest: Cancer stem cells in therapeutic resistance and angiogenesis. *J. Clin. Oncol.* **2008**, *26*, 2839–2845. [CrossRef] [PubMed]

40. Al-Hajj, M.; Wicha, M.S.; Benito-Hernandez, A.; Morrison, S.J.; Clarke, M.F. Prospective identification of tumorigenic breast cancer cells. *Proc. Natl. Acad. Sci. USA* **2003**, *100*, 3983–3988. [CrossRef] [PubMed]

41. Bartsch, R.; Wenzel, C.; Steger, G.G. Trastuzumab in the management of early and advanced stage breast cancer. *Biologics* **2007**, *1*, 19–31. [PubMed]

42. Vici, P.; Colucci, G.; Gebbia, V.; Amodio, A.; Giotta, F.; Belli, F.; Conti, F.; Gebbia, N.; Pezzella, G.; Valerio, M.R. First-line treatment with epirubicin and vinorelbine in metastatic breast cancer. *J. Clin. Oncol.* **2002**, *20*, 2689–2694. [CrossRef] [PubMed]

43. Holliday, D.L.; Speirs, V. Choosing the right cell line for breast cancer research. *Breast Cancer Res.* **2011**, *13*, 215. [CrossRef] [PubMed]

44. Eisen, M.B.; Brown, P.O. DNA arrays for analysis of gene expression. *Methods Enzymol.* **1999**, *303*, 179–205. [PubMed]

45. Brenton, J.D.; Carey, L.A.; Ahmed, A.A.; Caldas, C. Molecular classification and molecular forecasting of breast cancer: Ready for clinical application? *J. Clin. Oncol.* **2005**, *23*, 7350–7360. [CrossRef] [PubMed]

46. Parker, J.S.; Mullins, M.; Cheang, M.C.; Leung, S.; Voduc, D.; Vickery, T.; Davies, S.; Fauron, C.; He, X.; Hu, Z. Supervised risk predictor of breast cancer based on intrinsic subtypes. *J. Clin. Oncol.* **2009**, *27*, 1160–1167. [CrossRef] [PubMed]

47. Tang, Y.; Wang, Y.; Kiani, M.F.; Wang, B. Classification, treatment strategy, and associated drug resistance in breast cancer. *Clin. Breast Cancer* **2016**. [CrossRef] [PubMed]

48. Sotiriou, C.; Pusztai, L. Gene-expression signatures in breast cancer. *N. Engl. J. Med.* **2009**, *360*, 790–800. [CrossRef] [PubMed]

49. Mitri, Z.; Constantine, T.; O'Regan, R. The HER2 receptor in breast cancer: Pathophysiology, clinical use, and new advances in therapy. *Chemother. Res. Pract.* **2012**, *2012*, 743193. [CrossRef] [PubMed]

50. Carey, L.A.; Dees, E.C.; Sawyer, L.; Gatti, L.; Moore, D.T.; Collichio, F.; Ollila, D.W.; Sartor, C.I.; Graham, M.L.; Perou, C.M. The triple negative paradox: Primary tumor chemosensitivity of breast cancer subtypes. *Clin. Cancer Res.* **2007**, *13*, 2329–2334. [CrossRef] [PubMed]

51. Sirohi, B.; Arnedos, M.; Popat, S.; Ashley, S.; Nerurkar, A.; Walsh, G.; Johnston, S.; Smith, I. Platinum-based chemotherapy in triple-negative breast cancer. *Ann. Oncol.* **2008**, *19*, 1847–1852. [CrossRef] [PubMed]

52. Anders, C.; Carey, L.A. Understanding and treating triple-negative breast cancer. *Oncology* **2008**, *22*, 1233. [PubMed]

53. Fedele, P.; Calvani, N.; Marino, A.; Orlando, L.; Schiavone, P.; Quaranta, A.; Cinieri, S. Targeted agents to reverse resistance to endocrine therapy in metastatic breast cancer: Where are we now and where are we going? *Crit. Rev. Oncol. Hematol.* **2012**, *84*, 243–251. [CrossRef] [PubMed]

54. Vinson, J.A.; Su, X.; Zubik, L.; Bose, P. Phenol antioxidant quantity and quality in foods: Fruits. *J. Agric. Food Chem.* **2001**, *49*, 5315–5321. [CrossRef] [PubMed]

55. Scalbert, A.; Williamson, G. Dietary intake and bioavailability of polyphenols. *J. Nutr.* **2000**, *130*, 2073S–2085S. [PubMed]

56. Parisi, O.; Puoci, F.; Restuccia, D.; Farina, G.; Iemma, F.; Picci, N. Polyphenols and their formulations: Different strategies to overcome the drawbacks associated with their poor stability and bioavailability. *Polyphen. Hum. Health Dis.* **2014**, *4*, 29–45.

57. Yang, C.S.; Lee, M.J.; Chen, L.; Yang, G.Y. Polyphenols as inhibitors of carcinogenesis. *Environ. Health Perspect.* **1997**, *105*, 971. [CrossRef] [PubMed]

58. Dehkharghanian, M.; Lacroix, M.; Vijayalakshmi, M.A. Antioxidant properties of green tea polyphenols encapsulated in caseinate beads. *Dairy Sci. Technol.* **2009**, *89*, 485–499. [CrossRef]

59. Baydar, N.G.; Sagdic, O.; Ozkan, G.; Cetin, S. Determination of antibacterial effects and total phenolic contents of grape (*Vitis vinifera* L.) seed extracts. *Int. J. Food Sci. Technol.* **2006**, *41*, 799–804. [CrossRef]

60. Jung, H.J.; Hwang, I.A.; Sung, W.S.; Kang, H.; Kang, B.S.; Seu, Y.B.; Lee, D.G. Fungicidal effect of resveratrol on human infectious fungi. *Arch. Pharm. Res.* **2005**, *28*, 557–560. [CrossRef] [PubMed]

61. Chávez, J.H.; Leal, P.C.; Yunes, R.A.; Nunes, R.J.; Barardi, C.R.; Pinto, A.R.; Simões, C.M.; Zanetti, C.R. Evaluation of antiviral activity of phenolic compounds and derivatives against rabies virus. *Vet. Microbiol.* **2006**, *116*, 53–59. [CrossRef] [PubMed]

62. Hudson, T.S.; Hartle, D.K.; Hursting, S.D.; Nunez, N.P.; Wang, T.T.; Young, H.A.; Arany, P.; Green, J.E. Inhibition of prostate cancer growth by muscadine grape skin extract and resveratrol through distinct mechanisms. *Cancer Res.* **2007**, *67*, 8396–8405. [CrossRef] [PubMed]

63. Lazzè, M.C.; Pizzala, R.; Gutiérrez Pecharromán, F.J.; Gatòn Garnica, P.; Antolín Rodríguez, J.M.; Fabris, N.; Bianchi, L. Grape waste extract obtained by supercritical fluid extraction contains bioactive antioxidant molecules and induces antiproliferative effects in human colon adenocarcinoma cells. *J. Med. Food* **2009**, *12*, 561–568. [CrossRef] [PubMed]

64. Aquilano, K.; Baldelli, S.; Rotilio, G.; Ciriolo, M.R. Role of nitric oxide synthases in parkinson's disease: A review on the antioxidant and anti-inflammatory activity of polyphenols. *Neurochem. Res.* **2008**, *33*, 2416–2426. [CrossRef] [PubMed]

65. Nichols, J.A.; Katiyar, S.K. Skin photoprotection by natural polyphenols: Anti-inflammatory, antioxidant and DNA repair mechanisms. *Arch. Dermatol. Res.* **2010**, *302*, 71–83. [CrossRef] [PubMed]

66. Gamet-Payrastre, L.; Manenti, S.; Gratacap, M.P.; Tulliez, J.; Chap, H.; Payrastre, B. Flavonoids and the inhibition of PKC and PI 3-kinase. *Gen. Pharmacol. Vasc. Syst.* **1999**, *32*, 279–286. [CrossRef]

67. Richard, T.; Lefeuvre, D.; Descendit, A.; Quideau, S.; Monti, J. Recognition characters in peptide-polyphenol complex formation. *Biochim. Biophys. Acta Gen. Subj.* **2006**, *1760*, 951–958. [CrossRef] [PubMed]

68. Duthie, G.G.; Duthie, S.J.; Kyle, J.A. Plant polyphenols in cancer and heart disease: Implications as nutritional antioxidants. *Nutr. Res. Rev.* **2000**, *13*, 79–106. [CrossRef] [PubMed]

69. Andrade, R.G.; Ginani, J.S.; Lopes, G.K.; Dutra, F.; Alonso, A.; Hermes-Lima, M. Tannic acid inhibits in vitro iron-dependent free radical formation. *Biochimie* **2006**, *88*, 1287–1296. [CrossRef] [PubMed]

70. Baechler, B.J.; Nita, F.; Jones, L.; Frestedt, J.L. A novel liquid multi-phytonutrient supplement demonstrates DNA-protective effects. *Plant Foods Hum. Nutr.* **2009**, *64*, 81–85. [CrossRef] [PubMed]

71. Adlercreutz, H. Phyto-oestrogens and cancer. *Lancet Oncol.* **2002**, *3*, 364–373. [CrossRef]

72. Quideau, S.; Deffieux, D.; Douat-Casassus, C.; Pouységu, L. Plant polyphenols: Chemical properties, biological activities, and synthesis. *Angew. Chem. Int. Ed.* **2011**, *50*, 586–621. [CrossRef] [PubMed]

73. Scalbert, A.; Manach, C.; Morand, C.; Rémésy, C.; Jiménez, L. Dietary polyphenols and the prevention of diseases. *Crit. Rev. Food Sci. Nutr.* **2005**, *45*, 287–306. [CrossRef] [PubMed]

74. García-Lafuente, A.; Guillamón, E.; Villares, A.; Rostagno, M.A.; Martínez, J.A. Flavonoids as anti-inflammatory agents: Implications in cancer and cardiovascular disease. *Inflamm. Res.* **2009**, *58*, 537–552. [CrossRef] [PubMed]

75. Thomasset, S.C.; Berry, D.P.; Garcea, G.; Marczylo, T.; Steward, W.P.; Gescher, A.J. Dietary polyphenolic phytochemicals—Promising cancer chemopreventive agents in humans? A review of their clinical properties. *Int. J. Cancer* **2007**, *120*, 451–458. [CrossRef] [PubMed]

76. Barnes, S.; Prasain, J.; D'Alessandro, T.; Arabshahi, A.; Botting, N.; Lila, M.A.; Jackson, G.; Janle, E.M.; Weaver, C.M. The metabolism and analysis of isoflavones and other dietary polyphenols in foods and biological systems. *Food Funct.* **2011**, *2*, 235–244. [CrossRef] [PubMed]

77. Erdman, J.W.; Balentine, D.; Arab, L.; Beecher, G.; Dwyer, J.T.; Folts, J.; Harnly, J.; Hollman, P.; Keen, C.L.; Mazza, G. Flavonoids and heart health: Proceedings of the ILSI North America Flavonoids Workshop, May 31–June 1, 2005, Washington, DC. *J. Nutr.* **2007**, *137*, 718S–737S. [PubMed]

78. Maru, G.; Kumar, G.; Ghantasala, S.; Tajpara, P. *Polyphenol-Mediated in Vivo Cellular Responses during Carcinogenesis Polyphenols in Human Health and Disease*; Academic Press: Cambridge, MA, USA, 2014.

79. Lee, E.R.; Kang, Y.J.; Choi, H.Y.; Kang, G.H.; Kim, J.H.; Kim, B.W.; Han, Y.S.; Nah, S.Y.; Paik, H.D.; Park, Y.S. Induction of apoptotic cell death by synthetic naringenin derivatives in human lung epithelial carcinoma a549 cells. *Biol. Pharm. Bull.* **2007**, *30*, 2394–2398. [CrossRef] [PubMed]

80. Lee, E.R.; Kang, G.H.; Cho, S.G. Effect of flavonoids on human health: Old subjects but new challenges. *Recent Pat. Biotechnol.* **2007**, *1*, 139–150. [CrossRef] [PubMed]

81. Kim, B.W.; Lee, E.R.; Min, H.M.; Jeong, H.S.; Ahn, J.Y.; Kim, J.H.; Choi, H.Y.; Choi, H.; Kim, E.Y.; Park, S.P. Sustained ERK activation is involved in the kaempferol-induced apoptosis of breast cancer cells and is more evident under 3-D culture condition. *Cancer Biol. Ther.* **2008**, *7*, 1080–1089. [CrossRef] [PubMed]

82. Kim, J.H.; Song, M.; Kang, G.H.; Lee, E.R.; Choi, H.Y.; Lee, C.; Kim, J.H.; Kim, Y.; Koo, B.N.; Cho, S.G. Combined treatment of 3-hydroxyflavone and imatinib mesylate increases apoptotic cell death of imatinib mesylate-resistant leukemia cells. *Leuk. Res.* **2012**, *36*, 1157–1164. [CrossRef] [PubMed]

83. Lee, E.R.; Kim, J.H.; Choi, H.Y.; Jeon, K.; Cho, S.G. Cytoprotective effect of eriodictyol in UV-irradiated keratinocytes via phosphatase-dependent modulation of both the p38 MAPK and Akt signaling pathways. *Cell. Physiol. Biochem.* **2011**, *27*, 513–524. [CrossRef] [PubMed]

84. Dayem, A.A.; Choi, H.Y.; Kim, Y.B.; Cho, S.G. Antiviral effect of methylated flavonol isorhamnetin against influenza. *PLoS ONE* **2015**, *10*, e0121610. [CrossRef] [PubMed]

85. Scalbert, A.; Johnson, I.T.; Saltmarsh, M. Polyphenols: Antioxidants and beyond. *Am. J. Clin. Nutr.* **2005**, *81*, 215S–217S. [PubMed]

86. Birt, D.F.; Hendrich, S.; Wang, W. Dietary agents in cancer prevention: Flavonoids and isoflavonoids. *Pharmacol. Ther.* **2001**, *90*, 157–177. [CrossRef]

87. Kris-Etherton, P.M.; Keen, C.L. Evidence that the antioxidant flavonoids in tea and cocoa are beneficial for cardiovascular health. *Curr. Opin. Lipidol.* **2002**, *13*, 41–49. [CrossRef] [PubMed]

88. Kalinowska, M.; Bielawska, A.; Lewandowska-Siwkiewicz, H.; Priebe, W.; Lewandowski, W. Apples: Content of phenolic compounds vs. Variety, part of apple and cultivation model, extraction of phenolic compounds, biological properties. *Plant Physiol. Biochem.* **2014**, *84*, 169–188. [CrossRef] [PubMed]

89. Kondratyuk, T.P.; Pezzuto, J.M. Natural product polyphenols of relevance to human health. *Pharm. Biol.* **2004**, *42*, 46–63. [CrossRef]

90. Vitaglione, P.; Napolitano, A.; Fogliano, V. Cereal dietary fibre: A natural functional ingredient to deliver phenolic compounds into the gut. *Trends Food Sci. Technol.* **2008**, *19*, 451–463. [CrossRef]

91. Fogliano, V.; Corollaro, M.L.; Vitaglione, P.; Napolitano, A.; Ferracane, R.; Travaglia, F.; Arlorio, M.; Costabile, A.; Klinder, A.; Gibson, G. In vitro bioaccessibility and gut biotransformation of polyphenols present in the water-insoluble cocoa fraction. *Med. Nutr. Food Res.* **2011**, *55*, S44–S55. [CrossRef] [PubMed]

92. Marín, L.; Miguélez, E.M.; Villar, C.J.; Lombó, F. Bioavailability of dietary polyphenols and gut microbiota metabolism: Antimicrobial properties. *BioMed Res. Int.* **2015**, *2015*, 905215. [CrossRef] [PubMed]

93. Bang, S.H.; Hyun, Y.J.; Shim, J.; Hong, S.W.; Kim, D.H. Metabolism of rutin and poncirin by human intestinal microbiota and cloning of their metabolizing α-l-rhamnosidase from bifidobacterium dentium. *J. Microbiol. Biotechnol.* **2015**, *25*, 18–25. [CrossRef] [PubMed]

94. Day, A.J.; Cañada, F.J.; Díaz, J.C.; Kroon, P.A.; Mclauchlan, R.; Faulds, C.B.; Plumb, G.W.; Morgan, M.R.; Williamson, G. Dietary flavonoid and isoflavone glycosides are hydrolysed by the lactase site of lactase phlorizin hydrolase. *FEBS Lett.* **2000**, *468*, 166–170. [CrossRef]

95. Gee, J.M.; DuPont, M.S.; Day, A.J.; Plumb, G.W.; Williamson, G.; Johnson, I.T. Intestinal transport of quercetin glycosides in rats involves both deglycosylation and interaction with the hexose transport pathway. *J. Nutr.* **2000**, *130*, 2765–2771. [PubMed]

96. Nakagawa, K.; Okuda, S.; Miyazawa, T. Dose-dependent incorporation of tea catechins, (–)-epigallocatechin-3-gallate and (–)-epigallocatechin, into human plasma. *Biosci. Biotechnol. Biochem.* **1997**, *61*, 1981–1985. [CrossRef] [PubMed]

97. Filomeni, G.; De Zio, D.; Cecconi, F. Oxidative stress and autophagy: The clash between damage and metabolic needs. *Cell Death Differ.* **2015**, *22*, 377–388. [CrossRef] [PubMed]

98. Liang, X.H.; Jackson, S.; Seaman, M.; Brown, K.; Kempkes, B.; Hibshoosh, H.; Levine, B. Induction of autophagy and inhibition of tumorigenesis by beclin 1. *Nature* **1999**, *402*, 672–676. [PubMed]

99. Aita, V.M.; Liang, X.H.; Murty, V.; Pincus, D.L.; Yu, W.; Cayanis, E.; Kalachikov, S.; Gilliam, T.C.; Levine, B. Cloning and genomic organization of beclin 1, a candidate tumor suppressor gene on chromosome 17q21. *Genomics* **1999**, *59*, 59–65. [CrossRef] [PubMed]

100. Dilova, I.; Easlon, E.; Lin, S.J. Calorie restriction and the nutrient sensing signaling pathways. *Cell. Med. Life Sci.* **2007**, *64*, 752–767. [CrossRef] [PubMed]

101. Trepanowski, J.F.; Canale, R.E.; Marshall, K.E.; Kabir, M.M.; Bloomer, R.J. Impact of caloric and dietary restriction regimens on markers of health and longevity in humans and animals: A summary of available findings. *Nutr. J.* **2011**, *10*, 1. [CrossRef] [PubMed]

102. Inoki, K.; Zhu, T.; Guan, K.L. TSC2 mediates cellular energy response to control cell growth and survival. *Cell* **2003**, *115*, 577–590. [CrossRef]

103. Gwinn, D.M.; Shackelford, D.B.; Egan, D.F.; Mihaylova, M.M.; Mery, A.; Vasquez, D.S.; Turk, B.E.; Shaw, R.J. AMPK phosphorylation of raptor mediates a metabolic checkpoint. *Med. Cell* **2008**, *30*, 214–226. [CrossRef] [PubMed]

104. Jung, C.H.; Jun, C.B.; Ro, S.H.; Kim, Y.M.; Otto, N.M.; Cao, J.; Kundu, M.; Kim, D.H. ULK-Atg13-FIP200 complexes mediate mtor signaling to the autophagy machinery. *Med. Biol. Cell* **2009**, *20*, 1992–2003. [CrossRef] [PubMed]

105. Baur, J.A.; Pearson, K.J.; Price, N.L.; Jamieson, H.A.; Lerin, C.; Kalra, A.; Prabhu, V.V.; Allard, J.S.; Lopez-Lluch, G.; Lewis, K. Resveratrol improves health and survival of mice on a high-calorie diet. *Nature* **2006**, *444*, 337–342. [CrossRef] [PubMed]

106. Morselli, E.; Maiuri, M.C.; Markaki, M.; Megalou, E.; Pasparaki, A.; Palikaras, K.; Criollo, A.; Galluzzi, L.; Malik, S.A.; Vitale, I. The life span-prolonging effect of sirtuin-1 is mediated by autophagy. *Autophagy* **2010**, *6*, 186–188. [CrossRef] [PubMed]

107. Ng, F.; Tang, B.L. Sirtuins' modulation of autophagy. *J. Cell. Physiol.* **2013**, *228*, 2262–2270. [CrossRef] [PubMed]

108. Chung, S.; Yao, H.; Caito, S.; Hwang, J.W.; Arunachalam, G.; Rahman, I. Regulation of sirt1 in cellular functions: Role of polyphenols. *Arch. Biochem. Biophys.* **2010**, *501*, 79–90. [CrossRef] [PubMed]

109. Opipari, A.W.; Tan, L.; Boitano, A.E.; Sorenson, D.R.; Aurora, A.; Liu, J.R. Resveratrol-induced autophagocytosis in ovarian cancer cells. *Cancer Res.* **2004**, *64*, 696–703. [CrossRef] [PubMed]

110. Carbó, N.; Costelli, P.; Baccino, F.M.; López-Soriano, F.J.; Argilés, J.M. Resveratrol, a natural product present in wine, decreases tumour growth in a rat tumour model. *Biochem. Biophys. Res. Commun.* **1999**, *254*, 739–743. [CrossRef] [PubMed]

111. Baur, J.A.; Sinclair, D.A. Therapeutic potential of resveratrol: The in vivo evidence. *Nat. Rev. Drug Discov.* **2006**, *5*, 493–506. [CrossRef] [PubMed]

112. Signorelli, P.; Ghidoni, R. Resveratrol as an anticancer nutrient: Molecular basis, open questions and promises. *J. Nutr. Biochem.* **2005**, *16*, 449–466. [CrossRef] [PubMed]

113. Trincheri, N.F.; Follo, C.; Nicotra, G.; Peracchio, C.; Castino, R.; Isidoro, C. Resveratrol-induced apoptosis depends on the lipid kinase activity of vps34 and on the formation of autophagolysosomes. *Carcinogenesis* **2008**, *29*, 381–389. [CrossRef] [PubMed]

114. Armour, S.M.; Baur, J.A.; Hsieh, S.N.; Land-Bracha, A.; Thomas, S.M.; Sinclair, D.A. Inhibition of mammalian s6 kinase by resveratrol suppresses autophagy. *Aging* **2009**, *1*, 515–528. [CrossRef] [PubMed]

115. Scarlatti, F.; Maffei, R.; Beau, I.; Codogno, P.; Ghidoni, R. Role of non-canonical beclin 1-independent autophagy in cell death induced by resveratrol in human breast cancer cells. *Cell Death Differ.* **2008**, *15*, 1318–1329. [CrossRef] [PubMed]

116. Kim, Y.; Choi, B.T.; Lee, Y.T.; Park, D.I.; Rhee, S.H.; Park, K.Y.; Choi, Y.H. Resveratrol inhibits cell proliferation and induces apoptosis of human breast carcinoma MCF-7 cells. *Oncol. Rep.* **2004**, *11*, 441–446. [CrossRef] [PubMed]

117. Roy, S.K.; Chen, Q.; Fu, J.; Shankar, S.; Srivastava, R.K. Resveratrol inhibits growth of orthotopic pancreatic tumors through activation of foxo transcription factors. *PLoS ONE* **2011**, *6*, e25166. [CrossRef] [PubMed]

118. Back, J.H.; Zhu, Y.; Calabro, A.; Queenan, C.; Kim, A.S.; Arbesman, J.; Kim, A.L. Resveratrol-mediated downregulation of rictor attenuates autophagic process and suppresses UV induced skin carcinogenesis. *Photochem. Photobiol.* **2012**, *88*, 1165–1172. [CrossRef] [PubMed]

119. Hwang, J.T.; Kwak, D.W.; Lin, S.K.; Kim, H.M.; Kim, Y.M.; Park, O.J. Resveratrol induces apoptosis in chemoresistant cancer cells via modulation of AMPK signaling pathway. *Ann. N. Y. Acad. Sci.* **2007**, *1095*, 441–448. [CrossRef] [PubMed]

120. Miki, H.; Uehara, N.; Kimura, A.; Sasaki, T.; Yuri, T.; Yoshizawa, K.; Tsubura, A. Resveratrol induces apoptosis via ros-triggered autophagy in human colon cancer cells. *Int. J. Oncol.* **2012**, *40*, 1020–1028. [PubMed]

121. Puissant, A.; Auberger, P. AMPK-and p62/SQSTM1-dependent autophagy mediate resveratrol-induced cell death in chronic myelogenous leukemia. *Autophagy* **2010**, *6*, 655–657. [CrossRef] [PubMed]

122. Saller, R.; Brignoli, R.; Melzer, J.; Meier, R. An updated systematic review with meta-analysis for the clinical evidence of silymarin. *Forsch. Komplement. Res. Complement. Med.* **2008**, *15*, 9–20. [CrossRef] [PubMed]

123. Lu, P.; Mamiya, T.; Lu, L.; Mouri, A.; Zou, L.; Nagai, T.; Hiramatsu, M.; Ikejima, T.; Nabeshima, T. Silibinin prevents amyloid β peptide-induced memory impairment and oxidative stress in mice. *Br. J. Pharmacol.* **2009**, *157*, 1270–1277. [CrossRef] [PubMed]

124. Marrazzo, G.; Bosco, P.; La Delia, F.; Scapagnini, G.; Di Giacomo, C.; Malaguarnera, M.; Galvano, F.; Nicolosi, A.; Volti, G.L. Neuroprotective effect of silibinin in diabetic mice. *Neurosci. Lett.* **2011**, *504*, 252–256. [CrossRef] [PubMed]

125. Singh, R.P.; Agarwal, R. Mechanisms and preclinical efficacy of silibinin in preventing skin cancer. *Eur. J. Cancer* **2005**, *41*, 1969–1979. [CrossRef] [PubMed]

126. Singh, R.P.; Agarwal, R. Prostate cancer chemoprevention by silibinin: Bench to bedside. *Mol. Carcinogen.* **2006**, *45*, 436–442. [CrossRef] [PubMed]

127. Tyagi, A.; Singh, R.P.; Ramasamy, K.; Raina, K.; Redente, E.F.; Dwyer-Nield, L.D.; Radcliffe, R.A.; Malkinson, A.M.; Agarwal, R. Growth inhibition and regression of lung tumors by silibinin: Modulation of angiogenesis by macrophage-associated cytokines and nuclear factor-κb and signal transducers and activators of transcription 3. *Cancer Prev. Res.* **2009**, *2*, 74–83. [CrossRef] [PubMed]

128. Kauntz, H.; Bousserouel, S.; Gossé, F.; Raul, F. Silibinin triggers apoptotic signaling pathways and autophagic survival response in human colon adenocarcinoma cells and their derived metastatic cells. *Apoptosis* **2011**, *16*, 1042–1053. [CrossRef] [PubMed]

129. Duan, W.; Jin, X.; Li, Q.; Tashiro, S.I.; Onodera, S.; Ikejima, T. Silibinin induced autophagic and apoptotic cell death in HT1080 cells through a reactive oxygen species pathway. *J. Pharmacol. Sci.* **2010**, *113*, 48–56. [CrossRef] [PubMed]

130. Fan, S.; Li, L.; Chen, S.; Yu, Y.; Qi, M.; Tashiro, S.I.; Onodera, S.; Ikejima, T. Silibinin induced-autophagic and apoptotic death is associated with an increase in reactive oxygen and nitrogen species in hela cells. *Free Radic. Res.* **2011**, *45*, 1307–1324. [CrossRef] [PubMed]

131. Mira, L.; Silva, M.; Manso, C. Scavenging of reactive oxygen species by silibinin dihemisuccinate. *Biochem. Pharmacol.* **1994**, *48*, 753–759. [CrossRef]

132. Jiang, K.; Wang, W.; Jin, X.; Wang, Z.; Ji, Z.; Meng, G. Silibinin, a natural flavonoid, induces autophagy via ROS-dependent mitochondrial dysfunction and loss of ATP involving BNIP3 in human MCF7 breast cancer cells. *Oncol. Rep.* **2015**, *33*, 2711–2718. [CrossRef] [PubMed]

133. Zheng, N.; Zhang, P.; Huang, H.; Liu, W.; Hayashi, T.; Zang, L.; Zhang, Y.; Liu, L.; Xia, M.; Tashiro, S.I. Erα down-regulation plays a key role in silibinin-induced autophagy and apoptosis in human breast cancer MCF-7 cells. *J. Pharmacol. Sci.* **2015**, *128*, 97–107. [CrossRef] [PubMed]

134. Boots, A.W.; Haenen, G.R.; Bast, A. Health effects of quercetin: From antioxidant to nutraceutical. *Eur. J. Pharmacol.* **2008**, *585*, 325–337. [CrossRef] [PubMed]

135. Ferry, D.R.; Smith, A.; Malkhandi, J.; Fyfe, D.W.; Anderson, D.; Baker, J.; Kerr, D. Phase I clinical trial of the flavonoid quercetin: Pharmacokinetics and evidence for in vivo tyrosine kinase inhibition. *Clin. Cancer Res.* **1996**, *2*, 659–668. [PubMed]

136. Aalinkeel, R.; Bindukumar, B.; Reynolds, J.L.; Sykes, D.E.; Mahajan, S.D.; Chadha, K.C.; Schwartz, S.A. The dietary bioflavonoid, quercetin, selectively induces apoptosis of prostate cancer cells by down-regulating the expression of heat shock protein 90. *Prostate* **2008**, *68*, 1773–1789. [CrossRef] [PubMed]

137. Borska, S.; Drag-Zalesinska, M.; Wysocka, T.; Sopel, M.; Dumanska, M.; Zabel, M.; Dziegiel, P. Antiproliferative and pro-apoptotic effects of quercetin on human pancreatic carcinoma cell lines EPP85–181P and EPP85–181RDB. *Folia Histochem. Cytobiol.* **2010**, *48*, 222–229. [CrossRef] [PubMed]

138. Choi, E.J.; Bae, S.M.; Ahn, W.S. Antiproliferative effects of quercetin through cell cycle arrest and apoptosis in human breast cancer MDA-MB-453 cells. *Arch. Pharm. Res.* **2008**, *31*, 1281–1285. [CrossRef] [PubMed]

139. Conklin, C.M.; Bechberger, J.F.; MacFabe, D.; Guthrie, N.; Kurowska, E.M.; Naus, C.C. Genistein and quercetin increase connexin43 and suppress growth of breast cancer cells. *Carcinogenesis* **2006**, *28*, 93–100. [CrossRef] [PubMed]

140. Klappan, A.K.; Hones, S.; Mylonas, I.; Brüning, A. Proteasome inhibition by quercetin triggers macroautophagy and blocks mtor activity. *Histochem. Cell Biol.* **2012**, *137*, 25–36. [CrossRef] [PubMed]

141. Wang, K.; Liu, R.; Li, J.; Mao, J.; Lei, Y.; Wu, J.; Zeng, J.; Zhang, T.; Wu, H.; Chen, L. Quercetin induces protective autophagy in gastric cancer cells: Involvement of Akt-mTOR-and hypoxia-induced factor 1α-mediated signaling. *Autophagy* **2011**, *7*, 966–978. [CrossRef] [PubMed]

142. Polkowski, K.; Popiołkiewicz, J.; Krzeczyński, P.; Ramza, J.; Pucko, W.; Zegrocka-Stendel, O.; Boryski, J.; Skierski, J.S.; Mazurek, A.P.; Grynkiewicz, G. Cytostatic and cytotoxic activity of synthetic genistein glycosides against human cancer cell lines. *Cancer Lett.* **2004**, *203*, 59–69. [CrossRef] [PubMed]

143. Yu, Z.; Li, W.; Liu, F. Inhibition of proliferation and induction of apoptosis by genistein in colon cancer HT-29 cells. *Cancer Lett.* **2004**, *215*, 159–166. [CrossRef] [PubMed]

144. Ouchi, H.; Ishiguro, H.; Ikeda, N.; Hori, M.; Kubota, Y.; Uemura, H. Genistein induces cell growth inhibition in prostate cancer through the suppression of telomerase activity. *Int. J. Urol.* **2005**, *12*, 73–80. [CrossRef] [PubMed]

145. Li, Y.; Upadhyay, S.; Bhuiyan, M.; Sarkar, F.H. Induction of apoptosis in breast cancer cells MDA-MB-231 by genistein. *Oncogene* **1999**, *18*, 3166–3172. [CrossRef] [PubMed]

146. Gossner, G.; Choi, M.; Tan, L.; Fogoros, S.; Griffith, K.A.; Kuenker, M.; Liu, J.R. Genistein-induced apoptosis and autophagocytosis in ovarian cancer cells. *Gynecol. Oncol.* **2007**, *105*, 23–30. [CrossRef] [PubMed]

147. Houslay, M.D.; Christian, F. P62 (SQSTM1) forms part of a novel, reversible aggregate containing a specific conformer of the camp degrading phosphodiesterase, PDE4A4. *Autophagy* **2010**, *6*, 1198–1200. [CrossRef] [PubMed]

148. Christian, F.; Anthony, D.F.; Vadrevu, S.; Riddell, T.; Day, J.P.; McLeod, R.; Adams, D.R.; Baillie, G.S.; Houslay, M.D. P62 (SQSTM1) and cyclic amp phosphodiesterase-4A4 (PDE4A4) locate to a novel, reversible protein aggregate with links to autophagy and proteasome degradation pathways. *Cell Signal.* **2010**, *22*, 1576–1596. [CrossRef] [PubMed]

149. Dhillon, N.; Aggarwal, B.B.; Newman, R.A.; Wolff, R.A.; Kunnumakkara, A.B.; Abbruzzese, J.L.; Ng, C.S.; Badmaev, V.; Kurzrock, R. Phase ii trial of curcumin in patients with advanced pancreatic cancer. *Clin. Cancer Res.* **2008**, *14*, 4491–4499. [CrossRef] [PubMed]

150. Sharma, R.A.; Euden, S.A.; Platton, S.L.; Cooke, D.N.; Shafayat, A.; Hewitt, H.R.; Marczylo, T.H.; Morgan, B.; Hemingway, D.; Plummer, S.M. Phase i clinical trial of oral curcumin biomarkers of systemic activity and compliance. *Clin. Cancer Res.* **2004**, *10*, 6847–6854. [CrossRef] [PubMed]
151. Zhuang, W.; Long, L.; Zheng, B.; Ji, W.; Yang, N.; Zhang, Q.; Liang, Z. Curcumin promotes differentiation of glioma-initiating cells by inducing autophagy. *Cancer Sci.* **2012**, *103*, 684–690. [CrossRef] [PubMed]
152. Chadalapaka, G.; Jutooru, I.; Burghardt, R.; Safe, S. Drugs that target specificity proteins downregulate epidermal growth factor receptor in bladder cancer cells. *Mol. Cancer Res.* **2010**, *8*, 739–750. [CrossRef] [PubMed]
153. Han, J.; Pan, X.Y.; Xu, Y.; Xiao, Y.; An, Y.; Tie, L.; Pan, Y.; Li, X.J. Curcumin induces autophagy to protect vascular endothelial cell survival from oxidative stress damage. *Autophagy* **2012**, *8*, 812–825. [CrossRef] [PubMed]
154. Lee, Y.J.; Kim, N.Y.; Suh, Y.A.; Lee, C. Involvement of ROS in curcumin-induced autophagic cell death. *Korean J. Physiol. Pharmacol.* **2011**, *15*, 1–7. [CrossRef] [PubMed]
155. Aoki, H.; Takada, Y.; Kondo, S.; Sawaya, R.; Aggarwal, B.B.; Kondo, Y. Evidence that curcumin suppresses the growth of malignant gliomas in vitro and in vivo through induction of autophagy: Role of Akt and extracellular signal-regulated kinase signaling pathways. *Med. Pharmacol.* **2007**, *72*, 29–39. [CrossRef] [PubMed]
156. Pan, W.; Yang, H.; Cao, C.; Song, X.; Wallin, B.; Kivlin, R.; Lu, S.; Hu, G.; Di, W.; Wan, Y. AMPK mediates curcumin-induced cell death in CaOV3 ovarian cancer cells. *Oncol. Rep.* **2008**, *20*, 1553–1559. [PubMed]
157. Kim, J.Y.; Cho, T.J.; Woo, B.H.; Choi, K.U.; Lee, C.H.; Ryu, M.H.; Park, H.R. Curcumin-induced autophagy contributes to the decreased survival of oral cancer cells. *Arch. Oral Biol.* **2012**, *57*, 1018–1025. [CrossRef] [PubMed]
158. Shinojima, N.; Yokoyama, T.; Kondo, Y.; Kondo, S. Roles of the Akt/mTOR/p70S6K and ERK1/2 signaling pathways in curcumin-induced autophagy. *Autophagy* **2007**, *3*, 635–637. [CrossRef] [PubMed]
159. Jia, Y.L.; Li, J.; Qin, Z.H.; Liang, Z.Q. Autophagic and apoptotic mechanisms of curcumin-induced death in K562 cells. *J. Asian Natl. Prod. Res.* **2009**, *11*, 918–928. [CrossRef] [PubMed]
160. Gschwendt, M.; Muller, H.; Kielbassa, K.; Zang, R.; Kittstein, W.; Rincke, G.; Marks, F. Rottlerin, a novel protein kinase inhibitor. *Biochem. Biophys. Res. Commun.* **1994**, *199*, 93–98. [CrossRef] [PubMed]
161. Soltoff, S.P. Rottlerin: An inappropriate and ineffective inhibitor of PKCδ. *Trends Pharmacol. Sci.* **2007**, *28*, 453–458. [CrossRef] [PubMed]
162. Springael, C.; Thomas, S.; Rahmouni, S.; Vandamme, A.; Goldman, M.; Willems, F.; Vosters, O. Rottlerin inhibits human T cell responses. *Biochem. Pharmacol.* **2007**, *73*, 515–525. [CrossRef] [PubMed]
163. Zeng, H.; Lozinskaya, I.M.; Lin, Z.; Willette, R.N.; Brooks, D.P.; Xu, X. Mallotoxin is a novel human ether-a-go-go-related gene (hERG) potassium channel activator. *J. Pharmacol. Exp. Ther.* **2006**, *319*, 957–962. [CrossRef] [PubMed]
164. Zhang, D.; Anantharam, V.; Kanthasamy, A.; Kanthasamy, A.G. Neuroprotective effect of protein kinase cδ inhibitor rottlerin in cell culture and animal models of parkinson's disease. *J. Pharmacol. Exp. Ther.* **2007**, *322*, 913–922. [CrossRef] [PubMed]
165. Guimarães, E.L.; Empsen, C.; Geerts, A.; van Grunsven, L.A. Advanced glycation end products induce production of reactive oxygen species via the activation of NADPH oxidase in murine hepatic stellate cells. *J. Hepatol.* **2010**, *52*, 389–397. [CrossRef] [PubMed]
166. Mizuguchi, H.; Terao, T.; Kitai, M.; Ikeda, M.; Yoshimura, Y.; Das, A.K.; Kitamura, Y.; Takeda, N.; Fukui, H. Involvement of protein kinase Cdelta/extracellular signal-regulated kinase/poly (ADP-ribose) polymerase-1 (PARP-1) signaling pathway in histamine-induced up-regulation of histamine $H_1$ receptor gene expression in Hela cells. *J. Biol. Chem.* **2011**, *286*, 30542–30551. [CrossRef] [PubMed]
167. Sharma, V. A polyphenolic compound rottlerin demonstrates significant in vitro cytotoxicity against human cancer cell lines: Isolation and characterization from the fruits of *Mallotus philippinensis*. *J. Plant Biochem. Biotechnol.* **2011**, *20*, 190–195. [CrossRef]

168. Mann, A.P.; Verma, A.; Sethi, G.; Manavathi, B.; Wang, H.; Fok, J.Y.; Kunnumakkara, A.B.; Kumar, R.; Aggarwal, B.B.; Mehta, K. Overexpression of tissue transglutaminase leads to constitutive activation of nuclear factor-kappaB in cancer cells: Delineation of a novel pathway. *Cancer Res.* **2006**, *66*, 8788–8795. [CrossRef] [PubMed]

169. Fabre, C.; Carvalho, G.; Tasdemir, E.; Braun, T.; Ades, L.; Grosjean, J.; Boehrer, S.; Metivier, D.; Souquere, S.; Pierron, G. NF-kappaB inhibition sensitizes to starvation-induced cell death in high-risk myelodysplastic syndrome and acute myeloid leukemia. *Oncogene* **2007**, *26*, 4071–4083. [CrossRef] [PubMed]

170. Akar, U.; Ozpolat, B.; Mehta, K.; Fok, J.; Kondo, Y.; Lopez-Berestein, G. Tissue transglutaminase inhibits autophagy in pancreatic cancer cells. *Mol. Cancer Res.* **2007**, *5*, 241–249. [CrossRef] [PubMed]

171. Singh, B.N.; Kumar, D.; Shankar, S.; Srivastava, R.K. Rottlerin induces autophagy which leads to apoptotic cell death through inhibition of PI3K/Akt/mTOR pathway in human pancreatic cancer stem cells. *Biochem. Pharmacol.* **2012**, *84*, 1154–1163. [CrossRef] [PubMed]

172. Balgi, A.D.; Fonseca, B.D.; Donohue, E.; Tsang, T.C.; Lajoie, P.; Proud, C.G.; Nabi, I.R.; Roberge, M. Screen for chemical modulators of autophagy reveals novel therapeutic inhibitors of mTORC1 signaling. *PLoS ONE* **2009**, *4*, e7124. [CrossRef] [PubMed]

173. Li, M.J.; Yin, Y.C.; Wang, J.; Jiang, Y.F. Green tea compounds in breast cancer prevention and treatment. *World J. Clin. Oncol.* **2014**, *5*, 520–528. [CrossRef] [PubMed]

174. Harper, C.E.; Patel, B.B.; Wang, J.; Arabshahi, A.; Eltoum, I.A.; Lamartiniere, C.A. Resveratrol suppresses prostate cancer progression in transgenic mice. *Carcinogenesis* **2007**, *28*, 1946–1953. [CrossRef] [PubMed]

175. Trincheri, N.F.; Nicotra, G.; Follo, C.; Castino, R.; Isidoro, C. Resveratrol induces cell death in colorectal cancer cells by a novel pathway involving lysosomal cathepsin D. *Carcinogenesis* **2007**, *28*, 922–931. [CrossRef] [PubMed]

176. Rodrigo, R.; Gil-Becerra, D. Implications of polyphenols on endogenous antioxidant defense systems in human diseases. In *Polyphenols in Human Health Disease*; Elsevier: Amsterdam, The Netherlands, 2014; pp. 201–207.

177. Wang, H.; Cao, G.; Prior, R.L. Total antioxidant capacity of fruits. *J. Agric. Food Chem.* **1996**, *44*, 701–705. [CrossRef]

178. Bhattacharyya, A.; Chattopadhyay, R.; Mitra, S.; Crowe, S.E. Oxidative stress: An essential factor in the pathogenesis of gastrointestinal mucosal diseases. *Physiol. Rev.* **2014**, *94*, 329–354. [CrossRef] [PubMed]

179. Pham-Huy, L.A.; He, H.; Pham-Huy, C. Free radicals, antioxidants in disease and health. *Int. J. Biomed. Sci.* **2008**, *4*, 89–96. [PubMed]

180. Perron, N.R.; Brumaghim, J.L. A review of the antioxidant mechanisms of polyphenol compounds related to iron binding. *Cell Biochem. Biophys.* **2009**, *53*, 75–100. [CrossRef] [PubMed]

181. Guo, J.J.; Hsieh, H.Y.; Hu, C.H. Chain-breaking activity of carotenes in lipid peroxidation: A theoretical study. *J. Phys. Chem. B* **2009**, *113*, 15699–15708. [CrossRef] [PubMed]

182. Pietta, P.G. Flavonoids as antioxidants. *J. Natl. Prod.* **2000**, *63*, 1035–1042. [CrossRef]

183. Tsao, R.; Li, H. Antioxidant properties in vitro and in vivo: Realistic assessments of efficacy of plant extracts. *CAB Rev.* **2012**, *7*, 9.

184. Rice-Evans, C.A.; Miller, N.J.; Paganga, G. Structure-antioxidant activity relationships of flavonoids and phenolic acids. *Free Radic. Biol. Med.* **1996**, *20*, 933–956. [CrossRef]

185. Chuang, C.C.; McIntosh, M.K. Potential mechanisms by which polyphenol-rich grapes prevent obesity-mediated inflammation and metabolic diseases. *Annu. Rev. Nutr.* **2011**, *31*, 155–176. [CrossRef] [PubMed]

186. Zhou, B.; Wu, L.M.; Yang, L.; Liu, Z.L. Evidence for α-tocopherol regeneration reaction of green tea polyphenols in SDS micelles. *Free Radic. Biol. Med.* **2005**, *38*, 78–84. [CrossRef] [PubMed]

187. Tsao, R. Chemistry and biochemistry of dietary polyphenols. *Nutrients* **2010**, *2*, 1231–1246. [CrossRef] [PubMed]

188. Van Acker, S.A.; van den Berg, D.J.; Tromp, M.N.; Griffioen, D.H.; van Bennekom, W.P.; van der Vijgh, W.J.; Bast, A. Structural aspects of antioxidant activity of flavonoids. *Free Radic. Biol. Med.* **1996**, *20*, 331–342. [CrossRef]

189. Göçer, H.; Gülçin, İ. Caffeic acid phenethyl ester (CAPE): Correlation of structure and antioxidant properties. *Int. J. Food Sci. Nutr.* **2011**, *62*, 821–825. [CrossRef] [PubMed]

190. Mishra, P.; Kale, R.; Kar, A. Chemoprevention of mammary tumorigenesis and chemomodulation of the antioxidative enzymes and peroxidative damage in prepubertal Sprague Dawley rats by Biochanin A. *Mol. Cell. Biochem.* **2008**, *312*, 1–9. [CrossRef] [PubMed]

191. Singh, B.; Shoulson, R.; Chatterjee, A.; Ronghe, A.; Bhat, N.K.; Dim, D.C.; Bhat, H.K. Resveratrol inhibits estrogen-induced breast carcinogenesis through induction of NRF2-mediated protective pathways. *Carcinogenesis* **2014**, *35*, 1872–1880. [CrossRef] [PubMed]

192. Yang, C.S.; Li, G.; Yang, Z.; Guan, F.; Chen, A.; Ju, J. Cancer prevention by tocopherols and tea polyphenols. *Cancer Lett.* **2013**, *334*, 79–85. [CrossRef] [PubMed]

193. Hsieh, T.C.; Wu, J.M. Suppression of cell proliferation and gene expression by combinatorial synergy of EGCG, resveratrol and γ-tocotrienol in estrogen receptor-positive MCF-7 breast cancer cells. *Int. J. Oncol.* **2008**, *33*, 851–859. [PubMed]

194. Nadal-Serrano, M.; Pons, D.G.; Sastre-Serra, J.; del Mar Blanquer-Rosselló, M.; Roca, P.; Oliver, J. Genistein modulates oxidative stress in breast cancer cell lines according to ERA/ERB ratio: Effects on mitochondrial functionality, sirtuins, uncoupling protein 2 and antioxidant enzymes. *Int. J. Biochem. Cell Biol.* **2013**, *45*, 2045–2051. [CrossRef] [PubMed]

195. Chen, B.; Zhang, Y.; Wang, Y.; Rao, J.; Jiang, X.; Xu, Z. Curcumin inhibits proliferation of breast cancer cells through Nrf2-mediated down-regulation of Fen1 expression. *J. Steroid Biochem. Mol. Biol.* **2014**, *143*, 11–18. [CrossRef] [PubMed]

196. Siddiqui, M.A.; Ahamed, M.; Ahmad, J.; Khan, M.M.; Musarrat, J.; Al-Khedhairy, A.A.; Alrokayan, S.A. Nickel oxide nanoparticles induce cytotoxicity, oxidative stress and apoptosis in cultured human cells that is abrogated by the dietary antioxidant curcumin. *Food Chem. Toxicol.* **2012**, *50*, 641–647. [CrossRef] [PubMed]

197. Azam, S.; Hadi, N.; Khan, N.U.; Hadi, S.M. Prooxidant property of green tea polyphenols epicatechin and epigallocatechin-3-gallate: Implications for anticancer properties. *Toxicol. in Vitro* **2004**, *18*, 555–561. [CrossRef] [PubMed]

198. Bouayed, J.; Bohn, T. Exogenous antioxidants—Double-edged swords in cellular redox state: Health beneficial effects at physiologic doses versus deleterious effects at high doses. *Oxid. Med. Cell. Longev.* **2010**, *3*, 228–237. [CrossRef] [PubMed]

199. Wätjen, W.; Michels, G.; Steffan, B.; Niering, P.; Chovolou, Y.; Kampkötter, A.; Tran-Thi, Q.H.; Proksch, P.; Kahl, R. Low concentrations of flavonoids are protective in rat H4IIE cells whereas high concentrations cause DNA damage and apoptosis. *J. Nutr.* **2005**, *135*, 525–531. [PubMed]

200. Sandoval-Acuña, C.; Ferreira, J.; Speisky, H. Polyphenols and mitochondria: An update on their increasingly emerging ROS-scavenging independent actions. *Arch. Biochem. Biophys.* **2014**, *559*, 75–90. [CrossRef] [PubMed]

201. Perron, N.R.; García, C.R.; Pinzón, J.R.; Chaur, M.N.; Brumaghim, J.L. Antioxidant and prooxidant effects of polyphenol compounds on copper-mediated DNA damage. *J. Inorg. Biochem.* **2011**, *105*, 745–753. [CrossRef] [PubMed]

202. Ullah, M.F.; Ahmad, A.; Zubair, H.; Khan, H.Y.; Wang, Z.; Sarkar, F.H.; Hadi, S.M. Soy isoflavone genistein induces cell death in breast cancer cells through mobilization of endogenous copper ions and generation of reactive oxygen species. *Mol. Nutr. Food Res.* **2011**, *55*, 553–559. [CrossRef] [PubMed]

203. Singh, D.V.; Agarwal, S.; Singh, P.; Godbole, M.M.; Misra, K. Curcumin conjugates induce apoptosis via a mitochondrion dependent pathway in MCF-7 and MDA-MB-231 cell lines. *Asian Pac. J. Cancer Prev.* **2013**, *14*, 5797–5804. [CrossRef] [PubMed]

204. Braicu, C.; Pilecki, V.; Balacescu, O.; Irimie, A.; Berindan Neagoe, I. The relationships between biological activities and structure of flavan-3-ols. *Int. J. Mol. Sci.* **2011**, *12*, 9342–9353. [CrossRef] [PubMed]

205. Balkwill, F.; Mantovani, A. Inflammation and cancer: Back to virchow? *Lancet* **2001**, *357*, 539–545. [CrossRef]

206. Flossmann, E.; Rothwell, P.M. Effect of aspirin on long-term risk of colorectal cancer: Consistent evidence from randomised and observational studies. *Lancet* **2007**, *369*, 1603–1613. [CrossRef]

207. Chan, A.T.; Ogino, S.; Fuchs, C.S. Aspirin and the risk of colorectal cancer in relation to the expression of COX-2. *N. Engl. J. Med.* **2007**, *356*, 2131–2142. [CrossRef] [PubMed]

208. Anderson, W.F.; Schairer, C.; Chen, B.E.; Hance, K.W.; Levine, P.H. Epidemiology of inflammatory breast cancer (IBC). *Breast Dis.* **2005**, *22*, 9–23. [CrossRef] [PubMed]

209. Hance, K.W.; Anderson, W.F.; Devesa, S.S.; Young, H.A.; Levine, P.H. Trends in inflammatory breast carcinoma incidence and survival: The surveillance, epidemiology, and end results program at the national cancer institute. *J. Natl. Cancer Inst.* **2005**, *97*, 966–975. [CrossRef] [PubMed]

210. Kanaya, N.; Adams, L.; Takasaki, A.; Chen, S. Whole blueberry powder inhibits metastasis of triple negative breast cancer in a xenograft mouse model through modulation of inflammatory cytokines. *Nutr. Cancer* **2014**, *66*, 242–248. [CrossRef] [PubMed]

211. Vuong, T.; Mallet, J.F.; Ouzounova, M.; Rahbar, S.; Hernandez-Vargas, H.; Herceg, Z.; Matar, C. Role of a polyphenol-enriched preparation on chemoprevention of mammary carcinoma through cancer stem cells and inflammatory pathways modulation. *J. Transl. Med.* **2016**, *14*, 13. [CrossRef] [PubMed]

212. Biswas, S.K.; McClure, D.; Jimenez, L.A.; Megson, I.L.; Rahman, I. Curcumin induces glutathione biosynthesis and inhibits NF-κB activation and interleukin-8 release in alveolar epithelial cells: Mechanism of free radical scavenging activity. *Antioxid. Redox Signal.* **2005**, *7*, 32–41. [CrossRef] [PubMed]

213. Gerhäuser, C.; Klimo, K.; Heiss, E.; Neumann, I.; Gamal-Eldeen, A.; Knauft, J.; Liu, G.Y.; Sitthimonchai, S.; Frank, N. Mechanism-based in vitro screening of potential cancer chemopreventive agents. *Mutat. Res.* **2003**, *523–524*, 163–172. [CrossRef]

214. Wadsworth, T.L.; Koop, D.R. Effects of the wine polyphenolics quercetin and resveratrol on pro-inflammatory cytokine expression in raw 264.7 macrophages. *Biochem. Pharmacol.* **1999**, *57*, 941–949. [CrossRef]

215. Lawrence, T. The nuclear factor NF-κB pathway in inflammation. *Cold Spring Harb. Perspect. Biol.* **2009**, *1*, a001651. [CrossRef] [PubMed]

216. Dannenberg, A.J.; Subbaramaiah, K. Targeting cyclooxygenase-2 in human neoplasia: Rationale and promise. *Cancer Cell* **2003**, *4*, 431–436. [CrossRef]

217. Mackenzie, G.G.; Oteiza, P.I. Modulation of transcription factor NF-κB in Hodgkin's lymphoma cell lines: Effect of (−)-epicatechin. *Free Radic. Res.* **2006**, *40*, 1086–1094. [CrossRef] [PubMed]

218. Mackenzie, G.G.; Carrasquedo, F.; Delfino, J.M.; Keen, C.L.; Fraga, C.G.; Oteiza, P.I. Epicatechin, catechin, and dimeric procyanidins inhibit PMA-induced NF-κB activation at multiple steps in Jurkat T cells. *FASEB J.* **2004**, *18*, 167–169. [PubMed]

219. Divya, C.S.; Pillai, M.R. Antitumor action of curcumin in human papillomavirus associated cells involves downregulation of viral oncogenes, prevention of NFkB and AP-1 translocation, and modulation of apoptosis. *Mol. Carcinogen.* **2006**, *45*, 320–332. [CrossRef] [PubMed]

220. Wahyudi, S.; Sargowo, D. Green tea polyphenols inhibit oxidized LDL-induced NF-kB activation in human umbilical vein endothelial cells. *Acta Med. Indones.* **2007**, *39*, 66–70. [PubMed]

221. Granado-Serrano, A.B.; Martín, M.Á.; Bravo, L.; Goya, L.; Ramos, S. Quercetin attenuates TNF-induced inflammation in hepatic cells by inhibiting the NF-κB pathway. *Nutr. Cancer* **2012**, *64*, 588–598. [CrossRef] [PubMed]

222. Estrov, Z.; Shishodia, S.; Faderl, S.; Harris, D.; Van, Q.; Kantarjian, H.M.; Talpaz, M.; Aggarwal, B.B. Resveratrol blocks interleukin-1β–induced activation of the nuclear transcription factor NF-κB, inhibits proliferation, causes S-phase arrest, and induces apoptosis of acute myeloid leukemia cells. *Blood* **2003**, *102*, 987–995. [CrossRef] [PubMed]

223. Bachmeier, B.E.; Nerlich, A.G.; Iancu, C.M.; Cilli, M.; Schleicher, E.; Vené, R.; Dell'Eva, R.; Jochum, M.; Albini, A.; Pfeffer, U. The chemopreventive polyphenol curcumin prevents hematogenous breast cancer metastases in immunodeficient mice. *Cell. Physiol. Biochem.* **2007**, *19*, 137–152. [CrossRef] [PubMed]

224. Bachmeier, B.E.; Mohrenz, I.V.; Mirisola, V.; Schleicher, E.; Romeo, F.; Höhneke, C.; Jochum, M.; Nerlich, A.G.; Pfeffer, U. Curcumin downregulates the inflammatory cytokines CXCL1 and -2 in breast cancer cells via NFκB. *Carcinogenesis* **2008**, *29*, 779–789. [CrossRef] [PubMed]

225. Singh, B.N.; Shankar, S.; Srivastava, R.K. Green tea catechin, epigallocatechin-3-gallate (EGCG): Mechanisms, perspectives and clinical applications. *Biochem. Pharmacol.* **2011**, *82*, 1807–1821. [CrossRef] [PubMed]

226. Chung, S.S.; Vadgama, J.V. Curcumin and epigallocatechin gallate inhibit the cancer stem cell phenotype via down-regulation of STAT3–NFκB signaling. *Anticancer Res.* **2015**, *35*, 39–46. [PubMed]

227. Lamy, S.; Akla, N.; Ouanouki, A.; Lord-Dufour, S.; Béliveau, R. Diet-derived polyphenols inhibit angiogenesis by modulating the interleukin-6/STAT3 pathway. *Exp. Cell Res.* **2012**, *318*, 1586–1596. [CrossRef] [PubMed]

228. Zhao, X.; Sun, X.; Li, X.L. Expression and clinical significance of STAT3, P-STAT3, and VEGF-C in small cell lung cancer. *Asian Pac. J. Cancer Prev.* **2012**, *13*, 2873–2877. [CrossRef] [PubMed]

229. Bosch-Barrera, J.; Menendez, J.A. Silibinin and STAT3: A natural way of targeting transcription factors for cancer therapy. *Cancer Treat. Rev.* **2015**, *41*, 540–546. [CrossRef] [PubMed]

230. Monteiro, R.; Calhau, C.; Pinheiro-Silva, S.; Guerreiro, S.; Gärtner, F.; Azevedo, I.; Soares, R. Xanthohumol inhibits inflammatory factor production and angiogenesis in breast cancer xenografts. *J. Cell. Biochem.* **2008**, *104*, 1699–1707. [CrossRef] [PubMed]

231. Schneider, H.; Mueck, A.; Kuhl, H. IARC monographs program on carcinogenicity of combined hormonal contraceptives and menopausal therapy. *Climacteric* **2005**, *8*, 311–316. [CrossRef] [PubMed]

232. Miller, W.; Dixon, J. Local endocrine effects of aromatase inhibitors within the breast. *J. Steroid Biochem. Mol. Biol.* **2001**, *79*, 93–102. [CrossRef]

233. Czajka-Oraniec, I.; Simpson, E.R. Aromatase research and its clinical significance. *Endokrynol. Pol.* **2010**, *61*, 126–134. [PubMed]

234. Jiao, J.; Xiang, H.; Liao, Q. Recent advancement in nonsteroidal aromatase inhibitors for treatment of estrogen-dependent breast cancer. *Curr. Med. Chem.* **2010**, *17*, 3476–3487. [CrossRef] [PubMed]

235. Wang, T.; You, Q.; Huang, F.S.-G.; Xiang, H. Recent advances in selective estrogen receptor modulators for breast cancer. *Mini Rev. Med. Chem.* **2009**, *9*, 1191–1201. [CrossRef] [PubMed]

236. Jefferson, W.N.; Padilla-Banks, E.; Newbold, R.R. Adverse effects on female development and reproduction in CD-1 mice following neonatal exposure to the phytoestrogen genistein at environmentally relevant doses. *Biol. Reprod.* **2005**, *73*, 798–806. [CrossRef]

237. Pearce, S.T.; Jordan, V.C. The biological role of oestrogen receptors α and β in cancer. *Crit. Rev. Oncol. Hematol.* **2004**, *50*, 3–22. [CrossRef] [PubMed]

238. Nemenoff, R.A.; Winn, R.A. Role of nuclear receptors in lung tumourigenesis. *Eur. J. Cancer* **2005**, *41*, 2561–2568. [CrossRef] [PubMed]

239. Hsieh, R.W.; Rajan, S.S.; Sharma, S.K.; Guo, Y.; DeSombre, E.R.; Mrksich, M.; Greene, G.L. Identification of ligands with bicyclic scaffolds provides insights into mechanisms of estrogen receptor subtype selectivity. *J. Biol. Chem.* **2006**, *281*, 17909–17919. [CrossRef] [PubMed]

240. Barnes, S. Effect of genistein on in vitro and in vivo models of cancer. *J. Nutr.* **1995**, *125*, 777S–783S.

241. Kuiper, G.G.; Lemmen, J.G.; Carlsson, B.; Corton, J.C.; Safe, S.H.; van Der Saag, P.T.; van Der Burg, B.; Gustafsson, J.A. Interaction of estrogenic chemicals and phytoestrogens with estrogen receptor β. *Endocrinology* **1998**, *139*, 4252–4263. [PubMed]

242. Yoshimaru, T.; Komatsu, M.; Tashiro, E.; Imoto, M.; Osada, H.; Miyoshi, Y.; Honda, J.; Sasa, M.; Katagiri, T. Xanthohumol suppresses oestrogen-signalling in breast cancer through the inhibition of BIG3-PHB2 interactions. *Sci. Rep.* **2014**, *4*, 7355. [CrossRef] [PubMed]

243. Papoutsi, Z.; Kassi, E.; Tsiapara, A.; Fokialakis, N.; Chrousos, G.P.; Moutsatsou, P. Evaluation of estrogenic/antiestrogenic activity of ellagic acid via the estrogen receptor subtypes ERα and ERβ. *J. Agric. Food Chem.* **2005**, *53*, 7715–7720. [CrossRef] [PubMed]

244. Aiyer, H.S.; Gupta, R.C. Berries and ellagic acid prevent estrogen-induced mammary tumorigenesis by modulating enzymes of estrogen metabolism. *Cancer Prev. Res.* **2010**, *3*, 727–737. [CrossRef] [PubMed]

245. Nandhakumar, R.; Salini, K.; Devaraj, S.N. Morin augments anticarcinogenic and antiproliferative efficacy against 7, 12-dimethylbenz (a)-anthracene induced experimental mammary carcinogenesis. *Med. Cell. Biochem.* **2012**, *364*, 79–92. [CrossRef] [PubMed]

246. Fang, H.; Tong, W.; Shi, L.M.; Blair, R.; Perkins, R.; Branham, W.; Hass, B.S.; Xie, Q.; Dial, S.L.; Moland, C.L. Structure-activity relationships for a large diverse set of natural, synthetic, and environmental estrogens. *Chem. Res. Toxicol.* **2001**, *14*, 280–294. [CrossRef] [PubMed]

247. Wang, L.M.; Xie, K.P.; Huo, H.N.; Shang, F.; Zou, W.; Xie, M.J. Luteolin inhibits proliferation induced by IGF-1 pathway dependent ERα in human breast cancer MCF-7 cells. *Asian Pac. J. Cancer Prev.* **2012**, *13*, 1431–1437. [CrossRef] [PubMed]

248. Chen, F.P.; Chien, M.H. Phytoestrogens induce apoptosis through a mitochondria/caspase pathway in human breast cancer cells. *Climacteric* **2014**, *17*, 385–392. [CrossRef] [PubMed]

249. Huang, C.; Lee, S.Y.; Lin, C.L.; Tu, T.H.; Chen, L.H.; Chen, Y.J.; Huang, H.C. Co-treatment with quercetin and 1, 2, 3, 4, 6-penta-O-galloyl-β-d-glucose causes cell cycle arrest and apoptosis in human breast cancer MDA-MB-231 and AU565 cells. *J. Agric. Food Chem.* **2013**, *61*, 6430–6445. [CrossRef] [PubMed]

250. Le Corre, L.; Chalabi, N.; Delort, L.; Bignon, Y.J.; Bernard-Gallon, D.J. Differential expression of genes induced by resveratrol in human breast cancer cell lines. *Nutr. Cancer* **2006**, *56*, 193–203. [CrossRef] [PubMed]

251. Zeng, L.; Holly, J.M.; Perks, C.M. Effects of physiological levels of the green tea extract epigallocatechin-3-gallate on breast cancer cells. *Front. Endocrinol.* **2014**, *5*, 61. [CrossRef] [PubMed]

252. Messina, M.; Nagata, C.; Wu, A.H. Estimated asian adult soy protein and isoflavone intakes. *Nutr. Cancer* **2006**, *55*, 1–12. [CrossRef] [PubMed]

253. Wang, T.T.; Sathyamoorthy, N.; Phang, J.M. Molecular effects of genistein on estrogen receptor mediated pathways. *Carcinogenesis* **1996**, *17*, 271–275. [CrossRef] [PubMed]

254. Oseni, T.; Patel, R.; Pyle, J.; Jordan, V.C. Selective estrogen receptor modulators and phytoestrogens. *Planta Med.* **2008**, *74*, 1656–1665. [CrossRef] [PubMed]

255. Patisaul, H.B.; Jefferson, W. The pros and cons of phytoestrogens. *Front. Neuroendocrinol.* **2010**, *31*, 400–419. [CrossRef] [PubMed]

256. Simpson, E.R. Aromatase: Biologic Relevance of Tissue-Specific Expression. *Semin. Reprod. Med.* **2004**, *22*, 11–23. [PubMed]

257. Ghosh, D.; Griswold, J.; Erman, M.; Pangborn, W. Structural basis for androgen specificity and oestrogen synthesis in human aromatase. *Nature* **2009**, *457*, 219–223. [CrossRef] [PubMed]

258. Kudachkar, R.; O'Regan, R.M. Aromatase inhibitors as adjuvant therapy for postmenopausal patients with early stage breast cancer. *CA Cancer J. Clin.* **2005**, *55*, 145–163. [CrossRef] [PubMed]

259. Kim, M.J.; Woo, S.J.; Yoon, C.H.; Lee, J.S.; An, S.; Choi, Y.H.; Hwang, S.G.; Yoon, G.; Lee, S.J. Involvement of autophagy in oncogenic K-Ras-induced malignant cell transformation. *J. Biol. Chem.* **2011**, *286*, 12924–12932. [CrossRef] [PubMed]

260. Balunas, M.J.; Su, B.; Brueggemeier, R.W.; Kinghorn, A.D. Natural products as aromatase inhibitors. *Anti-Cancer Agents Med. Chem.* **2008**, *8*, 646–682. [CrossRef] [PubMed]

261. Brueggemeier, R.W.; Hackett, J.C.; Diaz-Cruz, E.S. Aromatase inhibitors in the treatment of breast cancer. *Endocr. Rev.* **2005**, *26*, 331–345. [CrossRef] [PubMed]

262. Kao, Y.C.; Zhou, C.; Sherman, M.; Laughton, C.A.; Chen, S. Molecular basis of the inhibition of human aromatase (estrogen synthetase) by flavone and isoflavone phytoestrogens: A site-directed mutagenesis study. *Environ. Health Perspect.* **1998**, *106*, 85–92. [CrossRef] [PubMed]

263. Wang, Y.; Gho, W.M.; Chan, F.L.; Chen, S.; Leung, L.K. The red clover (*Trifolium pratense*) isoflavone biochanin a inhibits aromatase activity and expression. *Br. J. Nutr.* **2008**, *99*, 303–310. [CrossRef] [PubMed]

264. Ye, L.; Gho, W.M.; Chan, F.L.; Chen, S.; Leung, L.K. Dietary administration of the licorice flavonoid isoliquiritigenin deters the growth of MCF-7 cells overexpressing aromatase. *Int. J. Cancer* **2009**, *124*, 1028–1036. [CrossRef] [PubMed]

265. Li, F.; Ye, L.; Lin, S.M.; Leung, L.K. Dietary flavones and flavonones display differential effects on aromatase (CYP19) transcription in the breast cancer cells MCF-7. *Mol. Cell. Endocrinol.* **2011**, *344*, 51–58. [CrossRef] [PubMed]

266. Li, F.; Wong, T.Y.; Lin, S.M.; Chow, S.; Cheung, W.H.; Chan, F.L.; Chen, S.; Leung, L.K. Coadministering luteolin minimizes the side effects of the aromatase inhibitor letrozole. *J. Pharmacol. Exp. Ther.* **2014**, *351*, 270–277. [CrossRef] [PubMed]

267. Ji, J.Z.; Lao, K.J.; Hu, J.; Pang, T.; Jiang, Z.Z.; Yuan, H.L.; Miao, J.S.; Chen, X.; Ning, S.S.; Xiang, H. Discovery of novel aromatase inhibitors using a homogeneous time-resolved fluorescence assay. *Acta Pharmacol. Sin.* **2014**, *35*, 1082–1092. [CrossRef] [PubMed]

268. González-Sarrías, A.; Ma, H.; Edmonds, M.E.; Seeram, N.P. Maple polyphenols, ginnalins A–C, induce S-and G2/M-cell cycle arrest in colon and breast cancer cells mediated by decreasing cyclins A and D1 levels. *Food Chem.* **2013**, *136*, 636–642. [CrossRef] [PubMed]

269. Liang, Y.C.; Lin-Shiau, S.Y.; Chen, C.F.; Lin, J.K. Inhibition of cyclin-dependent kinases 2 and 4 activities as well as induction of cdk inhibitors p21 and p27 during growth arrest of human breast carcinoma cells by (−)-epigallocatechin-3-gallate. *J. Cell. Biochem.* **1999**, *75*, 1–12. [CrossRef]

270. Mawson, A.; Lai, A.; Carroll, J.S.; Sergio, C.M.; Mitchell, C.J.; Sarcevic, B. Estrogen and insulin/IGF-1 cooperatively stimulate cell cycle progression in MCF-7 breast cancer cells through differential regulation of c-Myc and cyclin D1. *Mol. Cell. Endocrinol.* **2005**, *229*, 161–173. [CrossRef] [PubMed]

271. Li, J.; Zhu, F.; Lubet, R.A.; De Luca, A.; Grubbs, C.; Ericson, M.E.; D'Alessio, A.; Normanno, N.; Dong, Z.; Bode, A.M. Quercetin-3-methyl ether inhibits lapatinib-sensitive and -resistant breast cancer cell growth by inducing G2/M arrest and apoptosis. *Mol. Carcinogen.* **2013**, *52*, 134–143. [CrossRef] [PubMed]

272. Choi, J.A.; Kim, J.Y.; Lee, J.Y.; Kang, C.M.; Kwon, H.J.; Yoo, Y.D.; Kim, T.W.; Lee, Y.S.; Lee, S.J. Induction of cell cycle arrest and apoptosis in human breast cancer cells by quercetin. *Int. J. Oncol.* **2001**, *19*, 837–844. [CrossRef] [PubMed]

273. Chou, C.C.; Yang, J.S.; Lu, H.F.; Ip, S.W.; Lo, C.; Wu, C.C.; Lin, J.P.; Tang, N.Y.; Chung, J.G.; Chou, M.J. Quercetin-mediated cell cycle arrest and apoptosis involving activation of a caspase cascade through the mitochondrial pathway in human breast cancer MCF-7 cells. *Arch. Pharm. Res.* **2010**, *33*, 1181–1191. [CrossRef] [PubMed]

274. Hsieh, T.C.; Wong, C.; John Bennett, D.; Wu, J.M. Regulation of p53 and cell proliferation by resveratrol and its derivatives in breast cancer cells: An in silico and biochemical approach targeting integrin $\alpha v \beta 3$. *Int. J. Cancer* **2011**, *129*, 2732–2743. [CrossRef] [PubMed]

275. Simon, A.; Allais, D.; Duroux, J.; Basly, J.; Durand-Fontanier, S.; Delage, C. Inhibitory effect of curcuminoids on MCF-7 cell proliferation and structure–activity relationships. *Cancer Lett.* **1998**, *129*, 111–116. [CrossRef]

276. Choudhuri, T.; Pal, S.; Agarwal, M.L.; Das, T.; Sa, G. Curcumin induces apoptosis in human breast cancer cells through p53-dependent bax induction. *FEBS Lett.* **2002**, *512*, 334–340. [CrossRef]

277. Banerjee, M.; Singh, P.; Panda, D. Curcumin suppresses the dynamic instability of microtubules, activates the mitotic checkpoint and induces apoptosis in MCF-7 cells. *FEBS J.* **2010**, *277*, 3437–3448. [CrossRef] [PubMed]

278. Choi, E.J.; Kim, G.H. Apigenin causes G(2)/m arrest associated with the modulation of p21(Cip1) and Cdc2 and activates p53-dependent apoptosis pathway in human breast cancer SK-BR-3 cells. *J. Nutr. Biochem.* **2009**, *20*, 285–290. [CrossRef] [PubMed]

279. Umeda, D.; Tachibana, H.; Yamada, K. Epigallocatechin-3-*O*-gallate disrupts stress fibers and the contractile ring by reducing myosin regulatory light chain phosphorylation mediated through the target molecule 67kDa laminin receptor. *Biochem. Biophys. Res. Commun.* **2005**, *333*, 628–635. [CrossRef] [PubMed]

280. Elmore, S. Apoptosis: A review of programmed cell death. *Toxicol. Pathol.* **2007**, *35*, 495–516. [CrossRef] [PubMed]

281. Chien, S.Y.; Wu, Y.C.; Chung, J.G.; Yang, J.S.; Lu, H.F.; Tsou, M.F.; Wood, W.; Kuo, S.J.; Chen, D.R. Quercetin-induced apoptosis acts through mitochondrial-and caspase-3-dependent pathways in human breast cancer MDA-MB-231 cells. *Hum. Exp. Toxicol.* **2009**, *28*, 493–503. [CrossRef] [PubMed]

282. Seo, H.S.; Ku, J.M.; Choi, H.S.; Woo, J.K.; Jang, B.H.; Go, H.; Shin, Y.C.; Ko, S.G. Apigenin induces caspase-dependent apoptosis by inhibiting signal transducer and activator of transcription 3 signaling in HER2-overexpressing SKBR3 breast cancer cells. *Mol. Med. Rep.* **2015**, *12*, 2977–2984. [PubMed]

283. Thangapazham, R.L.; Passi, N.; Maheshwari, R.K. Green tea polyphenol and epigallocatechin gallate induce apoptosis and inhibit invasion in human breast cancer cells. *Cancer Biol. Ther.* **2007**, *6*, 1938–1943. [CrossRef] [PubMed]

284. Clément, M.V.; Hirpara, J.L.; Chawdhury, S.H.; Pervaiz, S. Chemopreventive agent resveratrol, a natural product derived from grapes, triggers CD95 signaling-dependent apoptosis in human tumor cells. *Blood* **1998**, *92*, 996–1002. [PubMed]

285. Alkhalaf, M. Resveratrol-induced apoptosis is associated with activation of p53 and inhibition of protein translation in T47D human breast cancer cells. *Pharmacology* **2007**, *80*, 134–143. [CrossRef] [PubMed]

286. Alkhalaf, M.; El-Mowafy, A.; Renno, W.; Rachid, O.; Ali, A.; Al-Attyiah, R. Resveratrol-induced apoptosis in human breast cancer cells is mediated primarily through the caspase-3-dependent pathway. *Arch. Med. Res.* **2008**, *39*, 162–168. [CrossRef] [PubMed]

287. Kotha, A.; Sekharam, M.; Cilenti, L.; Siddiquee, K.; Khaled, A.; Zervos, A.S.; Carter, B.; Turkson, J.; Jove, R. Resveratrol inhibits Src and Stat3 signaling and induces the apoptosis of malignant cells containing activated Stat3 protein. *Mol. Cancer Ther.* **2006**, *5*, 621–629. [CrossRef] [PubMed]

288. Sakamoto, T.; Horiguchi, H.; Oguma, E.; Kayama, F. Effects of diverse dietary phytoestrogens on cell growth, cell cycle and apoptosis in estrogen-receptor-positive breast cancer cells. *J. Nutr. Biochem.* **2010**, *21*, 856–864. [CrossRef] [PubMed]

289. Chen, J.; Duan, Y.; Zhang, X.; Ye, Y.; Ge, B.; Chen, J. Genistein induces apoptosis by the inactivation of the IGF-1R/p-Akt signaling pathway in MCF-7 human breast cancer cells. *Food Funct.* **2015**, *6*, 995–1000. [CrossRef] [PubMed]

290. Yang, P.M.; Tseng, H.H.; Peng, C.W.; Chen, W.S.; Chiu, S.J. Dietary flavonoid fisetin targets caspase-3-deficient human breast cancer MCF-7 cells by induction of caspase-7-associated apoptosis and inhibition of autophagy. *Int. J. Oncol.* **2012**, *40*, 469. [PubMed]

291. Gottesman, M.M. Mechanisms of cancer drug resistance. *Annu. Rev. Med.* **2002**, *53*, 615–627. [CrossRef] [PubMed]

292. Dean, M.; Fojo, T.; Bates, S. Tumour stem cells and drug resistance. *Nat. Rev. Cancer* **2005**, *5*, 275–284. [CrossRef] [PubMed]

293. Gottesman, M.M.; Fojo, T.; Bates, S.E. Multidrug resistance in cancer: Role of ATP–dependent transporters. *Nat. Rev. Cancer* **2002**, *2*, 48–58. [CrossRef] [PubMed]

294. Jodoin, J.; Demeule, M.; Béliveau, R. Inhibition of the multidrug resistance P-glycoprotein activity by green tea polyphenols. *Biochim. Biophys. Acta* **2002**, *1542*, 149–159. [CrossRef]

295. Wu, C.P.; Calcagno, A.M.; Hladky, S.B.; Ambudkar, S.V.; Barrand, M.A. Modulatory effects of plant phenols on human multidrug-resistance proteins 1, 4 and 5 (ABCC1, 4 and 5). *FEBS J.* **2005**, *272*, 4725–4740. [CrossRef] [PubMed]

296. Choi, B.H.; Kim, C.G.; Lim, Y.; Shin, S.Y.; Lee, Y.H. Curcumin down-regulates the multidrug-resistance *mdr1b* gene by inhibiting the PI3K/Akt/NFκB pathway. *Cancer Lett.* **2008**, *259*, 111–118. [CrossRef] [PubMed]

297. Harbottle, A.; Daly, A.K.; Atherton, K.; Campbell, F.C. Role of glutathione S-transferase p1, P-glycoprotein and multidrug resistance-associated protein 1 in acquired doxorubicin resistance. *Int. J. Cancer* **2001**, *92*, 777–783. [CrossRef] [PubMed]

298. O'Connor, M.L.; Xiang, D.; Shigdar, S.; Macdonald, J.; Li, Y.; Wang, T.; Pu, C.; Wang, Z.; Qiao, L.; Duan, W. Cancer stem cells: A contentious hypothesis now moving forward. *Cancer Lett.* **2014**, *344*, 180–187. [CrossRef] [PubMed]

299. Camerlingo, R.; Ferraro, G.A.; De Francesco, F.; Romano, M.; Nicoletti, G.; Di Bonito, M.; Rinaldo, M.; D'Andrea, F.; Pirozzi, G. The role of CD44+/CD24-/low biomarker for screening, diagnosis and monitoring of breast cancer. *Oncol. Rep.* **2014**, *31*, 1127–1132. [PubMed]

300. Valkenburg, K.C.; Graveel, C.R.; Zylstra-Diegel, C.R.; Zhong, Z.; Williams, B.O. Wnt/β-catenin signaling in normal and cancer stem cells. *Cancers* **2011**, *3*, 2050–2079. [CrossRef] [PubMed]

301. Ingham, P.W.; McMahon, A.P. Hedgehog signaling in animal development: Paradigms and principles. *Genes Dev.* **2001**, *15*, 3059–3087. [CrossRef] [PubMed]

302. McMahon, A.P.; Ingham, P.W.; Tabin, C.J. 1 Developmental roles and clinical significance of hedgehog signaling. *Curr. Top. Dev. Biol.* **2003**, *53*, 1–114. [PubMed]

303. Murone, M.; Rosenthal, A.; de Sauvage, F.J. Sonic hedgehog signaling by the patched-smoothened receptor complex. *Curr. Biol.* **1999**, *9*, 76–84. [CrossRef]

304. Liu, S.; Dontu, G.; Mantle, I.D.; Patel, S.; Ahn, N.S.; Jackson, K.W.; Suri, P.; Wicha, M.S. Hedgehog signaling and Bmi-1 regulate self-renewal of normal and malignant human mammary stem cells. *Cancer Res.* **2006**, *66*, 6063–6071. [CrossRef] [PubMed]

305. Ehtesham, M.; Sarangi, A.; Valadez, J.; Chanthaphaychith, S.; Becher, M.; Abel, T.; Thompson, R.; Cooper, M. Ligand-dependent activation of the hedgehog pathway in glioma progenitor cells. *Oncogene* **2007**, *26*, 5752–5761. [CrossRef] [PubMed]

306. Peacock, C.D.; Wang, Q.; Gesell, G.S.; Corcoran-Schwartz, I.M.; Jones, E.; Kim, J.; Devereux, W.L.; Rhodes, J.T.; Huff, C.A.; Beachy, P.A. Hedgehog signaling maintains a tumor stem cell compartment in multiple myeloma. *Proc. Natl. Acad. Sci. USA* **2007**, *104*, 4048–4053. [CrossRef] [PubMed]

307. Zhang, C.; Li, C.; He, F.; Cai, Y.; Yang, H. Identification of CD44+ CD24+ gastric cancer stem cells. *J. Cancer Res. Clin. Oncol.* **2011**, *137*, 1679–1686. [CrossRef] [PubMed]

308. Ng, J.M.; Curran, T. The hedgehog's tale: Developing strategies for targeting cancer. *Nat. Rev. Cancer* **2011**, *11*, 493–501. [CrossRef] [PubMed]

309. Feldmann, G.; Dhara, S.; Fendrich, V.; Bedja, D.; Beaty, R.; Mullendore, M.; Karikari, C.; Alvarez, H.; Iacobuzio-Donahue, C.; Jimeno, A. Blockade of hedgehog signaling inhibits pancreatic cancer invasion and metastases: A new paradigm for combination therapy in solid cancers. *Cancer Res.* **2007**, *67*, 2187–2196. [CrossRef] [PubMed]

310. Fan, P.; Fan, S.; Wang, H.; Mao, J.; Shi, Y.; Ibrahim, M.M.; Ma, W.; Yu, X.; Hou, Z.; Wang, B.; et al. Genistein decreases the breast cancer stem-like cell population through hedgehog pathway. *Stem Cell Res. Ther.* **2013**, *4*, 146. [CrossRef] [PubMed]

311. Bray, S.J. Notch signalling: A simple pathway becomes complex. *Nat. Rev. Mol. Cell Biol.* **2006**, *7*, 678–689. [CrossRef] [PubMed]

312. Ishii, H.; Iwatsuki, M.; Ieta, K.; Ohta, D.; Haraguchi, N.; Mimori, K.; Mori, M. Cancer stem cells and chemoradiation resistance. *Cancer Sci.* **2008**, *99*, 1871–1877. [CrossRef] [PubMed]

313. Cecchinato, V.; Chiaramonte, R.; Nizzardo, M.; Cristofaro, B.; Basile, A.; Sherbet, G.V.; Comi, P. Resveratrol-induced apoptosis in human T-cell acute lymphoblastic leukaemia MOLT-4 cells. *Biochem. Pharmacol.* **2007**, *74*, 1568–1574. [CrossRef] [PubMed]

314. Liu, S.; Dontu, G.; Wicha, M.S. Mammary stem cells, self-renewal pathways, and carcinogenesis. *Breast Cancer Res.* **2005**, *7*, 86–95. [CrossRef] [PubMed]

315. Clevers, H. Wnt/β-catenin signaling in development and disease. *Cell* **2006**, *127*, 469–480. [CrossRef] [PubMed]

316. Kim, J.; Zhang, X.; Rieger-Christ, K.M.; Summerhayes, I.C.; Wazer, D.E.; Paulson, K.E.; Yee, A.S. Suppression of Wnt signaling by the green tea compound (–)-epigallocatechin 3-gallate (EGCG) in invasive breast cancer cells. Requirement of the transcriptional repressor HBP1. *J. Biol. Chem.* **2006**, *281*, 10865–10875. [CrossRef] [PubMed]

317. Ju, J.; Hong, J.; Zhou, J.N.; Pan, Z.; Bose, M.; Liao, J.; Yang, G.Y.; Liu, Y.Y.; Hou, Z.; Lin, Y. Inhibition of intestinal tumorigenesis in Apcmin/+ mice by (–)-epigallocatechin-3-gallate, the major catechin in green tea. *Cancer Res.* **2005**, *65*, 10623–10631. [CrossRef] [PubMed]

318. Jaiswal, A.S.; Marlow, B.P.; Gupta, N.; Narayan, S. Beta-catenin-mediated transactivation and cell–cell adhesion pathways are important in curcumin (diferuylmethane)-induced growth arrest and apoptosis in colon cancer cells. *Oncogene* **2002**, *21*, 0414–0427. [CrossRef] [PubMed]

319. Clarke, J.D.; Dashwood, R.H.; Ho, E. Multi-targeted prevention of cancer by sulforaphane. *Cancer Lett.* **2008**, *269*, 291–304. [CrossRef] [PubMed]

320. Kallifatidis, G.; Rausch, V.; Baumann, B.; Apel, A.; Beckermann, B.M.; Groth, A.; Mattern, J.; Li, Z.; Kolb, A.; Moldenhauer, G. Sulforaphane targets pancreatic tumour-initiating cells by NF-κB-induced antiapoptotic signalling. *Gut* **2009**, *58*, 949–963. [CrossRef] [PubMed]

321. Li, Y.; Zhang, T.; Korkaya, H.; Liu, S.; Lee, H.F.; Newman, B.; Yu, Y.; Clouthier, S.G.; Schwartz, S.J.; Wicha, M.S. Sulforaphane, a dietary component of broccoli/broccoli sprouts, inhibits breast cancer stem cells. *Clin. Cancer Res.* **2010**, *16*, 2580–2590. [CrossRef] [PubMed]

322. Park, S.Y.; Kim, G.Y.; Bae, S.J.; Yoo, Y.H.; Choi, Y.H. Induction of apoptosis by isothiocyanate sulforaphane in human cervical carcinoma HeLa and hepatocarcinoma HepG2 cells through activation of caspase-3. *Oncol. Rep.* **2007**, *18*, 181–187. [CrossRef] [PubMed]

323. Pradeep, C.; Kuttan, G. Effect of piperine on the inhibition of lung metastasis induced B16F-10 melanoma cells in mice. *Clin. Exp. Metastasis* **2002**, *19*, 703–708. [CrossRef] [PubMed]

324. Kakarala, M.; Brenner, D.E.; Korkaya, H.; Cheng, C.; Tazi, K.; Ginestier, C.; Liu, S.; Dontu, G.; Wicha, M.S. Targeting breast stem cells with the cancer preventive compounds curcumin and piperine. *Breast Cancer Res. Treat.* **2010**, *122*, 777–785. [CrossRef] [PubMed]

325. Zhang, Y.; Piao, B.; Zhang, Y.; Hua, B.; Hou, W.; Xu, W.; Qi, X.; Zhu, X.; Pei, Y.; Lin, H. Oxymatrine diminishes the side population and inhibits the expression of β-catenin in MCF-7 breast cancer cells. *Med. Oncol.* **2011**, *28* (Suppl. 1), S99–S107. [CrossRef] [PubMed]

326. Mortensen, M.; Soilleux, E.J.; Djordjevic, G.; Tripp, R.; Lutteropp, M.; Sadighi-Akha, E.; Stranks, A.J.; Glanville, J.; Knight, S.; Jacobsen, S.-E.W. The autophagy protein Atg7 is essential for hematopoietic stem cell maintenance. *J. Exp. Med.* **2011**, *208*, 455–467. [CrossRef] [PubMed]

327. Gong, C.; Song, E.; Codogno, P.; Mehrpour, M. The roles of BECN1 and autophagy in cancer are context dependent. *Autophagy* **2012**, *8*, 1853–1855. [CrossRef] [PubMed]

328. Galavotti, S.; Bartesaghi, S.; Faccenda, D.; Shaked-Rabi, M.; Sanzone, S.; McEvoy, A.; Dinsdale, D.; Condorelli, F.; Brandner, S.; Campanella, M. The autophagy-associated factors DRAM1 and p62 regulate cell migration and invasion in glioblastoma stem cells. *Oncogene* **2013**, *32*, 699–712. [CrossRef] [PubMed]

329. Kumar, D.; Shankar, S.; Srivastava, R.K. Rottlerin-induced autophagy leads to the apoptosis in breast cancer stem cells: Molecular mechanisms. *Mol. Cancer* **2013**, *12*, 171. [CrossRef] [PubMed]

330. Fu, Y.; Chang, H.; Peng, X.; Bai, Q.; Yi, L.; Zhou, Y.; Zhu, J.; Mi, M. Resveratrol inhibits breast cancer stem-like cells and induces autophagy via suppressing Wnt/β-catenin signaling pathway. *PLoS ONE* **2014**, *9*, e102535. [CrossRef] [PubMed]

331. Singh, A.; Settleman, J. EMT, cancer stem cells and drug resistance: An emerging axis of evil in the war on cancer. *Oncogene* **2010**, *29*, 4741–4751. [CrossRef] [PubMed]

332. Polyak, K.; Weinberg, R.A. Transitions between epithelial and mesenchymal states: Acquisition of malignant and stem cell traits. *Nat. Rev. Cancer* **2009**, *9*, 265–273. [CrossRef] [PubMed]

333. Hugo, H.; Ackland, M.L.; Blick, T.; Lawrence, M.G.; Clements, J.A.; Williams, E.D.; Thompson, E.W. Epithelial-mesenchymal and mesenchymal-epithelial transitions in carcinoma progression. *J. Cell. Physiol.* **2007**, *213*, 374–383. [CrossRef] [PubMed]

334. Thiery, J.P.; Sleeman, J.P. Complex networks orchestrate epithelial–mesenchymal transitions. *Nat. Rev. Mol. Cell Biol.* **2006**, *7*, 131–142. [CrossRef] [PubMed]

335. Min, C.; Eddy, S.F.; Sherr, D.H.; Sonenshein, G.E. NF-κB and epithelial to mesenchymal transition of cancer. *J. Cell. Biochem.* **2008**, *104*, 733–744. [CrossRef] [PubMed]

336. Shi, X.P.; Miao, S.; Wu, Y.; Zhang, W.; Zhang, X.F.; Ma, H.Z.; Xin, H.L.; Feng, J.; Wen, A.D.; Li, Y. Resveratrol sensitizes tamoxifen in antiestrogen-resistant breast cancer cells with epithelial-mesenchymal transition features. *Int. J. Mol. Sci.* **2013**, *14*, 15655–15668. [CrossRef] [PubMed]

337. Vergara, D.; Valente, C.M.; Tinelli, A.; Siciliano, C.; Lorusso, V.; Acierno, R.; Giovinazzo, G.; Santino, A.; Storelli, C.; Maffia, M. Resveratrol inhibits the epidermal growth factor-induced epithelial mesenchymal transition in MCF-7 cells. *Cancer Lett.* **2011**, *310*, 1–8. [CrossRef] [PubMed]

338. Chung, H.; Choi, H.S.; Seo, E.K.; Kang, D.H.; Oh, E.S. Baicalin and baicalein inhibit transforming growth factor-β1-mediated epithelial-mesenchymal transition in human breast epithelial cells. *Biochem. Biophys. Res. Commun.* **2015**, *458*, 707–713. [CrossRef] [PubMed]

339. Yang, B.; Huang, J.; Xiang, T.; Yin, X.; Luo, X.; Huang, J.; Luo, F.; Li, H.; Li, H.; Ren, G. Chrysin inhibits metastatic potential of human triple-negative breast cancer cells by modulating matrix metalloproteinase-10, epithelial to mesenchymal transition, and PI3K/Akt signaling pathway. *J. Appl. Toxicol.* **2014**, *34*, 105–112. [CrossRef] [PubMed]

340. Nagaraj, G.; Ellis, M.J.; Ma, C.X. The natural history of hormone receptor-positive breast cancer: Attempting to decipher an intriguing concept. *Oncology* **2012**, *26*, 696–697, 700. [PubMed]

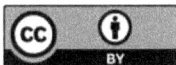

**MDPI**

*Review*

# The Anticancer Properties of *Herba Epimedii* and Its Main Bioactive Componentsicariin and Icariside II

Meixia Chen [1], Jinfeng Wu [2], Qingli Luo [1], Shuming Mo [1], Yubao Lyu [1], Ying Wei [1] and Jingcheng Dong [1,*]

[1]  Department of Integrative Medicine, Huashan Hospital, Fudan University, Shanghai 200040, China; cmx023@126.com (M.C.); qingqingluo2010@163.com (Q.L.); moshuming0703@163.com (S.M.); lvyubao80313@163.com (Y.L.); weiying_acup@126.com (Y.W.)

[2]  Department of Dermatology, Huashan Hospital, Fudan University, Shanghai 200040, China; wujinfeng21@163.com

*   Correspondence: jcdong2004@126.com; Tel.: +86-21-5288-8301

Received: 15 July 2016; Accepted: 2 September 2016; Published: 13 September 2016

**Abstract:** Cancer is one of the leading causes of deaths worldwide. Compounds derived from traditional Chinese medicines have been an important source of anticancer drugs and adjuvant agents to potentiate the efficacy of chemotherapeutic drugs and improve the side effects of chemotherapy. *Herba Epimedii* is one of most popular herbs used in China traditionally for the treatment of multiple diseases, including osteoporosis, sexual dysfunction, hypertension and common inflammatory diseases. Studies show *Herba Epimedii* also possesses anticancer activity. Flavonol glycosides icariin and icariside II are the main bioactive components of *Herba Epimedii*. They have been found to possess anticancer activities against various human cancer cell lines in vitro and mouse tumor models in vivo via their effects on multiple biological pathways, including cell cycle regulation, apoptosis, angiogenesis, and metastasis, and a variety of signaling pathways including JAK2-STAT3, MAPK-ERK, and PI3k-Akt-mTOR. The review is aimed to provide an overview of the current research results supporting their therapeutic effects and to highlight the molecular targets and action mechanisms.

**Keywords:** anticancer properties; *Herba Epimedii*; icariin; icariside II

## 1. Introduction

Cancer is a complex genetic disease involving abnormal cell growth and is continue to be one of the major causes of deaths in both developed and developing countries [1]. According to statistics, there are approximately 14.1 million new cancer cases and 8.2 million deaths in 2012 [2]. It is estimated that new cancer cases will increase to 20 million by 2025. Cancer has been recognized as one of the most crucial health problems all over the world due to its great increased incidence and significant mortality.

Plants have a long history of use in the treatment of cancer and it is reported that more than 3000 plant species have been used [3,4]. The search for anticancer drugs from plant sources started as early as the 1950s, and at present over 60% of anticancer drugs currently used are derived directly or indirectly from natural sources, including plants, marine organisms and micro-organisms [5,6]. One of the successful stories is the discovery and development of the vinca alkaloids, vinblastine and vincristine, isolated from *Catharanthusroseus G. Don* (Apocynaceae) [7], which are the first plant-derived anticancer agents applied to clinical use for the treatment of various cancers [8,9].

*Herba Epimedii* (Common name: Yin-yang-huo in China, Figure 1) is the dried leaf of *Epimedium brevicornu* Maxim., *Epimedium sagittatum* (Sieb. EtZucc.) Maxim., *Epimedium pubescens* Maxim. or *Epimedium koreanum* Nakaias as recorded in the Chinese Pharmacopoeia (Figure 1) [10]. There are more than 40 kinds of *Epimedium* plants all over the world, mainly distributed in the southwest and central regions of China, although some are found in the temperate and subtropical regions of Asia, Middle East as well as Europe [11]. *Herba Epimedii* has been recorded in the Chinese medical classics *Shen Nong Ben Cao Jing* 400 years ago and has been used in various traditional Chinese formulations. The herb is believed to "nourishing the kidney and reinforcing the Yang" and is proven to have remarkably therapeutic activities. In China and Japan, *Herba Epimedii* alone, or in the formulations, have been widely used for treatment of osteoporosis [12,13], sexual dysfunction [14], hypertension [15] and common inflammatory diseases, such as chronic obstructive pulmonary disease [16]. In addition, *Herba Epimedii* has been shown to exert anticancer effect on cancer cell lines in vitro and also in vivo in mouse tumor model [17].

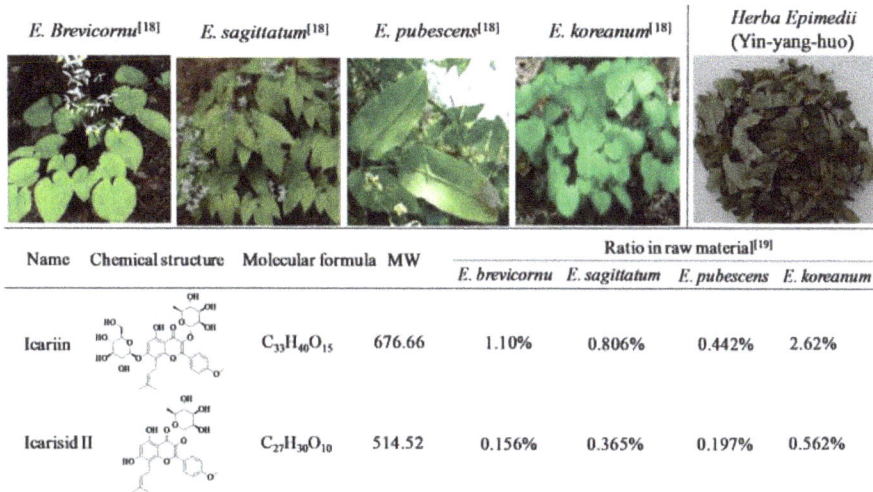

| Name | Chemical structure | Molecular formula | MW | Ratio in raw material[19] | | | |
|------|-------------------|-------------------|-----|----------------------------|---|---|---|
| | | | | *E. brevicornu* | *E. sagittatum* | *E. pubescens* | *E. koreanum* |
| Icariin | | $C_{33}H_{40}O_{15}$ | 676.66 | 1.10% | 0.806% | 0.442% | 2.62% |
| Icarisid II | | $C_{27}H_{30}O_{10}$ | 514.52 | 0.156% | 0.365% | 0.197% | 0.562% |

**Figure 1.** Natural sources and chemical structures of icariin and icariside II [18,19]. Herba Epimedii is made up of the dried leaves of *E. brevicornu*, *E. sagittatum*, *E. pubescens* or *E. koreanum*.

More than 260 constituents have been detected from Herba Epimedii with 141 flavonoids, 31 lignins and multiple other kinds of compounds [11], and the flavonoid glycosides have been confirmed to be the fundamental pharmacologically active constituents [20]. Icariin (Figure 1) is the major active constituent and has been chosen as the chemical marker for quality control of *Herba Epimedii* in Chinese Pharmacopeia. It is specified that the contents of icariin and the total flavonoids are no less than 0.5% and 5.0%, respectively [10]. Icariin has been found to possess a variety of pharmacological activities, including anti-osteoporosis [21], anti-inflammatory [22,23], antioxidant [24], antihepatotoxic [25], antidepressant [26] and neuroprotective effects [27]. It was also demonstrated to improve sexual disorder and to protect against cardiac ischemia/reperfusion injury [28,29] and atherosclerosis [30]. Besides, icariin was reported to exhibit anticancer activity against a series of human cancer cell lines.

Icariside II (Figure 1), another active flavonoid glycoside derived from *Herba Epimedii*, is the major pharmacological metabolite of icariin in vivo and has been reported to be obtained from icariin through enzymatic hydrolysis [31]. Icariside II has been shown to promote osteogenic differentiation of bone marrow derived stromal cells [32]. It shows protective effects on cognitive deficits [33] and cerebral ischemia-reperfusion injury [34] at least in part due to the inhibition of NF-kappaB. Additionally, icariside II has also been demonstrated to possess cytotoxic and cytostatic activities against various cancer cell lines.

The topic of this review will emphasize on the antitumor activities of *Herba Epimudii* and its two main active constituents and the mechanisms of action discovered so far.

## 2. Anticancer Effects of *Herba Epimedii* in Vitro and in Vivo

Recent studies showed that *Herba Epimedii* could restrain the proliferation of human breast cancer cell lines in vitro as well as inhibit tumor growth in rat model of bone metastasis from breast cancer. The antiproliferative activities of the ethanol extracts from *Herba Epimedii* on two different types of human breast cancer cells were investigated [35]. The 95% ethanol extract significantly inhibited the proliferation of human breast cancer MCF-7 cells in the range of 100–800 µg/mL in a dose dependent manner with an $IC_{50}$ of 528 µg/mL after 72 h treatment. The 70% ethanol extract exhibited a certain activity on the growth of MCF-7 cells, whereas the 20% and 40% ethanol extracts showed no significant antiproliferation activity. The four different ethanol extracts of *Herba Epimedii* showed no obvious antiproliferative activity on human breast cancer MDA-MB-231 cells. In the rat model of bone metastasis from breast cancer, significant increase of 50% Paw withdrawn threshold (50% PWT) and reduction of tumor sizes were observed after oral administration of the decoction of *Herba Epimedii* at a dose of 5 g/kg daily for 20 days. In addition, the bone structural mineral density (BMD) and bone mineral capacity (BMC) were significantly enhanced [36]. In another study, it was found that the *Epimedium sagittatum* extract inhibited the proliferation of various hepatoma and leukemia cell lines, including SK-Hep1, PLC/PRF/5, K562, U937, P3H1 and Raji, with $IC_{50}$ values of 15, 57, 74, 221, 40 and 80 µg/mL, respectively, whereas it showed no inhibition effects to HepG2 and Hep3B cell lines ($IC_{50}$ > 500 µg/mL). The Hep3B was found to be less sensitive to the extract compared with other cell lines, consistent with the reported result that cells with the p53 gene deleted, just like Hep3B cell line, were more resistant to drugs [17].

## 3. Anticancer Effects of Icariin and Icariside II in Vitro and in Vivo

As for anticancer effects, studies have been performed in various human cancer cell lines. Icariin and icariside are proved to inhibit the growth of human cancer cells in vitro through intervening with multiple signaling pathways which are crucial to tumor growth, progression, invasion and apoptosis. Different concentrations of icariin and icariside II were used in the studies, depending on the types of cancer cell lines. The anticancer activity of icariin and icariside II and the molecular targets on various cancer cell lines were summarized in Table 1.

Table 1. Effects and molecular targets of icariin and icariside II on different cancer cell lines.

| Cancer Types | Components | Cell Lines | Concentrations Con. Range | Concentrations IC-50 | Effects and Molecular Targets | Reference |
|---|---|---|---|---|---|---|
| Hepatocellular carcinoma | Icariin | HepG2 | 10 μM | NA | G0/G1↑, S↓, Bcl-2↓ | [37] |
| | Icariin | SMMC-7721 | 5–20 μM | around 10 μM | cleaved caspase-3/9↑, mitochondria cytochrome c↓, cytosol cytochrome c↑, cleaved PARP1↑, XIAP↓, MMP↓, Bcl-2↓, Bax↑, p-JNK↑, ROS↑ | [38] |
| Prostate carcinoma | Icariin | PC-3 | 30 μM | NA | Cyclin D1↓, CDK4↓ | [39] |
| | Icariside II | PC-3 | 0–40 μM | around 20 μM | MMP↓, cleaved caspase-3/8/9↑, cleaved PARP↑, COX-2↓, iNOS↓, VEGF↓, PGE₂↓ | [40] |
| Esophageal cancer | Icariin | EC109 | 20–80 μM | 106.13 μM (12 h); 73.65 μM (24 h); 38.59 μM (36 h) | cleaved caspase-9↑, ROS↑, NADPH oxidase activity↑, GSH↓, GRP78↑, ATF4↑, CHOP↑, p-PERK↑, p-eIF2α↑, Bcl2↓, PUMA↑ | [41] |
| | Icariin | TE1 | 20–80 μM | 115.29 μM (12 h); 76.77 μM (24 h); 42.21 μM (36 h) | | |
| Ovarian cancer | Icariin | A2780 | 13–50 μM | NA | caspase-3 activity↑, miR-21↓ PTEN↑ RECK↑ Bcl-2↓ | [42] |
| Lung cancer | Icariin | A549 | 25–100 μM | 118.25 μM (12 h); 86.21 μM (24 h); 56.8 μM (36 h) | ROS↑, caspase 3 activity↑, GSH↓, ERS-related molecules↑(p-PERK, ATF6, GRP78, p-eIF2a, and CHOP), Bcl-2↓, PUMA↑ | [43] |
| | Icariside II | A549 | 0–20 μM | NA | vimentin↓, N-cadherin↓, NF-κB↓, p-IκB↓, p65/IκB↑, p-Akt↓ p-GSK-3β↓ | [44] |
| | Icariside II | H1299 | 0–20 μM | NA | | |
| | Icariin | B16 | 20–200 μg/mL | 84.3μg/mL (72 h) | procaspase-9↓ cleaved caspase-9↑ | [45] |
| Melanoma | Icariin | A375 | 0–100 μM | 10.6 μM | G0/G1 phase↑, S↓, G2/M arrest↑, cyclin E↓, CDK2↓, cyclin B1↓, P-CDK1↓, ROS↑, p-p38↑, p-p53↑, p21↑, cleaved caspase-3↑, survivin↓, p-STAT3↓, p-ERK↓, cleaved PARP↑ | [46–48] |
| | Icariside II | SK-MEL-5 | 0–100 μM | 11.1 μM | | |
| Leydig cell tumor | Icariin | MLTC-1 | 12.5–100 μg/mL | 50 μg/mL (48 h) | S↓, Bcl-2↓, Bax↑, cytochrome c↑, cleaved caspase-3/9↑, piwil4↓ | [49] |
| Gastric adenocarcinoma | Icariin | BGC-823 | 20–200 μg/mL | 128 μg/mL | Rac1↓, VASP↓ | [50] |
| Medulloblastoma | Icariin | Daoy | NA | NA | Cyclin A↓, CDK2↓, Cyclin B1↓, cleaved caspase-3↑, cleaved caspase-9↑, PARP↑, Bcl-2↓ | [51] |
| | Icariin | D341 | NA | NA | | |

**Table 1.** *Cont.*

| Cancer Types | Components | Cell Lines | Concentrations | | Effects and Molecular Targets | Reference |
|---|---|---|---|---|---|---|
| | | | Con. Range | IC$_{50}$ | | |
| Sarcoma | Icariside II | U2OS | 0–30 μM | NA | 4E-BP1↑, mTORC1↓, p-S6K(Thr389)↓, p-S6(Ser235/236)↓, p-4E-BP1 (Ser65)↓ | [52] |
| | | SW1353 | 0–20 μM | NA | | |
| | | S180 | 0–20 μM | NA | | |
| Hepatoblastoma | Icariside II | HepG2 | 0–30 μM | NA | Δψ$_m$↓, ROS↑, Bax/Bcl-2↑, cleaved-Bid↑, LAMP1↑, LMP↑, cleaved caspase-8/9/7/3↑, PARP↑, LC3B-II↑, SQSTM1↑ | [53] |
| Osteosarcoma | Icariside II | MG-63 | 10–35 μM | NA | p-EGFR↓, p-PI3K↓, p-Akt↓, p-PDK↓, p-Raf↓, p-mTOR↓, p-PDK1↓, p-PRAS40↓, p-GSK↓, p-ERK↓ | [54] |
| | | Saos-2 | 10–35 μM | NA | | |
| | | HOS | 0–10 μM | NA | HIF-1α↓, VEGF↓, uPAR↓, ADM↓, MMP2↓, Glut4↓, MCT4↓, aldolase A↓, enolase 1↓ | [55] |
| Epidermoid carcinoma | Icariside II | A431 cell line | 0–100 μM | NA | cleaved caspase 9↑, cleaved PARP↑ caspase 9↓, PARP↓, p-STAT3↓, p-ERK↓, p-AKT↓, p-EGFR↑↓ | [56] |
| Acute myeloid leukemia | Icariside II | U937 | 0–50 μM | NA | cleaved PARP↑, procaspase 3↓, Bcl-2↓, Bcl-X$_L$↓, survivin↓, COX-2↓, p-STAT3↓, p-JAK2↓, p-Src↓ | [57] |
| Breast cancer | Icariside II | MCF-7 | 0–100 μM | 72.73 μM (24 h) | MMP↓, cleaved caspase-3/7/8/9↑, cleaved PARP↑, Δψ$_m$↓, cytosol cyto c↑, cytosol AIF↑, mitochondrial cyto c↓, mitochondria AIF↓, Fas↑, FADD↑, Bcl-x$_L$↑, Bax↑, Bim$_L$↑ | [58] |
| | | | | 57.98 μM (48 h) | | |
| | | | | 50.95 μM (72 h) | | |
| | | | | 37.75 μM (96 h) | | |
| | | MDA-MB-231 | 0–100 μM | 97.14 μM (24 h) | | |
| | | | | 62.75 μM (48 h) | | |
| | | | | 42.40 μM (72 h) | | |
| | | | | 38.65 μM (96 h) | | |
| Multiple myeloma | Icariside II | U266 | 0–100 μM | NA | p-STAT3↓, p-JAK2↓, p-c-Src↓, SHP-1↑, PTEN↑, cyclin D1↓, Bcl-2↓, Bcl-x$_L$↓, survivin↓ VEGF↓, COX-2↓, cleaved caspase-3↑, p-PARP↑ | [59] |

NA, not applicable; ↑, up-regulation; ↓, down-regulation.

Icariin and icariside II have been demonstrated to exhibit in vivo suppressive effects both on tumor weight and tumor volume on a variety of mouse tumor models without obvious side effects (Table 2). Intraperitoneal administration of icariin at the doses of 15–150 mg/kg significantly inhibited tumor growth in xenografted mice models with almost no or very low toxicity to animals. Oral administration of 65 mg/kg icariin was shown to inhibit the growth of melanoma tumor and to inhibit the metastasis of B16 melanoma cells, and the lifespan was apparently pro-longed [45]. At the doses of 10–100 mg/kg, icariside II resulted in significant decrease in tumor weight and volume in cancer cell bearing mice models. All these data suggested that icariin and icariside II indeed have therapeutic potential against cancers.

**Table 2.** In vivo evaluation of icariin and icariside II in mouse tumor models.

| Components | Tumor Models | Transplantation | Treatment | Results | Reference |
|---|---|---|---|---|---|
| Icariin | Esophageal cancer EC109 | Subcutaneous injection | Given by i.p. 60 and 120 mg/kg every day for 20 days | Significantly inhibit tumor growth | [41] |
| Icariin | Lung adenocarcinoma A549 | Subcutaneous injection | Given by i.p. 100 or 150 mg/kg (5 days/week) for 4 weeks | Significantly inhibit tumor growth | [43] |
| Icariin | Melanoma B16 | Subcutaneous injection into the right flank | Given by p.o. 65 mg/kg every day for 20 days | Apparently inhibit tumor growth | [45] |
| Icariin | Mammary carcinoma 4 T1-Neu | Subcutaneous inoculation tumor bearing mice | Given by i.p. 100 mg/kg three times a week starting on day 7 until day 28 | 61% reduction of tumor growth | [60] |
| Icariin | Hepatoma SMMC-7721 | Subcutaneous injectioninto the armpit | Given by i.p. 15, 30, and 60 mg/kg every day for 20 days | 38.7%, 54.7%, and 69.9% inhibition in tumor volume, respectively | [38] |
| Icariin | Hepatoma HepG2 | Subcutaneous injection | Given by i.g. 80 mg/kg for 35 days | 55.6% inhibition in tumor weight; 47.2% inhibition in tumor volume | [61] |
| Icariside II | Sarcoma S180 | Subcutaneous injection into the right armpit | Given by i.v. 10, 20, 30 mg/kg everyday for 9 days | 33.0%, 51.3%, and 62.6% reduction in tumor weight, respectively | [52] |
| Icariside II | Lung cancer A549 | Subcutaneous injection into the flank area | Given by i.v. 30 and 60 mg/kg once every 3 days for 24 consecutive days | Strongly suppress tumor volume | [44] |
| Icariside II | Liver carcinoma H22 | Inoculation | Given by i.v.10, 20, 30 mg/kg everyday for 9 days | Inhibit tumor growth | [53] |
| Icariside II | Sarcoma S180 | Subcutaneous injection into the right flanks | Given by i.p. 10, 20 and 30 mg/kg everyday for 10 days | Inhibit tumor proliferation | [54] |
| Icariside II | Melanoma B16 | Subcutaneous injection into the right flank | Given by i.p. 50 mg/kg and 100 mg/kg 3 times for a week | 41% and 49% decrease in tumor volume | [47] |

## 4. Icariin and Icariside II as Adjuvant Therapy

While icariin and icariside II as single agent exhibited antitumor activities towards diverse human cancers, their potentials of potentiating the antitumor activity of a variety of chemotherapeutic drugs as adjuvant agents have shown perspectives in recent years. The combination treatment with the natural bioactive components and the chemotherapeutic drugs could facilitate chemotherapy for patients with cancers and provide a higher efficacy remedy.

Icariin has been shown to potentiate the antitumor activity of arsenic trioxide, temozolomide, doxorubicin, 5-fluorouracil and gemcitabine on a variety of human cancer cell lines, including acute promyelocytic leukemia, glioblastomamultiforme, hepatocellular carcinoma, osteosarcoma, colorectal cancer and gallbladder cancer cell lines, as well as in xenograft murine models (Table 3).

Nutrients **2016**, *8*, 563

Table 3. Icariin and icariside II used as adjuvant agents in combination with chemotherapeutic drugs.

| Component | Chemotherapeutic Drugs | Cancer Types | Cell Lines | Tumor Models | Molecular Targets | Reference |
|---|---|---|---|---|---|---|
| Icariin | Temozolomide | Glioblastomamultiforme | U87MG | | NF-κB↓ | [62] |
| Icariin | Arsenic Trioxide | Acute promyelocytic leukemia | HL-60 | | ROS↑ | [63,64] |
| | | Hepatocellular carcinoma | NB4 | Xenograft murine model (HepG2) | ROS↑ NF-κB↓cyclin D1↓ Bcl-2↓Bcl-xL↓ COX-2↓survivin↓ VEGF↓ | |
| | | | SMMC-7721 | | | |
| | | | HepG2 | | | |
| Icariin | Doxorubicin | Osteosarcoma | MG-63/DOX | | MDR1↓ PI3K/Akt pathway↓ | [65] |
| Icariin | 5-Fluorouracil | Colorectal cancer | HT29 | Xenograft murine model (HCT116) | NF-κB↓ cyclin D1↓ caspase-8↑ caspase-9↑ caspase-3↑Bax↑ PARP↑Bcl-xL↑ | [66] |
| | | | HCT116 | | | |
| Icariin | Gemcitabine | Gallbladder cancer | GBC-SD | Xenograft murine model (GBC-SD) | NF-κB↓ caspase-3↑ G0/G1 phase arrest↑ Bcl-2↓Bcl-xL↓ | [67] |
| | | | SGC-996 | | | |
| Icariside II | Paclitaxel | Melanoma | A375 | | TLR4 MyD88-ERK↓ caspase-3↑ IL-8 ↓ VEGF↓ | [48] |
| Icariside II | Bortezomib | Multiple myeloma | U266 | | STAT3↓ JAK2↓ c-Src↓ SHP-1↓ PTEN↓ Bcl-2↓Bcl-xL↓survivin↓cyclin D1↓ COX-2↓ VEGF↓ | [59] |
| | Thalidomide | | U266 | | | |

The empty cells under tumor model indicates the studies are performed on cells (in vitro) rather than on tumor models (in vivo). ↑, up-regulation; ↓, down-regulation.

Arsenic trioxide (ATO), a traditional Chinese medicine, has been wildly used for the treatment of acute myeloid leukemia (AML) since 1970s in China and has been recommended as the front-line agent. In addition, ATO has exhibited antitumor activity against various solid tumor cell lines. Icariin has demonstrated to potentiate the antitumor activity of ATO in treating AML and hepatocellular carcinoma, at least partially correlated with the increase in the accumulation of intracellular reactive oxygen species (ROS). Of note, the sensitivity of APL cell line NB4 to ATO dues to the reduced glutathione content and the increased ROS production. Adjuvant agent, which promotes the accumulation of ROS, such as icariin, could potentiate the antitumor activity of ATO against APL [63]. Moreover, co-treatment with ATO and icariin resulted in a significant inhibition of tumor growth in xenograft murine model of Hep G2 compared to the treatment with either agent alone by promoting the generation of ROS and suppressing NF-κB without systemic toxicity [64].

Icariin potentiated the anti-tumor activity of temozolimide in glioblastomamultiforme cell line U87MG [62]. The cytotoxicity of doxorubin was enhanced by icariin via the inhibition of ABC1 and down regulation of PI3K/Akt pathway [65]. The combination of icariin and 5-fluorouracil led to the inhibition of tumor growth by suppressing NF-κB activity [66]. Icariin also potentiated the anti-tumor activity of gemcitabine in the treatment of gallbladder cancer by inhibiting NF-κB [67].

Icariside II has been demonstrated an increased inhibitory effect on human melanoma cells and multiple myeloma U266 cells when combined with paclitaxel and bortezomib/thalidomide, respectively (Table 3).

Paclitaxel is a widely used cancer chemotherapeutic drug and exhibits antitumor activity in a variety of human malignancies. It was revealed to induce the activation of the toll-like receptor 4 (TLR4) signaling pathway, which was functionally associated with tumor growth, invasion and chemoresistance [68]. Inhibition of the activation of TLR4-MyD88 has been considered as a novel approach for reversing chemoresistance of paclitaxel. Data from our laboratory demonstrated that Icariside II enhanced paclitaxel-induced apoptosis in human melanoma cells, which might be due to its inhibition on paclitaxel-induced activation of TLR4-MyD88-ERK signaling [48].

Bortezomib (a proteasome inhibitor) and thalidomide (an inhibitor of TNF expression) have been reported to be used for the treatment of multiple myeloma patients. Icariside II has been found to induce the suppression of survival proteins such as Bcl-xL and surviving as well as cleavages of PARP and caspase-3. Co-treatment of icariside II with bortezomib or thalidomide significantly improved the cytotoxic effects of bortezomib and thalidomide from 25% and 20% to 60% and 50% in U266 cells, respectively, accompanied by the further increase of caspase-3 activation and PARP cleavage [59].

Icariin and icariside II have played an excellent adjuvant effects without causing systemic toxicity in the chemotherapeutic treatment of several tumors by interfering with multiple molecular targets in tumor cells. They might be considered as the potential candidates for treating tumors in combination with common chemotherapeutic drugs, thus contributing to the development of the successful therapeutic strategies.

## 5. Molecular Mechanisms of Anticancer Activity of Icariin and Icariside II

Multiple studies have been performed to investigate the mechanisms by which icariin and icariside II exert their anti-tumor effects. The mechanisms are comprehensive and diverse, involving the regulation of a variety of targets, which play a particularly important role in the process of tumor proliferation, invasion, angiogenesis, metastasis and apoptosis. Besides the effects of icariin and icariside II on numerous signaling proteins and transcription factors, they also regulate the stages of the tumor cells by inhibiting proliferation and inducing apoptosis. In addition, they could play their anti-tumor effect through improving the tumor inflammatory microenvironment (Figure 2). Icariin and icariside II might be considered as potential chemotherapeutic agents for the treatment of various human cancers due to their multiple targets on the cell growth processes.

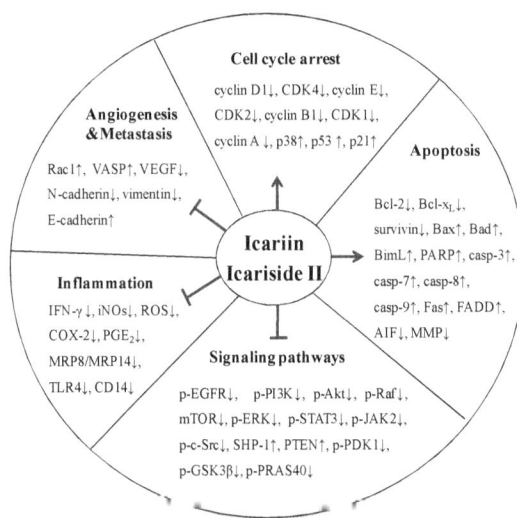

**Figure 2.** Overview of the anti-cancer effects of icariin and icariside II. Icariin and icariside II stimulate the cell cycle arrest via upregulation of p38, p53, and p21. Icariin and icariside II are involved in the induction of apoptosis and inhibit tumor angiogenesis and metastasis via suppression of multiple signaling pathways. They also have anti-inflammatory effects via downregulation of several factors, such as IFN-γ, iNOs, and COX-2, (← activation; ⊥ inhibition; ↑, up-regulation; ↓, down-regulation).

## 5.1. Effect on Cell Cycle Regulation

Cell division is divided into two stages: Mitosis (M) and the interlude between two M phases, including G1, S, and G2 phases. In addition, cells in G1 can enter a resting state called G0 just before the DNA replication [69,70]. In normal cells, the cell cycle is a highly regulated event, which is accurately regulated by cyclin dependent kinases (CDKs). The CDKs interact with various corresponding cyclins to form active complexes to ensure that the process at each stage is completely accomplished [71]. Tumor suppressor gene p53 is a vital cell cycle checkpoint regulator at the G1/S and G2/M checkpoints and serves to monitor the accuracy of vital events [72,73]. p38 MARK activation leads to the accumulation of p53 and the p53-induced cell cycle arrest is primarily mediated by the activation of p21 [74].

As shown in Figure 3, there are five active CDKs during the cell cycle, CDK2, CDK4 and CDK6 for G1, CDK2 for S, and CDK1 for both G2 and M. The complexes of cyclin D with CDK4 or CDK6 promote the progression through G1, cyclin E/CDK2 activates G1 into S, cyclin A/CDK2 promotes S progression, cyclin A/CDK1 activates G2 into M, while cyclin B/CDK1 stimulates the mitotic phase [75]. Disorders in the regulatory control of cell cycle could lead to the formation of tumors, characterized by the unlimited cell proliferation and abnormal apoptosis. Overexpression of cyclin D1 has been recognized as one of the distinct features in many types of human tumors [76]. Suppression of deregulated cell cycle progression in cancer cells by inhibiting the activities of CDKs or the cyclins have been considered as an effective strategy to inhibit the proliferation of the tumors [77].

Icariin has been reported to arrest the cell cycle at G0/G1 phase on the HepG2 cells. Icariin treatment for 72 h significantly increased the proportion of cells in G0/G1 phase, while the proportion of cells in S phases was remarkably lower (21.07%, $p < 0.01$) than that of the control group (28.62%) (Figure 3) [37]. Icariin also showed a weak G1 phase arrest accompanied by a mitochondrial transmembrane potential drop by decreasing cyclin D1 and CDK4 in human prostate carcinoma PC-3 cell line [39]. In another report, icariin stimulated S phase arrest in medulloblastoma cells by regulating the cell cycle regulators cyclin A, CDK2 and cyclin B1 [51].

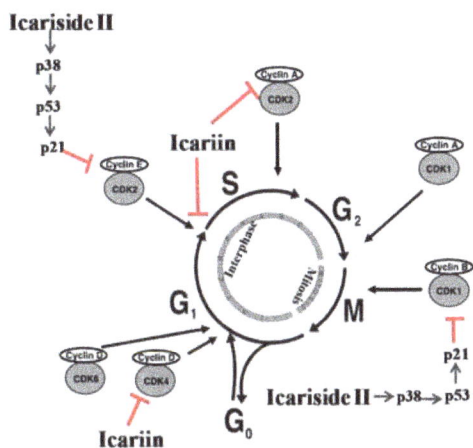

**Figure 3.** The cell cycle arrest induced by icariin and icariside II. Icariin and icariside II stimulate cell cycle arrest via suppression of the CDKs and cyclins at different stages, ($\leftarrow$ activation; $\perp$ inhibition).

Our study demonstrated that icariside II induced cell cycle arrest at G0/G1 and G2/M phases in A375 human melanoma cell line (Figure 3). After treatment with icariside II at a series of concentrations 0, 25, 50 and 100 μM, the percentage of cells in G0/G1 phase significantly increased with the increase of icariside II concentration and peaked at 100 μM (69.51%), as compared to the control group (44.01%). The cell cycle arrest of A375 cells at G0/G1 phase was found to be correlated with the decreased expression of cyclin E and CDK2, and the arrest at G2/M phase was associated with decreased expression of cyclin B1/CDK1 complex. It was determined that IS inhibits cell proliferation and induces cell cycle arrest through the generation of reactive oxygen species and activation of p38 and p53. These findings were further supported by the evidence that pretreatment with N-acetyl-L-cysteine, SB203580 or pifithrin-α significantly blocked icariside II-induced reduction of cell viability, increase of cell death and cell cycle arrest. Crucially, it was confirmed that these effects were mediated at least in part by activating the ROS-p38-p53 pathway [46].

## 5.2. Effect on Apoptosis

Apoptosis occurs normally during development to maintain the cell population in normal tissues or occurs as a defense mechanism to selectively eliminate the defective or unwanted cells which are damaged by disease [78]. It has been recognized as a necessary complementary to proliferation and plays a vital role in the development and regulation of the immune system, as well as the removal of damaged cells, and what's more, the disruption of apoptosis is implicated in tumors development [79].

It is well established that there are two main apoptotic pathways: The extrinsic (receptor mediated) and the intrinsic (mitochondrial mediated) signaling pathway (Figure 4). The extrinsic signaling pathway is initiated by the ligation of ligands and corresponding death receptors of the tumor necrosis factor (TNF) receptor subfamily, such as FasL/FasR and TNF-α/TNFR1 [80]. The formation of death-inducing signaling complex (DISC) leads to the autocatalytic activation of procaspase-8 [81]. The intrinsic apoptotic pathway is triggered by cellular stress factors including the negative signals involving the absence of some growth factors, hormones and cytokines and positive signals, including radiation, toxins, hypoxia, viral infections, and free radicals. These stimuli at on the mitochondrial membrane and result in change of themitochondrial permeability transition (MPT), loss of the mitochondrialtransmembrane potential and release of the pro-apopto ticproteins such as cytochrome c and apoptosis inducing factor (AIF) from mitochondria into the cytosol [82]. The released cytochrome c activates Apaf-1 and procaspase-9, resulting in the formation of apopto some [83]. The mitochondrial mediated apoptotic pathway is regulated by the members of the Bcl-2 family proteins [84], which are reported to be implicated with the tumor suppressor protein p53 and comprise two groups of proteins with the opposite function, the anti-apoptotic proteins (e.g., Bcl-2, Bcl-x and Bcl-$x_L$) and the pro-apoptotic proteins (e.g., Bax, Bid, Bak, Bim and Bik) [85]. The extrinsic pathway can be linked with the intrinsic pathway through caspase-8 by inducing the activation of Bid, in turn, acting on the mitochondrial membrane leading to the release of cytochrome c (Figure 4) [86].

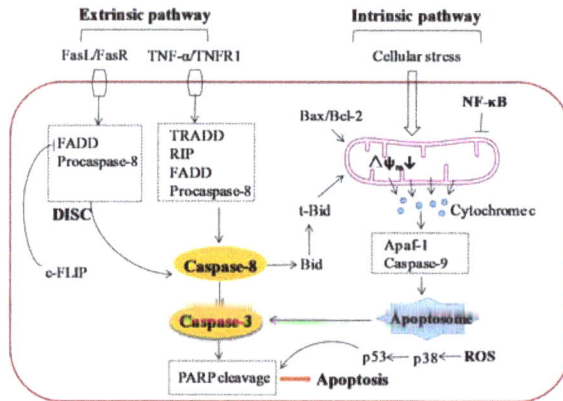

**Figure 4.** Apoptosis signaling pathways induced by icariin and icariside II. Icariin and icariside II induce apoptosis of tumor cells through two pathways, extrinsic (receptor-mediated) pathway and intrinsic (mitochondria-mediated) pathway. The binding of TNF-α with TNFR1 leads to the formation of TRADD and RIP, then the two factors combine with FADD and procaspase-8, which are resulted from FasL/FasR pathway, leading to the formation of death inducing signaling complex (DISC) and activating caspase-8. Activated caspase-8 stimulates the downstream caspase-3 and PARP, resulting in apoptosis, or cleaves Bid, which is the link between extrinsic pathway and intrinsic pathway, leading to the activation of intrinsic pathway. The cellular stress, activation of t-Bid, or modulation of Bax/Bcl-2 result in the downregulation of mitochondrial membrane potential and subsequent release of cytochrome c. Once released to cytosol, cytochrome c interacts with Apaf-1, resulting in the activation of caspase-9, which then activates caspase-3 resulting in cell death. Activation of NF-κB leads to the activation of several anti-apoptotic factors, which subsequently block the mitochondria-mediated pathway. Tumor cells produce ROS at higher levels, leading to the activation of p38 and p53, and subsequent apoptosis, (← activation; ⊥ inhibition).

Multiple studies have shown that icariin and icariside II can selectively kill cancer cells without apparent toxicity on normal cells by inducing apoptosis in many cancers, including hepatocellular carcinoma, prostate carcinoma, esophageal squamous cell carcinoma, ovarian cancer, lung cancer, melanoma, leydig cell tumor, gastric adenocarcinoma, promyelocytic leukemia, sarcoma, hepatoblastoma, medulloblastoma, osteosarcoma, epidermoid carcinoma, acute myeloid leukemia, breast cancer, and multiple myeloma. It seems that icariin and icariside II induce apoptosis via both extrinsic (caspase induced) and intrinsic (mitochondrial induced) signaling pathways.

Icariside II has been reported to increase the expression of Fas and the Fas-associated death domain (FADD) without changing the level of Daxx, which is also an Fas binding protein inducing apoptosis by activating the JNK pathway, and activate caspase-8 and caspase-3 in MCF-7 breast cancer cells, indicating the involvement of extrinsic apoptosis pathway [58]. It was speculated that the apoptosis induced by icariside II might be occurred by stimulating Fas/FADD signaling independently of FasL and subsequently activating caspase-8. Moreover, the extrinsic signaling pathway might exert its effects on the icariside II-treated MCF-7 cells independent of the intrinsic pathway for the absence truncated Bid (tBid), which is the key molecule linking the two apoptosis pathways.

Several studies have revealed that icariin and icariside II exert their anti-tumor effects by inducing apoptosis via mitochondrial induced signaling pathway, mainly characterized by the loss of mithchondrial membrane potential, release of cytochrome c, activation of caspase-9, caspase-3 and PARP, and elevation of intracellular reactive oxygen species (ROS), which played vital role in cell apoptosis (Table 1). In addition, icariside II has also been shown to induce the release of the apoptosis-inducing factor (AIF) and cytochrome c, and the activation of caspase-9, which are characteristic features of intrinsic apoptosis pathway [58].

Nuclear factor-kappaB (NF-κB), an inducible transcription factor, and its downstream genes were suggested to play an important role in cell proliferation, invasion, apoptosis and chemoresistance [87]. Recent studies have shown that icariin exhibits antitumor activity and potentiates the antitumor effect of several chemotherapeutic drugs via down-regulation of NF-κB in various human cancer cells, generally accompanied by the down-regulation of Bcl-2 and Bcl-x$_L$ [62,64,66,67]. Icariside II has been shown to prohibit invasion of lung cancer A549 and H1299 cells through suppression of Akt/NF-κB pathway [44].

*5.3. Effect on Angiogenesis and Metastasis*

The formation of new blood vessel is one of the key factors responsible for tumor growth and metastasis, not only supply nutrients for the metabolic needs of rapidly proliferating cancer cells but also provide conditions for cancer spread, resulting in malignant tumor growth, invasion and metastasis. Microvascular density in primary tumors is implicated in the numbers of tumor cells entered into the circulation in many tumors. Angiogenesis is regulated by multiple pro-angiogenic genes and signaling molecules including vascular endothelial growth factor (VEGF), basic fibroblast growth factor (bFGF), epidermal growth factor (EGF), platelet-derived growth factors (PDGF), angiopoetin (Ang), hypoxia-inducible factors, and matrix metal oproteinases [88].

Icariin has been shown to significantly prohibit the proliferation of vascular smooth muscle cells (VSMCs) and the activation of ERK1/2. Moreover, icariin also induced G1/S phase cell cycle arrest and decreased the expression of PCNA in VSMCs [89]. Based on these results, it was proposed that the inhibitory effect of icariin on the proliferation of VSMCs might be responsible for the suppression of tumor metastasis.

Effects of icariin and icariside II treatments on the adhesion and metastasis have been investigated in various human tumor cells, including esophageal carcinoma EC109 and TE1 [41], gastric adenocarcinoma BGC-823 [50], and lung cancer A549 and H1299 cell lines [44].

The adhesion and migration of icariin-treated EC109 and TE1 cells were evaluated after incubation in 15 μM ICA for 24 h [41]. The cell adhesion ratio decreased significantly to 47.23% ± 8.97% of that of the control in EC109 cells and 45.98% ± 6.72% of that of the control in TE1 cells, respectively ($p < 0.05$). Similarly, the scratch wound distance significantly increased by 159.23% ± 13.27% in EC109 cells and 179.26% ± 15.14% in TE1 cells, respectively ($p < 0.05$) [41]. Icariin was also reported to significantly inhibit tumor cells migration and invasion of human gastric adenocarcinoma cell line BGC-823 via the down-regulation of Rac1 and VASP [50]. The combination of icariin and the selective siRNA targeting Rac1 and VASP promoted the inhibitory effects. In addition, transfection with Rac1 plasmids pcDNA3-EGFP-Rac1-Q61L resulted in the improvement of expression levels of both Rac1 and VASP. Based on these results, it could be concluded that icariin inhibit the tumor cell invasion and migration through the Rac1-dependent VASP pathway [50]. A study has showed that icariside II prohibited the migration and epithelial-mesenchymal transition (EMT) via the inhibition of N-cadherin and vimentin up-regulation, and E-cadherin down-regulation induced by THP-1-CM in lung cancer A549 and H1299 cells [44].

*5.4. Effect on Multiple Signaling Pathways*

Multiple signaling pathways played vital role in cell survival, apoptosis and metastasis. Targeting various signaling pathways has been considered as a successful option in the treatment of cancer for its potential to avoid drug resistance, which is one of the major drawbacks of most anticancer drugs. Epidermal growth factor receptor (EGFR) is overexpressed in various types of human cancers and its expression is implicated with poor clinical prognosis [90]. Several small molecular kinase inhibitors and antibodies targeting on EGFR have been approved by FDA to treat diverse types of tumors. Activated EGFR recruits a variety of downstream signaling molecules, leading to the activation of major signaling pathways such as JAK2-STAT3, MAPK-ERK, and PI3k-Akt-mTOR, which play vital role in tumor growth, progression, and survival [91].

The inhibitory effects of icariside II on EGFR signaling have been investigated in human epidermoid carcinoma A431 cells [56] and in human osteosarcoma MG-63 and Saos-2 cells [54]. In our study, icariside II was found to inhibit the cell viability of A431 cells, accompanied by the decrease of phosphorylated EGFR. Pretreatment with LY294002 (a phosphatidylinositol 3-kinase (PI3K) inhibitor), EGF (an EGFR agonist) and AG1478 (an EGFR inhibitor) partially reversed the icariside II-induced decrease in cell viability, indicating icariside II effectively inhibited the EGF-induced activation of the EGFR pathway [56]. Icariside II was also found to decrease cell proliferation in MG-63 and Saos-2 cells by inactivating EGFR/mTOR signaling pathway and the decreased cell viability could be reversed partially by the pretreatment of EGF [54].

STAT3 is activated in a broad spectrum of human cancers, such as prostate cancers [92], breast cancer [93], and nasopharyngeal carcinoma [94], and has been implicated as a potential therapeutic target for multiple human cancers. Icariside II exhibited inhibitory effect on STAT3 signaling pathway in human melanoma A375 and SK-MEL-5 cells [47], epidermoid carcinoma A431 cells [56], acute myeloid leukemia U937 cells [57] and multiple myeloma U266 cells [59].

The phosphorylation of STATs is principally mediated via the activation of non-receptor protein tyrosine kinases called as JAK. Data from our laboratory showed that Icariside II dramatically inhibited the proliferation of melanoma A375 and SK-MEL-5 cells in vivo and in vitro by inhibiting the activation of the JAK-STAT3 and MAPK pathways but promoting an unsustained activation peak of the PI3K-AKT pathway [47]. Moreover, we also found icariside II induced apoptosis through inhibition of EGF-induced activation of STAT3 in A431 cells [56]. In U937 and U266 cells, Icariside II decreased the phosphorylation of JAK2 and c-Src, the upstream activators of the STAT pathway, and increased the expression of PTPs such as PTEN and protein tyrosine phosphatase (PTP) SH2 domain-containing phosphatase (SHP)-1 [57,59]. Sodium pervanadate (a PTP inhibitor) prevented Icariside II-induced apoptosis as well as STAT3 inactivation in U937 cells. Furthermore, silencing SHP-1 using specific siRNA significantly blocked STAT3 inactivation and apoptosis induced by Icariside II in U937 cells. All these results support a key role of SHP-1 in the suppression of STAT signaling pathways. In addition, icariside II was proved to reduce the level of STAT3 in MDA-MB-231 (breast adenocarcinoma) and DU145 (prostate carcinoma) cells, in which STAT3 is constitutively active [57].

The mitogen-activated protein kinase (MAPK-ERK, also known as Raf-MEK-ERK) pathway consisted several signal factors and the extracellular signal-regulated kinase-1 and 2 (ERK1/2) are extremely important in human cancers, which then activate ERK [95]. The importance of MAPK-ERK pathways in cancer progression and proliferation has been supported by Shield et al. [96]. Icariside II has been shown to inhibit the activation of ERK in melanoma A375 cells [47,48] and epidermoid carcinoma A431 cells [56]. Our data showed that icariside II treatment could effectively inhibit paclitaxel-induced activation of TLR4-MyD88-ERK signaling pathway in human melanoma A375 cells, which is proposed to be a novel target for reversing chemoresistance to paclitaxel. What's more, icariside II decreased cell proliferation and inactivated Raf-MEK-ERK signaling in osteosarcoma MG-63 and Saos-2 cells [54].

Phosphatidylinostinositol-3-kinase/protein kinase B (PI3K-AKT) signaling was found to play a key role in cell proliferation and is overexpressed in multiple human cancers [97]. As the downstream of PI3K-AKT, the mammalian target of rapamycin (mTOR), is a master growth regulator that senses the presence of growth factors by regulating p70S6K and 4E-binding protein 1 (4E-BP1) [98]. Icariside II, a natural mTOR inhibitor, was found to decrease the phosphorylation of PI3K-PDK1 and dephosphorylated Akt at Thr308 and Ser473 in osteosarcoma MG-63 and Saos-2 cells [54]. Akt activates mTOR by relieving proline-rich Akt substrate 40 (PRAS40)-mediated inhibition of mTOR. In addition, icariside II activated GSK3β, the direct target of Akt, by dephosphorylation atSer9, weakening the stability of transcription factors and cycle-related proteins. The suppression of icariside II on the phosphorylation of PI3K, Akt, PRAS40 was approved by mice bearing osteosarcoma sarcoma-180 cells. In conclusion, icariside II treatment moderated EGF-induced activation of PI3K/Akt/PRAS40 pathway in vitro as well as in vivo [54]. Icariside II was also shown to suppress aberrant energy homeostasis in osteosarcoma U2OS, fibrosarcoma S180 and chondrosarcoma SW1535 cells via suppression of mTORC1 by regulating mTORC1-4E-BP1 axis, suggesting a potential application of icariside II in sarcoma therapy [52]. In addition, icariin was reported to enhance cytotoxicity of doxorubin in the human osteosarcoma doxorubicin (DOX)-resistant MG-63/DOX cell line through down-regulation of PI3K-Akt pathway [65].

*5.5. Anti-Inflammatory Activity*

The hypothesis that chronic inflammation promoted cancer development and progression is strongly supported by the findings that individuals with chronic inflammation of the specific organ are significantly more susceptible to some organ-specific cancers [99]. The induction of myeloid suppressor cells (MDSC), one of the major factors mediating tumor-associated immune suppression, undermines the immune surveillance, thereby providing an environment favorable for tumor growth and allowing proliferation of malignant cells [100]. If inflammation facilitates tumor progression through the induction of more suppressive MDSCby signaling through the toll-like receptor 4 (TLR4) pathway, then it is possible that a decreased pro-inflammatory microenvironment may reduce the potency of MDSC. Data from our laboratory showed that icariin treatment reduced the expression of MRP8/MRP14 and TLR4 on human PBMCs [60]. Administration of icariin inhibited the tumor growth in 4T1-Neu tumor-bearing mice by reducing splenic MDSC accumulation and activation restoration of the functionality of effector CD8+ Tcells [60]. Furthermore, icariin significantly decreased the amounts of nitric oxide and reactive oxygen species in MDSC in vivo. Further, we saw a restoration of IFN-γ production by CD8+T cells and the drops of nitric oxide and reactive oxygen species in tumor bearing mice.

Recent findings demonstrated that cyclooxygenase-2 (COX-2) is over-expressed in various cancers, including pancreatic cancer [101], gastric carcinoma [102], and prostate cancer [103]. Prostaglandin $E_2$ (PGE$_2$), the proflammatory product of elevated COX-2, has been shown to play a crucial role in the progression of malignant tumor. Since COX-2 is increased in inflammatory microenvironment, it is considered as a molecular target for cancer prevention and treatment.

The mechanism of icariside II induced apoptosis in hormone-independent prostate carcinoma PC-3 cells was studied in association with COX-2 [40]. Data showed that Icariside II exerted cytotoxicity with IC$_{50}$ of approximately 20 μM on PC-3 cells. Furthermore, icariside II induced apoptosis via the suppression of COX-2, inducible NO synthase (iNOS), vascular endothelial growth factor (VEGF) and mitochondrial membrane potential, release of cytochrome c, and activation of caspase-8, -9 and, -3 expressions, and cleaved PARP. Moreover, exogeneous PGE2 inhibited PARP cleavage and knockdown of COX-2 enhanced PARP cleavage. These results indicated that icariside II induced mitochondrial dependent apoptosis by initiating the inhibition of COX-2/PGE2 pathway in PC-3 prostate [40]. The apoptosis induced by icariside II in acute myeloid leukemia U937 and multiple myeloma U266 was also found to be associated with the decrease of COX-2 [57,59].

# 6. Conclusions

A renewed interest emerges in the study of alternative and less toxic remedies for the treatment of many diseases, including cancer. Maximizing efficacy and minimizing side-effects has been recognized as the major goal of the treatment of cancers. *Herba Epimedii* has been traditionally used in clinical due to its multi-purpose activity and low toxicity. Collective data indicate that icariin and icariside II are the main bioactive components of *Herba Epimedii* and are potential anticancer agents towards a broad spectrum of human cancers. They exhibit broad toxicity to various types of human cancer cells by interfering with multiple mechanisms, inhibiting multiple signaling pathways, as well as regulating inflammatory microenvironment. Moreover, icariin and icariside II could be used as chemotherapeutic adjuvant agents in combination with standard drugs to improve the treatment effects and avoid drug resistance. In view of these demonstrated effects, icariin and icariside II could be potential therapeutic intervention agents alone or in combination with current chemotherapeutic drugs for cancers.

**Acknowledgments:** This work was funded by grant from Development Project of Shanghai Peak Disciplines-Integrative medicine (20150407), The Academy of Integrative Medicine of Fudan University, National Natural Science Foundation of China (81173390), and Shanghai Health and Family Planning Commission (ZYSNXD-CC-HPGC-JD-015).

**Author Contributions:** Jinfeng Wu and Qingli Luo performed the searching strategy, Meixia Chen analyzed the information and wrote the paper, Shuming Mo and YubaoLv conducted the Figures, Ying Wei revised and proofed the manuscript, Jingcheng Dong revised the manuscript and approved for submission.

**Conflicts of Interest:** The authors declare no conflict of interest.

# References

1. Siegel, R.L.; Miller, K.D.; Jemal, A. Cancer statiotioo, 2016 *CA Cancer J. Clin.* **2016**, *66*, 7–30. [CrossRef] [PubMed]
2. Ferlay, J.; Soerjomataram, I.; Dikshit, R.; Eser, S.; Mathers, C.; Rebelo, M.; Parkin, D.M.; Forman, D.; Bray, F. Cancer incidence and mortality worldwide: Sources, methods and major patterns in GLOBOCAN 2012. *Int. J. Cancer* **2015**, *136*, E359–E386. [CrossRef] [PubMed]
3. Graham, J.G.; Quinn, M.L.; Fabricant, D.S.; Farnsworth, N.R. Plants used against cancer-an extension of Jonathan Hartwell. *J. Ethnopharmacol.* **2000**, *73*, 347–377. [CrossRef]
4. Amin, A.R.; Kucuk, O.; Khuri, F.R.; Shin, D.M. Perspectives for cancer prevention with natural compounds. *J. Clin. Oncol.* **2009**, *27*, 2712–2725. [CrossRef] [PubMed]
5. Zhang, X.; Chen, L.X.; Ouyang, L.; Cheng, Y.; Liu, B. Plant natural compounds: Targeting pathways of autophagy as anti-cancer therapeutic agents. *Cell Prolif.* **2012**, *45*, 466–476. [CrossRef] [PubMed]
6. Cragg, G.M.; Newman, D.J. Plants as a source of anti-cancer agents. *J. Ethnopharmacol.* **2005**, *100*, 72–79. [CrossRef] [PubMed]
7. Kumar, A.; Patil, D.; Rajamohanan, P.R.; Ahmad, A. Isolation, purification and characterization of vinblastine and vincristine from endophytic fungus Fusarium oxysporum isolated from Catharanthus roseus. *PLoS ONE* **2013**, *8*, e71805. [CrossRef] [PubMed]
8. Nemeth, L.; Somfai, S.; Gal, F.; Kellner, B. Comparative studies concerning the tumour inhibition and the toxicology of vinblastine and vincristine. *Neoplasma* **1970**, *17*, 345–347. [PubMed]
9. Cipriani, D. Clinical experience with vinblastine and vincristine. *Cancro* **1968**, *21*, 185–189. [PubMed]
10. Editorial Committee of China Pharmacopoeia. *The Chinese Pharmacopoeia, Part I*, 2015 ed.; China Chemical Industry Press: Beijing, China, 2015; p. 486.
11. Ma, H.; He, X.; Yang, Y.; Li, M.; Hao, D.; Jia, Z. The genus Epimedium: An ethnopharmacological and phytochemical review. *J. Ethnopharmacol.* **2011**, *134*, 519–541. [CrossRef] [PubMed]
12. Xie, F.; Wu, C.F.; Lai, W.P.; Yang, X.J.; Cheung, P.Y.; Yao, X.S.; Leung, P.C.; Wong, M.S. The osteoprotective effect of Herba epimedii (HEP) extract in vivo and in vitro. *Evid. Based Complement. Altern. Med.* **2005**, *2*, 353–361. [CrossRef] [PubMed]
13. Wang, L.; Li, Y.; Guo, Y.; Ma, R.; Fu, M.; Niu, J.; Gao, S.; Zhang, D. Herba Epimedii: An Ancient Chinese Herbal Medicine in the Prevention and Treatment of Osteoporosis. *Curr. Pharm. Des.* **2016**, *22*, 328–349. [CrossRef] [PubMed]
14. Niu, R. Action of the drug Herba Epimedii on testosterone of the mouse plasma and its accessory sexual organ before and after processing. *China J. Chin. Mater. Med.* **1989**, *14*, 530–574.
15. Yu, L.; Li, H.; Huang, G.; Bai, Y.; Dong, Y. Clinical observations on treatment of 120 cases of coronary heart disease with herba epimedii. *J. Tradit. Chin. Med.* **1992**, *12*, 30–34. [PubMed]
16. Zhao, Y.L.; Song, H.R.; Fei, J.X.; Liang, Y.; Zhang, B.H.; Liu, Q.P.; Wang, J.; Hu, P. The effects of Chinese yam-epimedium mixture on respiratory function and quality of life in patients with chronic obstructive pulmonary disease. *J. Tradit. Chin. Med.* **2012**, *32*, 203–207. [CrossRef]

17. Lin, C.C.; Ng, L.T.; Hsu, F.F.; Shieh, D.E.; Chiang, L.C. Cytotoxic effects of Coptis chinensis and Epimedium sagittatum extracts and their major constituents (berberine, coptisine and icariin) on hepatoma and leukaemia cell growth. *Clin. Exp. Pharmacol. Physiol.* **2004**, *31*, 65–69. [CrossRef] [PubMed]

18. Khan, M.; Maryam, A.; Qazi, J.I.; Ma, T. Targeting Apoptosis and Multiple Signaling Pathways with Icariside II in Cancer Cells. *Int. J. Biol. Sci.* **2015**, *11*, 1100–1112. [CrossRef] [PubMed]

19. Huang, H.; Liang, M.; Zhang, X.; Zhang, C.; Shen, Z.; Zhang, W. Simultaneous determination of nine flavonoids and qualitative evaluation of Herba Epimedii by high performance liquid chromatography with ultraviolet detection. *J. Sep. Sci.* **2007**, *30*, 3207–3213. [CrossRef] [PubMed]

20. Pei, L.K.; Guo, B.L. A review on research of raw material and cut crude drug of Herba epimedii in last ten years. *China J. Chin. Mater. Med.* **2007**, *32*, 466–471.

21. Xie, X.; Pei, F.; Wang, H.; Tan, Z.; Yang, Z.; Kang, P. Icariin: A promising osteoinductive compound for repairing bone defect and osteonecrosis. *J. Biomater. Appl.* **2015**, *30*, 290–299. [CrossRef] [PubMed]

22. Wei, Y.; Liu, B.; Sun, J.; Lv, Y.; Luo, Q.; Liu, F.; Dong, J. Regulation of Th17/Treg function contributes to the attenuation of chronic airway inflammation by icariin in ovalbumin-induced murine asthma model. *Immunobiology* **2015**, *220*, 789–797. [CrossRef] [PubMed]

23. Chen, S.R.; Xu, X.Z.; Wang, Y.H.; Chen, J.W.; Xu, S.W.; Gu, L.Q.; Liu, P.Q. Icariin derivative inhibits inflammation through suppression of p38 mitogen-activated protein kinase and nuclear factor-kappaB pathways. *Biol. Pharm. Bull.* **2010**, *33*, 1307–1313. [CrossRef] [PubMed]

24. Xiong, W.; Chen, Y.; Wang, Y.; Liu, J. Roles of the antioxidant properties of icariin and its phosphorylated derivative in the protection against duck virus hepatitis. *BMC Vet. Res.* **2014**, *10*. [CrossRef] [PubMed]

25. Lee, M.K.; Choi, Y.J.; Sung, S.H.; Shin, D.I.; Kim, J.W.; Kim, Y.C. Antihepatotoxic activity of icariin, a major constituent of Epimedium koreanum. *Planta Med.* **1995**, *61*, 523–526. [CrossRef] [PubMed]

26. Liu, B.; Xu, C.; Wu, X.; Liu, F.; Du, Y.; Sun, J.; Tao, J.; Dong, J. Icariin exerts an antidepressant effect in an unpredictable chronic mild stress model of depression in rats and is associated with the regulation of hippocampal neuroinflammation. *Neuroscience* **2015**, *294*, 193–205. [CrossRef] [PubMed]

27. Liu, B.; Zhang, H.; Xu, C.; Yang, G.; Tao, J.; Huang, J.; Wu, J.; Duan, X.; Cao, Y.; Dong, J. Neuroprotective effects of icariin on corticosterone-induced apoptosis in primary cultured rat hippocampal neurons. *Brain Res.* **2011**, *1375*, 59–67. [CrossRef] [PubMed]

28. Meng, X.; Pei, H.; Lan, C. Icariin Exerts Protective Effect Against Myocardial Ischemia/Reperfusion Injury in Rats. *Cell Biochem. Biophys.* **2015**, *73*, 229–235. [CrossRef] [PubMed]

29. Zhai, M.; He, L.; Ju, X.; Shao, L.; Li, G.; Zhang, Y.; Liu, Y.; Zhao, H. Icariin Acts as a Potential Agent for Preventing Cardiac Ischemia/Reperfusion Injury. *Cell Biochem. Biophys.* **2015**, *72*, 589–597. [CrossRef] [PubMed]

30. Hu, Y.; Liu, K.; Yan, M.; Zhang, Y.; Wang, Y.; Ren, L. Effects and mechanisms of icariin on atherosclerosis. *Int. J. Clin. Exp. Med.* **2015**, *8*, 3585–3589. [PubMed]

31. Xia, Q.; Xu, D.; Huang, Z.; Liu, J.; Wang, X.; Wang, X.; Liu, S. Preparation of icariside II from icariin by enzymatic hydrolysis method. *Fitoterapia* **2010**, *81*, 437–442. [CrossRef] [PubMed]

32. Luo, G.; Gu, F.; Zhang, Y.; Liu, T.; Guo, P.; Huang, Y. Icariside II promotes osteogenic differentiation of bone marrow stromal cells in beagle canine. *Int. J. Clin. Exp. Pathol.* **2015**, *8*, 4367–4377. [PubMed]

33. Yin, C.; Deng, Y.; Gao, J.; Li, X.; Liu, Y.; Gong, Q. Icariside II, a novel phosphodiesterase-5 inhibitor, attenuates streptozotocin-induced cognitive deficits in rats. *Neuroscience* **2016**, *328*, 69–79. [CrossRef] [PubMed]

34. Deng, Y.; Xiong, D.; Yin, C.; Liu, B.; Shi, J.; Gong, Q. Icariside II protects against cerebral ischemia-reperfusion injury in rats via nuclear factor-kappaB inhibition and peroxisome proliferator-activated receptor up-regulation. *Neurochem. Int.* **2016**, *96*, 56–61. [CrossRef] [PubMed]

35. Chen, X.; Tang, L.; Li, Q. Antiproliferative activities of alcohol extracts of Herba Epimedii and Cortex Fraxini on breast cancer cell proliferation: In vitro study. *China Pharm.* **2007**, *18*, 1124–1127.

36. Yao, X.; Jia, L.Q.; Tan, H.Y.; Gao, F.Y.; Cui, J.; Li, H. Effects of Epimedium on rat tumor growth and bone destruction of breast cancer rats with bone metastasis. *Beijing J. Trad. Chin. Med.* **2008**, *27*, 882–884.

37. Wang, Z.M.; Song, N.; Ren, Y.L. Anti-proliferative and cytoskeleton-disruptive effects of icariin on HepG2 cells. *Mol. Med. Rep.* **2015**, *12*, 6815–6820. [CrossRef] [PubMed]

38. Li, S.; Dong, P.; Wang, J.; Zhang, J.; Gu, J.; Wu, X.; Wu, W.; Fei, X.; Zhang, Z.; Wang, Y.; et al. Icariin, a natural flavonol glycoside, induces apoptosis in human hepatoma SMMC-7721 cells via a ROS/JNK-dependent mitochondrial pathway. *Cancer Lett.* **2010**, *298*, 222–230. [CrossRef] [PubMed]

39. Huang, X.; Zhu, D.; Lou, Y. A novel anticancer agent, icaritin, induced cell growth inhibition, G1 arrest and mitochondrial transmembrane potential drop in human prostate carcinoma PC-3 cells. *Eur. J. Pharmacol.* **2007**, *564*, 26–36. [CrossRef] [PubMed]

40. Lee, K.S.; Lee, H.J.; Ahn, K.S.; Kim, S.H.; Nam, D.; Kim, D.K.; Choi, D.Y.; Ahn, K.S.; Lu, J.; Kim, S.H. Cyclooxygenase-2/prostaglandin E2 pathway mediates icariside II induced apoptosis in human PC-3 prostate cancer cells. *Cancer Lett.* **2009**, *280*, 93–100. [CrossRef] [PubMed]

41. Fan, C.; Yang, Y.; Liu, Y.; Jiang, S.; Di, S.; Hu, W.; Ma, Z.; Li, T.; Zhu, Y.; Xin, Z.; et al. Icariin displays anticancer activity against human esophageal cancer cells via regulating endoplasmic reticulum stress-mediated apoptotic signaling. *Sci. Rep.* **2016**, *6*. [CrossRef] [PubMed]

42. Li, J.; Jiang, K.; Zhao, F. Icariin regulates the proliferation and apoptosis of human ovarian cancer cells through microRNA-21 by targeting PTEN, RECK and Bcl-2. *Oncol. Rep.* **2015**, *33*, 2829–2836. [CrossRef] [PubMed]

43. Di, S.; Fan, C.; Yang, Y.; Jiang, S.; Liang, M.; Wu, G.; Wang, B.; Xin, Z.; Hu, W.; Zhu, Y.; et al. Activation of endoplasmic reticulum stress is involved in the activity of icariin against human lung adenocarcinoma cells. *Apoptosis* **2015**, *20*, 1229–1241. [CrossRef] [PubMed]

44. Song, J.; Feng, L.; Zhong, R.; Xia, Z.; Zhang, L.; Cui, L.; Yan, H.; Jia, X.; Zhang, Z. Icariside II inhibits the EMT of NSCLC cells in inflammatory microenvironment via down-regulation of Akt/NF-kappaB signaling pathway. *Mol. Carcinog.* **2016**. [CrossRef] [PubMed]

45. Li, X.; Sun, J.; Hu, S.; Liu, J. Icariin Induced B16 Melanoma Tumor Cells Apoptosis, Suppressed Tumor Growth and Metastasis. *Iran. J. Public Health* **2014**, *43*, 847–848. [PubMed]

46. Wu, J.; Song, T.; Liu, S.; Li, X.; Li, G.; Xu, J. Icariside II inhibits cell proliferation and induces cell cycle arrest through the ROS-p38-p53 signaling pathway in A375 human melanoma cells. *Mol. Med. Rep.* **2015**, *11*, 410–416. [CrossRef] [PubMed]

47. Wu, J.; Xu, J.; Eksioglu, E.A.; Chen, X.; Zhou, J.; Fortenbery, N.; Wei, S.; Dong, J. Icariside II induces apoptosis of melanoma cells through the downregulation of survival pathways. *Nutr. Cancer* **2013**, *65*, 110–117. [CrossRef] [PubMed]

48. Wu, J.; Guan, M.; Wong, P.F.; Yu, H.; Dong, J.; Xu, J. Icariside II potentiates paclitaxel-induced apoptosis in human melanoma A375 cells by inhibiting TLR4 signaling pathway. *Food Chem. Toxicol.* **2012**, *50*, 3019–3024. [CrossRef] [PubMed]

49. Wang, Q.; Hao, J.; Pu, J.; Zhao, L.; Lu, Z.; Hu, J.; Yu, Q.; Wang, Y.; Xie, Y.; Li, G. Icariin induces apoptosis in mouse MLTC-10 Leydig tumor cells through activation of the mitochondrial pathway and down-regulation of the expression of piwil4. *Int. J. Oncol.* **2011**, *39*, 973–980. [PubMed]

50. Wang, Y.; Dong, H.; Zhu, M.; Ou, Y.; Zhang, J.; Luo, H.; Luo, R.; Wu, J.; Mao, M.; Liu, X.; et al. Icariin exerts negative effects on human gastric cancer cell invasion and migration by vasodilator-stimulated phosphoprotein via Rac1 pathway. *Eur. J. Pharmacol.* **2010**, *635*, 40–48. [CrossRef] [PubMed]

51. Sun, Y.; Sun, X.H.; Fan, W.J.; Jiang, X.M.; Li, A.W. Icariin induces S-phase arrest and apoptosis in medulloblastoma cells. *Cell Mol. Biol.* **2016**, *62*, 123–129. [PubMed]

52. Zhang, C.; Yang, L.; Geng, Y.D.; An, F.L.; Xia, Y.Z.; Guo, C.; Luo, J.G.; Zhang, L.Y.; Guo, Q.L.; Kong, L.Y. Icariside II, a natural mTOR inhibitor, disrupts aberrant energy homeostasis via suppressing mTORC1–4E-BP1 axis in sarcoma cells. *Oncotarget* **2016**. [CrossRef] [PubMed]

53. Geng, Y.D.; Zhang, C.; Shi, Y.M.; Xia, Y.Z.; Guo, C.; Yang, L.; Kong, L.Y. Icariside II-induced mitochondrion and lysosome mediated apoptosis is counterbalanced by an autophagic salvage response in hepatoblastoma. *Cancer Lett.* **2015**, *366*, 19–31. [CrossRef] [PubMed]

54. Geng, Y.D.; Yang, L.; Zhang, C.; Kong, L.Y. Blockade of epidermal growth factor receptor/mammalian target of rapamycin pathway by Icariside II results in reduced cell proliferation of osteosarcoma cells. *Food Chem. Toxicol.* **2014**, *73*, 7–16. [CrossRef] [PubMed]

55. Choi, H.J.; Eun, J.S.; Kim, D.K.; Li, R.H.; Shin, T.Y.; Park, H.; Cho, N.P.; Soh, Y. Icariside II from Epimedium koreanum inhibits hypoxia-inducible factor-1alpha in human osteosarcoma cells. *Eur. J. Pharmacol.* **2008**, *579*, 58–65. [CrossRef] [PubMed]

56. Wu, J.; Zuo, F.; Du, J.; Wong, P.F.; Qin, H.; Xu, J. Icariside II induces apoptosis via inhibition of the EGFR pathways in A431 human epidermoid carcinoma cells. *Mol. Med. Rep.* **2013**, *8*, 597–602. [PubMed]

57. Kang, S.H.; Jeong, S.J.; Kim, S.H.; Kim, J.H.; Jung, J.H.; Koh, W.; Kim, J.H.; Kim, D.K.; Chen, C.Y.; Kim, S.H. Icariside II induces apoptosis in U937 acute myeloid leukemia cells: Role of inactivation of STAT3-related signaling. *PLoS ONE* **2012**, *7*, e28706. [CrossRef] [PubMed]

58. Huang, C.; Chen, X.; Guo, B.; Huang, W.; Shen, T.; Sun, X.; Xiao, P.; Zhou, Q. Induction of apoptosis by Icariside II through extrinsic and intrinsic signaling pathways in human breast cancer MCF7 cells. *Biosci. Biotechnol. Biochem.* **2012**, *76*, 1322–1328. [CrossRef] [PubMed]

59. Kim, S.H.; Ahn, K.S.; Jeong, S.J.; Kwon, T.R.; Jung, J.H.; Yun, S.M.; Han, I.; Lee, S.G.; Kim, D.K.; Kang, M.; et al. Janus activated kinase 2/signal transducer and activator of transcription 3 pathway mediates icariside II-induced apoptosis in U266 multiple myeloma cells. *Eur. J. Pharmacol.* **2011**, *654*, 10–16. [CrossRef] [PubMed]

60. Zhou, J.; Wu, J.; Chen, X.; Fortenbery, N.; Eksioglu, E.; Kodumudi, K.N.; Pk, E.B.; Dong, J.; Djeu, J.Y.; Wei, S. Icariin and its derivative, ICT, exert anti-inflammatory, anti-tumor effects, and modulate myeloid derived suppressive cells (MDSCs) functions. *Int. Immunopharmacol.* **2011**, *11*, 890–898. [CrossRef] [PubMed]

61. Yang, J.X.; Fichtner, I.; Becker, M.; Lemm, M.; Wang, X.M. Anti-proliferative efficacy of icariin on HepG2 hepatoma and its possible mechanism of action. *Am. J. Chin. Med.* **2009**, *37*, 1153–1165. [CrossRef] [PubMed]

62. Yang, L.; Wang, Y.; Guo, H.; Guo, M. Synergistic Anti-Cancer Effects of Icariin and Temozolomide in Glioblastoma. *Cell Biochem. Biophys.* **2015**, *71*, 1379–1385. [CrossRef] [PubMed]

63. Wang, Z.; Zhang, H.; Dai, L.; Song, T.; Li, P.; Liu, Y.; Wang, L. Arsenic Trioxide and Icariin Show Synergistic Anti-leukemic Activity. *Cell Biochem. Biophys.* **2015**, *73*, 213–219. [CrossRef] [PubMed]

64. Li, W.; Wang, M.; Wang, L.; Ji, S.; Zhang, J.; Zhang, C. Icariin synergizes with arsenic trioxide to suppress human hepatocellular carcinoma. *Cell Biochem. Biophys.* **2014**, *68*, 427–436. [CrossRef] [PubMed]

65. Wang, Z.; Yang, L.; Xia, Y.; Guo, C.; Kong, L. Icariin enhances cytotoxicity of doxorubicin in human multidrug-resistant osteosarcoma cells by inhibition of ABCB1 and down-regulation of the PI3K/Akt pathway. *Biol. Pharm. Bull.* **2015**, *38*, 277–284. [CrossRef] [PubMed]

66. Shi, D.B.; Li, X.X.; Zheng, H.T.; Li, D.W.; Cai, G.X.; Peng, J.J.; Gu, W.L.; Guan, Z.Q.; Xu, Y.; Cai, S.J. Icariin-mediated inhibition of NF-kappaB activity enhances the in vitro and in vivo antitumour effect of 5-fluorouracil in colorectal cancer. *Cell Biochem. Biophys.* **2014**, *69*, 523–530. [CrossRef] [PubMed]

67. Zhang, D.C.; Liu, J.L.; Ding, Y.B.; Xia, J.G.; Chen, G.Y. Icariin potentiates the antitumor activity of gemcitabine in gallbladder cancer by suppressing NF-kappaB. *Acta Pharmacol. Sin.* **2013**, *34*, 301–308. [CrossRef] [PubMed]

68. Kelly, M.G.; Alvero, A.B.; Chen, R.; Silasi, D.A.; Abrahams, V.M.; Chan, S.; Visintin, I.; Rutherford, T.; Mor, G. TLR-4 signaling promotes tumor growth and paclitaxel chemoresistance in ovarian cancer. *Cancer Res.* **2006**, *66*, 3859–3868. [CrossRef] [PubMed]

69. Nurse, P.; Masui, Y.; Hartwell, L. Understanding the cell cycle. *Nat. Med.* **1998**, *4*, 1103–1106. [CrossRef] [PubMed]

70. Sa, G.; Das, T. Anti cancer effects of curcumin: Cycle of life and death. *Cell Div.* **2008**, *3*, 14. [CrossRef] [PubMed]

71. Elledge, S.J. Cell cycle checkpoints: Preventing an identity crisis. *Science* **1996**, *274*, 1664–1672. [CrossRef] [PubMed]

72. Leonard, C.J.; Canman, C.E.; Kastan, M.B. The role of p53 in cell-cycle control and apoptosis: Implications for cancer. *Important Adv. Oncol.* **1995**, *121*, 33–42.

73. Kastan, M.B.; Canman, C.E.; Leonard, C.J. P53, cell cycle control and apoptosis: Implications for cancer. *Cancer Metastasis Rev.* **1995**, *14*, 3–15. [CrossRef] [PubMed]

74. Bulavin, D.V.; Saito, S.; Hollander, M.C.; Sakaguchi, K.; Anderson, C.W.; Appella, E.; Fornace, A.J., Jr. Phosphorylation of human p53 by p38 kinase coordinates N-terminal phosphorylation and apoptosis in response to UV radiation. *EMBO J.* **1999**, *18*, 6845–6854. [CrossRef] [PubMed]

75. Vermeulen, K.; Van Bockstaele, D.R.; Berneman, Z.N. The cell cycle: A review of regulation, deregulation and therapeutic targets in cancer. *Cell Prolif.* **2003**, *36*, 131–149. [CrossRef] [PubMed]

76. Hall, M.; Peters, G. Genetic alterations of cyclins, cyclin-dependent kinases, and Cdk inhibitors in human cancer. *Adv. Cancer Res.* **1996**, *68*, 67–108. [PubMed]

77. Noble, M.; Barrett, P.; Endicott, J.; Johnson, L.; McDonnell, J.; Robertson, G.; Zawaira, A. Exploiting structural principles to design cyclin-dependent kinase inhibitors. *Biochim. Biophys. Acta* **2005**, *1754*, 58–64. [CrossRef] [PubMed]

78. Elmore, S. Apoptosis: A review of programmed cell death. *Toxicol. Pathol.* **2007**, *35*, 495–516. [CrossRef] [PubMed]

79. Cotter, T.G. Apoptosis and cancer: The genesis of a research field. *Nat. Rev. Cancer* **2009**, *9*, 501–507. [CrossRef] [PubMed]

80. Ashkenazi, A.; Dixit, V.M. Death receptors: Signaling and modulation. *Science* **1998**, *281*, 1305–1308. [CrossRef] [PubMed]

81. Kischkel, F.C.; Hellbardt, S.; Behrmann, I.; Germer, M.; Pawlita, M.; Krammer, P.H.; Peter, M.E. Cytotoxicity-Dependent Apo-1 (Fas/Cd95)-Associated Proteins Form a Death-Inducing Signaling Complex (Disc) with the Receptor. *EMBO. J.* **1995**, *14*, 5579–5588. [PubMed]

82. Saelens, X.; Festjens, N.; Vande Walle, L.; van Gurp, M.; van Loo, G.; Vandenabeele, P. Toxic proteins released from mitochondria in cell death. *Oncogene* **2004**, *23*, 2861–2874. [CrossRef] [PubMed]

83. Chinnaiyan, A.M. The apoptosome: Heart and soul of the cell death machine. *Neoplasia.* **1999**, *1*, 5–15. [CrossRef] [PubMed]

84. Cory, S.; Adams, J.M. The Bcl2 family: Regulators of the cellular life-or-death switch. *Nat. Rev. Cancer.* **2002**, *2*, 647–656. [CrossRef] [PubMed]

85. Schuler, M.; Green, D.R. Mechanisms of p53-dependent apoptosis. *Biochem. Soc. Trans.* **2001**, *29*, 684–688. [CrossRef] [PubMed]

86. Igney, F.H.; Krammer, P.H. Death and anti-death: Tumour resistance to apoptosis. *Nat. Rev. Cancer* **2002**, *2*, 277–288. [CrossRef] [PubMed]

87. Aggarwal, B.B. Nuclear factor-kappaB: The enemy within. *Cancer Cell* **2004**, *6*, 203–208. [CrossRef] [PubMed]

88. Cao, Y.; Liu, Q. Therapeutic targets of multiple angiogenic factors for the treatment of cancer and metastasis. *Adv. Cancer Res.* **2007**, *97*, 203–224. [PubMed]

89. Hu, Y.; Liu, K.; Yan, M.; Zhang, Y.; Wang, Y.; Ren, L. Icariin inhibits oxidized low-density lipoprotein-induced proliferation of vascular smooth muscle cells by suppressing activation of extracellular signal-regulated kinase 1/2 and expression of proliferating cell nuclear antigen. *Mol. Med. Rep.* **2016**, *13*, 2899–2903. [PubMed]

90. Ekstrand, A.J.; Sugawa, N.; James, C.D.; Collins, V.P. Amplified and rearranged epidermal growth factor receptor genes in human glioblastomas reveal deletions of sequences encoding portions of the *N*- and/or *C*-terminal tails. *Proc. Natl. Acad. Sci. USA* **1992**, *89*, 4309–4313. [CrossRef] [PubMed]

91. Han, W.; Lo, H.W. Landscape of EGFR signaling network in human cancers: Biology and therapeutic response in relation to receptor subcellular locations. *Cancer Lett.* **2012**, *318*, 124–134. [CrossRef] [PubMed]

92. Mora, L.B.; Buettner, R.; Seigne, J.; Diaz, J.; Ahmad, N.; Garcia, R.; Bowman, T.; Falcone, R.; Fairclough, R.; Cantor, A.; et al. Constitutive activation of Stat3 in human prostate tumors and cell lines: Direct inhibition of Stat3 signaling induces apoptosis of prostate cancer cells. *Cancer Res.* **2002**, *62*, 6659–6666. [PubMed]

93. Dolled-Filhart, M.; Camp, R.L.; Kowalski, D.P.; Smith, B.L.; Rimm, D.L. Tissue microarray analysis of signal transducers and activators of transcription 3 (Stat3) and phospho-Stat3 (Tyr705) in node-negative breast cancer shows nuclear localization is associated with a better prognosis. *Clin. Cancer Res.* **2003**, *9*, 594–600. [PubMed]

94. Hsiao, J.R.; Jin, Y.T.; Tsai, S.T.; Shiau, A.L.; Wu, C.L.; Su, W.C. Constitutive activation of STAT3 and STAT5 is present in the majority of nasopharyngeal carcinoma and correlates with better prognosis. *Brit. J. Cancer* **2003**, *89*, 344–349. [CrossRef] [PubMed]

95. Santarpia, L.; Lippman, S.M.; El-Naggar, A.K. Targeting the MAPK-RAS-RAF signaling pathway in cancer therapy. *Expert. Opin. Ther. Targets* **2012**, *16*, 103–119. [CrossRef] [PubMed]

96. Shields, J.M.; Pruitt, K.; McFall, A.; Shaub, A.; Der, C.J. Understanding Ras: 'It ain't over 'til it's over'. *Trends Cell Biol.* **2000**, *10*, 147–154. [CrossRef]

97. Liu, P.; Cheng, H.; Roberts, T.M.; Zhao, J.J. Targeting the phosphoinositide 3-kinase pathway in cancer. *Nat. Rev. Drug Discov.* **2009**, *8*, 627–644. [CrossRef] [PubMed]

98. Guertin, D.A.; Sabatini, D.M. Defining the role of mTOR in cancer. *Cancer Cell* **2007**, *12*, 9–22. [CrossRef] [PubMed]

99. Shacter, E.; Weitzman, S.A. Chronic inflammation and cancer. *Oncology* **2002**, *16*, 217–229. [PubMed]

100. Bunt, S.K.; Sinha, P.; Clements, V.K.; Leips, J.; Ostrand-Rosenberg, S. Inflammation induces myeloid-derived suppressor cells that facilitate tumor progression. *J. Immunol.* **2006**, *176*, 284–290. [CrossRef] [PubMed]

101. Armstrong, L.; Davydova, J.; Brown, E.; Han, J.; Yamamoto, M.; Vickers, S.M. Delivery of interferon alpha using a novel Cox2-controlled adenovirus for pancreatic cancer therapy. *Surgery* **2012**, *152*, 114–122. [CrossRef] [PubMed]

102. Ristimaki, A.; Honkanen, N.; Jankala, H.; Sipponen, P.; Harkonen, M. Expression of cyclooxygenase-2 in human gastric carcinoma. *Cancer Res.* **1997**, *57*, 1276–1280. [PubMed]

103. Basler, J.W.; Piazza, G.A. Nonsteroidal anti-inflammatory drugs and cyclooxygenase-2 selective inhibitors for prostate cancer chemoprevention. *J. Urol.* **2004**, *171*, S59–S63. [CrossRef] [PubMed]

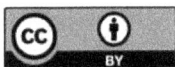

*nutrients*

MDPI

*Review*

# Anticancer Efficacy of Polyphenols and Their Combinations

Aleksandra Niedzwiecki *, Mohd Waheed Roomi, Tatiana Kalinovsky and Matthias Rath

Dr. Rath Research Institute, 1260 Memorex Drive, Santa Clara, CA 95050, USA; w.roomi@drrath.com (M.W.R.);
t.kalinovksy@drrath.com (T.K.); m.rath@drrath.com (M.R.)
* Correspondence: author@drrath.com; Tel.: +1-408-807-5564

Received: 15 July 2016; Accepted: 1 September 2016; Published: 9 September 2016

**Abstract:** Polyphenols, found abundantly in plants, display many anticarcinogenic properties including their inhibitory effects on cancer cell proliferation, tumor growth, angiogenesis, metastasis, and inflammation as well as inducing apoptosis. In addition, they can modulate immune system response and protect normal cells against free radicals damage. Most investigations on anticancer mechanisms of polyphenols were conducted with individual compounds. However, several studies, including ours, have indicated that anti-cancer efficacy and scope of action can be further enhanced by combining them synergistically with chemically similar or different compounds. While most studies investigated the anti-cancer effects of combinations of two or three compounds, we used more comprehensive mixtures of specific polyphenols and mixtures of polyphenols with vitamins, amino acids and other micronutrients. The mixture containing quercetin, curcumin, green tea, cruciferex, and resveratrol (PB) demonstrated significant inhibition of the growth of Fanconi anemia head and neck squamous cell carcinoma and dose-dependent inhibition of cell proliferation, matrix metalloproteinase (MMP)-2 and -9 secretion, cell migration and invasion through Matrigel. PB was found effective in inhibition of fibrosarcoma HT-1080 and melanoma A2058 cell proliferation, MMP-2 and -9 expression, invasion through Matrigel and inducing apoptosis, important parameters for cancer prevention. A combination of polyphenols (quercetin and green tea extract) with vitamin C, amino acids and other micronutrients (EPQ) demonstrated significant suppression of ovarian cancer ES-2 xenograft tumor growth and suppression of ovarian tumor growth and lung metastasis from IP injection of ovarian cancer A-2780 cells. The EPQ mixture without quercetin (NM) also has shown potent anticancer activity in vivo and in vitro in a few dozen cancer cell lines by inhibiting tumor growth and metastasis, MMP-2 and -9 secretion, invasion, angiogenesis, and cell growth as well as induction of apoptosis. The presence of vitamin C, amino acids and other micronutrients could enhance inhibitory effect of epigallocatechin gallate (EGCG) on secretion of MMPs. In addition, enrichment of NM with quercetin (EPQ mix) enhanced anticancer activity of NM in vivo. In conclusion, polyphenols, especially in combination with other polyphenols or micronutrients, have been shown to be effective against multiple targets in cancer development and progression, and should be considered as safe and effective approaches in cancer prevention and therapy.

**Keywords:** polyphenols; tumor growth; metastasis; Matrigel invasion

## 1. Introduction

Polyphenols comprise a diverse group of secondary metabolites abundant in plants, where they play key roles in regulating growth, metabolism, protecting against UV radiation and various pathogens. More than 8000 polyphenolic compounds have been identified in various plant species. Polyphenols have been subjected to numerous studies, investigating their potential health benefits, including protection against oxidative stress, cardiovascular disease, diabetes, asthma, neurodegenerative disease and even aging [1]. Particular interest in these naturally occurring plant components has been kindled by the search for new chemopreventive agents that are more effective and less toxic than conventional therapies. As such, this group of substances has been studied for anticarcinogenic properties, such as modulating cell proliferation, tumor growth, angiogenesis, metastasis, inflammation and apoptosis [2,3].

Polyphenols are classified based on the number of phenol rings and the structural elements that bind these rings to one another. The groups include: phenolic acids, stilbenes, lignans, and flavonoids. Flavonoids, which have both antioxidant and anti-inflammatory properties, are found in fruits, vegetables, legumes, red wine, and green tea. They are subdivided into six classes: flavonols, flavones, isoflavones, flavanones, anthocyanidins, and flavanols (catechins and proanthocyanidins) [4]. Flavonols, the most ubiquitous flavonoids in foods, are generally present at relatively low concentrations. Quercetin and kaempferol are the main representatives, and their richest sources are onions, curly kale, leeks, broccoli, and blueberries [4].

Flavones, consisting mainly of glycosides of luteolin and apigenin, are less common than flavonols in fruit and vegetables; parsley and celery are the main edible sources of flavones [4]. Flavanones, present in tomatoes and certain aromatic plants such as mint, are present in high concentrations only in citrus fruit. Isoflavones, flavonoids with structural similarities to estrogens, have the ability to bind to estrogen receptors, and thus are classified as phytoestrogens. They are found almost exclusively in leguminous plants. Flavanols occur as catechins (a monomer form) and proanthocyanidins (the polymer form).

Catechins are found in many types of fruit, red wine, green tea and chocolate. Gallocatechin, epigallocatechin, and epigallocatechin gallate (EGCG) are found in teas, seeds of leguminous plants and grapes [5,6]. Green tea, a rich source, contains up to 200 mg catechins in a cup of tea [7]. Flavanols are not glycosylated in foods as are other classes of flavonoids; thus tea epicatechins remain very stable when exposed to heat under acidic pH. Only 15% of these substances are degraded after 7 h in boiling water at pH 5 [8].

Among phenolic acids, hydroxybenzoic acids are found in tea and more common hydroxycinnamic acids are found in cinnamon, coffee, blueberries, kiwis, plums, apples, and cherries [4]. These acids are mostly found as glycosylated derivatives of esters of quinic acid, shikimic acid and tartaric acid [4]. Ferrulic acid is the most abundant phenolic acid found in cereal grains and in wheat; it may represent up to about 90% polyphenols [9].

Stilbenes are found in low quantities in our diet, which may be not sufficient to exercise significant health effects; larger quantities can be provided in concentrated extracts or in the form of purified compounds. Resveratrol is a key stilbene, found especially in red wine and peanuts, which has been extensively studied for its anticarcinogenic and other health effects [10].

Lignans are found in flax seeds, legumes, cereals, grains, fruits, algae, and certain vegetables [4]. Their concentration in linseed is about 1000 times as high as in other food sources [11]. Plant lignin, secoisolariciresinol diglycoside (SDG) and its metabolites have shown promise in reducing carcinogenic tumors, in particular hormone-sensitive ones such as breast, endometrium and prostate tumors [12].

## 2. Aspects Associated with Bioavailability of Polyphenols

Bioavailability defines the amount of nutrient that is digested, absorbed and metabolized in normal biochemical pathways. Most polyphenols are present in food in the form of esters, glycosides or polymers, and are metabolized by a common pathway. Before absorption, most polyphenols have to be hydrolyzed by intestinal enzymes or microflora present in colon. Only aglycones can be absorbed via the small intestine [13]. Subsequently, during absorption, polyphenols undergo extensive modification by conjugation in the intestinal cells and further processing in the liver through methylation, sulfation and glucuronidation [13]. Therefore, their forms detected in the blood and tissues differ from the ones present in food. In addition, the most biologically active polyphenols are not necessarily the most common ones in the diet.

Metabolic activity of polyphenols is dependent on intrinsic activity, relative absorption from the intestine, rate of metabolism and of elimination. In addition, digestive or hepatic metabolic activity may render the metabolites that reach the blood and target organs to differ in biological activity from their native form. Polyphenol metabolites circulate in the blood bound to proteins, mainly albumin, with binding affinity largely defined by their structural properties [14]. Protein binding can affect the rate of their delivery to cells and tissues.

Polyphenols are able to penetrate tissues, in particular the intestine and liver, where they are metabolized. Their excretion occurs through urine (mainly small conjugates) and more extensively conjugated metabolites are secreted in bile. It appears that the amount of metabolite in urine roughly corresponds to its maximum concentration in plasma. It is quite high for citrus fruit flavanones and decreases from isoflavones to flavonols. Thus, understanding polyphenol bioavailability is essential for determining their health effects.

## 3. Antitumor Effects of Select Polyphenols

Development of cancer is a multi-stage process that involves initiation, promotion and progression. Dietary polyphenols can affect and modulate multiple diverse biochemical processes and pathways involved in carcinogenesis [15]. In addition, they can act as biological response modifiers supporting immune system function, as well as protecting living cells against damage from free radicals. Although polyphenols in fruits and vegetables are widely implicated in cancer prevention, few protective effects of individual compounds have been firmly confirmed in clinical trials due to differences in dosing, timing and other confounding factors.

Several cancer preventive mechanisms have been identified as affected by polyphenols, including prevention of oxidation, detoxification of xenobiotics, induction of apoptosis, as well as estrogenic/anti-estrogenic activity, stimulating effects on immune system function, anti-inflammatory properties and their effects on the cellular signaling system. Among these are effects on nuclear factors, such as NF-κB or activator protein 1 (AP-1), which play central roles in cellular signaling cascades, regulating DNA transcription, gene expression in response to different stimuli, cell proliferation and survival [16,17]. Most investigations have been conducted with individual polyphenols in order to increase our understanding of biological and cellular mechanisms of their anticancer efficacy. However, final effects of these compounds are largely influenced by their interactions with other natural components, both at the cellular and organ levels. These aspects have been rarely evaluated and studied. Below we will discuss key studies investigating anti-cancer effects of individual polyphenols, as well as their efficacy when used in various combinations, the approach which has been promoted in our research.

### 3.1. Curcumin

This active ingredient of a rhizome of turmeric has been known for its anti-oxidant properties and many health benefits. It has been demonstrated in different cancer models that curcumin can inhibit cellular proliferation and angiogenesis, block cell cycle progression in tumor cells, and induce apoptosis [18–20]. Aoki et al. demonstrated inhibition of glioma cell xenograft tumor growth by curcumin [21]. Studies by Anand indicate that in addition to modulating cancer cell proliferation, angiogenesis and inducing apoptosis, curcumin can affect cancer invasion, and metastasis [22]. The anti-cancer efficacy of curcumin may involve a variety of mechanisms. Study of pancreatic cancer in nude mice has shown that curcumin can suppress pancreatic cancer cell proliferation and angiogenesis by inhibiting NF-kB-regulated gene products such as cyclin D1, cmyc, Bcl-2, Bcl-xL, and apoptosis protein-1, COX-2, MMP, and vascular endothelial growth factor (VEGF) [18]. Various studies, including the use of lung models, point to curcumin affecting the mechanisms involving inhibition of the signal transducer and activation of transcription Stat3 pathways [23], as well as matrix metalloproteinases and VEGF [18].

Curcumin's anti-tumor effects may also be due to its interactions with arachidonate metabolism and in vivo anti-angiogenic properties [24]. Some studies indicate curcumin interacts with vitamin D receptors, which would explain its preventive properties against colon cancer where vitamin D has strong anti-cancer effects [25]. Curcumin also appears to work in synergy with isoflavones in suppressing prostate specific antigen (PSA) production in prostate cells [26]. Gupta et al. have reviewed clinical trial research on curcumin and have concluded that curcumin, either alone or in combination with other agents, has demonstrated potential against various cancers, including colorectal, pancreatic, breast, prostate, lung, multiple myeloma, and head and neck squamous cell carcinoma [27]. Overall, chemoprevention and anticancer effects of curcumin are multimodal and complex. Molecular pathways and targets modulated by curcumin have been discussed in details in other review articles [28,29].

### 3.2. Quercetin

Cancer preventive effects of quercetin include induction of cell cycle arrest, apoptosis and antioxidant functions [30]. Induction of apoptosis by quercetin in cancer cells during different cell cycle stages without affecting normal cells has been documented in various cancers in vivo and in vitro [30]. Quercetin has been reported to reduce both the risk and progression of cancer through their free radical scavenging activity [31,32]. It protects cells from oxidative stress, inflammation, and DNA damage due to its antioxidant properties and modulates growth of many cancer cell lines by blocking cell cycle progression and tumor cell proliferation and by inducing apoptosis [33–36]. In addition, quercetin provided protection against liver cancer development in rats injected with a cancer inducer [37]. Furthermore, injection of quercetin directly into breast tumors led to a significant reduction of their mass [38]. Epidemiological studies report that intake of quercetin-rich food reduced the risk of gastric cancer by 43% [31] and colon cancer by 32% [39]. Consumption of quercetin was also reported to reduce lung cancer risk by 51% and even in heavy smokers by 65% [32]. Intravenous administration of quercetin in patients with different types of cancer demonstrated decreased activity of the enzyme tyrosine kinase, an enzyme required for tumor growth, in nine of 11 patients [40]. There is a growing interest among scientists in exploring synergistic interactions of quercetin with standard chemotherapeutics. Both in vitro and in vivo studies have shown that quercetin can potentiate the efficacy of concomitant drugs by enhancing their bioavailability and accumulation, and by sensitizing cancer cells to these chemotherapeutics [41]. From a clinical perspective, this would allow dose reduction of toxic drugs, thereby alleviating their severe side effects.

### 3.3. Resveratrol

Resveratrol has demonstrated to be effective in preventing all stages of cancer development and has been found effective in most cancers including prostate, breast, stomach, colon, lung, thyroid and pancreatic cancer cell lines [42]. Bishayee et al. reported that resveratrol can affect carcinogenesis by modulating signal transduction pathways that control cell division and growth, apoptosis, inflammation, angiogenesis and metastasis [43]. In vivo, resveratrol has shown efficacy in preventing and treating skin, esophageal, intestinal, and colon tumors [44]. Various anti-cancer cellular mechanisms of resveratrol have been suggested, including inhibition of angiogenesis, metastasis and induction of apoptosis [38]. Resveratrol has been studied in patients with colon cancer to evaluate the pharmacokinetic and metabolite profiles in these patients [45]. In addition, resveratrol studied in healthy volunteers demonstrated that it is well tolerated and modulates enzyme systems involved in carcinogen activation and detoxification [46]. Resveratrol has promising anti-cancer potential but, because of its poor bioavailability, the best efficacy has been limited to tumors it can come into direct contact with (e.g., skin cancers or gastrointestinal tract cancers).

*3.4. Cruciferous Plant Extracts*

Cruciferous vegetables of the *Brassica* genus, such as broccoli, cabbage, cauliflower and others contain a number of nutrients and phytochemicals with cancer preventive properties, including carotenoids, chlorophyll and fibers. Their unique anti-cancer characteristic relates to being a source of large quantities of sulfur containing natural compounds known as glucosinolates [47]. After hydrolysis they form bioactive isothiocyanates and indole-3-carbinol [48,49]. By 2011 more than 132 glucosinolates with their unique hydrolysis products had been identified in plants [50]. Epidemiological evidence suggests that high intake of cruciferous vegetables can lower risk of some cancers, including colon and lung cancers [48]. Numerous in vitro and in vivo studies suggest that dietary compounds from cruciferous plants may have potent chemopreventive properties by acting through different molecular mechanisms [51–56]. This includes many studies, which have shown that cruciferous vegetables can help prevent the onset and inhibit the progression of colon, breast, prostate, thyroid, cervical, and other cancers [57–66]. It has been shown that cruciferous bioactive components can facilitate detoxification and excretion of carcinogens, protect against oxidative stress, inhibit cancer cell proliferation and increase apoptosis, resulting in inhibition of tumor growth [67].

*3.5. Green Tea*

Green tea extract, rich in catechins, has been subjected to numerous studies and shown to modulate cancer cell growth, metastasis, angiogenesis, and other aspects of cancer progression by affecting different mechanisms [68–73]. The four principal tea catechins are epicatechin (EC), epicatechin-3-gallate (ECG), epigallocatechin (EGC) and epigallocatechin-3-gallate (EGCG) [74]. It has been shown that three of these catechins, EGCG, EGC and ECG, have anticancer preventive activity, and that their combination with an inactive EC has synergistic effect on prostate cancer cells PC-9, by inducing apoptosis and inhibiting proliferation [75].

The most studied of all green tea catechins in relation to cancer is EGCG, which is found at the highest concentration in green tea (10%–15%) [75]. Gupta et al. demonstrated that EGCG potently induced apoptosis and suppressed cell growth in vitro by modulating expression of cell cycle regulatory proteins, activating killer caspases, and suppressing activation of NF-κB [76]. Harakeh et al. demonstrated the anti-proliferative and pro-apoptotic effects of EGCG in HTLV-1-positive and -negative cells. These effects included down-regulation of TGF-alpha, up-regulation of TGF-beta2, increased cell distribution in pre-G(1) phase and upregulation of p53, Bax and p21 proteins expression while down-regulating Bcl-2alpha [73]. EGCG was reported to control and promote IL-23 dependent DNA repair, enhance cytotoxic T-cell activities and block cancer development by inhibiting carcinogenic signal transduction pathways [77]. EGCG was also shown to modulate several biological pathways, including growth factor-mediated pathway, the mitogen activated protein kinase-dependent pathway, and ubiquitin/proteasome degradation pathways [78]. Clinically, in a study of over 8000 individuals, daily consumption of green tea demonstrated delayed cancer onset; furthermore, breast cancer patients experienced a lower recurrence rate and longer remission [75]. Another clinical study found that oral ingestion of EGCG (200 mg per os) for 12 weeks was effective in patients with human papilloma virus-infected cervical lesions [79].

While EGCG is the most studied catechin in cancer, the in vitro study in human pancreatic ductal adenocarcinoma (PDAC) cells showed that two minor green tea catechins, ECG and EG, had much stronger anti proliferative and anti-inflammatory effects, including inhibition of NF-κB, IL8 and uPA, than EGCG [80].

Epigallocatechin gallate (EGCG) has poor bioavailability in rats and humans due to oxidation, metabolism and its efflux. In addition, specific interactions with other polyphenolic compounds can modulate its metabolic efficacy. However, a study by Kale et al. [81] showed that green tea extract consumed together with onion, which is rich in quercetin, can significantly enhance bioavailability of EGCG in humans. Wang et al. confirmed this effect, showing that quercetin affects EGCG by decreasing its methylation [82]. EGCG-quercetin interactions resulted in enhanced anti-proliferative effects of EGCG in androgen-dependent and androgen-independent prostate cancer cells [83]. EGCG bioavailability is affected by numerous compounds as its consumption with cereal and milk resulted in lower EGCG blood levels [84]. This indicates that proper selection of compounds and their combinations are important in achieving the desired biological effect.

## 4. Benefits of Nutrient Combinations—Pleiotropic Effects

Numerous in vitro and in vivo studies provide support for use of polyphenols in cancer prevention by applying them in combinations with other micronutrients for achieving pleiotropic effects. As mentioned previously, one of major problems with using polyphenols as anticancer agents individually is their poor bioavailability in the human body. In addition, their interactions with other natural compounds in a diet may hinder or complicate consistency of their efficacy [85]. Therefore, specifically designed combinations of several polyphenols or combinations of polyphenols with other natural agents aimed at defined biological targets will expand metabolic effects of constituents of such mixtures in controlled and reproducible ways. In addition, proper combinations of micronutrients enable use of lower doses of individual components without compromising their efficacy, rather than expanding the scope of cellular mechanisms affected. This novel approach opens up a possibility of developing more effective strategies against various human pathologies, including cancer.

Several in vitro and in vivo studies have shown that combinations of two or three polyphenols were more effective in inhibiting cancer growth than treatment with a single compound. Our research has demonstrated that multi-nutrient combinations, through their reciprocal interactions, including synergy, can modulate bioavailability of natural compounds and exercise pleiotropic effects by affecting multiple metabolic pathways involved in carcinogenesis simultaneously. Below we present a few examples of specific and effective anti-cancer nutrient mixtures. They include a combination of different polyphenols and combinations of polyphenols with vitamins and other micronutrients, which were selected to specifically target defined key cellular mechanisms involved in carcinogenesis.

### 4.1. Anticancer Effects of a Combination of Different Polyphenols

Several studies investigated the efficacy of mixtures containing two or three different polyphenols. These include combinations of EGCG with quercetin in prostate cancer cells [86,87], and EGCG with resveratrol in prostate cancer cell lines [88] and breast cancer MCF-7 cell line [89]. Combinations studied also included curcumin with EGCG and EC in lung cancer cell lines [90,91], curcumin with EGCG in human B-cell chronic leukemia [92] and in xenograft mouse models implanted with MDA-MB-231 breast cancer cells [93] and lung A549 cells [91]. Piao et al. [94] demonstrated anti-cancer effects of a tri-nutrient combination composed of curcumin, resveratrol and epicatechin gallate on cell viability, clonogenic survival, apoptosis and tumor growth in HPV-positive head and neck squamous cell carcinoma.

These findings indicate that more comprehensive mixtures of nutrients with similar or complementary anti-cancer mechanisms would allow for enhanced complementary or synergistic interactions between these compounds, thereby expanding different cancer mechanisms simultaneously and in a controlled fashion. Therefore, we combined the compounds previously investigated in combinations and cruciferous extract in order to enhance and expand their anti-cancer mechanisms through additive and synergistic effects. This mixture of nutrients (PB) included: quercetin, 400 mg; Cruciferex™ (prioprietary extract from cabbage, cauliflower, broccoli and carrots), 400 mg; turmeric root extract containing 95% curcuminoids, 300 mg; resveratrol, 50 mg; and standardized green tea extract (80% polyphenols), 300 mg. See Table 1 for summary of PB studies using in vitro and in vivo approaches. These included human Fanconi anemia head and neck squamous cell carcinoma (HNSCC), which with acute myeloid leukemia, are the major causes of mortality and morbidity in Fanconi anemia patients. We found that nude mice injected with OHSU-974 cells and subsequently fed a diet supplemented with 1% PB demonstrated inhibition of tumor growth by 67.6% ($p < 0.0001$) and tumor burden by 63.6% ($p < 0.0001$) [95]. In vitro study demonstrated dose-dependent inhibition of OSHU-974 cell proliferation, with cell toxicity detected at 27% ($p = 0.0003$) and 48% ($p = 0.0004$) at PB concentrations of 75 and 100 µg/mL, respectively [95]. These cells constitutively secrete matrix metalloproteinase (MMP)-2 and, after stimulation by phorbyl 12-myristate (PMA), also MMP-9. The secretion of MMPs by both stimulated and unstimulated cells was suppressed by PB in a dose-dependent manner, with total block of both at 50 µg/mL, which is below PB's toxicity level [95]. This concentration was also effective in inhibiting cancer cell migration (by scratch test) and invasion through Matrigel, apparently not related to cell toxicity, as no visible morphological changes were detected at this and lower concentrations [95].

**Table 1.** Anticancer effect of polyphenol mixture containing quercetin, curcumin, green tea, Cruciferex™, and resveratrol (PB) on cancer cell lines.

| Cancer Cell Line and in Vivo Design | Tumor Growth Inhibition | In Vitro Inhibition |
|---|---|---|
| FA HNSCC Athymic male nude mice injected SQ with $3 \times 10^6$ OSHU-974 cells Control group fed regular murine diet and PB group diet supplemented with PB 1% × 4 weeks [95] | Tumor weight by 67.6% ($p < 0.0001$) Tumor burden by 63.6% | Cell proliferation inhibited by 48% at 100 µg/mL PB; MMP-2 and -9 completely blocked at 50 µg/mL PB; cell migration and Matrigel invasion blocked at 50 µg/mL PB |
| Fibrosarcoma HT-1080 [96] | N/A | HT-1080 cell proliferation inhibited by 80% at 50 µg/mL PB; MMP-2 and -9 completely blocked at 50 µg/mL PB; Matrigel invasion blocked at 25 µg/mL PB; induction of dose-dependent apoptosis |
| Melanoma A-2058 [97] | N/A | A-2058 cell proliferation inhibited by 80% at 25 µg/mL PB; MMP-2 and -9 completely blocked at 50 µg/mL PB; Matrigel invasion blocked at 50 µg/mL PB; induction of dose-dependent apoptosis |

The inhibitory effects of PB were also observed in fibrosarcoma, which is an aggressive and highly metastatic cancer of connective tissue, and in melanoma, which causes the majority of skin cancer-related deaths, secondary to metastasis. The in vitro studies used human fibrosarcoma cell line HT-1080 [96] and melanoma A2058 cells [97]. The study showed that PB inhibited cell proliferation of human fibrosarcoma cells by 60% at 25 µg/mL and 80% at 50 µg/mL, and inhibited both MMP-2 and -9 secretion in a dose-dependent manner, with total inhibition at 50 µg/mL [96]. At PB concentration of 25 µg/mL, invasion of HT-1080 cells through Matrigel was totally blocked [96]. Melanoma cells were more sensitive to PB, as their proliferation was inhibited by 80% at 25 ug/mL and MMP-2 and -9 secretion and Matrigel cell invasion blocked completely at 50 µg/mL, indicating strong anti-invasive properties of this polyphenol mixture [97]. PB also induced cell apoptosis in both cell lines in a dose-dependent fashion.

### 4.2. Anticancer Effects of Combinations of Polyphenols, with Vitamins and Other Compounds

Combinations of polyphenols with mixtures of vitamins, amino acids and other micronutrients are rarely utilized in cancer research. We initiated this multi-targeted approach over a decade ago, demonstrating that a combination of EGCG with specific micronutrients showed anti-proliferative and anti-invasive effects in human breast (MDA-MB-231), colon (HCT 116) and melanoma (A-2058) cancer cells [98]. The investigated combination included EGCG from green tea together with ascorbic acid, lysine, proline, arginine, *N*-acetyl cysteine, selenium, copper and manganese. This mixture, designated as NM, was tested in vitro and in vivo against a few dozen human cancer cell lines. The composition of this specific micronutrient mixture exemplifies the importance of extracellular matrix-mediated processes in developing a general strategy of effective control of cancer. While most of natural compound combinations target intracellular regulatory mechanisms of tumorigenesis, our approach expands it to include connective tissue integrity as a common element involved in tumor growth, invasion and metastasis. The role of this natural anti-cancer barrier is frequently overlooked in therapeutic approaches to cancer. However, all critical metabolic steps in cancer require degradation of basement membrane and extracellular matrix components as the physical barrier restraining growth, migration and invasion of tumor cells. Increased activity of proteinases, such as MMPs and plasmin, accompanied by down-regulation of their natural inhibitors has been correlated with aggressiveness of cancer and angiogenesis, associated with neovascularization of tumors [99,100]. This new approach to curbing cancer growth by strengthening the connective tissue in the body was introduced by Rath in the 1990s [101]. This can be achieved with micronutrients essential for the synthesis and structure of connective tissue (vitamin C, lysine, proline, and copper manganese) and inhibitors of enzymatic breakdown of collagen facilitated by malignant cells (i.e., lysine). In addition to its essential role in collagen production, vitamin C has shown to be an effective anti-cancer agent (pro-oxidant effects) [102,103] and in cancer prevention (antioxidant effects) [104]. The presence of polyphenols in this mixture, in addition to selenium, *N*-acetylcysteine and arginine allows for expanding biological targets and enhancing several cellular mechanisms important in controlling cancer, such as immune system function. The mixture was formulated in two variants in regard to its polyphenol components: including both EGCG and quercetin (EPQ) and containing EGCG (NM) as the sole polyphenol. Both compositions were tested against several human and murine cancer cell lines both in vivo and in vitro.

### 4.2.1. EGCG in Combination with Vitamin C, Amino Acids and Other Micronutrients

The multiple aspects of anticancer efficacy of the combination of green tea extract rich in EGCG with ascorbic acid, lysine, proline, arginine, *N*-acetylcysteine, selenium, copper and manganese (NM) on several cancer cell lines in vivo and in vitro were presented in a review article [105].

This unique mixture demonstrated potent, significant suppression of hepatic and pulmonary metastasis in a murine model resulting in significant reduction in tumor size and tumor burden in all human cancer cell lines tested. In vitro studies demonstrated that NM was very effective in inhibition of cell proliferation (by MTT assay), MMP secretion (by gelatinase zymography), cell invasion (through Matrigel), cell migration (by scratch test), angiogenesis (VEGF and other angiogenic models), induction of apoptosis (by live green caspase) and induction of pro-apoptotic genes in many diverse cancer cell lines. A more recent study conducted with the NM mixture illustrates its efficacy against multiple parameters of cancer growth and progression in vivo and in vitro. We used an orthotopic breast cancer model to evaluate the development of tumors and metastasis, challenging mice with breast cancer 4T1 cells into the mammary pad, and also studied in vitro activity of NM on cell proliferation, MMP secretion, cell migration and invasion [106]. See Table 2 for summary of results. In contrast to human tumor cell models, murine tumor cell models often metastasize more effectively and display metastatic characteristics more similar to those observed in cancer patients. The 4T1 mammary carcinoma model was chosen since the primary tumor grows in the anatomically correct site and, as in human breast cancer, 4T1 metastatic disease develops spontaneously from the primary tumor. In addition, metastatic spread of 4T1 metastases to other organs and the draining lymph nodes is similar to that of human mammary cancer. The results showed that NM inhibited tumor weight and burden by 50% ($p = 0.02$) and 53.4% ($p < 0.0001$), respectively, and metastasis, by reducing mean number of colonies by 87% ($p < 0.0001$) and mean weight of lungs by 60% ($p = 0.0001$) compared to Control mice [106]. Metastasis to liver, spleen, kidney and heart was significantly reduced with NM supplementation [106].

**Table 2.** Anticancer effect of the combination of green tea extract with ascorbic acid, lysine, proline, arginine, *N*-acetyl cysteine, selenium, copper and manganese (NM) on breast 4T1 tumor [106].

| Tumor Cell Line/In Vivo Design | Tumor Growth and Metastasis | In Vitro Results |
|---|---|---|
| Orthotopic injection of $5 \times 10^5$ breast cancer 4T1 cells into the mammary pad of Balb C mice Control group fed regular murine diet and NM group diet supplemented with NM 0.5% × 4 weeks | Tumor weight reduced by 50% ($p = 0.02$) and tumor burden by 53.4% ($p < 0.0001$) in NM mice compared to Control mice Lung metastasis inhibited by 87% ($p < 0.0001$) in NM mice compared to Control mice Mean weight of lungs reduced by 60% ($p = 0.0001$) Metastasis to liver, spleen, kidney and heart significantly reduced in NM group compared to Control | Cell proliferation reduced by 50% at 250 μg/mL NM MMP-2 and -9 completely blocked at 1000 μg/mL NM Cell migration and Matrigel invasion blocked at 250 μg/mL NM |

4.2.2. Inhibitory Effects of EGCG Applied Individually, and in Combination with Other Micronutrients on MMPs

In a previous study, we compared the anticancer effects of EGCG alone, in green tea and in combinations with micronutrients on the critical aspect of malignancy. Since type IV collagenase matrix metalloproteinases, especially MMP-2 and MMP-9, have been found to promote invasion and metastasis of malignant tumors, we investigated the relative inhibitory effects in MMP-2 and -9 by EGCG, the main polyphenol in green tea extract (GTE) to that of GTE and to that of NM as a whole using four cancer cell lines expressing MMP-2, MMP-9 or both, to determine if there is an additive or synergistic effect from combinations of these agents [107]. The cell lines tested included human fibrosarcoma (HT-1080), hepatocellular carcinoma (SK-Hep-1), glioblastoma (T-98G) and uterine leiomyosarcoma (SK-UT-1). The cells were also treated with PMA 100 ng/mL to study enhanced expression of MMP-9. Secretion of MMPs was assessed by gelatinase zymography. Fibrosarcoma and hepatocellular carcinoma cells expressed both MMP-2 and MMP-9, glioblastoma cells MMP-2 and PMA-induced MMP-9, and uterine leimyosarcoma cells only PMA-induced MMP-9. NM was the most potent dose-dependent inhibitor of MMPs, followed by green tea extract and EGCG. See Table 3 for summary of results. These results suggest the enhanced efficacy of nutrients working in synergy to modulate complex pathways such as MMP expression.

**Table 3.** Comparative cumulative expression of MMP-2 and -9 in cell lines treated with epigallocatechin gallate (EGCG), green tea extract (GTE) and the nutrient mixture (NM) [107].

|  | EGCG | GTE | NM | EGCG + PMA | GTE + PMA | NM + PMA |
|---|---|---|---|---|---|---|
| | | | Fibrosarcoma HT-1080 | | | |
| MMP-2 | 7.88 | 7.47 | 3.29 | 0.21 | 0.20 | 0 |
| MMP-9 | 5.74 | 3.02 | 1.58 | 209.06 | 139.84 | 93.54 |
| | | | Hepatocellular carcinoma Sk-Hep-1 | | | |
| MMP-2 | 1.21 | 1.10 | 0 | 0.77 | 0.55 | 0.29 |
| MMP-9 | 256.51 | 187.28 | 26.59 | 611.90 | 593.80 | 508.28 |
| | | | Glioblastoma T-98G | | | |
| MMP-2 | 109.97 | 86.63 | 65.84 | 178.16 | 140.09 | 53.20 |
| MMP-9 | 0.37 | 0.37 | 0.10 | 92.69 | 82.67 | 52.50 |
| | | | Uterine leimyosarcoma SK-UT-1 | | | |
| MMP-2 | 0 | 0 | 0 | 51.36 | 49.97 | 34.30 |
| MMP-9 | 0 | 0 | 0 | 87.42 | 87.30 | 77.95 |

4.2.3. Quercetin in Enhancing the Micronutrient Mixture Efficacy in Established Breast Cancer Tumors

We observed that including quercetin in the nutrient mixture containing EGCG has beneficial effects when administered to rats at early stages of breast tumor growth. Breast tumors were induced by IP administration of *N*-methyl-*N*-nitrosourea to Wistar rats [108]. After tumors were evident in all rats, the animals were divided into groups and fed one of the following regimens for 60 days: control diet; 30 mg green tea extract alone; 30 mg green tea extract in combination with NM; or a diet containing 30 mg of green tea extract, NM and quercetin. The results showed that tumor size/rat was significantly lower in all supplemented groups than in the Control group. The rats on the diet containing NM and quercetin showed significantly lower values for tumor incidence, mean tumor volume and mean tumor weight compared to the Control, the green tea extract and the NM groups [108]. Rats in the Control group developed 24 carcinomas (mostly of grade III severity), contrasted with six carcinomas (all of which were of grade II severity) in the NM supplemented group containing quercetin. The incidence, mean tumor volume and mean tumor weight of the green tea extract group alone (2.0, 7.27 cc, and 5.33 g, respectively) were higher than those of the NM group (1.4, 3.39 cc, and 1.71 g, respectively), and that was greater than that of the quercetin + NM group (1.0, 2.69 cc, and 1.35 g, respectively); however, the differences did not reach statistical significance. Higher anti-cancer efficacy of the mixture in the presence of quercetin might be related to its effects on EGCG bioavailability, as the results showed that administration of EGCG in the mixture with vitamins, amino acids and trace element (NM) resulted in a modest increase of its plasma concentration to 45.81 ng/mL from 35.84 ng/mL with EGCG administered alone. The enrichment of this mixture with quercetin resulted in increased plasma EGCG level to 65.94 ng/mL.

### 4.2.4. Anticancer Effects of EGCG plus Quercetin in the Micronutrient Mixture

The studies presented below illustrate the anti-cancer potential of EGCG and quercetin in combination with the micronutrient mixture against ovarian cancer using two different cell lines (ES-2 and A-2780) [109,110]. See Table 4 for summary of results. EPQ contains the following nutrients in the relative amounts indicated: vitamin C (as ascorbic acid and as Mg, Ca ascorbates, and ascorbyl palmitate) 700 mg; L-lysine 1000 mg; L-proline 750 mg; L-arginine 500 mg; *N*-acetyl cysteine 200 mg; standardized green tea extract (80% polyphenol) 1000 mg; quercetin as quercetin dihydrate, from *Saphora japonica* 50 mg; selenium 30 µg; copper 2 mg; manganese 1 mg.

**Table 4.** Anticancer effect of mixture containing polyphenols quercetin and green tea extract with ascorbic acid, lysine, proline, arginine, *N*-acetyl cysteine, selenium, copper and manganese (EPQ).

| Cancer Cell Line and In Vivo Design | Tumor Growth and Metastasis Inhibition | In Vitro Inhibition |
|---|---|---|
| Athymic female mice inoculated subcutaneously with $3 \times 10^6$ ovarian ES-2 cells Control group fed regular murine diet and EPQ group diet supplemented with EPQ 0.5% × 4 weeks [109] | Tumor weight reduced by 59.2% ($p < 0.0001$) and tumor burden by 59.7% $p < 0.0001$) in EPQ mice | ES-2 cell proliferation inhibited by 35% at 1000 µg/mL EPQ; MMP-2 virtual total block at 1000 µg/mL EPQ; cell migration and Matrigel invasion blocked at 500 µg/mL EPQ |
| Athymic female mice inoculated intraperitoneally with $2 \times 10^6$ ovarian A-2780 cells Control group fed regular murine diet and EPQ group diet supplemented with EPQ 0.5% × 4 weeks [110] | Incidence of ovarian tumors reduced to 1 small tumor in EPQ group contrasted with Control group mice which all developed large ovarian tumors; tumor growth suppressed by 87% ($p < 0.0001$); lung metastasis completely suppressed in EPQ mice, but 100% present in Control mice | A-2780 cell proliferation inhibited by 80% at 1000 µg/mL EPQ; MMP-9 virtual total block at 250 µg/mL EPQ; Matrigel invasion blocked at 250 µg/mL EPQ |

Epithelial ovarian carcinoma is the leading cause of death from gynecological malignancy due to metastasis and recurrence. Our previous publication on athymic female mice inoculated with ES-2 ovarian cancer cells showed that dietary intake of EPQ (0.5%, w/w) inhibited weight and burden of tumors by 59.2% ($p < 0.0001$) and 59.7% ($p < 0.0001$), respectively [109] (see Figure 1). A subsequent study on ovarian carcinoma used IP injection of ovarian cancer A-2780 cells into athymic female mice and focused on ovarian tumor growth and lung metastasis [110]. In the A-2780 study, all Control mice developed large ovarian tumors, whereas five out of six mice in the EPQ group developed no tumors, and one, only a small tumor [110]. EPQ suppressed tumor growth by 87% ($p < 0.0001$). In addition, all animals in the Control group had lung metastasis while, in contrast, no metastasis was observed in the EPQ group of mice [110]. In vitro, the effects of EPQ on cell proliferation, MMP secretion, invasion through Matrigel, migration by scratch test and morphology were evaluated in ES-2 [109] and A2780 [110] cells. EPQ exhibited 35% toxicity over the control in ES-2 cells [109] and 80% in A-2780 cells [110] at 1000 µg/mL concentration. ES-2 cells demonstrated only MMP-2, with and without PMA, which was inhibited by EPQ in a dose dependent fashion, with near total inhibition at 1000 µg/mL [109]. A-2780 cells demonstrated only MMP-9 expression, which EPQ inhibited in a dose dependent fashion, with virtual total block at 250 µg/mL concentration [110]. Migration of ES-2 cells by scratch test and invasion through Matrigel were inhibited in a dose dependent manner with total block of invasion and migration at 500 µg/mL [109]. Invasion through Matrigel of A-2780 cells was completely inhibited by EPQ at 250 µg/mL [110]. H&E staining showed no morphological changes below 500 µg/mL EPQ in A-2780 cells [110] and below 1000 µg/mL EPQ in ES-2 cells [109]. See Table 4 for summary of results.

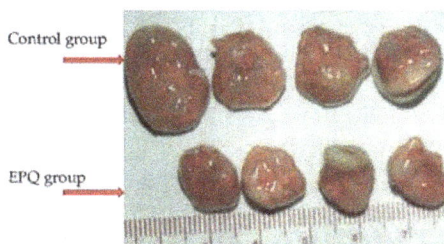

**Figure 1.** Gross photographs of representative tumors from Control and EPQ groups of mice inoculated with ovarian cancer ES-2 cells. Mean tumor weight and burden of EPQ group tumors were inhibited by 59.2% ($p < 0.0001$) and 59.7% ($p < 0.0001$) compared to Control group, respectively.

An earlier study investigated the efficacy of a combination of polyphenols, quercetin and green tea, on prostate cancer xenograft tumor growth. The results confirmed the synergistic effects of this nutrient combination resulting in tumor growth inhibition by 45%, compared to 15% with quercetin and 21% with green tea only [111]. Although the experimental design and tumor type differed in the Wang studies from our research, both investigations point out to enhance anticancer effects of various nutrient combinations and the importance of connective tissue in confining tumor growth and metastasis.

## 5. Conclusions

Current cancer therapies based on chemotherapy and radiation are associated with significant side effects. Therefore, there is an urgent need for developing alternate or adjuvant approaches. Polyphenolic compounds, which are abundant from dietary sources, show great promise in cancer treatment, especially considering their safe use. Due to their ability to modulate multiple biological mechanisms involved in cancer initiation and progression, they offer more comprehensive therapeutic effects than single drugs. Bioavailability, as well as curative and preventive properties of these nutrients, can be enhanced and expanded in combination therapies that include natural compounds of the same or different chemical class. Combinations of polyphenols with micronutrients essential for maintaining integrity and stability of extracellular matrix offer expanded anti-cancer benefits. They include targeting complementary metabolic pathways important in curtailing cancer invasion and metastasis. Therefore, future research directions should expand to using natural compounds, especially in combinations, as safe, effective and affordable therapeutic approaches to cancer.

**Acknowledgments:** The research study was funded by Dr. Rath Health Foundation (Santa Clara, CA, USA), a non-profit organization.

**Author Contributions:** This review was written by A.N., M.W.R., T.K. and M.R.

**Conflicts of Interest:** The authors declare no conflict of interest.

## References

1. Scalbert, A.; Manach, C.; Morand, C.; Rémésy, C.; Jime'nez, L. Dietary polyphenols and the prevention of diseases. *Crit. Rev. Food Sci. Nutr.* **2005**, *45*, 287–306. [CrossRef] [PubMed]
2. Ramos, S. Cancer chemoprevention and chemotherapy: Dietary polyphenols and signaling pathways. *Mol. Nutr. Food Res.* **2008**, *52*, 507–526. [CrossRef] [PubMed]
3. Fantini, M.; Benvenuto, M.; Masuelli, L.; Frajese, G.V.; Tresoldi, I.; Modesti, A.; Bei, R. In vitro and in vivo antitumoral effects of combinations of polyphenols, or polyphenols and anticancer drugs: Perspectives on cancer treatment. *Int. J. Mol. Sci.* **2015**, *16*, 9236–9282. [CrossRef] [PubMed]
4. Manach, C.; Scalbert, A.; Morand, C.; Rémésy, C.; Jime'nez, L. Polyphenols: Food sources and bioavailability. *Am. J. Clin. Nutr.* **2004**, *79*, 727–747. [PubMed]

5.  Arts, I.C.W.; van de Putte, B.; Hollman, P.C.H. Catechin contents of foods commonly consumed in The Netherlands. Fruits, vegetables, staple foods, and processed foods. *J. Agric. Food Chem.* **2000**, *48*, 1746–1751. [CrossRef] [PubMed]
6.  Arts, I.C.; van de Putte, B.; Hollman, P.C.H. Catechin contents of foods commonly consumed in The Netherlands. Tea, wine, fruit juices, and chocolate milk. *J. Agric. Food Chem.* **2000**, *48*, 1752–1757. [CrossRef] [PubMed]
7.  Lakenbrink, C.; Lapczynski, S.; Maiwald, B.; Engelhardt, U.H. Flavonoids and other polyphenols in consumer brews of tea and other caffeinated beverages. *J. Agric. Food Chem.* **2000**, *48*, 2848–2852. [CrossRef] [PubMed]
8.  Zhu, Q.Y.; Zhang, A.Q.; Tsang, D.; Huang, Y.; Chen, Z.Y. Stability of green tea catechins. *J. Agric. Food Chem.* **1997**, *45*, 4624–4628. [CrossRef]
9.  Lempereur, I.; Rouau, X.; Abecassis, J. Genetic and agronomic variation in arabinoxylan and ferulic acid contents of durum wheat (Triticum durum L) grain and its milling fractions. *J. Cereal Sci.* **1999**, *25*, 103–110. [CrossRef]
10. Bhat, K.P.; Pezzuto, J.M. Cancer chemopreventive activity of resveratrol. *Ann. N. Y. Acad. Sci.* **2002**, *957*, 210–229. [CrossRef] [PubMed]
11. Adlercreutz, H.; Mazur, W. Phyto-oestrogens and western diseases. *Ann. Med.* **1997**, *29*, 95–120. [CrossRef] [PubMed]
12. Touré, A.; Xuemin, X. Flax lignans: Source, biosynthesis, metabolism, antioxidant activity, bio-active components, and health benefits. *Compr. Rev. Food Sci. Food Saf.* **2010**, *9*, 261–269. [CrossRef]
13. Scalbert, A.; Williamson, G. Dietary intake and bioavailability of polyphenols. *J. Nutr.* **2000**, *130*, 2073S–2085S. [PubMed]
14. Bogaards, I.J.P.; van Ommen, B.; Falke, H.E.; Willems, M.I.; van Bladeren, P.J. Glutathione S-transferase subunit induction patterns of Brussel sprouts, allyl isothiocyanate and goitrin in rat liver and small intestinal mucosa: A new approach for the identification of inducing xenobiotics. *Food Chem. Toxicol.* **1990**, *28*, 81–88. [CrossRef]
15. Han, X.; Shen, T.; Lou, H. Dietary polyphenols and their biological significance. *Int. J. Mol. Sci.* **2007**, *8*, 950–988. [CrossRef]
16. Shen, S.Q.; Zhang, Y.; Xiang, J.J.; Xiong, C.L. Protective effect of curcumin against liver warm ischemia/reperfusion injury in rat model is associated with regulation of heat shock protein and antioxidant enzymes. *World J. Gastroenterol.* **2007**, *13*, 1953–1961. [CrossRef] [PubMed]
17. Chen, C.; Yu, R.; Owuor, E.D.; Kong, A.N. Activation of antioxidant response element (ARE), mitogen-activated protein kinases (MAPKs) and caspases by major green tea polyphenol components during cell survival and death. *Arch. Pharm. Res.* **2000**, *23*, 605–612. [CrossRef] [PubMed]
18. Kunnumakkara, A.B.; Guha, S.; Krishnan, S.; Diagaradjane, P.; Gelovani, J.; Aggarwal, B.B. Curcumin potentiates antitumor activity of gemcitabine in an orthotopic model of pancreatic cancer through suppression of proliferation, angiogenesis, and inhibition of nuclear factor kappa B-regulated gene products. *Cancer Res.* **2007**, *67*, 3853–3861. [CrossRef] [PubMed]
19. Collett, G.P.; Campbell, F.C. Curcumin induces c-jun N-terminal kinase-dependent apoptosis in HCT116 human colon cancer cells. *Carcinogenesis* **2004**, *25*, 2183–2189. [CrossRef] [PubMed]
20. Anto, R.J.; Mukhopadhyay, A.; Denning, K.; Aggarwal, B.B. Curcumin (diferuloylmethane) induces apoptosis through activation of caspase-8, BID cleavage and cytochrome c release: Its suppression by ectopic expression of Bcl-2 and Bcl-xL. *Carcinogenesis* **2002**, *23*, 143–150. [CrossRef] [PubMed]
21. Aoki, H.; Takada, Y.; Kondo, S.; Sawaya, R.; Aggarwal, B.; Kondo, Y. Evidence that curcumin suppresses the growth of malignant gliomas in vitro and in vivo through induction of autophagy: Role of Akt and ERK signaling pathways. *Mol. Pharmacol.* **2007**, *72*, 29–39. [CrossRef] [PubMed]
22. Anand, P.; Sundaram, C.; Jhurani, S.; Kunnumakkara, A.B.; Aggarwal, B.B. Curcumin and cancer: An 'old-age' disease with an 'age-old' solution. *Cancer Lett.* **2008**, *267*, 133–164. [CrossRef] [PubMed]
23. Alexandrov, M.G.; Song, L.J.; Altiok, S.; Gray, J.; Haura, E.B.; Kumar, N.B. Curcumin: A novel Stat3 pathway inhibitor for chemoprevention of lung cancer. *Eur. J. Cancer Prev.* **2012**, *21*, 407–412. [CrossRef] [PubMed]
24. Ng, T.P.; Chiam, P.C.; Lee, T.; Chua, H.C.; Lim, L.; Kua, E.H. Curry consumption and cognitive function in the elderly. *Am. J. Epidemiol.* **2006**, *164*, 898–906. [CrossRef] [PubMed]

25. Bartik, L.; Whitfield, G.K.; Kaczmarska, M.; Lowmiller, C.L.; Moffet, E.W.; Furmick, J.K.; Hernandez, Z.; Haussler, C.A.; Haussler, M.R.; Jurutka, P.W. Curcumin: A novel nutritionally derived ligand of the vitamin D receptor with implications for colon cancer. *J. Nutr. Biochem.* **2010**, *21*, 1153–1161. [CrossRef] [PubMed]

26. Ide, H.; Tokiwa, S.; Sakamaki, K.; Nishio, K.; Isotani, S.; Muto, S.; Hama, T.; Masuda, H.; Horie, S. Combined inhibitory effect of soy flavones and curcumin on the production of prostate specific antigen. *Prostate* **2010**, *70*, 1127–1133. [CrossRef] [PubMed]

27. Gupta, S.C.; Patchva, S.; Aggarwal, B.B. Therapeutic roles of curcumin: Lessons learned from clinical trials. *AAPS J.* **2013**, *15*, 195–218. [CrossRef] [PubMed]

28. Ravindran, J.; Prasad, S.; Aggrawal, B.B. Curcumin and cancer cells: How many ways can curry kill tumor cells selectively? *AAPS J.* **2009**, *11*, 495–510. [CrossRef] [PubMed]

29. Shanmugam, M.K.; Rane, G.; Kanchi, M.M. The multifaceted role of curcumin in cancer prevention and treatment. *Molecules* **2015**, *20*, 2728–2769. [CrossRef] [PubMed]

30. Gibellini, L.; Pinti, M.; Nasi, M.; Montagna, J.P.; De Biasi, S.; Roat, E.; Bertoncelli, L.; Cooper, E.L.; Cossarizza, A. Quercetin and cancer chemoprevention. *Evid. Based Complement. Alternat. Med.* **2011**, *2011*, 591356. [CrossRef] [PubMed]

31. Ekstrom, A.M.; Serafini, M.; Nyren, O.; Wolk, A.; Bosetti, C.; Bellocco, R. Dietary quercetin intake and risk of gastric cancer: Results from a population-based study in Sweden. *Ann. Oncol.* **2011**, *22*, 438–443. [CrossRef] [PubMed]

32. Lam, T.K.; Rotunno, M.; Lubin, J.H.; Wacholder, S.; Consonni, D.; Pesatori, A.C.; Bertazzi, P.A.; Chanock, S.J.; Burdette, L.; Goldstein, A.M.; et al. Dietary quercetin, quercetin-gene interaction, metabolic gene expression in lung tissue and lung cancer risk. *Carcinogenesis* **2010**, *31*, 634–642. [CrossRef] [PubMed]

33. Jeong, J.H.; An, J.Y.; Kwon, Y.T.; Rhee, J.G.; Lee, Y.G. Effects of low dose quercetin: Cancer cell-specific inhibition of cell cycle progression. *J. Cell. Biochem.* **2009**, *106*, 73–82. [CrossRef] [PubMed]

34. Yang, J.H.; Hsia, T.C.; Kuo, H.M.; Chou, P.D.; Chou, C.C.; Wei, Y.H.; Chung, J.G. Inhibition of lung cancer cell growth by quercetin glucuronides via G 2/M arrest and induction of apoptosis. *Drug Metab. Dispos.* **2006**, *34*, 296–304. [CrossRef] [PubMed]

35. Nair, H.K.; Rao, K.V.K.; Aalinkeel, R.; Mahajan, S.; Chawda, R.; Schwartz, S.A. Inhibition of prostate cancer cell colony formation by the flavonoid quercetin correlates with modulation of specific regulatory genes. *Clin. Diagn. Lab. Immunol.* **2004**, *11*, 63–69. [CrossRef] [PubMed]

36. Mu, C.; Jia, P.; Yan, Z.; Liu, X.; Li, X.; Liu, H. Quercetin induces cell cycle G1 arrest through elevating Cdk inhibitors p21 and p27 in human hepatoma cell line (HepG2). *Methods Find. Exp. Clin. Pharmacol.* **2007**, *29*, 179–183. [CrossRef] [PubMed]

37. Seufi, A.M.; Ibrahim, S.S.; Elmagrahby, T.K.; Hafez, E.E. Preventive effect of the flavonoid, quercetin, on hepatic cancer in rats via oxidant/antioxidant activity: Molecular and histological evidences. *J. Exp. Clin. Cancer Res.* **2009**, *28*, 80. [CrossRef] [PubMed]

38. Devipriya, S.; Ganapthy, V.; Shyamaladevi, C.S. Suppression of tumor growth and invasion in 9,10 dimethyl benz (a) anthracene induced mammary carcinoma by the plant bioflavonoid quercetin. *Chem-Biol. Interact.* **2006**, *162*, 106–113. [CrossRef] [PubMed]

39. Theodoratou, E.; Kyle, J.; Cetnarskyj, R.; Farrington, S.M.; Tenesa, A.; Barnetson, R.; Porteous, M.; Dunlop, M.; Campbell, H. Dietary flavonoids and the risk of colorectal cancer. *Cancer Epidemiol. Biomark. Prev.* **2007**, *16*, 684–693. [CrossRef] [PubMed]

40. Ferry, D.R.; Smith, A.; Malkhandi, J.; Fyfe, D.W.; de Takats, P.G.; Anderson, D.; Baker, J.; Kerr, D.J. Phase I clinical trial of the flavonoid quercetin: Pharmacokinetics and evidence for in vivo tyrosine kinase inhibition. *Clin. Cancer Res.* **1996**, *2*, 659–668. [PubMed]

41. Miles, S.L.; McFarland, M.; Niles, R.M. Molecular and physiological actions of quercetin: Need for clinical trials to assess its benefits in human disease. *Nutr. Rev.* **2014**, *72*, 720–734. [CrossRef] [PubMed]

42. Udenigwe, C.C.; Ramprasath, V.R.; Aluko, R.E.; Jones, P.J. Potential of resveratrol in anticancer and anti-inflammatory therapy. *Nutr. Rev.* **2008**, *66*, 445–454. [CrossRef] [PubMed]

43. Bishayee, A. Cancer prevention and treatment with resveratrol: From rodent studies to clinical trials. *Cancer Prev. Res.* **2009**, *2*, 409–418. [CrossRef] [PubMed]

44. Kukreja, A.; Waddhwa, N.; Tiwari, A. Therapeutic role of resveratrol and piceatannol in disease prevention. *J. Blood Disord. Transf.* **2014**, *5*, 1–6. [CrossRef]

45. Patel, K.R.; Brown, V.A.; Jones, D.J.L.; Britton, R.G.; Hemingway, D.; Miller, A.S.; West, K.P.; Booth, T.D.; Perloff, M.; Crowell, J.A.; et al. Clinical pharmacology of resveratrol and its metabolites in colorectal cancer patients. *Cancer Res.* **2010**, *70*, 7392–7399. [CrossRef] [PubMed]

46. Chow, H.H.S.; Garland, L.L.; Hsu, C.H.; Vining, D.R.; Chew, W.M.; Miller, J.A.; Perloff, M.; Crowell, J.A.; Alberts, D.S. Resveratrol modulates drug- and carcinogen-metabolizing enzymes in a healthy volunteer study. *Cancer Prev. Res.* **2010**, *3*, 1168–1175. [CrossRef] [PubMed]

47. Drewnowski, A.; Gomez-Carneros, C. Bitter taste, phytonutrients and the consumer: A review. *Am. J. Clin. Nutr.* **2000**, *72*, 1424–1435. [PubMed]

48. Hidgon, J.V.; Delage, B.; Williams, D.E.; Dashwood, R.H. Cruciferous vegetables and human cancer risk: Epidemiologic evidence and mechanistic basis. *Pharmacol. Res.* **2007**, *55*, 224–236.

49. Holst, B.; Williamson, G. A critical review of the bioavailability of glucosinolates and related compounds. *Nat. Proc. Rep.* **2004**, *21*, 425–447. [CrossRef] [PubMed]

50. Agerbirk, N.; Olsen, C.E. Glucosinolate structures in evolution. *Phytochemistry* **2012**, *77*, 16–45. [CrossRef] [PubMed]

51. Kandala, P.K.; Srivastava, S.K. DIMming ovarian cancer growth. *Curr. Drug Targets* **2012**, *13*, 1869–1875. [CrossRef] [PubMed]

52. Bradlow, H.L. Indole-3-carbinol as a chemopreventive agent in breast and prostate cancer. *In Vivo* **2008**, *22*, 441–116. [PubMed]

53. Beaver, L.M.; Yu, T.W.; Sokolowski, E.I.; Williams, D.E.; Dashwood, R.H.; Ho, E. 3,3′-diindolylmethane, but not indole-3-carbinol, inhibits histone deacetylase activity in prostate cancer cells. *Toxicol. Appl. Pharmacol.* **2012**, *263*, 345–351. [CrossRef] [PubMed]

54. Sepkovic, D.W.; Raucci, L.; Stein, J.; Carlisle, A.D.; Auborn, K.; Ksieski, H.B.; Nyirenda, T.; Bradlow, H.L. 3,3′-Diindolylmethane increases serum interferon-γ levels in the K14-HPV16 transgenic mouse model for cervical cancer. *In Vivo* **2012**, *26*, 207–211. [PubMed]

55. Chinni, S.R.; Li, Y.; Upadhyay, S.; Koppolu, P.K.; Sarkar, F.H. Indole-3-carbinol (I3C) induced cell growth inhibition, G1 cell cycle arrest and apoptosis in prostate cancer cells. *Oncogene* **2001**, *20*, 2927–2937. [CrossRef] [PubMed]

56. Li, Y.; Li, X.; Sarkar, F.H. Gene expression profiles of IC3 and DIM-treated PC3 human prostate cancer dells determined by cDNA microarray analysis. *J. Nutr.* **2003**, *133*, 1011–1019. [PubMed]

57. Aggarwal, B.B.; Ichikawa, H. Molecular targets and anticancer potential of indole-3-carbinol and its derivatives. *Cell Cycle* **2005**, *4*, 1201–1215. [CrossRef] [PubMed]

58. Sarkar, F.H.; Li, Y. Indole-3-carbinol and prostate cancer. *J. Nutr.* **2004**, *134*, 3493S–8349S. [PubMed]

59. Plate, A.Y.; Gallaher, D.D. Effects of indole-3-carbinol and phenethyl isothiocyanate on colon carcinogenesis induced by azoxymethane in rats. *Carcinogenesis* **2006**, *27*, 287–292. [CrossRef] [PubMed]

60. Tadi, K.; Chang, Y.; Ashok, B.T.; Chen, Y.; Moscatello, A.; Schaefer, S.D.; Schantz, S.P.; Policastro, A.J.; Geliebter, J.; Tiwari, R.K. 3,3′-Diindolylmethane, a cruciferous vegetable derived synthetic anti-proliferative compound in thyroid disease. *Biochem. Biophys. Res. Commun.* **2005**, *337*, 1019–1025. [CrossRef] [PubMed]

61. Kim, Y.S.; Milner, J.A. Targets for indole-3-carbinol in cancer prevention. *J. Nutr. Biochem.* **2005**, *16*, 65–73. [CrossRef] [PubMed]

62. Brew, C.T.; Aronchik, I.; Hsu, J.C.; Sheen, J.H.; Dickson, R.B.; Bjeldanes, L.F.; Firestone, G.L. Indole-3-carbinol activates the ATM signaling pathway independent of DNA damage to stabilize p53 and induce G1 arrest of human mammary epithelial cells. *Int. J. Cancer* **2006**, *118*, 857–868. [CrossRef] [PubMed]

63. Chang, X.; Tou, J.C.; Hong, C.; Chen, Y.; Moscatello, A.; Schaefer, S.D.; Schantz, S.P.; Policastro, A.J.; Geliebter, J.; Tiwari, R.K. 3,3′-Diindolylmethane inhibits angiogenesis and the growth of transplantable human breast carcinoma in athymic mice. *Carcinogenesis* **2005**, *26*, 771–778. [CrossRef] [PubMed]

64. Shukla, Y.; Kalra, N.; Katiyar, S.; Siddiqui, I.A.; Arora, A. Chemopreventive effect of indole-3-carbinol on induction of preneoplastic altered hepatic foci. *Nutr. Cancer* **2004**, *50*, 214–220. [CrossRef] [PubMed]

65. Garikapaty, V.P.; Ashok, B.T.; Chen, Y.G.; Mittelman, A.; Iatropoulos, M.; Tiwari, R.K. Anti-carcinogenic and anti-metastatic properties of indole-3-carbinol in prostate cancer. *Oncol. Rep.* **2005**, *13*, 89–93. [CrossRef] [PubMed]

66. Bonnesen, C.; Eggleston, I.M.; Hayes, J.D. Dietary indoles and isothiocyanates that are generated from cruciferous vegetables can both stimulate apoptosis and confer protection against DNA damage in human colon cell lines. *Cancer Res.* **2001**, *61*, 6120–6130. [PubMed]

67. Keck, A.S.; Finley, J.W. Cruciferous vegetables: Cancer protective mechanisms of glucosinolate hydrolysis products and selenium. *Integr. Cancer Ther.* **2004**, *3*, 5–12. [CrossRef] [PubMed]

68. Valcic, S.; Timmermann, B.N.; Alberts, D.S.; Wächter, G.A.; Krutzsch, M.; Wymer, J.; Guillén, J.M. Inhibitory effect of six green tea catechins and caffeine on the growth of four selected human tumor cell lines. *Anticancer Drugs* **1996**, *7*, 461–468. [CrossRef] [PubMed]

69. Mukhtar, H.; Ahmad, N. Tea polyphenols: Prevention of cancer and optimizing health. *Am. J. Clin. Nutr.* **2000**, *71*, S1698–S1702, discussion S1703–S1704.

70. Yang, G.Y.; Liao, J.; Kim, K.; Yurkow, E.J.; Yang, C.S. Inhibition of growth and induction of apoptosis in human cancer cell lines by tea polyphenols. *Carcinogenesis* **1998**, *19*, 611–616. [CrossRef] [PubMed]

71. Taniguchi, S.; Fujiki, H.; Kobayashi, H.; Go, H.; Miyado, K.; Sadano, H.; Shimokawa, R. Effect of (−)-epigallocatechin gallate, the main constituent of green tea, on lung metastasis with mouse B16 melanoma cell lines. *Cancer Lett.* **1992**, *65*, 51–54. [CrossRef]

72. Hara, Y. *Green Tea: Health Benefits and Applications*; Marcel Dekker: New York, NY, USA, 2001.

73. Harakeh, S.; Abu-El-Ardat, K.; Diab-Assaf, M.; Niedzwiecki, A.; El-Sabban, M.; Rath, M. Epigallocatechin-3-gallate induces apoptosis and cell cycle arrest in HTLV-1-positive and -negative leukemia cells. *Med. Oncol.* **2008**, *25*, 30–39. [CrossRef] [PubMed]

74. Cabrera, C.; Gimenez, R.; Lopez, M.C. Determination of tea components with antioxidant activity. *J. Agric. Food Chem.* **2003**, *53*, 4427–4435. [CrossRef] [PubMed]

75. Fujiki, H.; Suganuma, M.; Okabe, S.; Sueoka, E.; Suga, K.; Imai, K.; Nakachi, K.; Kimura, S. Mechanistic findings of green tea as cancer preventive for humans. *Proc. Soc. Exp. Biol. Med.* **1999**, *220*, 225–228. [CrossRef] [PubMed]

76. Gupta, S.; Hastak, K.; Afaq, F.; Ahmad, N.; Mukhtar, H. Essential role of caspases in epigallocatechin-3-gallate-mediated inhibition of nuclear factor kappa B and induction of apoptosis. *Oncogene* **2004**, *23*, 2507–2522. [CrossRef] [PubMed]

77. Ahmed, S.; Wang, N.; Lalonde, M.; Goldberg, V.M.; Haqqi, T.M. Green tea polyphenol epigallocatechin-3-gallate (EGCG) differentially inhibits interleukin-1 beta-induced expression of matrix metalloproteinase-1 and -13 in human chondrocytes. *J. Pharmacol. Exp. Ther.* **2004**, *308*, 767–773. [CrossRef] [PubMed]

78. Khan, N.; Afaq, F.; Saleem, M.; Ahmad, N.; Mukhtar, H. Targeting multiple signaling pathways by green tea polyphenol (−)-epigallocatechin-3-gallate. *Cancer Res.* **2006**, *66*, 2500–2505. [CrossRef] [PubMed]

79. Ahn, W.S.; Yoo, J.; Huh, S.W.; Kim, C.K.; Lee, J.M.; Namkoong, S.E.; Bae, S.M.; Lee, I.P. Protective effects of green tea extracts (polyphenon E and EGCG) on human cervical lesions. *Eur. J. Cancer Prev.* **2003**, *12*, 383–390. [CrossRef] [PubMed]

80. Kurbitz, C.; Heise, D.; Redmer, T.; Goumas, F.; Arlt, A.; Lemke, J.; Rimbach, G.; Kalthoff, H.; Trauzold, A. Epicatechin gallate and catechin gallate are superior to epigallocatechin gallate in growth suppression and anti-inflammatory activities in pancreatic tumor cells. *Cancer Sci.* **2011**, *102*, 728–734. [CrossRef] [PubMed]

81. Kale, A.; Gawande, S.; Kotwal, S.; Netke, S.; Roomi, W.; Ivanov, V.; Niedzwiecki, A.; Rath, M. Studies on the effects of oral administration of nutrient mixture, quercetin and red onions on the bioavailability of epigallocatechin gallate from green tea extract. *Phytother. Res.* **2010**, *24*, S48–S55. [CrossRef] [PubMed]

82. Wang, P.; Herber, D.; Henning, S.M. Quercetin increased bioavailability and decreased methylation of green tea polyphenols in vitro and in vivo. *Food Funct.* **2012**, *3*, 635–642. [CrossRef] [PubMed]

83. Wang, P.; Herber, D.; Henning, S.M. Quercetin increased antiproliferative activity of green tea polyphenol (−)-epigallocatechin gallate in prostate cancer cells. *Nutr. Cancer* **2012**, *64*, 580–587. [CrossRef] [PubMed]

84. Naumovsky, N.; Blades, B.L.; Roach, P.D. Food inhibits the oral bioavailability of the major green tea antioxidant epigallocatechin gallate in humans. *Antioxidants* **2015**, *4*, 373–393. [CrossRef] [PubMed]

85. Williamson, G.; Manach, C. Bioavailability and bioefficacy of polyphenols in humans. II. Review of 93 intervention studies. *Am. J. Clin. Nutr.* **2005**, *81*, 243S–255S. [PubMed]

86. Hsieh, T.C.; Wu, J.M. Targeting CWR22Rv1 prostate cancer cell proliferation and gene expression by combinations of the phytochemicals, EGCG, genistein and quercetin. *Anticancer Res.* **2009**, *29*, 4025–4032. [PubMed]

87. Tang, S.N.; Singh, C.; Nall, D.; Meeker, D.; Shankar, S.; Srivastava, R.K. The dietary bioflavonoid quercetin synergizes with epigallocatechin gallate (EGCG) to inhibit prostate cancer stem cell characterstic, invasion migration and epithelial-mesenchymal transition. *J. Mol. Signal.* **2010**, *5*, 14. [CrossRef] [PubMed]

88. Ahmad, K.A.; Harris, N.H.; Johnson, A.D.; Lindvall, H.C.; Wang, G.; Ahmed, K. Protein kinase CK2 modulates apoptosis induced by resveratrol and epigallocatechin gallate in prostate cancer cells. *Mol. Cancer Ther.* **2007**, *6*, 1006–1012. [CrossRef] [PubMed]

89. Hsieh, T.C.; Wu, J.M. Suppression of cell proliferation and gene expression by combinatorial synergy of EGCG, resveratrol and gamma-tocotrienol in estrogen positive MCF-7 breast cancer cells. *Int. J. Oncol.* **2008**, *33*, 851–859. [PubMed]

90. Saha, A.; Kuzuhara, T.; Echigo, N.; Suganuma, M.; Fujiki, H. New role of (−)epicatechin in enhancing the induction of growth inhibition and apoptosis in human lung cancer cells by curcumin. *Cancer Prev. Res.* **2010**, *3*, 953–962. [CrossRef] [PubMed]

91. Zhou, D.H.; Wang, X.; Yang, M.; Shi, X.; Huang, W.; Feng, Q. Combination of low concentration of (−)epigallocatechin gallate (EGCG) and curcumin strongly suppresses the growth of non small cell lung cancer in vitro and in vivo through causing cell cycle arrest. *Int. J. Mol. Sci.* **2013**, *14*, 12023–12036. [CrossRef] [PubMed]

92. Ghosh, A.K.; Kay, N.E.; Secreto, C.R.; Shanafelt, T.D. Curcumin inhibits prosurvival pathways in chronic lymphocytic leukemia B cells and may overcome their stromal protection in combination with EGCG. *Clin. Cancer Res.* **2009**, *15*, 1250–1258. [CrossRef] [PubMed]

93. Somers-Edgar, T.J.; Scandlyn, M.J.; Stuart, E.C.; Le Nedelec, M.J.; Valentine, S.P.; Rosengren, R.J. The combination of epigallocatechin gallate and curcumin suppresses ER alpha-breast cancer cell growth in vitro and in vivo. *Int. J. Cancer* **2008**, *122*, 1966–1971. [CrossRef] [PubMed]

94. Piao, L.; Mukherjee, S.; Chang, Q.; Xie, X.; Li, H.; Castellanos, M.R.; Banerjee, P.; Iqbal, H.; Ivancic, R.; Wang, X.; et al. TriCurin, a novel formulation of curcumin, epicatechin gallate and resveratrol, inhibits the tumorigenicity of human papillomavirus-positive head and neck squamous cell carcinoma. *Oncotarget* **2016**. [CrossRef] [PubMed]

95. Roomi, M.W.; Kalinovsky, T.; Roomi, N.W.; Niedzwiecki, A.; Rath, M. In vitro and in vivo inhibition of human Fanconi anemia head and neck squamous carcinoma by a phytonutrient combination. *Int. J. Oncol.* **2015**, *46*, 2261–2266. [CrossRef] [PubMed]

96. Roomi, M.W.; Jariwalla, N.; Roomi, N.W.; Rath, M.; Niedzwiecki, A. Abstract 1500: A novel nutrient mixture exhibits antitumor activity in human fibrosarcoma cell line HT-1080. In Proceedings of the 102nd Annual Meeting of the AACR, Orlando, FL, USA, 2–6 April 2011.

97. Roomi, M.W.; Siddiqui, S.; Roomi, N.W.; Niedzwiecki, A.; Rath, M. Abstract 1503: Anti-cancer effects of a nutrient mixture in human melanoma cells A2058: Inhibition of cell proliferation, MMP expression, invasion and apoptosis. In Proceedings of the 102nd Annual Meeting of the AACR, Orlando, FL, USA, 2–6 April 2011.

98. Netke, S.P.; Roomi, M.W.; Ivanov, V.; Niedzwiecki, A.; Rath, M. A specific combination of ascorbic acid, lysine, proline and epigallocatechin gallate inhibits proliferation and extracellular matrix invasion of various human cancer cell lines. *Res. Commun. Pharmacol. Toxicol. Emerg. Drugs* **2003**, *8*, IV37–IV49.

99. Stetler-Stevenson, W.G. The role of matrix metalloproteinases in tumor invasion, metastasis and angiogenesis. *Surg. Oncol. Clin. N. Am.* **2001**, *10*, 383–392. [PubMed]

100. Dano, K.; Andreasen, P.A.; Grondahl-Hansen, J.; Kristensen, P.; Nielsen, L.S.; Skriver, L. Plasminogen activators, tissue degradation and cancer. *Adv. Cancer Res.* **1985**, *44*, 139–266. [PubMed]

101. Rath, M.; Pauling, L. Plasmin-induced proteolysis and the role of apoprotein(a), lysine and synthetic analogs. *Orthomol. Med.* **1992**, *7*, 17–23.

102. Park, S. The effects of high concentrations of vitamin on cancer cells. *Nutrients* **2013**, *5*, 3496–3505. [CrossRef] [PubMed]

103. Chen, Q.; Espey, M.G.; Krishna, M.C.; Mitchell, J.B.; Corpe, C.P.; Buettner, G.R.; Shacter, E.; Levine, M. Pharmacologic ascorbic acid concentrations selectively kill cancer cells: Action as a pro-drug to deliver hydrogen peroxide to tissues. *Proc. Natl. Acad. Sci. USA* **2005**, *102*, 13604–13609. [CrossRef] [PubMed]

104. Lutsenko, E.A.; Carcamo, J.M.; Golde, D.W. Vitamin C prevents DNA mutation induced by oxidative stress. *J. Biol. Chem.* **2001**, *277*, 16895–16899. [CrossRef] [PubMed]

105. Niedzwiecki, A.; Roomi, M.W.; Kalinovsky, T.; Rath, M. Micronutrient synergy—A new tool in effective control of metastasis and other key mechanisms of cancer. *Cancer Metastasis Rev.* **2010**, *29*, 529–543. [CrossRef] [PubMed]

106. Roomi, M.W.; Kalinovsky, T.; Roomi, N.M.; Cha, J.; Rath, M.; Niedzwiecki, A. In vivo and in vitro effects of a nutrient mixture on breast 4T1 cancer progression. *Int. J. Oncol.* **2014**, *44*, 1933–1944. [PubMed]

107. Roomi, M.W.; Monterrey, J.C.; Kalinovsky, T.; Rath, M.; Niedzwiecki, A. Comparative effects of EGCG, green tea, and a nutrient mixture on the patterns of MMP-2 and MMP-9 expression in cancer cell lines. *Oncol. Rep.* **2010**, *24*, 747–757. [PubMed]
108. Kale, A.; Gawande, S.; Kotwal, S.; Netke, S.; Roomi, M.W.; Ivanov, V.; Niedzwiecki, A.; Rath, M. A combination of green tea extract, specific nutrient mixture and quercetin: An effective intervention treatment for the regression of *N*-methyl-*N*-nitrosourea (MNU)-induced mammary tumors in Wistar rats. *Oncol. Lett.* **2010**, *1*, 313–317. [PubMed]
109. Roomi, M.W.; Kalinovsky, T.; Niedzwiecki, A.; Rath, M. A nutrient mixture modulates ovarian ES-2 cancer progression by inhibiting xenograft tumor growth and cellular MMP secretion, migration and invasion. *Int. J. Clin. Exp. Med.* **2016**, *9*, 814–822.
110. Roomi, M.W.; Niedzwiecki, A.; Rath, M. Abstract 4053: A unique nutrient mixture suppresses ovarian cancer growth of A-2780 by inhibiting invasion and MMP-9 secretion. In Proceedings of the 107th Annual Meeting of the AACR, New Orleans, LA, USA, 16–20 April 2016.
111. Wang, P.; Vadgama, J.V.; Said, J.W.; Magyar, C.E.; Doan, N.; Heber, D.; Henning, S.M. Enhanced inhibition of prostate cancer xenograft tumor growth by combining quercetin and green tea. *J. Nutr. Biochem.* **2014**, *25*, 73–80. [CrossRef] [PubMed]

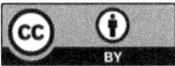

*nutrients*

MDPI

*Review*

# Reducing Breast Cancer Recurrence: The Role of Dietary Polyphenolics

Andrea J. Braakhuis [1,*], Peta Campion [1] and Karen S. Bishop [2]

[1] Discipline of Nutrition and Dietetics, FM & HS, University of Auckland, Private Bag 92019, Auckland 1142, New Zealand; pcam131@aucklanduni.ac.nz

[2] Auckland Cancer Society Research Center, FM & HS, University of Auckland, Private Bag 92019, Auckland 1142, New Zealand; kbishop@auckland.ac.nz

* Correspondance: a.braakhuis@auckland.ac.nz; Tel.: +64-992-362-51

Received: 25 July 2016; Accepted: 31 August 2016; Published: 6 September 2016

**Abstract:** Evidence from numerous observational and clinical studies suggest that polyphenolic phytochemicals such as phenolic acids in olive oil, flavonols in tea, chocolate and grapes, and isoflavones in soy products reduce the risk of breast cancer. A dietary food pattern naturally rich in polyphenols is the Mediterranean diet and evidence suggests those of Mediterranean descent have a lower breast cancer incidence. Whilst dietary polyphenols have been the subject of breast cancer risk-reduction, this review will focus on the clinical effects of polyphenols on reducing recurrence. Overall, we recommend breast cancer patients consume a diet naturally high in flavonol polyphenols including tea, vegetables (onion, broccoli), and fruit (apples, citrus). At least five servings of vegetables and fruit daily appear protective. Moderate soy protein consumption (5–10 g daily) and the Mediterranean dietary pattern show the most promise for breast cancer patients. In this review, we present an overview of clinical trials on supplementary polyphenols of dietary patterns rich in polyphenols on breast cancer recurrence, mechanistic data, and novel delivery systems currently being researched.

**Keywords:** polyphenols; breast cancer; human trials

## 1. Introduction

Breast cancer is the most commonly diagnosed cancer in females worldwide [1]. Diet-related factors are thought to account for around 30% of all cancer in developed countries, with breast cancer being no exception. Obesity, a lack of physical activity, and, to a lesser extent, alcohol increase the risk of breast cancer [2], whereas consumption of vegetables, fruits, legumes, grains, and green tea appear to be protective [3]. In particular, several plant components especially phytochemicals may protect against DNA damage and block specific carcinogen pathways. There are a multitude of in vitro studies outlining the effect specific dietary components have on breast cancer; however, interpretation and clinical application of such studies is problematic, as cell-based studies fail to account for human absorption and metabolism. Presently, there are very few evidence-based nutrition guidelines for breast cancer survivors to follow and many are confused about nutrition support post-diagnosis. Secondary prevention or adjunct therapy through dietary intervention is a cost-effective alternative for preventing the large burden of healthcare associated with breast cancer treatment. In the past decade, epidemiologic and preclinical evidence suggest that polyphenolic phytochemicals present in many plant foods possess chemo-preventive properties against breast cancer [2]. Epidemiological data suggests dietary patterns naturally rich in polyphenols are protective against breast cancer. Whilst data on the nutritional aspect of cancer prevention and the reduction of risk are important, the degree to which the outcomes that can be applied to reducing cancer recurrence is questionable. Increasing evidence suggests that diets providing a variety of polyphenols are useful with regard to breast cancer prevention and cessation.

The health benefits of polyphenols have been linked mostly to their antioxidant effects. Although this is an important contributor, polyphenol phytochemicals also interact with other pathways, especially receptor signalling. Polyphenols have been reported to reduce inflammation and cancer recurrence by (a) acting as an antioxidant or increasing antioxidant gene or protein expression; (b) decreasing cancer cell proliferation; (c) blocking pro-inflammatory cytokines or endotoxin-mediated kinases and transcription factors involved in cancer progression; (d) increasing histone deacetylase activity; or (e) activating transcription factors that antagonize chronic inflammation [4,5]. Polyphenol phytochemicals can interfere with both estrogen receptor (ER) and tyrosine kinase receptor (TKR) signalling, thereby inducing apoptotic and/or autophagy cell death. Estrogen receptors are central to the development of primary and secondary breast cancers. Estrogen binds membrane-initiated steroid signalling (MISS) or TKR to initiate a cascade of effects via estrogen response elements (ERE), AP-1, SP1, and other transcription factors to activate pro-apoptotic genes [6]. There are some indications that polyphenols can bind ER with varying affinities. Thus, it is clear that targeting these ER pathways using dietary polyphenols may affect the development of both primary and secondary breast cancer. The importance of other dietary factors, including meat, fibre, and vitamins, is not yet clear [7]. There has been interest in the potential of naturally occurring cancer chemo-preventive agents, such as polyphenols, to curb the increasing burden of breast cancer treatment [8,9]. Dietary polyphenols may support current medical treatment options to improve prognosis.

This article reviews the current literature on breast cancer clinical trials of polyphenolic phytochemicals with an aim to identify potential nutritional strategies for breast cancer patients, post-diagnosis.

## 2. Methods

The current review discusses the evidence on dietary polyphenols and food patterns naturally high in polyphenols and breast cancer recurrence or relevant biomarkers. In selecting the literature to review, studies that addressed the prognosis and recurrence of breast cancer in survivors were identified. Inclusion criteria included any breast cancer stage and type, human trials only, and intervention commenced after breast cancer diagnosis. Particular attention has been given to human randomised control trials and observational studies on breast cancer survivors. Studies included in Table 1 were human data and must have investigated polyphenol-rich dietary intake or supplements. For inclusion, our definition of a "polyphenol rich diet" were those investigating vegetables (onion, broccoli) and fruit (apples, citrus). Articles from any date of publication or language were considered. PubMed, Google Scholar, and PEN—Practice-Based Nutrition Database—were searched using various key terms, including "breast cancer", "nutrition", "polyphenol", and "human". Abstracts were reviewed for relevant material.

**Table 1.** Clinical studies of polyphenols in breast cancer patients. Table includes human studies only and those with a dietary or supplemental intervention. Abbreviations: BCa—Breast cancer.

| Author, Year | Research Design/Assessment/Outcome Measure | Participants | Summary Outcome |
|---|---|---|---|
| Rock, Natarajan et al., 2009 [10] | Design; Observational. Assessed intake of vegetables, fruit and fibre. Outcome: Time to secondary BCa cancer event | 3043 early-mid diagnosed BCa patients | Greater intake of fruit and vegetables naturally high in polyphenols and carotenoids, was associated with improved likelihood of breast cancer–free survival regardless of study group assignment. HR = 0.67 |

**Table 1.** *Cont.*

| Author, Year | Research Design/Assessment/Outcome Measure | Participants | Summary Outcome |
|---|---|---|---|
| Mignone, Giovannucci et al., 2009 [11] | Design: Observational. Assessed dietary intake of fruit and vegetable consumption. Outcome: risk of breast cancer | 5707 BCa patients; 6389 Controls | A high consumption of fruit and vegetables naturally high in polyphenols and carotenoids may reduce the risk of premenopausal but not postmenopausal breast cancer, particularly among smokers |
| Baglietto, Krishnan et al., 2011 [12] | Design: Observational. Assessed dietary intake patterns. Outcome: Risk of invasive breast cancer | 20,967 women of which 815 develop invasive BCa | A dietary pattern rich in fruit and salad might protect against invasive breast cancer and that the effect might be stronger for ER- and PR-negative tumours |
| Pierce, J.P., Natarajan, L., Caan, B.J. et al., 2007 [13] | Design: Intervention Education to promote 5 servings of fruit and vegetable. Outcome: Time to secondary BCa event | 1537 Bca patients; 1551 controls | Among survivors of early stage breast cancer, adoption of a diet that was very high in vegetables, fruit, and fibre and low in fat did not reduce additional breast cancer events or mortality during a 7.3-year follow-up period. Unfortunately, the control group also received written education material |
| Sartippour M.R., Rao J.Y., Apple S., Wu et al., 2004 [14] | Design: Intervention. 200 mg isoflavones for 2-weeks. Assessment: Direct breast tissue samples from patients were assessed for cancer growth | 17 BCa patients; 26 Controls | No change in apoptosis/mitosis ratio |
| DiSilvestro R.A., Goodman, J., Dy, E., Lavalle, G. 2005 [15] | Design: Intervention. 138 mg isoflavones for 24-days. Assessment: Blood samples were assessed for oxidative status | 7 BCa patients, crossover design | Increased SOD activity. No change in oxidative stress markers |
| Inoue, M., Tajima, K., Mizutani, M. et al., 2001 [16] | Design: Observational. Assessment: Consumption of green tea | 1160 women of which 133 develop BCa | 3+ cups of green tea daily was associated with lower BCa recurrence in early stages (HR = 0.69, 95% CI 0.47–1.00) |

## 3. Discussion

### 3.1. Dietary Amelioration of Inflammation Associated with Breast Cancer

Many studies suggest that low-grade inflammation is mitigated by healthy dietary habits, such as polyphenols and the Mediterranean food pattern, resulting in lower circulating concentrations of inflammatory markers [17]. Western-type or meat-based patterns are positively associated with low-grade inflammation [18]. Among the components of a healthy diet, whole grains, vegetables and fruits, and fish are all associated with lower inflammation, and a limited number of observational studies suggested a pro-inflammatory action of diets rich in saturated fatty acids or trans-monounsaturated fats [19]. The association between inflammation and cancer has been reported elsewhere [20], citing major mediators nuclear factor kappa B (NF-κB), tumour necrosis factor (TNF), and cyclooxygenase-2 (COX-2), given the combined role in inflammation, cell proliferation, angiogenesis, and metastasis. Inhibition of COX-2 thus blocking the inhibition cascade may be an important mechanism by which polyphenols exert benefit to the breast cancer patient. The consumption of polyphenol-rich foods is thought to have an effect in modulating low-grade inflammation [21].

The inflammatory environment that promotes breast cancer tumour growth links to obesity and metabolic syndrome. Women who gain weight in adulthood and overweight postmenopausal women have a greater risk for breast cancer than lean women [22]. However, there are inconsistencies regarding the effect modification of menopausal status. In contrast, evidence exists showing that overweight and obesity is associated with reduced risk in premenopausal women [23]. Metabolic syndrome (clinically defined as having three of the following factors: Abdominal obesity, hypertension, hyperglycemia, high triglycerides, or low HDL cholesterol [24] has been associated with a 2.6 times higher risk of breast cancer in postmenopausal women [25]. It can be deduced that a range of factors, including age, hormone levels, and obesity and overweight, affect breast cancer risk. Because overweight and obesity are powerful modifiable risk factors [26], interventions, including dietary intervention, should be investigated further. Whilst clear evidence links metabolic syndrome with increased risk of breast cancer, it is also clear that post-diagnosis weight gain occurs in 50%–95% of patients and is associated with poor prognosis. Excess weight gain is associated with elevated inflammatory markers, against which polyphenols may protect.

According to a study conducted on rats, dietary supplementation of a high-fat diet and polyphenols led to dramatic changes in gut microbial community structure [27]. Cranberry polyphenols protected mice on a high-fat, high-sucrose diet against oxidative stress, inflammation, weight gain, and markers of metabolic syndrome [28]. Chronic low-grade inflammation promoted by an individual's diet and their functioning gut microbiota may influence cancer progression.

Dietary polyphenols may protect against breast cancer progression, despite limited absorption and digestion, raising questions about their mechanism of action. As discussed, polyphenols appear to alter gut microbiota in rats and mice and has also been demonstrated in human studies. It was found that a moderate intake of red wine had positive effects on the composition of the gut microbiota and a reduction in the inflammatory markers [29]. Polyphenols may assist the breast cancer patient by minimizing weight gain, improving the inflammatory profile and altering gut microbiota activity, thus reducing tumour growth.

### 3.2. Antioxidant Action of Polyphenolics

Polyphenols are secondary metabolites of plants and are generally involved in defense against ultraviolet radiation or aggression due to their physiological effects and structure [30]. Many of the biological actions of polyphenols have been attributed to their antioxidant properties; however, recent research has suggested that polyphenols may affect several cellular pathways, thereby exerting a pleiotropic effect [31]. Cellular pathways initiated by polyphenols may delay and reduce the carcinogenic processes in breast tissue [32,33]. Oxidative stress is known to alter the cellular redox status, resulting in altered gene expression by the activation of several redox-sensitive transcription factors. This signaling cascade affects both cell growth and cell death. An increased rate of reactive oxygen species (ROS) production occurs in highly proliferative cancer cells, owing to oncogenic mutations that promote aberrant metabolism. The ability of dietary polyphenols to modulate cellular signal transduction pathways, through the activation or repression of multiple redox-sensitive transcription factors, has been claimed for their potential therapeutic use as chemo-preventive agents [34].

Red wine polyphenols reduce breast cancer cell proliferation in a dose-dependent manner by specifically targeting steroid receptors and modifying the production of ROS [4]. However, it should be noted that it would not be prudent to advise the breast cancer patient to consume alcohol, given the potentially damaging effects. Phenolic phytochemicals have a strong antioxidant potential due to the hydroxyl groups associated with their aromatic rings. Phenolic phytochemicals have been shown to increase the levels of anti-inflammatory genes such as superoxide dismutase (SOD), glutathione peroxidase (GPx), and heme oxygenase (HO)-1 via activation of the transcription factor nuclear factor-erythroid 2 (NF-E2)-related factor 2 (Nrf2). Thus, polyphenols have an inherent capacity to reduce ROS and other free radicals, thereby preventing their activation of oxidative stress and inflammation [35]. Polyphenols are effective free radical scavengers and their antioxidant properties should not be overlooked. In a recent meta-analysis of data from 7500 participants, those who reported a high polyphenol intake, especially of stilbenes and lignans, showed a reduced risk of overall mortality compared to those with lower intakes [36]. Polyphenols where found to be protective against chronic disease, implying a change in oxidative status. The antioxidant properties of polyphenols are thought to delay and to fight the carcinogenic processes in breast tissue [32,33]. Further studies will likely provide additional insights into the mechanism of redox control of breast cancer. Whilst polyphenols appear to reduce oxidative stress, the degree to which breast cancer prognosis is improved is unclear.

### 3.3. Polyphenols Protect DNA from the Carcinogen-Induced Damage

Chronic activation of inflammatory processes is widely regarded as an enabling characteristic towards the development of cancer. We know that chronic inflammation can drive tumour growth and the production of ROS [37]. In turn, ROS can cause DNA damage. Production of ROS, together with deficiencies in the capacity to repair DNA (genotype dependent), can interact to increase carcinogenic capabilities [37,38]. Base-excision repair genes, such as *XRCC1* G399A [37] and *OGG1* C326G, are associated with reduced repair of DNA lesions associated with ROS [39].

The mutagen sensitivity assay (MSA) can be used as a marker of the ability of DNA to respond to and repair DNA damage and hence it has been used to test response to mutagens and bioactives [38]. The Comet and Micronucleus assays have also been extensively used to determine the extent of DNA strand breaks and repair [40–42], and there are a number of other methods, including RAD1 focus formation [43], PCR, and the TUNEL assay, as well as numerous others [44].

Germline mutations in DNA mismatch repair genes (*BRCA1*, *BRCA2*, *CHEK2*, *ERCC4*, *FAAP100*, and *TP53BP1*, amongst others) are associated with breast cancer susceptibility [45,46]. In some cases, it may be possible to modify diet to help decrease the risk of breast cancer and breast cancer recurrence [45]. In a study of triple negative breast cancer (TNBC) patients, Lee et al. assessed 16 single nucleotide polymorphisms (SNPs) associated with DNA repair [45]. The authors found that the risk of TNBC was associated with six of the SNPs and that this risk was modified by zinc, folate, and β-carotene levels such that low levels increased risk [45]. These effects were additive. In other studies, it has been reported that high plasma levels of β-carotene, or the consumption of a carotenoid rich diet, were associated with lower levels of breast cancer or breast cancer recurrence [10,11] or a reduction in oxidative stress in those previously treated for breast cancer [47]. Others found that diets rich in fruits and salads, a food pattern traditionally high in polyphenols, was associated with a reduced risk of breast cancer, particularly estrogen and progesterone receptor negative breast cancers [12].

Polyphenols can act as pro- and anti-oxidants, depending on the experimental or environmental conditions [41], and may modify the interaction between carcinogenic capabilities and breast cancer risk. In addition, polyphenols may enhance repair or change methylation status of promoter regions to favour DNA repair, or protect against DNA damage. Adams et al. found that polyphenols from blueberries inhibited cell proliferation and cell migration in human TNBC cell lines [48] and decreased tumour size and inhibited metastasis in a TNBC xenograft study in mice [49]. Similarly, Meeran et al. assessed the effect of Epigallocatechin-3-gallate (EGCG) and sulforaphane, an isothiocynate derived predominantly from plants of the order Brassicales and known to have strong chemo-preventative and anti-inflammatory properties on breast cancer cell lines [50,51]. They found that sulforaphane and EGCG inhibited cell proliferation, telomerase activity, and *human telomerase reverse transcriptase* (*hTERT*) gene expression [50,51]. *hTERT* is widely expressed in cancers, but not in normal cells, and downregulation of *hTERT* in breast cancer can lead to the inhibition of cell proliferation and the induction of apoptosis. Food or dietary compound induced changes in *hTERT* expression, which, in many cases, are due to epigenetic modifications [50–52].

### 3.4. Dietary Sources of Polyphenols

Following the systematic search, a small subset of polyphenol types emerged as having human-derived evidence with regard to breast cancer recurrence. This review focuses on the human-derived evidence on breast cancer, and we focus the discussion on phenolic acids, flavonols, and isoflavones. Whilst cell line data on polyphenols such as curcumin and resveratrol are promising, very little has been conducted in human clinical trials.

### 3.4.1. Phenolic Acids

One of the major dietary sources of dietary phenolic is olive oil, which contains caffeic, oleuropein, and hydroxytyrosol, amongst others. Previous research attributes the health effects of olive oil to its high content in oleic acid. Nowadays, the health benefits of olive oil are also attributed to its phenolic content, namely olepurenoil [53]. Researchers have indicated that the antioxidant capacity of polyphenols in olive oil may reduce the risk of developing cardiovascular diseases and cancer [54].

Studies have indicated that the biological activity of polyphenols in olive oil is higher when they are part of the diet than when these molecules are administered as food supplements [54,55]. The processing of olive oil also determines the variability and availability of polyphenol content in this product. The polyphenol content of olive oil is important, not only for the delivery of compounds with strong anti-oxidant capacity, but also because it exists in conjunction with fatty acids that are potentially oxidised [54]. The phenolic composition of olive oils varies in quantity and quality depending on the olive variety, the age of the tree, and the agricultural techniques used in cultivation.

Recent data suggest a polyphenolic compound found in olive oil, known as oleocanthal, can selectively kill cancerous breast cells while leaving healthy cells intact [56]. Oleocanthal ruptures the lysosome of cancerous cells by inhibiting acid sphingomyelinase activity, which destabilizes the interaction between proteins required for lysosomal membrane stability [56]. The ruptured cell renders the cancer to usual enzymatic degradation and programmed cell death. Further research is needed to confirm findings in human trials, but results are promising. Researchers suggest those on a Mediterranean diet may benefit from the higher consumption of olive oil [56].

Coffee contains numerous compounds, potentially beneficial as well as harmful. With regard to breast cancer, coffee drinking may even have a protective effect. Coffee contains various polyphenols, which inhibit harmful oxidation processes in the body, while the latter include acrylamide, whose high intake in daily diet may have carcinogenic action [57]. In mechanistic cell studies, coffee polyphenols change the expression of STAT5B and ATF-2 modifying cyclin D1 levels in cancer cells [58]. Whilst in vitro studies suggest coffee may offer protection against breast cancer, the overall effect requires clarification, given the paucity of clinical trials.

### 3.4.2. Flavonols

Flavonols are the major polyphenolic sub-group of flavonoids, which are present in tea, onions, broccoli, and various common fruits. Example polyphenol flavonols include quercetin, kaempferol, myricetin, and isorhamnetin, with an estimated intake of 12.9 mg/day in a typical Western diet [59].

Flavonols may act through anti-oxidant, pro-oxidant, anti-estrogenic, cell signalling pathway modulation, or mitochondrial toxicity to inhibit breast carcinogenesis. One study investigating the effect of flavonols of breast cancer risk reported a risk ratio of 0.94 (0.72, 1.22; *p*-value for test of trend = 0.54) for the sum of flavonol-rich foods. Among the major food sources of flavonols, a significant inverse association with the intake of beans or lentils was reported, but not with tea, onions, apples, string beans, broccoli, green pepper, or blueberries [60]. Despite no overall association between intake of flavonols and risk of breast cancer, there was an inverse association with the intake of beans or lentils. In contrast, a recent meta-analysis of flavonoid intake and breast cancer risk suggested that dietary flavonols and flavones, but not other flavonoid subclasses or total flavonoids, was associated with a decreased risk of breast cancer, especially among post-menopausal women [59]. Given the large range in polyphenols present in the flavonol sub-group, definitive recommendations are difficult; however, it is safe to assume a diet high in beans and legumes and a range of flavonols including onions, apples, citrus, tea, and broccoli are likely to be protective.

### 3.4.3. Isoflavones

Estrogen is believed to play a role in breast cancer development and progression, and any nutritional intervention that blocks the production or reduces the hormone action is likely to be effective in improving clinical outcomes in breast cancer survivors. Soy food consumption has been attributed to protection against breast cancer, primarily because of the soybean isoflavones (genistein, daidzein, and glycitein), which are natural estrogen receptor modulators. In vitro studies show that genistein inhibits the growth of breast cancer cells, including hormone-dependent and independent cell types at higher concentrations (10–50 µmol/L), while stimulating growth at lower concentrations (<10 µmol/L) [61]. Whilst the structure of soy isoflavones mimics estrogen, the majority of human research fails to detect any clinically relevant estrogenic activity, as determined by estradiol, estrone, and sex hormone binding globulin [62]. In one of the key human intervention studies on soy protein, results were stratified by the amount of soy consumed and showed a dose-response relationship between decreasing risk of breast cancer with an increased soy food intake, translating to a 16% risk reduction per 10 mg of daily isoflavone consumed [63]. However, concerns remain regarding optimal dose of soy foods to ensure improved survival in breast cancer sufferers, and further clinical trials are needed. Soybeans contain a number of anticarcinogens, suggesting that consumption may protect against breast cancer, with non-fermented products such as tofu and soymilk showing more promise.

Unfortunately, clinical outcomes in animal and human epidemiological studies are varied, with 65% of studies reporting no effect or slightly protective against breast cancer risk. A recent review demonstrated the protective effect soy consumption has on breast cancer development, recurrence, and mortality [62]. At this stage, soy phytoestrogens require further research [64]. The protective association of soy food appears more pronounced in postmenopausal women. However, the reduced risk of recurrence results should be interpreted with caution given the modest effect and wide confidence intervals for most studies and the lack of dose response relationship in one positive study.

Both the breast cancer treatment drug Tamoxifen and dietary phytoestrogens bind estrogen receptors, and many have theorised that soy consumption will reduce drug efficacy. In a study on investigating the association of soy food consumption and survival in breast cancer sufferers, women in the highest soy food intake groups had the lowest mortality and recurrence rate compared with women in the lowest intake group, regardless of tamoxifen use. Among women whose soy intake was in the highest quartile, tamoxifen did not confer additional health benefits [65]. Based on this limited epidemiological data, it follows that moderate soy protein consumption (5–10 g/day) in combination with Tamoxifen use represents the optimal treatment combination for relevant breast cancer patients.

Within nutrition science, the critical concept of food synergy recognises that nutrients exist in a purposeful biological sense within foods, delivering them in combinations that reflect biological functionality [66]. Thus, while it is difficult to separate out the effects of foods within a total diet, it is also difficult to study the effects of nutrients and bioactive substances in the isolation of foods [67].

*3.5. Polyphenol-Rich Dietary Pattern and Breast Cancer Progression*

The Mediterranean diet has been shown to reduce body weight by 4.4% over a year and improve the inflammatory profile in cardiac and diabetic groups. Given the tendency for breast cancer survivors to gain weight and risk metabolic syndrome, the Mediterranean diet may assist with weight loss and provide specific benefits over and above the usual low-fat, healthy diet intervention. The Mediterranean diet is a plant-based dietary pattern characterized by a high intake of olive oil, legumes, whole grains, fruit, vegetables, nuts, seeds, fish, and is rich in dietary polyphenols. The diet has been linked to a decreased risk of developing breast cancer [48]. The Mediterranean diet contains a wide range of various polyphenols, particularly from nuts, fruit, and coffee [68], and represents a potential population approach to increasing the intake of polyphenols. Epidemiological evidence strongly suggests that long-term consumption of diets rich in plant polyphenols, much like that of the Mediterranean diet, can offer protection against development of major chronic and neurodegenerative diseases [69,70]. Suggested mechanisms through which the Mediterranean diet may impact breast cancer initiation and proliferation include increased insulin sensitivity and reduction of excess insulin production, anti-inflammatory and antioxidant effects of the diet, high fibre content, and an association with reduced risk of excess weight gain and obesity [48]. The health benefits of the Mediterranean diet are likely a synergistic effect of weight loss, polyphenol intake, and improved glycemic control.

There are three main randomised trials investigating the effect of following a Mediterranean diet pattern and the prognosis following treatment for breast cancer. The results, however, are mixed. In 2007, The Women's Healthy Eating and Living (WHEL) Randomised Trial found that a diet high in vegetable, fruit, and fibre and low in fat intake did not reduce additional breast cancer events or mortality over a relatively long follow-up period [13]. These results are at odds with the Women's Intervention Nutrition Study (WINS), a randomised trial that focused on a low-fat diet and weight loss, reporting that this diet was associated with longer relapse-free survival of breast cancer patients [71]. Follow up times and differences in menopausal status between studies may explain outcomes. Difficulties in ascertaining the polyphenol content of these diets make conclusions regarding efficacy difficult.

Another reason for the difference in the results of these trials may be that, in WINS, the women lost weight in the randomised group, whereas those women in the WHEL study had an iso-caloric diet by design, and the women in the intervention group gained around 1 kg. The results from previous observational studies suggesting calorie reduction and weight loss are beneficial in breast cancer prognosis may add context to this situation and show why the results of the WHEL study were to no effect. Such an interpretation is verified by the relatively consistent observations that overweight and obese breast cancer patients have a worse prognosis than lean patients [1,72–74]. The Mediterranean diet has been shown to support weight loss in participants and as such may offer multiple benefits in polyphenol intake and weight loss.

The most recent randomised trial investigating the effects of a Mediterranean macrobiotic lifestyle on breast cancer prognosis is the DIANA-5 trial [75]. It demonstrated that dietary modification based on Mediterranean and macrobiotic dietary principles can reduce body weight, and the bioavailability of sex hormones and growth factors may promote tumour growth [76,77]. The diet consisted of low consumption of fats, refined carbohydrates and animal products, and the high consumption of whole grain cereals, legumes, and vegetables.

Chemotherapy works to significantly decrease recurrences and improve survival in women with early breast cancer, but a major side effect is weight gain which, as discussed, is associated with a poorer prognosis [78]. The trial showed this specific diet significantly decreases body weight and waist circumference, thereby improving insulin sensitivity [79]. Like the WINS trial, only post-menopausal women were included in the study. The results may have differed for pre-menopausal women if they were also included.

Overall, the DIANA-5 trial has the potential to provide a clear answer to the hypothesis that a comprehensive modification of diet can lead to a longer event-free survival among women after breast cancer treatment [75]. Intervention has been shown to be effective in changing lifestyle in terms of diet and weight loss. Combined with other modifiable factors, a Mediterranean diet that focuses on weight loss and reducing insulin resistance may have substantial benefits for women previously treated for breast cancer. All of these studies have pieced together components that warrant further investigation to the role of a Mediterranean-based diet and breast cancer prognosis, event-free survival, and mortality.

### 3.6. Disease Characteristics and Biomarkers

A reduction in breast cancer incidence and mortality is the gold standard criteria for success in a clinical trial; however, this approach is expensive and ethically difficult to implement. The use of surrogate breast cancer biomarkers is an appealing alternative. Breast cancer biomarkers useful for investigating the efficacy of polyphenols include specific oncogenic pathways (e.g., COX-2, or prostaglandin E2, a product of COX mediated catalysis), levels of circulating disease related proteins, such as ostrodial or estrogen, changes in breast cancer histology and cytology, genomic alterations

A major challenge in the treatment of breast cancer is its high heterogeneity from patient to patient, which initiated its classification into three major molecular subtypes—estrogen receptors (ER), progesterone receptors (PR), and HER2, hormone receptor positive with luminal A (ER+PR+HER2−) and luminal B (ER+PR+HER2+) phenotypes, HER2 positive (ER−PR−HER2+), and triple negative/basal-like (ER−PR−HER2−) [80–82]. About 70% of breast cancers are estrogen receptor positive [83]. Recent data suggest that molecular subtypes differ substantially in the intracellular pathways responsible for cell growth and metastatic spread, suggesting a wide array of potential molecular targets of polyphenols [84]. The efficacy of polyphenolic therapy is likely to differ pending the breast cancer stage and subtype.

### 3.7. Epigenetic Potential of Polyphenolic Phytochemicals

Epigenetics refers to heritable changes in DNA that are involved in the control of gene expression. Epigenetic mechanisms include changes in DNA methylation, histone modification, and non-coding RNAs [84]. While epigenetic characteristics are sometimes inherited they can also be modified by environmental and dietary factors. Inflammatory pathways can trigger epigenetic switches from nontransformed to metastatic cancer cells via signalling involving NF κB and STAT3 transcription factors, microRNAs (Lin28 and let 7), and IL-6 cytokines [85]. Moreover, the polyphenols resveratrol and quercetin decreased miRNA-155 and inhibited NF κB-involved inflammation in a cancer cell line study. Increasing evidence suggests polyphenols are capable of influencing epigenetic characteristics relevant to cancer progression. It is beyond the scope of this review to outline all the research of all aspects of the epigenetic potential of polyphenols; other reviews have been completed [85]. Of the more notable epigenetic modification by polyphenols, epigenetically modified genes can be restored, inactivated methylated genes can be demethylated, and histone complexes can be rendered transcriptionally active by dietary intervention. Common to cancer initiation is the inhibition of tumour suppressor genes by DNA methylation of transcription factors. DNA methyltransferase (DNMT) inhibitors can undergo such methylation, which polyphenols have been demonstrated to reverse [86].

Polyphenols can also alter heritable gene expression, activity of epigenetic machinery and decreases micro-RNAs related to inflammation and cancer growth. So far, it is not clear whether the occasional or typical dietary intake of polyphenols results in long-term epigenetic regulation of gene expression, downstream chemo-preventative effects, or both.

### 3.8. Bioavailability of Polyphenols

Biological properties of polyphenols depend on their bioavailability. The chemical structure of polyphenols determines their rate and extent of intestinal absorption, as well as the nature of the metabolites circulating in the plasma. For most flavonoids absorbed in the small intestine, the plasma concentration rapidly decreases (elimination half-life period of 1–2 h). The elimination half-life period for quercetin is much higher (24 h) probably due to its particularly high affinity for plasma albumin [87]. Flavonols, isoflavones, flavones, and anthocyanins are usually glycosylated. Following high-dose polyphenol administration, metabolism occurs primarily in the liver, whereas, when smaller doses were administered, metabolism took place first at the intestinal mucosa, the liver playing a secondary role to further modify the conjugated polyphenol. This implies that the intestine is an important site for metabolism of food-derived polyphenols [88]. Intestinal microbiological fermentation decreases the bioavailability of the many polyphenols; however, it also gives rise to metabolites that may be more bioactive than the native polyphenols [88]. Metabolic responses based on dose also suggest that any potential benefit will vary based on the polyphenol dose used. Studies on ideal dose and delivery route are needed.

To circumvent poor bioavailability of polyphenols, a current area of promising research is using nanotechnology. One such nanotechnology, titled "Nano emulsions", are a class of extremely small droplets that allow polyphenol phytochemicals to be transported through the cell membranes more easily, resulting in an increased concentration in plasma and improved bioavailability. Curcumin Nano emulsions show 85% inhibition of 12-*O*-Tetradecanoylphorbol-13-acetate (TPA)-induced mouse ear inflammation as well as the inhibition of cyclin D1 expression. In addition, dibenzoylmethane (DBM) Nano emulsions improve oral bioavailability of curcumin 3-fold, compared with the conventional DBM emulsions [89]. The degree to which improved bioavailability improves survival in breast cancer patients is still to be determined, as there is likely a dose-response that is still to be ascertained.

*3.9. Limitations (Toxicity, Bioavailability, Challenges and Weaknesses Associated with Human Trials, etc.)*

Several factors have been proposed to explain differences observed between the positive effects of polyphenol consumption reported in epidemiological studies and the unclear to negative findings reported in intervention trials with supplements. These factors include the following: (1) differing doses of administered compounds; (2) additive or synergistic effects, such as those between polyphenols and other antioxidants, present in whole foods but not in supplements; and (3) differences in bioavailability and metabolism [88]. Results from randomised clinical trials vary to those of in vitro studies largely as a result of these factors.

With any human dietary study, interpreting outcomes and defining appropriate dietary recommendations can be extremely difficult. Studies typically involve many methodological considerations such as dietary pattern differences across populations, accurately measuring food intake, biological mechanisms, genetic variations, food definitions, bias, and other confounding factors [90]. Adding further complication is that many studies between cancer and diet provide weak associations, whereby confounding factors, exposure misclassification, and other biases, even modest ones, can have a large impact on the overall conclusions [91]. To best answer questions regarding efficacy of dietary polyphenols, in vitro studies of polyphenol metabolites should be followed up with human clinical trials and we would recommend that further studies use placebo controlled, double-blind trials that extend over many years with a sufficient sample size. Unfortunately, such studies are expensive to conduct.

## 4. Conclusions

Whilst recognizing the broad nature of investigating the efficacy of polyphenols for breast cancer patients, we can conclude the following based on clinical and observational studies. Early diagnosed breast cancer patients should consume at least five servings of vegetables and fruit, and we recommend those high in flavonols such as onions, broccoli, apples, and citrus, amongst others. Both green and black tea consumption is protective, with 3+ cups of green tea being particularly helpful. We would recommend women diagnosed with breast cancer to adopt a moderate soy protein consumption (5–10 g/day) from non-fermented soy products such as soymilk and tofu.

The Mediterranean diet appears useful in assisting with weight control and improving metabolic syndrome. It is a dietary pattern naturally high in legumes and olive oil, both of which have been independently reported to improve in vitro and in vivo breast cancer recurrence and biomarkers of disease. Foods rich in polyphenols are the preferred methods of delivery over supplements, until more is known. Further research should include specific dietary foods in large randomized control trials, which, the authors recognize, are expensive to conduct.

**Author Contributions:** A.B. designed the concept, conducted the search, wrote the majority of the paper and managed the authors; K.B. wrote key sections of the paper; P.C. wrote sections and managed the reference list.

**Conflicts of Interest:** The authors declare no conflict of interest.

## References

1.    Hauner, H.; Hauner, D. The Impact of Nutrition on the Development and Prognosis of Breast Cancer. *Breast Care (Basel)* **2010**, *5*, 377–381. [CrossRef] [PubMed]

2. Key, T.J.; Allen, N.E.; Spencer, E.A.; Travis, R.C. The effect of diet on risk of cancer. *Lancet* **2002**, *360*, 861–868. [CrossRef]
3. Gandini, S.; Merzenich, H.; Robertson, C.; Boyle, P. Meta-analysis of studies on breast cancer risk and diet: The role of fruit and vegetable consumption and the intake of associated micronutrients. *Eur. J. Cancer* **2000**, *36*, 636–646. [CrossRef]
4. Damianaki, A.; Bakogeorgou, E.; Kampa, M.; Notas, G.; Hatzoglou, A.; Panagiotou, S.; Gemetzi, C.; Kouroumalis, E.; Martin, P.M.; Castanas, E. Potent inhibitory action of red wine polyphenols on human breast cancer cells. *J. Cell. Biochem.* **2000**, *78*, 429–441. [CrossRef]
5. Williamson, G.; Manach, C. Bioavailability and bioefficacy of polyphenols in humans. II. Review of 93 intervention studies. *Am. J. Clin. Nutr.* **2005**, *81*, S243–S255.
6. Aiyer, H.S.; Warri, A.M.; Woode, D.R.; Hilakivi-Clarke, L.; Clarke, R. Influence of berry polyphenols on receptor signaling and cell-death pathways: Implications for breast cancer prevention. *J. Agric. Food Chem.* **2012**, *60*, 5693–5708. [CrossRef] [PubMed]
7. Abdulla, M.; Gruber, P. Role of diet modification in cancer prevention. *Biofactors* **2000**, *12*, 45–51. [CrossRef] [PubMed]
8. Lambert, J.D.; Yang, C.S. Mechanisms of cancer prevention by tea constituents. *J. Nutr.* **2003**, *133*, S3262–S3267.
9. Spagnuolo, C.; Russo, G.L.; Orhan, I.E.; Habtemariam, S.; Daglia, M.; Sureda, A.; Nabavi, S.F.; Devi, K.P.; Loizzo, M.R.; Tundis, R.; et al. Genistein and cancer: Current status, challenges, and future directions. *Adv. Nutr.* **2015**, *6*, 408–419. [CrossRef] [PubMed]
10. Rock, C.L.; Natarajan, L.; Pu, M.; Thomson, C.A.; Flatt, S.W.; Caan, B.J.; Gold, E.B.; Al-Delaimy, W.K.; Newman, V.A.; Hajek, R.A.; et al. Longitudinal biological exposure to carotenoids is associated with breast cancer-free survival in the Women's Healthy Eating and Living Study. *Cancer Epidemiol. Biomark. Prev.* **2009**, *18*, 486–494. [CrossRef] [PubMed]
11. Mignone, L.I.; Giovannucci, E.; Newcomb, P.A.; Titus-Ernstoff, L.; Trentham-Dietz, A.; Hampton, J.M.; Willet, W.C.; Egan, K.M. Dietary carotenoids and the risk of invasive breast cancer. *Int. J. Cancer* **2009**, *124*, 2929–2937. [CrossRef] [PubMed]
12. Baglietto, L.; Krishnan, K.; Severi, G.; Hodge, A.; Brinkman, M.; English, D.R.; McLean, C.; Hopper, J.L.; Giles, G.G. Dietary patterns and risk of breast cancer. *Br. J. Cancer* **2011**, *104*, 524–531. [CrossRef] [PubMed]
13. Pierce, J.P.; Natarajan, L.; Caan, B.J.; Parker, B.A.; Greenberg, E.R.; Flatt, S.W.; Rock, C.L.; Kealey, S.; Al-Delaimy, W.K.; Bardwell, W.A.; et al. Influence of a diet very high in vegetables, fruit, and fiber and low in fat on prognosis following treatment for breast cancer: The Women's Healthy Eating and Living (WHEL) randomized trial. *JAMA* **2007**, *298*, 289–298. [CrossRef] [PubMed]
14. Sartippour, M.R.; Rao, J.Y.; Apple, S.; Wu, D.; Henning, S.; Wang, H.; Elashoff, R.; Rubio, R.; Heber, D.; Brooks, M.N. A pilot clinical study of short-term isoflavone supplements in breast cancer patients. *Nutr. Cancer* **2004**, *49*, 59–65. [CrossRef] [PubMed]
15. DiSilvestro, R.A.; Goodman, J.; Dy, E.; Lavalle, G. Soy isoflavone supplementation elevates erythrocyte superoxide dismutase, but not plasma ceruloplasmin in postmenopausal breast cancer survivors. *Breast Cancer Res. Treat.* **2005**, *89*, 251–255. [CrossRef] [PubMed]
16. Inoue, M.; Tajima, K.; Mizutani, M.; Iwata, H.; Iwase, T.; Miura, S.; Hirose, K.; Hamajima, N.; Tominaga, S. Regular consumption of green tea and the risk of breast cancer recurrence: Follow-up study from the Hospital-based Epidemiologic Research Program at Aichi Cancer Center (HERPACC), Japan. *Cancer Lett.* **2001**, *167*, 175–182. [CrossRef]
17. Centritto, F.; Iacoviello, L.; di Giuseppe, R.; De Curtis, A.; Costanzo, S.; Zito, F.; Grioni, S.; Sieri, S.; Donati, M.B.; de Gaetano, G.; et al. Dietary patterns, cardiovascular risk factors and C-reactive protein in a healthy Italian population. *Nutr. Metab. Cardiovasc. Dis.* **2009**, *19*, 697–706. [CrossRef] [PubMed]
18. Barbaresko, J.; Koch, M.; Schulze, M.B.; Nothlings, U. Dietary pattern analysis and biomarkers of low-grade inflammation: A systematic literature review. *Nutr. Rev.* **2013**, *71*, 511–527. [CrossRef] [PubMed]
19. Calder, P.C.; Ahluwalia, N.; Brouns, F.; Buetler, T.; Clement, K.; Cunningham, K.; Esposito, K.; Jonsson, L.S.; Kolb, H.; Lansink, M.; et al. Dietary factors and low-grade inflammation in relation to overweight and obesity. *Br. J. Nutr.* **2011**, *106*, S5–S78. [CrossRef] [PubMed]
20. Ramos, S. Cancer chemoprevention and chemotherapy: Dietary polyphenols and signalling pathways. *Mol. Nutr. Food Res.* **2008**, *52*, 507–526. [CrossRef] [PubMed]

21. Bonaccio, M.; Pounis, G.; Cerletti, C.; Donati, M.B.; Iacoviello, L.; de Gaetano, G. Mediterranean diet, dietary polyphenols and low-grade inflammation: Results from the moli-sani study. *Br. J. Clin. Pharmacol.* **2016**. [CrossRef] [PubMed]

22. Lahmann, P.H.; Schulz, M.; Hoffmann, K.; Boeing, H.; Tjonneland, A.; Olsen, A.; Overvad, K.; Key, T.J.; Allen, N.E.; Khaw, K.T.; et al. Long-term weight change and breast cancer risk: The European prospective investigation into cancer and nutrition (EPIC). *Br. J. Cancer* **2005**, *93*, 582–589. [CrossRef] [PubMed]

23. National Cancer Institute. United States of America: Obesity and Cancer Risk, 2012. Available online: http://www.cancer.gov/about-cancer/causes-prevention/risk/obesity/obesity-fact-sheet (accessed on 20 June 2016).

24. Expert Panel on Detection, Evaluation and Treatment of High Cholesterol in Adults. Executive Summary of the Third Report of the National Cholesterol Education Program (NCEP) Expert Panel on Detection, Evaluation and Treatment of High Blood Cholesterol in Adults (Adult Treatment Panel III). *J. Am. Med. Assoc.* **2001**, *285*, 2486–2497.

25. Agnoli, C.; Berrino, F.; Abagnato, C.A.; Muti, P.; Panico, S.; Crosignani, P.; Krogh, V. Metabolic syndrome and postmenopausal breast cancer in the ORDET cohort: A nested case-control study. *Nutr. Metab. Cardiovasc. Dis.* **2010**, *20*, 41–48. [CrossRef] [PubMed]

26. Chan, D.S.; Vieira, A.R.; Aune, D.; Bandera, E.V.; Greenwood, D.C.; McTiernan, A.; Navarro-Rosenblatt, D.; Thune, I.; Vieira, R.; Norat, T. Body mass index and survival in women with breast cancer-systematic literature review and meta-analysis of 82 follow-up studies. *Ann. Oncol.* **2014**, *25*, 1901–1914. [CrossRef] [PubMed]

27. Roopchand, D.E.; Carmody, R.N.; Kuhn, P.; Moskal, K.; Rojas-Silva, P.; Turnbaugh, P.J.; Raskin, I. Dietary Polyphenols Promote Growth of the Gut Bacterium Akkermansia muciniphila and Attenuate High-Fat Diet-Induced Metabolic Syndrome. *Diabetes* **2015**, *64*, 2847–2858. [CrossRef] [PubMed]

28. Anhe, F.F.; Roy, D.; Pilon, G.; Dudonne, S.; Matamoros, S.; Varin, T.V.; Garofalo, C.; Moine, Q.; Desjardins, Y.; Levy, E.; et al. A polyphenol-rich cranberry extract protects from diet-induced obesity, insulin resistance and intestinal inflammation in association with increased *Akkermansia* spp. population in the gut microbiota of mice. *Gut* **2015**, *64*, 872–883. [CrossRef] [PubMed]

29. Moreno-Indias, I.; Sanchez-Alcoholado, L.; Perez-Martinez, P.; Andres-Lacueva, C.; Cardona, F.; Tinahones, F.; Queipo-Ortuno, M.I. Red wine polyphenols modulate fecal microbiota and reduce markers of the metabolic syndrome in obese patients. *Food Funct.* **2016**, *7*, 1775–1787. [CrossRef] [PubMed]

30. Ramos, S. Effects of dietary flavonoids on apoptotic pathways related to cancer chemoprevention. *J. Nutr. Biochem.* **2007**, *18*, 427–442. [CrossRef] [PubMed]

31. Maraldi, T.; Vauzour, D.; Angeloni, C. Dietary polyphenols and their effects on cell biochemistry and pathophysiology 2013. *Oxid. Med. Cell. Longev.* **2014**, *2014*, 576363. [CrossRef] [PubMed]

32. Varinska, L.; Gal, P.; Mojzisova, G.; Mirossay, L.; Mojzis, J. Soy and breast cancer: Focus on angiogenesis. *Int. J. Mol. Sci.* **2015**, *16*, 11728–11749. [CrossRef] [PubMed]

33. Yang, C.S.; Lambert, J.D.; Sang, S. Antioxidative and anti-carcinogenic activities of tea polyphenols. *Arch. Toxicol.* **2009**, *83*, 11–21. [CrossRef] [PubMed]

34. Di Domenico, F.; Foppoli, C.; Coccia, R.; Perluigi, M. Antioxidants in cervical cancer: Chemopreventive and chemotherapeutic effects of polyphenols. *Biochim. Biophys. Acta* **2012**, *1822*, 737–747. [CrossRef] [PubMed]

35. Rahman, I.; Biswas, S.K.; Kirkham, P.A. Regulation of inflammation and redox signaling by dietary polyphenols. *Biochem. Pharmacol.* **2006**, *72*, 1439–1452. [CrossRef] [PubMed]

36. Duell, E.J.; Millikan, R.C.; Pittman, G.S.; Winkel, S.; Lunn, R.M.; Tse, C.K.; Eaton, A.; Mohrenweiser, H.W.; Newman, B.; Bell, D.A. Polymorphisms in the DNA repair gene XRCC1 and breast cancer. *Cancer Epidemiol. Biomark. Prev.* **2001**, *10*, 217–222.

37. Tresserra-Rimbau, A.; Rimm, E.B.; Medina-Remon, A.; Martinez-Gonzalez, M.A.; Lopex-Sabeter, M.C.; Covas, M.I.; Corella, D.; Salas-Salvado, J.; Gomez-Gracia, E.; Lapetra, J.; et al. Polyphenol intake and mortality risk: A re-analysis of the PREDIMED trial. *BMC Med.* **2014**, *12*, 77–89. [CrossRef] [PubMed]

38. Kosti, O.; Byrne, C.; Meeker, K.L.; Watkins, K.M.; Loffredo, C.A.; Shields, P.G.; Schwartz, M.D.; Willey, S.C.; Cocilovo, C.; Zheng, Y.L. Mutagen sensitivity, tobacco smoking and breast cancer risk: A case-control study. *Carcinogenesis* **2010**, *31*, 654–659. [CrossRef] [PubMed]

39. Songserm, N.; Promthet, S.; Pientong, C.; Ekalaksananan, T.; Chopjitt, P.; Wiangnon, S. Gene-environment interaction involved in cholangiocarcinoma in the Thai population: Polymorphisms of DNA repair genes, smoking and use of alcohol. *BMJ Open* **2014**, *4*, e005447. [CrossRef] [PubMed]

40. Collins, A.R. The comet assay for DNA damage and repair: Principles, applications, and limitations. *Mol. Biotechnol.* **2004**, *26*, 249–261. [CrossRef]

41. Rodeiro, I.; Delgado, R.; Garrido, G. Effects of a Mangifera indica L. stem bark extract and mangiferin on radiation-induced DNA damage in human lymphocytes and lymphoblastoid cells. *Cell Prolif.* **2014**, *47*, 48–55. [CrossRef] [PubMed]

42. Bishop, K.S.; Erdrich, S.; Karunasinghe, N.; Han, D.Y.; Zhu, S.; Jesuthasan, A.; Ferguson, L.R. An investigation into the association between DNA damage and dietary fatty acid in men with prostate cancer. *Nutrients* **2015**, *7*, 405–422. [CrossRef] [PubMed]

43. Powell, S.N.; Riaz, N.; Mutter, W.; Ng, C.K.Y.; Delsite, R.; Piscuoglio, S.; King, T.A.; Martelotto, L.; Sakr, R.; Brogi, E.; et al. Abstract S4–03: A functional assay for homologous recombination (HR) DNA repair and whole exome sequencing reveal that HR-defective sporadic breast cancers are enriched for genetic alterations in DNA repair genes. *Cancer Res.* **2016**, *76*. [CrossRef]

44. Kumari, S.; Rastogi, R.; Singh, K.; Singh, S.; Sinha, R. DNA damage: Detection strategies. *EXCLI J.* **2008**, *7*, 44–62.

45. Lee, E.; Levine, E.A.; Franco, V.I.; Allen, G.O.; Gong, F.; Zhang, Y.; Hu, J.J. Combined genetic and nutritional risk models of triple negative breast cancer. *Nutr. Cancer* **2014**, *66*, 955–963. [CrossRef] [PubMed]

46. Campeau, P.M.; Foulkes, W.D.; Tischkowitz, M.D. Hereditary breast cancer: New genetic developments, new therapeutic avenues. *Hum. Genet.* **2008**, *124*, 31–42. [CrossRef] [PubMed]

47. Thomson, C.A.; Stendell-Hollis, N.R.; Rock, C.L.; Cussler, E.C.; Flatt, S.W.; Pierce, J.P. Plasma and dietary carotenoids are associated with reduced oxidative stress in women previously treated for breast cancer. *Cancer Epidemiol. Biomark. Prev.* **2007**, *16*, 2008–2015. [CrossRef] [PubMed]

48. Adams, L.S.; Phung, S.; Yee, N.; Seeram, N.P.; Li, L.; Chen, S. Blueberry phytochemicals inhibit growth and metastatic potential of MDA-MB-231 breast cancer cells through modulation of the phosphatidylinositol 3-kinase pathway. *Cancer Res.* **2010**, *70*, 3594–3605. [CrossRef] [PubMed]

49. Adams, L.S.; Kanaya, N.; Phung, S.; Liu, Z.; Chen, S. Whole blueberry powder modulates the growth and metastasis of MDA-MB-231 triple negative breast tumors in nude mice. *J. Nutr.* **2011**, *141*, 1805–1812. [CrossRef] [PubMed]

50. Meeran, S.M.; Patel, S.N.; Tollefsbol, T.O. Sulforaphane causes epigenetic repression of hTERT expression in human breast cancer cell lines. *PLoS ONE* **2010**, *5*, e11457. [CrossRef] [PubMed]

51. Meeran, S.M.; Patel, S.N.; Chan, T.H.; Tollefsbol, T.O. A novel prodrug of epigallocatechin-3-gallate: Differential epigenetic hTERT repression in human breast cancer cells. *Cancer Prev. Res. (Phila.)* **2011**, *4*, 1243–1254. [CrossRef] [PubMed]

52. Meeran, S.M.; Patel, S.N.; Li, Y.; Shukla, S.; Tollefsbol, T.O. Bioactive dietary supplements reactivate ER expression in ER-negative breast cancer cells by active chromatin modifications. *PLoS ONE* **2012**, *7*, e37748. [CrossRef] [PubMed]

53. Martin-Pelaez, S.; Covas, M.I.; Fito, M.; Kusar, A.; Pravst, I. Health effects of olive oil polyphenols: Recent advances and possibilities for the use of health claims. *Mol. Nutr. Food Res.* **2013**, *57*, 760–771. [CrossRef] [PubMed]

54. De la Torre-Robles, A.; Rivas, A.; Lorenzo-Tovar, M.L.; Monteagudo, C.; Mariscal-Arcas, M.; Olea-Serrano, F. Estimation of the intake of phenol compounds from virgin olive oil of a population from southern Spain. *Food Addit. Contam. Part A Chem. Anal. Control Expo. Risk Assess.* **2014**, *31*, 1460–1469. [CrossRef] [PubMed]

55. Covas, M.I.; Nyyssonen, K.; Poulsen, H.E.; Kaikkonen, J.; Zunft, H.J.; Kiesewetter, H.; Gaddi, A.; de la Torre, R.; Mursu, J.; Baumler, H.; et al. The effect of polyphenols in olive oil on heart disease risk factors: A randomized trial. *Ann. Intern. Med.* **2006**, *145*, 333–341. [CrossRef] [PubMed]

56. LeGendre, O.; Breslin, P.A.; Foster, D.A. (−)-Oleocanthal rapidly and selectively induces cancer cell death via lysosomal membrane permeabilization. *Mol. Cell. Oncol.* **2015**, *2*, e1006077. [CrossRef] [PubMed]

57. Wierzejska, R. Coffee consumption vs. cancer risk—A review of scientific data. *Rocz. Panstwowego Zakladu Hig.* **2015**, *66*, 293–298.

58. Oleaga, C.; Ciudad, C.J.; Noe, V.; Izquierdo-Pulido, M. Coffee polyphenols change the expression of STAT5B and ATF-2 modifying cyclin D1 levels in cancer cells. *Oxid. Med. Cell. Longev.* **2012**, *2012*, 390385. [CrossRef] [PubMed]

59. Cui, L.; Liu, X.; Tian, Y.; Xie, C.; Li, Q.; Cui, H.; Sun, C. Flavonoids, flavonoid subclasses and breast cancer risk: A meta-analysis of epidemiologic studies. *PLoS ONE* **2013**, *8*, e54318.

60. Adebamowo, C.A.; Cho, E.; Sampson, L.; Katan, M.B.; Spiegelman, D.; Willett, W.C.; Holmes, M.D. Dietary flavonols and flavonol-rich foods intake and the risk of breast cancer. *Int. J. Cancer* **2005**, *114*, 628–633. [CrossRef] [PubMed]

61. Constantinou, A.; Huberman, E. Genistein as an inducer of tumor cell differentiation: Possible mechanisms of action. *Proc. Soc. Exp. Biol. Med.* **1995**, *208*, 109–115. [CrossRef] [PubMed]

62. Fritz, H.; Seely, D.; Flower, G.; Skidmore, B.; Fernandes, R.; Vadeboncoeur, S.; Kennedy, D.; Cooley, K.; Wong, R.; Sagar, S.; et al. Soy, red clover, and isoflavones and breast cancer: A systematic review. *PLoS ONE* **2013**, *8*, e81968. [CrossRef] [PubMed]

63. Shike, M.; Doane, A.S.; Russo, L.; Cabal, R.; Reis-Filho, J.S.; Gerald, W.; Cody, H.; Khanin, R.; Bromberg, J.; Norton, L. The effects of soy supplementation on gene expression in breast cancer: A randomized placebo-controlled study. *J. Natl. Cancer Inst.* **2014**, *106*. [CrossRef] [PubMed]

64. Messina, M.J.; Persky, V.; Setchell, K.D.; Barnes, S. Soy intake and cancer risk: A review of the in vitro and in vivo data. *Nutr. Cancer* **1994**, *21*, 113–131. [CrossRef] [PubMed]

65. Shu, X.O.; Zheng, Y.; Cai, H.; Gu, K.; Chen, Z.; Zheng, W.; Lu, W. Soy food intake and breast cancer survival. *JAMA* **2009**, *302*, 2437–2443. [CrossRef] [PubMed]

66. Jacobs, D.R., Jr.; Gross, M.D.; Tapsell, L.C. Food synergy: An operational concept for understanding nutrition. *Am. J. Clin. Nutr.* **2009**, *89*, S1543–S1548. [CrossRef] [PubMed]

67. Tapsell, L.C. Foods and food components in the Mediterranean diet: Supporting overall effects. *BMC Med.* **2014**, *12*. [CrossRef] [PubMed]

68. Saura-Calixto, F.; Goni, I. Antioxidant capacity of the Spanish Mediterranean Diet. *Food Chem.* **2006**, *94*, 442–447. [CrossRef]

69. Arts, I.C.; Hollman, P.C. Polyphenols and disease risk in epidemiologic studies. *Am. J. Clin. Nutr.* **2005**, *81*, S317–S325.

70. Scalbert, A.; Manach, C.; Morand, C.; Remesy, C.; Jimenez, L. Dietary polyphenols and the prevention of diseases. *Crit. Rev. Food Sci. Nutr.* **2005**, *45*, 287–306. [CrossRef] [PubMed]

71. Chlebowski, R.T.; Blackburn, G.L.; Thomson, C.A.; Nixon, D.W.; Shapiro, A.; Hoy, M.K.; Goodman, M.T.; Giuliano, A.E.; Karanja, N.; McAndrew, P.; et al. Dietary fat reduction and breast cancer outcome: Interim efficacy results from the Women's Intervention Nutrition Study. *J. Natl. Cancer Inst.* **2006**, *98*, 1767–1776. [CrossRef] [PubMed]

72. Hauner, D.; Hauner, H. Metabolic syndrome and breast cancer: Is there a link? *Breast Care (Basel)* **2014**, *9*, 277–281. [CrossRef] [PubMed]

73. McTiernan, A.; Irwin, M.; Vongruenigen, V. Weight, physical activity, diet, and prognosis in breast and gynecologic cancers. *J. Clin. Oncol.* **2010**, *28*, 4074–4080. [CrossRef] [PubMed]

74. Protani, M.; Coory, M.; Martin, J.H. Effect of obesity on survival of women with breast cancer: Systematic review and meta-analysis. *Breast Cancer Res. Treat.* **2010**, *123*, 627–635. [CrossRef] [PubMed]

75. Villarini, A.; Pasanisi, P.; Traina, A.; Mano, M.P.; Bonanni, B.; Panico, S.; Scipioni, C.; Galasso, R.; Paduos, A.; Simeoni, M.; et al. Lifestyle and breast cancer recurrences: The DIANA-5 trial. *Tumori* **2012**, *98*, 1–18. [PubMed]

76. Berrino, F.; Bellati, C.; Secreto, G.; Camerini, E.; Pala, V.; Panico, S.; Allegro, G.; Kaaks, R. Reducing bioavailable sex hormones through a comprehensive change in diet: The diet and androgens (DIANA) randomized trial. *Cancer Epidemiol. Biomark. Prev.* **2001**, *10*, 25–33.

77. Berrino, F.; Villarini, A.; De Petris, M.; Raimondi, M.; Pasanisi, P. Adjuvant diet to improve hormonal and metabolic factors affecting breast cancer prognosis. *Ann. N. Y. Acad. Sci.* **2006**, *1089*, 110–118. [CrossRef] [PubMed]

78. Villarini, A.; Pasanisi, P.; Raimondi, M.; Gargano, G.; Bruno, E.; Morelli, D.; Evangelista, A.; Curtosi, P.; Berrino, F. Preventing weight gain during adjuvant chemotherapy for breast cancer: A dietary intervention study. *Breast Cancer Res. Treat.* **2012**, *135*, 581–589. [CrossRef] [PubMed]

79. Dahabreh, I.J.; Linardou, H.; Siannis, F.; Fountzilas, G.; Murray, S. Trastuzumab in the adjuvant treatment of early-stage breast cancer: A systematic review and meta-analysis of randomized controlled trials. *Oncologist* **2008**, *13*, 620–630. [CrossRef] [PubMed]

80. Engstrom, M.J.; Opdahl, S.; Hagen, A.I.; Romundstad, P.R.; Akslen, L.A.; Haugen, O.A.; Vatten, L.J.; Bofin, A.M. Molecular subtypes, histopathological grade and survival in a historic cohort of breast cancer patients. *Breast Cancer Res. Treat.* **2013**, *140*, 463–473. [CrossRef] [PubMed]

81. Schnitt, S.J. Classification and prognosis of invasive breast cancer: From morphology to molecular taxonomy. *Mod. Pathol.* **2010**, *23*, S60–S64. [CrossRef] [PubMed]

82. Staaf, J.; Ringner, M. Making breast cancer molecular subtypes robust? *J. Natl. Cancer Inst.* **2014**, *107*. [CrossRef] [PubMed]

83. Jonat, W.; Pritchard, K.I.; Sainsbury, R.; Klijn, J.G. Trends in endocrine therapy and chemotherapy for early breast cancer: A focus on the premenopausal patient. *J. Cancer Res. Clin. Oncol.* **2006**, *132*, 275–286. [CrossRef] [PubMed]

84. Jenkins, E.O.; Deal, A.M.; Anders, C.K.; Prat, A.; Perou, C.M.; Carey, L.A.; Muss, H.B. Age-specific changes in intrinsic breast cancer subtypes: A focus on older women. *Oncologist* **2014**, *19*, 1076–1083. [CrossRef] [PubMed]

85. Vanden Berghe, W. Epigenetic impact of dietary polyphenols in cancer chemoprevention: Lifelong remodeling of our epigenomes. *Pharmacol. Res.* **2012**, *65*, 565–576. [CrossRef] [PubMed]

86. Link, A.; Balaguer, F.; Shen, Y.; Lozano, J.J.; Leung, H.C.; Boland, C.R.; Goel, A. Curcumin modulates DNA methylation in colorectal cancer cells. *PLoS ONE* **2013**, *8*, e57709. [CrossRef] [PubMed]

87. Tapiero, H.; Tew, K.D.; Ba, G.N.; Mathe, G. Polyphenols: Do they play a role in the prevention of human pathologies? *Biomed. Pharmacother.* **2002**, *56*, 200–207. [CrossRef]

88. Bohn, T. Dietary factors affecting polyphenol bioavailability. *Nutr. Rev.* **2014**, *72*, 429–452. [CrossRef] [PubMed]

89. Huang, Q.; Yu, H.; Ru, Q. Bioavailability and delivery of nutraceuticals using nanotechnology. *J. Food Sci.* **2010**, *75*, R50–R57. [CrossRef] [PubMed]

90. Miller, P.E.; Alexander, D.D.; Weed, D.L. Uncertainty of results in nutritional epidemiology. *Nutr. Today* **2014**, *49*, 147–152. [CrossRef]

91. Alexander, D.D.; Weed, D.L.; Miller, P.E.; Mohamed, M.A. Red Meat and Colorectal Cancer: A Quantitative Update on the State of the Epidemiologic Science. *J. Am. Coll. Nutr.* **2015**, *34*, 521–543. [CrossRef] [PubMed]

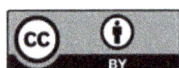

*nutrients*

MDPI

*Review*

# Molecular Targets Underlying the Anticancer Effects of Quercetin: An Update

Fazlullah Khan [1,2], Kamal Niaz [1,2], Faheem Maqbool [1,2], Fatima Ismail Hassan [1,2], Mohammad Abdollahi [1,2,*], Kalyan C. Nagulapalli Venkata [3], Seyed Mohammad Nabavi [4] and Anupam Bishayee [3,*]

1   Pharmaceutical Sciences Research Center, International Campus, Tehran University of Medical Sciences, Tehran 1417614411, Iran; fazlullahdr@gmail.com (F.K.); kamalniaz1989@gmail.com (K.N.); faheemthepharmacist@gmail.com (F.M.) pharm.fatee@yahoo.com (F.I.H.)
2   Department of Toxicology and Pharmacology, Faculty of Pharmacy, Tehran University of Medical Sciences, Tehran 1417614411, Iran
3   Department of Pharmaceutical Sciences, College of Pharmacy, Larkin Health Sciences Institute, Miami, FL 33169, USA; kvenkata@Ularkin.org
4   Applied Biotechnology Research Center, Baqiyatallah University of Medical Sciences, Tehran 1435916471, Iran; nabavi208@gmail.com
*   Correspondence: Mohammad.Abdollahi@UToronto.Ca or Mohammad@TUMS.Ac.Ir (M.A.); abishayee@Ularkin.org or abishayee@gmail.com (A.B.); Tel.: +98-216-959-104 (M.A.); +1-305-760-7511 (A.B.)

Received: 23 July 2016; Accepted: 22 August 2016; Published: 29 August 2016

**Abstract:** Quercetin, a medicinally important member of the flavonoid family, is one of the most prominent dietary antioxidants. It is present in a variety of foods—including fruits, vegetables, tea, wine, as well as other dietary supplements—and is responsible for various health benefits. Numerous pharmacological effects of quercetin include protection against diseases, such as osteoporosis, certain forms of malignant tumors, and pulmonary and cardiovascular disorders. Quercetin has the special ability of scavenging highly reactive species, such as hydrogen peroxide, superoxide anion, and hydroxyl radicals. These oxygen radicals are called reactive oxygen species, which can cause oxidative damage to cellular components, such as proteins, lipids, and deoxyribonucleic acid. Various oxygen radicals play important roles in pathophysiological and degenerative processes, such as aging. Subsequently, several studies have been performed to evaluate possible advantageous health effects of quercetin and to collect scientific evidence for these beneficial health claims. These studies also gather data in order to evaluate the exact mechanism(s) of action and toxicological effects of quercetin. The purpose of this review is to present and critically analyze molecular pathways underlying the anticancer effects of quercetin. Current limitations and future directions of research on this bioactive dietary polyphenol are also critically discussed.

**Keywords:** quercetin; cancer prevention; diet; bioavailability; DNA damage; polyphenols

## 1. Introduction

During the last decade, the proportion of scientific studies based on non-nutritive components of diet has increased. Such components are present in diet and have the ability to protect the body from the harmful effects of degenerative diseases, cancer, and cardiovascular ailments. Carotenoids and flavonoids, two distinct groups of phytochemicals, represent valuable constituents of food. Other dietary agents—such as phytoalexins, phenolic acids, indole-3-carbinol, and organosulfur compounds—are also important phytochemicals with interesting biological activities [1,2]. Phytochemicals are generally present in a variety of foods, fruits, vegetables, beverages, and many other food products and medicinally important herbal preparations. The important point that brings the attention of the scientists towards the naturally occurring compounds for the purpose of testing is the presence of numerous phytochemicals existing in plant-derived foods. There are a wide variety of biological activities which are still unknown for the majority of these compounds [3]. Plant-derived phytochemicals activate various cell signaling pathways that play key roles in the prevention of physiological disorders in the body, which are mainly responsible for the development of cancers, neurodegenerative and cardiovascular diseases [4,5]. Various scientific studies conducted on experimental animal models for the assessment of the exact mechanisms through which phytochemicals exert their actions provide a good and valuable description of how food supplements containing abundant amounts of phytochemicals exhibit protective roles against degenerative disorders [6]. It is noteworthy to find out that such plant-derived medicinally important constituents have the ability to demonstrate preventive and protective measures against pathological disorders.

Flavonoids are mostly present in nature in the form of benzo-γ-pyrone derivatives. These compounds are mostly present in a variety of plants, vegetables, and flowers. Flavonoids have diverse structural frameworks and play important roles in the body's defense system. The beneficial effects of flavonoid-rich foods have been demonstrated by various studies [7]. Data collected from different clinical trials have tried to underscore the exact mode of action exerted by flavonoids. There is a need to evaluate new possible ways to understand the beneficial activities associated with the consumption of flavonoid-rich food in order to advance our knowledge about the possible beneficial action of plant extracts. There are 4000 types of different flavonoids found in nature with diverse subcategories, such as flavones, isoflavones, flavonones, and chalcones. Flavonoids possess important biological activities, such as anti-inflammatory, antioxidant, hepatoprotective, and antimicrobial properties [8].

Quercetin is a key member of the polyphenol family and is largely found in various vegetables and fruits, such as capers, lovage, dill, cilantro, onions, various berries (e.g., chokeberries, cranberries, and lingonberries), and apples. Quercetin is well known for its anticarcinogenic potential. The anticancer property of quercetin is due to various cell signaling mechanisms and its ability to inhibit enzymes responsible for the activation of carcinogens. Moreover, quercetin exerts anticancer effect by binding to cellular receptors and proteins [9,10].

Several previous publications [11–16] present an excellent overview of research related to the therapeutic application of quercetin in cancer prevention and treatment. Nevertheless, there exists a need for a systematic, up-to-date, and critical evaluation of literature to understand biochemical and molecular mechanisms of the anticancer action of quercetin. In this review article, first we focused on chemical reactivity of quercetin and related analogs. Secondly, we discussed the molecular targets as well as signaling pathways implicated in anticancer and cancer preventive potential of quercetin. Thirdly, we presented epidemiological evidences regarding quercetin consumption and cancer occurrence. Finally, we discussed future directions of research to understand the full potential of quercetin in cancer prevention and treatment.

## 2. Bibliographic Search

The scientific information gathered in this review was collected by widespread search of several electronic databases, including PubMed, Scopus, Medline, Web of Science, EBASE, and Google Scholar. The criteria for the exclusion of articles was the language of reports being other than English, reports with unavailable abstracts, studies related to quercetin effects apart from its anticancer profile, and studies which showed the linkage between cancer and cancer risk factors, such as tobacco smoking and alcohol consumption. Various appropriate articles not indexed by PubMed were also considered, and 27 such reports which fulfilled the criteria for inclusion were further recovered from Google Scholar. Therefore, the total number of included articles in this review is 127 (Figure 1).

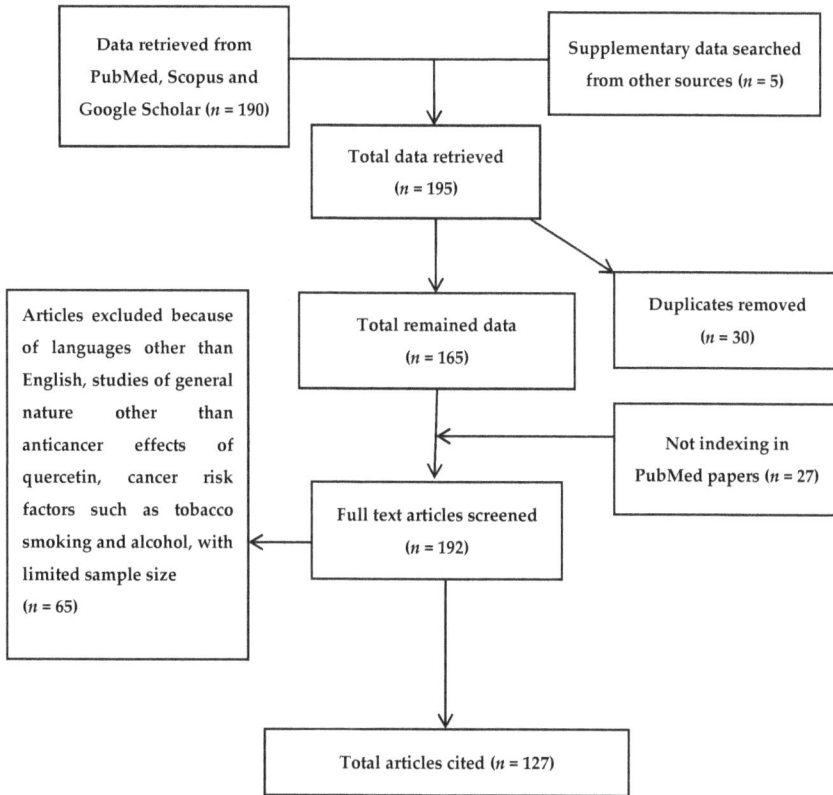

**Figure 1.** Flow diagram of included studies. The number of citations and resource materials that have been screened, excluded and/or included in this review is indicated in parenthesis.

## 3. Chemistry of Quercetin and Its Analogs

Quercetin is a polyphenolic secondary metabolite that belongs to the flavonol class of flavonoids. It is characterized by a benzo-($\gamma$)-pyrone skeletal structure with C6-C3-C6 carbon framework, consisting of two benzene rings, A and B, linked by a three-carbon pyrone ring C as shown in Figure 2 [17]. Quercetin is referred to as pentahydroxyflavonol due to the presence of five hydroxyl groups on its flavonol skeletal framework at 3, 3′, 4′, 5, and 7 carbons [12]. The wide range of biochemical and pharmacological activities of quercetin and its metabolites is due to the relative substitution of various functional groups on the flavonol molecule [18].

Phytochemical investigations of various plant extracts have revealed that quercetin can exist in a free state as an aglycone, or as its derivative by conjugating with: (1) carbohydrates as quercetin glycosides, (2) lipids as prenylated quercetin, (3) alcohols as quercetin ethers, and (4) a sulfate group as quercetin sulfate [19].

Quercetin glycosides are formed through the *O*-glycosidic bond between a sugar and the hydroxyl group of quercetin molecule, and the general glycosylation site on the quercetin molecule is at the 3-hydroxyl position. However, glycosylation of other hydroxyl groups has also been reported [20]. The sugar moieties can be monosaccharides, disaccharides, or polysaccharides, and the most common carbohydrate substituents are glucose, galactose, rhamnose, and xylose. Isoquercetin, hyperoside, quercitrin, and rutin are a few of the most abundant and well-studied quercetin glycosides (Figure 2) [21].

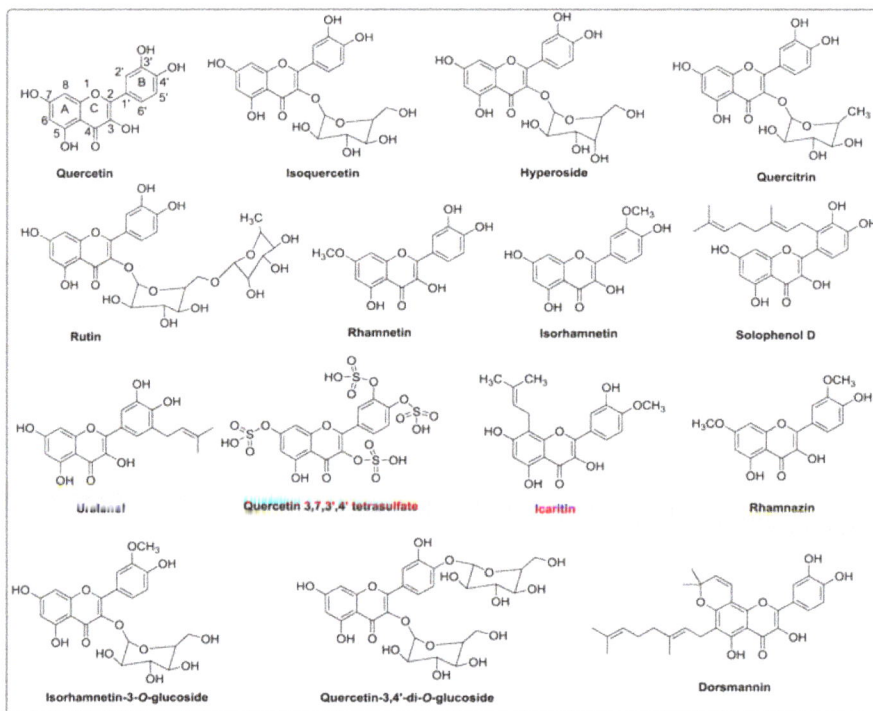

**Figure 2.** Structures of quercetin and its derivatives [19–24].

Quercetin methyl ethers are one of the most widely studied natural pigments, and they are formed through the conjugation of the quercetin hydroxyl group with alcohol, generally methanol. Quercetin ethers can exist in various configurations, from mono-ethers to penta-ethers, with substitution on all the hydroxyl groups of quercetin molecule. Rhamnetin, isorhamnetin, and rhamnazin are a few representatives of quercetin ether analogs [19].

Prenylflavonols are an important group of molecules belonging to the flavonol subclass. They are well-known for their wide range of biological activities, such as antioxidant, antibacterial, anti-inflammatory, and anticancer properties [22]. Structurally, in C-prenylflavonols, prenyl groups are attached to the carbon atom of the flavonol skeleton. In the past few years, prenylated quercetin analogs, such as solophenol D and uralenol, have gained a lot of attention due to their antibacterial properties. It has been reported that prenylation may enhance the biological functions of quercetin by increasing its hydrophobicity and bioavailability [23,24].

In addition to the sugar, lipid, and alcohol derivatives, quercetin also exists as sulfate conjugate in nature. Quercetin 3,7,3′,4′-tetrasulfate, isolated from the leaves *Flaveria bidentis*, has shown remarkable anticoagulant properties [25]. The multisubstituted derivatives, such as icaritin, isorhamnetin 3-*O*-glucoside, quercetin-3,4′-di-*O*-glucoside, and dorsmannin, can form from the combination of same or different functional groups. The number and nature of these functional group substitutions have profound effects on the physicochemical properties and biological effects of quercetin analogs [26].

The best described biochemical property of quercetin is its ability to act as an antioxidant. The antioxidant activity and free radical scavenging properties of quercetin are attributed to its chemical structure [27]. There are three important structural features: (1) catechol functionality (ortho-dihydroxyl) on B ring, (2) a $\Delta^2$ double bond adjacent to a 4-oxo group in pyrone C ring, and (3) hydroxyl groups at C-3 and C-5 carbons in the benzopyrone AC ring [28]. The structural variables—such as configuration, substitution, and number of hydroxyl groups—greatly influence the mechanisms involved in antioxidant activity, like their ability to scavenge radical species and their ability to chelate metals [29].

Quercetin also inhibits the lipid peroxidation process, a common consequence of oxidative stress, and consequently protects against lipid membrane damage [30]. Due to its lower redox potential, quercetin is able to reduce highly oxidizing free radicals, such as superoxide and peroxide radicals. Because of its ability to chelate metal ions, quercetin can inhibit the generation of free radicals [28].

## 4. Bioavailability and Metabolism of Quercetin

In order to estimate the efficacy of quercetin in terms of its anticarcinogenic effect, it is important to understand the bioavailability of quercetin as well as its intestinal absorption and metabolism conversion rate. When quercetin was administered intravenously to rodents, it immediately disappeared from the plasma. It was evident from this experiment that quercetin was rapidly metabolized and eliminated from the body through urine and no evidence was observed regarding the storage of quercetin inside the tissues and body fluids. Previously, there was a common belief about the excretion of quercetin into feces without being absorbed by the intestine, but it is evident from recent studies that an excessive amount of quercetin found in foods is likely to be absorbed from the intestine and subsequently converted to its respective metabolites [31]. In the transportation of the metabolites of quercetin, the body's lymphatic system is also involved [32]. Repeated intake of onion resulted in accumulation of quercetin metabolites in various tissues and blood, which reached a total plasma concentration of 0.6 μM after 1 week. Hence, it is important to keep the plasma quercetin metabolite concentration at an acceptable and significant level [33].

It is evident from studies conducted recently that the metabolites of quercetin were rapidly distributed among various organs at low levels after intake of dietary quercetin for a long time [34]. It is also evident that regular consumption of dietary quercetin results in the storage of metabolites throughout the body [35]. Generally, the conversion of quercetin to its metabolic derivatives decreases its free radical scavenging activity, but there are some metabolic derivatives of quercetin, which are capable of removing the reactive species from the body. Moreover, during the process of inflammation, quercetin-3-glucuronide is metabolized, resulting in the accumulation of quercetin aglycone [36]. Recent studies showed that glucuronide, a more active form of aglycone metabolite of quercetin, was used for the incorporation into macrophages [34]. This study showed those actions of quercetin metabolites which are mostly site-specific in nature and are recommended for inflammatory conditions. The modified forms of quercetin are present in human blood and stored in inactive forms, which are further converted into active residues and ultimately converted into the active constituents to exert their actions at specific target sites.

## 5. Protective Effects of Quercetin

Quercetin and its metabolites are crucial due to their physiological functions as well as their role in the elimination of cancerous cells. Therefore, it is important to further investigate this specialized aspect of quercetin in terms of protection against cancer and other degenerative disorders, as these ailments are the leading causes of death throughout the world.

It was investigated recently that by influencing the pentose phosphate pathway with the production of CYP450, the preventive environment for cytochrome c-mediated apoptosis can be maintained. This cytochrome is an important part of the electron transport chain and is released from mitochondria during the apoptosis process. Therefore, the cancerous cells keep constant control over cell death through the release of cytochrome c [37]. These metabolic changes are important for the survival of cells for a longer time and also for the spreading of cancer cells [38]. Various studies have been performed to evaluate the pharmacological actions of quercetin in biological systems in order to investigate the precise mode of action of quercetin [39,40]. Therefore, it is evident from these studies that quercetin and its metabolites, which are present in various plants, play crucial roles in the protection against cancer and oxidative stress. When PC-12 cells were treated with nerve growth factor (NGF), the cells ceased to multiply and began to extend branching varicose processes similar to those produced by sympathetic neurons in primary cell culture [41]. Quercetin exhibited NGF-like action when it came in contact with PC-12 cells. Quercetin also causes cell differentiation similar to that caused by NGF [42]. Although the exact mechanism is still unclear, the well-characterized NGF-inducing capacity is more likely related to the differentiation-inducing effects of quercetin [43]. The protective effects of quercetin have also been observed in primary cultures [39]. Quercetin increased the rate of survival of cells when it was administered 24 h before the oxidative stress. In a cell culture model, it was reported that quercetin internalization into neurons happened rapidly, and a neuroprotective pathway involved Nrf2-dependent variation of the GSH redox system was observed [44].

When the aqueous quercetin was administered in experimental animals, there was a significant reduction in brain ischemic lesions [45]. Quercetin has been used in a variety of studies to evaluate its protective effects. In one study, the anticancer effects of quercetin were studied in animal models. The investigators examined the physiological changes after they administered colchicine by intracerebroventricular route [46].

In a similar study, quercetin was administered to mice for a period of seven days through intraperitoneal (i.p.) route. After administration of quercetin, memory improvement was observed in mice [47]. In this study the developmental changes were linked with the inhibition of cyclooxygenase 2 enzyme. It was observed that there was a noteworthy improvement in the learning ability of mice in comparison with the control group of mice [48]. Quercetin also increased the activity of superoxide dismutase (SOD) and lowered the level of malondialdehyde. Quercetin and other flavonoids acted as prodrugs and were metabolized into active hydroxyphenyl acetic acid metabolites by microflora in the intestine [49]. The protective effects of quercetin were observed in rats with known evidence of cerebral ischemia [50]. By administering two consecutive doses of quercetin, the memory problem in rats—which was induced by repeated cerebral ischemia—was improved and the level of cell death was reduced in the region I of hippocampus proper area (CA1). In another study, when quercetin was administered through i.p. route to rats with spinal cord injuries for a period of 10 days, half of the rats started walking [51].

In a study evaluating the penetration of quercetin across the blood–brain barrier, it was observed that quercetin induced various changes within different brain regions based on an in situ brain perfusion model in rats [52].

## 6. Molecular Mechanisms of Quercetin

Quercetin is used for therapeutic purposes in various disorders due to its antioxidant capability The reactive oxygen species (ROS) scavenging activity is attributed to a change in $OH^-$ ions, which has a relation to electron exchange [53]. Catechol oxidative agents, such as semiquinones and quinones formed due to quercetin, alter redox homeostasis and inhibit primary positive effects [27]. In vitro study predicted that due to this special feature quercetin has a protective role in the nervous system. In the current scenario, the neuroprotective activity of quercetin cannot be ignored and additional in vivo studies should be investigated with different humanized animal models to translate the efficacy. Quercetin exerts its antioxidant activity by competitively inhibiting the xanthine oxidase enzyme and noncompetitively blocking the xanthine dehydrogenase enzyme. The inhibitory capabilities are due to its flavonoid structure rather than to its antioxidant potential [54].

### 6.1. HMGB1 Signaling Pathway

High-mobility group box protein 1 (HMGB1) is a nuclear protein which is highly preserved. It is secreted by the action of macrophages previously activated and it works as a crucial "late" facilitator of fatal endotoxemia and sepsis formation [55]. The HMGB1 protein, which is present outside the cell, can motivate the release of tumor necrosis factor-α (TNF-α), interleukin-1β (IL-1β), and other inflammatory mediators from monocytes [55,56]. Quercetin stimulates the inhibition of HMGB1-induced TNF-α and IL-1β mRNA expression, which suggests that quercetin modulates cell signaling that in turn regulates the action of proinflammatory cytokines. The activation of mitogen-activated protein kinase (MAPK) signaling pathway is a significant step in the HMGB1-induced gene expression process, which causes the release of inflammatory cytokines—such as TNF-α, and IL-1β—inside macrophages, neutrophils, and endothelial cells. HMGB1-induced cytokine release partially interferes with MAPK pathways. HMGB1 or lipopolysaccharides (LPS) time-dependently induce phosphorylation of p38, c-Jun N–terminal kinase, and extracellular signal-regulated kinase in macrophages. Quercetin considerably inhibits HMGB1- or LPS-induced phosphorylation of each kinase [57]. Apart from MAPK activation, the nuclear factor-κB (NF-κB) signal transduction pathway is also involved in HMGB1-induced cellular activation, and NF-κB-dependent transcriptional activity is very important for cytokine expression [58,59]. In cells, NF-κB subunits (p50 and p65) exist as inactive trimers in the cytosol through the interaction with IκBα, which is the most important member of the IκB family [60]. Quercetin significantly inhibits IκBα degradation and nuclear translocation of NF-κB p65. Therefore, after stimulation with HMGB1 or LPS, p65, the key activator of NF-κB-regulated transcription, becomes available to NF-κB-regulated genes in the nucleus and nuclear localization is most effectively inhibited by quercetin.

*6.2. Thymic Stromal Lymphopoietin (TSLP) Activation*

The level of TSLP, which is an epithelial-derived cytokine with a role in T helper (Th) cells' Type-2 immunity, is considerably increased in human skin as well as blood. The TSLP signaling process is initiated through proteins, including 1L-7 chain of receptor, which has potential to enhance the B lymphocyte activation and dendritic cells [61]. Primary skin keratinocytes are mostly responsible for expressing the TSLP in smooth muscle and lung connective tissues. TSLP contributes its main biological role by influencing various cells [62]. It is evident that TSLP has the potential to activate both CD4+ T and CD8+ cells along with other B lymphocytes' differentiation, which in turn promotes the release and activation of chemokines. Additionally, it can enhance the secretory mechanism of the Th2 cytokines from mast cells. During the binding of TSLP with respective receptors, various signaling pathways are activated [63]. It has been reported in a recent study that due to the activation of these receptors, there is a marked promotion in the phosphorylation process of Janus kinase-signal transducers and activators of transcription (JAK-STAT) signaling, which further causes skin inflammation [64]. Thus, targeting the above signaling pathway is a viable approach to design a treatment plan for various inflammatory diseases, including cancer.

*6.3. JAK-STAT Signaling Pathway*

JAK-STAT signaling pathway is a typical signal transduction pathway for various types of inflammatory cytokines and growth regulatory factors. The binding of ligands to their respective receptors leads to the activation of JAK, which further increases the phosphorylation process and hence leads to the activation of STAT. The STATs, which are already activated, enter the nucleus, where they start the regulation of gene expression [65]. Studies have shown that the activated mast cells stimulate the formation of the Th2 cytokines and decrease the secretory mechanism of Th1 cytokines. JAK-STAT signaling is activated by mast cells, which in turn activate the IL-13 production in the Th2 cell line [66].

Quercetin has the ability to actively inhibit the JAK-STAT signaling pathway in various inflammatory disorders. Furthermore, treatment of activated T cells with quercetin in vitro inhibited the interleukin-12 (IL-12)-induced phosphorylation of JAK2, tyrosine kinase-2 (TYK2), STAT3, and STAT4, which result in decreased levels of T cell propagation and Th1 variation [67]. Therefore, these anti-inflammatory and antiapoptotic properties of quercetin have a key role in the reduction of cancer by controlling the toll-like receptor-2 (TLR2) and JAK2/STAT3 pathway and causing the inhibition of STAT3 tyrosine phosphorylation within inflammatory cells [68]. Pretreatment of cholangiocarcinoma cells with quercetin inhibited the cytokine-mediated upregulation of inducible nitric oxide synthase (iNOS) and expression of intercellular adhesion molecule-1 (ICAM-1) in the

JAK/STAT cascade pathway. Also, quercetin blocked the activation of inflammatory cytokine interleukin-6 and interferon-γ [69]. It was reported that LPS-induced STAT1 activation was inhibited by quercetin in combination with its profound inhibitory effects on iNOS and NF-κB expression, which are persistently involved in activation of interleukin-2 (IL-2) as shown in Figure 3 [70].

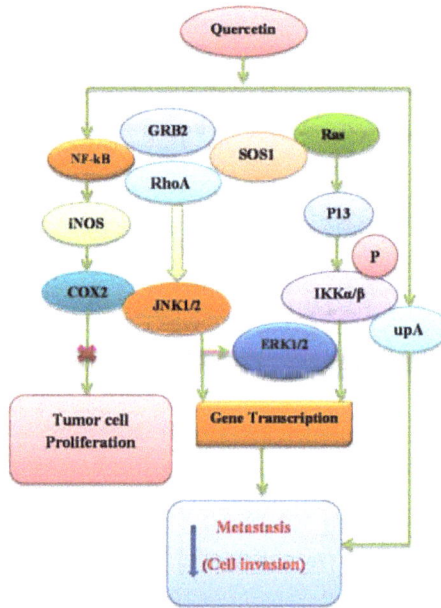

**Figure 3.** Anticancer pathways and mechanisms of quercetin.

## 7. Anticancer Effects of Quercetin

Vegetables and fruits are rich sources of phytochemicals with significant potential to prevent cancer due to the presence of abundant antioxidants. Among polyphenols, quercetin is the most important and naturally occurring cancer-preventing agent. The importance of dietary quercetin is due to its antioxidant potential and anti-inflammatory effects [47]. The cancer preventive and therapeutic effects of quercetin have been demonstrated through in vitro (Table 1) as well as in vivo (Table 2) experimental findings.

**Table 1.** In vitro anticancer effects of quercetin and its analogs.

| Compound tested | Cell lines | Effects | Mechanisms | References |
|---|---|---|---|---|
| Quercetin | MCF-7, HCC1937, SK-Br3, 4T1, MDA-MB-231 | Induced apoptosis | ↑Bcl-2,↓Bax expression,↓Her-2, inhibition of PI3K-Akt pathway | [71] |
| Quercetin | MIA PaCa-2, BxPC-3 | Inhibited proliferation | ↓Her-2, regulation of Wnt/β-catenin | [72] |
| Quercetin | CX-1, SW480, HT-29, HCT116 | Inhibited proliferation | ↓HIF-1κ, regulation of Wnt/β-catenin | [73] |
| Quercetin | LNCaP, PC-3 | Inhibited proliferation | ↓VEGF secretion, ↓mRNA levels | [74] |
| Quercetin | HepG2 | Inhibited proliferation | ↓PI3K,↓PKC | [75] |

Table 1. *Cont.*

| Compound tested | Cell lines | Effects | Mechanisms | References |
|---|---|---|---|---|
| Rutin | ACC | Inhibited proliferation | ↓PI3K,↓Akt,↓IKK-α,↓NF-κB | [76] |
| Rutin | SKOV3 | Inhibited cell growth | ↓Cyclin D1 | [77] |
| Rutin | HeLa | Inhibited cell growth | ↑p53,↓NF-κB | [78] |
| Quercetin | A549 | Inhibited cell growth | ↓cdk1,↓cyclin B | [79] |
| Quercetin | JB6 P+ | Inhibited cell migration | Regulation of p13K/Akt | [5] |
| Quercetin | U373MG | Inhibited cell migration | ↑caspase-7,↑JNK,↑p53 | [80] |

Quercetin, when used in pharmacologically safe doses, inhibits the phosphatidylinositol 3-kinase (PI3K)-Akt/PKB (protein kinase B) pathway in cancer cells [81]. Both Raf and MAPK/extracellular signal-regulated kinase (ERK) kinase (MEK) act as direct targets for quercetin, leading to the potential to decrease MEK1 activity more powerfully when compared to PD098059, which is a specific MEK inhibitor. Quercetin donates a hydrogen bond to the main amide group of Ser-212, which is known to stabilize the inactive conformation of the activated loop of MEK1 [82]. When a dose of 10 g quercetin/kg was administered to rats for 11 weeks, physiological changes were observed inside the rats' colons. This study indicated that quercetin extensively downregulated the potential oncogenic MAPK signaling in vivo [83]. Various in vitro studies have demonstrated that quercetin plays a key role in cancer prevention and tumor suppression in different cell lines [84]. The doses of quercetin that showed anticancer effects in vitro were ranging from 3 to 50 μM [85]. The cancer prevention properties of quercetin in vivo studies have been confirmed in colon cancer [11]. Furthermore, quercetin has been shown to exhibit anticancer effects in melanoma [86]. The inhibition of tumor growth by quercetin was evaluated when it was administered as a food supplement to experimental models. However, contradictory results have been reported in the literature [87].

Table 2. In vivo anticancer effects of quercetin and its analogs.

| Compound tested | Animal models | Effects | Mechanisms | Dose | Duration | References |
|---|---|---|---|---|---|---|
| Quercetin | FemaleCF1 mice | Retarded tumor growth | ↓PCNA; ↑mmu-miR-205-5P | 8 g/kg/day (diet) | 42 days | [88] |
| Quercetin | Male F344 rats | Inhibited tumor growth | ↓EphA2;↓PI3K; ↓MMP-2;↓MMP-9 | 100 mg/kg (i.p.) | 18 days | [89] |
| Rutin | Male F344 rats | Suppressed tumor growth | ↓ACF | 25 mg/kg (i.p.) | 28 days | [89] |
| Quercetin | Female CD-1 mice | Inhibited tumor nodule formation | ↓papilloma | 3–6 mg/kg (p.o.) | 14 days | [90] |
| Quercetin | Male Swiss mice | Inhibited tumor nodule formation | ↓AD | 6 mg/kg (i.p.) | 2 times/ week 21 days | [91] |
| Quercetin | Female Sprague-Dawley rats | Reduced tumor volume | ↓ADC | 17.5 mg/kg (i.v.) | 2 times/ week for 24 days | [92] |

i.p., intraperitoneal; i.v., intravenous; p.o., per os.

## 7.1. Binding Ability of Quercetin to SEK1–JNK1/2 and MEK1–ERK1/2

Studies have shown that various pathways are the possible molecular targets of quercetin to inhibit inflammatory responses as shown in Figure 3. Quercetin chemically binds to protein kinase as evidenced by the bead-bound pull-down assay, which has been recognized as a potent screening tool. Quercetin binds with SAPK/ERK kinase 1 (SEK1), c-Jun *N*-terminal kinase 1/2 (JNK1/2), MEK1 and ERK1/2 [93].

Several studies have provided useful evidences that there are many hydrogen bonds between different hydroxyl groups of quercetin and amino acid residues of SEK1–JNK1/2 and MEK1–ERK1/2. The ERK1/2 is part of a MAPK cascade, which consists of consecutively functioning kinases, such as Raf, MEK, and ERK1/2 [94]. The active ERK1/2 induces reprogramming events related to gene expression by actively phosphorylating diverse intracellular molecular target proteins and other transcription factors, and hence potentiates cellular growth, spreading, and antiapoptotic properties.

## 7.2. Cellular Senescence Induction and Telomerase Inhibition

It is a process of irreversible cell aging that occurs in most of the normal cells in response to the restriction of telomerase enzymes or due to changes in the three-dimensional structure of telomerase. The cellular death activity is also associated with oncogenic activation or stress caused by oxidation [95]. The process of senescence induction by phytochemicals is a new alternative approach to chemoprevention. In a recent study, it was confirmed that both quercetin and resveratrol induced the cell death process even in very low doses in cells which showed resistance to glioma formation [96]. Despite the fact that there was no proper identification of a molecular target, there was a marked decrease in Akt phosphorylation. In the senescence induction process, quercetin also targeted the telomerase induction in eluding the replicate immortality.

Telomerases are specialized DNA polymerases having the ability to join the repeating parts of the telomerase enzymes with the ends of the DNA strands. The enzyme telomerase is significantly expressed at certain intervals in the majority of the cells, including the excessively proliferating human cells. The presence of telomerase activity is closely related to cell death resistance [95]. Quercetin and other polyphenols, including epigallocatechin-3-gallate (EGCG), inhibit the activity of telomerase in a cell-free system. The telomerase inhibitory effect was confirmed using adenocarcinoma and breast carcinoma patients [97].

## 7.3. Cell Death Induction Activity

Programmed cell death is an important mechanism which is activated to eliminate cancer cells in the body [95]. There are extrinsic and intrinsic pathways which control the cell death activity in the body, and these pathways are under the influence of cytokines, which act by binding with tumor necrosis factor receptors (TNF-R). The cytokines are large molecules which are mostly involved in the development of immunity [98].

Quercetin bypasses the cell damage resistance through various mechanisms. One example of quercetin action is evident in lymphocytic leukemia cell line. Quercetin is introduced to the body with minimum toxic concentrations to induce the apoptotic process. From this study, it is evident that quercetin induces the apoptotic process when combined with antibodies for the enhancement of immunity [99].

At molecular levels, quercetin acts by lowering the ROS inside the cell. This property of scavenging free radical species is a unique function of quercetin among flavonoid derivatives [100]. Apoptosis-inducing activity of quercetin has been confirmed in leukemia and also in cells which are resistant to TNF-related apoptosis-inducing ligand (TRAIL)-induced apoptosis [101].

### 7.4. Interactions of Quercetin with Cellular Receptors

Quercetin binds with different receptors present throughout the body and shows its anticancer properties. In a recent study, it was concluded that both Raf and MEK are molecular targets of quercetin in the prevention and treatment of cancer [102]. Whether quercetin has direct interactions with cell receptors is still unclear, but there are reports that aryl hydrocarbon receptor (AhR) is a known molecular target receptor for the majority of flavonoids, including quercetin. The AhR receptor is a ligand-gated transcription factor which is activated by the interaction with synthetic and natural chemicals [45,103]. Similarly, AhR is responsible for the regulation and expression of cytochrome P-450 (CYP) 1 family, and this family is fully capable of activating procarcinogens. In the biotransformation of polycyclic aromatic hydrocarbons (PAHs) to metabolites, which are carcinogenic in nature, the CYP1 family members are actively involved [104]. The process of biotransformation is closely associated with cancer development in the lung. Also, a high level of CYP1 is responsible for colon cancer, a major cause of cancer-related death [105].

Quercetin inhibits the transformation of AhR and protects the cells from the toxicity induced by dioxins [106]. The $IC_{50}$ values of quercetin 3-$O$-$\beta$-D-glucuronide and quercetin 4'-$O$-$\beta$-D-glucuronide were 42.6 and 181 $\mu$M, respectively. It is indicated from this result that aglycones have stronger antagonistic activity than glucuronides and other metabolites. Quercetin also blocks the biotransformation of AhR in rat hepatocytes. It is noteworthy that the inhibitory effect of quercetin is much stronger than the effects of $\alpha$-naphthoflavone, a well-known antagonist for AhR [107]. It is evident from these results that quercetin is a strong antagonist for AhR and hence exerts its pharmacological effects against carcinogenicity developed by PAHs. Quercetin also interacts with other receptors, which are involved in the prevention of cancer, but the exact mechanism is still unclear [108]. Quercetin has no role in the increase or decrease and distribution of estrogen receptors-beta isoforms in breast cancer [109]. Quercetin has been shown to possess inhibitory effects in human prostate cancer, and this effect is linked to the expression of androgen receptors [110]. It has been suggested in a recent report that a transcription factor is involved in quercetin-mediated inhibition of androgenic receptor [111].

### 7.5. Signal Transduction Modification

There are various reports which document modulatory effects of quercetin and other flavonoids on signal transduction pathways. The use of quercetin enhances the cell death process in HepG2 human hepatoma cells. There are two mechanisms involved in this process; one is the activation of caspase-3 and caspase-9, but not caspase-8. The other mechanism involves an increase in the translocation of proapoptotic Bax to the membrane of mitochondria [112]. In a similar study, it has been shown that quercetin causes the cleavage of polymerase and also potentiates the upregulation of Bax (Figure 4). Quercetin decreases the levels of key oncogenic protein Ras in cancer cells and blocks the cell proliferation and survival [113].

Quercetin has been shown to cause changes in apoptosis in mesangial cells by inhibiting the activation of JNK and other ERKs pathways. It is also clear that there is no significant effect on the level of p38 MAPK [114]. In a similar study, it is reported that quercetin caused the inhibition of phosphorylation of p38 and Bcl2. This property of quercetin is useful as it may stop the apoptotic process [115]. The action of quercetin may be considered as short-term or long-term. The short-term effect causes scavenging of free radicals and it is mostly antioxidative and antiapoptotic in nature, while the long term effect is pro-oxidative [116]. The proapoptotic action of quercetin is linked mostly to a decreased level of glutamate-stimulating hormones (GSH). It is evident that GSH plays an important role in determining the antioxidant nature of flavonoids. The action of quercetin may depend upon the concentrations of quercetin in cell culture medium [117].

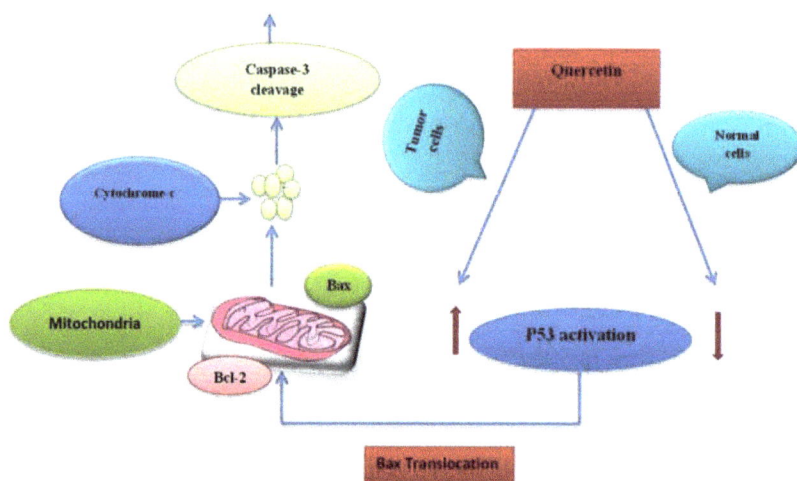

**Figure 4.** Modulation of mitochondrial apoptotic signaling pathways by quercetin. Quercetin induces p53 activation resulting in upregulation of Bax and downregulation of Bcl-2 in tumor cells. This leads to caspase activation and ultimately apoptotic cell death.

How to determine the accurate mechanism through which quercetin exerts its effect in controlling the signal transduction pathway is still unclear. There are few studies on the mechanisms of action of quercetin, and the specific targets of quercetin are not well known [118]. Apart from the findings mentioned above, it has been reported that the MEK/ERK pathway is activated by quercetin during the process of programmed cell death in human lung cancer. This contradiction may be because of the basic difference in investigational conditions, including the use of various cell lines [119]. Quercetin is important in the regulation of signal transduction pathways, and such pathways are crucial in the production of inflammatory mediators. Quercetin also decreases the LPS formation of cytokinase, and this enzyme causes the inhibition of iNOS by further suppressing ERK and p38 MAPK [120]. Moreover, quercetin significantly reduces the half-life of Ras protein, which is oncogenic in nature, but no significant action was reported when the cells were treated with proteasome inhibitor [113].

## 8. Epidemiological Studies about Quercetin

Emerging studies suggest that intake of fruits and vegetables decrease the risk of human carcinomas, including colon, breast, bladder, stomach, and lung cancer [121]. A plethora of phytochemicals present in plant-based food products are consumed by humans on a daily basis. However, it is still unknown which one among these phytoconstituents is responsible for protective action against cancer. The most studied phytochemicals for anticancer potential are flavonoids [122]. A few studies indicate an opposite relation among the dietary consumption of polyphenols and cancer risk [123]. However, Hertog and his coworkers [124] assert that there is no association between the intake of flavonol or flavone derivatives and cancer-related mortality rates.

Regarding quercetin, an opposite co-relation exists between the consumption of quercetin found in foods and the development of lung cancer caused by smoking [125]. A recent multiethnic clinical study has provided evidence about the cancer preventive effects of quercetin in the progression of pancreatic cancer in individuals who were chain smokers and nonsmokers. However, the effect was more pronounced in smokers compared to nonsmokers, as quercetin imparted its antioxidant activity in smokers who had increased oxidative stress relative to nonsmokers [126]. It is evident from many studies that quercetin has beneficial effects against cancer risks. In a study, Gates and coworkers [127] evaluated the relationship between the intake of quercetin and the incidence rate of the ovarian cancer among the nursing staff. The data collected from these results revealed that quercetin intake had a nonsignificant 29% decrease in ovarian cancer risk compared to women with the lowest intake of quercetin.

## 9. Conclusion and Future Perspectives

The studies presented here suggest the potential effects of quercetin in cancer therapy. Numerous in vitro and in vivo experiments have shown various mechanisms of action that could suppress multiple oncogenic signaling pathways. Quercetin is safe with no reported toxicity when applied for the treatment of human cancer. Since quercetin and its derivatives have great benefits, it is the need of the hour to investigate further the effects of these molecules in the prevention and intervention of cancer. However, there is still no conclusive evidence regarding its exact mode of action in order to enhance its clinical application in the treatment of human cancer. Therefore, the future perspective of research should concentrate on the evaluation of quercetin's precise mechanisms of action. Similarly, it is necessary to perform more clinical studies on the efficacy and bioavailability of quercetin in biological systems for the future use in human population, especially in the treatment of cancer. Moreover, the conversions of quercetin to its metabolites must be considered while assessing the efficacy and bioavailability of quercetin for further pharmacological use. The conjugation of xenobiotics with quercetin alters the reactivity of quercetin, but there are some metabolites of quercetin in conjugated form which showed beneficial biological activities. It is important to investigate further mechanisms of action of quercetin, especially in terms of suppressing carcinogenicity in rodents. The results obtained from the current epidemiological studies shows that there is shortage of evidence of quercetin intake for the prevention of human cancer. There is a need to conduct further epidemiological studies to evaluate the role of quercetin in human cancer prevention. Updating the database related to dietary flavonoids will deliver significant information for future epidemiological studies. The use of quercetin in the field of pharmaceuticals is limited because of its poor water solubility and oral bioavailability. In order to enhance the solubility and bioavailability of quercetin inside human body, various scientific approaches have been taken into consideration, including the application of novel drug delivery systems such as nanoparticles and liposomes. These and additional approaches may help us to understand the full potential of quercetin in cancer prevention and therapy.

**Acknowledgments:** This article is the outcome of an in-house financially non-supported study.

**Author Contributions:** All authors have directly participated in the planning or drafting of the manuscript and read and approved the final version.

**Conflicts of Interest:** The authors declare no conflict of interest.

## References

1.  Surh, Y.J. Cancer chemoprevention with dietary phytochemicals. *Nat. Rev. Cancer* **2003**, *3*, 768–780. [CrossRef] [PubMed]
2.  Russo, G.L. Ins and outs of dietary phytochemicals in cancer chemoprevention. *Biochem. Pharmacol.* **2007**, *74*, 533–544. [CrossRef] [PubMed]
3.  Kris-Etherton, P.; Lefevre, M.; Beecher, G.; Gross, M.; Keen, C.; Etherton, T. Bioactive compounds in nutrition and health-research methodologies for establishing biological function: The antioxidant and anti-inflammatory effects of flavonoids on atherosclerosis. *Annu. Rev. Nutr.* **2004**, *24*, 511–538. [CrossRef] [PubMed]
4.  Kim, J.; Lee, H.J.; Lee, K.W. Naturally occurring phytochemicals for the prevention of Alzheimer's disease. *J. Neurochem.* **2010**, *112*, 1415–1430. [CrossRef] [PubMed]
5.  Lee, K.W.; Bode, A.M.; Dong, Z. Molecular targets of phytochemicals for cancer prevention. *Nat. Rev. Cancer* **2011**, *11*, 211–218. [CrossRef] [PubMed]
6.  Crowe, F.L.; Roddam, A.W.; Key, T.J.; Appleby, P.N.; Overvad, K.; Jakobsen, M.U.; Tjønneland, A.; Hansen, L.; Boeing, H.; Weikert, C. Fruit and vegetable intake and mortality from ischaemic heart disease: Results from

the European Prospective Investigation into Cancer and Nutrition (EPIC)-Heart study. *Eur. Heart J.* **2011**, *32*, 1235–1243. [CrossRef] [PubMed]

7.   Benavente-Garcia, O.; Castillo, J. Update on uses and properties of citrus flavonoids: New findings in anticancer, cardiovascular, and anti-inflammatory activity. *J. Agric. Food. Chem.* **2008**, *56*, 6185–6205. [CrossRef] [PubMed]

8.   Kanadaswami, C.; Lee, L.T.; Lee, P.P.; Hwang, J.J.; Ke, F.C.; Huang, Y.T.; Lee, M.T. The antitumor activities of flavonoids. *In Vivo* **2005**, *19*, 895–909.

9.   Canivenc-Lavier, M.C.; Vernevaut, M.F.; Totis, M.; Siess, M.H.; Magdalou, J.; Suschetet, M. Comparative effects of flavonoids and model inducers on drug-metabolizing enzymes in rat liver. *Toxicology* **1996**, *114*, 19–27. [CrossRef]

10.  Shih, H.; Pickwell, G.V.; Quattrochi, L.C. Differential effects of flavonoid compounds on tumor promoter-induced activation of the human CYP1A2 enhancer. *Arch. Biochem.* **2000**, *373*, 287–294. [CrossRef] [PubMed]

11.  Murakami, A.; Ashida, H.; Terao, J. Multitargeted cancer prevention by quercetin. *Cancer Lett.* **2008**, *269*, 315–325. [CrossRef] [PubMed]

12.  Mendoza-Wilson, A.M.; Glossman-Mitnik, D. CHIH-DFT determination of the molecular structure, infrared and ultraviolet spectra of the flavonoid quercetin. *J. Mol. Struc. Theochem.* **2004**, *681*, 71–76. [CrossRef]

13.  Mendoza, E.; Burd, R. Quercetin as a systemic chemopreventative agent: Structural and functional mechanisms. *Mini. Rev. Med. Chem.* **2011**, *11*, 1216–1221. [CrossRef] [PubMed]

14.  Russo, G.L.; Russo, M.; Spagnuolo, C.; Tedesco, I.; Bilotto, S.; Iannitti, R.; Palumbo, R. Quercetin: A pleiotropic kinase inhibitor against cancer. In *Advances in Nutrition and Cancer*; Springer: Berlin/Heidelberg, Geramny, 2014; pp. 185–205.

15.  Sak, K. Site-specific anticancer effects of dietary flavonoid quercetin. *Nutr. Cancer* **2014**, *66*, 177–193. [CrossRef] [PubMed]

16.  Brito, A.F.; Ribeiro, M.; Abrantes, A.M.; Pires, A.S.; Teixo, R.J.; Tralhao, G.J.; Botelho, M.F. Quercetin in Cancer Treatment, Alone or in Combination with Conventional Therapeutics? *Curr. Med. Chem.* **2015**, *22*, 3025–3039. [CrossRef] [PubMed]

17.  Cook, N.; Samman, S. Flavonoids, chemistry, metabolism, cardioprotective effects, and dietary sources. *J. Nutr. Biochem.* **1996**, *7*, 66–76. [CrossRef]

18.  Materska, M. Quercetin and its derivatives: Chemical structure and bioactivity—A review. *Pol. J. Food Nutr. Sci.* **2008**, *58*, 407–413.

19.  Williams, C.A.; Grayer, R.J. Anthocyanins and other flavonoids. *Nat. Prod. Rep.* **2004**, *21*, 539–573. [CrossRef] [PubMed]

20.  Biesaga, M.; Pyrzynska, K. Analytical procedures for determination of quercetin and its glycosides in plant material. *Crit. Rev. Chem.* **2009**, *39*, 95–107. [CrossRef]

21.  Hollman, P.C.; Bijsman, M.N.; van Gameren, Y.; Cnossen, E.P.; de Vries, J.H.; Katan, M.B. The sugar moiety is a major determinant of the absorption of dietary flavonoid glycosides in man. *Free Radic. Res.* **1999**, *31*, 569–573. [CrossRef] [PubMed]

22.  Chen, X.; Mukwaya, E.; Wong, M.; Zhang, Y. A systematic review on biological activities of prenylated flavonoids. *Pharm. Biol.* **2014**, *52*, 655–660. [CrossRef] [PubMed]

23.  Inui, S.; Hosoya, T.; Shimamura, Y.; Masuda, S.; Ogawa, T.; Kobayashi, H.; Shirafuji, K.; Moli, R.T.; Kozone, I.; Shin-ya, K.; et al. Solophenols B–D and Solomonin: New Prenylated Polyphenols Isolated from Propolis Collected from The Solomon Islands and Their Antibacterial Activity. *J. Agric. Food Chem.* **2012**, *60*, 11765–11770. [CrossRef] [PubMed]

24.  Jia, S.; Ma, C.; Wang, J. Studies on flavonoid constituents isolated from the leaves of *Glycyrrhiza uralensis* Fisch. *Acta Pharm. Sin.* **1989**, *25*, 758–762.

25.  De Santiago, O.P.; Juliani, H. Isolation of quercetin 3,7,3′,4′-tetrasulphate from *Flaveria bidentis* L. Otto Kuntze. *Experientia* **1972**, *28*, 380–381. [CrossRef]

26.  Dastagir, G.; Hussain, F.; Khan, A.A. Antibacterial activity of some selected plants of family Zygophyllaceae and Euphorbiaceae. *J. Med. Plants Res.* **2012**, *6*, 5360–5368.

27.  Boots, A.W.; Haenen, G.R.; Bast, A. Health effects of quercetin: From antioxidant to nutraceutical. *Eur. J. Pharmacol.* **2008**, *585*, 325–337. [CrossRef] [PubMed]

28. Heim, K.E.; Tagliaferro, A.R.; Bobilya, D.J. Flavonoid antioxidants: Chemistry, metabolism and structure-activity relationships. *J. Nutr. Biochem.* **2002**, *13*, 572–584. [CrossRef]
29. Dangles, O.; Dufoura, C.; Fargeixa, G. Inhibition of lipid peroxidation by quercetin and quercetin derivatives: Antioxidant and prooxidant effects. *J. Chem. Soc. Perkin Trans.* **2000**, *2*, 1215–1222. [CrossRef]
30. Heijnen, C.G.; Haenen, G.R.; Minou Oostveen, R.; Stalpers, E.M.; Bast, A. Protection of flavonoids against lipid peroxidation: The structure activity relationship revisited. *Free Radic. Res.* **2002**, *36*, 575–581. [CrossRef] [PubMed]
31. Murota, K.; Shimizu, S.; Miyamoto, S.; Izumi, T.; Obata, A.; Kikuchi, M.; Terao, J. Unique uptake and transport of isoflavone aglycones by human intestinal Caco-2 cells: Comparison of isoflavonoids and flavonoids. *J. Nutr.* **2002**, *132*, 1956–1961. [PubMed]
32. Terao, J.; Kawai, Y.; Murota, K. Vegetable flavonoids and cardiovascular disease. *Asia Pac. J. Clin. Nutr.* **2008**, *17*, 291–293. [PubMed]
33. Moon, J.-H.; Nakata, R.; Oshima, S.; Inakuma, T.; Terao, J. Accumulation of quercetin conjugates in blood plasma after the short-term ingestion of onion by women. *Am. J. Physiol. Regul. Integr. Comp. Physiol.* **2000**, *279*, 461–467.
34. Shimoi, K.; Saka, N.; Nozawa, R.; Sato, M.; Amano, I.; Nakayama, T.; Kinae, N. Deglucuronidation of a flavonoid, luteolin monoglucuronide, during inflammation. *Drug Metab. Dispos.* **2001**, *29*, 1521–1524. [PubMed]
35. De Boer, V.C.; Dihal, A.A.; van der Woude, H.; Arts, I.C.; Wolffram, S.; Alink, G.M.; Rietjens, I.M.C.M.; Keijer, J.; Hollman, P.C.H. Tissue distribution of quercetin in rats and pigs. *J. Nutr.* **2005**, *135*, 1718–1725. [PubMed]
36. Kawai, Y.; Nishikawa, T.; Shiba, Y.; Saito, S.; Murota, K.; Shibata, N.; Kobayashi, M.; Kanayama, M.; Uchida, K.; Terao, J. Macrophage as a target of quercetin glucuronides in human atherosclerotic arteries implication in the anti-atherosclerotic mechanism of dietary flavonoids. *J. Biol. Chem.* **2008**, *283*, 9424–9434. [CrossRef] [PubMed]
37. Ahangarpour, A.; Eskandari, M.; Vaezlari, A. Effect of aqueous and hydroalcoholic extract of Beberis vulgaris on insulin secretion from islets of langerhans isolated from male mice. *Armaghane Danesh* **2012**, *17*, 289–298.
38. Ruckenstuhl, C.; Büttner, S.; Carmona-Gutierrez, D.; Eisenberg, T.; Kroemer, G.; Sigrist, S.J.; Fröhlich, K.U.; Madeo, F. The Warburg effect suppresses oxidative stress induced apoptosis in a yeast model for cancer. *PLoS ONE* **2009**, *4*, 4592. [CrossRef]
39. Dajas, F.; Arredondo, F.; Echeverry, C.; Ferreira, M.; Morquio, A.; Rivera, F. Flavonoids and the brain: Evidences and putative mechanisms for a protective capacity. *Curr. Neuropharmacol.* **2005**, *3*, 193–205. [CrossRef]
40. Ossola, B.; Kääriäinen, T.M.; Männistö, P.T. The multiple faces of quercetin in neuroprotection. *Expert Opin. Drug Saf.* **2009**, *8*, 397–409. [CrossRef] [PubMed]
41. Greene, L.A.; Tischler, A.S. Establishment of a noradrenergic clonal line of rat adrenal pheochromocytoma cells which respond to nerve growth factor. *Proc. Natl. Acad. Sci. USA* **1976**, *73*, 2424–2428. [CrossRef] [PubMed]
42. Blasina, M.; Vaamonde, L.; Morquio, A.; Echeverry, C.; Arredondo, F.; Dajas, F. Differentiation induced by *Achyrocline satureioides* (Lam) infusion in PC12 cells. *Phytother. Res.* **2009**, *23*, 1263–1269. [CrossRef] [PubMed]
43. Rydén, M.; Hempstead, B.; Ibáñez, C.F. Differential modulation of neuron survival during development by nerve growth factor binding to the p75 neurotrophin receptor. *J. Biol. Chem.* **1997**, *272*, 16322–16328. [CrossRef] [PubMed]
44. Arredondo, F.; Echeverry, C.; Abin-Carriquiry, J.A.; Blasina, F.; Antúnez, K.; Jones, D.P.; Go, Y.M.; Liang, Y.L.; Dajas, F. After cellular internalization, quercetin causes Nrf2 nuclear translocation, increases glutathione levels, and prevents neuronal death against an oxidative insult. *Free Radic. Biol. Med.* **2010**, *49*, 738–747. [CrossRef] [PubMed]
45. Dajas, F.; Rivera, F.; Blasina, F.; Arredondo, F.; Echeverry, C.; Lafon, L.; Morquio, A.; Heizen, H. Cell culture protection and in vivo neuroprotective capacity of flavonoids. *Neurotox. Res.* **2003**, *5*, 425–432. [CrossRef] [PubMed]
46. Kumar, A.; Sehgal, N.; Kumar, P.; Padi, S.; Naidu, P. Protective effect of quercetin against ICV colchicine-induced cognitive dysfunctions and oxidative damage in rats. *Phytother. Res.* **2008**, *22*, 1563–1569. [CrossRef] [PubMed]

47. Patil, C.S.; Singh, V.P.; Satyanarayan, P.; Jain, N.K.; Singh, A.; Kulkarni, S.K. Protective effect of flavonoids against aging-and lipopolysaccharide-induced cognitive impairment in mice. *Pharmacology* **2003**, *69*, 59–67. [CrossRef] [PubMed]

48. Lu, J.; Zheng, Y.L.; Luo, L.; Wu, D.M.; Sun, D.X.; Feng, Y.J. Quercetin reverses D-galactose induced neurotoxicity in mouse brain. *Behav. Brain Res.* **2006**, *171*, 251–260. [CrossRef] [PubMed]

49. Vissiennon, C.; Nieber, K.; Kelber, O.; Butterweck, V. Route of administration determines the anxiolytic activity of the flavonols kaempferol, quercetin and myricetin—Are they prodrugs? *J. Nutr. Biochem.* **2012**, *23*, 733–740. [CrossRef] [PubMed]

50. Pu, F.; Mishima, K.; Irie, K.; Motohashi, K.; Tanaka, Y.; Orito, K.; Egawa, T.; Kitamura, Y.; Egashira, N.; Iwasaki, K. Neuroprotective effects of quercetin and rutin on spatial memory impairment in an 8-arm radial maze task and neuronal death induced by repeated cerebral ischemia in rats. *J. Pharmacol. Sci.* **2007**, *104*, 329–334. [CrossRef] [PubMed]

51. Schültke, E.; Kamencic, H.; Skihar, V.; Griebel, R.; Juurlink, B. Quercetin in an animal model of spinal cord compression injury: Correlation of treatment duration with recovery of motor function. *Spinal Cord* **2010**, *48*, 112–117. [CrossRef] [PubMed]

52. Youdim, K.A.; Shukitt-Hale, B.; Joseph, J.A. Flavonoids and the brain: Interactions at the blood-brain barrier and their physiological effects on the central nervous system. *Free Radic. Biol. Med.* **2004**, *37*, 1683–1693. [CrossRef] [PubMed]

53. Boots, A.W.; Haenen, G.R.; den Hartog, G.J.; Bast, A. Oxidative damage shifts from lipid peroxidation to thiol arylation by catechol-containing antioxidants. *Biochim. Biophys. Acta* **2002**, *1583*, 279–284. [CrossRef]

54. Bindoli, A.; Valente, M.; Cavallini, L. Inhibitory action of quercetin on xanthine oxidase and xanthine dehydrogenase activity. *Pharmacol. Res. Commun.* **1985**, *17*, 831–839. [CrossRef]

55. Rendon-Mitchell, B.; Ochani, M.; Li, J.; Han, J.; Wang, H.; Yang, H.; Susarla, S.; Czura, C.; Mitchell, R.A.; Chen, G. IFN-γ induces high mobility group box 1 protein release partly through a TNF-dependent mechanism. *J. Immunol.* **2003**, *170*, 3890–3897. [CrossRef] [PubMed]

56. Andersson, U.; Wang, H.; Palmblad, K.; Aveberger, A.C.; Bloom, O.; Erlandsson-Harris, H.; Janson, A.; Kokkola, R.; Zhang, M.; Yang, H.; et al. High mobility group 1 protein (HMG-1) stimulates proinflammatory cytokine synthesis in human monocytes. *J. Exp. Med.* **2000**, *192*, 565–570. [CrossRef] [PubMed]

57. Degryse, B.; Bonaldi, T.; Scaffidi, P.; Müller, S.; Resnati, M.; Sanvito, F.; Arrigoni, G.; Bianchi, M.E. The high mobility group (HMG) boxes of the nuclear protein HMG1 induce chemotaxis and cytoskeleton reorganization in rat smooth muscle cells. *J. Cell Biol.* **2001**, *152*, 1197–1206. [CrossRef] [PubMed]

58. Park, J.S.; Svetkauskaite, D.; He, Q.; Kim, J.Y.; Strassheim, D.; Ishizaka, A.; Abraham, E. Involvement of toll-like receptors 2 and 4 in cellular activation by high mobility group box 1 protein. *J. Biol. Chem.* **2004**, *279*, 7370–7377. [CrossRef] [PubMed]

59. Kokkola, R.; Andersson, A.; Mullins, G.; Östberg, T.; Treutiger, C.J.; Arnold, B.; Nawroth, P.; Andersson, U.; Harris, R.A.; Harris, H.E. RAGE is the major receptor for the proinflammatory activity of HMGB1 in rodent macrophages. *Scand. J. Immunol.* **2005**, *61*, 1–9. [CrossRef] [PubMed]

60. Luo, J.L.; Kamata, H.; Karin, M. IKK/NF-κB signaling: Balancing life and death—A new approach to cancer therapy. *J. Clin. Investig.* **2005**, *115*, 2625–2632. [CrossRef] [PubMed]

61. Briot, A.; Deraison, C.; Lacroix, M.; Bonnart, C.; Robin, A.; Besson, C.; Dubus, P.; Hovnanian, A. Kallikrein 5 induces atopic dermatitis-like lesions through PAR2-mediated thymic stromal lymphopoietin expression in Netherton syndrome. *J. Exp. Med.* **2009**, *206*, 1135–1147. [CrossRef] [PubMed]

62. Wilson, S.R.; Thé, L.; Batia, L.M.; Beattie, K.; Katibah, G.E.; McClain, S.P.; Pellegrino, M.; Estandian, D.; Bautista, D. The epithelial cell-derived atopic dermatitis cytokine TSLP activates neurons to induce itch. *Cell* **2013**, *155*, 285–295. [CrossRef] [PubMed]

63. Zhong, J.; Sharma, J.; Raju, R.; Palapetta, S.M.; Prasad, T.K.; Huang, T.C.; Yoda, A.; Tyner, J.W.; Bodegom, D.V.; Weinstock, D.M. TSLP signaling pathway map: A platform for analysis of TSLP-mediated signaling. *Database* **2014**, *2014*. [CrossRef] [PubMed]

64. Arima, K.; Watanabe, N.; Hanabuchi, S.; Chang, M.; Sun, S.C.; Liu, Y.J. Distinct signal codes generate dendritic cell functional plasticity. *Sci. Signal.* **2010**, *3*, 165. [CrossRef] [PubMed]

65. Bao, L.; Zhang, H.; Chan, L.S. The involvement of the JAK-STAT signaling pathway in chronic inflammatory skin disease atopic dermatitis. *JAK-STAT* **2013**, *2*, 24137. [CrossRef] [PubMed]

66. Horr, B.; Borck, H.; Thurmond, R.; Grösch, S.; Diel, F. STAT1 phosphorylation and cleavage is regulated by the histamine (H4) receptor in human atopic and non-atopic lymphocytes. *Int. Immunopharmacol.* **2006**, *6*, 1577–1585. [CrossRef] [PubMed]

67. Muthian, G.; Bright, J.J. Quercetin, a flavonoid phytoestrogen, ameliorates experimental allergic encephalomyelitis by blocking IL-12 signaling through JAK-STAT pathway in T lymphocyte. *J. Clin. Immunol.* **2004**, *24*, 542–552. [CrossRef] [PubMed]

68. Liao, Y.R.; Lin, J.Y. Quercetin, but not its metabolite quercetin-3-glucuronide, exerts prophylactic immunostimulatory activity and therapeutic antiinflammatory effects on lipopolysaccharide-treated mouse peritoneal macrophages ex vivo. *J. Agric. Food Chem.* **2014**, *62*, 2872–2880. [CrossRef] [PubMed]

69. Senggunprai, L.; Kukongviriyapan, V.; Prawan, A.; Kukongviriyapan, U. Quercetin and EGCG exhibit chemopreventive effects in cholangiocarcinoma cells via suppression of JAK/STAT signaling pathway. *Phytother. Res.* **2014**, *28*, 841–848. [CrossRef] [PubMed]

70. Hämäläinen, M.; Nieminen, R.; Vuorela, P.; Heinonen, M.; Moilanen, E. Anti-inflammatory effects of flavonoids: Genistein, kaempferol, quercetin, and daidzein inhibit STAT-1 and NF-κB activations, whereas flavone, isorhamnetin, naringenin, and pelargonidin inhibit only NF-κB activation along with their inhibitory effect on iNOS expression and NO production in activated macrophages. *Mediators Inflamm.* **2007**, *2007*, 45673. [PubMed]

71. Duo, J.; Ying, G.; Wang, G.W.; Zhang, L. Quercetin inhibits human breast cancer cell proliferation and induces apoptosis via Bcl-2 and Bax regulation. *Mol. Med. Rep.* **2012**, *5*, 1453–1456. [PubMed]

72. Kim, H.; Seo, E.M.; Sharma, A.R.; Ganbold, B.; Park, J.; Sharma, G.; Kang, Y.H.; Song, D.K.; Lee, S.S.; Nam, J.S. Regulation of Wnt signaling activity for growth suppression induced by quercetin in 4T1 murine mammary cancer cells. *Int. J. Oncol.* **2013**, *43*, 1319–1325. [PubMed]

73. Shan, B.E.; Wang, M.X.; Li, R.Q. Quercetin inhibit human SW480 colon cancer growth in association with inhibition of cyclin D1 and survivin expression through Wnt/β-catenin signaling pathway. *Cancer Investig.* **2009**, *27*, 604–612. [CrossRef] [PubMed]

74. Bhat, F.A.; Sharmila, G.; Balakrishnan, S.; Arunkumar, R.; Elumalai, P.; Suganya, S.; Raja, S.P.; Srinivasan, N.; Arunakaran, J. Quercetin reverses EGF-induced epithelial to mesenchymal transition and invasiveness in prostate cancer (PC-3) cell line via EGFR/PI3K/Akt pathway. *J. Nutr. Biochem.* **2014**, *25*, 1132–1139. [CrossRef] [PubMed]

75. Maurya, A.K.; Vinayak, M. Anticarcinogenic action of quercetin by downregulation of phosphatidylinositol 3-kinase (PI3K) and protein kinase C (PKC) via induction of p53 in hepatocellular carcinoma (HepG2) cell line. *Mol. Biol. Rep.* **2015**, *42*, 1419–1429. [CrossRef] [PubMed]

76. Sun, Z.J.; Chen, G.; Hu, X.; Zhang, W.; Liu, Y.; Zhu, L.X.; Zhou, Q.; Zhao, Y.F. Activation of PI3K/Akt/IKK-α/NF-κB signaling pathway is required for the apoptosis-evasion in human salivary adenoid cystic carcinoma: Its inhibition by quercetin. *Apoptosis* **2010**, *15*, 850–863. [CrossRef] [PubMed]

77. Catanzaro, D.; Ragazzi, E.; Vianello, C.; Caparrotta, L.; Montopoli, M. Effect of Quercetin on Cell Cycle and Cyclin Expression in Ovarian Carcinoma and Osteosarcoma Cell Lines. *Nat. Prod. Commun.* **2015**, *10*, 1365–1368. [PubMed]

78. Priyadarsini, R.V.; Murugan, R.S.; Maitreyi, S.; Ramalingam, K.; Karunagaran, D.; Nagini, S. The flavonoid quercetin induces cell cycle arrest and mitochondria-mediated apoptosis in human cervical cancer (HeLa) cells through p53 induction and NF-κB inhibition. *Eur. J. Pharmacol.* **2010**, *649*, 84–91. [CrossRef] [PubMed]

79. Yeh, S.L.; Yeh, C.L.; Chan, S.T.; Chuang, C.H. Plasma rich in quercetin metabolites induces G2/M arrest by upregulating PPAR-γ expression in human A549 lung cancer cells. *Planta Med.* **2011**, *77*, 992–998. [CrossRef] [PubMed]

80. Kim, H.; Moon, J.Y.; Ahn, K.S.; Cho, S.K. Quercetin induces mitochondrial mediated apoptosis and protective autophagy in human glioblastoma U373MG cells. *Oxid. Med. Cell Longev.* **2013**, *2013*, 596496. [CrossRef] [PubMed]

81. Gulati, N.; Laudet, B.; Zohrabian, V.M.; Murali, R.; Jhanwar, M.U. The antiproliferative effect of Quercetin in cancer cells is mediated via inhibition of the PI3K-Akt/PKB pathway. *Anticancer Res.* **2006**, *26*, 1177–1181. [PubMed]

82. Lee, D.H.; Lee, Y.J. Quercetin suppresses hypoxia-induced accumulation of hypoxia-inducible factor-1α (HIF-1α) through inhibiting protein synthesis. *J. Cell. Biochem.* **2008**, *105*, 546–553. [CrossRef] [PubMed]

83. Dihal, A.A.; van der Woude, H.; Hendriksen, P.J.; Charif, H.; Dekker, L.J.; IJsselstijn, L.; De Boer, V.C.J.; Alink, G.M.; Burgers, P.C.; Rietjens, I.M.C.M. Transcriptome and proteome profiling of colon mucosa from quercetin fed F344 rats point to tumor preventive mechanisms, increased mitochondrial fatty acid degradation and decreased glycolysis. *Proteomics* **2008**, *8*, 45–61. [CrossRef] [PubMed]

84. Braganhol, E.; Zamin, L.L.; Canedo, A.D.; Horn, F.; Tamajusuku, A.S.; Wink, M.R.; Salbego, C.; Battastini, A.M. Antiproliferative effect of quercetin in the human U138MG glioma cell line. *Anticancer Drugs* **2006**, *17*, 663–671. [CrossRef] [PubMed]

85. Lamson, D.W.; Brignall, M.S. Antioxidants and cancer, part 3: Quercetin. *Altern. Med. Rev. J. Clin. Ther.* **2000**, *5*, 196–208.

86. Caltagirone, S.; Rossi, C.; Poggi, A.; Ranelletti, F.O.; Natali, P.G.; Brunetti, M.; Aiello, F.B.; Piantelli, M. Flavonoids apigenin and quercetin inhibit melanoma growth and metastatic potential. *Int. J. Cancer* **2000**, *87*, 595–600. [CrossRef]

87. Yang, C.S.; Landau, J.M.; Huang, M.T.; Newmark, H.L. Inhibition of carcinogenesis by dietary polyphenolic compounds. *Annu. Rev. Nutr.* **2001**, *21*, 381–406. [CrossRef] [PubMed]

88. Deschner, E.E.; Ruperto, J.; Wong, G.; Newmark, H.L. Quercetin and rutin as inhibitors of azoxymethanol-induced colonic neoplasia. *Carcinogenesis* **1991**, *12*, 1193–1196. [CrossRef] [PubMed]

89. Dihal, A.A.; de Boer, V.C.; van der Woude, H.; Tilburgs, C.; Bruijntjes, J.P.; Alink, G.M.; Rietjens, I.M.; Woutersen, R.A.; Stierum, R.H. Quercetin, but not its glycosidated conjugate rutin, inhibits azoxymethane-induced colorectal carcinogenesis in F344 rats. *J. Nutr.* **2006**, *136*, 2862–2867. [PubMed]

90. Kato, R.; Nakadate, T.; Yamamoto, S.; Sugimura, T. Inhibition of 12-O-tetradecanoylphorbol-13-acetate-induced tumor promotion and ornithine decarboxylase activity by quercetin: Possible involvement of lipoxygenase inhibition. *Carcinogenesis* **1983**, *4*, 1301–1305. [CrossRef] [PubMed]

91. Khanduja, K.; Gandhi, R.; Pathania, V.; Syal, N. Prevention of N-nitrosodiethylamine-induced lung tumorigenesis by ellagic acid and quercetin in mice. *Food Chem. Toxicol.* **1999**, *37*, 313–318. [CrossRef]

92. Verma, A.K.; Johnson, J.A.; Gould, M.N.; Tanner, M.A. Inhibition of 7, 12-dimethylbenz (a) anthracene-and N-nitrosomethylurea-induced rat mammary cancer by dietary flavonol quercetin. *Cancer Res.* **1988**, *48*, 5754–5758. [PubMed]

93. Kumamoto, T.; Fujii, M.; Hou, D.X. Akt is a direct target for myricetin to inhibit cell transformation. *Mol. Cell. Biochem.* **2009**, *332*, 33–41. [CrossRef] [PubMed]

94. Raman, M.; Chen, W.; Cobb, M. Differential regulation and properties of MAPKs. *Oncogene* **2007**, *26*, 3100–3112. [CrossRef] [PubMed]

95. Hanahan, D.; Weinberg, R.A. Hallmarks of cancer: The next generation. *Cell* **2011**, *144*, 646–674. [CrossRef] [PubMed]

96. Zamin, L.L.; Filippi-Chiela, E.C.; Dillenburg-Pilla, P.; Horn, F.; Salbego, C.; Lenz, G. Resveratrol and quercetin cooperate to induce senescence-like growth arrest in C6 rat glioma cells. *Cancer Sci.* **2009**, *100*, 1655–1662. [CrossRef] [PubMed]

97. Cosan, D.T.; Soyocak, A.; Basaran, A.; Degirmenci, İ.; Gunes, H.V.; Sahin, F.M. Effects of various agents on DNA fragmentation and telomerase enzyme activities in adenocarcinoma cell lines. *Mol. Biol. Rep.* **2011**, *38*, 2463–2469. [CrossRef] [PubMed]

98. Russo, M.; Mupo, A.; Spagnuolo, C.; Russo, G.L. Exploring death receptor pathways as selective targets in cancer therapy. *Biochem. Pharmacol.* **2010**, *80*, 674–682. [CrossRef] [PubMed]

99. Russo, M.; Palumbo, R.; Mupo, A.; Tosto, M.; Iacomino, G.; Scognamiglio, A.; Tedesco, I.; Galano, G.; Russo, G.L. Flavonoid quercetin sensitizes a CD95-resistant cell line to apoptosis by activating protein kinase Cα. *Oncogene* **2003**, *22*, 3330–3342. [CrossRef] [PubMed]

100. Russo, M.; Palumbo, R.; Tedesco, I.; Mazzarella, G.; Russo, P.; Iacomino, G.; Russo, G.L. Quercetin and anti-CD95 (Fas/Apo1) enhance apoptosis in HPB-ALL cell line. *FEBS Lett.* **1999**, *462*, 322–328. [CrossRef]

101. Russo, M.; Nigro, P.; Rosiello, R.; D'Arienzo, R.; Russo, G. Quercetin enhances CD95-and TRAIL-induced apoptosis in leukemia cell lines. *Leukemia* **2007**, *21*, 1130–1133. [CrossRef] [PubMed]

102. Lee, K.W.; Kang, N.J.; Heo, Y.S.; Rogozin, E.A.; Pugliese, A.; Hwang, M.K.; Bowden, G.T.; Bode, A.M.; Lee, H.J.; Dong, Z. Raf and MEK protein kinases are direct molecular targets for the chemopreventive effect of quercetin, a major flavonol in red wine. *Cancer Res.* **2008**, *68*, 946–955. [CrossRef] [PubMed]

103. Denison, M.S.; Pandini, A.; Nagy, S.R.; Baldwin, E.P.; Bonati, L. Ligand binding and activation of the Ah receptor. *Chem. Biol. Interact.* **2002**, *141*, 3–24. [CrossRef]

104. Guengerich, F.P.; Shimada, T. Oxidation of toxic and carcinogenic chemicals by human cytochrome P-450 enzymes. *Chem. Res. Toxicol.* **1991**, *4*, 391–407. [CrossRef] [PubMed]

105. Moon, Y.J.; Wang, X.; Morris, M.E. Dietary flavonoids: Effects on xenobiotic and carcinogen metabolism. *Toxicol. in Vitro* **2006**, *20*, 187–210. [CrossRef] [PubMed]

106. Ashida, H.; Fukuda, I.; Yamashita, T.; Kanazawa, K. Flavones and flavonols at dietary levels inhibit a transformation of aryl hydrocarbon receptor induced by dioxin. *FEBS Lett.* **2000**, *476*, 213–217. [CrossRef]

107. Fukuda, I.; Ashida, H. Suppressive effects of flavonoids on activation of the aryl hydrocarbon receptor induced by dioxins. In *ACS Symposium Series*; Oxford University Press: Cary, NC, USA, 2008; Volume 993, pp. 369–374.

108. Van Der Woude, H.; Ter Veld, M.G.; Jacobs, N.; Van Der Saag, P.T.; Murk, A.J.; Rietjens, I.M. The stimulation of cell proliferation by quercetin is mediated by the estrogen receptor. *Mol. Nutr. Food Res.* **2005**, *49*, 763–771. [CrossRef] [PubMed]

109. Cappelletti, V.; Miodini, P.; Di Fronzo, G.; Daidone, M.G. Modulation of estrogen receptor-β isoforms by phytoestrogens in breast cancer cells. *Int. J. Oncol.* **2006**, *28*, 1185–1191. [CrossRef] [PubMed]

110. Xing, N.; Chen, Y.; Mitchell, S.H.; Young, C.Y. Quercetin inhibits the expression and function of the androgen receptor in LNCaP prostate cancer cells. *Carcinogenesis* **2001**, *22*, 409–414. [CrossRef] [PubMed]

111. Yuan, H.; Gong, A.; Young, C.Y. Involvement of transcription factor Sp1 in quercetin-mediated inhibitory effect on the androgen receptor in human prostate cancer cells. *Carcinogenesis* **2005**, *26*, 793–801. [CrossRef] [PubMed]

112. Duraj, J.; Zazrivcova, K.; Bodo, J.; Sulikova, M.; Sedlak, J. Flavonoid quercetin, but not apigenin or luteolin, induced apoptosis in human myeloid leukemia cells and their resistant variants. *Neoplasma* **2004**, *52*, 273–279.

113. Psahoulia, F.H.; Moumtzi, S.; Roberts, M.L.; Sasazuki, T.; Shirasawa, S.; Pintzas, A. Quercetin mediates preferential degradation of oncogenic Ras and causes autophagy in Ha-RAS-transformed human colon cells. *Carcinogenesis* **2007**, *28*, 1021–1031. [CrossRef] [PubMed]

114. Ishikawa, Y.; Kitamura, M. Anti-apoptotic effect of quercetin: Intervention in the JNK-and ERK-mediated apoptotic pathways. *Kidney Int.* **2000**, *58*, 1078–1087. [CrossRef] [PubMed]

115. Marone, M.; D'Andrilli, G.; Das, N.; Ferlini, C.; Chatterjee, S.; Scambia, G. Quercetin abrogates taxol-mediated signaling by inhibiting multiple kinases. *Exp. Cell Res.* **2001**, *270*, 1–12. [CrossRef] [PubMed]

116. Ferraresi, R.; Troiano, L.; Roat, E.; Lugli, E.; Nemes, E.; Nasi, M.; Pinti, M.; Fernandez, M.I.; Cooper, E.L.; Cossarizza, A. Essential requirement of reduced glutathione (GSH) for the anti-oxidant effect of the flavonoid quercetin. *Free Radic. Res.* **2005**, *39*, 1249–1258. [CrossRef] [PubMed]

117. Robaszkiewicz, A.; Balcerczyk, A.; Bartosz, G. Antioxidative and prooxidative effects of quercetin on A549 cells. *Cell Biol. Int.* **2007**, *31*, 1245–1250. [CrossRef] [PubMed]

118. Zebisch, A.; Czernilofsky, A.P.; Keri, G.; Smigelskaite, J.; Sill, H.; Troppmair, J. Signaling through RAS-RAF-MEK-ERK: From basics to bedside. *Curr. Med. Chem.* **2007**, *14*, 601–623. [CrossRef] [PubMed]

119. Nguyen, T.; Tran, E.; Nguyen, T.; Do, P.; Huynh, T.; Huynh, H. The role of activated MEK-ERK pathway in quercetin-induced growth inhibition and apoptosis in A549 lung cancer cells. *Carcinogenesis* **2004**, *25*, 647–659. [CrossRef] [PubMed]

120. Cho, S.Y.; Park, S.J.; Kwon, M.J.; Jeong, T.S.; Bok, S.H.; Choi, W.Y.; Jeong, W.I.; Ryu, S.Y.; Do, S.H.; Lee, C.S. Quercetin suppresses proinflammatory cytokines production through MAP kinases and NF-κB pathway in lipopolysaccharide-stimulated macrophage. *Mol. Cell. Biochem.* **2003**, *243*, 153–160. [CrossRef] [PubMed]

121. Ross, J.A.; Kasum, C.M. Dietary flavonoids: Bioavailability, metabolic effects, and safety. *Annu. Rev. Nutr.* **2002**, *22*, 19–34. [CrossRef] [PubMed]

122. Neuhouser, M.L. Review: Dietary flavonoids and cancer risk: Evidence from human population studies. *Nutr. Cancer* **2004**, *50*, 1–7. [CrossRef] [PubMed]

123. Hirvonen, T.; Virtamo, J.; Korhonen, P.; Albanes, D.; Pietinen, P. Flavonol and flavone intake and the risk of cancer in male smokers (Finland). *Cancer Causes Control* **2001**, *12*, 797–802. [CrossRef]

124. Hertog, M.G.; Hollman, P.C.; Katan, M.B.; Kromhout, D. Intake of potentially anticarcinogenic flavonoids and their determinants in adults in The Netherlands. *Nutr. Cancer* **1993**, *20*, 21–29. [CrossRef] [PubMed]

125. Stefani, E.D.; Boffetta, P.; Deneo-Pellegrini, H.; Mendilaharsu, M.; Carzoglio, J.C.; Ronco, A.; Olivera, L. Dietary antioxidants and lung cancer risk: A case-control study in Uruguay. *Nutr. Cancer* **1999**, *34*, 100–110. [CrossRef] [PubMed]

126. Nöthlings, U.; Murphy, S.P.; Wilkens, L.R.; Henderson, B.E.; Kolonel, L.N. Flavonols and pancreatic cancer risk the multiethnic cohort study. *Am. J. Epidemiol.* **2007**, *166*, 924–931. [CrossRef] [PubMed]

127. Gates, M.A.; Tworoger, S.S.; Hecht, J.L.; De Vivo, I.; Rosner, B.; Hankinson, S.E. A prospective study of dietary flavonoid intake and incidence of epithelial ovarian cancer. *Int. J. Cancer* **2007**, *121*, 2225–2232. [CrossRef] [PubMed]

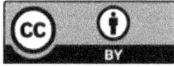

*nutrients*

MDPI

*Review*

# Natural Polyphenols for Prevention and Treatment of Cancer

Yue Zhou [1], Jie Zheng [1], Ya Li [1], Dong-Ping Xu [1], Sha Li [2], Yu-Ming Chen [1] and Hua-Bin Li [1,3,*]

[1]  Guangdong Provincial Key Laboratory of Food, Nutrition and Health, School of Public Health, Sun Yat-sen University, Guangzhou 510080, China; zhouyue3@mail2.sysu.edu.cn (Y.Z.); zhengj37@mail2.sysu.edu.cn (J.Z.); liya28@mail2.sysu.edu.cn (Y.L.); xudp@mail2.sysu.edu.cn (D.-P.X.); chenyum@mail.sysu.edu.cn (Y.-M.C.)
[2]  School of Chinese Medicine, The University of Hong Kong, Hong Kong, China; u3003781@connect.hku.hk
[3]  South China Sea Bioresource Exploitation and Utilization Collaborative Innovation Center, Sun Yat-sen University, Guangzhou 510006, China
*  Correspondence: lihuabin@mail.sysu.edu.cn; Tel.: +86-20-8733-2391

Received: 15 June 2016; Accepted: 12 August 2016; Published: 22 August 2016

**Abstract:** There is much epidemiological evidence that a diet rich in fruits and vegetables could lower the risk of certain cancers. The effect has been attributed, in part, to natural polyphenols. Besides, numerous studies have demonstrated that natural polyphenols could be used for the prevention and treatment of cancer. Potential mechanisms included antioxidant, anti-inflammation as well as the modulation of multiple molecular events involved in carcinogenesis. The current review summarized the anticancer efficacy of major polyphenol classes (flavonoids, phenolic acids, lignans and stilbenes) and discussed the potential mechanisms of action, which were based on epidemiological, in vitro, in vivo and clinical studies within the past five years.

**Keywords:** polyphenol; flavonoid; anticancer; antioxidant; anti-inflammation

## 1. Introduction

Globally, there were approximately 14.1 million new cancer cases in 2012, and the number was estimated to reach 25 million in 2032. Aside from the high incidence, cancer is also one of the leading causes of death. In 2012 alone, there were about 8.2 million cancer-related deaths, which were mainly attributed to lung, gastric, colorectal, liver, breast, prostate and cervical cancer [1]. The situation urges the research of cancer prevention and treatment. In the last two decades, the anticancer effects of natural polyphenols have become a hot topic in many laboratories. Meanwhile, polyphenols are potential candidates for the discovery of anticancer drugs. Polyphenols are defined as compounds having at least one aromatic ring with one or more hydroxyl functional groups attached. Natural polyphenols refer to a large group of plant secondary metabolites ranging from small molecules to highly polymerized compounds [2]. Polyphenols are widely present in foods and beverages of plant origins (e.g., fruits, vegetables, spices, soy, nuts, tea and wine) [3–5]. Based on chemical structures, natural polyphenols can be divided into five classes, including flavonoids, phenolic acids, lignans, stilbenes and other polyphenols. Flavonoids and phenolic acids are the most common classes, and account for about 60% and 30% of all natural polyphenols, respectively (Table 1) [6]. A plethora of studies have documented the anticancer effects of natural polyphenols [7–11]. Noteworthy examples include anthocyanins from blueberries, epigallocatechin gallate (EGCG) from green tea, resveratrol from red wine and isoflavones from soy. The anticancer efficacy of natural polyphenols has largely been attributed to their potent antioxidant and anti-inflammatory activities as well as their abilities to modulate molecular targets and signaling pathways, which were associated with cell survival, proliferation, differentiation, migration, angiogenesis, hormone activities, detoxification enzymes, immune responses, etc. [12,13].

The present review summarized recent discoveries about the anti-carcinogenic properties of natural polyphenols and discussed the mechanisms of action, which were based on evidence from epidemiological studies, laboratory experiments and clinical trials.

**Table 1.** The classification of natural polyphenols.

| Classification | | Representative Members | Major Dietary Sources |
|---|---|---|---|
| flavonoids | anthocyanins | delphinidin, pelargonidin, cyanidin, malvidin | berries, grapes, cherries, plums, pomegranates |
| | flavanols | epicatechin, epigallocatechin, EGCG, procyanidins | apples, pears, legumes, tea, cocoa, wine |
| | flavanones | hesperidin, naringenin | citrus fruits |
| | flavones | apigenin, chrysin, luteolin, | parsley, celery, orange, onions, tea, honey, spices |
| | flavonols | quercetin, kaempferol, myricetin, isorhamnetin, galangin | berries, apples, broccoli, beans, tea |
| | isoflavonoids | genistein, daidzein | soy |
| phenolic acids | hydroxybenzoic acid | ellagic acid, gallic acid | pomegranate, grapes, berries, walnuts, chocolate, wine, green tea |
| | hydroxycinnamic acid | ferulic acid, chlorogenic acid | coffee, cereal grains |
| lignans | | sesamin, secoisolariciresinol diglucoside | flaxseeds, sesame |
| stilbenes | | resveratrol, pterostilbene, piceatannol | grapes, berries, red wine |

## 2. Epidemiological Studies

Evidence from epidemiological studies is inconsistent, especially when considering the results of prospective cohort studies (Table 2). A case-control study in Canada reported favorable effects of a high dietary intake of total flavonoids on lung cancer risks [14]. Apart from this, in a Korean study, for women, the intake of total flavonoids, as well as flavones and anthocyanidins, was inversely associated with the risk of gastric cancer [15]. However, another study in America found no significant association between flavonoids intake and the incidence or survival of gastric cancer [16]. For colorectal cancer, a meta-analysis showed protective roles of high dietary isoflavone intake [17]. Besides, a Spanish case-control study suggested that the dietary intake of total flavonoids (especially certain subclasses) and lignans might decrease colorectal cancer risks [18]. However, large prospective cohorts showed that high habitual consumption of flavonoids could not protect against colorectal cancer [19]. In addition, the Fukuoka study reported no association between total dietary polyphenols and colorectal cancer risks [20]. For hepatocellular carcinoma (HCC), the European Prospective Investigation into Cancer and Nutrition suggested that a high intake of dietary flavanols, but not total flavonoids, might modestly decrease HCC risks [21,22]. In addition, according to a meta-analysis, the risk of breast cancer was reduced in women with a high intake of flavonols and flavones [23]. Studies also suggested that soy isoflavone intake reduced breast cancer risk for Asian women, which was more potent for post-menopausal women (OR 0.46, 95% CI 0.28–0.78) than for premenopausal women (OR 0.63, 95% CI 0.50–0.80). However, for women in Western countries, no significant association could be found, which might due to low levels of isoflavone consumption in the Western population [24,25]. In addition, the estrogen receptor (ER) status might modify the association. For example, a U.S. prospective cohort study showed that a modest inverse trend existed for dietary flavanols intake and the risk of ER-negative breast cancer, but not ER-positive cancer [26]. For prostate cancer, data from a Netherlands cohort study showed that dietary flavonoid intake was correlated with decreased risks of advanced stage prostate cancer but not overall or non-advanced prostate cancer [27]. On the contrary, in a prospective cohort study, the intake of total flavonoids as well as flavan-3-ols, isoflavones, and proanthocyanidins, increased prostate cancer risks [28].

It should be noted that the assessment of polyphenol intakes in many epidemiological studies was based on food questionnaires, which could not provide the exact composition of foods. Therefore, it might be difficult for them to reflect the real impact of natural polyphenols on cancer. In this case, the experimental study in cell culture or animal modes might be a more direct way to assess the anticancer efficacy of natural polyphenols as well as to examine the possible mechanisms involved in this process.

**Table 2.** Dietary polyphenol intake and cancer risks.

| Cancer | Polyphenols | Study Type | Risk Estimates (95% CI) | References |
|--------|-------------|------------|-------------------------|------------|
| lung cancer | flavonoids | case-control study | 0.63 (0.47–0.85) | [14] |
| gastric cancer | flavonoids | case-control study | no significant association | [16] |
|  | flavonoids | case-control study | 0.33 (0.15–0.73) | [15] |
| colorectal cancer | flavonoids | cohort study | no significant association | [19] |
|  | flavonoids and lignans | case-control study | total flavonoids 0.59 (0.35–0.99); lignans 0.59 (0.34–0.99) | [18] |
|  | polyphenols | case-control study | no significant association | [20] |
|  | isoflavones | meta-analysis | 0.76 (0.59–0.98) | [17] |
| HCC | flavanols | cohort study | 0.62 (0.33–0.99) | [22] |
| breast cancer | flavonoids | meta-analysis | flavonols 0.88 (0.80–0.98); flavones 0.83 (0.76–0.91); no significant association for total flavonoids or other subclasses | [23] |
|  | isoflavones | meta-analysis | 0.68 (0.52–0.89) | [25] |
|  | flavanols | cohort study | 0.81 (0.67–0.97) | [26] |
|  | flavonoids | cohort study | 1.15 (1.04–1.27) | [28] |
| prostate cancer | flavonoids | cohort study | total catechin 0.73 (0.57–0.95); epicatechin 0.74 (0.57–0.95); kaempferol 0.78 (0.61–1.00); myricetin 0.71 (0.55–0.91) | [27] |

## 3. Experimental Studies

Accumulating evidence from laboratory studies has supported the anticancer properties of natural polyphenols. Given the vast number of studies, a search of PubMed and Web of Science was conducted to identify relevant peer-reviewed articles published in English within 5 years.

### 3.1. Anthocyanins

Anthocyanins (Figure 1), which occur ubiquitously throughout the plant kingdom, are the basis for the bright attractive red, blue and purple colors of fruits and vegetables. In plants, anthocyanins are usually glycosylated with glucose, galactose, arabinose, rutinose, etc. The aglycone forms are known as anthocyanidin, including cyanidin, delphinidin, peonidin, petunidin, pelargonidin, and malvidin [29].

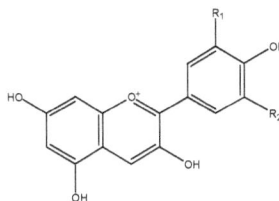

**Figure 1.** The chemical structures of cyanidin ($R_1$ = OH, $R_2$ = H), delphinidin ($R_1$ = $R_2$ = OH), peonidin ($R_1$ = OCH3, $R_2$ = H), petunidin ($R_1$ = OCH3, $R_2$ = OH), pelargonidin ($R_1$ = $R_2$ = H) and malvidin ($R_1$ = $R_2$ = OCH3).

Among anthocyanins, delphinidin possesses strong anticancer activities. Studies have shown that delphinidin treatment induced apoptosis and cell cycle arrest in several types of cancer. This effect might be due to suppression of the NF-κB pathway [30,31]. The over-expression of human epidermal growth factor receptor 2 (HER2) is usually associated with poor prognosis. A study found that two anthocyanins extracted from black rice, peonidin-3-glucoside and cyaniding-3-glucoside, could induce apoptosis and selectively decrease cell proliferation and tumor growth of HER2 positive breast cancer [32]. In addition, peonidin-3-glucoside treatment significantly suppressed invasion and metastasis of lung cancer cells by down-regulating the matrix metalloproteinase (MMP) [33]. In similar ways, cyanidin-3-O-sambubioside from *Acanthopanax sessiliflorus* fruit inhibited angiogenesis and invasion of breast cancer cells [34]. Though anthocyanins are usually considered as antioxidants, a study showed that certain anthocyanins (cyanidin and delphinidin) exhibited oxidative stress-based cytotoxicity to colorectal cancer cells [35]. Another study evaluated the impact of chemical structures on chemopreventive activities of anthocyanins in colon cancer cells. Data indicated that nonacylated monoglycosylated anthocyanins were more potent in inhibiting cancer cell growth, while anthocyanins with pelargonidin aglycone and triglycosylation were weak [36]. On the other hand, it was suggested that a mixture of different anthocyanins might be better than a single one in cancer treatment. For example, a combination of sub-optimal concentration of anthocyanidins synergistically suppressed the growth of lung cancer cells. Meanwhile, in a mice model of lung cancer, a mixture of anthocyanidins from bilberry (0.5 mg/mouse) or delphinidin (1.5 mg/mouse) all inhibited tumor growth, and the effective concentration of delphinidin in the mixture was eight-fold lower than the purified compound [7].

### 3.2. Xanthohumol

Xanthohumol (Figure 2) is a major prenylated chalcone isolated from hops (*Humulus lupulus*). The compound can also be found in beer, but to a much less extent. In some cancers, the xanthohumol-induced cell death was accompanied by apoptosis and S phase cell cycle arrest [37,38]. A study suggested that the apoptosis induced by treatment of xanthohumol (10–40 μM) to HepG2 liver cancer cells was due to modulation of the NF-κB/p53 signaling pathway [39]. Another study reported that xanthohumol treatment (>5 μM) mediated anticancer activity in human liver cancer cells through suppression of the Notch1 signaling pathway [40]. In addition, xanthohumol could block the estrogen signaling pathway. By doing so, it selectively suppressed the growth of ERα-positive breast cancer both in vitro and in vivo [41]. Cysteine X Cysteine chemokine receptor 4 (CXCR4) is over-expressed in many cancers and mediates metastasis of cancer cells to sites expressing its cognate ligand CXCL12. A study demonstrated that xanthohumol treatment dose- and time-dependently decreased expression of CXCR4, thus inhibiting cell invasion induced by CXCL12 in breast and colon cancer cells [42]. In another study, by promoting production of reactive oxygen species (ROS), xanthohumol treatment inhibited the progression of advanced tumor and the growth of poorly differentiated prostate cancer in the transgenic mice [43].

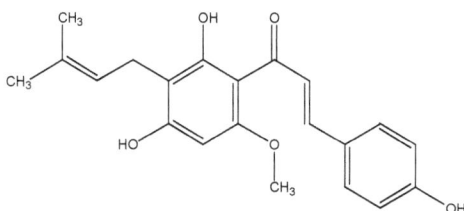

**Figure 2.** The chemical structure of xanthohumol.

### 3.3. Flavanols

Flavanols, also known as flavan-3-ols, have the most complex structures among subclasses of flavonoid. Flavanols include simple monomers (catechins) as well as oligomers and polymers, the latter two are known as proanthocyanidins or condensed tannins. Flavanols can be commonly found in foodstuffs [29].

#### 3.3.1. EGCG

Smoking is a well-established risk factor of lung cancer. A study showed that EGCG (Figure 3) treatment suppressed nicotine-induced migration and invasion of A549 lung cancer cells in vitro as well as in mice through inhibiting angiogenesis and epithelial-mesenchymal transition (EMT) [9]. The effects of EGCG varied with dose. In CL1-5 lung cancer cells, at concentration of 5–20 μM, EGCG effectively suppressed the invasion and migration through suppressing MMP-2 expression. While at higher concentration (>20 μM), it exhibited anti-proliferation activities through induction of $G_2/M$ cell cycle arrest but not apoptosis [44]. Another study found that several gastric cancer cell lines were sensitive to EGCG (100 μM) induced apoptosis due to inhibition of survivin, a potent anti-apoptotic protein [45]. Many signaling pathways might be affected by EGCG treatment. A study showed that EGCG (20 μM) exerted anti-proliferative effects in gastric cancer cell by preventing the β-catenin oncogenic signaling pathway [46]. Another study on colon cancer suggested that the Akt, extracellular signal-related kinase (ERK) 1/2 and alternative p38MAPK signaling pathways were involved in the chemopreventive effects of EGCG [47]. Besides, there is a growing interest in cancer epigenetics in recent years mainly due to the reversibility of epigenetic alterations. Major epigenetic alterations involve DNA methylation, histone modifications and miRNAs [48]. The combination of EGCG and sodium butyrate inhibited DNA methyltransferases and class I histone deacetylases (HDACs) in colorectal cancer cells, thus modulating global DNA methylation and histone modifications [49]. In addition, the cancer stem cell plays a key role in chemoresistance and recurrence. Both in vitro and in vivo studies showed that EGCG could suppress cancer stem cell growth of colorectal cancer as well as breast cancer [50,51]. The anticancer activities of EGCG might involve modulation of hormone activities. It is known that exposure to estrogen is an important risk factor of breast cancer. A study found that EGCG (1 μM) could suppress estrogen (estradiol, E2)-induced breast cancer cell proliferation [52]. In addition, EGCG treatment down-regulated ERα in ER$^+$/PR$^+$ breast cancer cells [53]. Treatment of EGCG (20 μM) also inhibited metastasis of breast cancer cells by restoring the balance between MMP and the tissue inhibitor of matrix metalloproteinase (TIMP). Mechanistic studies suggested that the epigenetic induction of TIMP-3 was a key event in this process, which involved modifying the enhancer of zeste homolog 2 and HDAC1 [54]. Androgen deprivation is a main therapy for prostate cancer. It was reported that EGCG could functionally antagonize androgen, leading to suppression of prostate cancer growth both in vitro and in vivo [55].

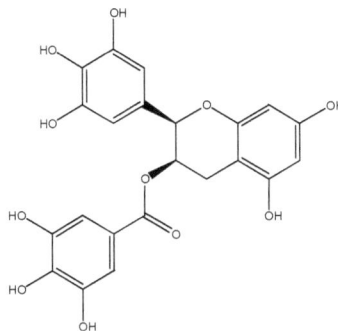

**Figure 3.** The chemical structure of EGCG.

### 3.3.2. Procyanidins

A study suggested that procyanidin C1 from Cinnamomi cortex might be able to prevent TGF-β-induced EMT in the A549 lung cancer cells [56]. Another study found that hexmer form of procyanidins from cocoa inhibited the proliferation (50 and 100 μM), induced apoptosis and $G_2/M$ cell cycle arrest in several colorectal cancer cells, which was possibly mediated by the Akt pathway [57]. Procyanidins from Japanese quince also showed pro-apoptotic effects on Caco-2 colon cancer cells, with the oligomer enriched extract showing a more potent pro-apoptotic activity [58]. Besides, data shows that in breast cancer cells, treatment of procyanidins from evening primrose (25–100 μM gallic acid equivalents) decreased cell viability by promoting apoptosis and reduced cell invasion by suppressing angiogenesis propensity [59].

### 3.4. Flavanones

Flavanones (Figure 4) are abundant in citrus fruits, especially the solid parts of fruit. Major flavanones are naringenin from grapefruit and hesperetin from oranges [2].

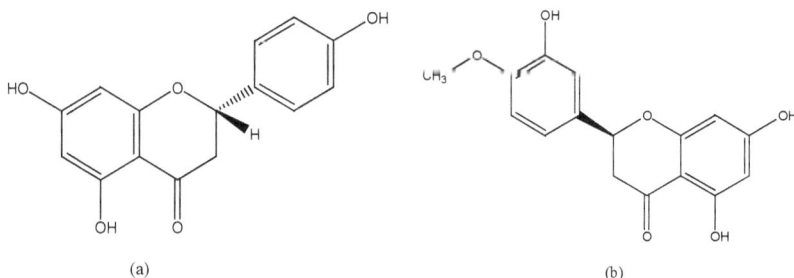

(a)                                                      (b)

**Figure 4.** The chemical structures of naringenin (**a**) and hesperetin (**b**).

### 3.4.1. Naringenin

In A549 lung cancer cells, naringenin treatment enhanced TRAIL-mediated apoptosis by up-regulating the expression of death receptor 5 [60]. Besides, in SGC-7901 gastric cancer cells, naringenin treatment inhibited cancer cell proliferation, invasion, and migration and induced apoptosis, which might be related to its inhibition of the Akt signaling pathway [61]. Another study in colon cancer cells suggested that the pro-apoptotic activity of naringenin was mediated by the p38-dependent pathway [62]. In HCC cells, naringenin could suppress TPA-induced cancer cell invasion by down-regulating multiple signaling pathways, such as the NF-κB pathway, the ERK and c-Jun N-terminal kinase (JNK) signaling pathway [63]. Besides, naringenin treatment to HepG2 liver cancer cells induced mitochondrial-mediated apoptosis and cell cycle arrest through up-regulation of p53 [64]. In breast cancer cells, naringenin demonstrated anti-estrogenic activity in estrogen-rich status and estrogenic activity in estrogen-deficient status [65]. In addition, oral administration of naringenin suppressed breast cancer metastases after surgery by modulating the host immunity [66].

### 3.4.2. Hesperetin

In gastric cancer cells, hesperetin treatment (100–400 μM) decreased cell proliferation and induced mitochondria-mediated apoptosis via promoting intracellular ROS accumulation. Meanwhile, the compound (i.p. 20–40 mg/kg thrice a week) significantly suppressed the growth of xenograft tumors in mice model of gastric cancer [67]. Besides, dietary hesperetin showed anti-proliferative activities against chemical-induced colon carcinogenesis. Oral supplements of hesperetin (20 mg/kg/day) reduced the proliferating cell nuclear antigen, the formation of aberrant crypt foci induced by 1,2-dimethylhydrazine in rat [68]. In breast cancer cells, hesperetin (40–200 μM) induced growth inhibition also involved mitochondria-mediated apoptosis, increased ROS and activation of ASK1/JNK pathway [69]. Cancer cells usually have high levels of glucose uptake and metabolism, which plays an important role in tumor growth. A study suggested that the anti-proliferative effects of hesperetin (50–100 μM) on breast cancer were possibly due to the suppression of glucose uptake [70]. Another study found that hesperetin treatment ($IC_{50}$ 40–90 μM) decreased proliferation and induced apoptosis in PC-3 prostate cancer cells, which was likely mediated by inhibition of the NF-κB pathway [71]. In addition, hesperetin ($IC_{50}$ 650 μM) exhibited potential anticancer effects on cervical cancer cells through the induction of both extrinsic and intrinsic apoptosis [72].

### 3.5. Flavones

Flavones (Figure 5) in food are usually the glycosides of apigenin and luteolin. Important dietary sources of flavones are parsley and celery [2].

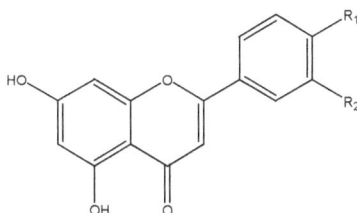

**Figure 5.** The chemical structures of apigenin ($R_1$ = OH, $R_2$ = H), chrysin ($R_1$ = $R_2$ = H) and luteolin ($R_1$ = $R_2$ = OH).

### 3.5.1. Apigenin

Apigenin is a common flavonoid widely distributed in plant-based food, such as orange, parsley, onions, tea and wheat sprouts [73]. In H460 lung cancer cells, treatment of apigenin (40–160 μM) induced apoptosis and DNA damage, which was accompanied by increased production of ROS and $Ca^{2+}$ as well as a change of the Bax/Bcl-2 ratio [74]. Apigenin (20 μg/mL) also induced apoptosis in gastric cancer cells, especially in the undifferentiated gastric cancer cells, while showed little cytotoxicity to normal gastric cells [75]. *Helicobacter pylori* infection is known to cause ulcers and is possibly linked to gastric cancer. Atrophic gastritis was suggested to be a critical step in *Helicobacter pylori*-induced carcinogenesis. A study found that apigenin administration (30–60 mg/kg/week) could prevent *Helicobacter pylori*-induced atrophic gastritis as well as gastric cancer development in Mongolian gerbils [76]. Additionally, apigenin treatment (20–120 μM) suppressed proliferation, invasion and migration of several colorectal cancer cell lines. The compound (50 mg/kg) also inhibited tumor growth and metastasis in the orthotopic colorectal cancer model [77].

About 20% of breast cancer cases are HER2-positive, with amplification of human epidermal growth factor receptor (HER2) or over-expression of HER2 protein. These cancers are usually more aggressive and more resistant to hormone treatment than other types of breast cancer. A study found that apigenin treatment (20–100 μM) significantly suppressed growth and caused apoptosis in HER2-positive breast cancer cells, which was possibly mediated by inhibition of the signal transducer and activator of transcription 3 (STAT3) signaling pathway [78]. Another study reported anticancer effects of apigenin on MDA-MB-231 breast cancer cells in vitro (10–40 μM) and in vivo (5 and 25 mg/kg). Possible mechanisms included induction of $G_2$/M cell cycle arrest and epigenetic alterations. Apigenin inhibited HDACs, which induced acetylation of histone H3 in the p21[WAF1/CIP1] promoter region, leading to enhanced transcription of p21[WAF1/CIP1] [79]. Similar epigenetic effects were also found in prostate cancer. Apigenin inhibited HDACs, especially HDAC1 and HDAC3 expression. In this way apigenin treatment (20–40 μM) induced cell cycle arrest and apoptosis in prostate cancer cells and markedly inhibited tumor growth in mice (oral administration: 20 and

50 µg/mouse/day) [80]. In addition, apigenin treatment to mice (20 and 50 µg/mouse/day) markedly decreased tumor volumes of the prostate, inhibited angiogenesis and completely prevented distant organ metastasis, which at least in part, was mediated by the PI3K/Akt/Forkhead box O (FoxO) signaling pathway [81].

### 3.5.2. Chrysin

Chrysin is a naturally occurring flavone present in honey and propolis as well as the passion flower (*Passiflora caerulea*), and has displayed a variety of bioactivities, such as antioxidant, anti-inflammatory and anticancer activities [82]. AMPK activation is associated with cancer cell apoptosis. A study suggested that AMPK activation might be involved in the growth inhibition and apoptosis induced by chrysin treatment (10 µM) in lung cancer cells, and ROS might be a key regulator in this process [83]. Chrysin (50–100 µM) also exhibited chemopreventive effects in colorectal cancer cells, mainly as a result of TNF-mediated apoptotic cell death, and the aryl hydrocarbon receptor, a transcriptional factor, seemed to modulate this process [84]. Besides, in human triple-negative breast cancer cells, chrysin treatment (5, 10 and 20 µM) dose-dependently inhibited the potential of cancer cells to invasion and migration by down-regulating MMP-10, EMT and the PI3K/Akt signaling pathway [82].

### 3.5.3. Luteolin

Luteolin is abundant in artichoke as well as several spices, including sage, thyme and oregano. In A549 lung cancer cells, luteolin exhibited significant cytotoxic effects (IC$_{50}$ 40.2 µM) through induction of G$_2$ cell cycle arrest and apoptosis. The apoptosis was induced in a mitochondria-dependent pathway and was associated with activation of JNK and inhibition of NF-κB (p65) translocation [85]. The micro-environment around cancer cells is highly involved in cancer progression. It was reported that luteolin (1–10 µM) effectively suppressed IL-4 induced polarization of tumor-associated macrophages (major components of cancer cell micro-environment) and consequently inhibited monocyte recruitment and migration of Lewis lung cancer cells [86]. Hypoxia is another important component of cancer micro-environment. In non-small lung cancer cells, high levels of hypoxia are usually related to EMT. Luteolin treatment (5–50 µM) to non-small lung cancer cells could inhibit hypoxia-induced EMT as well as cell viability, proliferation and motility. The effect was at least partly through suppressing the expression of integrin β1 and FAK [87]. More importantly, luteolin administration (i.p. 10 and 30 mg/kg/day) effectively suppressed tumor growth in a lung cancer mice model with EGF receptor mutation and drug resistance [88].

In a human gastric cancer xenograft model, luteolin treatment (i.p. 10 mg/kg/day) significantly suppressed tumor growth, without causing apparent toxicity or weight loss [89]. Luteolin treatment (20–100 µM) also exhibited cytotoxic effect on several colon cancer cell lines through induction of apoptosis and cell cycle arrest. Meantime, the same treatment exerted no evident toxicity on normal differentiated enterocytes [90,91]. These effects of luteolin might be associated with down-regulation of the IGF-1-mediated PI3K/Akt and ERK1/2 pathways, and suppression of synthesis of sphingosine-1-phosphate and ceramide traffic [90,91]. Besides, it was indicated that ERα was a possible target of luteolin. By down-regulating the expression of ERα, luteolin treatment (10–40 µM) suppressed IGF-1-mediated PI3K/Akt pathway, leading to growth inhibition of MCF-7 breast cancer cells accompanied by cell cycle arrest and apoptosis [92]. In the MDA-MB-231 ER-negative breast cancer cells, luteolin treatment also induced cell cycle arrest and apoptosis possibly mediated by EGFR. In addition, luteolin-supplemented diet (0.01% or 0.05%) effectively reduced tumor burden in mice inoculated with MDA-MB-231 cells [93]. Besides, in LNCaP prostate cancer cells, luteolin treatment (30 µM) arrested the cell cycle at G$_1$/S phase, induced cell apoptosis and inhibited cell invasion. The possible mechanism might be down-regulated expression of prostate-specific antigen by luteolin [94].

## 3.6. Flavonols

Flavonols (Figure 6) are probably the most widely distributed flavonoids in foods, but they are usually present at relatively low concentrations [2]. Representatives of this subclass are quercetin, kaempferol, myricetin, galangin and isorhamnetin.

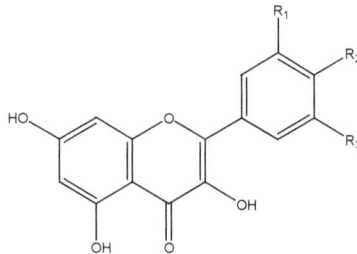

**Figure 6.** The chemical structures of quercetin ($R_1$ = H, $R_2$ = $R_3$ = OH), kaempferol ($R_1$ = $R_3$ = H, $R_2$ = OH), myricetin ($R_1$ = $R_2$ = $R_3$ = OH), galangin ($R_1$ = $R_2$ = $R_3$ = H) and isorhamnetin ($R_1$ = H, $R_2$ = OH, $R_3$ = OCH3).

### 3.6.1. Quercetin

Quercetin treatment ($IC_{50}$ 2.30 ± 0.26 µM) to A549 lung cancer cells induced growth inhibition via apoptosis. In similar ways, quercetin (8.4 mg/kg) inhibited the growth of transplanted lung cancer in nude mice [95]. On the other hand, though exposure of gastric cancer cells to quercetin ($IC_{50}$ 40 and 160 µM in two cell lines respectively) led to pronounced apoptosis, the treatment also induced protective autophagy, which impaired the anticancer effects of quercetin [96]. AMPK-mediated signaling pathway, which participates in regulation of energy homeostasis, is important for the adaptive responses of cancer cells and might be critical for the effects of quercetin. A study found that quercetin treatment (i.p. 50 mg/kg/day) significantly decreased tumor volume in the HCT116 colon cancer xenograft model by reducing AMPK activity. Similarly, by inhibiting AMPK, the apoptosis induced by quercetin (100 µM) was more pronounced under hypoxic conditions than normoxic conditions in HCT116 colon cancer cells [97]. Besides, in a mouse model of colorectal cancer, dietary quercetin supplementation (25 mg/kg/day) alleviated several symptoms of cachexia such as body weight, grip strength and muscle mass [98]. Another study found that quercetin treatment (0.05–0.15 mM) to HCC cells effectively inhibited proliferation and induced apoptosis through up-regulation of Bad and Bax, and concomitant down-regulating Bcl-2 and survivin. Importantly, quercetin (i.p. 40 mg/kg/day) also exhibited excellent inhibition effects on tumor growth in mice [99].

The exposure of MCF-7 breast cancer cells to quercetin (50–200 µM) caused a dose- and time-dependent decrease of proliferation through induction of apoptosis, which was accompanied by up-regulation of Bax and down-regulation of Bcl-2 [100]. The inhibition of insulin receptor signaling by quercetin (100 µM) also impairs proliferation of MDA-MB-231 breast cancer cells. Quercetin feeding (50 µg/mouse/day) resulted in a significant decrease of tumor growth in mice model of breast cancer [101]. In another study, quercetin (1–100 µM) inhibited breast cancer cells growth and migration via reversing EMT, which was linked with the modulation of β-catenin as well as its target genes (e.g., cyclin D1 and c-Myc) [102]. VEGFR2-mediated pathway participates in the angiogenesis in cancer development. Quercetin (34 mg/kg/day) inhibited angiogenesis of breast cancer xenograft in mice, which was performed through suppressing this pathway [103]. Besides, dietary quercetin (200 mg/kg body weight thrice a week) protected against prostate carcinogenesis induced by hormone (testosterone) and carcinogen (*N*-methyl-*N*-nitrosourea) in rats [104]. In another preclinical rat model of prostate cancer, oral administration of quercetin (200 mg/kg/day) prevented cancer development by down-regulating the cell survival, proliferative and anti-apoptotic proteins [105]. In HeLa cervical cancer cells, quercetin treatment ($110.38 \pm 0.66$ µM) led to ROS accumulation to induce apoptosis and $G_2/M$ cell cycle arrest [106].

### 3.6.2. Kaempferol

Kaempferol is a natural flavonol broadly distributed in apples, strawberries, broccoli and beans, and exhibits a wide range of beneficial properties, such as cardioprotective, anti-diabetic, and anti-allergic effects [107]. In A549 lung cancer cells, kaempferol treatment inhibited TGF-β1-induced EMT and migration through suppressing the phosphorylation of smad3 mediated by Akt1 [107]. Another study reported that kaempferol treatment exhibited significant anti-proliferative effects on MKN28 and SGC7901 gastric cancer cells without apparent cytotoxicity to normal gastric epithelial cells. The possible mechanism might be induction of apoptosis and $G_2/M$ cell cycle arrest. More importantly, administration of kaempferol suppressed gastric cancer growth in vivo [108]. In HT-29 colon cancer cells, the treatment of kaempferol (0–60 µM) provoked apoptosis by activating the death receptor pathway and mitochondrial pathway [109]. Another study in SK-HEP-1 human liver cancer cells found $G_2/M$ cell cycle arrest and autophagy following kaempferol treatment, which might be the result of the modulation of CDK1/cyclin B expression and AMPK and AKT signaling pathways [110]. Kaempferol induced apoptosis in MCF-7 breast cancer cells [111]. In the same cell line, treatment of kaempferol (100 µM) also significantly suppressed glucose uptake mediated by GLUT1, which might be another mechanism underlying its anti-proliferative effects [112]. Besides, both in vitro and in vivo study revealed that kaempferol could prevent breast cancer induced by 17β-estradiol or triclosn, an exogenous estrogen [113]. Kaempferol treatment also inhibited breast cell invasion through down-regulating the expression and activity of MMP-9 by blocking the PKCδ/MAPK/AP-1 cascades [114].

### 3.6.3. Myricetin

Myricetin is rich in berries, walnuts and herbs. Myricetin treatment to gastric cancer cells exhibited anti-proliferative effects by inducing apoptosis and cell cycle arrest [115]. In HCT-15 human colon cancer cells, myricetin treatment induced apoptotic cell death by modulating the Bax/Bcl-2-dependent pathway [116]. Similarly, myricetin also decreased the expression of anti-apoptotic survivin and Bcl-2 and increased the expression of pro-apoptotic Bax in HCC cells and in vivo [117].

### 3.6.4. Galangin

Galangin is a naturally occurring flavonoid rich in oregano as well as in *Alpinis officinarum*, a common spice in Asia. Galangin treatment (50–200 µM) to SNU-484 human gastric cancer cells dose- and time-dependently inhibited cell proliferation through induction of apoptosis [118]. Besides, in hepG2 liver cancer cells, galangin treatment (10–30 µM) significantly inhibited chemical-induced cell invasion and metastasis by modulating the PKC/ERK pathway [119]. Another study suggested that galangin (79.8–134 µM) could promote ER stress to suppress the proliferation of HCC cells [120].

### 3.6.5. Isorhamnetin

Isorhamnetin is a natural flavonoid rich in fruits and vegetables as well as tea, and is also an immediate metabolite of quercetin, which has drawn attention for its excellent anti-inflammatory and anticancer activities [121,122].

Treatment of isorhamnetin to A549 lung cancer cells induced apoptotic cell death, which was accompanied by the up-regulation of capase-3, Bax, p53 and the down-regulation of Bcl-2, cyclin D1 and PCNA protein. More importantly, isorhamnetin administration to tumor-bearing mice significantly suppressed tumor growth [123]. Additionally, isorhamnetin suppressed gastric cancer proliferation and invasion, and induced apoptosis by modulating the peroxisome proliferator-activated receptor γ (PPAR γ)-mediated pathway in vitro and in vivo [124]. Another study investigated the anti-proliferative activity of isorhamnetin in several human colorectal cancer cell lines (HT29, HCT116 and SW480), and found that the compound inhibited proliferation of all tested cancer cells by blocking the PI3K/Akt/mTOR pathway [125]. Both in vitro and in vivo experiments suggested that the anticancer property of isorhamnetin in colon cancer involved inhibition of inflammation as well as oncogenic Src activity and consequential loss of nuclear β-catenin [126]. Another study documented the anti-proliferative and pro-apoptotic activities of isorhamnetin in breast cancer cells, which was probably mediated by the Akt and MAPK kinase signaling pathways [121]. Besides, in MDA-MB-231 breast cancer cells, isorhamnetin treatment significantly suppressed cell invasion by down-regulating MMP-2 and MMP-9, which might be associated with the inhibition of p38 MAPK and STAT3 [122].

### 3.7. Isoflavones

Due to structural similarities to estrogen, isoflavones (Figure 7) have been classified as phytoestrogen, another important class of phytochemicals. Genistein and daidzein from soy are representative members of this subclass [2].

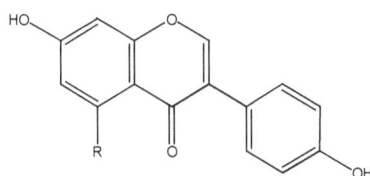

**Figure 7.** The chemical structures of daidzein (R = H) and genistein (R = OH).

### 3.7.1. Daidzein

Data indicated that daidzein was an apoptosis inducer in liver cancer cells and treatment of daidzein (200–600 μM) caused mitochondrial-dependent apoptosis mediated by the Bcl-2 family [127]. In an in vitro study, daidzein (50 μM) as well as its metabolites R-equol and S-equol, suppressed the invasion of MDA-MB-231 human breast cancer cells at least partly through the down-regulation of MMP-2 expression [128]. However, another study reported that daidzein treatment (3–10 μM) up-regulated proto-oncogene BRF2 in ER-positive breast cancer cells but not ER-negative cells. Female mice treated with a high-isoflavone commercial diet showed significantly increased BRF2 expression [129].

### 3.7.2. Genistein

Genistein is the most abundant isoflavonoid contained in soy as well as soy products and is also a major active component of hormonal supplements for menopausal women [10]. In H446 lung cancer cells, genistein treatment (25–75 μM) effectively suppressed the cell proliferation and migration, which was accompanied by induction of apoptosis and $G_2/M$ cell cycle arrest. Importantly, the treatment also suppressed the expression of Forehead box protein M1 and its target genes regulating cell cycle or apoptosis, such as survivin, cyclin B1 and Cdc25. Therefore, the effects of genistein were at least partly mediated by Forkhead box protein M1 [130]. In addition, genistein treatment (15 μM) to gastric cancer cells suppressed the cancer cell stem-like abilities, includingself-renewal, drug resistance and carcinogenicity, which might be due to down-regulation of stemness related genes as well as drug resistance gene ABCG2. Meantime, genistein (i.p. 1.5 mg/kg/day) significantly decreased the weight and size of gastric cancer inoculated in nude mice [131]. Besides, genistein (25–100 μM) exhibited anti-proliferative and pro-apoptotic effects on colon cancer cells. The study indicated that inhibition of oncogenic miR-95, Akt and SGK as well as phosphorylation of Akt could be involved in these anticancer effects. Moreover, genistein treatment (i.p. 20, 50, 80 mg/kg/day) to mice significantly decreased the weight and size of transplanted colorectal cancer [132]. Oral administration of genistein also inhibited angiogenesis and suppressed metastasis of colorectal cancer to distant organs in mice [133].

According to in vitro studies, the anticancer effects of genistein on colorectal cancer might involve the suppression of Wnt, NF-κB signaling pathways [134,135]. Additionally, in nude mice inoculated with liver cancer cells, oral administration of genistein (50 mg/kg/day) significantly suppressed the intrahepatic metastasis [136].

Genistein treatment (5, 10 or 20 μM) elicited growth inhibition of MDA-MB-231 breast cancer cells, which was accompanied by apoptosis and $G_2$/M cell cycle arrest. This effect might be mediated by down-regulation of the NF-κB activity via the Notch-1 pathway [137]. In MCf-7 breast cancer cells, genistein treatment (15 and 30 μM) also inhibited cell growth, induced apoptosis and decreased the $CD44^+CD24^-$ cancer stem cells. Importantly, genistein (i.p. 20 and 50 mg/kg/day) could also target breast cancer stem cells to reduce the volume and weight of xenograft tumors in nude mice. The effects might be correlated with down-regulation of Hedgehog-Gli1 signaling pathway [138]. However, some studies found that genistein has adverse effects on breast cancer treatment. A study suggested that the ERα/ERβ ratio could be a determinant of genistein functions in breast cancer. In breast cancer with a low ERα/ERβ ratio (e.g., T4D7 cells), genistein treatment might be harmless or even beneficial, while in breast cancer with a high ratio (e.g., MCF-7 cells), the treatment might be counterproductive [139]. Genistein (10 μM) could also affect the expression and function of ATP-binding cassette drug transporters in breast cancer cells. The effect resulted in an increase of efflux and resistance of chemotherapeutic drugs (doxorubicin and mitoxantrone) in MCF-7 cells [10]. Moreover, in athymic mice model of breast cancer, a low dose long-term treatment of genistein (≤500 ppm) led to tumor growth as well as more aggressive and advanced phenotypes [140]. Genistein was also reported to have different effects on prostate cancer cells. In LAPC-4 cells with wild androgen receptor, genistein treatment (0.5–50 μM) dose dependently suppressed cell proliferation and androgen receptor. However, in LNCaP cells with T877A mutant androgen receptor, genistein promoted cancer cell growth and androgen receptor at physiological concentration (0.5–5 μM), but showed inhibitory activities at higher concentration. Similar biphasic activities of genistein were also observed in PC-3 cells transfected with androgen receptor mutants [141]. In addition, the exposure of HeLa cervical cancer cells to genistein ($IC_{50}$ 100 μM) led to growth inhibition mediated by apoptosis and $G_2$/M cell cycle arrest and suppressed cell migration by modulating MMP-9 and TIMP-1 [142].

### 3.8. Phenolic Acids

Phenolic acids (Figure 8) can be mainly classified into two groups, hydroxybenzoic acid and hydroxycinnamic acid. Hydroxybenzoic acids present in few edible plants and are not considered to be of high nutritional interest. The other group is more common in food, but its consumption is highly variable, depending on intake of coffee [2].

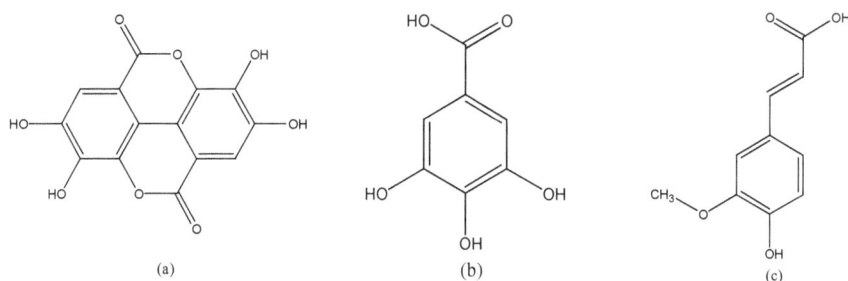

**Figure 8.** The chemical structures of (**a**) ellagic acid; (**b**) gallic acid and (**c**) ferulic acid.

### 3.8.1. Ellagic Acid

Ellagic acid is a dietary flavonoid abundantly in pomegranate, grapes, strawberries and walnuts [143]. Ellagic acid (50–200 μM) exerted anti-proliferative and pro-apoptotic effects in colon cancer cell lines in a concentration dependent manner [144]. Besides, in a chemical-induced liver cancer rat model, oral administration of ellagic acid (30 mg/kg/day) normalized the permeability of mitochondrial outer membrane and alleviated inflammation-mediated cancer cell proliferation [145]. Ellagic acid (10–40 µg/mL) also showed growth inhibitory effects on MCF-7 breast cancer cells, which was accompanied by $G_0/G_1$ cell cycle arrest. The modulation of the TGF-β/Smads signaling pathway was suggested to be the potential mechanism [143]. Furthermore, exposure to ellagic acid (i.p. 50 and 100 mg/kg/day) suppressed tumor growth and angiogenesis in mice implanted with breast cancer cells [146]. In another study, non-cytotoxic dose of ellagic acid (25 and 50 µM) to androgen independent prostate cancer cells markedly suppressed the cell invasion and motility. The effect might be the result of down-regulation of MMPs [147]. Besides, at higher dose (10–100 µM), ellagic acid treatment was found to induce growth inhibition and caspase-dependent apoptosis in PC3 prostate cancer cells in a dose responsive manner [148].

### 3.8.2. Gallic Acid

Gallic acid is widely distributed in plant-based food in free forms as well as part of hydrolyzable tannins. Blackberry, raspberry, walnuts, chocolate, wine, green tea and vinegar are rich sources of the compound. Gallic acid possesses various pharmacological activities, such as anti-microbial, anti-inflammatory and anticancer activities [149,150]. Exposure to gallic acid (3.5 µM) inhibited migration of AGS gastric cancer cells, which was possibly mediated by up-regulation of RhoB as well as down-regulation of AKT/small GTPase signals and NF-κB activity. In addition to this, compared with the control, feeding with gallic acid solution (0.25% and 0.5%) significantly decreased tumor size and weight in mice models of gastric cancer [151]. The ROS-dependent pro-apoptotic effects of gallic acid led to decreased viability of different cancer cells, such as HCT-15 colon cancer cells (200 µM) and LNCaP prostate cancer cells (80 µg/mL) [149,152]. Besides, gallic acid treatment selectively inhibited growth of liver cancer cells through the mitochondria-mediated apoptotic pathways ($IC_{50}$ for cancer cells 28.5 ± 1.6 µg/mL and 22.1 ± 1.4 µg/mL, for normal human hepatocytes 80.9 ± 4.6 µg/mL) [153]. Studies on MCF-7 breast cancer cells also showed that gallic acid treatment inhibited cell proliferation ($IC_{50}$ 80.5 µM) and induced apoptosis via both the extrinsic and intrinsic pathways [150]. Additionally, exposure to gallic acid (25 and 50 µM) suppressed the invasion and migration of PC-3 prostate cancer cells through down-regulation of MMP-2 and MMP-9 [154]. In another study, gallic acid (50, 100, and 200 µM) in PC-3 prostate cancer cells provoked DNA damage and inhibited expression of DNA repair genes, which contributed to gallic-induced growth inhibition [155]. Treatment with gallic acid (10–40 µg/mL) decreased cell viability, proliferation, invasion and angiogenesis HeLa and HTB-35 cervical cancer cells, but showed less cytotoxicity on normal cells (HUVEC), indicating a potential role of the compound in cervical cancer treatment [156].

### 3.8.3. Ferulic Acid

The main dietary sources of ferulic acid are cereal grains, particularly the outer parts of grain. The compound has attracted great attention due to its therapeutic activities against various diseases, such as cancer, cardiovascular and neurodegenerative diseases [157,158].

It was reported that ferulic acid was a pro-oxidant at high concentration or in the presence of metal ions such as copper. Since the increased level of copper was observed in many cancers, and cancer cells are usually under greater oxidative stress than normal cells, the pro-oxidant ability of ferulic acid might lead to selective cytotoxicity to cancer cells [157]. Ferulic acid (10 µg/mL) also decreased cell viability and enhanced efficacy of radiotherapy in two cervical cancer cell lines (HeLa and ME-180), possibly through promotion of ROS [159]. Another study on prostate cancer found that the effects of ferulic acid varied with cell types. Ferulic acid treatment caused cell cycle arrest in PC-3 cells ($IC_{50}$ 300 µM), and led to apoptosis in LNCaP cells ($IC_{50}$ 500 µM) [158].

### 3.9. Lignans

Lignans (Figure 9) are widely present in plants, such as flaxseed, sesame, and seeds of *Arctium lappa*. Secoisolariciresinol diglucoside (SDG) is a natural lignan rich in flaxseed, and can be converted into more biologically active lignans (enterodiol and enterolactone) by human colon bacteria. These lignans are structurally similar to estradiol; thus, they may have anticancer effects for hormone-related cancers, such as breast, prostate and colon cancer. For example, SDG was reported to possess selective estrogen receptor modulating effects and display anti-estrogenic activity in a high estrogen environment. Treatment with SDG (100 ppm in diet) normalized some biomarkers changed by carcinogen in mammary gland tissue of mice [160]. In another study, enterolactone modulated expression of genes involved in cell proliferation and cell cycle of MDA-MB-231 breast cancer cells (IC$_{50}$ 261.9 ± 10.5 µM) [161].

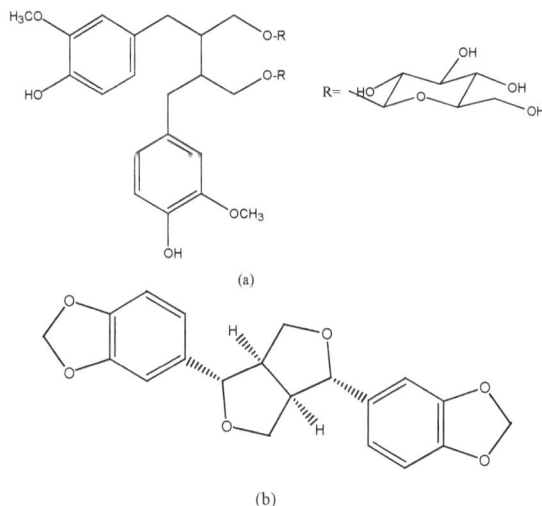

**Figure 9.** The chemical structures of (**a**) Secoisolariciresinol diglucoside and (**b**) sesamin.

Sesamin is a major lipid soluble lignan from sesame oil. Sesamin treatment (1, 10 and 50 µM) dose-dependently decreased cell viability and increased apoptosis in MCF-7 breast cancer cells. The lignan (10–100 µM) also inhibited the pro-angiogenic activity of macrophages in MCF-7 cells by down-regulating VEGF and MMP-9 [162]. Besides, it was suggested that STAT3 played an important role in sesamin (25–125 µM) induced G$_2$/M cell cycle arrest and apoptosis in HepG2 cells [163]. Sesamin (10–100 µg/mL) could suppress lipopolysaccharide-induced proliferation and invasion of PC3 prostate cancer cells by modulating the p38-MAPK and NF-κB signaling pathways. Likewise, sesamin pretreatment (10 mg/kg every three days, injection) suppressed PC3 cells-derived tumor growth triggered by lipopolysaccharide in mice [164].

### 3.10. Stilbenes

Natural stilbenes (Figure 10) are another important group of polyphenols. Though they only exist in a limited group of plant families, the prominent health benefits of resveratrol, an important member of this class, have attracted a lot of studies into natural stilbenes.

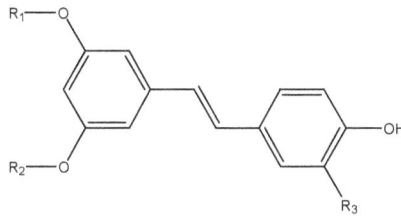

**Figure 10.** The chemical structures of resveratrol ($R_1 = R_2 = R_3 = H$), pterostilbene ($R_1 = R_2 = CH3$, $R_3 = OH$), piceatannol ($R_1 = R_2 = H$, $R_3 = OH$).

### 3.10.1. Resveratrol

Resveratrol is predominantly found in red wine, grapes and berries. X-ray repair cross complement group 1 (XRCC1) participates in base excision repair. It was reported that resveratrol treatment (5–50 μM) could suppress XRCC1 expression, thus leading to enhanced chemosensitivity to etoposide (a topoisomerase II inhibitor) of human non-small-cell lung cancer cell lines [165]. Besides, it was reported that 20 μM resveratrol treatment significantly suppressed invasion and metastasis of A549 lung cancer cells by inhibiting EMT [11].

In gastric cancer cells, resveratrol treatment (25 and 50 μM) arrested cancer cells in the $G_1$ phase, resulting in senescence instead of apoptosis. In similar ways, resveratrol (40 mg/kg/day) inhibited gastric cancer development in nude mice [166]. However, at higher concentrations (50–200 μM), resveratrol induced DNA damage and apoptosis in human gastric adenocarcinoma cells via promoting generation of ROS [167]. Resveratrol induced apoptosis in different colon cancer cell lines via modulating diverse targets. For example, resveratrol induced caspase-8 and -3 dependent apoptosis via ROS-triggered autophagy in HT-29 ($IC_{50}$ 150 μM) and COLO 201 ($IC_{50}$ 75 μM) human colon cancer cells [168]. A study reported that the indirect DNA-damaging effects of resveratrol (30 μM) in colon cancer cells were mainly caused by overproduction of ROS [169]. Another study suggested that the DNA damage induced by resveratrol (25 μM) was due to topoisomerase II poisoning rather than promoting ROS production [170]. Besides, resveratrol (50 μM) suppressed expression of multi-drug resistance protein 1 (MDR1) and drug efflux in drug-resistant colorectal cancer cells [171]. Activating mutations in Kras contribute to sporadic colorectal cancer. An in vivo study found that dietary supplements of resveratrol (equivalent to 105 and 210 mg daily for humans) protected against formation and growth of colorectal cancer by suppressing expression of Kras [172]. In addition, in colorectal cancer patients, following oral administration of resveratrol, high concentrations of resveratrol conjugates (mainly RSV-3-*O*-sulfate, RSV-3-*O*-glucuronide and RSV-4′-*O*-glucuronide) were found in the colorectum. Mixture of these conjugates exhibited synergistic anticancer effects by inducing DNA damage and apoptosis in human colorectal cancer cells. Therefore, despite the low bioavailability of resveratrol, the anti-carcinogenic properties could also be achieved by its main metabolites [173]. Cancer stem cells possess the ability to self-renew and are important for tumor generation. Three signaling pathways regulated the self-renewal of breast cancer stem cells are Wnt, Notch and Hedgehog. It was reported that resveratrol could inhibit the Wnt/β-catenin signaling pathway in breast cancer stem cells. Accordingly, resveratrol treatment (i.v. 100 mg/kg/day) to mice significantly suppressed tumor growth as well as the breast cancer stem cells in primary xenografts [174]. Resveratrol is also a powerful chemopreventive agent against liver cancer. At low concentration, resveratrol treatment (25–100 μM) inhibited metastasis of HCC cells and decreased expression of urokinase-type plasminogen activator (u-PA), which involved down-regulation of the SP-1 signaling pathway [175]. Besides, in *N*-nitrosodiethylamine treated rat, the oral administration of resveratrol (20 mg/kg/day) either at early or advanced stages of liver carcinogenesis was equally effective, possibly mediated by apoptosis [176]. In androgen independent prostate cancer cells, resveratrol treatment (25–100 μM) induced autophagy-mediated cell death [177]. In addition, oral administration of resveratrol (30 mg/kg thrice a week) to mice inhibited proliferation, induced apoptosis, and suppressed angiogenesis and metastasis of prostate cancer [178]. In several cervical cancer cells, resveratrol treatment (150–250 μM) caused cell cycle arrest and apoptosis [179].

### 3.10.2. Pterostilbene

Pterostilbene is a natural dimethoxylated analog of resveratrol mainly found in blueberries. The hydroxyl group substitution with methoxyl groups gives pterostilbene greater lipophilicity, oral bioavailability and biological half-life than resveratrol.

Pinostilbene is a major metabolite of pterostilbene in the colon of mice. At physiologically relevant concentrations (20 and 40 μM), it significantly inhibited cell growth, and induced apoptosis and S phase arrest of human colon cancer cells. Therefore, pinostilbene might be important for the anticancer effects of orally administered pterostilbene [180]. In addition, pterostilbene treatment (25–75 μM) was able to induce apoptosis in breast cancer cells via Bax activation and over-expression [181]. MicroRNAs (miRNAs) are small non-coding RNAs, which control post-transcriptional expression of genes. It was suggested that miRNAs are highly involved in the development of cancer [48]. A study reported that pterostilbene treatment inhibited EMT and metastasis of breast cancer cells (2.5–10 μM). Mechanistic investigations also showed an up-regulation of miR-205 following pterostilbene treatment, which inhibited the Src/Fak signaling and suppressed tumor growth and metastasis in MDA-MD-231-bearing NOD/SCID mice (i.p. 10 mg/kg thrice a week) [182]. Another study found that pterostilbene treatment selectively killed breast cancer stem cells (IC$_{50}$ 25 μM) and sensitized these cells to chemotherapeutic drug paclitaxel [183]. Besides, pterostilbene treatment (80 μM) activated AMPK in both p53 positive and negative human prostate cancer cells, but the cell fate following AMPK activation was affected by p53 status. In p53 positive LNCaP cells, pterostilbene caused G$_1$ cell cycle arrest by increasing p53 expression, while in p53 negative PC3 cells, pterostilbene treatment induced apoptosis [184]. In another study, pterostilbene (i.p. 50 mg/kg/day) inhibited tumor growth in mice models of prostate cancer [185].

### 3.10.3. Piceatannol

Piceatannol is a hydroxylated analog of resveratrol present in a variety of foods, for example, grapes, berries, passion fruit, and white tea. In colorectal cancer cells, piceatannol treatment (30 μM) induced apoptosis by up-regulating miR-129, and thus down-regulating Bcl-2, which is a known target of miR-129 [186]. Besides, in prostate cancer cells, treatment with piceatannol (25 and 50 μM) inhibited proliferation, and induced cell cycle arrest and apoptosis, which might be associated with down-regulated mTOR [187]. Piceatannol was also a potential anti-invasive and anti-metastasis agent on prostate cancer cells. The oral administration of piceatannol (20 mg/kg/day) significantly suppressed the metastasis of prostate cancer to lung in mice [188].

The anticancer activities and potential mechanisms of the polyphenols reviewed in this section were summarized in Table 3 and Figure 11. Due to the critical role of cancer stem cells in cancer development and treatment, the anti-cancer stem cell effects of polyphenols were summarized in Table 4. It should be noted that curcumin is not discussed in this section because it has been extensively reviewed [189–191]. Besides, the bioavailability of many polyphenols is low, which might hamper their application in cancer treatment (Table 5) [6].

**Table 3.** The in vitro and in vivo anticancer activities of natural polyphenols.

| Polyphenol | Study Type | Dose | Main Effects | References |
|---|---|---|---|---|
| **Lung Cancer** | | | | |
| peonidin-3-glucoside | in vitro | 10–40 μM | inhibiting cancer cell invasion, motility, secretion of MMPs and u-PA | [33] |
| anthocyanidins | in vivo | 0.5 mg/mouse | inhibiting tumor growth | [7] |
| xanthohumol | in vitro | 14–42 μM | inducing apoptosis and cell cycle arrest | [38] |
| EGCG | in vitro | 5–20 μM | suppressing cancer cell invasion, migration, MMP-2 | [44] |
| EGCG | in vivo | NA [1] | suppressing nicotine-induced angiogenesis | [9] |
| procyanidin C1 | in vitro | 1.25–40 μg/mL | inhibiting TGF-β-induced EMT | [56] |
| naringenin | in vitro | 100 μM | enhancing TRAIL-mediated apoptosis | [60] |
| apigenin | in vitro | 40–160 μM | inducing apoptosis and DNA damage | [74] |
| chrysin | in vitro | 10 μM | inducing apoptosis, AMPK activation, ROS | [83] |
| luteolin | in vitro | 5–50 μM | inducing apoptosis, cell cycle arrest, inhibiting monocyte recruitment, migration, EMT | [85–87] |
| luteolin | in vivo | 10–30 mg/kg | suppressing tumor growth | [88] |
| quercetin | in vivo | 8.4 mg/kg | suppressing tumor growth | [95] |
| kaempferol | in vitro | 10–50 μM | inhibiting TGF-β1-induced EMT and migration | [107] |
| isorhamnetin | in vivo | NA | suppressing tumor growth | [123] |
| genistein | in vitro | 25–75 μM | suppressing cancer cell proliferation and migration, accompanied by apoptosis and cell cycle arrest | [130] |
| resveratrol | in vitro | 5–50 μM | decreasing XRCC1 expression, enhancing chemosensitivity, suppressing invasion, metastasis | [13,165] |
| **Gastric Cancer** | | | | |
| EGCG | in vitro | 20–100 μM | inducing apoptosis, down-regulating survivin, the β-catenin signaling pathway | [45,46] |
| naringenin | in vitro | 20–80 μM | inducing apoptosis, inhibiting cancer cell proliferation, invasion, migration and the AKT pathway | [61] |
| hesperetin | in vivo | 20–40 mg/kg | suppressing tumor growth | [67] |
| apigenin | in vitro | 20 μg/mL | inducing apoptosis | [75] |
| apigenin | in vivo | 30–60 mg/kg | preventing *Helicobacter pylori*-induced atrophic gastritis and carcinogenesis | [76] |
| luteolin | in vivo | 10 mg/kg | suppressing tumor growth | [89] |
| quercetin | in vitro | 40–160 μM | inducing apoptosis and protective autophagy | [96] |
| kaempferol | in vivo | 20 mg/kg | suppressing tumor growth | [108] |
| myricetin | in vitro | 20–40 μM | inducing apoptosis and cell cycle arrest | [115] |
| galangin | in vitro | 50–200 μM | inducing apoptosis | [118] |
| isorhamnetin | in vivo | 1 mg/kg | increasing PPAR-γ, decreasing Bcl-2 and CD31 | [124] |
| gallic acid | in vivo | 0.25% and 0.5% in water | decreasing tumor size and weight | [151] |
| resveratrol | in vitro | 50–200 μM | inducing apoptosis, DNA damage, ROS production | [167] |
| resveratrol | in vivo | 40 mg/kg | suppressing tumor growth | [166] |

Table 3. *Cont.*

| Polyphenol | Study Type | Dose | Main Effects | References |
|---|---|---|---|---|
| **Colorectal Cancer** | | | | |
| delphinidin | in vitro | 30–240 μM | inducing apoptosis, cell cycle arrest, oxidative stress | [30] |
| cyanidin | in vitro | 100 μM | inducing oxidative stress | [35] |
| EGCG | in vitro | 1–50 μM | inducing epigenetic alteration, apoptosis, MAPK and Akt pathways activation | [47,49] |
| procyanidins | in vitro | 50 and 100 μM | inducing apoptosis and cell cycle arrest | [57] |
| naringenin | in vitro | 50–200 μM | inducing apoptosis | [62] |
| hesperetin | in vivo | 20 mg/kg | suppressing chemical-induced carcinogenesis | [68] |
| apigenin | in vivo | 50 mg/kg | inhibiting tumor growth and metastasis | [77] |
| chrysin | in vitro | 50–100 μM | inducing TNF-mediated apoptotic cell death | [84] |
| luteolin | in vitro | 20-100 μM | inducing apoptosis and cell cycle arrest | [90] |
| quercetin | in vivo | 25–50 mg/kg | suppressing tumor growth by reducing AMPK activity and alleviating cachexia symptoms | [97,98] |
| kaempferol | in vitro | 0–60 μM | inducing apoptosis | [109] |
| myricetin | in vitro | NA | inducing apoptosis | [116] |
| isorhamnetin | in vivo | 200 g/kg in diet | suppressing mortality, tumor number, tumor burden and chemical-induced inflammatory responses | [126] |
| genistein | in vivo | 20–80 mg/kg | decreasing the weight and size of transplanted tumor, inhibiting angiogenesis and metastasis | [132,133] |
| ellagic acid | in vitro | 50–200 μM | inducing apoptosis | [144] |
| gallic acid | in vitro | 200 μM | inducing apoptosis | [149] |
| resveratrol | in vitro | 25–150 μM | inducing apoptosis, DNA damage and suppressing drug resistance | [168–171] |
| resveratrol | in vivo | equal to 105 and 210 mg for human | suppressing tumor development by modulation of Kras | [172] |
| piceatannol | in vitro | 30 μM | inducing apoptosis mediated by miR-129 | [186] |
| **Liver Cancer** | | | | |
| xanthohumol | in vitro | 5–40 μM | inducing apoptosis, modulating the NF-κB/p53 and the Notch1 signaling pathways | [39,40] |
| naringenin | in vitro | 25–200 μM | suppressing TPA-induced cancer cell invasion, inducing apoptosis and cell cycle arrest | [63,64] |
| quercetin | in vivo | 40 mg/kg | suppressing tumor growth | [99] |
| kaempferol | in vitro | 25–100 μM | inducing cell cycle arrest and autophagy | [110] |
| myricetin | in vivo | 100 mg/kg | suppressing chemical-induced carcinogenesis | [117] |
| galangin | in vitro | 10–134 μM | inhibiting chemical-induced cell invasion, metastasis, promoting ER stress | [119,120] |
| daidzein | in vitro | 200–600 μM | inducing apoptosis | [127] |
| genistein | in vivo | 50 mg/kg | suppressing the intrahepatic metastasis | [136] |
| ellagic acid | in vivo | 30 mg/kg | suppressing chemical-induced carcinogenesis | [145] |
| gallic acid | in vitro | 22.1–28.5 μg/mL | inducing apoptosis | [153] |
| sesamin | in vitro | 25–125 μM | inducing apoptosis and cell cycle arrest mediated by STAT3 | [163] |

**Table 3.** *Cont.*

| Polyphenol | Study Type | Dose | Main Effects | References |
|---|---|---|---|---|
| **Liver Cancer** | | | | |
| resveratrol | in vitro | 25–100 μM | inhibiting metastasis, decreasing expression of u-PA, down-regulating the SP-1 signaling pathway | [175] |
| resveratrol | in vivo | 20 mg/kg | suppressing chemical-induced carcinogenesis | [176] |
| **Breast Cancer** | | | | |
| anthocyanins | in vivo | 6 mg/kg | suppressing the growth of HER2-positive tumor | [32] |
| cyanidin-3-O-sambubioside | in vitro | 1–30 μM | inhibiting angiogenesis and invasion | [34] |
| xanthohumol | in vitro | NA | decreasing expression of CXCR4, inhibiting cell invasion induced by CXCL12 | [42] |
| xanthohumol | in vivo | 0.3 and 1.0 mg/kg | blocking the estrogen singling pathway, selectively suppressing the growth of ERα-positive breast cancer | [41] |
| EGCG | in vitro | 1–40 μM | suppressing estrogen-induced cancer cell proliferation, down-regulating ERα, inhibiting metastasis by restoring the balance between MMP and TIMP | [52–54] |
| procyanidins | in vitro | 25–100 μM | inducing apoptosis, reducing invasion, angiogenesis | [59] |
| naringenin | in vivo | 100 mg/kg | suppressing lung metastases by the host immunity | [66] |
| hesperetin | in vitro | 40–200 μM | inducing apoptosis, ROS production and activation of ASK1/JNK pathway, suppressing glucose uptake | [69,70] |
| apigenin | in vitro | 20–100 μM | suppressing growth and causing apoptosis possibly mediated by the STAT3 signaling pathway | [78] |
| apigenin | in vivo | 5–25 mg/kg | inducing cell cycle arrest through epigenetic change | [79] |
| chrysin | in vitro | 5–20 μM | inhibiting cancer cell invasion and migration | [84] |
| luteolin | in vitro | 10–40 μM | down-regulating ERα expression, inducing apoptosis and cell cycle arrest | [92] |
| luteolin | in vivo | 0.01%–0.05% in diet | reducing tumor burden | [93] |
| quercetin | in vitro | 1–200 μM | inducing apoptosis, suppressing the insulin receptor signaling and EMT | [100–102] |
| quercetin | in vivo | 34 mg/kg | inhibiting angiogenesis | [103] |
| kaempferol | in vitro | 100 μM | inducing apoptosis and suppressing glucose uptake | [111,112] |
| kaempferol | in vivo | 100 mg/kg | preventing cancer development induced by estrogen | [113] |
| isorhamnetin | in vitro | 10–40 μM | inhibiting cancer cell adhesion, migration, invasion | [122] |
| daidzein | in vitro | 3–50 μM | decreasing invasion, MMP-2 expression, up-regulating proto-oncogene BRF2 in ER-positive cancer cells | [128,129] |
| genistein | in vitro | 5–20 μM | inducing apoptosis, cell cycle arrest, increasing drug resistance | [10,137] |
| genistein | in vivo | ≤500 ppm | enhancing tumor growth | [140] |
| ellagic acid | in vitro | 10–40 μg/mL | inducing cell cycle arrest | [143] |

**Table 3.** *Cont.*

| Polyphenol | Study Type | Dose | Main Effects | References |
|---|---|---|---|---|
| **Breast Cancer** | | | | |
| ellagic acid | in vivo | 50–100 mg/kg | suppressing tumor growth and angiogenesis | [146] |
| gallic acid | in vitro | 80.5 μM | inducing apoptosis | [150] |
| SDG | in vivo | 100 ppm in diet | normalizing some biomarkers changed by carcinogen | [160] |
| enterolactone | in vitro | 261.9 ± 10.5 μM | modulating expression of genes involved in cell proliferation and cell cycle | [161] |
| sesamin | in vitro | 1–100 μM | inducing apoptosis and inhibiting the pro-angiogenic activity of macrophages | [162] |
| pterostilbene | in vitro | 25–75 μM | inducing apoptosis | [181] |
| pterostilbene | in vivo | 10 mg/kg | suppressing tumor growth and metastasis | [182] |
| **Prostate Cancer** | | | | |
| delphinidin | in vitro | 3–90 μM | inducing apoptosis and cell cycle arrest | [31] |
| xanthohumol | in vivo | 50 μg/mouse | suppressing tumor growth and progression | [43] |
| EGCG | in vivo | 1 mg 3×/week | antagonizing androgen, suppressing tumor growth | [55] |
| hesperetin | in vitro | 40–90 μM | inducing apoptosis, inhibiting the NF-κB pathway | [71] |
| apigenin | in vivo | 20 and 50 μg/mouse | suppressing tumor growth, angiogenesis, metastasis | [81] |
| luteolin | in vitro | 30 μM | inducing apoptosis, cell cycle arrest, inhibiting invasion | [94] |
| quercetin | in vivo | 200 mg/kg | inhibiting carcinogenesis induced by hormone and carcinogen | [104] |
| genistein | in vitro | 0.5–50 μM | different effects dependent on androgen receptor | [141] |
| ellagic acid | in vitro | 10–100 μM | inducing apoptosis, inhibiting cell invasion, motility | [147,148] |
| gallic acid | in vitro | 25–200 μM | provoking DNA damage, down-regulating DNA repair genes, invasion and migration | [154,155] |
| ferulic acid | in vitro | 300–500 μM | inducing apoptosis and cell cycle arrest | [158] |
| sesamin | in vivo | 10 mg/kg | suppressed tumor growth induced by LPS | [164] |
| resveratrol | in vitro | 25–100 μM | inducing autophagy-mediated cell death | [177] |
| resveratrol | in vivo | 30 mg/kg | inducing apoptosis, suppressing angiogenesis and metastasis | [178] |
| pterostilbene | in vitro | 80 μM | inducing apoptosis and cell cycle arrest | [184] |
| pterostilbene | in vivo | 50 mg/kg | suppressing tumor growth | [185] |
| piceatannol | in vitro | 25 and 50 μM | inducing apoptosis and cell cycle arrest | [187] |
| piceatannol | in vivo | 20 mg/kg | suppressing lung metastasis | [188] |
| **Cervical Cancer** | | | | |
| hesperetin | in vitro | 650 μM | inducing apoptosis | [72] |
| quercetin | in vitro | 110.38 μM | inducing apoptosis and cell cycle arrest | [106] |
| genistein | in vitro | 100 μM | inducing apoptosis, cell cycle arrest, suppressing cell migration | [142] |
| gallic acid | in vitro | 10–40 μg/mL | decreasing cell proliferation, invasion, angiogenesis | [156] |
| ferulic acid | in vitro | 10 μg/mL | enhancing efficacy of radiotherapy | [159] |
| resveratrol | in vitro | 150–250 μM | inducing apoptosis and cell cycle arrest | [179] |

[1] NA, stands for not available.

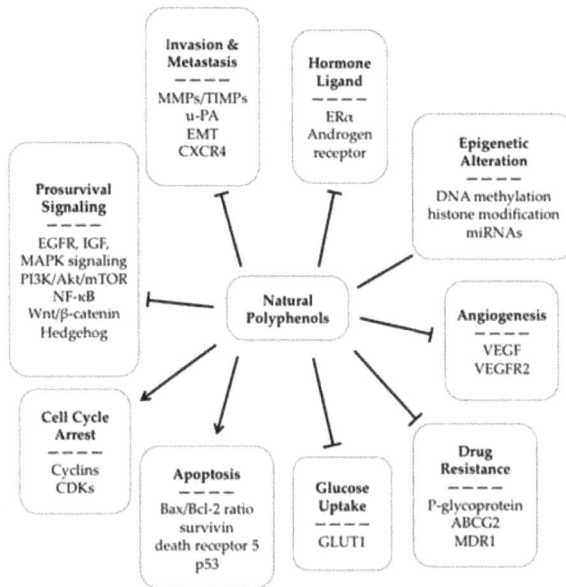

**Figure 11.** Mechanisms of the anticancer activities of natural polyphenols → stands for activation, – for regulation, ⊥ for inhibition.

**Table 4.** The anti-cancer stem cell effects of polyphenols.

| Compound | Cancer | Study Type | Dose | Effect | References |
|---|---|---|---|---|---|
| EGCG | colorectal cancer | in vivo | 100 μM | Inhibiting tumor growth of spheroid-derived cancer stem cell xenografts | [50] |
| | breast cancer | in vivo | 16.5 mg/kg | decreasing tumor growth, the expression of VEGF-D and peritumoral lymphatic vessel density | [51] |
| genistein | gastric cancer | in vivo | 1.5 mg/kg | decreasing tumor weight and size | [131] |
| | breast cancer | in vivo | 20–50 mg/kg | targeting breast cancer stem cells to reduce the growth of xenograft tumors and inhibiting the Hedgehog-Gli1 signaling pathway | [138] |
| resveratrol | breast cancer | in vivo | 100 mg/kg | inhibited the Wnt/β-catenin signaling pathway, tumor growth and cancer stem cells | [174] |
| pterostilbene | breast cancer | in vitro | 25 μM | decreasing cancer stem cells and drug resistance | [183] |

Table 5. The bioavailability of some natural polyphenols.

| Compound | Subject | Treatment | Urine Concentration | Plasm Concentration |
|---|---|---|---|---|
| anthocyanins | human | black berries 200 g (960 μmol) * | total urinary excretion of anthocyanin metabolites 0.160% | NA |
| EGCG | human | 2 mg/kg | NA | mean Cmax 0.09 μmol/L, Tmax 2 h |
| naringenin | human | fresh orange segments 150 g (11.8 mg/150 g fresh weight) * | mean urinary excretion 12.5% | mean Cmax 0.08 μmol/L, Tmax 5.88 h |
| hesperetin | human | fresh orange segments 150 g (79.7 mg/150 g fresh weight) * | mean urinary excretion 4.53% | mean Cmax 0.09 μmol/L, Tmax 7 h |
| quercetin | human | dry shallot skin 1.4 mg/kg (4.93 μmol/g fresh weight) * | NA | mean Cmax 3.95 μmol/L, Tmax 2.78 h |
| isorhamnetin | rat | 0.25 mg/kg | NA | mean Cmax 0.18 μmol/L, Tmax 8 h |
| daidzein | human | soy milk 750 mL/day (5.4 mg/250 mL) * | 148.35 μmol/24 h after 5 days | 196.1 nmol/L after 5 days |
| genistein | human | soy milk 750 mL/day (16.98 mg/250 mL) * | 2077.7 μmol/24 h after 5 days | 797.04 nmol/L after 5 days |
| ellagic acid | human | freeze-dried black raspberry 45 g/day (0.3 mg/g dry weight) * | NA | mean Cmax 0.01 μmol/L, Tmax 1.98 h |
| gallic acid | human | grape skin extract 18 g (0.7 mg/g dry weight) * | 5.9 μmol after 24 h | NA |
| ferulic acid | rat | 5.15 mg/kg | mean urinary excretion 43.4% | mean Cmax 1.68 μmol/L, Tmax 1 h |
| resveratrol | human | 1 mg/kg trans-resveratrol | mean urinary excretion 26% | 0.75 μg/mL after 1.5 h |

* Indicates content of the compound in food; NA, stands for not available.

## 4. Clinical Trials

Though numerous studies have demonstrated that natural polyphenol could be potential candidates for anticancer therapy, clinical studies in this area are relatively few and the therapeutic efficacy is sometimes non-significant. A review of early clinical investigations on polyphenolic phytochemicals suggested tea polyphenols could be used for the prevention of premalignancy, but evidence was less convincing for curcumin and soy isoflavones [192]. Table 6 summarized some clinical evidence about the use of natural polyphenol in cancer treatment. The clinical trials in this section were identified from the PubMed database using the MeSH term "neoplasms" combined with "polyphenols".

Table 6. Summary of clinical trials with polyphenols in various cancers.

| Subject | Treatment | Outcome | References |
|---|---|---|---|
| 54 patients with localized prostate cancer | synthetic genistein (30 mg) daily for 3–6 weeks | decreasing level of serum prostate specific antigen (PSA) | [193] |
| 158 men aged 50–75 with rising prostate specific antigen | isoflavone (60 mg) daily for 12 months | reducing prostate cancer incidence for patients aged 65 or more | [194] |
| 86 patients with localized prostate cancer | soy isoflavone (80 mg total isoflavones, 51 mg aglucon units) daily for 6 weeks | no significant change in serum hormone levels, total cholesterol, or PSA | [195] |
| 10 breast cancer patients undergoing radiotherapy | EGCG (400 mg) thrice daily for 2–8 weeks | enhancing efficacy of radiotherapy | [196] |

**Table 6.** *Cont.*

| Subject | Treatment | Outcome | References |
| --- | --- | --- | --- |
| 147 patients with prostate cancer | flaxseed (30 mg) daily for 30 days | significant inverse association between total urinary enterolignans and enterolactone and Ki67 in the tumor tissue | [197] |
| 87 patients with resected colorectal cancer or polypectomy | flavonoid mixture (20 mg apigenin and 20 mg EGCG) for 3–4 years | reducing recurrence rate of colon neoplasia in patients with resected colon cancer | [198] |
| 5 familial adenomatous polyposis patients with colectomy | curcumin (480 mg) and quercetin (20 mg) thrice daily for 6 months | reducing polyp number and size from baseline without appreciable toxicity | [199] |
| 85 patients with prostate cancer | isoflavones (40 mg) and curcumin (100 mg) daily for 6 months | decreasing level of serum PSA | [200] |
| 44 smokers with 8 or more aberrant crypt foci | curcumin (2 or 4 g) daily for 30 days | decreasing number of aberrant crypt foci | [201] |
| 126 patients with colorectal cancer | curcumin (360 mg) thrice daily for 10–30 days | increasing body weight and expression of p53, suppressing serum level of TNF-$\alpha$ | [202] |

## 5. Conclusions

The epidemiological studies about the relationship between dietary polyphenol consumption and cancer risks yielded different results. The difficult in assessing intake of dietary polyphenols and the diversity of polyphenols might contribute to the inconsistent results. On the other hand, the vast majority of laboratory studies supported anticancer activities of natural polyphenols, such as anthocyanins, EGCG, resveratrol and curcumin. The mechanisms of action mainly included modulation of molecular events and signaling pathways associated with cell survival, proliferation, differentiation, migration, angiogenesis, hormone activities, detoxification enzymes, immune responses, etc. Besides, the anticancer effects of polyphenol varied with cancer types, cell lines and doses. It is of note that some polyphenols, such as genistein and daidzein, have been suggested to have adverse effects on hormone-related cancer. Therefore, the use of these polyphenols in cancer treatment should be cautious. In addition, clinical trials about the anticancer actions of polyphenol are limited. In the future, more epidemiological studies employing biomarkers of polyphenols are needed to assess the impact of dietary polyphenols on cancer risks. Besides, the anticancer activities of more polyphenols need to be assessed and compared, and the mechanisms of action require further study. Larger, randomized clinical trials need to be carried out to provide more reliable evidence. Additionally, the bioavailability of polyphenols should be evaluated and improved. Special attention should be paid to the safety of polyphenols.

**Acknowledgments:** This work was supported by the National Natural Science Foundation of China (No. 81372976), Key Project of Guangdong Provincial Science and Technology Program (No. 2014B020205002), and the Hundred-Talents Scheme of Sun Yat-sen University.

**Author Contributions:** Yue Zhou, Sha Li and Hua-Bin Li conceived this paper; Yue Zhou, Jie Zheng, Ya Li and Dong-Ping Xu wrote this paper; and Sha Li, Yu-Ming Chen and Hua-Bin Li revised the paper.

**Conflicts of Interest:** The authors declare no conflict of interest.

## References

1. WHO | Cancer. Available online: http://www.who.int/mediacentre/factsheets/fs297/en/ (accessed on 17 May 2016).

2.  Manach, C.; Scalbert, A.; Morand, C.; Remesy, C.; Jimenez, L. Polyphenols: Food sources and bioavailability. *Am. J. Clin. Nutr.* **2004**, *79*, 727–747. [PubMed]
3.  Zhou, Y.; Li, Y.; Zhou, T.; Zheng, J.; Li, S.; Li, H.B. Dietary natural products for prevention and treatment of liver cancer. *Nutrients* **2016**, *8*, 156. [CrossRef] [PubMed]
4.  Fu, L.; Xu, B.T.; Xu, X.R.; Qin, X.S.; Gan, R.Y.; Li, H.B. Antioxidant capacities and total phenolic contents of 56 wild fruits from South China. *Molecules* **2010**, *15*, 8602–8617. [CrossRef] [PubMed]
5.  Deng, G.F.; Lin, X.; Xu, X.R.; Gao, L.; Xie, J.; Li, H.B. Antioxidant capacities and total phenolic contents of 56 vegetables. *J. Funct. Foods* **2013**, *5*, 260–266. [CrossRef]
6.  Neveu, V.; Perez-Jimenez, J.; Vos, F.; Crespy, V.; du Chaffaut, L.; Mennen, L.; Knox, C.; Eisner, R.; Cruz, J.; Wishart, D.; et al. Phenol-Explorer: An online comprehensive database on polyphenol contents in foods. *Database* **2010**, *2010*, 24. [CrossRef] [PubMed]
7.  Kausar, H.; Jeyabalan, J.; Aqil, F.; Chabba, D.; Sidana, J.; Singh, I.P.; Gupta, R.C. Berry anthocyanidins synergistically suppress growth and invasive potential of human non-small-cell lung cancer cells. *Cancer Lett.* **2012**, *325*, 54–62. [CrossRef] [PubMed]
8.  Li, A.N.; Li, S.; Zhang, Y.; Xu, X.R.; Chen, Y.; Li, H.B. Resources and biological activities of Natural Polyphenols. *Nutrients* **2014**, *6*, 6020–6047. [CrossRef] [PubMed]
9.  Shi, J.; Liu, F.; Zhang, W.; Liu, X.; Lin, B.; Tang, X. Epigallocatechin-3-gallate inhibits nicotine-induced migration and invasion by the suppression of angiogenesis and epithelial-mesenchymal transition in non-small cell lung cancer cells. *Oncol. Rep.* **2015**, *33*, 2972–2980. [CrossRef] [PubMed]
10. Rigalli, J.P.; Tocchetti, G.N.; Arana, M.R.; Villanueva, S.S.; Catania, V.A.; Theile, D.; Ruiz, M.L.; Weiss, J. The phytoestrogen genistein enhances multidrug resistance in breast cancer cell lines by translational regulation of ABC transporters. *Cancer Lett.* **2016**, *376*, 165–172. [CrossRef] [PubMed]
11. Wang, H.; Zhang, H.; Tang, L.; Chen, H.; Wu, C.; Zhao, M.; Yang, Y.; Chen, X.; Liu, G. Resveratrol inhibits TGF-beta1-induced epithelial-to-mesenchymal transition and suppresses lung cancer invasion and metastasis. *Toxicology* **2013**, *303*, 139–146. [CrossRef] [PubMed]
12. Li, F.; Li, S.; Li, H.B.; Deng, G.F.; Ling, W.H.; Xu, X.R. Antiproliferative activities of tea and herbal infusions. *Food Funct.* **2013**, *4*, 530–538. [CrossRef] [PubMed]
13. Li, F.; Li, S.; Li, H.; Deng, G.; Ling, W.; Wu, S.; Xu, X.; Chen, F. Antiproliferative activity of peels, pulps and seeds of 61 fruits. *J. Funct. Foods* **2013**, *5*, 1298–1309. [CrossRef]
14. Christensen, K.Y.; Naidu, A.; Parent, M.E.; Pintos, J.; Abrahamowicz, M.; Siemiatycki, J.; Koushik, A. The risk of lung cancer related to dietary intake of flavonoids. *Nutr. Cancer* **2012**, *64*, 964–974. [CrossRef] [PubMed]
15. Woo, H.D.; Lee, J.; Choi, I.J.; Kim, C.G.; Lee, J.Y.; Kwon, O.; Kim, J. Dietary flavonoids and gastric cancer risk in a Korean population. *Nutrients* **2014**, *6*, 4961–4973. [CrossRef] [PubMed]
16. Petrick, J.L.; Steck, S.E.; Bradshaw, P.T.; Trivers, K.F.; Abrahamson, P.E.; Engel, L.S.; He, K.; Chow, W.H.; Mayne, S.T.; Risch, H.A.; et al. Dietary intake of flavonoids and oesophageal and gastric cancer: Incidence and survival in the United States of America (USA). *Br. J. Cancer* **2015**, *112*, 1291–1300. [CrossRef] [PubMed]
17. Tse, G.; Eslick, G.D. Soy and isoflavone consumption and risk of gastrointestinal cancer: A systematic review and meta-analysis. *Eur. J. Nutr.* **2016**, *55*, 63–73. [CrossRef] [PubMed]
18. Zamora-Ros, R.; Not, C.; Guino, E.; Lujan-Barroso, L.; Garcia, R.M.; Biondo, S.; Salazar, R.; Moreno, V. Association between habitual dietary flavonoid and lignan intake and colorectal cancer in a Spanish case-control study (the Bellvitge Colorectal Cancer Study). *Cancer Causes Control* **2013**, *24*, 549–557. [CrossRef] [PubMed]
19. Nimptsch, K.; Zhang, X.; Cassidy, A.; Song, M.; O'Reilly, E.J.; Lin, J.H.; Pischon, T.; Rimm, E.B.; Willett, W.C.; Fuchs, C.S.; et al. Habitual intake of flavonoid subclasses and risk of colorectal cancer in 2 large prospective cohorts. *Am. J. Clin. Nutr.* **2016**, *103*, 184–191. [CrossRef] [PubMed]
20. Wang, Z.J.; Ohnaka, K.; Morita, M.; Toyomura, K.; Kono, S.; Ueki, T.; Tanaka, M.; Kakeji, Y.; Maehara, Y.; Okamura, T.; et al. Dietary polyphenols and colorectal cancer risk: The Fukuoka colorectal cancer study. *World J. Gastroenterol.* **2013**, *19*, 2683–2690. [CrossRef] [PubMed]
21. Zamora-Ros, R.; Agudo, A.; Lujan-Barroso, L.; Romieu, I.; Ferrari, P.; Knaze, V.; Bueno-de-Mesquita, H.B.; Leenders, M.; Travis, R.C.; Navarro, C.; et al. Dietary flavonoid and lignan intake and gastric adenocarcinoma risk in the European Prospective Investigation into Cancer and Nutrition (EPIC) study. *Am. J. Clin. Nutr.* **2012**, *96*, 1398–1408. [CrossRef] [PubMed]

22. Zamora-Ros, R.; Fedirko, V.; Trichopoulou, A.; Gonzalez, C.A.; Bamia, C.; Trepo, E.; Nothlings, U.; Duarte-Salles, T.; Serafini, M.; Bredsdorff, L.; et al. Dietary flavonoid, lignan and antioxidant capacity and risk of hepatocellular carcinoma in the European prospective investigation into cancer and nutrition study. *Int. J. Cancer* **2013**, *133*, 2429–2443. [CrossRef] [PubMed]

23. Hui, C.; Qi, X.; Qianyong, Z.; Xiaoli, P.; Jundong, Z.; Mantian, M. Flavonoids, flavonoid subclasses and breast cancer risk: A meta-analysis of epidemiologic studies. *PLoS ONE* **2013**, *8*, e54318. [CrossRef] [PubMed]

24. Chen, M.; Rao, Y.; Zheng, Y.; Wei, S.; Li, Y.; Guo, T.; Yin, P. Association between soy isoflavone intake and breast cancer risk for pre- and post-menopausal women: A meta-analysis of epidemiological studies. *PLoS ONE* **2014**, *9*, e89288. [CrossRef] [PubMed]

25. Xie, Q.; Chen, M.L.; Qin, Y.; Zhang, Q.Y.; Xu, H.X.; Zhou, Y.; Mi, M.T.; Zhu, J.D. Isoflavone consumption and risk of breast cancer: A dose-response meta-analysis of observational studies. *Asia Pac. J. Clin. Nutr.* **2013**, *22*, 118–127. [PubMed]

26. Wang, Y.; Gapstur, S.M.; Gaudet, M.M.; Peterson, J.J.; Dwyer, J.T.; McCullough, M.L. Evidence for an association of dietary flavonoid intake with breast cancer risk by estrogen receptor status is limited. *J. Nutr.* **2014**, *144*, 1603–1611. [CrossRef] [PubMed]

27. Geybels, M.S.; Verhage, B.A.; Arts, I.C.; van Schooten, F.J.; Goldbohm, R.A.; van den Brandt, P.A. Dietary flavonoid intake, black tea consumption, and risk of overall and advanced stage prostate cancer. *Am. J. Epidemiol.* **2013**, *177*, 1388–1398. [CrossRef] [PubMed]

28. Wang, Y.; Stevens, V.L.; Shah, R.; Peterson, J.J.; Dwyer, J.T.; Gapstur, S.M.; McCullough, M.L. Dietary flavonoid and proanthocyanidin intakes and prostate cancer risk in a prospective cohort of US men. *Am. J. Epidemiol.* **2014**, *179*, 974–986. [CrossRef] [PubMed]

29. Crozier, A.; Jaganath, I.B.; Clifford, M.N. Dietary phenolics: Chemistry, bioavailability and effects on health. *Nat. Prod. Rep.* **2009**, *26*, 1001–1043. [CrossRef] [PubMed]

30. Yun, J.M.; Afaq, F.; Khan, N.; Mukhtar, H. Delphinidin, an anthocyanidin in pigmented fruits and vegetables, induces apoptosis and cell cycle arrest in human colon cancer HCT116 cells. *Mol. Carcinog.* **2009**, *48*, 260–270. [CrossRef] [PubMed]

31. Bin, H.B.; Asim, M.; Siddiqui, I.A.; Adhami, V.M.; Murtaza, I.; Mukhtar, H. Delphinidin, a dietary anthocyanidin in pigmented fruits and vegetables: A new weapon to blunt prostate cancer growth. *Cell Cycle* **2008**, *7*, 3320–3326.

32. Liu, W.; Xu, J.; Wu, S.; Liu, Y.; Yu, X.; Chen, J.; Tang, X.; Wang, Z.; Zhu, X.; Li, X. Selective anti-proliferation of HER2-positive breast cancer cells by anthocyanins identified by high-throughput screening. *PLoS ONE* **2013**, *8*, e81586. [CrossRef] [PubMed]

33. Ho, M.L.; Chen, P.N.; Chu, S.C.; Kuo, D.Y.; Kuo, W.H.; Chen, J.Y.; Hsieh, Y.S. Peonidin 3-glucoside inhibits lung cancer metastasis by downregulation of proteinases activities and MAPK pathway. *Nutr. Cancer* **2010**, *62*, 505–516. [CrossRef] [PubMed]

34. Lee, S.J.; Hong, S.; Yoo, S.H.; Kim, G.W. Cyanidin-3-*O*-sambubioside from *Acanthopanax sessiliflorus* fruit inhibits metastasis by downregulating MMP-9 in breast cancer cells MDA-MB-231. *Planta Med.* **2013**, *79*, 1636–1640. [CrossRef] [PubMed]

35. Cvorovic, J.; Tramer, F.; Granzotto, M.; Candussio, L.; Decorti, G.; Passamonti, S. Oxidative stress-based cytotoxicity of delphinidin and cyanidin in colon cancer cells. *Arch. Biochem. Biophys.* **2010**, *501*, 151–157. [CrossRef] [PubMed]

36. Jing, P.; Bomser, J.A.; Schwartz, S.J.; He, J.; Magnuson, B.A.; Giusti, M.M. Structure-function relationships of anthocyanins from various anthocyanin-rich extracts on the inhibition of colon cancer cell growth. *J. Agric. Food Chem.* **2008**, *56*, 9391–9398. [CrossRef] [PubMed]

37. Yong, W.K.; Abd, M.S. Xanthohumol induces growth inhibition and apoptosis in ca ski human cervical cancer cells. *Evid.-Based Complement. Altern. Med.* **2015**, *2015*, 921306. [CrossRef] [PubMed]

38. Yong, W.K.; Ho, Y.F.; Malek, S.N. Xanthohumol induces apoptosis and S phase cell cycle arrest in A549 non-small cell lung cancer cells. *Pharmacogn. Mag.* **2015**, *11*, S275–S283. [PubMed]

39. Zhao, X.; Jiang, K.; Liang, B.; Huang, X. Anticancer effect of xanthohumol induces growth inhibition and apoptosis of human liver cancer through NF-kappaB/p53-apoptosis signaling pathway. *Oncol. Rep.* **2016**, *35*, 669–675. [PubMed]

40. Kunnimalaiyaan, S.; Sokolowski, K.M.; Balamurugan, M.; Gamblin, T.C.; Kunnimalaiyaan, M. Xanthohumol inhibits Notch signaling and induces apoptosis in hepatocellular carcinoma. *PLoS ONE* **2015**, *10*, e127464. [CrossRef] [PubMed]

41. Yoshimaru, T.; Komatsu, M.; Tashiro, E.; Imoto, M.; Osada, H.; Miyoshi, Y.; Honda, J.; Sasa, M.; Katagiri, T. Xanthohumol suppresses oestrogen-signalling in breast cancer through the inhibition of BIG3-PHB2 interactions. *Sci. Rep.* **2014**, *4*, 7355. [CrossRef] [PubMed]

42. Wang, Y.; Chen, Y.; Wang, J.; Chen, J.; Aggarwal, B.B.; Pang, X.; Liu, M. Xanthohumol, a prenylated chalcone derived from hops, suppresses cancer cell invasion through inhibiting the expression of CXCR4 chemokine receptor. *Curr. Mol. Med.* **2012**, *12*, 153–162. [CrossRef] [PubMed]

43. Vene, R.; Benelli, R.; Minghelli, S.; Astigiano, S.; Tosetti, F.; Ferrari, N. Xanthohumol impairs human prostate cancer cell growth and invasion and diminishes the incidence and progression of advanced tumors in TRAMP mice. *Mol. Med.* **2012**, *18*, 1292–1302. [CrossRef] [PubMed]

44. Deng, Y.T.; Lin, J.K. EGCG inhibits the invasion of highly invasive CL1-5 lung cancer cells through suppressing MMP-2 expression via JNK signaling and induces G2/M arrest. *J. Agric. Food Chem.* **2011**, *59*, 13318–13327. [CrossRef] [PubMed]

45. Onoda, C.; Kuribayashi, K.; Nirasawa, S.; Tsuji, N.; Tanaka, M.; Kobayashi, D.; Watanabe, N. (−)-Epigallocatechin-3-gallate induces apoptosis in gastric cancer cell lines by down-regulating survivin expression. *Int. J. Oncol.* **2011**, *38*, 1403–1408. [PubMed]

46. Tanaka, T.; Ishii, T.; Mizuno, D.; Mori, T.; Yamaji, R.; Nakamura, Y.; Kumazawa, S.; Nakayama, T.; Akagawa, M. (−)-Epigallocatechin-3-gallate suppresses growth of AZ521 human gastric cancer cells by targeting the DEAD-box RNA helicase p68. *Free Radic. Biol. Med.* **2011**, *50*, 1324–1335. [CrossRef] [PubMed]

47. Cerezo-Guisado, M.I.; Zur, R.; Lorenzo, M.J.; Risco, A.; Martin-Serrano, M.A.; Alvarez-Barrientos, A.; Cuenda, A.; Centeno, F. Implication of Akt, ERK1/2 and alternative p38MAPK signalling pathways in human colon cancer cell apoptosis induced by green tea EGCG. *Food Chem. Toxicol.* **2015**, *84*, 125–132. [CrossRef] [PubMed]

48. Thakur, V.S.; Deb, G.; Babcook, M.A.; Gupta, S. Plant phytochemicals as epigenetic modulators: Role in cancer chemoprevention. *AAPS J.* **2014**, *16*, 151–163. [CrossRef] [PubMed]

49. Saldanha, S.N.; Kala, R.; Tollefsbol, T.O. Molecular mechanisms for inhibition of colon cancer cells by combined epigenetic-modulating epigallocatechin gallate and sodium butyrate. *Exp. Cell Res.* **2014**, *324*, 40–53. [CrossRef] [PubMed]

50. Toden, S.; Tran, H.M.; Tovar-Camargo, O.A.; Okugawa, Y.; Goel, A. Epigallocatechin-3-gallate targets cancer stem-like cells and enhances 5-fluorouracil chemosensitivity in colorectal cancer. *Oncotarget* **2016**, *7*, 16158–16171. [CrossRef] [PubMed]

51. Mineva, N.D.; Paulson, K.E.; Naber, S.P.; Yee, A.S.; Sonenshein, G.E. Epigallocatechin-3-gallate inhibits stem-like inflammatory breast cancer cells. *PLoS ONE* **2013**, *8*, e73464.

52. Tu, S.H.; Ku, C.Y.; Ho, C.T.; Chen, C.S.; Huang, C.S.; Lee, C.H.; Chen, L.C.; Pan, M.H.; Chang, H.W.; Chang, C.H.; et al. Tea polyphenol (−)-epigallocatechin-3-gallate inhibits nicotine- and estrogen-induced alpha9-nicotinic acetylcholine receptor upregulation in human breast cancer cells. *Mol. Nutr. Food Res.* **2011**, *55*, 455–466. [CrossRef] [PubMed]

53. De Amicis, F.; Russo, A.; Avena, P.; Santoro, M.; Vivacqua, A.; Bonofiglio, D.; Mauro, L.; Aquila, S.; Tramontano, D.; Fuqua, S.A.; et al. In vitro mechanism for downregulation of ER-alpha expression by epigallocatechin gallate in ER+/PR+ human breast cancer cells. *Mol. Nutr. Food Res.* **2013**, *57*, 840–853. [CrossRef] [PubMed]

54. Deb, G.; Thakur, V.S.; Limaye, A.M.; Gupta, S. Epigenetic induction of tissue inhibitor of matrix metalloproteinase-3 by green tea polyphenols in breast cancer cells. *Mol. Carcinog.* **2015**, *54*, 485–499. [CrossRef] [PubMed]

55. Siddiqui, I.A.; Asim, M.; Hafeez, B.B.; Adhami, V.M.; Tarapore, R.S.; Mukhtar, H. Green tea polyphenol EGCG blunts androgen receptor function in prostate cancer. *FASEB J.* **2011**, *25*, 1198–1207. [CrossRef] [PubMed]

56. Kin, R.; Kato, S.; Kaneto, N.; Sakurai, H.; Hayakawa, Y.; Li, F.; Tanaka, K.; Saiki, I.; Yokoyama, S. Procyanidin C1 from Cinnamomi Cortex inhibits TGF-beta-induced epithelial-to-mesenchymal transition in the A549 lung cancer cell line. *Int. J. Oncol.* **2013**, *43*, 1901–1906. [PubMed]

57. Choy, Y.Y.; Fraga, M.; Mackenzie, G.G.; Waterhouse, A.L.; Cremonini, E.; Oteiza, P.I. The PI3K/Akt pathway is involved in procyanidin-mediated suppression of human colorectal cancer cell growth. *Mol. Carcinog.* **2016**. [CrossRef] [PubMed]

58. Gorlach, S.; Wagner, W.; Podsedek, A.; Szewczyk, K.; Koziolkiewicz, M.; Dastych, J. Procyanidins from Japanese quince (*Chaenomeles japonica*) fruit induce apoptosis in human colon cancer Caco-2 cells in a degree of polymerization-dependent manner. *Nutr. Cancer* **2011**, *63*, 1348–1360. [CrossRef] [PubMed]

59. Lewandowska, U.; Szewczyk, K.; Owczarek, K.; Hrabec, Z.; Podsedek, A.; Sosnowska, D.; Hrabec, E. Procyanidins from evening primrose (*Oenothera paradoxa*) defatted seeds inhibit invasiveness of breast cancer cells and modulate the expression of selected genes involved in angiogenesis, metastasis, and apoptosis. *Nutr. Cancer* **2013**, *65*, 1219–1231. [CrossRef] [PubMed]

60. Jin, C.Y.; Park, C.; Hwang, H.J.; Kim, G.Y.; Choi, B.T.; Kim, W.J.; Choi, Y.H. Naringenin up-regulates the expression of death receptor 5 and enhances TRAIL-induced apoptosis in human lung cancer A549 cells. *Mol. Nutr. Food Res.* **2011**, *55*, 300–309. [CrossRef] [PubMed]

61. Bao, L.; Liu, F.; Guo, H.B.; Li, Y.; Tan, B.B.; Zhang, W.X.; Peng, Y.H. Naringenin inhibits proliferation, migration, and invasion as well as induces apoptosis of gastric cancer SGC7901 cell line by downregulation of AKT pathway. *Tumour Biol.* **2016**. [CrossRef] [PubMed]

62. Song, H.M.; Park, G.H.; Eo, H.J.; Jeong, J.B. Naringenin-Mediated ATF3 Expression Contributes to Apoptosis in Human Colon Cancer. *Biomol. Ther. (Seoul)* **2016**, *24*, 140–146. [CrossRef] [PubMed]

63. Yen, H.R.; Liu, C.J.; Yeh, C.C. Naringenin suppresses TPA-induced tumor invasion by suppressing multiple signal transduction pathways in human hepatocellular carcinoma cells. *Chem. Biol. Interact.* **2015**, *235*, 1–9. [CrossRef] [PubMed]

64. Arul, D.; Subramanian, P. Naringenin (citrus flavonone) induces growth inhibition, cell cycle arrest and apoptosis in human hepatocellular carcinoma cells. *Pathol. Oncol. Res.* **2013**, *19*, 763–770. [CrossRef] [PubMed]

65. Kim, S.; Park, T.I. Naringenin: A partial agonist on estrogen receptor in T47D-KBluc breast cancer cells. *Int. J. Clin. Exp. Med.* **2013**, *6*, 890–899. [PubMed]

66. Qin, L.; Jin, L.; Lu, L.; Lu, X.; Zhang, C.; Zhang, F.; Liang, W. Naringenin reduces lung metastasis in a breast cancer resection model. *Protein Cell* **2011**, *2*, 507–516. [CrossRef] [PubMed]

67. Zhang, J.; Wu, D.; Vikash; Song, J.; Wang, J.; Yi, J.; Dong, W. Hesperetin induces the apoptosis of gastric cancer cells via activating mitochondrial pathway by increasing reactive oxygen species. *Dig. Dis. Sci.* **2015**, *60*, 2985–2995. [CrossRef] [PubMed]

68. Aranganathan, S.; Nalini, N. Antiproliferative efficacy of hesperetin (citrus flavanoid) in 1,2-dimethylhydrazine-induced colon cancer. *Phytother. Res.* **2013**, *27*, 999–1005. [CrossRef] [PubMed]

69. Palit, S.; Kar, S.; Sharma, G.; Das, P.K. Hesperetin induces apoptosis in breast carcinoma by triggering accumulation of ROS and activation of ASK1/JNK pathway. *J. Cell. Physiol.* **2015**, *230*, 1729–1739. [CrossRef] [PubMed]

70. Yang, Y.; Wolfram, J.; Boom, K.; Fang, X.; Shen, H.; Ferrari, M. Hesperetin impairs glucose uptake and inhibits proliferation of breast cancer cells. *Cell Biochem. Funct.* **2013**, *31*, 374–379. [CrossRef] [PubMed]

71. Sambantham, S.; Radha, M.; Paramasivam, A.; Anandan, B.; Malathi, R.; Chandra, S.R.; Jayaraman, G. Molecular mechanism underlying hesperetin-induced apoptosis by in silico analysis and in prostate cancer PC-3 cells. *Asian Pac. J. Cancer Prev.* **2013**, *14*, 4347–4352. [CrossRef] [PubMed]

72. Alshatwi, A.A.; Ramesh, E.; Periasamy, V.S.; Subash-Babu, P. The apoptotic effect of hesperetin on human cervical cancer cells is mediated through cell cycle arrest, death receptor, and mitochondrial pathways. *Fundam. Clin. Pharmacol.* **2013**, *27*, 581–592. [CrossRef] [PubMed]

73. Zhu, Y.; Wu, J.; Li, S.; Wang, X.; Liang, Z.; Xu, X.; Xu, X.; Hu, Z.; Lin, Y.; Chen, H.; et al. Apigenin inhibits migration and invasion via modulation of epithelial mesenchymal transition in prostate cancer. *Mol. Med. Rep.* **2015**, *11*, 1004–1008. [CrossRef] [PubMed]

74. Lu, H.F.; Chie, Y.J.; Yang, M.S.; Lu, K.W.; Fu, J.J.; Yang, J.S.; Chen, H.Y.; Hsia, T.C.; Ma, C.Y.; Ip, S.W.; et al. Apigenin induces apoptosis in human lung cancer H460 cells through caspase- and mitochondria-dependent pathways. *Hum. Exp. Toxicol.* **2011**, *30*, 1053–1061. [CrossRef] [PubMed]

75. Chen, J.; Chen, J.; Li, Z.; Liu, C.; Yin, L. The apoptotic effect of apigenin on human gastric carcinoma cells through mitochondrial signal pathway. *Tumor Biol.* **2014**, *35*, 7719–7726. [CrossRef] [PubMed]

76. Kuo, C.H.; Weng, B.C.; Wu, C.C.; Yang, S.F.; Wu, D.C.; Wang, Y.C. Apigenin has anti-atrophic gastritis and anti-gastric cancer progression effects in Helicobacter pylori-infected Mongolian gerbils. *J. Ethnopharmacol.* **2014**, *151*, 1031–1039. [CrossRef] [PubMed]

77. Chunhua, L.; Donglan, L.; Xiuqiong, F.; Lihua, Z.; Qin, F.; Yawei, L.; Liang, Z.; Ge, W.; Linlin, J.; Ping, Z.; et al. Apigenin up-regulates transgelin and inhibits invasion and migration of colorectal cancer through decreased phosphorylation of AKT. *J. Nutr. Biochem.* **2013**, *24*, 1766–1775. [CrossRef] [PubMed]

78. Seo, H.S.; Jo, J.K.; Ku, J.M.; Choi, H.S.; Choi, Y.K.; Woo, J.K.; Kim, H.I.; Kang, S.Y.; Lee, K.M.; Nam, K.W.; et al. Induction of caspase-dependent extrinsic apoptosis by apigenin through inhibition of signal transducer and activator of transcription 3 (STAT3) signalling in HER2-overexpressing BT-474 breast cancer cells. *Biosci. Rep.* **2015**, *35*, e00276. [CrossRef] [PubMed]

79. Tseng, T.H.; Chien, M.H.; Lin, W.L.; Wen, Y.C.; Chow, J.M.; Chen, C.K.; Kuo, T.C.; Lee, W.J. Inhibition of MDA-MB-231 breast cancer cell proliferation and tumor growth by apigenin through induction of G2/M arrest and histone H3 acetylation-mediated p21 expression. *Environ. Toxicol.* **2016**. [CrossRef] [PubMed]

80. Pandey, M.; Kaur, P.; Shukla, S.; Abbas, A.; Fu, P.; Gupta, S. Plant flavone apigenin inhibits HDAC and remodels chromatin to induce growth arrest and apoptosis in human prostate cancer cells: In vitro and in vivo study. *Mol. Carcinog.* **2012**, *51*, 952–962. [CrossRef] [PubMed]

81. Shukla, S.; Bhaskaran, N.; Babcook, M.A.; Fu, P.; Maclennan, G.T.; Gupta, S. Apigenin inhibits prostate cancer progression in TRAMP mice via targeting PI3K/Akt/FoxO pathway. *Carcinogenesis* **2014**, *35*, 452–460. [CrossRef] [PubMed]

82. Yang, B.; Huang, J.; Xiang, T.; Yin, X.; Luo, X.; Huang, J.; Luo, F.; Li, H.; Li, H.; Ren, G. Chrysin inhibits metastatic potential of human triple-negative breast cancer cells by modulating matrix metalloproteinase-10, epithelial to mesenchymal transition, and PI3K/Akt signaling pathway. *J. Appl. Toxicol.* **2014**, *34*, 105–112. [CrossRef] [PubMed]

83. Shao, J.J.; Zhang, A.P.; Qin, W.; Zheng, L.; Zhu, Y.F.; Chen, X. AMP-activated protein kinase (AMPK) activation is involved in chrysin-induced growth inhibition and apoptosis in cultured A549 lung cancer cells. *Biochem. Biophys. Res. Commun.* **2012**, *423*, 448–453. [CrossRef] [PubMed]

84. Ronnekleiv-Kelly, S.M.; Nukaya, M.; Diaz-Diaz, C.J.; Megna, B.W.; Carney, P.R.; Geiger, P.G.; Kennedy, G.D. Aryl hydrocarbon receptor-dependent apoptotic cell death induced by the flavonoid chrysin in human colorectal cancer cells. *Cancer Lett.* **2016**, *370*, 91–99. [CrossRef] [PubMed]

85. Cai, X.; Ye, T.; Liu, C.; Lu, W.; Lu, M.; Zhang, J.; Wang, M.; Cao, P. Luteolin induced G2 phase cell cycle arrest and apoptosis on non-small cell lung cancer cells. *Toxicol. Vitro* **2011**, *25*, 1385–1391. [CrossRef] [PubMed]

86. Choi, H.J.; Choi, H.J.; Chung, T.W.; Ha, K.T. Luteolin inhibits recruitment of monocytes and migration of Lewis lung carcinoma cells by suppressing chemokine (C-C motif) ligand 2 expression in tumor-associated macrophage. *Biochem. Biophys. Res. Commun.* **2016**, *470*, 101–106. [CrossRef] [PubMed]

87. Ruan, J.; Zhang, L.; Yan, L.; Liu, Y.; Yue, Z.; Chen, L.; Wang, A.Y.; Chen, W.; Zheng, S.; Wang, S.; et al. Inhibition of hypoxia-induced epithelial mesenchymal transition by luteolin in non-small cell lung cancer cells. *Mol. Med. Rep.* **2012**, *6*, 232–238. [PubMed]

88. Hong, Z.; Cao, X.; Li, N.; Zhang, Y.; Lan, L.; Zhou, Y.; Pan, X.; Shen, L.; Yin, Z.; Luo, L. Luteolin is effective in the non-small cell lung cancer model with L858R/T790M EGF receptor mutation and erlotinib resistance. *Br. J. Pharmacol.* **2014**, *171*, 2842–2853. [CrossRef] [PubMed]

89. Lu, J.; Li, G.; He, K.; Jiang, W.; Xu, C.; Li, Z.; Wang, H.; Wang, W.; Wang, H.; Teng, X.; et al. Luteolin exerts a marked antitumor effect in cMet-overexpressing patient-derived tumor xenograft models of gastric cancer. *J. Transl. Med.* **2015**, *13*, 42. [CrossRef] [PubMed]

90. Lim, D.Y.; Cho, H.J.; Kim, J.; Nho, C.W.; Lee, K.W.; Park, J.H. Luteolin decreases IGF-II production and downregulates insulin-like growth factor-I receptor signaling in HT-29 human colon cancer cells. *BMC Gastroenterol.* **2012**, *12*, 9. [CrossRef] [PubMed]

91. Abdel, H.L.; Di Vito, C.; Marfia, G.; Ferraretto, A.; Tringali, C.; Viani, P.; Riboni, L. Sphingosine Kinase 2 and Ceramide Transport as Key Targets of the Natural Flavonoid Luteolin to Induce Apoptosis in Colon Cancer Cells. *PLoS ONE* **2015**, *10*, e143384. [CrossRef] [PubMed]

92. Wang, L.M.; Xie, K.P.; Huo, H.N.; Shang, F.; Zou, W.; Xie, M.J. Luteolin inhibits proliferation induced by IGF-1 pathway dependent ERalpha in human breast cancer MCF-7 cells. *Asian Pac. J. Cancer Prev.* **2012**, *13*, 1431–1437. [CrossRef] [PubMed]

93. Lee, E.J.; Oh, S.Y.; Sung, M.K. Luteolin exerts anti-tumor activity through the suppression of epidermal growth factor receptor-mediated pathway in MDA-MB-231 ER-negative breast cancer cells. *Food Chem. Toxicol.* **2012**, *50*, 4136–4143. [CrossRef] [PubMed]

94. Tsui, K.H.; Chung, L.C.; Feng, T.H.; Chang, P.L.; Juang, H.H. Upregulation of prostate-derived Ets factor by luteolin causes inhibition of cell proliferation and cell invasion in prostate carcinoma cells. *Int. J. Cancer* **2012**, *130*, 2812–2823. [CrossRef] [PubMed]

95. Zheng, S.Y.; Li, Y.; Jiang, D.; Zhao, J.; Ge, J.F. Anticancer effect and apoptosis induction by quercetin in the human lung cancer cell line A-549. *Mol. Med. Rep.* **2012**, *5*, 822–826. [CrossRef] [PubMed]

96. Wang, K.; Liu, R.; Li, J.; Mao, J.; Lei, Y.; Wu, J.; Zeng, J.; Zhang, T.; Wu, H.; Chen, L.; et al. Quercetin induces protective autophagy in gastric cancer cells: Involvement of Akt-mTOR- and hypoxia-induced factor 1alpha-mediated signaling. *Autophagy* **2011**, *7*, 966–978. [CrossRef] [PubMed]

97. Kim, H.S.; Wannatung, T.; Lee, S.; Yang, W.K.; Chung, S.H.; Lim, J.S.; Choe, W.; Kang, I.; Kim, S.S.; Ha, J. Quercetin enhances hypoxia-mediated apoptosis via direct inhibition of AMPK activity in HCT116 colon cancer. *Apoptosis* **2012**, *17*, 938–949. [CrossRef] [PubMed]

98. Velazquez, K.T.; Enos, R.T.; Narsale, A.A.; Puppa, M.J.; Davis, J.M.; Murphy, E.A.; Carson, J.A. Quercetin supplementation attenuates the progression of cancer cachexia in ApcMin/+ mice. *J. Nutr.* **2014**, *144*, 868–875. [CrossRef] [PubMed]

99. Dai, W.; Gao, Q.; Qiu, J.; Yuan, J.; Wu, G.; Shen, G. Quercetin induces apoptosis and enhances 5-FU therapeutic efficacy in hepatocellular carcinoma. *Tumor Biol.* **2015**, *5*, 6307–6313. [CrossRef] [PubMed]

100. Duo, J.; Ying, G.G.; Wang, G.W.; Zhang, L. Quercetin inhibits human breast cancer cell proliferation and induces apoptosis via Bcl-2 and Bax regulation. *Mol. Med. Rep.* **2012**, *5*, 1453–1456. [PubMed]

101. Wang, F.; Yang, Y. Quercetin suppresses insulin receptor signaling through inhibition of the insulin ligand-receptor binding and therefore impairs cancer cell proliferation. *Biochem. Biophys. Res. Commun.* **2014**, *452*, 1028–1033. [CrossRef] [PubMed]

102. Srinivasan, A.; Thangavel, C.; Liu, Y.; Shoyele, S.; Den, R.B.; Selvakumar, P.; Lakshmikuttyamma, A. Quercetin regulates beta-catenin signaling and reduces the migration of triple negative breast cancer. *Mol. Carcinog.* **2016**, *55*, 743–756. [CrossRef] [PubMed]

103. Zhao, X.; Wang, Q.; Yang, S.; Chen, C.; Li, X.; Liu, J.; Zou, Z.; Cai, D. Quercetin inhibits angiogenesis by targeting calcineurin in the xenograft model of human breast cancer. *Eur. J. Pharmacol.* **2016**, *781*, 60–68. [CrossRef] [PubMed]

104. Sharmila, G.; Athirai, T.; Kiruthiga, B.; Senthilkumar, K.; Elumalai, P.; Arunkumar, R.; Arunakaran, J. Chemopreventive effect of quercetin in MNU and testosterone induced prostate cancer of Sprague-Dawley rats. *Nutr. Cancer* **2014**, *66*, 38–46. [CrossRef] [PubMed]

105. Sharmila, G.; Bhat, F.A.; Arunkumar, R.; Elumalai, P.; Raja, S.P.; Senthilkumar, K.; Arunakaran, J. Chemopreventive effect of quercetin, a natural dietary flavonoid on prostate cancer in in vivo model. *Clin. Nutr.* **2014**, *33*, 718–726. [CrossRef] [PubMed]

106. Bishayee, K.; Ghosh, S.; Mukherjee, A.; Sadhukhan, R.; Mondal, J.; Khuda-Bukhsh, A.R. Quercetin induces cytochrome-c release and ROS accumulation to promote apoptosis and arrest the cell cycle in $G_2/M$, in cervical carcinoma: Signal cascade and drug-DNA interaction. *Cell Prolif.* **2013**, *46*, 153–163. [CrossRef] [PubMed]

107. Jo, E.; Park, S.J.; Choi, Y.S.; Jeon, W.K.; Kim, B.C. Kaempferol suppresses transforming growth factor-beta1-induced epithelial-to-mesenchymal transition and migration of A549 lung cancer cells by inhibiting Akt1-mediated phosphorylation of smad3 at threonine-179. *Neoplasia* **2015**, *17*, 525–537. [CrossRef] [PubMed]

108. Song, H.; Bao, J.; Wei, Y.; Chen, Y.; Mao, X.; Li, J.; Yang, Z.; Xue, Y. Kaempferol inhibits gastric cancer tumor growth: An in vitro and in vivo study. *Oncol. Rep.* **2015**, *33*, 868–874. [CrossRef] [PubMed]

109. Lee, H.S.; Cho, H.J.; Yu, R.; Lee, K.W.; Chun, H.S.; Park, J.H. Mechanisms underlying apoptosis-inducing effects of Kaempferol in HT-29 human colon cancer cells. *Int. J. Mol. Sci.* **2014**, *15*, 2722–2737. [CrossRef] [PubMed]

110. Huang, W.W.; Tsai, S.C.; Peng, S.F.; Lin, M.W.; Chiang, J.H.; Chiu, Y.J.; Fushiya, S.; Tseng, M.T.; Yang, J.S. Kaempferol induces autophagy through AMPK and AKT signaling molecules and causes G2/M arrest via downregulation of CDK1/cyclin B in SK-HEP-1 human hepatic cancer cells. *Int. J. Oncol.* **2013**, *42*, 2069–2077. [PubMed]

111. Liao, W.; Chen, L.; Ma, X.; Jiao, R.; Li, X.; Wang, Y. Protective effects of kaempferol against reactive oxygen species-induced hemolysis and its antiproliferative activity on human cancer cells. *Eur. J. Med. Chem.* **2016**, *114*, 24–32. [CrossRef] [PubMed]

112. Azevedo, C.; Correia-Branco, A.; Araujo, J.R.; Guimaraes, J.T.; Keating, E.; Martel, F. The chemopreventive effect of the dietary compound kaempferol on the MCF-7 human breast cancer cell line is dependent on inhibition of glucose cellular uptake. *Nutr. Cancer* **2015**, *67*, 504–513. [CrossRef] [PubMed]

113. Kim, S.H.; Hwang, K.A.; Choi, K.C. Treatment with kaempferol suppresses breast cancer cell growth caused by estrogen and triclosan in cellular and xenograft breast cancer models. *J. Nutr. Biochem.* **2016**, *28*, 70–82. [CrossRef] [PubMed]

114. Li, C.; Zhao, Y.; Yang, D.; Yu, Y.; Guo, H.; Zhao, Z.; Zhang, B.; Yin, X. Inhibitory effects of kaempferol on the invasion of human breast carcinoma cells by downregulating the expression and activity of matrix metalloproteinase-9. *Biochem. Cell. Biol.* **2015**, *93*, 16–27. [CrossRef] [PubMed]

115. Feng, J.; Chen, X.; Wang, Y.; Du, Y.; Sun, Q.; Zang, W.; Zhao, G. Myricetin inhibits proliferation and induces apoptosis and cell cycle arrest in gastric cancer cells. *Mol. Cell. Biochem.* **2015**, *408*, 163–170. [CrossRef] [PubMed]

116. Kim, M.E.; Ha, T.K.; Yoon, J.H.; Lee, J.S. Myricetin induces cell death of human colon cancer cells via BAX/BCL2-dependent pathway. *Anticancer Res.* **2014**, *34*, 701–706. [PubMed]

117. Iyer, S.C.; Gopal, A.; Halagowder, D. Myricetin induces apoptosis by inhibiting P21 activated kinase 1 (PAK1) signaling cascade in hepatocellular carcinoma. *Mol. Cell. Biochem.* **2015**, *407*, 223–237. [CrossRef]

118. Kim, D.A.; Jeon, Y.K.; Nam, M.J. Galangin induces apoptosis in gastric cancer cells via regulation of ubiquitin carboxy-terminal hydrolase isozyme L1 and glutathione S-transferase P. *Food Chem. Toxicol.* **2012**, *50*, 684–688. [CrossRef] [PubMed]

119. Chien, S.T.; Shi, M.D.; Lee, Y.C.; Te, C.C.; Shih, Y.W. Galangin, a novel dietary flavonoid, attenuates metastatic feature via PKC/ERK signaling pathway in TPA-treated liver cancer HepG2 cells. *Cancer Cell Int.* **2015**, *15*, 15. [CrossRef] [PubMed]

120. Su, L.; Chen, X.; Wu, J.; Lin, B.; Zhang, H.; Lan, L.; Luo, H. Galangin inhibits proliferation of hepatocellular carcinoma cells by inducing endoplasmic reticulum stress. *Food Chem. Toxicol.* **2013**, *62*, 810–816. [CrossRef] [PubMed]

121. Hu, S.; Huang, L.; Meng, L.; Sun, H.; Zhang, W.; Xu, Y. Isorhamnetin inhibits cell proliferation and induces apoptosis in breast cancer via Akt and mitogenactivated protein kinase kinase signaling pathways. *Mol. Med. Rep.* **2015**, *12*, 6745–6751. [PubMed]

122. Li, C.; Yang, D.; Zhao, Y.; Qiu, Y.; Cao, X.; Yu, Y.; Guo, H.; Gu, X.; Yin, X. Inhibitory effects of isorhamnetin on the invasion of human breast carcinoma cells by downregulating the expression and activity of matrix metalloproteinase-2/9. *Nutr. Cancer* **2015**, *67*, 1191–1200. [CrossRef] [PubMed]

123. Li, Q.; Ren, F.Q.; Yang, C.L.; Zhou, L.M.; Liu, Y.Y.; Xiao, J.; Zhu, L.; Wang, Z.G. Anti-proliferation effects of isorhamnetin on lung cancer cells in vitro and in vivo. *Asian Pac. J. Cancer Prev.* **2015**, *16*, 3035–3042. [CrossRef] [PubMed]

124. Ramachandran, L.; Manu, K.A.; Shanmugam, M.K.; Li, F.; Siveen, K.S.; Vali, S.; Kapoor, S.; Abbasi, T.; Surana, R.; Smoot, D.T.; et al. Isorhamnetin inhibits proliferation and invasion and induces apoptosis through the modulation of peroxisome proliferator-activated receptor gamma activation pathway in gastric cancer. *J. Biol. Chem.* **2012**, *287*, 38028–38040. [CrossRef] [PubMed]

125. Li, C.; Yang, X.; Chen, C.; Cai, S.; Hu, J. Isorhamnetin suppresses colon cancer cell growth through the PI3KAktmTOR pathway. *Mol. Med. Rep.* **2014**, *9*, 935–940. [PubMed]

126. Saud, S.M.; Young, M.R.; Jones-Hall, Y.L.; Ileva, L.; Evbuomwan, M.O.; Wise, J.; Colburn, N.H.; Kim, Y.S.; Bobe, G. Chemopreventive activity of plant flavonoid isorhamnetin in colorectal cancer is mediated by oncogenic Src and beta-catenin. *Cancer Res.* **2013**, *73*, 5473–5484. [CrossRef] [PubMed]

127. Park, H.J.; Jeon, Y.K.; You, D.H.; Nam, M.J. Daidzein causes cytochrome c-mediated apoptosis via the Bcl-2 family in human hepatic cancer cells. *Food Chem. Toxicol.* **2013**, *60*, 542–549. [CrossRef] [PubMed]

128. Magee, P.J.; Allsopp, P.; Samaletdin, A.; Rowland, I.R. Daidzein, R-(+)equol and S-(−)equol inhibit the invasion of MDA-MB-231 breast cancer cells potentially via the down-regulation of matrix metalloproteinase-2. *Eur. J. Nutr.* **2014**, *53*, 345–350. [CrossRef] [PubMed]

129. Koo, J.; Cabarcas-Petroski, S.; Petrie, J.L.; Diette, N.; White, R.J.; Schramm, L. Induction of proto-oncogene BRF2 in breast cancer cells by the dietary soybean isoflavone daidzein. *BMC Cancer* **2015**, *15*, 905. [CrossRef] [PubMed]

130. Tian, T.; Li, J.; Li, B.; Wang, Y.; Li, M.; Ma, D.; Wang, X. Genistein exhibits anti-cancer effects via down-regulating FoxM1 in H446 small-cell lung cancer cells. *Tumor Biol.* **2014**, *35*, 4137–4145. [CrossRef] [PubMed]

131. Huang, W.; Wan, C.; Luo, Q.; Huang, Z.; Luo, Q. Genistein-inhibited cancer stem cell-like properties and reduced chemoresistance of gastric cancer. *Int. J. Mol. Sci.* **2014**, *15*, 3432–3443. [CrossRef] [PubMed]

132. Qin, J.; Teng, J.; Zhu, Z.; Chen, J.; Huang, W.J. Genistein induces activation of the mitochondrial apoptosis pathway by inhibiting phosphorylation of Akt in colorectal cancer cells. *Pharm. Biol.* **2016**, *54*, 74–79. [CrossRef] [PubMed]

133. Xiao, X.; Liu, Z.; Wang, R.; Wang, J.; Zhang, S.; Cai, X.; Wu, K.; Bergan, R.C.; Xu, L.; Fan, D. Genistein suppresses FLT4 and inhibits human colorectal cancer metastasis. *Oncotarget* **2015**, *6*, 3225–3239. [CrossRef] [PubMed]

134. Luo, Y.; Wang, S.X.; Zhou, Z.Q.; Wang, Z.; Zhang, Y.G.; Zhang, Y.; Zhao, P. Apoptotic effect of genistein on human colon cancer cells via inhibiting the nuclear factor-kappa B (NF-kappaB) pathway. *Tumor Biol.* **2014**, *35*, 11483–11488. [CrossRef] [PubMed]

135. Lepri, S.R.; Zanelatto, L.C.; Da, S.P.; Sartori, D.; Ribeiro, L.R.; Mantovani, M.S. Effects of genistein and daidzein on cell proliferation kinetics in HT29 colon cancer cells: The expression of CTNNBIP1 (beta-catenin), APC (adenomatous polyposis coli) and BIRC5 (survivin). *Hum. Cell* **2014**, *27*, 78–84. [CrossRef] [PubMed]

136. Dai, W.; Wang, F.; He, L.; Lin, C.; Wu, S.; Chen, P.; Zhang, Y.; Shen, M.; Wu, D.; Wang, C.; et al. Genistein inhibits hepatocellular carcinoma cell migration by reversing the epithelial-mesenchymal transition: Partial mediation by the transcription factor NFAT1. *Mol. Carcinog.* **2015**, *54*, 301–311. [CrossRef] [PubMed]

137. Pan, H.; Zhou, W.; He, W.; Liu, X.; Ding, Q.; Ling, L.; Zha, X.; Wang, S. Genistein inhibits MDA-MB-231 triple-negative breast cancer cell growth by inhibiting NF-kappaB activity via the Notch-1 pathway. *Int. J. Mol. Med.* **2012**, *30*, 337–343. [PubMed]

138. Fan, P.; Fan, S.; Wang, H.; Mao, J.; Shi, Y.; Ibrahim, M.M.; Ma, W.; Yu, X.; Hou, Z.; Wang, B.; et al. Genistein decreases the breast cancer stem-like cell population through Hedgehog pathway. *Stem Cell Res. Ther.* **2013**, *4*, 146. [CrossRef] [PubMed]

139. Pons, D.G.; Nadal-Serrano, M.; Torrens-Mas, M.; Oliver, J.; Roca, P. The phytoestrogen genistein affects breast cancer cells treatment depending on the ERalpha/ERbeta ratio. *J. Cell. Biochem.* **2016**, *117*, 218–229. [CrossRef] [PubMed]

140. Andrade, J.E.; Ju, Y.H.; Baker, C.; Doerge, D.R.; Helferich, W.G. Long-term exposure to dietary sources of genistein induces estrogen-independence in the human breast cancer (MCF-7) xenograft model. *Mol. Nutr. Food Res.* **2015**, *59*, 413–423. [CrossRef] [PubMed]

141. Mahmoud, A.M.; Zhu, T.; Parray, A.; Siddique, H.R.; Yang, W.; Saleem, M.; Bosland, M.C. Differential effects of genistein on prostate cancer cells depend on mutational status of the androgen receptor. *PLoS ONE* **2013**, *8*, e78479. [CrossRef] [PubMed]

142. Hussain, A.; Harish, G.; Prabhu, S.A.; Mohsin, J.; Khan, M.A.; Rizvi, T.A.; Sharma, C. Inhibitory effect of genistein on the invasive potential of human cervical cancer cells via modulation of matrix metalloproteinase-9 and tissue inhibitors of matrix metalloproteinase-1 expression. *Cancer Epidemiol.* **2012**, *36*, e387–e393. [CrossRef] [PubMed]

143. Chen, H.S.; Bai, M.H.; Zhang, T.; Li, G.D.; Liu, M. Ellagic acid induces cell cycle arrest and apoptosis through TGF-beta/Smad3 signaling pathway in human breast cancer MCF-7 cells. *Int. J. Oncol.* **2015**, *46*, 1730–1738. [PubMed]

144. Yousef, A.I.; El-Masry, O.S.; Abdel, M.M. Impact of cellular genetic make-up on colorectal cancer cell lines response to ellagic acid: Implications of small interfering RNA. *Asian Pac. J. Cancer Prev.* **2016**, *17*, 743–748. [CrossRef] [PubMed]

145. Srigopalram, S.; Jayraaj, I.A.; Kaleeswaran, B.; Balamurugan, K.; Ranjithkumar, M.; Kumar, T.S.; Park, J.I.; Nou, I.S. Ellagic acid normalizes mitochondrial outer membrane permeabilization and attenuates inflammation-mediated cell proliferation in experimental liver cancer. *Appl. Biochem. Biotechnol.* **2014**, *173*, 2254–2266. [CrossRef] [PubMed]

146. Wang, N.; Wang, Z.Y.; Mo, S.L.; Loo, T.Y.; Wang, D.M.; Luo, H.B.; Yang, D.P.; Chen, Y.L.; Shen, J.G.; Chen, J.P. Ellagic acid, a phenolic compound, exerts anti-angiogenesis effects via VEGFR-2 signaling pathway in breast cancer. *Breast Cancer Res. Treat.* **2012**, *134*, 943–955. [CrossRef] [PubMed]

147. Pitchakarn, P.; Chewonarin, T.; Ogawa, K.; Suzuki, S.; Asamoto, M.; Takahashi, S.; Shirai, T.; Limtrakul, P. Ellagic acid inhibits migration and invasion by prostate cancer cell lines. *Asian Pac. J. Cancer Prev.* **2013**, *14*, 2859–2863. [CrossRef] [PubMed]

148. Malik, A.; Afaq, S.; Shahid, M.; Akhtar, K.; Assiri, A. Influence of ellagic acid on prostate cancer cell proliferation: A caspase-dependent pathway. *Asian Pac. J. Trop. Med.* **2011**, *4*, 550–555. [CrossRef]

149. Subramanian, A.P.; Jaganathan, S.K.; Mandal, M.; Supriyanto, E.; Muhamad, I.I. Gallic acid induced apoptotic events in HCT-15 colon cancer cells. *World J. Gastroenterol.* **2016**, *22*, 3952–3961. [CrossRef] [PubMed]

150. Wang, K.; Zhu, X.; Zhang, K.; Zhu, L.; Zhou, F. Investigation of gallic acid induced anticancer effect in human breast carcinoma MCF-7 cells. *J. Biochem. Mol. Toxicol.* **2014**, *28*, 387–393. [CrossRef] [PubMed]

151. Ho, H.H.; Chang, C.S.; Ho, W.C.; Liao, S.Y.; Lin, W.L.; Wang, C.J. Gallic acid inhibits gastric cancer cells metastasis and invasive growth via increased expression of RhoB, downregulation of AKT/small GTPase signals and inhibition of NF-kappaB activity. *Toxicol. Appl. Pharmacol.* **2013**, *266*, 76–85. [CrossRef] [PubMed]

152. Russell, L.J.; Mazzio, E.; Badisa, R.B.; Zhu, Z.P.; Agharahimi, M.; Oriaku, E.T.; Goodman, C.B. Autoxidation of gallic acid induces ROS-dependent death in human prostate cancer LNCaP cells. *Anticancer Res.* **2012**, *32*, 1595–1602. [PubMed]

153. Sun, G.; Zhang, S.; Xie, Y.; Zhang, Z.; Zhao, W. Gallic acid as a selective anticancer agent that induces apoptosis in SMMC-7721 human hepatocellular carcinoma cells. *Oncol. Lett.* **2016**, *11*, 150–158. [CrossRef] [PubMed]

154. Liu, K.C.; Huang, A.C.; Wu, P.P.; Lin, H.Y.; Chueh, F.S.; Yang, J.S.; Lu, C.C.; Chiang, J.H.; Meng, M.; Chung, J.G. Gallic acid suppresses the migration and invasion of PC-3 human prostate cancer cells via inhibition of matrix metalloproteinase-2 and -9 signaling pathways. *Oncol. Rep.* **2011**, *26*, 177–184. [PubMed]

155. Liu, K.C.; Ho, H.C.; Huang, A.C.; Ji, B.C.; Lin, H.Y.; Chueh, F.S.; Yang, J.S.; Lu, C.C.; Chiang, J.H.; Meng, M.; et al. Gallic acid provokes DNA damage and suppresses DNA repair gene expression in human prostate cancer PC-3 cells. *Environ. Toxicol.* **2013**, *28*, 579–587. [CrossRef] [PubMed]

156. Zhao, B.; Hu, M. Gallic acid reduces cell viability, proliferation, invasion and angiogenesis in human cervical cancer cells. *Oncol. Lett.* **2013**, *6*, 1749–1755. [PubMed]

157. Sarwar, T.; Zafaryab, M.; Husain, M.A.; Ishqi, H.M.; Rehman, S.U.; Rizvi, M.M.; Tabish, M. Redox cycling of endogenous copper by ferulic acid leads to cellular DNA breakage and consequent cell death: A putative cancer chemotherapy mechanism. *Toxicol. Appl. Pharmacol.* **2015**, *289*, 251–261. [CrossRef] [PubMed]

158. Eroglu, C.; Secme, M.; Bagci, G.; Dodurga, Y. Assessment of the anticancer mechanism of ferulic acid via cell cycle and apoptotic pathways in human prostate cancer cell lines. *Tumor Biol.* **2015**, *36*, 9437–9446. [CrossRef] [PubMed]

159. Karthikeyan, S.; Kanimozhi, G.; Prasad, N.R.; Mahalakshmi, R. Radiosensitizing effect of ferulic acid on human cervical carcinoma cells in vitro. *Toxicol. Vitro* **2011**, *25*, 1366–1375. [CrossRef] [PubMed]

160. Delman, D.M.; Fabian, C.J.; Kimler, B.F.; Yeh, H.; Petroff, B.K. Effects of flaxseed lignan secoisolariciresinol diglucosideon preneoplastic biomarkers of cancer progression in a model of simultaneous breast and ovarian cancer development. *Nutr. Cancer* **2015**, *67*, 857–864. [CrossRef] [PubMed]

161. Xiong, X.Y.; Hu, X.J.; Li, Y.; Liu, C.M. Inhibitory effects of enterolactone on growth and metastasis in human breast cancer. *Nutr. Cancer* **2015**, *67*, 1324–1332. [CrossRef] [PubMed]

162. Lee, C.C.; Liu, K.J.; Wu, Y.C.; Lin, S.J.; Chang, C.C.; Huang, T.S. Sesamin inhibits macrophage-induced vascular endothelial growth factor and matrix metalloproteinase-9 expression and proangiogenic activity in breast cancer cells. *Inflammation* **2011**, *34*, 209–221. [CrossRef] [PubMed]

163. Deng, P.; Wang, C.; Chen, L.; Wang, C.; Du, Y.; Yan, X.; Chen, M.; Yang, G.; He, G. Sesamin induces cell cycle arrest and apoptosis through the inhibition of signal transducer and activator of transcription 3 signalling in human hepatocellular carcinoma cell line HepG2. *Biol. Pharm. Bull.* **2013**, *36*, 1540–1548. [CrossRef] [PubMed]

164. Xu, P.; Cai, F.; Liu, X.; Guo, L. Sesamin inhibits lipopolysaccharide-induced proliferation and invasion through the p38-MAPK and NF-kappaB signaling pathways in prostate cancer cells. *Oncol. Rep.* **2015**, *33*, 3117–3123. [PubMed]

165. Ko, J.C.; Syu, J.J.; Chen, J.C.; Wang, T.J.; Chang, P.Y.; Chen, C.Y.; Jian, Y.T.; Jian, Y.J.; Lin, Y.W. Resveratrol enhances etoposide-induced cytotoxicity through down-regulating ERK1/2 and AKT-Mediated X-ray repair cross-complement group 1 (XRCC1) protein expression in human non-small-cell lung cancer cells. *Basic Clin. Pharmacol. Toxicol.* **2015**, *117*, 383–391. [CrossRef] [PubMed]

166. Yang, Q.; Wang, B.; Zang, W.; Wang, X.; Liu, Z.; Li, W.; Jia, J. Resveratrol inhibits the growth of gastric cancer by inducing G1 phase arrest and senescence in a Sirt1-dependent manner. *PLoS ONE* **2013**, *8*, e70627. [CrossRef] [PubMed]

167. Wang, Z.; Li, W.; Meng, X.; Jia, B. Resveratrol induces gastric cancer cell apoptosis via reactive oxygen species, but independent of sirtuin1. *Clin. Exp. Pharmacol. Physiol.* **2012**, *39*, 227–232. [CrossRef]

168. Miki, H.; Uehara, N.; Kimura, A.; Sasaki, T.; Yuri, T.; Yoshizawa, K.; Tsubura, A. Resveratrol induces apoptosis via ROS-triggered autophagy in human colon cancer cells. *Int. J. Oncol.* **2012**, *40*, 1020–1028. [PubMed]

169. Colin, D.J.; Limagne, E.; Ragot, K.; Lizard, G.; Ghiringhelli, F.; Solary, E.; Chauffert, B.; Latruffe, N.; Delmas, D. The role of reactive oxygen species and subsequent DNA-damage response in the emergence of resistance towards resveratrol in colon cancer models. *Cell Death Dis.* **2014**, *5*, e1533. [CrossRef] [PubMed]

170. Demoulin, B.; Hermant, M.; Castrogiovanni, C.; Staudt, C.; Dumont, P. Resveratrol induces DNA damage in colon cancer cells by poisoning topoisomerase II and activates the ATM kinase to trigger p53-dependent apoptosis. *Toxicol. Vitro* **2015**, *29*, 1156–1165. [CrossRef] [PubMed]

171. Wang, Z.; Zhang, L.; Ni, Z.; Sun, J.; Gao, H.; Cheng, Z.; Xu, J.; Yin, P. Resveratrol induces AMPK-dependent MDR1 inhibition in colorectal cancer HCT116/L-OHP cells by preventing activation of NF-kappaB signaling and suppressing cAMP-responsive element transcriptional activity. *Tumor Biol.* **2015**, *36*, 9499–9510. [CrossRef] [PubMed]

172. Saud, S.M.; Li, W.; Morris, N.L.; Matter, M.S.; Colburn, N.H.; Kim, Y.S.; Young, M.R. Resveratrol prevents tumorigenesis in mouse model of Kras activated sporadic colorectal cancer by suppressing oncogenic Kras expression. *Carcinogenesis* **2014**, *35*, 2778–2786. [CrossRef] [PubMed]

173. Aires, V.; Limagne, E.; Cotte, A.K.; Latruffe, N.; Ghiringhelli, F.; Delmas, D. Resveratrol metabolites inhibit human metastatic colon cancer cells progression and synergize with chemotherapeutic drugs to induce cell death. *Mol. Nutr. Food Res.* **2013**, *57*, 1170–1181. [CrossRef] [PubMed]

174. Fu, Y.; Chang, H.; Peng, X.; Bai, Q.; Yi, L.; Zhou, Y.; Zhu, J.; Mi, M. Resveratrol inhibits breast cancer stem-like cells and induces autophagy via suppressing Wnt/beta-catenin signaling pathway. *PLoS ONE* **2014**, *9*, e102535.

175. Yeh, C.B.; Hsieh, M.J.; Lin, C.W.; Chiou, H.L.; Lin, P.Y.; Chen, T.Y.; Yang, S.F. The antimetastatic effects of resveratrol on hepatocellular carcinoma through the downregulation of a metastasis-associated protease by SP-1 modulation. *PLoS ONE* **2013**, *8*, e56661. [CrossRef] [PubMed]

176. Rajasekaran, D.; Elavarasan, J.; Sivalingam, M.; Ganapathy, E.; Kumar, A.; Kalpana, K.; Sakthisekaran, D. Resveratrol interferes with *N*-nitrosodiethylamine-induced hepatocellular carcinoma at early and advanced stages in male Wistar rats. *Mol. Med. Rep.* **2011**, *4*, 1211–1217. [PubMed]

177. Selvaraj, S.; Sun, Y.; Sukumaran, P.; Singh, B.B. Resveratrol activates autophagic cell death in prostate cancer cells via downregulation of STIM1 and the mTOR pathway. *Mol. Carcinog.* **2015**, *5*, 818–831. [CrossRef] [PubMed]

178. Ganapathy, S.; Chen, Q.; Singh, K.P.; Shankar, S.; Srivastava, R.K. Resveratrol enhances antitumor activity of TRAIL in prostate cancer xenografts through activation of FOXO transcription factor. *PLoS ONE* **2010**, *5*, e15627. [CrossRef] [PubMed]

179. Garcia-Zepeda, S.P.; Garcia-Villa, E.; Diaz-Chavez, J.; Hernandez-Pando, R.; Gariglio, P. Resveratrol induces cell death in cervical cancer cells through apoptosis and autophagy. *Eur. J. Cancer Prev.* **2013**, *22*, 577–584. [CrossRef] [PubMed]

180. Sun, Y.; Wu, X.; Cai, X.; Song, M.; Zheng, J.; Pan, C.; Qiu, P.; Zhang, L.; Zhou, S.; Tang, Z.; et al. Identification of pinostilbene as a major colonic metabolite of pterostilbene and its inhibitory effects on colon cancer cells. *Mol. Nutr. Food Res.* **2016**. [CrossRef] [PubMed]

181. Moon, D.; McCormack, D.; McDonald, D.; McFadden, D. Pterostilbene induces mitochondrially derived apoptosis in breast cancer cells in vitro. *J. Surg. Res.* **2013**, *180*, 208–215. [CrossRef] [PubMed]

182. Su, C.M.; Lee, W.H.; Wu, A.T.; Lin, Y.K.; Wang, L.S.; Wu, C.H.; Yeh, C.T. Pterostilbene inhibits triple-negative breast cancer metastasis via inducing microRNA-205 expression and negatively modulates epithelial-to-mesenchymal transition. *J. Nutr. Biochem.* **2015**, *26*, 675–685. [CrossRef] [PubMed]

183. Wu, C.H.; Hong, B.H.; Ho, C.T.; Yen, G.C. Targeting cancer stem cells in breast cancer: Potential anticancer properties of 6-shogaol and pterostilbene. *J. Agric. Food Chem.* **2015**, *63*, 2432–2441. [CrossRef] [PubMed]

184. Lin, V.C.; Tsai, Y.C.; Lin, J.N.; Fan, L.L.; Pan, M.H.; Ho, C.T.; Wu, J.Y.; Way, T.D. Activation of AMPK by pterostilbene suppresses lipogenesis and cell-cycle progression in p53 positive and negative human prostate cancer cells. *J. Agric. Food Chem.* **2012**, *60*, 6399–6407. [CrossRef] [PubMed]

185. Dhar, S.; Kumar, A.; Rimando, A.M.; Zhang, X.; Levenson, A.S. Resveratrol and pterostilbene epigenetically restore PTEN expression by targeting oncomiRs of the miR-17 family in prostate cancer. *Oncotarget* **2015**, *6*, 27214–27226. [CrossRef] [PubMed]

186. Zhang, H.; Jia, R.; Wang, C.; Hu, T.; Wang, F. Piceatannol promotes apoptosis via up-regulation of microRNA-129 expression in colorectal cancer cell lines. *Biochem. Biophys. Res. Commun.* **2014**, *452*, 775–781. [CrossRef] [PubMed]

187. Hsieh, T.C.; Lin, C.Y.; Lin, H.Y.; Wu, J.M. AKT/mTOR as novel targets of polyphenol piceatannol possibly contributing to inhibition of proliferation of cultured prostate cancer cells. *ISRN Urol.* **2012**, *2012*, 272697. [CrossRef] [PubMed]

188. Kwon, G.T.; Jung, J.I.; Song, H.R.; Woo, E.Y.; Jun, J.G.; Kim, J.K.; Her, S.; Park, J.H. Piceatannol inhibits migration and invasion of prostate cancer cells: Possible mediation by decreased interleukin-6 signaling. *J. Nutr. Biochem.* **2012**, *23*, 228–238. [CrossRef] [PubMed]

189. Devassy, J.G.; Nwachukwu, I.D.; Jones, P.J. Curcumin and cancer: Barriers to obtaining a health claim. *Nutr. Rev.* **2015**, *73*, 155–165. [CrossRef] [PubMed]

190. Vallianou, N.G.; Evangelopoulos, A.; Schizas, N.; Kazazis, C. Potential anticancer properties and mechanisms of action of curcumin. *Anticancer Res.* **2015**, *35*, 645–651. [PubMed]

191. Shanmugam, M.; Rane, G.; Kanchi, M.; Arfuso, F.; Chinnathambi, A.; Zayed, M.; Alharbi, S.; Tan, B.; Kumar, A.; Sethi, G. The Multifaceted Role of Curcumin in Cancer Prevention and Treatment. *Molecules* **2015**, *20*, 2728–2769. [CrossRef] [PubMed]

192. Thomasset, S.C.; Berry, D.P.; Garcea, G.; Marczylo, T.; Steward, W.P.; Gescher, A.J. Dietary polyphenolic phytochemicals—Promising cancer chemopreventive agents in humans? A review of their clinical properties. *Int. J. Cancer* **2007**, *120*, 451–458. [CrossRef] [PubMed]

193. Lazarevic, B.; Boezelijn, G.; Diep, L.M.; Kvernrod, K.; Ogren, O.; Ramberg, H.; Moen, A.; Wessel, N.; Berg, R.E.; Egge-Jacobsen, W.; et al. Efficacy and safety of short-term genistein intervention in patients with localized prostate cancer prior to radical prostatectomy: A randomized, placebo-controlled, double-blind Phase 2 clinical trial. *Nutr. Cancer* **2011**, *63*, 889–898. [CrossRef] [PubMed]

194. Miyanaga, N.; Akaza, H.; Hinotsu, S.; Fujioka, T.; Naito, S.; Namiki, M.; Takahashi, S.; Hirao, Y.; Horie, S.; Tsukamoto, T.; et al. Prostate cancer chemoprevention study: An investigative randomized control study using purified isoflavones in men with rising prostate-specific antigen. *Cancer Sci.* **2012**, *103*, 125–130. [CrossRef] [PubMed]

195. Hamilton-Reeves, J.M.; Banerjee, S.; Banerjee, S.K.; Holzbeierlein, J.M.; Thrasher, J.B.; Kambhampati, S.; Keighley, J.; Van Veldhuizen, P. Short-term soy isoflavone intervention in patients with localized prostate cancer: A randomized, double-blind, placebo-controlled trial. *PLoS ONE* **2013**, *8*, e68331.

196. Zhang, G.; Wang, Y.; Zhang, Y.; Wan, X.; Li, J.; Liu, K.; Wang, F.; Liu, K.; Liu, Q.; Yang, C.; et al. Anti-cancer activities of tea epigallocatechin-3-gallate in breast cancer patients under radiotherapy. *Curr. Mol. Med.* **2012**, *12*, 163–176. [CrossRef] [PubMed]

197. Azrad, M.; Vollmer, R.T.; Madden, J.; Dewhirst, M.; Polascik, T.J.; Snyder, D.C.; Ruffin, M.T.; Moul, J.W.; Brenner, D.E.; Demark-Wahnefried, W. Flaxseed-derived enterolactone is inversely associated with tumor cell proliferation in men with localized prostate cancer. *J. Med. Food* **2013**, *16*, 357–360. [CrossRef] [PubMed]

198. Hoensch, H.; Groh, B.; Edler, L.; Kirch, W. Prospective cohort comparison of flavonoid treatment in patients with resected colorectal cancer to prevent recurrence. *World J. Gastroenterol.* **2008**, *14*, 2187–2193. [CrossRef] [PubMed]

199. Cruz-Correa, M.; Shoskes, D.A.; Sanchez, P.; Zhao, R.; Hylind, L.M.; Wexner, S.D.; Giardiello, F.M. Combination treatment with curcumin and quercetin of adenomas in familial adenomatous polyposis. *Clin. Gastroenterol. Hepatol.* **2006**, *4*, 1035–1038. [CrossRef] [PubMed]

200. Ide, H.; Tokiwa, S.; Sakamaki, K.; Nishio, K.; Isotani, S.; Muto, S.; Hama, T.; Masuda, H.; Horie, S. Combined inhibitory effects of soy isoflavones and curcumin on the production of prostate-specific antigen. *Prostate* **2010**, *70*, 1127–1133. [CrossRef] [PubMed]

201. Carroll, R.E.; Benya, R.V.; Turgeon, D.K.; Vareed, S.; Neuman, M.; Rodriguez, L.; Kakarala, M.; Carpenter, P.M.; McLaren, C.; Meyskens, F.J.; et al. Phase IIa clinical trial of curcumin for the prevention of colorectal neoplasia. *Cancer Prev. Res.* **2011**, *4*, 354–364. [CrossRef] [PubMed]

202. He, Z.Y.; Shi, C.B.; Wen, H.; Li, F.L.; Wang, B.L.; Wang, J. Upregulation of p53 expression in patients with colorectal cancer by administration of curcumin. *Cancer Investig.* **2011**, *29*, 208–213. [CrossRef] [PubMed]

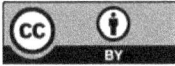

*nutrients*

MDPI

*Review*

# Evidence to Support the Anti-Cancer Effect of Olive Leaf Extract and Future Directions

Anna Boss [1,*], Karen S. Bishop [2], Gareth Marlow [1], Matthew P. G. Barnett [3] and Lynnette R. Ferguson [1,2]

[1] Discipline of Nutrition, FM & HS, University of Auckland Medical School, Private Bag 92019, Auckland 1142, New Zealand; MarlowG@cardiff.ac.uk (G.M.); l.ferguson@auckland.ac.nz (L.R.F.)
[2] Auckland Cancer Society Research Centre, FM & HS, University of Auckland Medical School, Private Bag 92019, Auckland 1142, New Zealand; k.bishop@auckland.ac.nz
[3] Food Nutrition & Health Team, Food & Bio-based Products Group, AgResearch Limited, Grasslands Research Centre, Tennent Drive, Palmerston North 4442, New Zealand; matthew.barnett@agresearch.co.nz
* Correspondence: abos517@aucklanduni.ac.nz; Tel.: +64-9923-6372

Received: 18 July 2016; Accepted: 16 August 2016; Published: 19 August 2016

**Abstract.** The traditional Mediterranean diet (MD) is associated with long life and lower prevalence of cardiovascular disease and cancers. The main components of this diet include high intake of fruit, vegetables, red wine, extra virgin olive oil (EVOO) and fish, low intake of dairy and red meat. Olive oil has gained support as a key effector of health benefits and there is evidence that this relates to the polyphenol content. Olive leaf extract (OLE) contains a higher quantity and variety of polyphenols than those found in EVOO. There are also important structural differences between polyphenols from olive leaf and those from olive fruit that may improve the capacity of OLE to enhance health outcomes. Olive polyphenols have been claimed to play an important protective role in cancer and other inflammation-related diseases. Both inflammatory and cancer cell models have shown that olive leaf polyphenols are anti-inflammatory and protect against DNA damage initiated by free radicals. The various bioactive properties of olive leaf polyphenols are a plausible explanation for the inhibition of progression and development of cancers. The pathways and signaling cascades manipulated include the NF-κB inflammatory response and the oxidative stress response, but the effects of these bioactive components may also result from their action as a phytoestrogen. Due to the similar structure of the olive polyphenols to oestrogens, these have been hypothesized to interact with oestrogen receptors, thereby reducing the prevalence and progression of hormone related cancers. Evidence for the protective effect of olive polyphenols for cancer in humans remains anecdotal and clinical trials are required to substantiate these claims idea. This review aims to amalgamate the current literature regarding bioavailability and mechanisms involved in the potential anti-cancer action of olive leaf polyphenols.

**Keywords:** olive leaf; oleuropein; oxidative stress; inflammation; Mediterranean diet; Cyclooxygenase-2

---

## 1. Introduction

Cancer is a group of diseases involving proliferation of mutated cells [1]. In 2012, over 14 million new cases of cancer were reported [2], triggering a push to further develop treatments and preventative strategies. Cancer is predominantly an age-related disease, therefore with better conditions of life and increased longevity it is likely to continue increasing in prevalence. However, there are clearly factors other than age that contribute to its development. The traditional Mediterranean diet (MD) has gained robust scientific support for providing protection against some cancers [3,4]. The MD has shown an ability to influence the inflammatory response, which plays a pivotal role in aging and in reducing its age-associated non-communicable diseases such as cancer. However, the mechanisms of action behind the effects of the MD on inflammation are not entirely clear [5–7]. It has been suggested that the NF-κB inflammatory response, eicosanoid pathways and oxidative stress via free radical formation, have been suggested to play a role in MD related health benefits [5,8,9]. The diet, as a whole, has shown a protective role in cancer, however, the distribution of people still consuming it is gradually receding due to the spread of the western-type urban society, globalization and consumption [10]. Because of this, it is important to understand whether any beneficial effects ascribed to the MD are due to a particular component of the diet, rather than the whole diet. As one example, polyphenol bioactive components have shown particular promise and have therefore been a research focus.

Extra virgin olive oil (EVOO) is typically used as a traditional component of the MD and has also been correlated with improved cardiovascular disease and cancer outcomes [11,12]. EVOO is manufactured by pressing olives to create a paste, which is churned to amalgamate oil droplets which are then extracted. There is a considerable variation in EVOO characteristics that can be attributed to the olive variety, the geographical location the olives were derived from [13] and the method of oil extraction [14]. Intake of both MD and EVOO has been shown to correlate with a reduced overall risk of cancer and is more specifically associated with reduced risk of cancers of the digestive system, prostate and breast [12].

EVOO is primarily a monounsaturated fatty acid (MUFA) in the form of oleic acid, with minor components including various phenolics [15]. It has been recognised that the polyphenol content plays an important role in health benefits. The European Food Safety Authority (EFSA) have approved the use of the general claim "olive oil polyphenols contribute to the protection of blood lipids from oxidative stress" when oil contains no less than 5 mg of hydroxytyrosol (HT) and its derivatives (such as tyrosol and oleuropein) per 20 mL OO [16] (Figure 1). There are several studies that have shown that EVOO with higher phenolic content provides stronger anti-inflammatory and antioxidant effects than OO with a lower phenolic content [17,18]. This suggests the phenolic component, rather than the fat in the oil, is the effector.

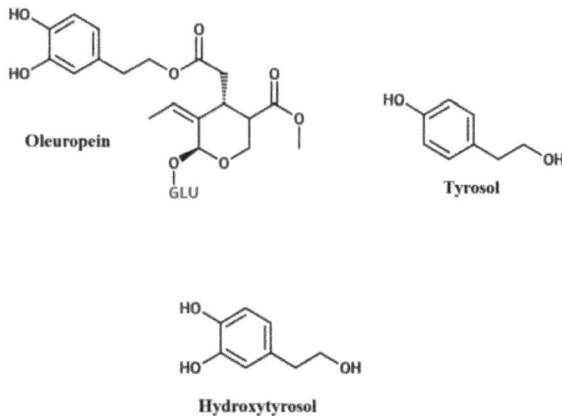

**Figure 1.** The olive polyphenol hydroxytyrosol and its derivatives, oleuropein and tyrosol (adapted from [19]).

Olive tree leaves (*Olea europaea*) are widely used in traditional medicine in the Mediterranean region [20]. In the Bible, the olive plant is referenced numerous times for its medicinal use [21]. The bioactive properties of the leaf have created a foundation for use as an antioxidant, anti-hypertensive, anti-atherogenic, anti-inflammatory, hypoglycemic, and hypocholesterolemic treatment [20]. Olive tree leaves contain similar polyphenols to those found in EVOO or the fruit itself, albeit at a much higher concentration [20,22]. Consequently, olive leaf extract (OLE) may hold an even greater potential than EVOO for improving health outcomes. During EVOO processing leaves can unintentionally be left in the mixture if the separation methods are inadequate, alternately leaves can also be added to EVOO mixtures to provide health benefits and improve flavor [23]. The addition of leaves increase the phenolic and chlorophyll content of the oil but also the organoleptic traits as measured in volunteer taste tests [24]. Components of OLE that are not detected in the oil from the fruit include several flavonoids, namely luteolin and apigenin, which have demonstrated anti-cancer properties [25–29]. In addition, the structure of phenolics differs between the olive fruit and leaf, with OLE containing a higher proportion with a glycoside moiety (Figure 2 and Table 1) [19]. The presence of a glucose molecule could play an important role in respect to both bioavailability and bioactive potential of the polyphenols, thereby impacting the health benefits for humans.

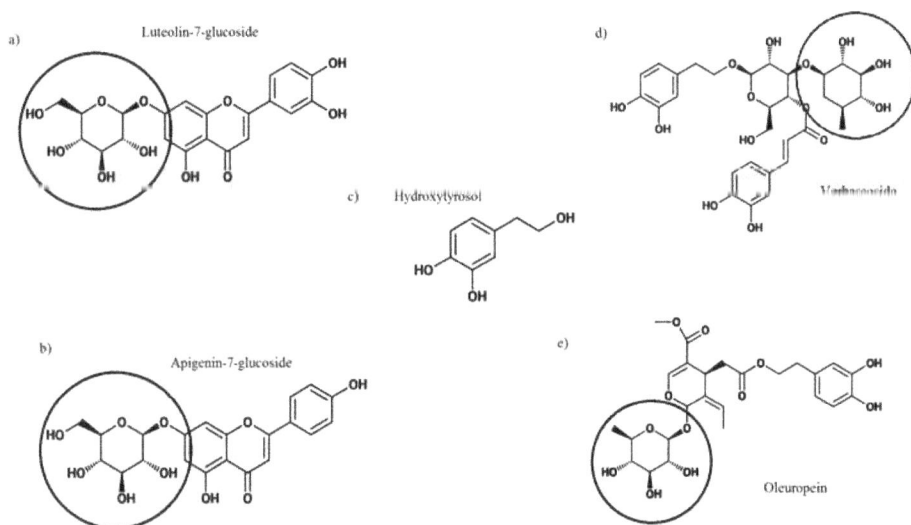

**Figure 2.** Most abundant phenolics present in OLE. Structures (**a**) and (**b**) are flavonoids. Structures (**d**) and (**e**) are esters of (**c**) which is a simple phenolic. The glucoside moieties are circled. This figure is adapted from [19].

**Table 1.** Comparison of phenolic compounds found in olive leaf extract and olive oil, with values reported in mg/kg [30]. Luteolin, apigenin, verbascoside and oleuropein all have a glucoside moiety. Values are an estimated range generated from a comprehensive review of the published literature.

| | Hydroxytyrosol | Oleuropein | Luteolin-7-Glucoside | Apigenin-7-Glucoside | Verbascoside | Oleuropein Aglycone | Reference |
|---|---|---|---|---|---|---|---|
| | 131.77 ± 32 | ND | ND | ND | ND | 17.24 ± 1.15 | [30] |
| Olive oil | 3.0 ± 0.2 | ND | ND | ND | 0.08 ± 0.02 | NM | [31] |
| mg/Kg | 12.5 | ND | NM | NM | NM | NM | [32] |
| | 4.3–9.9 | ND | 4.0–7.6 | 1.5–2.6 | ND | 67.7–136.4 | [33] |
| | 0.15–1.53 | ND | ND | ND | ND | 0.35–6.43 | [34] |
| | NM | 26,471.4 ± 1760.2 | 4208.9 ± 97.8 | 2333.1 ± 74.7 | 966.1 ± 18.1 | NM | [35] |
| Olive | ND | 19,050 ± 880 | 155 ± 10 | 207 ± 10 | 1428 ± 46 | NM | [31] |
| leaf | NM | 19,860 ± 54 | NM | NM | 200 ± 40 | NM | [36] |
| mg/Kg | NM | 22,610 ± 632 | 970 ± 43 | 1072 ± 38 | 488 ± 21 | NM | [37] |
| | NM | 5173–12,921 | 219–444 | 192–488 | 213–501 | NM | [38] |

Abbreviations: not detected: ND; not measured: NM.

Although there is a large body of research that has investigated the phenolic components of olive products and the benefits they provide to human health [39–42], there are currently no approved claims in regard to OLE. OLE not only contains a higher quantity and variety of polyphenols than those found in EVOO, but many of the polyphenols also contain a glucose moiety. This structural difference in the polyphenols may have important consequences by altering their capacity to improve health outcomes [43,44]. In previous work, OLE polyphenols have demonstrated the ability to inhibit proliferation of several cancer cell lines including pancreatic [45], leukaemia [46] and breast [28,47]. Cellular models for breast and prostate cancers have been inhibited by the olive polyphenols oleuropein and HT [48–51]. Importantly, oleuropein and HT have consistently been reported to discriminate between cancer and normal cells; inhibiting proliferation and inducing apoptosis only in cancer cells. The intake of polyphenols in observational studies is difficult to quantify and therefore assign effect and intervention studies in regards to cancer have not been carried out, therefore the relationship between polyphenols and cancer outcomes in humans has not been substantiated.

Research into the anti-cancer properties of olive polyphenols is abundant with a focus on the health effects of EVOO. Evidence suggests that the bioactive components of OLE, although similar to EVOO, may be more potent and therefore show more potential for improving health outcomes. This review aims to amalgamate the current literature regarding bioavailability and anti-cancer mechanisms involved in OLE polyphenol action. The literature identified for this review was found using the search engines PubMed-NCBI, Scopus and ScienceDirect with a combination of block searching and pearl-growing. Key words used for the search were olive leaf extract, polyphenols, cancer, oleuropein, hydroxytyrosol, Mediterranean diet, inflammation, and bioavailability. The key components from the research articles pivotal to this review have been summarized in Supplementary Table S1.

## 2. Olive Leaf Polyphenols

The Mediterranean region, where olive trees are predominantly grown, is characterized by extended periods of sunlight and high rates of pathogen and insect attack. To combat these stressors, olive trees synthesize high volumes of polyphenols which are largely stored in their thick leaves [52]. The concentration and variety of polyphenols present in the leaves will be influenced by many factors such as geographical location, cultivar of tree, and the age of the tree [49]. Polyphenols comprise multiple phenolic groups, each consisting of an aromatic ring with a varying number of hydroxyl groups [19]. The polyphenols predominantly occur in a conjugated form, with one or several sugars attached to the hydroxyl group [53]. The number and structure of phenol rings in a polyphenol are used for classification and will determine its bioactive properties. The main phenolic compounds are the secoiridoids (namely oleuropein) and flavonoids (Figure 2), these have shown the ability to influence human and animal inflammatory and metabolic biomarkers [41,54–56].

Secoiridoids are a group of compounds found exclusively in plants of the *Olearaceae* family, and make up the majority of olive polyphenols (~85% of olive leaf polyphenols) [57]. In OLE the secoiridoid, oleuropein is the most abundant polyphenol (Figure 2), while its derivatives oleuropein aglycone, oleoside, and ligstroside aglycone are also present at varying concentrations [19]. The research surrounding oleuropein is abundant. It has been associated with numerous health benefits including the ability to: lower blood pressure in rats [58], decrease plasma glucose concentrations in rats [55], inhibit the growth of microbes grown on agar plates [59], inhibit cultured parasitic protozoans [60] and has also shown the ability to induce apoptosis in cancer cell models: colorectal [61], breast ([61–63] and prostate [48]. Human trials looking into the effect of OLE on cancer do not yet exist.

Hydrolysis of oleuropein gives rise to oleuropein aglycone, elenolic acid, HT and a glucose molecule (Figure 3) [64]. HT is a phenolic alcohol and the second most abundant phenolic acid in olive leaf. Tyrosol is another phenolic acid derived from oleuropein, but is found in low concentrations in the leaf (Table 1). Other related compounds include verbascoside, which also has demonstrated anti-inflammatory, anti-oxidant and antineoplastic properties similar to the other olive leaf bioactives [65], as well as caffeic acid (220.5 ± 23.3 mg/kg) [35] and p-coumaric acid.

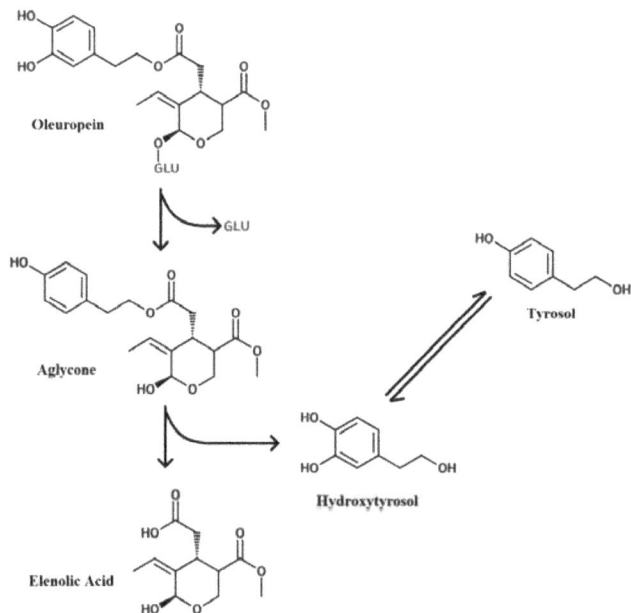

**Figure 3.** Glycosylation of oleuropein to its aglycone this gives rise to elenolic acid and hydroxytyrosol. Tyrosol in turn is hydrolysed from hydroxytyrosol (modified from Granados-Principal et al., 2010 [64]).

OLE consists of a number of flavonoids (~2% of olive leaf polyphenols) including luteolin, apigenin (Table 1), rutin (495.9 ± 12.2 mg/kg) [35], catechin (19.3–32.6 mg/g dried extract) [66] and diosmetin (8.70 mg/g dried extract) [22]. Luteolin is able to suppress inflammatory expression in macrophages and adipocytes [67]. Apigenin is present at relatively low concentrations within olive leaf, but it has also been linked to anti-inflammatory, anti-cancer and anti-oxidising properties [68].

Other components of OLE that occur in smaller concentrations include oleanolic acid [69], vanillin and vanillic acid, [59], as well as tocopherols and β carotene [70]. In human studies, α tocopherols have been correlated to lower prostate cancer mortality, but β carotene at high concentrations, has been correlated to increased mortality of lung cancer patients [71].

Thousands of phytochemicals with differing attributes have been identified and isolated, but a point which is often overlooked is that it can be a combination of compounds that induce health benefits [72–74]. Within plants, polyphenols are present in mixtures and not as independent compounds; the polyphenols have evolved together, generally for the purpose of deterring insect feeding and the levels of the different bioactives with these mixtures need to be considered when looking at bioactive properties for human health. While the evolutionary purpose for the polyphenol mixtures it not for human benefit, the nature of the mixtures may nevertheless be important for human health. Several studies have demonstrated that the phenolic compounds from OLE may display a synergistic effect when in the same proportions as occurring naturally in the olive leaf. The secoiridoids, flavonoids and other phenols in OLE provide a stronger anti-microbial and antioxidant effect when working together, as opposed to the phenolics independently [59,75,76]. Through the use of different antioxidant assays it was determined that OLE flavonoids, simple phenols and secoiridoids utilize different mechanisms to exert an anti-oxidant effect [75], which at least in part explains their additive effect.

### 3. Bioavailability of Olive Leaf Polyphenols

In nutrition, bioavailability refers to the amount of compound/nutrient extracted from a food or supplement that is capable of being absorbed and made available for physiological use by the body [77]. There are many factors that will influence the bioavailability of a compound including the vector, time taken for absorption, structure of compound/bioactive target or the individual person [78]. The matrix that the olive leaf is consumed and maintained may also have an impact on the bioavailability of the active components. The leaves can be consumed in tea, as a powder or in an extract form As an example, De Bock and co-authors demonstrated that the polyphenol derivatives measured in plasma differed when the OLE was administered as a safflower oil compared to a glycerol matrix [79].

The ability to produce health benefits in different organs throughout the body requires that the bioactive olive leaf polyphenols, or their metabolites, are able to infiltrate these areas. After an acute load of olive phenolic (3 g phenolic extract from olive cake/kg of body weight) extract in mice, samples demonstrated that phenolic derivatives and conjugates (oleuropein, tyrosol, HT and luteolin) were absorbed, metabolised and present in the plasma (oleuropein derivative: max 4 h: 24 nmol/L and HT: max 2 h: 5.2 nmol/L), the heart (luteolin derivative at 1 h: 0.47 nmol/g), kidney (luteolin derivative 1 h: 0.04 nmol/g, HT max 4 h: 3.8 nmol/g), testicles (olueropein derivative Cmax 2 h: 0.07 nmol/g and HT max 2 h: 2.7 nmol/g) and had even passed the blood brain barrier (olueropein derivative at 2 h: 2.8 nmol/g) [80].

The research looking into bioavailability of polyphenols from OLE in commercial glycerol formulations consistently show that oleuropein is bioavailable in humans but there is differing evidence regarding the metabolites found in plasma [79,81]. De Bock reported the primary metabolite recovered to be glucoronidated and sulphated HT [79]. In contrast, Kendall's group reported that no HT was detected in urine samples, but glucuronic acid conjugates, derived from oleuropein aglycone were detected [81]. In rats fed oleuropein, liquid chromatography-mass spectrometry (LC-MS) detected oleuropein, oleuropein aglycone, elenolic acid and HT both within faeces and urine at 24 h [82]. This demonstrates the stability of these compounds and therefore the potential ability to reach other parts of the body intact and in an active form.

Corona et al. (2006) reported HT and tyrosol traversed the perfused small intestine membrane of rats but oleuropein did not, and would therefore likely reach the large intestine intact [83]. Incubating with anaerobic human microbiota with olueropein resulted in rapid and extensive microbiota degradation of oleuropein to HT and other metabolites [83]. Specifically the gastrointestinal bacterium *Lactobacillus planatarum* has the ability to metabolize oleuropein to HT [84]. The microbiota acting to break down oleuropein to HT would have an important impact on bioavailability if oleuropein cannot traverse membranes, but HT and other metabolites can, as reported by Corona et al. 2006. Another study has since found that oleuropein orally administered to rats resulted in the production of oleuropein metabolites from the gastrointestinal tract as well as metabolites in the blood [82]. The most recent research looking into the metabolism of oleuropein verses oleuropein aglycone in rodents (5 mg phenol/kg/day) found that oleuropein resulted in the greatest bioavailabilty (measured by the highest content of HT excreted in urine) and a greater diversity of microbial metabolites due to its superior ability to reach the colon intact [44].

*Glycosylation of Polyphenols*

The glucose moiety that is present on many of the olive leaf polyphenols could have an important impact on their bioactive properties. The glucose molecule significantly increases the molar mass of the polyphenol; oleuropein is 540.51 g/mol, where the oleuropein aglycone is 394 g/mol. The glucose molecule may improve stability and bioavailability, and facilitate cell entry but it also may impede bioactive properties.

Through collection and processing methods of olives and leaves, different glycosylation enzymes are activated [85]. The transformation of oleuropein is dependent on the type of glycosylation enzyme acting (β-glucosidase, hemicellulase, tannase, neutral protease, cellulase, glucoamylase, papain, alkaline protease, amylase, β-glucanase) and this will result in varied concentrations and ratios of HT, oleuropein aglycone, elonolic acid and total phenolics [86,87]. The combination of polyphenols may improve the OLE biostability, insuring polyphenols are still present in the olive leaf extract when consumed by humans but also improving the polyphenols ability to reach different areas of the body intact. For example oxidoreductase enzymes reduce the abundance of oleuropein in OLE, but the presence of HT is able to inhibit their action [86].

Olive leaf polyphenols containing a glucose moiety have been suggested to play an important role in relation to cancer cell treatment. A study looking at oleuropein found removal of the glucose moiety reduced its ability to inhibit proliferation of cancer cells [43]. This indicated that the hydrophilic glucose may be enabling oleuropein to enter cells via GLUT transporters to create the anti-cancer affect. GLUT mRNA expression is often increased in cancer cells and is correlated to cancer progression [88]. The glucose moiety in oleuropein may facilitate its diffusion into these cells in precedence to normal cells and therefore result in a greater inhibitory effect on cancer versus normal cells. Another study has indicated that the olive flavonoid apigenin is able to reduce the expression of GLUT1 in prostate cancer cell lines thereby inhibiting proliferation of the cancer [29].

Another study looking at the effect of oleuropein (dissolved in water) verses oleuropein aglycone (dissolved in ethanol 100%) (6 to 100 μM) in MCF-7 found the aglycone to be more effective at reducing cell viability [89]. This would suggest that the glycoside is essential for anti-cancer effects.

Protective effects of the MD and EVOO against cancers, as discussed in the introduction, are primarily associated with cancers of the digestive system. This could be due to the bioavailability of the polyphenols, with the polyphenol constituents creating the anti-cancer effects not being able to reach other parts of the body to have an impact. Consequently if the glucose moiety, a prominent characteristic of olive leaf polyphenols improves bioavailability it may also improve protective effects for different cancers.

## 4. OLE and Evidence of the Ability of Olive Leaf Polyphenols to Scavenge Nitric Oxide and Quench Reactive Oxygen Species

Reactive oxygen species (ROS) and nitrogen species (NOS) are essential for cell function. They are involved in energy supply, detoxification, chemical signaling and immune response. However, when overproduced they can create stress by damaging DNA, lipids and proteins and they are widely accepted to play an important role in pathologies and aging [20,90]. Chronic disease is associated with oxidative stress, therefore an increased antioxidant intake or intake of compounds that enhance the body's own antioxidant system is expected to reduce the risk of these diseases. It was this hypothesis that has led to an increased interest in antioxidants and their bioactive properties. Phenolics are one group for which there is robust evidence supporting the health promoting effects of antioxidants. There is a general consensus that olive leaf phenolics have a strong ability to scavenge nitric oxide (NO) and quench ROS [91,92].

Antioxidant properties have been an important focus of research into polyphenols and are a widely accepted mechanism for their health benefits. However, it has been suggested that several constraints impede polyphenol in vivo scavenging of radicals, and that they would be inefficient at mounting an antioxidant defense [93]. Concerns that have been highlighted include bioavailability (the anti-oxidizing agent must reach these radicals in an active form to quench them) and kinetic constraints for antioxidant scavenging (radicals may actually react with other biological molecules such as DNA and lipids in the cell at the same rate as the antioxidants) [93]. This could mean that a very high concentration of polyphenols would need to be ingested to perceive any effect in humans. Instead it is suggested that antioxidant compounds, such as polyphenols, are able to activate transcription factors such as nuclear factor (erythroid-derived 2)-like 2 (Nrf2) that bind to the Electrophile Response Element (EpRE) and thereby transcribe genes for protective enzymes that provide the health benefits (Forman et al., 2014 and Figure 4). Several in vitro studies using humans cells and animal in vivo studies investigating olive polyphenols have supported Nrf2 activation and its consequential expression of protective genes [72,94]. Conversely, a recent human intervention study has shown no evidence of altered phase II enzyme expression (the downstream product of Nrf2 activation) in peripheral blood mononuclear cells following consumption of HT (5 mg and 25 mg per day in olive mill waste water) [95]. The olive mill waste water was tested to confirm oleuropein was not present.

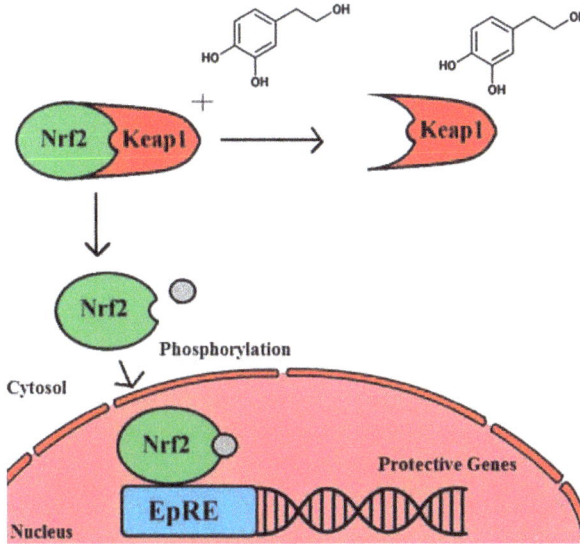

**Figure 4.** Polyphenol interaction with Nrf2 and activation of *EpRE* genes. The polyphenol (HT) reacts with Keap1 permitting Nrf2 to escape. Nrf2 requires phosphorylation before it is able to enter the nucleus. This schematic is modified from [93].

The Xenohormesis hypothesis suggests the stress-induced secondary metabolite production in plants is recognized by humans upon consumption, and these signals initiate stress response pathways [72,73]. Similarities in the human and plant extracellular signal-regulated kinase (ERK) pathways (these are able to activate many transcription factors and play an important role in cell regulation functions) show that polyphenols are able to activate pathways, such as AMP-activated protein kinase (AMPK) and hold the potential to modulate redox and mitochondrial signaling [96,97]. During eukaryotic evolution, glucose was the preferred carbon source. Rapid cell growth was the best way to utilize glucose, and AMPK activation provided the off switch mechanism in this process [72]. Therefore, AMPK activation (or similar pathways) could result in decreased ATP and increases in mitochondrial free radicals, implicating protection from chronic disease and aging [72]. Evidence for this theory was provided by microarray analysis of gene expression after EVOO treatment of breast cancer cells. These results demonstrated up-regulation of AMPK, and the top Canonical pathway regulated was the Nrf2 Mediated Oxidative stress pathway [72].

HT in vitro studies using human cell lines has been shown to up-regulate the expression of endogenous antioxidant genes (Heme Oxygenase 1 (HO-1), NAD(P)H-quinone oxidoreductase (NQO1), Glutathione (GSH)) via Nrf2 overexpression. The c-Jun N-terminal kinase (JNK) pathway plays an important role in inflammatory signaling. The JNK pathway was up-regulated following treatment with HT and inhibiting this pathway established its requirement for GSH and *p62* regulation. However, *HO-1* or *NQ-1* were unaffected [94]. p62 inactivates *Keap1*, increasing Nrf2 in the nucleus and consequently increasing the expression of oxidation defense enzyme genes [98]. Oleuropein in a human in vitro model has also been shown to activate Nrf2 and HO-1 expression [99]. However, in vivo human trials with HT have failed to find an up-regulation of phase 2 enzymes which are the by-product of EpRE and Nrf2 stimulation [95].

## 5. Olive Leaf Properties That Protect against Development and Progression of Cancer

Genetic changes are involved in the prevalence of cancers, however it is environmental and lifestyle factors such as obesity [100], unbalanced diet, tobacco, lack of exercise and alcohol consumption that account for the majority of the attributing cause [101]. Olive leaf contains strong anti-oxidants, it would be logical to conclude that these would help in mitigating the effect of genetic lesions that give rise to cancer. However, olive leaf has also attracted attention as a potential cancer treatment [28,46,102,103]. In previous work, olive leaf polyphenols have demonstrated the ability to inhibit the proliferation of several cancer cell lines including pancreatic [45], leukaemia [46], breast [28,47,49], prostate [48] and colorectal [61]. Importantly, oleuropein and HT have consistently been reported to discriminate between cancer and normal cells; inhibiting proliferation and inducing apoptosis only in cancer cells [48,49]. The challenge with relating the anti-cancer effects in cell models to in vivo arises when considering bioavailability of the polyphenols. This could explain why OO protective effects in humans show a strong association with cancers of the digestive system [12]. In other cancers OO phenolics has been suggested to act as phytoestrogens and anti-inflammatory agents, thus producing a protective effect.

A higher risk of breast cancer is linked to over-exposure to oestrogen [104,105] and growth of breast cancer can be stimulated by estradiol, which binds to the oestrogen receptor (ER). This receptor is an important biomarker and target for breast cancer prevention and treatment [106]. Work with breast cancer cell lines and OLE polyphenols have indicated potential mechanisms of action that include action as a phytoestrogen. Oleuropein and HT both possess an aromatic ring that is similar to that in estradiol, therefore these compounds are hypothesized to compete with oestrogens for receptor binding sites [50,107]. In the MCF-7 breast cancer cell line, HT and oleuropein (at doses between 10 and 75 µM) dose-dependently prevented cell proliferation through inhibition of the oestrogen activated ERK1/2 signaling pathway but did not show a direct effect on the mediation of ER gene expression [50]. It was later shown that oestrogen responses were also mediated by the GPER/GPER30 receptors, of which HT and oleuropein are agonists [108]. Despite both oestrogen and the polyphenols showing the same mechanism of receptor binding, they have opposite effects. Oestrogen leads to cell proliferation, while polyphenols lead to apoptosis or cell death. Both activate the ERK1/2 pathways but it has been proposed that the length of activation could influence the effect, with prolonged activation leading to apoptosis, and short-term to cell proliferation [108]. Sustained ERK activation has previously been demonstrated to result in inhibition of MCF-7 cell growth [109]. In vivo studies looking at olive leaf polyphenols also appear to support an anti-cancer effect. Oleuropein (125 mg/kg of diet) slowed tumor growth and inhibited cancer metastasis after MCF-7 cell xenograft establishment in mice [110]. OLE dissolved in water (150 and 225 mg/kg/day) reduced tumour volume and weight in mice after breast cancer xenograft [111].

The aromatase (CYP19) enzyme is the catalyst for the rate determining reaction in oestrogen synthesis. Inhibiting CYP19 effectively prevents oestrogen synthesis and because high levels of oestrogen are linked to breast cancer, this holds potential as a treatment [112]. A recent clinical study has shown that amylase inhibitors taken daily for 5 years were successfully able to reduce the incidence of breast cancer in high-risk postmenopausal women [113]. In MCF-7 cells, luteolin suppressed CYP19 transcription potentially via activator protein-1 (AP1) and C/EBP binding to the aromatase promoter [26].

The olive flavones apigenin and luteolin have been shown to act as aryl hydrocarbon receptor (AhR) antagonists in mouse cell lines [114]. Upon ligand binding, AhR is translocated to the nucleus where it activates response elements in the DNA sequence and consequent production of xenobiotic enzymes [115]. Other work has found that AhR in cancer cell lines acts as a tumour suppressor through diminished DNA replication and G0/G1 arrest [116]. Another study has reported that apigenin suppresses the growth of MCF-7 cells, inhibiting the NF-κB signaling pathway, the phosphorylation of IkBα, and nuclear translocation of p65 within the nucleus [27]. Apigenin was not found to inhibit cell survival signaling through mediators such as AKT, ERK, JNK, or p38, but it decreased STAT3 transcriptional activity in the cells, indicating that this compound induces growth-suppressive activity. The transcription factor STAT3 is more specifically involved in inflammatory signaling within cancer tumours and interacts with cytokines [117], thus by inhibiting STAT3, luteolin could also be having an anti-inflammatory effect. In another study oleuropein was cytotoxic to MDA-MB-231 and MCF-7 cells, avoiding damage to normal cells, with apoptosis taking place via induction of the mitochondrial pathway [49]. MCF-7 cell proliferation was inhibited by oleuropein at the S-phase of the cell cycle by an up-regulation of the p21 gene, and inhibition of NF-κB and its target D1 gene expression.

In PC3 and DU145 prostate cancer cell lines, HT has demonstrated the ability to interfere with cell proliferation [51]. HT also activated mitogen-activated protein kinase (MAPK), ERK, p38 MAPK and JNK. However, when inhibited by specific antagonists, HT was still able to inhibit cell growth. The authors concluded that HT was able to induce apoptosis in cancer cells via the generation of superoxide dismutase (SOD) and extracellular ROS.

Work using the prostate cancer cell lines, LNCaP and DU145, found that oleuropein was pro-oxidative, causing loss of viability, but in non-malignant cells (a benign hyperplastic prostatic epithelial cell line) oleuropein acted as an anti-oxidant [48]. The downstream products of EpRE activation were all increased with oleuropein; pAkt, y-glutamylcysteine (y-GCS), heme oxygenase-1 (HO-1) and ROS. Interference with pAkt was proposed as the mechanism enabling cell apoptosis in these prostate cancer cell lines [48].

### 5.1. Anti-Inflammatory Properties of Olive Leaf Polyphenols and Their Effects on Cancer

Inflammation is the natural defense mechanism against foreign threats, and its mechanisms are essential for survival. However, chronic inflammation, even at low levels, has been correlated to many health complications and age-associated diseases, including but not limited to cancer and cardiovascular disease [118]. The NF-κB signaling pathways play a pivotal role in inflammatory response and are an attractive target for preventing inflammation. NF-κB resides inactive within the cytoplasm due to the presence of IκB kinase, an inhibitor enzyme, therefore it can be activated very quickly to initiate cytokine and prostanoid production. There is strong evidence that olive polyphenols are able to interact with these pathways [119–121].

The cyclooxygenase 2 (COX-2) enzyme plays an important role in inflammation as the catalyst for the synthesis for prostanoids and hence an inflammatory response [122]. Cellular studies with OLE polyphenols have found a protective effect in relation to inflammation; a down-regulation of NO and COX-2 [120,123–125]. Inhibition of the Toll-like receptor (TLR) signaling induced by LPS was demonstrated not only by down-regulation of iNOS and COX2, but also by a decrease in ERK1/2, JNK and nuclear factor of kappa light polypeptide gene enhancer in B-cells inhibitor alpha (IκBα) phosphorylation in vitro after oleuropein treatment [120] (Figure 5). In down-regulating this pathway the pro-inflammatory enzymes interleukin 6 (IL-6) and interleukin 1β (IL-1β) and the gene AP-1 were also down-regulated. In human monocytes HT inhibited LPS induced COX-2 and prostanoid production, however, it increased TNF-α. In contrast in human cell models tyrosol down-regulated TNF-α and induced NF-κB, JNK and ERK phosphorylation and COX-2 expression [126] (Figure 5). Lastly the olive flavonoid luteolin regulated IL-1β induced COX-2 expression via ERK, JNK and NF-κB [127].

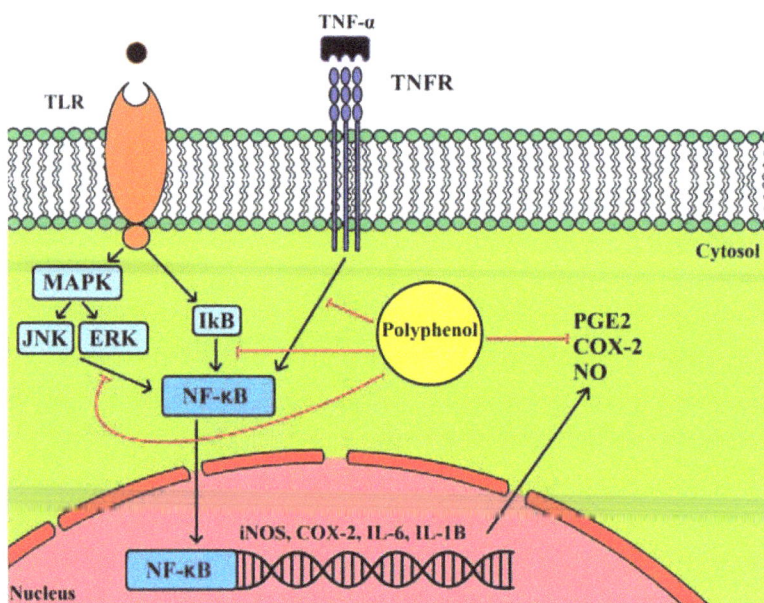

**Figure 5.** Olive leaf polyphenols may interact with gene and protein expression directly or via an interaction with receptors on the cell membrane. Toll-like receptor (TLR) and tumour necrosis factor receptor (TNFR) activation results in inflammatory gene expression (COX2, IL-6, IL-6 and IL-1β) and prostanoid production. This illustration shows the potential points at which OLE polyphenols could interact if able to enter the cell membrane.

### 5.2. Cancer, Inflammation and COX2 Expression

An overexpression of COX-2 has been linked to invasiveness of many cancers including human breast cancer [128,129], prostate [130] and colorectal [131]. Drugs that inhibit COX-2 enzymes are able to reduce the risk of breast cancer [132], and have pro-apoptotic effects in the MCF-7 cell line [133] and prostate cancer cell lines [134]. Luteolin, when administered with the COX-2 inhibitor celecoxib, created a synergistic effect in MCF-7 and three other breast cancer cell lines. Interestingly, the ERK1/2 levels were inhibited in the oestrogen receptor positive cell lines, but were increased in the negative cell lines [135]. Down-regulation of the phosphatidylinositide 3-kinase (P13K)/Akt pathway inhibits phosphorylated Akt levels, which in turn stimulates apoptosis. Phosphorylated Akt levels were decreased in all cell lines [135].

A review on breast cancer found all stages of cancer progression corresponded to COX-2 expression [129]. COX-2 is a down-stream product of NF-κB which was down-regulated in MCF-7 treated with oleuropein [49]. In mouse models, COX-2 driven prostaglandin E2 (PGE2) expression in mammary tissue led to an increase of *CYP19* and aromatase-catalysed oestrogen biosynthesis [136]. Samples taken from patients with breast cancer showed a correlation between transcription of *CYP19* and both gene and protein expressions of COX-2 and PGE2 [137]. In a previous study the authors hypothesized that HT and oleuropein were able to inhibit proliferation via competing for oestrogen binding sites [50]. These studies suggest that OLE polyphenols may be acting in MCF-7 to block oestrogen receptor binding and to inhibit COX-2 expression, which appears to down-regulate *CYP19* expression [136].

Another gene that COX-2 can regulate is p53. Work in human mammary tissue has demonstrated that COX-2 represses p53 transcription thereby inhibiting cell apoptosis [138] and it has since been demonstrated that p53 down-regulates aromatase expression in breast adipose stromal cells [139].

Work looking at the effects of oleuropein in MCF-7 has shown that it is able to induce apoptosis via up-regulating p53, and consequently the transcription of Bax/Bcl-2 apoptotic genes [62]. Other studies have also measured a change in p53 and Bax expression with oleuropein inhibition of cervical cancer cells [140] and p53 pathway up-regulation with oleuropein inhibition of colorectal cancer cells [61].

In vivo, luteolin (10 mg/kg/day) reduced both volume and weight of tumors in a prostate xenograft mouse model and in vitro, using the prostate cancer cells PC-3, it down-regulated VEGF phosphorylation of VEGF2 receptor and its downstream inflammatory markers IL-8 and IL-6 [25]. If VEGF is correlated to PGE2, as in the breast cancer models mentioned above, then it could be a downstream effect of COX-2 inhibition.

PGE2 expression pushes the immune response from a T-helper 1 (Th1) (including cells such as Natural killer (NK) cells) to a Th2 (such as mast cells) and Th17 mediated response, which is less effective at fighting off infections or protecting from cancer [141]. This potentiates acute, local inflammation driven by phagocytes, which is less aggressive than the Th1/Th17 response [141]. By down-regulating COX-2, the balance will shift back to Th1, which may improve immune-competence. For example COX-2 knock out in breast cancer cells inhibited tumour growth by enhancing T-cell survival and immune surveillance in tumours [142].

The tumour microenvironment has an important impact on tumour progression and metastasis, therefore its manipulation has been suggested as a target for cancer therapy [143]. It has been demonstrated in breast cancer MCF-7 cells that tumour associated macrophages are able to enhance COX-2 levels in the tumour. Conversely inhibiting COX-2 in macrophages was able to inhibit levels in the tumour [144]. In several human intervention studies with olive polyphenols, COX-2 expression in immune cells was down-regulated [145,146]. In cancer patients this could potentially lead to a down-regulation of COX-2 in tumours and thereby inhibit tumour progression. In other intervention studies the inflammatory markers NF-κB, p65, IKKβ, and IKKα [147] and NF-κB, IL-6 and IL-1β [148] have been down-regulated with olive polyphenols. These studies measured changes after single 40 mL doses of EVOO (containing the olive polyphenols), quantities achievable in an individual's standard diet.

### 5.3. Quinone Hypothesis for Anti-Cancer Properties of Olive Leaf

As quinones, olive leaf polyphenols could bind to the cysteine residues of NF-κB in cancer cells and manipulate gene expression. This would explain the observed gene expression in in vitro models [46,120,126]. A recent study has indicated olive leaf polyphenols in a quinone form could interact with Topoisomerase IIα [149]. The olive leaf polyphenols oleuropein, verbascoside, and HT were categorized by Vann et al. as Topoisomerase IIα poisons. Topoisomerase IIα is an enzyme essential for cell survival, catalysing the breaking and re-joining of the DNA helix to remove tangles and playing an important role in cell replication. Acting as Topoisomerase IIα poisons the polyphenols increased DNA cleavage, this effect was 10–100 times stronger in the presence of an oxidant [149]. This is consistent with the idea that the polyphenols have been transformed into quinone electrophiles, which are then able to bind to cysteine residues. This study also demonstrated that the olive leaf polyphenol tyrosol was unable to act as a poison consistent with its inability to form a quinone and bind to the cysteine residue within Topoisomerase IIα.

Although potentially dangerous in normal cells, Topisomerase IIα is an important target for cancer treatment. Due to the requirement of an oxidant environment, this might explain why no toxicity has been shown in normal cells in comparison to tumour cell models; the quinones were not formed.

### 6. Conclusions

There is strong evidence from cell models which demonstrates that olive polyphenols, and specifically the combination found in olive leaf, are able to modulate and interact with molecular pathways and in doing so may inhibit the progression and development of cancer. However, it is important to acknowledge that cell models are very different from the complex human body and applying these findings to cancer outcomes in humans is difficult.

Meta-analysis correlating the consumption of a MD and OO in humans to protection from digestive system, prostate and breast cancers [4,12], suggest that the effects may be constrained by bioavailability but also directs to a phytoestrogenic mechanism of action. Not only are the reduced risk of oestrogen related cancers in females correlated to protective effects of phytoestrogens, but a recent meta-analysis has correlated a lower risk of prostate cancer with phytoestrogen consumption [150].

The evidence suggests that olive polyphenols may act differently when in different combinations and at different concentrations. The presence of a glucose molecule, one factor that differentiates olive leaf polyphenols from OO polyphenols, is likely to affect the bioavailability and therefore bioactive properties. Changes to microbiota and microbiota-mediated degradation of polyphenols, demonstrate the glucose molecule has an effect.

Both cell models and human intervention studies demonstrate olive polyphenols are creating an anti-inflammatory change involving NF-κB inhibition. The down-stream products of NF-κB: including COX-2, IL-6, IL-8, IL-1β are expressed at lower levels creating a tumour micro-environment that no longer facilitates progression or development of cancers. This may account for the lower prevalence of cancer in people consuming a MD.

To answer the question "does OLE protect against cancer?" is difficult. Evidence is available in cell and animal models to support the conclusion that OLE does have beneficial effects and there is anecdotal evidence that olive polyphenols have a protective effect against cancer in humans. People consuming the MD have a lower prevalence of cancer, the MD consists of a high content of polyphenols, and olive leaf is an excellent source of many of these polyphenols. However, in order to prove that OLE improves cancer outcomes in humans, clinical trials would be required.

**Supplementary Materials:** The following are available online at http://www.mdpi.com/2072-6643/8/8/513/s1, Table S1: Olive leaf polyphenol treatment in different cancer models; in vivo and in vitro.

**Acknowledgments:** Funding was provided to Anna Boss from Comvita, New Zealand Limited, 234 Wilson Road South, Paengaroa, Te Puke 3189.

**Author Contributions:** All authors contributed to the preparation of this review article.

**Conflicts of Interest:** The authors declare no conflict of interest.

## Abbreviations

The following abbreviations are used in this manuscript:

| | |
|---|---|
| AhR | Aryl hydrocarbon receptor |
| AP1 | Activator protein-1 |
| EVOO | Extra Virgin Olive oil |
| HT | Hydroxytyrosol |
| JNK | c-Jun *N*-terminal kinase |
| MD | Mediterranean diet |
| MAPK | Mitogen-activated protein kinase |
| Nrf2 | Nuclear factor (erythroid-derived 2)-like 2 |
| NO | Nitric oxide |
| OLE | Olive leaf extract |
| OO | Olive oil |
| ROS | Reactive oxygen species |
| TLR | Toll-like receptor |

## References

1. Hanahan, D.; Weinberg, R.A. Hallmarks of cancer: The next generation. *Cell* **2011**, *144*, 646–674. [CrossRef] [PubMed]

2. Ferlay, J.; Soerjomataram, I.; Dikshit, R.; Eser, S.; Mathers, C.; Rebelo, M.; Parkin, D.M.; Forman, D.D.; Bray, F. Cancer incidence and mortality worldwide: Sources, methods and major patterns in GLOBOCAN 2012. *Int. J. Cancer* **2014**, *136*. [CrossRef] [PubMed]

3. Filomeno, M.; Bosetti, C.; Bidoli, E.; Levi, F.; Serraino, D.; Montella, M.; La Vecchia, C.; Tavani, A. Mediterranean diet and risk of endometrial cancer: A pooled analysis of three Italian case-control studies. *Br. J. Cancer* **2015**, *112*, 1816–1821. [CrossRef] [PubMed]

4. Schwingshackl, L.; Hoffmann, G. Does a Mediterranean-Type Diet Reduce Cancer Risk? *Curr. Nutr. Rep.* **2015**, *5*, 9–17. [CrossRef] [PubMed]

5. Ostan, R.; Lanzarini, C.; Pini, E.; Scurti, M.; Vianello, D.; Bertarelli, C.; Fabbri, C.; Izzi, M.; Palmas, G.; Biondi, F.; et al. Inflammaging and cancer: A challenge for the Mediterranean diet. *Nutrients* **2015**, *7*, 2589–2621. [CrossRef] [PubMed]

6. Marlow, G.; Ellett, S.; Ferguson, I.R.; Zhu, S.; Karunasinghe, N.; Jesuthasan, A.C.; Han, D.; Fraser, A.G.; Ferguson, L.R. Transcriptomics to study the effect of a Mediterranean-inspired diet on inflammation in Crohn's disease patients. *Hum. Genom.* **2013**, *7*, 24. [CrossRef] [PubMed]

7. Panunzio, M.F.; Caporizzi, R.; Antoniciello, A.; Cela, E.P.; Ferguson, L.R.; D'Ambrosio, P. Randomized, controlled nutrition education trial promotes a Mediterranean diet and improves anthropometric, dietary, and metabolic parameters in adults. *Ann. Ig. Med. Prev. Comunità* **2010**, *23*, 13–25.

8. Yubero-Serrano, E.M.; Delgado-Casado, N.; Delgado-Lista, J.; Perez-Martinez, P.; Tasset-Cuevas, I.; Santos-Gonzalez, M.; Caballero, J.; Garcia-Rios, A.; Marin, C.; Gutierrez-Mariscal, F.M.; et al. Postprandial antioxidant effect of the Mediterranean diet supplemented with coenzyme Q10 in elderly men and women. *Age (Dordr)* **2011**, *33*, 579–590. [CrossRef] [PubMed]

9. Camargo, A.; Delgado-Lista, J.; Garcia-Rios, A.; Cruz-Teno, C.; Yubero-Serrano, E.M.; Perez-Martinez, P.; Gutierrez-Mariscal, F.M.; Lora-Aguilar, P.; Rodriguez-Cantalejo, F.; Fuentes-Jimenez, F.; et al. Expression of proinflammatory, proatherogenic genes is reduced by the Mediterranean diet in elderly people. *Br. J. Nutr.* **2012**, *108*, 500–508. [CrossRef] [PubMed]

10. Renna, M.; Rinaldi, V.A.; Gonnella, M. The Mediterranean Diet between traditional foods and human health: The culinary example of Puglia (Southern Italy). *Int. J. Gastron. Food Sci.* **2015**, *2*, 63–71. [CrossRef]

11. Schwingshackl, L.; Hoffmann, G. Monounsaturated fatty acids, olive oil and health status: A systematic review and meta-analysis of cohort studies. *Lipids Health Dis.* **2014**, *13*, 154. [CrossRef] [PubMed]

12. Psaltopoulou, T.; Kosti, R.I.; Haidopoulos, D.; Dimopoulos, M.; Panagiotakos, D.B. Olive oil intake is inversely related to cancer prevalence: A systematic review and a meta-analysis of 13,800 patients and 23,340 controls in 19 observational studies. *Lipids Health Dis.* **2011**, *10*, 127. [CrossRef] [PubMed]

13. Portarena, S.; Baldacchini, C.; Brugnoli, E. Geographical discrimination of extra-virgin olive oils from the Italian coasts by combining stable isotope data and carotenoid content within a multivariate analysis. *Food Chem.* **2017**, *215*, 1–6. [CrossRef]

14. Jabeur, H.; Zribi, A.; Bouaziz, M. Changes in chemical and sensory characteristics of Chemlali extra-virgin olive oil as depending on filtration. *Eur. J. Lipid Sci. Technol.* **2016**. [CrossRef]

15. Aparicio, R.; Harwood, J. Handbook of Olive Oil: Analysis and Properties. Springer Science & Business Media, 2013. Available online: https://books.google.com/books?hl=en&lr=&id=gQrkBwAAQBAJ&pgis=1 (accessed on 8 March 2016).

16. EFSA Panel on Dietetic Products, N. and A. (NDA). Scientific Opinion on the Substantiation of health Claims Related to Polyphenols in Olive and Protection of LDL Particles from Oxidative damage (ID 1333, 1638, 1639, 1696, 2865), Maintenance of Normal Blood HDL Cholesterol Concentrations (ID 1639), Mainte. *EFSA J. 2011* **2011**, *9*. [CrossRef]

17. Farràs, M.; Valls, R.M.; Fernández-Castillejo, S.; Giralt, M.; Solà, R.; Subirana, I.; Motilva, M.-J.; Konstantinidou, V.; Covas, M.-I.; Fitó, M. Olive oil polyphenols enhance the expression of cholesterol efflux related genes in vivo in humans. A randomized controlled trial. *J. Nutr. Biochem.* **2013**, *24*, 1334–1339. [CrossRef] [PubMed]

18. Castañer, O.; Corella, D.; Covas, M.I.; Sorlí, J.V.; Subirana, I.; Flores-Mateo, G.; Nonell, L.; Bulló, M.; de la Torre, R.; Portolés, O.; et al. In vivo transcriptomic profile after a Mediterranean diet in high-cardiovascular risk patients: A randomized controlled trial. *Am. J. Clin. Nutr.* **2013**, *98*, 845–853. [CrossRef] [PubMed]

19. Lockyer, S.; Yaqoob, P.; Spencer, J.P.E.; Rowland, I. Olive leaf phenolics and cardiovascular risk reduction: Physiological effects and mechanisms of action. *Nutr. Aging* **2012**, *1*, 125–140.

20. El, S.N.; Karakaya, S. Olive tree (*Olea europaea*) leaves: Potential beneficial effects on human health. *Nutr. Rev.* **2009**, *67*, 632–638. [CrossRef] [PubMed]

21. Wren, R. Potter's New Cyclopaedia of Botanical Drugs and Preparations. 1994. Available online: https://scholar.google.co.nz/scholar?hl=en&q=R.C.+Wren+%28Ed.%29%2C+Potter%27s+New+Cyclopaedia+of+Botanical+Drugs+and+Preparations%2C+The+C.W.+Daniel%2C+Essex%2C+UK+%281994%29%2C+p.+20&btnG=&as_sdt=1%2C5&as_sdtp=#0 (accessed on 21 October 2015).

22. Ye, J.; Wang, C.; Chen, H.; Zhou, H. Variation Rule of Hydroxytyrosol Content in Olive Leaves. Available online: http://en.cnki.com.cn/Article_en/CJFDTOTAL-LCHX201102015.htm (accessed on 15 May 2015).

23. Mihailova, A.; Abbado, D.; Pedentchouk, N. Differences in *n*-alkane profiles between olives and olive leaves as potential indicators for the assessment of olive leaf presence in virgin olive oils. *Eur. J. Lipid Sci. Technol.* **2015**, *117*, 1480–1485. [CrossRef]

24. Nenadis, N.; Moutafidou, A.; Gerasopoulos, D.; Tsimidou, M.Z. Quality characteristics of olive leaf-olive oil preparations. *Eur. J. Lipid Sci. Technol.* **2010**, *112*, 1337–1344. [CrossRef]

25. Pratheeshkumar, P.; Son, Y.-O.; Budhraja, A.; Wang, X.; Ding, S.; Wang, L.; Hitron, A.; Lee, J.-C.; Kim, D.; Divya, S.P.; et al. Luteolin inhibits human prostate tumor growth by suppressing vascular endothelial growth factor receptor 2-mediated angiogenesis. *PLoS ONE* **2012**, *7*, e52279. [CrossRef] [PubMed]

26. Li, F.; Ye, L.; Lin, S.; Leung, L.K. Dietary flavones and flavonones display differential effects on aromatase (CYP19) transcription in the breast cancer cells MCF 7. *Mol. Cell. Endocrinol.* **2011**, *344*, 51–58. [CrossRef] [PubMed]

27. Seo, H.-S.; Choi, H.-S.; Kim, S.-R.; Choi, Y.K.; Woo, S.-M.; Shin, I.; Woo, J.-K.; Park, S.-Y.; Shin, Y.C.; Ko, S.-G.; et al. Apigenin induces apoptosis via extrinsic pathway, inducing p53 and inhibiting STAT3 and NFκB signaling in HER2-overexpressing breast cancer cells. *Mol. Cell. Biochem.* **2012**, *366*, 319–334. [CrossRef] [PubMed]

28. Barrajón-Catalán, E.; Taamalli, A.; Quirantes-Piné, R.; Roldan-Segura, C.; Arráez-Román, D.; Segura-Carretero, A.; Micol, V.; Zarrouk, M. Differential metabolomic analysis of the potential antiproliferative mechanism of olive leaf extract on the JIMT-1 breast cancer cell line. *J. Pharm. Biomed. Anal.* **2015**, *105*, 156–162. [CrossRef] [PubMed]

29. Gonzalez-Menendez, P.; Hevia, D.; Rodriguez-Garcia, A.; Mayo, J.C.; Sainz, R.M. Regulation of GLUT transporters by flavonoids in androgen-sensitive and -insensitive prostate cancer cells. *Endocrinology* **2014**, *155*, 3238–3250. [CrossRef] [PubMed]

30. Artajo, L.S.; Romero, M.P.; Motilva, M.J. Transfer of phenolic compounds during olive oil extraction in relation to ripening stage of the fruit. *J. Sci. Food Agric.* **2006**, *86*, 518–527. [CrossRef]

31. Luján, R.J.; Capote, F.P.; Marinas, A.; de Castro, M.D.L. Liquid chromatography/triple quadrupole tandem mass spectrometry with multiple reaction monitoring for optimal selection of transitions to evaluate nutraceuticals from olive-tree materials. *Rapid Commun. Mass Spectrom.* **2008**, *22*, 855–864. [CrossRef] [PubMed]

32. Flores, A.; Isabel, M.; Romero-González, R.; Frenich, G.; Vidal, A.; Martínez, L.J. Analysis of phenolic compounds in olive oil by solid-phase extraction and ultra high performance liquid chromatography-tandem mass spectrometry. *Food Chem.* **2012**, *134*, 2465–2472. [CrossRef] [PubMed]

33. Šarolić, M.; Gugić, M.; Friganović, E.; Tuberoso, C.; Jerković, I. Phytochemicals and Other Characteristics of Croatian Monovarietal Extra Virgin Olive Oils from Oblica, Lastovka and Levantinka Varieties. *Molecules* **2015**, *20*, 4395–4409. [CrossRef] [PubMed]

34. Rigane, G.; Ayadi, M.; Boukhris, M.; Sayadi, S.; Bouaziz, M. Characterisation and phenolic profiles of two rare olive oils from southern Tunisia: Dhokar and Gemri-Dhokar cultivars. *J. Sci. Food Agric.* **2013**, *93*, 527–534. [CrossRef] [PubMed]

35. Pereira, A.P.; Ferreira, I.C.; Marcelino, F.; Valentão, P.; Andrade, P.B.; Seabra, R.; Estevinho, L.; Bento, A.; Pereira, J.A. Phenolic Compounds and Antimicrobial Activity of Olive (*Olea europaea* L. Cv. Cobrançosa) Leaves. *Molecules* **2007**, *12*, 1153–1162. [CrossRef] [PubMed]

36. Aouidi, F.; Ayari, S.; Ferhi, H.; Roussos, S.; Hamdi, M. Gamma irradiation of air-dried olive leaves: Effective decontamination and impact on the antioxidative properties and on phenolic compounds. *Food Chem.* **2011**, *127*, 1105–1113. [CrossRef] [PubMed]

37. Japón-Luján, L.; Luque-Rodríguez, J.; Luque de Castro, M. Dynamic ultrasound-assisted extraction of oleuropein and related biophenols from olive leaves. *J. Chromatogr. A* **2006**, *1108*, 76–82. [CrossRef] [PubMed]

38. Japón-Luján, R.; Luque de Castro, M.D. Liquid-liquid extraction for the enrichment of edible oils with phenols from olive leaf extracts. *J. Agric. Food Chem.* **2008**, *56*, 2505–2511. [CrossRef] [PubMed]

39. Oliveras-López, M.-J.; Berná, G.; Jurado-Ruiz, E.; López-García de la Serrana, H.; Martín, F. Consumption of extra-virgin olive oil rich in phenolic compounds has beneficial antioxidant effects in healthy human adults. *J. Funct. Foods* **2014**, *10*, 475–484. [CrossRef]

40. Rosignoli, P.; Fuccelli, R.; Fabiani, R.; Servili, M.; Morozzi, G. Effect of olive oil phenols on the production of inflammatory mediators in freshly isolated human monocytes. *J. Nutr. Biochem.* **2013**, *24*, 1513–1519. [CrossRef] [PubMed]

41. Lockyer, S.; Rowland, I.; Spencer, J.P.E.; Yaqoob, P.; Stonehouse, W. Impact of phenolic-rich olive leaf extract on blood pressure, plasma lipids and inflammatory markers: A randomised controlled trial. *Eur. J. Nutr.* **2016**. [CrossRef] [PubMed]

42. Martín-Peláez, S.; Mosele, J.I.; Pizarro, N.; Farràs, M.; de la Torre, R.; Subirana, I.; Pérez-Cano, F.J.; Castañer, O.; Solà, R.; Fernandez-Castillejo, S.; et al. Effect of virgin olive oil and thyme phenolic compounds on blood lipid profile: implications of human gut microbiota. *Eur. J. Nutr.* **2015**. [CrossRef] [PubMed]

43. Hamdi, H.K.; Castellon, R. Oleuropein, a non-toxic olive iridoid, is an anti-tumor agent and cytoskeleton disruptor. *Biochem. Biophys. Res. Commun.* **2005**, *334*, 769–778. [CrossRef] [PubMed]

44. López de las Hazas, M.-C.; Piñol, C.; Macià, A.; Romero, M.-P.; Pedret, A.; Solà, R.; Rubió, L.; Motilva, M.-J. Differential absorption and metabolism of hydroxytyrosol and its precursors oleuropein and secoiridoids. *J. Funct. Foods* **2016**, *22*, 52–63. [CrossRef]

45. Goldsmith, C.D.; Vuong, Q.V.; Sadeqzadeh, E.; Stathopoulos, C.E.; Roach, P.D.; Scarlett, C.J. Phytochemical Properties and Anti-Proliferative Activity of *Olea europaea* L. Leaf Extracts against Pancreatic Cancer Cells. *Molecules* **2015**, *20*, 12992–3004. [CrossRef] [PubMed]

46. Samet, I.; Han, J.; Jlaiel, L.; Sayadi, S.; Isoda, H. Olive (*Olea europaea*) Leaf Extract Induces Apoptosis and Monocyte/Macrophage Differentiation in Human Chronic Myelogenous Leukemia K562 Cells: Insight into the Underlying Mechanism. *Oxid. Med. Cell. Longev.* **2014**, *2014*, 927619. [CrossRef] [PubMed]

47. Quirantes-Piné, R.; Zurek, G.; Barrajón-Catalán, E.; Bäßmann, C.; Micol, V.; Segura-Carretero, A.; Fernández-Gutiérrez, A. A metabolite-profiling approach to assess the uptake and metabolism of phenolic compounds from olive leaves in SKBR3 cells by HPLC-ESI-QTOF-MS. *J. Pharm. Biomed. Anal.* **2013**, *72*, 121–126. [CrossRef] [PubMed]

48. Acquaviva, R.; Di Giacomo, C.; Sorrenti, V.; Galvano, F.; Santangelo, R.; Cardile, V.; Gangia, S.; D'Orazio, N.; Abraham, N.G.; Vanella, L. Antiproliferative effect of oleuropein in prostate cell lines. *Int. J. Oncol.* **2012**, *41*, 31–38. [PubMed]

49. Elamin, M.H.; Daghestani, M.H.; Omer, S.A.; Elobeid, M.A.; Virk, P.; Al-Olayan, E.M.; Hassan, Z.K.; Mohammed, O.B.; Aboussekhra, A. Olive oil oleuropein has anti-breast cancer properties with higher efficiency on ER-negative cells. *Food Chem. Toxicol.* **2013**, *53*, 310–316. [CrossRef] [PubMed]

50. Sirianni, R.; Chimento, A.; De Luca, A.; Casaburi, I.; Rizza, P.; Onofrio, A.; Iacopetta, D.; Puoci, F.; Andò, S.; Maggiolini, M.; et al. Oleuropein and hydroxytyrosol inhibit MCF-7 breast cancer cell proliferation interfering with ERK1/2 activation. *Mol. Nutr. Food Res.* **2010**, *54*, 833–840. [CrossRef] [PubMed]

51. Luo, C.; Li, Y.; Wang, H.; Cui, Y.; Feng, Z.; Li, H.; Li, Y.; Wang, Y.; Wurtz, K.; Weber, P.; et al. Hydroxytyrosol promotes superoxide production and defects in autophagy leading to anti-proliferation and apoptosis on human prostate cancer cells. *Curr. Cancer Drug Targets* **2013**, *13*, 625–639. [CrossRef] [PubMed]

52. Erbay, Z.; Icier, F. A review of thin layer drying of foods: Theory, modeling, and experimental results. *Crit. Rev. Food Sci. Nutr.* **2010**, *50*, 441–464. [CrossRef] [PubMed]

53. Pandey, K.; Rizvi, S. Plant polyphenols as dietary antioxidants in human health and disease. *Oxid. Med. Cell. Longev.* **2009**, *2*, 270–278. [CrossRef] [PubMed]

54. de Bock, M.; Derraik, J.G.B.; Brennan, C.M.; Biggs, J.B.; Morgan, P.E.; Hodgkinson, S.C.; Hofman, P.L.; Cutfield, W.S. Olive (*Olea europaea* L.) leaf polyphenols improve insulin sensitivity in middle-aged overweight men: A randomized, placebo-controlled, crossover trial. *PLoS ONE* **2013**, *8*, e57622.

55. Jemai, H.; El Feki, A.; Sayadi, S. Antidiabetic and antioxidant effects of hydroxytyrosol and oleuropein from olive leaves in alloxan-diabetic rats. *J. Agric. Food Chem.* **2009**, *57*, 8798–8804. [CrossRef] [PubMed]

56. Kuem, N.; Song, S.J.; Yu, R.; Yun, J.W.; Park, T. Oleuropein attenuates visceral adiposity in high-fat diet-induced obese mice through the modulation of WNT10b- and galanin-mediated signalings. *Mol. Nutr. Food Res.* **2014**, *58*, 2166–2176. [CrossRef] [PubMed]

57. Bendini, A.; Cerretani, L.; Carrasco-Pancorbo, A.; Gómez-Caravaca, A.M.; Segura-Carretero, A.; Fernández-Gutiérrez, A.; Lercker, G. Phenolic Molecules in Virgin Olive Oils: A Survey of Their Sensory Properties, Health Effects, Antioxidant Activity and Analytical Methods. An Overview of the Last Decade Alessandra. *Molecules* **2007**, *12*, 1679–1719. [CrossRef] [PubMed]

58. Nekooeian, A.A.; Khalili, A.; Khosravi, M.B. Oleuropein offers cardioprotection in rats with simultaneous type 2 diabetes and renal hypertension. *Indian J. Pharmacol.* **2015**, *46*, 398–403. [CrossRef] [PubMed]

59. Lee, O.-H.; Lee, B.-Y. Antioxidant and antimicrobial activities of individual and combined phenolics in *Olea europaea* leaf extract. *Bioresour. Technol.* **2010**, *101*, 3751–3754. [CrossRef] [PubMed]

60. Elamin, M.H.; Al-Maliki, S.S. Leishmanicidal and apoptotic activities of oleuropein on Leishmania major. *Int. J. Clin. Pharmacol. Ther.* **2014**, *52*, 880–888. [CrossRef] [PubMed]

61. Cárdeno, A.; Sánchez-Hidalgo, M.; Rosillo, M.A.; Alarcón de la Lastra, C. Oleuropein, a secoiridoid derived from olive tree, inhibits the proliferation of human colorectal cancer cell through downregulation of HIF-1α. *Nutr. Cancer* **2013**, *65*, 147–156. [CrossRef] [PubMed]

62. Hassan, Z.K.; Elamin, M.H.; Omer, S.A.; Daghestani, M.H.; Al-Olayan, E.S.; Elobeid, M.A.; Virk, P. Oleuropein Induces Apoptosis Via the p53 Pathway in Breast Cancer Cells. *Asian Pac. J. Cancer Prev.* **2013**, *14*, 6739–6742. [CrossRef]

63. Han, J.; Talorete, T.P.N.; Yamada, P.; Isoda, H. Anti-proliferative and apoptotic effects of oleuropein and hydroxytyrosol on human breast cancer MCF-7 cells. *Cytotechnology* **2009**, *59*, 45–53. [CrossRef] [PubMed]

64. Granados-Principal, S.; Quiles, J.L.; Ramirez-Tortosa, C.L.; Sanchez-Rovira, P.; Ramirez-Tortosa, M.C. Hydroxytyrosol: from laboratory investigations to future clinical trials. *Nutr. Rev.* **2010**, *68*, 191–206. [CrossRef] [PubMed]

65. Alipieva, K.; Korkina, L.; Orhan, I.E.; Georgiev, M.I. Verbascoside—A review of its occurrence, (bio) synthesis and pharmacological significance. *Biotechnol. Adv.* **2014**, *32*, 1065–1076. [CrossRef] [PubMed]

66. Al-Rimawi, F.; Odeh, I.; Bisher, A.; Abbadi, J.; Qabbajeh, M. Effect of Geographical Region and Harvesting Date on Antioxidant Activity, Phenolic and Flavonoid Content of Olive Leaves. *J. Food Nutr. Res.* **2014**, *2*, 925–930. [CrossRef]

67. Ando, C.; Takahashi, N.; Hirai, S.; Nishimura, K.; Lin, S.; Uemura, T.; Goto, T.; Yu, R.; Nakagami, J.; Murakami, S.; et al. Luteolin, a food-derived flavonoid, suppresses adipocyte-dependent activation of macrophages by inhibiting JNK activation. *FEBS Lett.* **2009**, *583*, 3649–3654. [CrossRef] [PubMed]

68. Shukla, S.; Gupta, S. Apigenin: A promising molecule for cancer prevention. *Pharm. Res.* **2010**, *27*, 962–978. [CrossRef] [PubMed]

69. Guinda, Á.; Pérez-Camino, M.C.; Lanzón, A. Supplementation of oils with oleanolic acid from the olive leaf (*Olea europaea*). *Eur. J. Lipid Sci. Technol.* **2004**, *106*, 22–26. [CrossRef]

70. Tabera, J.; Guinda, A.; Ruiz-Rodríguez, A.; Señoráns, F.J.; Ibáñez, E.; Albi, T.; Reglero, G. Countercurrent supercritical fluid extraction and fractionation of high-added-value compounds from a hexane extract of olive leaves. *J. Agric. Food Chem.* **2004**, *52*, 4774–4779. [CrossRef] [PubMed]

71. Virtamo, J.; Taylor, P.R.; Kontto, J.; Männistö, S.; Utriainen, M.; Weinstein, S.J.; Huttunen, J.; Albanes, D. Effects of α-tocopherol and β-carotene supplementation on cancer incidence and mortality: 18-year postintervention follow-up of the Alpha-tocopherol, Beta-carotene Cancer Prevention Study. *Int. J. Cancer* **2014**, *135*, 178–185. [CrossRef] [PubMed]

72. Menendez, J.A.; Joven, J.; Aragonès, G.; Barrajón-Catalán, E.; Beltrán-Debón, R.; Borrás-Linares, I.; Camps, J.; Corominas-Faja, B.; Cufí, S.; Fernández-Arroyo, S.; et al. Xenohormetic and anti-aging activity of secoiridoid polyphenols present in extra virgin olive oil: A new family of gerosuppressant agents. *Cell Cycle* **2013**, *12*, 555–578. [CrossRef] [PubMed]

73. Joven, J.; Micol, V.; Segura-Carretero, A.; Alonso-Villaverde, C.; Menéndez, J.A. Polyphenols and the modulation of gene expression pathways: Can we eat our way out of the danger of chronic disease? *Crit. Rev. Food Sci. Nutr.* **2014**, *54*, 985–1001. [CrossRef] [PubMed]

74. Fardet, A.; Rock, E. The search for a new paradigm to study micronutrient and phytochemical bioavailability: From reductionism to holism. *Med. Hypotheses.* **2014**, *82*, 181–186. [CrossRef] [PubMed]

75. De Marino, S.; Festa, C.; Zollo, F.; Nini, A.; Antenucci, L.; Raimo, G.; Iorizzi, M. Antioxidant Activity and Chemical Components as Potential Anticancer Agents in the Olive Leaf (*Olea europaea L.* cv Leccino.) Decoction. *Anticancer. Agents Med. Chem.* **2014**, *14*, 1376–1385. [CrossRef] [PubMed]

76. Benavente-garcia, O.; Castillo, J.; Lorente, J.; Ortun, A. Antioxidant activity of phenolics extracted from *Olea europaea L.* leaves. *Food Chem.* **2000**, *68*, 457–462. [CrossRef]

77. Etcheverry, E.P.; Grusak, M.A.; Fleige, L.E. Application of in vitro bioaccessibility and bioavailability methods for calcium, carotenoids, folate, iron, magnesium, polyphenols, zinc, and vitamins B6, B12, D, and E. *Front. Physiol.* **2012**, *3*, 317. [CrossRef] [PubMed]

78. D'Archivio, M.; Filesi, C.; Varì, R.; Scazzocchio, B.; Masella, R. Bioavailability of the polyphenols: Status and controversies. *Int. J. Mol. Sci.* **2010**, *11*, 1321–1342. [CrossRef] [PubMed]

79. De Bock, M.; Thorstensen, E.B.; Derraik, J.G.B.; Henderson, H.V.; Hofman, P.L.; Cutfield, W.S. Human absorption and metabolism of oleuropein and hydroxytyrosol ingested as olive (*Olea europaea L.*) leaf extract. *Mol. Nutr. Food Res.* **2013**, *57*, 2079–2085. [CrossRef] [PubMed]

80. Serra, A.; Rubió, L.; Borràs, X.; Macià, A.; Romero, M.-P.; Motilva, M.-J. Distribution of olive oil phenolic compounds in rat tissues after administration of a phenolic extract from olive cake. *Mol. Nutr. Food Res.* **2012**, *56*, 486–496. [CrossRef] [PubMed]

81. Kendall, M.; Batterham, M.; Callahan, D.L.; Jardine, D.; Prenzler, P.D.; Robards, K.; Ryan, D. Randomized controlled study of the urinary excretion of biophenols following acute and chronic intake of olive leaf supplements. *Food Chem.* **2012**, *130*, 651–659. [CrossRef]

82. Lin, P.; Qian, W.; Wang, X.; Cao, L.; Li, S.; Qian, T. The biotransformation of oleuropein in rats. *Biomed. Chromatogr.* **2013**, *27*, 1162–1167. [CrossRef] [PubMed]

83. Corona, G.; Tzounis, X.; Assunta Dessì, M.; Deiana, M.; Debnam, E.S.; Visioli, F.; Spencer, J.P.E. The fate of olive oil polyphenols in the gastrointestinal tract: Implications of gastric and colonic microflora-dependent biotransformation. *Free Radic. Res.* **2006**, *40*, 647–658. [CrossRef] [PubMed]

84. Landete, J.M.; Curiel, J.A.; Rodríguez, H.; de las Rivas, B.; Muñoz, R. Study of the inhibitory activity of phenolic compounds found in olive products and their degradation by Lactobacillus plantarum strains. *Food Chem.* **2008**, *107*, 320–326. [CrossRef]

85. Ramírez, E.; Medina, E.; Brenes, M.; Romero, C. Endogenous enzymes involved in the transformation of oleuropein in Spanish table olive varieties. *J. Agric. Food Chem.* **2014**, *62*, 9569–9575. [CrossRef] [PubMed]

86. De Leonardis, A.; Macciola, V.; Cuomo, F.; Lopez, F. Evidence of oleuropein degradation by olive leaf protein extract. *Food Chem.* **2015**, *175*, 568–574. [CrossRef] [PubMed]

87. Yuan, J.-J.; Wang, C.-Z.; Ye, J.-Z.; Tao, R.; Zhang, Y.-S. Enzymatic hydrolysis of oleuropein from Olea europea (olive) leaf extract and antioxidant activities. *Molecules* **2015**, *20*, 2903–2921. [CrossRef] [PubMed]

88. Szablewski, L. Expression of glucose transporters in cancers. *Biochim. Biophys. Acta* **2013**, *1835*, 164–169. [CrossRef] [PubMed]

89. Menendez, J.A.; Vazquez-Martin, A.; Colomer, R.; Brunet, J.; Carrasco-Pancorbo, A.; Garcia-Villalba, R.; Fernandez-Gutierrez, A.; Segura-Carretero, A. Olive oil's bitter principle reverses acquired autoresistance to trastuzumab (Herceptin) in HER2-overexpressing breast cancer cells. *BMC Cancer* **2007**, *7*, 80. [CrossRef] [PubMed]

90. Murphy, M.P.; Holmgren, A.; Larsson, N.-G.; Halliwell, B.; Chang, C.J.; Kalyanaraman, B.; Rhee, S.G.; Thornalley, P.J.; Partridge, L.; Gems, D.; et al. Unraveling the biological roles of reactive oxygen species. *Cell Metab.* **2011**, *13*, 361–366. [CrossRef] [PubMed]

91. de la Puerta, R.; Domínguez, M.E.M.; Rúíz-Gutíerrez, V.; Flavill, J.A.; Hoult, J.R.S. Effects of virgin olive oil phenolics on scavenging of reactive nitrogen species and upon nitrergic neurotransmission. *Life Sci.* **2001**, *69*, 1213–1222. [CrossRef]

92. de la Puerta, R.; Ruiz Gutierrez, V.; Hoult, J.R. Inhibition of leukocyte 5-lipoxygenase by phenolics from virgin olive oil. *Biochem. Pharmacol.* **1999**, *57*, 445–449. [CrossRef]

93. Forman, H.J.; Davies, K.J.A.; Ursini, F. How do nutritional antioxidants really work: Nucleophilic tone and para-hormesis versus free radical scavenging in vivo. *Free Radic. Biol. Med.* **2014**, *66*, 24–35. [CrossRef] [PubMed]

94. Zou, X.; Feng, Z.; Li, Y.; Wang, Y.; Wertz, K.; Weber, P.; Fu, Y.; Liu, J. Stimulation of GSH synthesis to prevent oxidative stress-induced apoptosis by hydroxytyrosol in human retinal pigment epithelial cells: Activation of Nrf2 and JNK-p62/SQSTM1 pathways. *J. Nutr. Biochem.* **2012**, *23*, 994–1006. [CrossRef] [PubMed]

95. Crespo, M.C.; Tomé-Carneiro, J.; Burgos-Ramos, E.; Loria Kohen, V.; Espinosa, M.I.; Herranz, J.; Visioli, F. One-week administration of hydroxytyrosol to humans does not activate Phase II enzymes. *Pharmacol. Res.* **2015**, *95*, 132–137. [CrossRef] [PubMed]

96. Khanal, P.; Oh, W.-K.; Yun, H.J.; Namgoong, G.M.; Ahn, S.-G.; Kwon, S.-M.; Choi, H.-K.; Choi, H.S. p-HPEA-EDA, a phenolic compound of virgin olive oil, activates AMP-activated protein kinase to inhibit carcinogenesis. *Carcinogenesis* **2011**, *32*, 545–553. [CrossRef] [PubMed]

97. Zrelli, H.; Matsuoka, M.; Kitazaki, S.; Zarrouk, M.; Miyazaki, H. Hydroxytyrosol reduces intracellular reactive oxygen species levels in vascular endothelial cells by upregulating catalase expression through the AMPK-FOXO3a pathway. *Eur. J. Pharmacol.* **2011**, *660*, 275–282. [CrossRef] [PubMed]

98. Komatsu, M.; Kurokawa, H.; Waguri, S.; Taguchi, K.; Kobayashi, A.; Ichimura, Y.; Sou, Y.-S.; Ueno, I.; Sakamoto, A.; Tong, K.I.; et al. The selective autophagy substrate p62 activates the stress responsive transcription factor Nrf2 through inactivation of Keap1. *Nat. Cell Biol.* **2010**, *12*, 213–223. [CrossRef] [PubMed]

99. Parzonko, A.; Czerwińska, M.E.; Kiss, A.K.; Naruszewicz, M. Oleuropein and oleacein may restore biological functions of endothelial progenitor cells impaired by angiotensin II via activation of Nrf2/heme oxygenase-1 pathway. *Phytomedicine* **2013**, *20*, 1088–1094. [CrossRef] [PubMed]

100. Ligibel, J.A.; Alfano, C.M.; Courneya, K.S.; Demark-Wahnefried, W.; Burger, R.A.; Chlebowski, R.T.; Fabian, C.J.; Gucalp, A.; Hershman, D.L.; Hudson, M.M.; et al. American Society of Clinical Oncology position statement on obesity and cancer. *J. Clin. Oncol.* **2014**, *32*, 3568–3574. [CrossRef] [PubMed]

101. Anand, P.; Kunnumakkara, A.B.; Kunnumakara, A.B.; Sundaram, C.; Harikumar, K.B.; Tharakan, S.T.; Lai, O.S.; Sung, B.; Aggarwal, B.B. Cancer is a preventable disease that requires major lifestyle changes. *Pharm. Res.* **2008**, *25*, 2097–2116. [CrossRef] [PubMed]

102. Mijatovic, S.A.; Timotijevic, G.S.; Miljkovic, D.M.; Radovic, J.M.; Maksimovic-Ivanic, D.D.; Dekanski, D.P.; Stosic-Grujicic, S.D. Multiple antimelanoma potential of dry olive leaf extract. *Int. J. Cancer* **2011**, *128*, 1955–1965. [CrossRef] [PubMed]

103. Fares, R.; Bazzi, S.; Baydoun, S.E.; Abdel-Massih, R.M. The antioxidant and anti-proliferative activity of the Lebanese *Olea europaea* extract. *Plant Foods Hum. Nutr.* **2011**, *66*, 58–63. [CrossRef] [PubMed]

104. Kaaks, R. Endogenous hormone metabolism as an exposure marker in breast cancer chemoprevention studies. *IARC Sci. Publ.* **2001**, *154*, 149–162. [PubMed]

105. Key, T.; Appleby, P.; Barnes, I.; Reeves, G. Endogenous Hormones and Breast Cancer Collaborative Group. Endogenous sex hormones and breast cancer in postmenopausal women: Reanalysis of nine prospective studies. *J. Natl. Cancer Inst.* **2002**, *94*, 606–616. [PubMed]

106. Bartlett, J.M.S.; Brookes, C.L.; Robson, T.; van de Velde, C.J.H.; Billingham, L.J.; Campbell, F.M.; Grant, M.; Hasenburg, A.; Hille, E.T.M.; Kay, C.; et al. Estrogen receptor and progesterone receptor as predictive biomarkers of response to endocrine therapy: A prospectively powered pathology study in the Tamoxifen and Exemestane Adjuvant Multinational trial. *J. Clin. Oncol.* **2011**, *29*, 1531–1538. [CrossRef] [PubMed]

107. Carrera-González, M.P.; Ramírez-Expósito, M.J.; Mayas, M.D.; Martínez-Martos, J.M. Protective role of oleuropein and its metabolite hydroxytyrosol on cancer. *Trends Food Sci. Technol.* **2013**, *31*, 92–99. [CrossRef]

108. Chimento, A.; Casaburi, I.; Rosano, C.; Avena, P.; De Luca, A.; Campana, C.; Martire, E.; Santolla, M.F.; Maggiolini, M.; Pezzi, V.; et al. Oleuropein and hydroxytyrosol activate GPER/GPR30-dependent pathways leading to apoptosis of ER-negative SKBR3 breast cancer cells. *Mol. Nutr. Food Res.* **2014**, *58*, 478–489. [CrossRef] [PubMed]

109. Kim, B.-W.; Lee, E.-R.; Min, H.-M.; Jeong, H.-S.; Ahn, J.-Y.; Kim, J.-H.; Choi, H.-Y.; Choi, H.; Kim, E.Y.; Park, S.P.; et al. Sustained ERK activation is involved in the kaempferol-induced apoptosis of breast cancer cells and is more evident under 3-D culture condition. *Cancer Biol. Ther.* **2014**, *7*, 1080–1089. [CrossRef]

110. Sepporta, M.V.; Fuccelli, R.; Rosignoli, P.; Ricci, G.; Servili, M.; Morozzi, G.; Fabiani, R. Oleuropein inhibits tumour growth and metastases dissemination in ovariectomised nude mice with MCF-7 human breast tumour xenografts. *J. Funct. Foods.* **2014**, *8*, 269–273. [CrossRef]

111. Milanizadeh, S.; Bigdeli, M.R.; Rasoulian, B.; Amani, D. The Effects of Olive Leaf Extract on Antioxidant Enzymes Activity and Tumor Growth in Breast Cancer. *Thrita* **2014**, *3*. [CrossRef]

112. Osborne, C.; Tripathy, D. Aromatase inhibitors: Rationale and use in breast cancer. *Annu. Rev. Med.* **2005**, *56*, 103–116. [CrossRef] [PubMed]

113. Cuzick, J.; Sestak, I.; Forbes, J.F.; Dowsett, M.; Knox, J.; Cawthorn, S.; Saunders, C.; Roche, N.; Mansel, R.E.; von Minckwitz, G.; et al. Anastrozole for prevention of breast cancer in high-risk postmenopausal women (IBIS-II): An international, double-blind, randomised placebo-controlled trial. *Lancet* **2014**, *383*, 1041–1048. [CrossRef]

114. Amakura, Y.; Tsutsumi, T.; Sasaki, K.; Nakamura, M.; Yoshida, T.; Maitani, T. Influence of food polyphenols on aryl hydrocarbon receptor-signaling pathway estimated by in vitro bioassay. *Phytochemistry* **2008**, *69*, 3117–3130. [CrossRef] [PubMed]

115. Wakabayashi, N.; Slocum, S.L.; Skoko, J.J.; Shin, S.; Kensler, T.W. When NRF2 talks, who's listening? *Antioxid. Redox Signal.* **2010**, *13*, 1649–1663. [CrossRef] [PubMed]

116. Fan, Y.; Boivin, G.P.; Knudsen, E.S.; Nebert, D.W.; Xia, Y.; Puga, A. The aryl hydrocarbon receptor functions as a tumor suppressor of liver carcinogenesis. *Cancer Res.* **2010**, *70*, 212–220. [CrossRef] [PubMed]

117. Yang, L.; Karin, M. Roles of tumor suppressors in regulating tumor-associated inflammation. *Cell Death Differ.* **2014**, *21*, 1677–1686. [CrossRef] [PubMed]

118. Franceschi, C.; Campisi, J. Chronic inflammation (inflammaging) and its potential contribution to age-associated diseases. *J. Gerontol. A Biol. Sci. Med. Sci.* **2014**, *69* (Suppl 1), S4–S9. [CrossRef] [PubMed]

119. Killeen, M.J.; Linder, M.; Pontoniere, P.; Crea, R. NF-κβ signaling and chronic inflammatory diseases: Exploring the potential of natural products to drive new therapeutic opportunities. *Drug Discov. Today* **2014**, *19*, 373–378. [CrossRef] [PubMed]

120. Ryu, S.-J.; Choi, H.-S.; Yoon, K.-Y.; Lee, O.-H.; Kim, K.-J.; Lee, B.-Y. Oleuropein suppresses LPS-induced inflammatory responses in RAW 264.7 cell and zebrafish. *J. Agric. Food Chem.* **2015**, *63*, 2098–2105. [CrossRef] [PubMed]

121. Scoditti, E.; Nestola, A.; Massaro, M.; Calabriso, N.; Storelli, C.; De Caterina, R.; Carluccio, M.A. Hydroxytyrosol suppresses MMP-9 and COX-2 activity and expression in activated human monocytes via PKCα and PKCβ1 inhibition. *Atherosclerosis* **2014**, *232*, 17–24. [CrossRef] [PubMed]

122. Liu, B.; Qu, L.; Yan, S. Cyclooxygenase-2 promotes tumor growth and suppresses tumor immunity. *Cancer Cell Int.* **2015**, *15*, 106. [CrossRef] [PubMed]

123. Scoditti, E.; Calabriso, N.; Massaro, M.; Pellegrino, M.; Storelli, C.; Martines, G.; De Caterina, R.; Carluccio, M.A. Mediterranean diet polyphenols reduce inflammatory angiogenesis through MMP-9 and COX-2 inhibition in human vascular endothelial cells: A potentially protective mechanism in atherosclerotic vascular disease and cancer. *Arch. Biochem. Biophys.* **2012**, *527*, 81–89. [CrossRef] [PubMed]

124. Zhang, X.; Cao, J.; Zhong, L. Hydroxytyrosol inhibits pro-inflammatory cytokines, iNOS, and COX-2 expression in human monocytic cells. *Naunyn Schmied. Arch. Pharmacol.* **2009**, *379*, 581–586. [CrossRef] [PubMed]

125. Fuccelli, R.; Fabiani, R.; Sepporta, M.V.; Rosignoli, P. The hydroxytyrosol-dependent increase of TNF-α in LPS-activated human monocytes is mediated by PGE2 and adenylate cyclase activation. *Toxicol. Vitro* **2015**, *29*, 933–937. [CrossRef] [PubMed]

126. Lamy, S.; Ben Saad, A.; Zgheib, A.; Annabi, B. Olive oil compounds inhibit the paracrine regulation of TNF-α-induced endothelial cell migration through reduced glioblastoma cell cyclooxygenase-2 expression. *J. Nutr. Biochem.* **2015**, *27*, 136–145. [CrossRef] [PubMed]

127. Lamy, S.; Moldovan, P.L.; Ben Saad, A.; Annabi, B. Biphasic effects of luteolin on interleukin-1β-induced cyclooxygenase-2 expression in glioblastoma cells. *Biochim. Biophys. Acta* **2015**, *1853*, 126–135. [CrossRef] [PubMed]

128. Bocca, C.; Ievolella, M.; Autelli, R.; Motta, M.; Mosso, L.; Torchio, B.; Bozzo, F.; Cannito, S.; Paternostro, C.; Colombatto, S.; et al. Expression of COX-2 in human breast cancer cells as a critical determinant of epithelial-to-mesenchymal transition and invasiveness. *Expert Opin. Ther. Targets* **2014**, *18*, 121–135. [CrossRef] [PubMed]

129. Harris, R.E.; Casto, B.C.; Harris, Z.M. Cyclooxygenase-2 and the inflammogenesis of breast cancer. *World J. Clin. Oncol.* **2014**, *5*, 677–692. [CrossRef] [PubMed]

130. Bieniek, J.; Childress, C.; Swatski, M.D.; Yang, W. COX-2 inhibitors arrest prostate cancer cell cycle progression by down-regulation of kinetochore/centromere proteins. *Prostate* **2014**, *74*, 999–1011. [CrossRef] [PubMed]

131. Peng, L.; Zhou, Y.; Wang, Y.; Mou, H.; Zhao, Q. Prognostic significance of COX-2 immunohistochemical expression in colorectal cancer: A meta-analysis of the literature. *PLoS ONE* **2013**, *8*, e58891. [CrossRef] [PubMed]

132. Brasky, T.M.; Bonner, M.R.; Moysich, K.B.; Ambrosone, C.B.; Nie, J.; Tao, M.H.; Edge, S.B.; Kallakury, B.V.S.; Marian, C.; Trevisan, M.; et al. Non-steroidal anti-inflammatory drug (NSAID) use and breast cancer risk in the Western New York Exposures and Breast Cancer (WEB) Study. *Cancer Causes Control* **2010**, *21*, 1503–1512. [CrossRef] [PubMed]

133. Barnes, N.L.P.; Warnberg, F.; Farnie, G.; White, D.; Jiang, W.; Anderson, E.; Bundred, N.J. Cyclooxygenase-2 inhibition: Effects on tumour growth, cell cycling and lymphangiogenesis in a xenograft model of breast cancer. *Br. J. Cancer* **2007**, *96*, 575–582. [CrossRef] [PubMed]

134. Katkoori, V.R.; Manne, K.; Vital-Reyes, V.S.; Rodríguez-Burford, C.; Shanmugam, C.; Sthanam, M.; Manne, U.; Chatla, C.; Abdulkadir, S.A.; Grizzle, W.E. Selective COX-2 inhibitor (celecoxib) decreases cellular growth in prostate cancer cell lines independent of p53. *Biotech. Histochem.* **2013**, *88*, 38–46. [CrossRef] [PubMed]

135. Jeon, Y.W.; Ahn, Y.E.; Chung, W.S.; Choi, H.J.; Suh, Y.J. Synergistic effect between celecoxib and luteolin is dependent on estrogen receptor in human breast cancer cells. *Tumor Biol.* **2015**, *36*, 6349–6359. [CrossRef] [PubMed]

136. Subbaramaiah, K.; Howe, L.R.; Port, E.R.; Brogi, E.; Fishman, J.; Liu, C.H.; Hla, T.; Hudis, C.; Dannenberg, A.J. HER-2/neu status is a determinant of mammary aromatase activity in vivo: Evidence for a cyclooxygenase-2-dependent mechanism. *Cancer Res.* **2006**, *66*, 5504–5511. [CrossRef] [PubMed]

137. Subbaramaiah, K.; Morris, P.G.; Zhou, X.K.; Morrow, M.; Du, B.; Giri, D.; Kopelovich, L.; Hudis, C.A.; Dannenberg, A.J. Increased levels of COX-2 and prostaglandin E2 contribute to elevated aromatase expression in inflamed breast tissue of obese women. *Cancer Discov.* **2012**, *2*, 356–365. [CrossRef] [PubMed]

138. Choi, E.-M.; Heo, J.-I.; Oh, J.-Y.; Kim, Y.-M.; Ha, K.-S.; Kim, J.-I.; Han, J.A. COX-2 regulates p53 activity and inhibits DNA damage-induced apoptosis. *Biochem. Biophys. Res. Commun.* **2005**, *328*, 1107–1112. [CrossRef] [PubMed]

139. Wang, X.; Docanto, M.M.; Sasano, H.; Lo, C.; Simpson, E.R.; Brown, K.A. Prostaglandin E2 inhibits p53 in human breast adipose stromal cells: A novel mechanism for the regulation of aromatase in obesity and breast cancer. *Cancer Res.* **2015**, *75*, 645–655. [CrossRef] [PubMed]

140. Yao, J.; Wu, J.; Yang, X.; Yang, J.; Zhang, Y.; Du, L. Oleuropein Induced Apoptosis in HeLa Cells via a Mitochondrial Apoptotic Cascade Associated With Activation of the c-Jun NH2-Terminal Kinase. *J. Pharmacol. Sci.* **2014**, *125*, 300–311. [CrossRef] [PubMed]

141. Kalinski, P. Regulation of immune responses by prostaglandin E2. *J. Immunol.* **2012**, *188*, 21–28. [CrossRef] [PubMed]

142. Chen, E.P.; Markosyan, N.; Connolly, E.; Lawson, J.A.; Li, X.; Grant, G.R.; Grosser, T.; FitzGerald, G.A.; Smyth, E.M. Myeloid Cell COX-2 deletion reduces mammary tumor growth through enhanced cytotoxic T-lymphocyte function. *Carcinogenesis* **2014**, *35*, 1788–1797. [CrossRef] [PubMed]

143. Quail, D.F.; Joyce, J.A. Microenvironmental regulation of tumor progression and metastasis. *Nat. Med.* **2013**, *19*, 1423–1437. [CrossRef] [PubMed]

144. Li, H.; Yang, B.; Huang, J.; Lin, Y.; Xiang, T.; Wan, J.; Li, H.; Chouaib, S.; Ren, G. Cyclooxygenase-2 in tumor-associated macrophages promotes breast cancer cell survival by triggering a positive-feedback loop between macrophages and cancer cells. *Oncotarget* **2015**, *6*, 29637–29650. [PubMed]

145. Llorente-Cortés, V.; Estruch, R.; Mena, M.P.; Ros, E.; González, M.A.M.; Fitó, M.; Lamuela-Raventós, R.M.; Badimon, L. Effect of Mediterranean diet on the expression of pro-atherogenic genes in a population at high cardiovascular risk. *Atherosclerosis* **2010**, *208*, 442–450. [CrossRef] [PubMed]

146. Camargo, A.; Ruano, J.; Fernandez, J.M.; Parnell, L.D.; Jimenez, A.; Santos-Gonzalez, M.; Marin, C.; Perez-Martinez, P.; Uceda, M.; Lopez-Miranda, J.; et al. Gene expression changes in mononuclear cells in patients with metabolic syndrome after acute intake of phenol-rich virgin olive oil. *BMC Genom.* **2010**, *11*, 253. [CrossRef] [PubMed]

147. Perez-Herrera, P.; Delgado-Lista, J.; Torres-Sanchez, L.; Rangel-Zuñiga, O.; Camargo, A.; Moreno-Navarrete, J.; Garcia-Olid, B.; Quintana-Navarro, G.; Alcala-Diaz, J.; Muñoz-Lopez, C.; et al. The postprandial inflammatory response after ingestion of heated oils in obese persons is reduced by the presence of phenol compounds. *Mol. Nutr. Food Res.* **2012**, *56*, 510–514. [CrossRef] [PubMed]

148. Camargo, A.; Rangel-Zuñiga, O.A.; Haro, C.; Meza-Miranda, E.R.; Peña-Orihuela, P.; Meneses, M.E.; Marin, C.; Yubero-Serrano, E.M.; Perez-Martinez, P.; Delgado-Lista, J.; et al. Olive oil phenolic compounds decrease the postprandial inflammatory response by reducing postprandial plasma lipopolysaccharide levels. *Food Chem.* **2014**, *162*, 161–171. [CrossRef] [PubMed]

149. Vann, K.R.; Sedgeman, C.A.; Gopas, J.; Golan-Goldhirsh, A.; Osheroff, N. Effects of Olive Metabolites on DNA Cleavage Mediated by Human Type II Topoisomerases. *Biochemistry* **2015**, *54*, 4531–4541. [CrossRef] [PubMed]

150. He, J.; Wang, S.; Zhou, M.; Yu, W.; Zhang, Y.; He, X. Phytoestrogens and risk of prostate cancer: A meta-analysis of observational studies. *World J. Surg. Oncol.* **2015**, *13*, 231. [CrossRef] [PubMed]

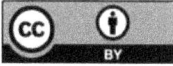

![nutrients logo] *nutrients*

MDPI

*Review*

# Suppressive Effects of Tea Catechins on Breast Cancer

Li-Ping Xiang [1,2], Ao Wang [2], Jian-Hui Ye [1], Xin-Qiang Zheng [1], Curt Anthony Polito [1], Jian-Liang Lu [1], Qing-Sheng Li [1] and Yue-Rong Liang [1,2,*]

[1]   Tea Research Institute, Zhejiang University, # 866 Yuhangtang Road, Hangzhou 310058, China;
     gzzyzj_2009@vip.sina.com (L.-P.X.); jianhuiye@zju.edu.cn (J.-H.Y.); xqzheng@zju.edu.cn (X.-Q.Z.);
     curtpolito@outlook.com (C.A.P.); jllu@zju.edu.cn (L.-J.L.); qsli@zju.edu.cn (Q.-S.L.)
[2]   National Tea and Tea product Quality Supervision and Inspection Center (Guizhou), Zunyi 563100, China;
     wangaocn@gmail.com
*   Correspondence: yrliang@zju.edu.cn; Tel./Fax: +86-571-889-82704

Received: 15 June 2016; Accepted: 22 July 2016; Published: 28 July 2016

**Abstract:** Tea leaf (*Camellia sinensis*) is rich in catechins, which endow tea with various health benefits. There are more than ten catechin compounds in tea, among which epigallocatechingallate (EGCG) is the most abundant. Epidemiological studies on the association between tea consumption and the risk of breast cancer were summarized, and the inhibitory effects of tea catechins on breast cancer, with EGCG as a representative compound, were reviewed in the present paper. The controversial results regarding the role of tea in breast cancer and areas for further study were discussed.

**Keywords:** *Camellia sinensis*; anticancer; antioxidant; signaling pathway; anti-proliferation; DNA methylation; metastasis

## 1. Introduction

Breast cancer is a common cancer in women. There were an estimated 1.7 million new cases (25% of all cancers in women) and 0.5 million cancer deaths (15% of all cancer deaths in women) in 2012 [1]. Though there have been great advances in the treatment of breast cancer, mortality from breast cancer is still high, and it is the second leading cause of cancer-related death among women in the United States [2]. Diet is considered to be an important factor preventing breast cancer [2,3].

Tea is one of the most popular beverages consumed all over the world. Tea leaves are rich in catechins, a group of polyphenols that endow tea with many health benefits. (−)-Epigallocatechingallate (EGCG), (−)-epicatechingallate (ECG), (−)-epigallocatechin (EGC), and (−)-epicatechin (EC) are the major catechins in fresh tea leaf, while more than ten catechins are usually detected in various kinds of processed teas, owing to the isomerization of epi-type catechins during tea processing [4]. Teas are classified into fully-fermented black tea, semi-fermented Oolong tea, and unfermented green tea, based on the degree of fermentation, during which catechins are oxidized. EGCG is the most abundant catechin in tea, and it accounts for more than 40% of total catechins in green tea leaves [5]. The total concentration of catechins is 58.0–183.9 mg/g in green tea [4], 74.8–105.7 mg/g in oolong tea [6], and 11.7–55.3 mg/g in black tea [7]. Green tea polyphenols (GTP) are considered to be a potential candidate for further development as a chemoprotective factor for the primary prevention of age-related eye diseases [8]. There have been epidemiological and in vitro studies regarding the association of tea consumption with depression among breast cancer survivors [9]. Drinking tea or green tea was not associated with overall breast cancer risk [10]. However, the effects of tea and its catechins on the prevention of breast cancer are still inconclusive and controversial [11,12]. The present review will highlight the recent advances in the effects of tea and its catechins on breast cancer, including epidemiological, in vivo, and in vitro studies. The controversial results from in vitro and in vivo studies, as well as directions for further study are also discussed in the present paper.

## 2. Epidemiological Evidence

As early as 1997, an epidemiological study carried out in Japan showed that drinking green tea had a potentially preventive effect on breast cancer, especially among women who drank more than 10 cups of green tea per day [13]. Many cohort studies or case-control studies on the association between tea consumption and breast cancer risk have been carried out since then. Cohort studies in China and the USA showed that habitual drinking of green tea was weakly associated with a decreased risk of breast cancer [14,15]. There was a time-dependent interaction between green tea consumption and age of breast cancer onset ($p$ for interaction = 0.03). Women who started drinking tea at the age of 25 or younger had a hazard ratio (HR) of 0.69 (95% confidence interval (CI): 0.41–1.17) to develop premenopausal breast cancer, compared with non-tea drinkers [16]. Tea drinking was also helpful to the treatment of breast cancer patients. Habitual tea-drinking (more than 100 g dried tea per month) was inversely associated with depression among patients who were diagnosed with stage 0 to III breast cancer, with odds ratio (OR) 0.39 and 95% CI ranging from 0.19 to 0.84 [9]. Drinking tea or green tea was not associated with overall breast cancer risk [10].

The association between tea consumption and decreased risk of breast cancer was also confirmed by population-based case-control studies carried out in China [10,12,17], the USA [18–20], and Singapore [21,22]. There were studies showing that green tea consumption significantly reduced the risk of breast cancer [18] and the women who drank three or more cups of tea per day had a 37% reduced breast cancer risk than their counterparts that did not drink tea [20]. Differences in the efficacy of tea consumption on breast cancer were observed between various populations. Among women with high-activity of the angiotensin-converting enzyme (ACE) genotype, green tea intake frequency significantly decreased the risk of breast cancer ($p$ = 0.039) [21]. Among women with low folate intake or high-activity MTHFR/TYMS (methylene tetrahydrofolate reductase /thymidylate synthetase) genotypes, green tea consumption was inversely associated with breast cancer risk [22], suggesting that folate pathway inhibition might be one of the mechanisms for the protection that green tea provides against breast cancer in humans. A significant association between regular tea consumption and lower risk for breast cancer [12] was observed among premenopausal Chinese women (OR = 0.62, 95% CI: 0.40–0.97) [10], but an increased risk was seen in postmenopausal women (OR = 1.40, 95% CI: 1.00–1.96) [10]. An inverse association between tea consumption and breast cancer was observed among younger women (less than 50 years old), which was consistent for in situ and invasive breast cancer and ductal and lobular breast cancer [20]. Combined intake of green tea and mushroom showed an additional decreased risk of breast cancer [17]. Table 1 lists the epidemiological evidence for the association between tea intake and the risk of breast cancer.

**Table 1.** Epidemiological evidence for the association between green tea intake and the risk of breast cancer.

| Type of Study | Location | Number of Subjects | Main Results | References |
|---|---|---|---|---|
| Population-based cohort study | Shanghai, China | 1399 women with breast cancer | Drinking tea regularly (>100 g dried tea per month) was inversely associated with overall depression. | Chen et al. (2010) [9] |
| Hospital-based case–control study | Hong Kong, China | Cases: 439 Controls: 434 | Habitual tea drinking was significantly associated with a lower risk for breast cancer in premenopausal women (OR = 0.62, 95%CI: 0.40–0.97). | Li et al. (2016) [10] |
| Case–control study | Southeast China | Cases: 1009 Controls: 1009 | Green tea consumption was associated with a reduced risk of breast cancer. | Zhang et al. (2007) [12] |
| Prospective cohort study | Saitama Prefecture, Japan | 9 years of follow-up study (71,248.5 person-years) | Drinking green tea had a potentially preventive effect on breast cancer | Imai et al. (1997) [13] |
| Population-based study | Shanghai, China | Cases: 3454 Controls: 3474 | Drinking green tea regularly was weakly associated with a decreased risk of breast cancer. | Shrubsole et al. (2009) [14] |
| Long-term cohort study (1980–2002) | Boston, USA | 85,987 female participants | There was a significant inverse association of caffeine intake with breast cancer among postmenopausal women | Ganmaa et al. (2008) [15] |
| Population-based cohort study | Shanghai, China | 74,942 Chinese women | Women who started drinking tea at 25 year of age or younger had a hazard ratio 0.69 (CI: 0.41–1.17) to develop premenopausal breast cancer, compared with non-tea drinkers | Dai et al. (2010) [16] |
| Case–control study | Southeast China | Cases: 1009 Controls: 1009 | Green tea intake was associated with decreased breast cancer risk in premenopausal and postmenopausal Chinese women, and there was an additional decreased risk from the joint effect of green tea and mushrooms | Zhang et al. (2009) [17] |
| Population-based, case–control study | Los Angeles, USA | Cases: 501 Controls: 594 | Green tea consumption showed a significantly reduced risk of breast cancer, while black tea consumption was not associated with the risk of breast cancer | Wu et al. (2003) [18] |
| Population-based case–control study | Massachusetts, USA | Cases: 5082 Controls: 4501 | Among women less than 50 years old, those who drank three or more cups of tea per day had a 37% reduced breast cancer risk compared to their counterparts that did not drink tea | Kumar et al. (2009) [20] |
| Nested case–control study | Singapore | Cases: 297 Controls: 665 | There was significant association between green tea intake frequency and decreased risk of breast cancer in the women with high-activity of angiotensin-converting enzyme (ACE) genotype ($p = 0.039$) | Yuan et al. (2005) [21] |
| Nested case–control study | Singapore | Cases: 380 Controls: 662 | Green tea intake was inversely associated with decreased breast cancer risk among women with low folate intake and high-activity MTHFR/TYMS genotypes | Inoue et al. (2008) [22] |
| Meta-analysis | Boston, USA | Cases: 5617 | Increased green tea consumption (>3 cups, day) was inversely associated with recurrence (Pooled RR = 0.73 95% CI: 0.56–0.96). An analysis of case–control studies of incidence suggested an inverse association with a pooled RR of 0.81 (95% CI 0.75, 0.88) while no association was found among cohort studies of incidence | Ogunleye et al. (2010) [23] |

## 3. Mechanism of Tea Catechins in Suppressing Breast Cancer

### 3.1. Suppressing Carcinogen-Induced ROS Elevation and DNA Damage

ROS (reactive oxygen species) are a group of chemically-reactive molecules, including hydrogen peroxide, superoxide anion radical, singlet oxygen, and hydroxyl radicals, which are crucially involved in multiple stages of carcinogenesis [24]. The anti-carcinogenic activity of tea catechins is considered to be related to their protection of DNA from ROS-induced damages by alleviating ROS stress. It was shown that short-term exposure of breast cancer cells to 4-(methylnitrosamino)-1-(3-pyridyl)-1-butanone (NNK) and benzo[a]pyrene (B[a]P) would increase the level of ROS, resulting in the activation of the extracellular signal-regulated kinase (ERK) pathway and subsequent induction of DNA damage [25]. In vitro [26] and in vivo [27] studies showed that tea catechins prevented breast carcinogenesis by alleviating ROS stress. Ten μg/mL EGCG suppressed chronically-induced cellular carcinogenesis by blocking carcinogen-induced ROS elevation [25]. Tea polyphenols, such as green tea catechins and black tea theaflavins, could inhibit DNA cleavage induced by the combination of hydrogen peroxide and cytochrome c [26]. Green tea catechins or black tea theaflavins delay mammary carcinogenesis in the TAg mouse model, which is accompanied by an antioxidant effect in the target organ, as reflected by levels of M1dG (malondialdehyde–deoxyganosine) adducts [27] which is a prevalent guanine adduct formed by a condensation reaction between guanosine. Furthermore, the combination of catechins with anticancer drugs such as tamoxifen (TAM) showed an etiological role in the abrogation of TAM-induced toxicity by relieving oxidative stress and biochemical perturbations [28].

The mechanism for the alleviation of ROS stress by catechins includes their increasing of the activity of anti-oxidases such as catalase, superoxide dismutase (SOD), and glutathione peroxidase (GHS-px) [29] directly scavenging ROS [25], preventing the iron-induced generation of hydroxyl free radicals via Haber–Weiss and Fenton reactions by chelating ferrous iron. The potent antioxidant and anti-inflammatory activities of EGCG are also beneficial to the modulation of mitochondrial functions, impacting mitochondrial bioenergetic control, cell cycle, and mitochondria-related apoptosis [30].

### 3.2. Regulating Cell Signaling Pathways

The PI3K/Akt/mTOR (phosphoinositide-3-kinase/protein kinase B/mammalian target of rapamycin) signaling pathway is a commonly activated signaling pathway in human cancer. The important nodes in this pathway are used as key therapeutic targets for cancer treatments. EGCG was confirmed to be an ATP-competitive inhibitor of both PI3K and mTOR in breast cancer cells MDA-MB-231, with $Ki$ values ranging 380 nM to 320 nM, respectively [30]. Molecular docking studies showed that EGCG binds well to the PI3K kinase domain active site, showing ATP-competitive activity [31]. Tumor-associated fatty acid synthase (FAS) is implicated in breast carcinoma and is connected to the epidermal growth factor receptor (EGFR) signaling pathway. Suppression of FAS in cancer cells may lead to growth inhibition and the apoptosis of breast cancer cells. EGCG suppressed EGFR signaling and downstream phosphatidylinositol 3-kinase (PI3K)/Akt activation in the MCF-7 breast cancer cell line, resulting in down-regulation of FAS expression. It is considered that EGCG may be useful in the chemoprevention of breast carcinoma in which FAS over-expression results from signaling of human epidermal growth factor receptor 2 (HER2) or/and HER3, two members of EGFR family [32]. Exposure to carcinogens such as 4-(methylnitrosamino)-1-(3-pyridyl)-1-butanone (NNK) and benzo[a]pyrene (B[a]P) will result in an elevation of ROS, leading to activation of the Raf-independent extracellular signal-regulated kinase (ERK) pathway, which will induce DNA damage. Green tea extract (GTE) was confirmed to inhibit the activation of the ERK pathway by blocking carcinogen-induced ROS elevation, resulting in the suppression of chronically-induced breast cell carcinogenesis [25]. Wnt (wingless integrated) proteins are a group of highly conserved secreted signaling molecules which play critical roles during embryonic development and in the regeneration of adult tissues. Mutations in Wnt genes or Wnt pathway components lead to developmental defects and many cancers are caused by abnormal Wnt signaling. EGCG induced HMG-box transcription factor 1 (HBP1) transcriptional repressor, resulting in blockage of the Wnt/β-catenin pathway and inhibition of both breast cancer cell tumorigenic proliferation and invasiveness [33]. Met, a hepatocyte growth factor (HGF) receptor, is a strong prognostic indicator of breast cancer patient outcome and survival. Therapies targeting Met will have beneficial clinic outcomes. Catechins with R1 galloyl and R2 hydroxyl groups had a strong ability to inhibit HGF/Met signaling and block invasive breast cancer [34].

### 3.3. Interacting with Target Proteins

Estrogen is associated with the initiation and growth of breast cancer due to its action on proto-oncogenes and breast cell proliferation [35]. The interactions between estrogen and its specific estrogen receptor (ERs) proteins are increasingly drawing research interest in breast cancer etiology and clinical therapy studies. The ERs are classified into nuclear ERs and membrane ERs [36,37]. ERα and ERβ are two important subtypes of nuclear ERs, and they are used as reference for clinical diagnosis and therapy decisions regarding breast cancer [35,37]. Synthetic ER antagonists were designed to occupy the ligand-binding pocket to block the access of estrogen to the ERs, which have been used clinically in the treatment of ER-positive breast cancer [37]. The interaction between catechins and ERs showed anti-estrogenic activity, and so catechins are considered for use as potential phytoestrogens to replace synthetic ER antagonists in clinical use [32,38,39]. EGCG could reactivate ERα expression in ERα-negative breast cancer cells by its remodeling effect on the chromatin structure of the ERα promoter through altering histone acetylation and methylation status [40]. These results support further preclinical and clinical evaluation of EGCG as a therapeutic option for ER-negative breast cancer. Furthermore, EGCG can bind with high affinity to many other target proteins in cancer cells, such as 70 kDa zeta-associated protein (Zap-70) [41], 67-kDa laminin receptor [42], phosphoinositide 3 kinase (PI3K) [31], Ras-GTPase activating protein (GAP), SH3 domain-binding protein 1 (G3BP1) [43], insulin-like growth factor 1 receptor (IGF-1R) [44], vimentin [45], Bcl-2 and Bcl-xL [46], GRP78 [47], and Fyn [48], resulting in the inhibition of breast cancer. EGCG interacts with target proteins via hydrogen bonding, during which the hydroxyl groups of EGCG serve as hydrogen bond donors.

### 3.4. Inhibiting DNA Methylation

DNA methylation is an important epigenetic mechanism for the inactivation of many genes related to tumor suppressors and DNA repair enzymes [49]. DNA methylation is catalyzed by specific DNA methyltransferase (DNMT) or catechol-*O*-methyltransferase (COMT), in which *S*-adenosyl-L-methionine (SAM) is the methyl donor. *S*-adenosyl-L-homocysteine (SAH)—a potent noncompetitive inhibitor of DNMTs—is formed when the methyl group of SAM combines with the DNA substrate. Recent studies showed that tea catechins inhibited human DNMT-mediated DNA methylation through two mechanisms—i.e., the direct inhibition of DNMTs by catechins and the indirect inhibition of DNMTs by increasing the SAH level. Their inhibitory potency is in the rank order of EGCG > ECG > EGC > EC, based on the concentration for 50% inhibition ($IC_{50}$) [50]. EGCG interacted with DNMT enzyme by forming hydrogen bonds with proline[1223], glutamate[1265], cysteine[1225], serine[1229], and arginine[1309] in the catalytic pocket of DNMT, and the B and D ring moieties of EGCG played important roles [51]. Synthetic analog of EGCG had the same effect on COMT as EGCG [52]. Methylated EGCG led to decreased proteasome-inhibitory activity and cancer-preventive effects of EGCG [53]. The suppressive effects of EGCG on DNA methylation were closely associated with its anti-tumor activity [54].

### 3.5. Inhibiting Tumor Angiogenesis

Angiogenesis, which is essential for tumor growth, can provide nutrients and oxygen for tumor growth [55]. Vascular endothelial growth factor (VEGF), the most effective angiogenesis factor, has been reported to stimulate endothelial cells in the proliferation of tumor blood vessels. Subsequently, the proliferation of endothelial cells prompts the formation of new blood vessels [55,56].

Thus, inhibiting angiogenesis would be conducive to tumor suppression. Tea catechins—especially EGCG—exert prominent antiangiogenic activity [57–59], which results in decreased breast cancer risk. Catechins could effectively inhibit VEGF expression in breast cancer cells, leading to the suppression of endothelial cell formation and angiogenesis. GTE or EGCG suppressed VEGF protein secretion by inhibiting VEGF promoter activity, resulting in decreased expression of VEGF transcript, c-jun transcript, c-fos transcript, and protein kinase C (PKC) [60].

The antiangiogenic mechanism of catechins is closely related to VEGF signaling intervention. The VEGF-induced angiogenesis signal pathway is initiated through a multi-component receptor complex composed of VEGF-2, β-bcatenin, VE-cadherin, and PI3-kinase. Catechins inhibited the formation of the multi-component receptor complex, resulting in the interference of VEGF signaling and the inhibition of endothelial cell formation [61].

### 3.6. Anti-Proliferation and Inducing Breast Cancer Cell Apoptosis

The mechanism of action of anticancer drugs is based on their ability to induce apoptosis in cancer cells. Tea catechins such as EGCG, gallocatechin gallate (GCG), and gallocatechin (GC) showed 100%, 97%, and 95% inhibition of breast cancer cell proliferation, respectively at a concentration of 50 μM, [62]. Tea catechins suppress proliferation and induce apoptosis of breast cancer cells via several pathways, including: (1) Inducing cell cycle arrest. The cell growth of human breast cancer cell line T47D was arrested at the G(2)/M phase in a dose-dependent manner by EGCG. The mechanism is that catechins phosphorylate c-jun N-terminal kinase/stress activated protein kinase (JNK/SAPK) and p38. The phosphorylated JNK/SAPK and p38 inhibit the phosphorylation of cell division cycle 2 (cdc2) and regulate the expression of cyclin A, cyclin B1, and cyclin-dependent kinase proteins, resulting in G(2) arrest [63]; (2) Promoting tumor protein P53 (TP53)/caspase-mediated apoptosis. Catechin hydrate (CH) is a strong antioxidant and an efficient scavenger of free radicals. CH exhibits anticancer effects by inhibiting the proliferation of breast cancer cells and inducing the apoptosis of cancer cells, partially through suppression of the expression of caspase-3, caspase-8, caspase-9, and TP53 [64]; (3) Down-regulating anti-apoptotic factors. Catechins such as catechin, GC, and catechin gallate (CG) induced breast cancer cell apoptosis by suppressing the expression of anti-apoptotic factors such as B cell lymphoma 2 (Bcl-2), Bcl-xL, and survivin, accompanied by the inhibition of NFκB, JAK/STAT, and PI3K pathways [65]. Oligonol—a catechin-rich preparation—triggered apoptosis in estrogen-responsive MCF-7 and estrogen-unresponsive MDA-MB-231 breast cancer cells through the modulation of pro-apoptotic Bcl-2 family proteins and MEK/ERK signaling pathway [66]; (4) Inhibiting fatty acid synthase (FAS). FAS is a breast cancer-associated enzyme connected to human epidermal growth factor receptor (HER). Suppression of FAS may lead to cancer cell apoptosis. EGCG down-regulated FAS by suppressing HER2 or/and HER3 signaling and downstream PI3K/Akt activation in the MCF-7 breast cancer cell line [32]; (5) Regulating NO/NOS system. Catechins ($10^{-7}$ M) inhibited proliferation of human breast cancer cell T47D, with cells being arrested at the S phase of cell cycle. The anti-proliferative activity of catechins is considered to be involved in the nitric oxide/nitric oxide synthase (NO/NOS) system because catechin treatment decreased NOS, resulting in NO reduction [67]. However, the role of NO in regulating the anti-proliferative effect of catechins is ambiguous, and the regulation mechanism of catechins on the NO/NOS system is not fully clear yet; (6) Inducing $Ca^{2+}$-associated apoptosis. EGCG induced an increase in endoplasmic reticulum calcium ($[Ca^{2+}]_{ER}$) and a decrease in cytosolic $Ca^{2+}$ by inhibiting Bcl-2 mediated $Ca^{2+}$ leakage from the endoplasmic reticulum in MCF-7 breast cancer cells [68]. EGCG acts via the signaling pathways related to cell membrane and endoplasmic reticulum stress to suppress cell proliferation or provoke apoptosis [69].

### 3.7. Anti-Metastasis of Breast Cancer Cells

The metastasis of cancer cells includes three key steps; i.e., adhesion, migration, and invasion. EGCG can effectively inhibit the invasion and migration of breast cancer cells, resulting in decreased lung and liver metastasis [70]. Tea catechins showed an inhibitory effect on the migratory and invasive potential of breast cancer cells [71,72]. Catechins inhibit metastasis by modulating the activity of proteolytic enzymes, regulating the signaling pathway and growth factor/receptor, suppressing the epithelial-to-mesenchymal transition (EMT) process and inhibiting angiogenesis [72,73].

Degradation of extracellular matrix components by matrix metalloproteinases (MMPs) and other proteolytic enzymes is critical in tumor invasion and metastasis behavior. Pro-MMP-2 is a proenzyme involved in the malignant progression of tumors. Membrane type-1 matrix metalloproteinase (MT1-MMP) cleaves the N-terminal prodomain of pro-MMP-2, which generates the active intermediate that is modified into the fully active enzyme MMP-2 afterwards. EGCG down-regulated MT1-MMP transcription, resulting in the inhibition of the MT1-MMP-driven migration of breast cancer cells [73]. Catechins can modulate the secretion of urokinase plasminogen activator (uPA), which is closely related to proteolytic enzymes in breast cancer cells and inhibits their invasive behavior by suppressing the transcription factors AP-1 and NF-κB [71]. EGCG can also remarkably attenuate lipopolysaccharide (LPS)-induced cell migration by a significant internalization of 67KD laminin receptor (67LR) [42,73].

EGCG also plays important roles in inhibiting tumor metastasis through the modulation of signaling pathways, including the modulation of β1 integrin-mediated signaling [74], down regulation of vasodilator-stimulated phosphoprotein (VASP) expression via the Rac1 pathway [72], enhancing the expression of α1-antitrypsin by regulating the PI3K/AKT pathway [75], and down-regulating the EGFR signaling pathway [76].

## 4. Inconsistent Results and Further Study Suggestions

### 4.1. Inconsistent Results

Although animal and in vitro studies showed that tea catechins were associated with a protective role against breast cancer, evidence from in vivo and human epidemiological studies is inconsistent. Increased green tea consumption (>3 cups/day) was inversely associated with recurrence (Pooled RR = 0.73, 95% CI: 0.56–0.96). An analysis of case–control studies investigating incidence suggested an inverse association, with a pooled RR of 0.81 (95% CI: 0.75, 0.88), while no association was found among cohort studies of incidence [23,77,78]. There are many factors leading to the controversial results.

First, the suppressive effects of tea on breast cancer differed between various kinds of tea. The reduction in breast cancer risk was usually associated with green tea consumption, rather than black tea consumption [10,11,15,17,79]. The major bioactive components in tea are catechins, especially EGCG. Black tea is a fully-fermented tea, and about 80% of tea catechins are oxidized and converted into orange and red tea pigments (theaflavins and thearubigins) during fermentation. This may explain why black tea consumption was not associated with the decreased risk of breast cancer.

Second, contradictory results arose from different populations investigated. An epidemiological study showed that daily tea consumption was significantly associated with a lower risk in the population of premenopausal women (OR = 0.62, 95% CI: 0.40–0.97), but an increased risk for breast cancer in the population of postmenopausal women (OR = 1.40, 95% CI: 1.00–1.96). The relationship between drinking green tea with the risk of breast cancer differed between ER-negative (OR = 1.22, 95% CI: 0.43–3.43) and ER-positive (OR = 0.61, 95% CI: 0.25–1.49) populations among postmenopausal women [10]. The observations of men and women gave different results. Tea drinking showed a strong association with increased risk for breast cancer in men, but no association with the development of breast cancer in women [80]. There was a significant association between the intake frequency of green tea and the decrease in risk of breast cancer among women with high-activity of the angiotensin-converting enzyme (ACE) genotype. However, no association was observed between the intake frequency of green tea and the risk of breast cancer among women with the low-activity ACE genotype [21]. These controversial results might be due to the differences in physiological status between various populations, which gave different responses to the bioactive components in tea.

Third, contradictory results between in vitro and in vivo studies arose from low bioavailability and biotransformation in vivo. When EGCG was incubated with rat liver microsomes at 1–100 μM for 30 min in vitro, EGCG selectively bound to COMT [81]. However, in vivo tests showed that supplementation with a high dose of EGCG does not impair the activity of COMT [82]. A bioavailability test using $^3$H-EGCG in mice revealed a wide distribution of radioactivity in target organs, including digestive tract, liver, lung, pancreas, mammary gland, brain, kidney, uterus, and ovary. However, radioactivity in the blood was low, being about 2% of total administered radioactivity at 6 h after administration, and the status was sustained for 24 h. However, 37.1% of total administered radioactivity was excreted in feces and 6.6% in urine within 24 h [83]. Chemical modification of tea catechins occurring in the digestive tract might lead to their low bioavailability. Under physiological conditions, COMT can metabolize EGCG to 4″-O-methyl-EGCG (MeEGCG) and 4′,4″-di-O-methyl-EGCG (DiMeEGCG), resulting in a reduction of the oral bioavailability of EGCG and reduced cancer-related biological activities of EGCG. Combination of EGCG and Tolcapone (TOL) (a COMT inhibitor) was found to improve the bioavailability of EGCG and to synergistically enhance the cancer suppressive effect of EGCG by inhibiting the COMT-mediated methylation of EGCG in vivo [84]. The authors deduced that the differences in the suppressive effect of catechins on breast cancer between various populations might be related to the differentiation in the bioavailability of catechins between different populations, owing to variations in physiological status.

### 4.2. Further Study Suggestions

Improvement of the bioavailability of the bioactive catechins will be an important research topic in the future. The development of methods to improve the stability of tea catechins will enhance their oral bioavailability. The usage of stabilizers and/or encapsulation of EGCG into particulate systems such as nanoparticles or microparticles can significantly increase its stability [85]. It was reported that encapsulation of tea extract in chitosan encapsulation in nanoparticles (NPs) was beneficial in stabilizing catechins including EGCG and catechin (C) in vivo, resulting in a significant improvement of their intestinal absorption [86]. Encapsulation of catechin and epicatechin (EC) in bovine serum albumin NPs (BSA-NPs) could also improve their stability and antioxidant potential in cell line A549 [87]. Antitumor activity of folate-conjugated chitosan-coated EGCG NPs (FCS-EGCG-NPs)—prepared by ionic gelation method using folic acid-modified carboxymethyl chitosan—gave a greater tumor inhibitory effect on cancer cells than free EGCG, especially in the cancer cells with a strong expression of folic acid receptors on the cell surface [88]. Loading EGCG in cationic lipid nanoparticles (LNs) is recognized as a promising strategy for prolonging EGCG release [89].

Developing complex formulations using various tea catechins and other bioactive components will also improve the stability and bioavailability of tea catechins. Although EC did not induce apoptosis of lung cancer cell line PC-9, co-treatment of EGCG with 100 μM EC reduced the $IC_{50}$ of EGCG from 60 μM to 15 μM, suggesting that EC enhanced the anti-cancer activity of EGCG [83]. The combination of 75 μM EGCG with the cancer preventive agent Sulindac (10 μM or 100 μM) induced apoptosis of PC-9 cells over 10 times more strongly than Sulindac alone [83]. The cellular accumulation of EC was increased by co-administrating with other catechins, especially gallated catechins [90]. Green tea catechins, formulated with xylitol and vitamin C and then encapsulated in g-cyclodextrin (g-CD) or coated with hydroxypropyl methyl cellulose phthalate (HPMCP), provided a synergistic effect to significantly enhance the intestinal absorption of catechins [91]. Encapsulation of hydrophilic catechin and hydrophobic curcumin within a water-in-oil-in-water (W/O/W) double emulsion by a two-step emulsification method significantly increased their stability in simulated gastrointestinal fluid and gave a four-fold augmentation in their bio-accessibility, compared to that of freely-suspended curcumin and catechin solutions [92]. When EGCG was loaded into hydrogel prepared by ionic interaction gelatin and γ-polyglutamic acid with ethylcarbodiimide as the crosslinker, EGCG was more stable in the harsh gastrointestinal tract environment than free EGCG [93].

However, encapsulated EGCG should be taken without food in order to maximize its systemic absorption, because the co-administration of EGCG with foods such as a light breakfast or strawberry sorbet reduced systemic or plasma EGCG [94].

## 5. Conclusions

Though the role of tea in breast cancer is uncertain, there have been many in vitro and in vivo studies showing the association between green tea consumption and the decreased risk of breast cancer. There are more than ten catechin compounds in tea, among which EGCG is the most abundant and shows the most active suppressing effects on breast cancer. Catechins are a group of natural antioxidants, and they suppress carcinogen-induced ROS and DNA damage by enhancing antioxidant enzymes, scavenging ROS, and promoting the repair of damaged DNA. Catechins such as EGCG regulate cell signaling pathways relating to breast carcinogenesis, such as PI3k/Akt/mTOR, EGFR, ERK, Wnt/β-catenin, and HGF/Met pathways. EGCG interacts with target proteins in the breast cancer cells, such as ERα, Zap-70, PI3K, G3BP1, IGF-1R, vimentin, Bcl-2, Bcl-xL, GRP78, and Fyn via hydrogen bonding, which plays a role in the inhibition of breast cancer. Catechins inhibit DNA methylation by suppressing DNMTs and increasing SAH levels. GTE or EGCG suppressed the secretion of VEGF protein by inhibiting VEGF promoter activity, resulting in the inhibition of tumor angiogenesis. Catechins suppress proliferation and induce apoptosis of breast cancer cells by inducing cell cycle arrest and $Ca^{2+}$-associated apoptosis, promoting TP53/caspase-mediated apoptosis, down-regulating anti-apoptotic factors, inhibiting FAS, and regulating the NO/NOS system. Tea catechins inhibit metastasis of breast cancer cells via the modulation of proteolytic enzymes, suppressing the EMT, and down-regulating MT1-MMP transcription (Figure 1).

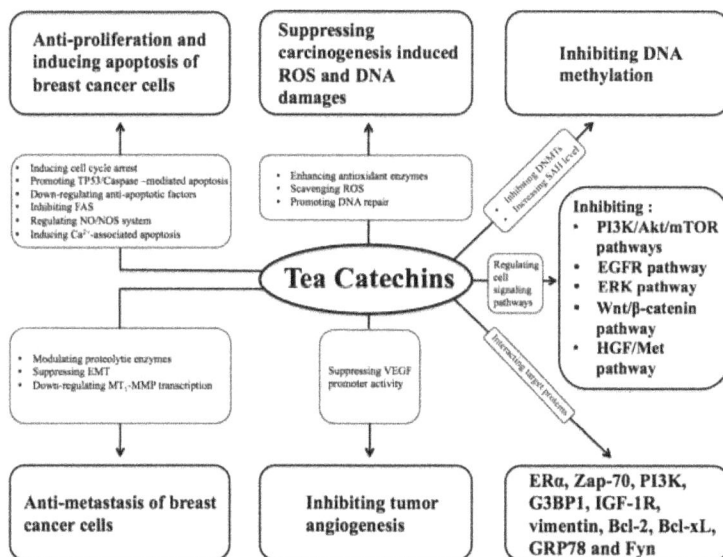

**Figure 1.** Effects of tea catechins on breast cancer. Akt: protein kinase B; DNMT: DNA methyltransferase; EGFR: epidermal growth factor receptor; EMT: epithelial-to-mesenchymal transition; ERα: estrogen receptor alpha; ERK: extracellular signal-regulated kinase; FAS: fatty acid synthase; G3BP1: SH3 domain-binding protein 1; HGF: hepatocyte growth factor; IGF-1R: insulin-like growth factor 1 receptor; MT1-MMP: membrane type-1 matrix metalloproteinase; mTOR: mammalian target of rapamycin; NO/NOS: nitric oxide/nitric oxide synthase; PI3K: phosphoinositide-3-kinase; ROS: reactive oxygen species; SAH: *S*-adenosyl-L-homocysteine; TP53: tumor protein P53; VEGF: vascular endothelial growth factor; Zap-70: 70 kDa zeta-associated protein.

The inconsistent results between in vitro and in vivo studies are considered to arise from the low oral bioavailability and the biotransformation of catechins in vivo. Further studies on the development of methods to stabilize catechins in the digestive tract and complex formulation with synergistic effects between catechins and other ingredients will be beneficial to improve oral bioavailability and anti-tumor effects of tea catechins. Overall, tea catechins show a potential role in suppressing breast cancer.

**Acknowledgments:** This work was financially supported by the Specialized Research Fund for the Doctoral Program of Higher Education of China (SRFDP No. 20110101110094).

**Author Contributions:** L.P. Xiang: Sections 2 and 3.5; A. Wang: Abstract and Section 3.7; J.H. Ye: Section 3.2; X.Q. Zheng: Section 3.1; C.A. Polito: Section 3.3 and English polishing; J.L. Lu: Section 3.4; Q.S. Li: 5. Conclusion and Figure 1; Y.R. Liang: Sections 1, 3.6, 4.1 and 4.2.

**Conflicts of Interest:** The authors declare no conflict of interest.

# References

1. Stewart, B.W.; Wild, C.P. *World Cancer Report 2014*; World Health Organization: French, 2014; Chapters 1.1 and 5.2; Available online: http://www.searo.who.int/publications/bookstore/documents/9283204298/en/ (accessed on 20 May 2016).
2. Kushi, L.H.; Doyle, C.; McCullough, M.; Rock, C.L.; Demark-Wahnefried, W.; Bandera, E.V.; Gapstur, S.; Patel, A.V.; Andrews, K.; Gansler, T. American cancer society guidelines on nutrition and physical activity for cancer prevention: Reducing the risk of cancer with healthy food choices and physical activity. *CA Cancer J. Clin.* **2012**, *62*, 30–67. [CrossRef] [PubMed]
3. Thomson, C.A. Diet and breast cancer: Understanding risks and benefits. *Nutr. Clin. Pract.* **2012**, *27*, 636–650. [CrossRef] [PubMed]
4. Liang, Y.R.; Ye, Q.; Jin, J.; Liang, H.; Lu, J.L.; Du, Y.Y.; Dong, J.J. Chemical and instrumental assessment of green tea sensory preference. *Int. Food Prop.* **2008**, *11*, 258–272. [CrossRef]
5. Dong, J.J.; Ye, J.H.; Lu, J.L.; Zheng, X.Q.; Liang, Y.R. Isolation of antioxidant catechins from green tea and its decaffeination. *Food Bioprod. Process.* **2011**, *89*, 62–66. [CrossRef]
6. Lin, S.Y.; Chen, Y.L.; Lee, C.L.; Cheng, C.Y.; Roan, S.F.; Chen, I.Z. Monitoring volatile compound profiles and chemical compositions during the process of manufacturing semi-fermented oolong tea. *J. Hortic. Sci. Biotechnol.* **2013**, *88*, 159–164. [CrossRef]
7. Liang, Y.R.; Lu, J.L.; Zhang, L.Y.; Wu, S.; Wu, Y. Estimation of black tea quality by analysis of chemical composition and colour difference of tea infusions. *Food Chem.* **2003**, *80*, 283–290. [CrossRef]
8. Xu, J.Y.; Wu, L.Y.; Zheng, X.Q.; Lu, J.L.; Wu, M.Y.; Liang, Y.R. Green tea polyphenols attenuating ultraviolet b-induced damage to human retinal pigment epithelial cells in vitro. *Invest. Ophthalmol. Vis. Sci.* **2010**, *51*, 6665–6670. [CrossRef] [PubMed]
9. Chen, X.; Lu, W.; Zheng, Y.; Gu, K.; Chen, Z.; Zheng, W.; Shu, X.O. Exercise, tea consumption, and depression among breast cancer survivors. *J. Clin. Oncol.* **2010**, *28*, 991–998. [CrossRef] [PubMed]
10. Li, M.; Tse, L.A.; Chan, W.C.; Kwok, C.H.; Leung, S.L.; Wu, C.; Yu, W.C.; Yu, I.T.S.; Yu, C.H.T.; Wang, F.; et al. Evaluation of breast cancer risk associated with tea consumption by menopausal and estrogen receptor status among Chinese women in Hong Kong. *Cancer Epidemiol.* **2016**, *40*, 73–78. [CrossRef] [PubMed]
11. Suzuki, Y.; Tsubono, Y.; Nakaya, N.; Suzuki, Y.; Koizumi, Y.; Tsuji, I. Green tea and the risk of breast cancer: Pooled analysis of two prospective studies in Japan. *Br. J. Cancer* **2004**, *90*, 1361–1363. [CrossRef] [PubMed]
12. Zhang, M.; Holman, C.D.A.J.; Huang, J.P.; Xie, X. Green tea and the prevention of breast cancer: A case-control study in Southeast China. *Carcinogenesis* **2007**, *28*, 1074–1078. [CrossRef] [PubMed]
13. Imai, K.; Suga, K.; Nakachi, K. Cancer-Preventive effects of drinking green tea among a Japanese population. *Prev. Med.* **1997**, *26*, 769–775. [CrossRef] [PubMed]
14. Shrubsole, M.J.; Lu, W.; Chen, Z.; Shu, X.O.; Zheng, Y.; Dai, Q.; Cai, Q.; Gu, K.; Ruan, Z.X.; Gao, Y.T.; et al. Drinking Green Tea Modestly Reduces Breast Cancer Risk. *J. Nutr.* **2009**, *139*, 310–316. [CrossRef] [PubMed]
15. Ganmaa, D.; Willett, W.C.; Li, T.Y.; Feskanich, D.; Dam, R.M.V.; Lopez-Garcia, E.; Hunter, D.J.; Holmes, M.D. Coffee, tea, caffeine and risk of breast cancer: A 22-year follow-up. *Int. J. Cancer* **2008**, *122*, 2071–2076. [CrossRef] [PubMed]

16. Dai, Q.; Shu, X.O.; Li, H.L.; Yang, G.; Shrubsole, M.J.; Cai, H.; Wen, W.Q.; Franke, A.; Gao, Y.T.; Zheng, W. Is green tea drinking associated with a later onset of breast cancer? *Ann. Epidemiol.* **2010**, *20*, 74–81. [CrossRef] [PubMed]

17. Zhang, M.; Huang, J.; Xie, X.; Holman, C.D.A.J. Dietary intakes of mushrooms and green tea combine to reduce the risk of breast cancer in Chinese women. *Int. J. Cancer* **2009**, *124*, 1404–1408. [CrossRef] [PubMed]

18. Wu, A.H.; Yu, M.C.; Tseng, C.C.; Hankin, J.; Pike, M.C. Green tea and risk of breast cancer in Asian Americans. *Int. J. Cancer* **2003**, *106*, 574–579. [CrossRef] [PubMed]

19. Wu, A.H.; Yu, M.C.; Tseng, C.C.; Pike, M.C. Body size, hormone therapy and risk of breast cancer in Asian-American women. *Int. J. Cancer* **2007**, *120*, 844–852. [CrossRef] [PubMed]

20. Kumar, N.; Titus-Ernstoff, L.; Newcomb, P.A.; Trentham-Dietz, A.; Anic, G.; Egani, K.M. Tea consumption and risk of breast cancer. *Cancer Epidemiol. Biomark.* **2009**, *18*, 341–345. [CrossRef] [PubMed]

21. Yuan, J.M.; Koh, W.P.; Sun, C.L.; Lee, J.P.; Yu, M.C. Green tea intake, ACE gene polymorphism and breast cancer risk among Chinese women in Singapore. *Carcinogenesis* **2005**, *26*, 1389–1394. [CrossRef] [PubMed]

22. Inoue, M.; Robien, K.; Wang, R.; Berg, D.J.V.D.; Koh, W.P.; Yu, M.C. Green tea intake, MTHFR/TYMS genotype and breast cancer risk: The Singapore Chinese Health Study. *Carcinogenesis* **2008**, *29*, 1967–1972. [CrossRef] [PubMed]

23. Ogunleye, A.A.; Xue, F.; Michels, K.B. Green tea consumption and breast cancer risk or recurrence: A meta-analysis. *Breast Cancer Res. Treat.* **2010**, *119*, 477–484. [CrossRef] [PubMed]

24. Guyton, K.Z.; Kensler, T.W. Oxidative mechanisms in carcinogenesis. *Br. Med. Bull.* **1993**, *49*, 523–544. [PubMed]

25. Rathore, K.; Choudhary, S.; Odoi, A.; Wang, H.C.R. Green tea catechin intervention of reactive oxygen species-mediated ERK pathway activation and chronically induced breast cell carcinogenesis. *Carcinogenesis* **2012**, *33*, 174–183. [CrossRef] [PubMed]

26. Ruch, R.J.; Cheng, S.J.; Klaunig, J.E. Prevention of cytotoxicity and inhibition of intercellular communication by antioxidant catechins isolated from Chinese green tea. *Carcinogenesis* **1989**, *10*, 1003–1008. [CrossRef] [PubMed]

27. Kaur, S.; Greaves, P.; Cooke, D.N.; Edwards, R.; Steward, W.P.; Gescher, A.J.; Marczylo, T.H. Breast cancer prevention by green tea catechins and black tea theaflavins in the C3(1) SV40 T,t antigen transgenic mouse model is accompanied by increased apoptosis and a decrease in oxidative DNA adducts. *J. Agric. Food Chem.* **2007**, *55*, 3378–3385. [CrossRef] [PubMed]

28. Parvez, S.; Tabassum, H.; Rehman, H.; Banerjee, B.D.; Athar, M.; Raisuddin, S. Catechin prevents tamoxifen-induced oxidative stress and biochemical perturbations in mice. *Toxicology* **2006**, *225*, 109–118. [CrossRef] [PubMed]

29. Abrahim, N.N.; Kanthimathi, M.S.; Abdul-Aziz, A. Piper betle shows antioxidant activities, inhibits MCF-7 cell proliferation and increases activities of catalase and superoxide dismutase. *BMC Complement. Altern. Med.* **2012**, *12*, 220–230. [CrossRef] [PubMed]

30. De Oliveira, M.R.; Nabavi, S.F.; Daglia, M.; Rastrell, L. Epigallocatechin gallate and mitochondria—A story of life and death. *Pharmacol. Res.* **2016**, *104*, 70–85. [CrossRef] [PubMed]

31. Van Aller, G.S.; Carson, J.D.; Tang, W.; Peng, H.; Zhao, L.; Copeland, R.A.; Tummino, P.J.; Luo, L. Epigallocatechingallate (EGCG), a major component of green tea, is a dual phosphoinositide-3-kinase/mTOR inhibitor. *Biochem. Biophys. Res. Commun.* **2011**, *406*, 194–199. [CrossRef] [PubMed]

32. Pan, M.H.; Lin, C.C.; Lin, J.K.; Chen, W.J. Tea polyphenol (−)-epigallocatechin 3-gallate suppresses heregulin-beta 1-induced fatty acid synthase expression in human breast cancer cells by inhibiting phosphatidylinositol 3-kinase/Akt and mitogen-activated protein kinase cascade signaling. *J. Agric. Food Chem.* **2007**, *55*, 5030–5037. [CrossRef] [PubMed]

33. Kim, J.Y.; Zhang, X.W.; Rieger-Christ, K.M.; Summerhayes, I.C.; Wazer, D.E.; Paulson, K.E.; Yee, A.S. Suppression of Wnt signaling by the green tea compound (−)-epigallocatechin 3-gallate (EGCG) in invasive breast cancer cells-Requirement of the transcriptional repressor HBP1. *J. Biol. Chem.* **2006**, *281*, 10865–10875. [CrossRef] [PubMed]

34. Bigelow, R.L.H.; Cardelli, J.A. The green tea catechins, (−)-epigallocatechin-3-gallate (EGCG) and (−)-epicatechin-3-gallate (ECG), inhibit HGF/Met signaling in immortalized and tumorigenic breast epithelial cells. *Oncogene* **2006**, *25*, 1922–1930. [CrossRef] [PubMed]

35.  Pike, M.C.; Spicer, D.V.; Dahmoush, L.; Press, M.F. Estrogens, progestogens, normal breast cell-proliferation, and breast-cancer risk. *Epidemiol. Rev.* **1992**, *15*, 17–35.

36.  Haldosen, L.A.; Zhao, C.Y.; Dahlman-Wright, K. Estrogen receptor beta in breast cancer. *Mol. Cell. Endocrinol.* **2014**, *382*, 665–672. [CrossRef] [PubMed]

37.  Heldring, N.; Pike, A.; Andersson, S.; Matthews, J.; Cheng, G.; Hartman, J.; Tujague, M.; Strom, A.; Treuter, E.; Warner, M.; et al. Estrogen receptors: How do they signal and what are their targets. *Physiol. Rev.* **2007**, *87*, 905–931. [CrossRef] [PubMed]

38.  Kuruto-Niwa, R.; Inoue, S.; Ogawa, S.; Muramatsu, M.; Nozawa, R. Effects of tea catechins on the ERE-regulated estrogenic activity. *J. Agric. Food Chem.* **2000**, *48*, 6355–6361. [CrossRef] [PubMed]

39.  Goodin, M.G.; Fertuck, K.C.; Zacharewski, T.R.; Rosengren, R.J. Estrogen receptor-mediated actions of polyphenoliccatechins in vivo and in vitro. *Toxicol. Sci.* **2002**, *69*, 354–361. [CrossRef] [PubMed]

40.  Li, Y.Y.; Yuan, Y.Y.; Meeran, S.M.; Tollefsbol, T.O. Synergistic epigenetic reactivation of estrogen receptor-alpha (ERα) by combined green tea polyphenol and histone deacetylase inhibitor in ER alpha-negative breast cancer cells. *Mol. Cancer* **2010**, *9*, 274. [CrossRef] [PubMed]

41.  Shim, J.H.; Choi, H.S.; Pugliese, A.; Lee, S.Y.; Chae, J.I.; Choi, B.Y.; Bode, A.M.; Dong, Z. (−)-Epigallocatechin gallate regulates CD3-mediated T cell receptor signaling in leukemia through the inhibition of ZAP-70 kinase. *J. Biol. Chem.* **2008**, *283*, 28370–28379. [CrossRef] [PubMed]

42.  Umeda, D.; Yano, S.; Yamada, K.; Tachibana, H. Green tea polyphenol epigallocatechin-3-gallate signaling pathway through 67-kDa laminin receptor. *J. Biol. Chem.* **2008**, *283*, 3050–3058. [CrossRef] [PubMed]

43.  Shim, J.H.; Su, Z.Y.; Chae, J.I.; Kim, D.J.; Zhu, F.; Ma, W.Y.; Bode, A.M.; Yang, C.S.; Dong, Z. Epigallocatechin gallate suppresses lung cancer cell growth through Ras-GTPase-activating protein SH3 domain-binding protein 1. *Cancer Prev. Res. (Phila)* **2010**, *3*, 670–679. [CrossRef] [PubMed]

44.  Li, M.; He, Z.; Ermakova, S.; Zheng, D.; Tang, F.; Cho, Y.Y.; Zhu, F.; Ma, W.Y.; Sham, Y.; Rogozin, E.A.; et al. Direct inhibition of insulin-like growth factor-I receptor kinase activity by (−)-epigallocatechin-3-gallate regulates cell transformation. *Cancer Epidemiol. Biomark. Prev.* **2007**, *16*, 598–605. [CrossRef] [PubMed]

45.  Ermakova, S.; Choi, B.Y.; Choi, H.S.; Kang, B.S.; Bode, A.M.; Dong, Z. The intermediate filament protein vimentin is a new target for epigallocatechin gallate. *J. Biol. Chem.* **2005**, *280*, 16882–16890. [CrossRef] [PubMed]

46.  Leone, M.; Zhai, D.; Sareth, S.; Kitada, S.; Reed, J.C.; Pellecchia, M. Cancer prevention by tea polyphenols is linked to their direct inhibition of antiapoptotic Bcl-2-family proteins. *Cancer Res.* **2003**, *63*, 8118–8121. [PubMed]

47.  Ermakova, S.P.; Kang, B.S.; Choi, B.Y.; Choi, H.S.; Schuster, T.F.; Ma, W.Y.; Bode, A.M.; Dong, Z. (-)-Epigallocatechin gallate overcomes resistance to etoposide-induced cell death by targeting the molecular chaperone glucose-regulated protein 78. *Cancer Res.* **2006**, *66*, 9260–9269. [CrossRef] [PubMed]

48.  He, Z.; Tang, F.; Ermakova, S.; Li, M.; Zhao, Q.; Cho, Y.Y.; Ma, W.Y.; Choi, H.S.; Bode, A.M.; Yang, C.S.; et al. Fyn is a novel target of (−)-epigallocatechin gallate in the inhibition of JB6 Cl41 cell transformation. *Mol. Carcinog.* **2008**, *47*, 172–183. [CrossRef] [PubMed]

49.  Jones, P.A.; Takai, D. The role of DNA methylation in mammalian epigenetics. *Science* **2001**, *293*, 1068–1070. [CrossRef] [PubMed]

50.  Lee, J.L.; Shim, J.Y.; Zhu, B.T. Mechanisms for the inhibition of DNA methyltransferases by tea catechins and bioflavonoids. *Mol. Pharmacol.* **2005**, *68*, 1018–1030. [CrossRef] [PubMed]

51.  Fang, M.Z.; Wang, Y.; Ai, N.; Hou, Z.; Sun, Y.; Lu, H.; Welsh, W.; Yang, C.S. Tea polyphenol (−)-epigallocatechin-3-gallate inhibits DNA methyltransferase and reactivates methylation-silenced genes in cancer cell lines. *Cancer Res.* **2003**, *63*, 7563–7570. [PubMed]

52.  Huo, C.; Yang, H.; Cui, Q.C.; Dou, Q.P.; Chan, T.H. Proteasome inhibition in human breast cancer cells with high catechol-o-methyltransferase activity by green tea polyphenol EGCG analog. *Bioorg. Med. Chem.* **2010**, *18*, 1252–1258. [CrossRef] [PubMed]

53.  Landis-Piwowar, K.R.; Wan, S.B.; Wiegand, R.A.; Kuhn, D.J.; Chan, T.H.; Dou, Q.P. Methylation suppresses the proteasome-inhibitory function of green tea polyphenols. *J. Cell. Physiol.* **2007**, *213*, 256–260. [CrossRef] [PubMed]

54.  Landis-Piwowar, K.R.; Chen, D.I.; Chan, T.H.; Dou, Q.P. Inhibition of catechol-O-methyltransferase activity in human breast cancer cells enhances the biological effect of the green tea polyphenol (−)-EGCG. *Oncol. Rep.* **2010**, *24*, 563–569. [PubMed]

55. Folkman, J. Angiogenesis in cancer, vascular, rheumatoid and other disease. *Nat. Med.* **1995**, *1*, 27–31. [CrossRef] [PubMed]

56. Ferrara, N.; Davis-Smyth, T. The biology of vascular endothelial growth factor. *Endocr. Rev.* **1997**, *18*, 4–25. [CrossRef] [PubMed]

57. Mukhtar, H.; Katiyar, S.K.; Agarwal, R. Green tea and skin-anticarcinogenic effects. *J. Invest. Dermatol.* **1994**, *102*, 3–7. [CrossRef] [PubMed]

58. Stoner, G.D.; Mukhtar, H. Polyphenols as cancer chemopreventive agents. *J. Cell. Biochem.* **1995**, *22*, 169–180. [CrossRef]

59. Tang, F.Y.; Meydani, M. Green tea catechins and vitamin E inhibit angiogenesis of human microvascular endothelial cells through suppression of IL-8 production. *Nutr. Cancer* **2001**, *41*, 119–125. [CrossRef] [PubMed]

60. Maryam, R.S.; Shao, Z.M.; David, H. Green tea inhibits vascular endothelial growth factor (VEGF) induction inhuman breast cancer cells. *J. Nutr.* **2002**, *132*, 2307–2311.

61. Shaun, K.R.; Guo, W.M.; Liu, L.P. Green tea catechin, epigallocatechin-3-gallate, inhibits vascular endothelial growth factor angiogenic signaling by disrupting the formation of a receptor complex. *J. Cancer* **2006**, *118*, 1635–1644.

62. Seeram, N.P.; Zhang, Y.; Nair, M.G. Inhibition of proliferation of human cancer cells and cyclooxygenase enzymes by anthocyanidins and catechins. *Nutr. Cancer* **2003**, *46*, 101–106. [CrossRef] [PubMed]

63. Deguchi, H.; Fujii, T.; Nakagawa, S.; Koga, T.; Shirouzu, K. Analysis of cell growth inhibitory effects of catechin through MAPK in human breast cancer cell line T47D. *Int. J. Oncol.* **2002**, *21*, 1301–1305. [CrossRef] [PubMed]

64. Alshatwi, A.A. Catechin hydrate suppresses MCF-7 proliferation through TP53/Caspase-mediated apoptosis. *J. Exp. Clin. Canc. Res.* **2010**, *29*, 2–9. [CrossRef] [PubMed]

65. Afsar, T.; Trembley, J.H.; Salomon, C.E.; Razak, S.; Khan, M.R.; Ahmed, K. Growth inhibition and apoptosis in cancer cells induced by polyphenolic compounds of *Acacia hydaspica*: Involvement of multiple signal transduction pathways. *Sci. Rep.* **2016**, *6*, 23077. [CrossRef] [PubMed]

66. Jo, E.H.; Lee, S.J.; Ahn, N.S.; Park, J.S.; Hwang, J.W.; Kim, S.H.; Aruoma, O.I.; Lee, Y.S.; Kang, K.S. Induction of apoptosis in MCF-7 and MDA-MB-231 breast cancer cells by Oligonol is mediated by Bcl-2 family regulation and MEK/ERK signaling. *Eur. J. Cancer Prev.* **2007**, *16*, 342–347. [CrossRef] [PubMed]

67. Nifli, A.P.; Kampa, M.; Alexaki, V.I.; Notas, G.; Castanas, E. Polyphenol interaction with the T47D human breast cancer cell line. *J. Dairy Res.* **2005**, *72*, 44–50. [CrossRef] [PubMed]

68. Palmer, A.E.; Jin, C.; Reed, J.C.; Tsien, R.Y. Bcl-2-Mediated alterations in endoplasmic reticulum Ca2t analyzed with an improved genetically encoded fluorescent sensor. *Proc. Natl. Acad. Sci. USA* **2004**, *101*, 17404–17409. [CrossRef] [PubMed]

69. Hsu, Y.C.; Liou, Y.M. The Anti-cancer effects of (−)-epigalocathine-3-gallate on the signaling pathways associated with membrane receptors in MCF-7 cells. *J. Cell. Physiol.* **2011**, *226*, 2721–2730. [CrossRef] [PubMed]

70. Luo, K.; Koa, C.H.; Yue, G.G.L.; Lee, J.K.M.; Li, K.K.; Lee, M.; Li, G.; Fung, K.P.; Leung, P.C.; Lau, C.B.S. Green tea (*Camellia sinensis*) extract inhibits both the metastasis and osteolytic components of mammary cancer 4T1 lesions in mice. *J. Nutr. Biochem.* **2014**, *25*, 395–403. [CrossRef] [PubMed]

71. Slivova, V.; Zaloga, G.; DeMichele, S.J.; Mukerji, P.; Huang, Y.S.; Siddiqui, R.; Harvey, K.; Valachovicova, T.; Sliva, D. Green tea polyphenols modulate secretion of urokinase plasminogen activator (uPA) and inhibit invasive behavior of breast cancer cells. *Nutr. Cancer* **2005**, *52*, 66–73. [CrossRef] [PubMed]

72. Zhang, Y.; Han, G.; Fan, B.; Zhou, Y.; Zhou, X.; Wei, L.; Zhang, J. Green tea (−)-epigallocatechin-3-gallate down-regulates VASP expression and inhibits breast cancer cell migration and invasion by attenuating Rac1 activity. *Eur. J. Pharmacol.* **2009**, *606*, 172–179. [CrossRef] [PubMed]

73. Annabi, B.; Lachambre, M.P.; Bousquet-Gagnon, N.; Page, M.; Gingras, D.; Beliveau, R. Green tea polyphenol (−)-epigallocatechin 3-gallate inhibits MMP-2 secretion and MT1-MMP-driven migration in glioblastoma cells. *Biochim. Biophys. Acta* **2002**, *1542*, 209–220. [CrossRef]

74. Sen, T.; Chatterjee, A. Epigallocatechin-3-gallate (EGCG) downregulates EGF-induced MMP-9 in breast cancer cells: Involvement of integrin receptor alpha 5 beta 1 in the process. *Eur. J. Nutr.* **2011**, *50*, 465–478. [CrossRef] [PubMed]

75. Xiaokaiti, Y.; Wu, H.M.; Chen, Y.; Yang, H.P.; Duan, J.H.; Li, X.; Pan, Y.; Tie, L.; Zhang, L.R.; Li, X.J. EGCG reverses human neutrophil elastase-induced migration in A549 cells by directly binding to HNE and by regulating alpha1-AT. *Sci. Rep.* **2015**, *5*, 11494. [CrossRef] [PubMed]

76. Farabegoli, F.; Papi, A.; Orlandi, M. (−)-Epigallocatechin-3-gallate down-regulates EGFR, MMP-2, MMP-9 and EMMPRIN and inhibits the invasion of MCF-7 tamoxifen-resistant cells. *Biosci. Rep.* **2010**, *31*, 99–108. [CrossRef] [PubMed]

77. Zhou, P.; Li, J.P.; Zhang, C. Green tea consumption and breast cancer risk: Three recent meta-analyses. *Breast Cancer Res. Treat.* **2011**, *127*, 581–582. [CrossRef] [PubMed]

78. Ogunleye, A.A.; Xue, F.; Michels, K.B. Green tea consumption and breast cancer risk: Three recent meta-analyses Rebuttal. *Breast Cancer Res. Treat.* **2011**, *127*, 583.

79. Baker, J.A.; Beehler, G.P.; Sawant, A.C.; Jayaprakash, V.; McCann, S.E.; Moysich, K.B. Consumption of coffee, but not black tea, is associated with decreased risk of premenopausal breast cancer. *J. Nutr.* **2006**, *136*, 166–171. [PubMed]

80. Rosenblatt, K.A.; Thomas, D.B.; Jimenez, L.M.; Fish, B.; McTiernan, A.; Stalsberg, H.; Stemhagen, A.; Thompson, W.D.; Curnen, M.G.M.; Satariano, W.; et al. The relationship between diet and breast cancer in men (United States). *Cancer Cause Control* **1999**, *10*, 107–113. [CrossRef]

81. Weng, Z.; Greenhaw, J.; Salminen, W.F.; Shi, Q. Mechanisms for epigallocatechin gallate induced inhibition of drug metabolizing enzymes in rat liver microsomes. *Toxicol. Lett.* **2012**, *214*, 328–338. [CrossRef] [PubMed]

82. Lorenz, M.; Paul, F.; Moobed, M.; Baumann, G.; Zimmermann, B.F.; Stangl, K.; Stangl, V. The activity of catechol-O-methyltransferase (COMT) is not impaired by high doses of epigallocatechin-3-gallate (EGCG) in vivo. *Eur. J. Pharmacol.* **2014**, *740*, 645–651. [CrossRef] [PubMed]

83. Suganuma, M.; Okabe, S.; Sueoka, N.; Sueoka, E.; Matsuyama, S.; Imai, K.; Nakachi, K.; Fujiki, H. Green tea and cancer chemoprevention. *Mutat. Res.* **1999**, *428*, 339–344. [CrossRef]

84. Forester, S.C.; Lambert, J.D. The catechol-O-methyltransferase inhibitor, tolcapone, increases the bioavailability of unmethylated (−)-epigallocatechin-3-gallate in mice. *J. Funct. Foods* **2015**, *17*, 183–188. [CrossRef] [PubMed]

85. Krupkova, O.; Ferguson, S.J.; Wuertz-Kozak, K. Stability of (−)-epigallocatechin gallate and its activity in liquid formulations and delivery systems. *J. Nutr. Biochem.* **2016**, *37*, 1–12. [CrossRef]

86. Dube, A.; Nicolazzo, J.A.; Larson, I. Chitosan nanoparticles enhance the intestinal absorption of the green tea catechins (+)-catechin and (−)-epigallocatechingallate. *Eur. J. Pharm. Sci.* **2014**, *41*, 219–225. [CrossRef] [PubMed]

87. Yadav, R.; Kumar, D.; Kumari, A.; Yadav, S.K. Encapsulation of catechin and epicatechin on BSA NPs improved their stability and antioxidant potential. *EXCLI J.* **2014**, *13*, 331–346. [PubMed]

88. Liang, J.; Cao, L.; Zhang, L.; Wan, X. Preparation, characterization, and in vitro antitumor activity of folate conjugated chitosan coated EGCG nanoparticles. *Food Sci. Biotechnol.* **2014**, *23*, 569–575. [CrossRef]

89. Fangueiro, J.F.; Calpena, A.C.; Clares, B.; Andreani, T.; Egea, M.A.; Veiga, F.J.; Garcia, M.L.; Silva, A.M.; Souto, E.B. Biopharmaceutical evaluation of epigallocatechin gallate-loaded cationic lipid nanoparticles (EGCG-LNs): In vivo, in vitro and ex vivo studies. *Int. J. Pharm.* **2016**, *502*, 161–169. [CrossRef] [PubMed]

90. Tagashira, T.; Choshi, T.; Hibino, S.; Kamishikiryou, J.; Sugihara, N. Influence of gallate and pyrogallol moieties on the intestinal absorption of (−)-epicatechin and (−)-epicatechingallate. *J. Food Sci.* **2012**, *77*, H208–H215. [CrossRef] [PubMed]

91. Naumovski, N.; Blades, B.L.; Roach, P.D. Food inhibits the oral bioavailability of the major green tea antioxidant epigallocatechingallate in humans. *Antioxidants* **2015**, *4*, 373–393. [CrossRef] [PubMed]

92. Son, Y.R.; Chung, J.H.; Ko, S.; Shim, S.M. Combinational enhancing effects of formulation and encapsulation on digestive stability and intestinal transport of green tea catechins. *J. Microencapsul.* **2016**, *33*, 183–190. [CrossRef] [PubMed]

93. Aditya, N.P.; Aditya, S.; Yang, H.; Kim, H.W.; Park, S.O.; Ko, S. Co-Delivery of hydrophobic curcumin and hydrophilic catechin by a water-in-oil-in-water double emulsion. *Food Chem.* **2015**, *173*, 7–13. [CrossRef] [PubMed]

94. Garcia, J.P.D.; Hsieh, M.F.; Doma, B.T.; Peruelo, D.C.; Chen, I.H.; Lee, H.M. Synthesis of gelatin-γ-polyglutamic acid-based hydrogel for the in vitro controlled release of epigallocatechin gallate (EGCG) from *Camellia sinensis*. *Polymers* **2014**, *6*, 39–58. [CrossRef]

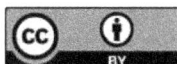

*nutrients*

MDPI

*Review*

# Curcumin AntiCancer Studies in Pancreatic Cancer

Sabrina Bimonte [1,*,†], Antonio Barbieri [2,*,†], Maddalena Leongito [1], Mauro Piccirillo [1], Aldo Giudice [3], Claudia Pivonello [4], Cristina de Angelis [5], Vincenza Granata [6], Raffaele Palaia [1] and Francesco Izzo [1]

[1]   Division of Abdominal Surgical Oncology, Hepatobiliary Unit, Istituto Nazionale per lo studio e la cura dei Tumori "Fondazione G. Pascale"—IRCCS—Via Mariano Semmola, Naples 80131, Italy; maddalenaleongito@virgilio.it (M.L.); mauropiccirillo73@libero.it (M.P.); r.palaia@istitutotumori.na.it (R.P.); f.izzo@istitutotumori.na.it (F.I.)

[2]   S.S.D Sperimentazione Animale, Istituto Nazionale per lo studio e la cura dei Tumori "Fondazione G. Pascale"—IRCCS, Naples 80131, Italy

[3]   Epidemiology Unit, Istituto Nazionale per lo studio e la cura dei Tumori "Fondazione G. Pascale"—IRCCS—Via Mariano Semmola, Naples 80131, Italy; aldo.giudice@libero.it

[4]   Dipartimento di Medicina Clinica e Chirurgia, Sezione di Endocrinologia, Università di Napoli Federico II, Naples 80131, Italy; cpivonello@gmail.com

[5]   I.O.S. & Coleman Srl, Naples 80011, Italy; cristinadeangelis83@hotmail.it

[6]   Division of Radiology, Istituto Nazionale per lo studio e la cura dei Tumori "Fondazione G. Pascale"—IRCCS—Via Mariano Semmola, Naples 80131, Italy; cinzia.granata80@libero.it

*   Correspondence: s.bimonte@istitutotumori.na.it (S.B.); a.barbieri@istitutotumori.na.it (A.B.); Tel.: +39-081-5903-221 (S.B.)

†   These authors contributed equally to this work.

Received: 23 May 2016; Accepted: 13 July 2016; Published: 16 July 2016

**Abstract:** Pancreatic cancer (PC) is one of the deadliest cancers worldwide. Surgical resection remains the only curative therapeutic treatment for this disease, although only the minority of patients can be resected due to late diagnosis. Systemic gemcitabine-based chemotherapy plus nab-paclitaxel are used as the gold-standard therapy for patients with advanced PC; although this treatment is associated with a better overall survival compared to the old treatment, many side effects and poor results are still present. Therefore, new alternative therapies have been considered for treatment of advanced PC. Several preclinical studies have demonstrated that curcumin, a naturally occurring polyphenolic compound, has anticancer effects against different types of cancer, including PC, by modulating many molecular targets. Regarding PC, in vitro studies have shown potent cytotoxic effects of curcumin on different PC cell lines including MiaPaCa-2, Panc-1, AsPC-1, and BxPC-3. In addition, in vivo studies on PC models have shown that the anti-proliferative effects of curcumin are caused by the inhibition of oxidative stress and angiogenesis and are due to the induction of apoptosis. On the basis of these results, several researchers tested the anticancer effects of curcumin in clinical trials, trying to overcome the poor bioavailability of this agent by developing new bioavailable forms of curcumin. In this article, we review the results of pre-clinical and clinical studies on the effects of curcumin in the treatment of PC.

**Keywords:** curcumin; natural compound; pancreatic cancer; therapy

## 1. Introduction

Pancreatic cancer is one of the deadliest cancer worldwide [1]. Surgical resection remains the only curative therapeutic treatment for this disease, although only the minority of patients can be resected due to late diagnosis [2]. Systemic gemcitabine-based chemotherapy has been used as the standard therapy for patients with advanced PC, although this treatment is associated with many side effects and poor overall survival [3,4]. In order to improve the overall survival of patients with PC, many studies combined the use of gemcitabine with different agents, although the results were not encouraging [5–11]. For these reasons, new alternative therapies involving natural compounds with minimal toxicity, such as curcumin, have been considered for treatment of PC. Curcumin, a naturally occurring polyphenolic compound, derives from turmeric (*Curcuma longa*). It has been commonly used as a food additive or dietary pigment and in traditional medicine [12–16]. Preclinical in vitro and in vivo studies have demonstrated that curcumin has several pharmacologic effects, including antioxidant, anti-inflammatory, and anticancer activities, in different types of cancer, including PC, by modulating multiple signaling pathways [15,17–44]. Taken together, these results suggest that curcumin can be considered a new therapeutic drug in PC treatment [45]. In addition it has many advantages for patients, such as safety and minimal toxicity. Several researchers tested the anticancer effects of curcumin in clinical trials, trying to overcome the poor bioavailability of this agent by developing new bioavailable forms of curcumin [15,46–57]. In this article, we review the results of pre-clinical and clinical studies on the effects of curcumin in the treatment of pancreatic cancer.

## 2. Effects of Curcumin in Treatment of PC

(a)  *In Vitro Studies: Dissecting the Molecular Mechanism Underlying the Antitumor Effects of Curcumin in PC Cell Growth*

Several preclinical studies showed that curcumin has antitumor effects by modulating multiple cell-signaling pathways in different types of cancers, including colorectal [28,33,58], pancreatic [17,18,22,27–31,34,35,42,43,59–67], breast [26], lung [32], hepatic [20], ovarian [25], head and neck [68], and prostate [24].

Regarding PC, in vitro studies on the effects of curcumin have been performed on different PC cells lines including MiaPaCa-2, MPanc-96, BxPC-3, Panc-1, AsPC-1, and L3.6pL. Results from these studies showed that the anti-proliferative effects of curcumin are mainly due to the inhibition of oxidative stress and angiogenesis and the induction of apoptosis [17,18,22,29,34,42,43,59,60,65,69–73]. The first report on the antitumor effect of curcumin in PC was described by Li et al. [17]. The authors demonstrated that curcumin down-regulated Nuclear factor kappa-light-chain-enhancer of activated B cells (NF-κB) and growth control molecules induced by NF-κB in human pancreatic cells in a time- and dose-dependent manner. These effects were accompanied by marked growth inhibition and apoptosis. Similar results were obtained by Wang et al. [22]. Then authors demonstrated that the Notch-1 signaling pathway was associated with NF-κB activity during curcumin-induced cell growth inhibition and apoptosis of pancreatic cells, suggesting that the down-regulation of Notch signaling by curcumin could represent a novel strategy for the treatment of patients with PC. In another study, it was demonstrated that curcumin treatment inhibited the proliferation of BxPC-3 human pancreatic cancer cells by DNA damage-mediated G2/M cell cycle arrest, by inhibition of cyclin B1/Cyclin-dependent kinase 1 (Cdk1) expression and by the activation of ataxia tel-angiectasia mutated (ATM)/Checkpoint kinase 1(Chk1)/Cell Division Cycle 25C (Cdc25C) [29]. Jutooru et al. showed that curcumin inhibited NF-κB expression and Panc-1 and L3.6pL cancer cell growth by down-regulation of the specificity protein Sp1 [59]. We also demonstrated that curcumin inhibited the proliferation and enhanced the apoptosis of MIA PaCa-2 cells, through the suppression of NF-κB-activation [18]. Recent findings showed that curcumin induced apoptosis in PC cells through the induction of forkhead box O1 (FOXO1) and the inhibition of the phosphatidylinositol 3-kinase/phosphatidylinositol 3-kinase (PI3K/Akt) pathway [43]. The antitumor role of curcumin in PC was also demonstrated by Diaz et al. in Panc-1 cells. The authors showed that curcumin induced pancreatic adenocarcinoma cell death via the reduction of the inhibitors of apoptosis (IAP) [42]. Finally, very recently, it was demonstrated that a small-molecule tolfenamic acid and dietary spice curcumin treatment enhanced the anti-proliferative effect in PC cells L3.6pl and MIA PaCa-2 through Sp1 suppression, NF-κB disruption of translocation to the nucleus and cell cycle phase distribution [34].

These results suggest that curcumin exerts its antitumor effect on PC by acting on different molecular mechanisms. Specifically, other studies showed that treatment of PC cells with curcumin has been associated with reduced migration and invasiveness of tumor cells, inhibition of cancer stem cell function, reversal of the epithelial-mesenchymal transition (EMT), and suppression of miR-221, Cyclooxygenase 2 (COX-2) and their effectors and pro-inflammatory cytokines [69,70]. In addition, it has been demonstrated that curcumin can also block signal transducer and activator of transcription 1 (STAT1) and signal transducer and activator of transcription 3 (STAT3) phosphorylation, and epidermal growth factor receptor (EGFR) and (neurogenic locus notch homolog protein-1) Notch-1 signaling pathways, which play important roles in pancreatic tumor growth [74]. It has been also demonstrated that siRNA/shRNA, small-molecule kinase inhibitors, and curcumin targeting these tumor stem cell markers and tumor suppressor miRNAs could be the perfect therapeutic agents for the treatment of PC [31,67,69,75–77] (Figure 1).

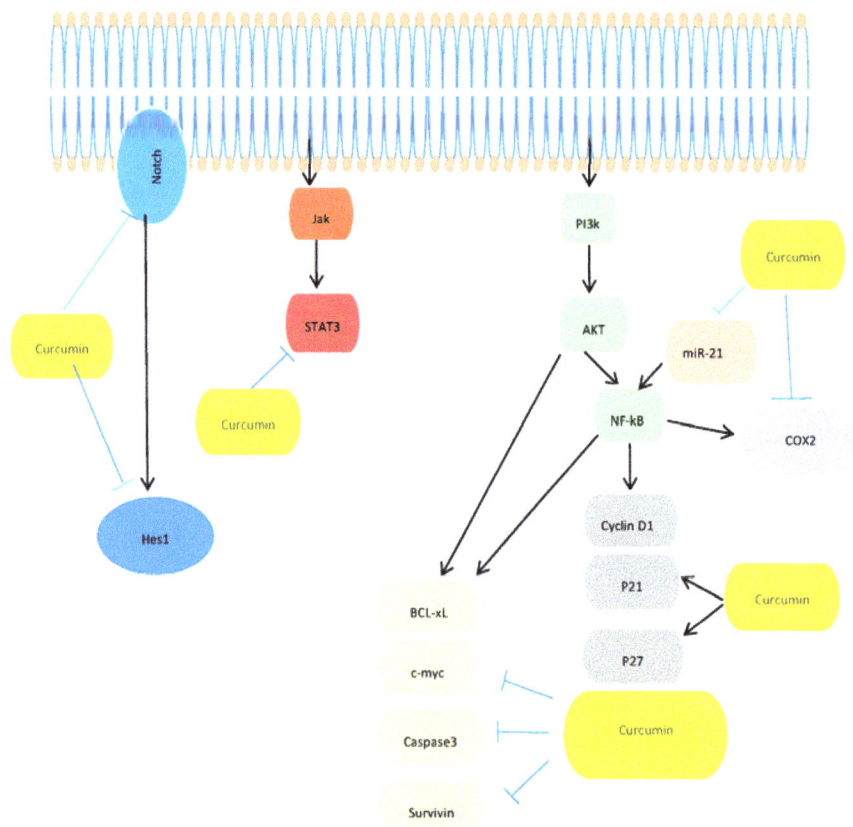

**Figure 1.** A schematization of molecular targets in PC regulated by curcumin. NF-κB: Nuclear factor kappa-light-chain-enhancer of activated B cells; COX2: Cyclooxygenase 2; Hes-1: Cyclin-dependent kinase 1; Akt: Protein kinase B; Stat3: Signal transducer and activator of transcription 3; PI3K: phosphatidylinositol 3-kinase; Notch-1: Neurogenic locus notch homolog protein-1; c-myc: C-mycproto-oncogene; Jak: Janus kinase. P21: Cyclin-dependent kinase inhibitor; P27: Cyclin-dependent kinase inhibitor; BCL-xL: B-cell lymphoma-extra large.

In order to ameliorate the aqueous solubility of curcumin, different derivatives of this compound or delivery system have been developed [78,79]. One curcumin analogue used in in vitro experiments is the 3,4-difluorobenzylidene curcumin (CDF). This compound has a higher tendency to accumulate in the pancreas than normal curcumin [74,80]. Although it has been demonstrated that CDF has cytotoxic effects on both resistant and nonresistant pancreatic tumor cell lines with respect to curcumin, this curcumin derivative still presents low aqueous solubility. To bypass this problem, researchers developed a new delivery system based on nanoparticles, such as hyaluronic acid (HA)-conjugated polyamidoamine dendrimers and hyaluronic acid (HA) and styrene-maleic acid-engineered nanomicelles of CDF. Results from studies performed with these systems gained improvements of aqueous solubility, stability, release profile and antitumor effects on PC cells lines with respect to unformulated CDF [56,63,81]. Table 1 summarizes the most relevant in vitro studies on the antitumor effect of curcumin in PC cells.

**Table 1.** A summary of in vitro studies on the role of curcumin in Pancreatic Cancer cell growth.

| Cell Lines | Dose of Curcumin (µM) | Molecular Targets | Reference |
|---|---|---|---|
| MiaPaCa-2; BxPC-3; Panc-1; MPanc-96 | ⩾25 | NF-κB↓;VEGF↓ | [71] |
| MiaPaCa-2 | 50 | NF-κB↓ | [18] |
| BxPC-3 | 2.5 | Cdk1↓; cyclin B1↓ | [29] |
| Panc-28; L3.6p | ⩾25 | NF-κB↓, Sp-1, Sp-3, Sp4↓ | [59] |
| Miapaca-E; Miapaca-M; BxPC-3 | ⩾4 | miR-220↑; miR-21↓ | [31] |
| Panc-1 | ⩾25 | IAP↓ | [42] |
| L3.6pl; MIA PaCa-2 | 5–25 | NF-κB↓, Sp-1, Sp-3, Sp4↓ | [34] |
| PANC-1 | 10–30 | Shh↓, GLI1↓, E-cadherin↓, vimentin↓ | [70] |

NF-κB: Nuclear factor kappa-light-chain-enhancer of activated B cells; VEGF: Vascular endothelial growth factor; Cdk1: Cyclin-dependent kinase 1; Sp-1: Specificity protein 1; Sp-3: Specificity protein 3; Sp4: Specificity protein 4; IAP: inhibitors of apoptosis; Shh: Sonic hedgehog, GLI1: Glioma-associated oncogene homologue 1; E-cadherin: Epithelial cadherin.

*(b)*   *In Vivo Studies: Effects of Curcumin in Mouse Model of PC*

The antitumor effect of curcumin and its analogues on PC has been demonstrated in in vivo experiments on mouse models of PC [18,27,59,71,74,82–88]. The first in vivo study was reported by Kunnumakara et al. [71]. The authors demonstrated that curcumin (1 g/kg orally) potentiated the antitumor activity of gemcitabine (25 mg/kg via intraperitoneal injection) in an orthotopic mouse model of PC [15] through the suppression of proliferation, angiogenesis, and inhibition of NF-κB-regulated gene products. Our research group also reported similar results. In fact, we demonstrated with the generation of an orthotropic mouse model of PC that tumors from mice injected with MIA PaCa-2 cells and placed on a diet containing curcumin at 0.6% for six weeks were smaller than those observed in controls. We also showed a down-regulation of the NF-κB-regulated gene products, suggesting that curcumin had great potential in the treatment of human PC, through the modulation of the NF-κB pathway [18]. Mach et al., in a xenograft human PC model, established the minimum effective dose (MED, 20 mg/kg) and optimal dosing schedule for liposomal curcumin [88]. In another study, the in vivo antitumorigenic activity of curcumin was investigated in athymic nude bearing L36pL cells as xenografts. The authors demonstrated that curcumin (dose of 100 mg/kg/days) inhibited tumor growth and tumor weight by down-regulation of the Sp transcription factor [59]. In order to potentiate the effects of curcumin on PC in vivo, several studies were performed using different forms of curcumin. Bao et al. demonstrated that CDF (2.5 mg/mouse/days; 5 mg/mouse/days; intragastric once daily for three weeks), an analogue of curcumin analogue, inhibited pancreatic tumor growth by switching on suppressor microRNAs and attenuating the expression of histone methyltransferase enhancer of zeste homolog 2, EZH2 [74]. Similar effects were reported for synthetic curcumin analogues EF31 and UBS109. The authors demonstrated, both in vitro and in vivo, that these analogues were potent DNA hypomethylating agents in PC [86]. The efficacy of liposomal curcumin in human PC was also reported by Ranjan et al. The authors showed that in xenograft tumors in nude mice, liposomal curcumin (20 mg/kg i.p. three times a week for four weeks) induced a suppression of tumor growth compared to untreated controls, indicating that this agent could be beneficial in patients with PC [85]. Similar results have been reported by recent studies in which the efficacy of curcuminoids and nanomicelles in treatment of PC was demonstrated [81,82]. It is important to underline that in all studies performed with curcumin derivatives and or a delivery system, the antitumor effects have been reported to be greater with respect to those observed with conventional curcumin. On the basis of these results, researchers tested the anticancer effects of curcumin in clinical trials, trying to overcome the poor bioavailability of this agent by developing new bioavailable forms of curcumin. Table 2 summarizes preclinical in vivo studies on the anticancer effects of curcumin against PC.

**Table 2.** Preclinical in vivo studies on the anticancer effects of curcumin against PC.

| Animal Models | Drug | Dose of Curcumin | Effects | Reference |
|---|---|---|---|---|
| Orthotopic mouse model (MIA PaCa-2 cells) | Curcumin + Gemcitabine | 1 g/kg (orally) | Suppression of proliferation, angiogenesis, and inhibition of NF-κB in tumors | [71] |
| Orthotopic mouse model (MIA PaCa-2 cells) | Curcumin | 0.6% for 6 weeks (dietary food) | Tumor growth inhibition and down regulation of the NF-κB-regulated gene products | [18] |
| Xenograft mouse model (L36pl cells) | Curcumin | 100 mg/kg/days | Tumor growth and Tumor weight inhibition | [59] |
| Orthotopic mouse model (MIA PaCa-2 cells) | CDF | 2.5 mg/mouse/days; 5 mg/mouse/days; intragastric once daily for 3 weeks | Tumor growth inhibition, reduced expression of EZH2 | [74] |
| Xenograft mouse model (MIA PaCa-2 cells) | Liposomal curcumin | 20 mg/kg i.p. three-times a week for four weeks | Tumor growth inhibition | [85] |

*(c)*   *Clinical Trials*

In order to translate the preclinical antitumor effects of curcumin into clinical practice, few clinical trials have been performed so far. Healthy volunteers and cancer patients were treated with curcumin, administered orally, in different clinical trials (phase I and pharmacokinetic studies). No dose-limiting toxicity (DLT) of up to at least 12 g/day was observed in patients, although nausea and diarrhea have been reported [48,89,90]. It was established that the daily oral dose of curcumin of 8 g or less is the most commonly used in clinical trials, due to its poor bioavailability.

Several phase II clinical trials on the antitumor effects of curcumin in PC were conducted [91–93]. Dhillon et al. conducted the first trial [91] and successfully tested the safety and the efficacy of curcumin used as a monotherapy in 25 patients of PC. Another group conducted a phase I/II clinical trial of curcumin in 21 patients with PC (resistant to gemcitabine-based chemotherapy), combining gemcitabine-based chemotherapy with curcumin treatment (8 g daily oral dose) [92]. Results from this study indicated that combination therapy using 8 g oral curcumin daily with gemcitabine-based chemotherapy was safe and feasible in patients with PC. Another interesting study tested the efficacy and feasibility of curcumin (8 g daily oral dose) in combination with gemcitabine monotherapy (standard dose and schedule) in 17 chemo-naive patients with PC. Differently from previous studies, increased gastrointestinal toxicity was observed in seven patients treated with this therapy, probably due to the elevated dose of curcumin combined with gemcitabine. For this reason, the dose of curcumin was reduced from 8 to 4 g [93]. From this study emerged the problem of the poor bioavailability of curcumin, which strongly limited its application in clinical practice. To solve this problem, new curcumin analogs and new drug delivery systems have been developed [46–55]. Interesting results have been reported by dose escalation and pharmacokinetic studies performed with Theracurcumin, a nanoparticle-based curcumin [55]. These studies demonstrated that the plasma curcumin levels observed after Theracurcumin ingestion were higher with respect to those obtained with conventional curcumin. The phase I clinical trial involving Theracurcumin (level 1 group: 200 mg oral/daily; level 2 group: 400 mg oral/daily) was conducted on 16 patients with PC resistant to gemcitabine-based chemotherapy [94]. The results from this study showed that repetitive systemic exposure to high concentrations of Theracurmin did not increase the incidence of side effects in cancer patients receiving gemcitabine-based chemotherapy, indicating that this agent could represent a new agent for PC treatments.

New clinical trials are needed to test the therapeutic effects of curcumin and its analogues in patients with PC.

## 3. Conclusions

Several preclinical studies have demonstrated that curcumin, a naturally occurring polyphenolic compound, has anticancer effects against different types of cancer, including PC, by modulating many molecular targets. On the basis of these results, several researchers tested the anticancer effects of curcumin in clinical trials, trying to overcome the poor bioavailability of this agent, which limited its clinical application. New bioavailable forms of curcumin have been developed and the results from clinical trials on patients with PC suggest that these agents could represent promising new treatments for PC, although more clinical studies will be still needed.

**Acknowledgments:** I.O.S. and Coleman Srl covered the costs for publication of this paper in OPEN access.

**Author Contributions:** The present review was mainly written by S.B., A.B. and F.I. and revised and edited by the rest of the authors. M.L., M.P.; A.G., C.D.A., C.V., V.G., R.P. prepared the tables and figure. S.B. and F.I. revised and confirmed the final version of the manuscript.

**Conflicts of Interest:** The authors declare no conflict of interest.

## Abbreviations

| | |
|---|---|
| PC | Pancreatic cancer |
| NF-κB | Nuclear factor kappa-light-chain-enhancer of activated B cells |
| Cdk1 | Cyclin-dependent kinase 1 |
| ATM | Ataxia tel-angiectasia |
| Chk1 | Checkpoint kinase 1 |
| Cdc25C | Cell division cycle 25C |
| FOXO1 | Forkhead box O1 |
| PI3K | Phosphatidylinositol 3-kinase |
| Akt | Phosphatidylinositol 3-kinase |
| Sp1 | Specificity protein |
| IAP | Inhibitors of apoptosis |
| EMT | epithelial-mesenchymal transition |
| STAT1 | Activator of transcription 1 |
| STAT3 | Signal transducer and activator of transcription 3 |
| EGFR | Epidermal growth factor receptor |
| Notch-1 | Neurogenic locus notch homolog protein-1 |
| COX2 | Cyclooxygenase 2 |
| Hes-1 | Cyclin-dependent kinase 1 |
| Akt | Protein kinase B |
| Stat3 | Signal transducer and activator of transcription 3 |
| PI3K | phosphatidylinositol 3-kinase |
| Notch-1 | Neurogenic locus notch homolog protein-1 |
| c-myc | C-mycproto-oncogene |
| Jak | Janus kinase |
| P21 | Cyclin-dependent kinase inhibitor |
| P27 | Cyclin-dependent kinase inhibitor |
| BCL-xL | B-cell lymphoma-extra large |
| CDF | 3, 4-difluorobenzylidene curcumin |
| HA | hyaluronic acid |
| Sp-3 | Specificity protein 3 |

| Sp4 | Specificity protein 4 |
| Shh | Sonic hedgehog |
| GLI1 | Glioma-associated oncogene homologue 1 |
| E-cadherin | Epithelial cadherin |
| EZH2 | enhancer of zeste homolog 2 |
| MED | minimum effective dose |
| DLT | dose-limiting toxicity |

## References

1. Siegel, R.; Naishadham, D.; Jemal, A. Cancer statistics, 2013. *CA Cancer J. Clin.* **2013**, *63*, 11–30. [CrossRef] [PubMed]
2. Stathis, A.; Moore, M.J. Advanced pancreatic carcinoma: Current treatment and future challenges. *Nat. Rev. Clin. Oncol.* **2010**, *7*, 163–172. [CrossRef] [PubMed]
3. Burris, H.A., 3rd; Moore, M.J.; Andersen, J.; Green, M.R.; Rothenberg, M.L.; Modiano, M.R.; Cripps, M.C.; Portenoy, R.K.; Storniolo, A.M.; Tarassoff, P.; et al. Improvements in survival and clinical benefit with gemcitabine as first-line therapy for patients with advanced pancreas cancer: A randomized trial. *J. Clin. Oncol.* **1997**, *15*, 2403–2413. [PubMed]
4. Berlin, J.D.; Catalano, P.; Thomas, J.P.; Kugler, J.W.; Haller, D.G.; Benson, A.B., 3rd. Phase III study of gemcitabine in combination with fluorouracil versus gemcitabine alone in patients with advanced pancreatic carcinoma: Eastern cooperative oncology group trial e2297. *J. Clin. Oncol.* **2002**, *20*, 3270–3275. [CrossRef] [PubMed]
5. Lima, C.M.R.; Green, M.R.; Rotche, R.; Miller, W.H., Jr.; Jeffrey, G.M.; Cisar, L.A.; Morganti, A.; Orlando, N.; Gruia, G.; Miller, L.L. Irinotecan plus gemcitabine results in no survival advantage compared with gemcitabine monotherapy in patients with locally advanced or metastatic pancreatic cancer despite increased tumor response rate. *J. Clin. Oncol.* **2004**, *22*, 3776–3783. [CrossRef] [PubMed]
6. Louvet, C.; Labianca, R.; Hammel, P.; Lledo, G.; Zampino, M.G.; Andre, T.; Zaniboni, A.; Ducreux, M.; Aitini, E.; Taieb, J.; et al. Gemcitabine in combination with oxaliplatin compared with gemcitabine alone in locally advanced or metastatic pancreatic cancer: Results of a gercor and giscad phase III trial. *J. Clin. Oncol.* **2005**, *23*, 3509–3516. [CrossRef] [PubMed]
7. Oettle, H.; Richards, D.; Ramanathan, R.K.; van Laethem, J.L.; Peeters, M.; Fuchs, M.; Zimmermann, A.; John, W.; Von Hoff, D.; Arning, M.; et al. A phase III trial of pemetrexed plus gemcitabine versus gemcitabine in patients with unresectable or metastatic pancreatic cancer. *Ann. Oncol.* **2005**, *16*, 1639–1645. [CrossRef] [PubMed]
8. Heinemann, V.; Quietzsch, D.; Gieseler, F.; Gonnermann, M.; Schonekas, H.; Rost, A.; Neuhaus, H.; Haag, C.; Clemens, M.; Heinrich, B.; et al. Randomized phase III trial of gemcitabine plus cisplatin compared with gemcitabine alone in advanced pancreatic cancer. *J. Clin. Oncol.* **2006**, *24*, 3946–3952. [CrossRef] [PubMed]
9. Herrmann, R.; Bodoky, G.; Ruhstaller, T.; Glimelius, B.; Bajetta, E.; Schuller, J.; Saletti, P.; Bauer, J.; Figer, A.; Pestalozzi, B.; et al. Gemcitabine plus capecitabine compared with gemcitabine alone in advanced pancreatic cancer: A randomized, multicenter, phase III trial of the swiss group for clinical cancer research and the central european cooperative oncology group. *J. Clin. Oncol.* **2007**, *25*, 2212–2217. [CrossRef] [PubMed]
10. Poplin, E.; Feng, Y.; Berlin, J.; Rothenberg, M.L.; Hochster, H.; Mitchell, E.; Alberts, S.; O'Dwyer, P.; Haller, D.; Catalano, P.; et al. Phase III, randomized study of gemcitabine and oxaliplatin versus gemcitabine (fixed-dose rate infusion) compared with gemcitabine (30-min infusion) in patients with pancreatic carcinoma e6201: A trial of the eastern cooperative oncology group. *J. Clin. Oncol.* **2009**, *27*, 3778–3785. [CrossRef] [PubMed]
11. Ueno, H.; Ioka, T.; Ikeda, M.; Ohkawa, S.; Yanagimoto, H.; Boku, N.; Fukutomi, A.; Sugimori, K.; Baba, H.; Yamao, K.; et al. Randomized phase III study of gemcitabine plus s-1, s-1 alone, or gemcitabine alone in patients with locally advanced and metastatic pancreatic cancer in Japan and Taiwan: Gest study. *J. Clin. Oncol.* **2013**, *31*, 1640–1648. [CrossRef] [PubMed]
12. Aggarwal, B.B.; Sundaram, C.; Malani, N.; Ichikawa, H. Curcumin: The Indian solid gold. *Adv. Exp. Med. Biol.* **2007**, *595*, 1–75. [PubMed]
13. Strimpakos, A.S.; Sharma, R.A. Curcumin: Preventive and therapeutic properties in laboratory studies and clinical trials. *Antioxid. Redox Signal.* **2008**, *10*, 511–545. [CrossRef] [PubMed]

14. Kanai, M. Therapeutic applications of curcumin for patients with pancreatic cancer. *World J. Gastroenterol.* **2014**, *20*, 9384–9391. [PubMed]

15. Pattanayak, R.; Basak, P.; Sen, S.; Bhattacharyya, M. Interaction of kras g-quadruplex with natural polyphenols: A spectroscopic analysis with molecular modeling. *Int. J. Biol. Macromol.* **2016**, *89*, 228–237. [CrossRef] [PubMed]

16. Perrone, D.; Ardito, F.; Giannatempo, G.; Dioguardi, M.; Troiano, G.; Lo Russo, L.; A, D.E.L.; Laino, L.; Lo Muzio, L. Biological and therapeutic activities, and anticancer properties of curcumin. *Exp. Ther. Med.* **2015**, *10*, 1615–1623. [CrossRef] [PubMed]

17. Li, L.; Aggarwal, B.B.; Shishodia, S.; Abbruzzese, J.; Kurzrock, R. Nuclear factor-kappaB and ikappaB kinase are constitutively active in human pancreatic cells, and their down-regulation by curcumin (diferuloylmethane) is associated with the suppression of proliferation and the induction of apoptosis. *Cancer* **2004**, *101*, 2351–2362. [CrossRef] [PubMed]

18. Bimonte, S.; Barbieri, A.; Palma, G.; Luciano, A.; Rea, D.; Arra, C. Curcumin inhibits tumor growth and angiogenesis in an orthotopic mouse model of human pancreatic cancer. *Biomed. Res. Int.* **2013**, *2013*, 810423. [CrossRef] [PubMed]

19. Bimonte, S.; Barbieri, A.; Palma, G.; Rea, D.; Luciano, A.; D'Aiuto, M.; Arra, C.; Izzo, F. Dissecting the role of curcumin in tumour growth and angiogenesis in mouse model of human breast cancer. *Biomed. Res. Int.* **2015**, *2015*, 878134. [CrossRef] [PubMed]

20. Notarbartolo, M.; Poma, P.; Perri, D.; Dusonchet, L.; Cervello, M.; D'Alessandro, N. Antitumor effects of curcumin, alone or in combination with cisplatin or doxorubicin, on human hepatic cancer cells. Analysis of their possible relationship to changes in Nf-kappaB activation levels and in iap gene expression. *Cancer Lett.* **2005**, *224*, 53–65. [CrossRef] [PubMed]

21. Tomita, M.; Kawakami, H.; Uchihara, J.N.; Okudaira, T.; Masuda, M.; Takasu, N.; Matsuda, T.; Ohta, T.; Tanaka, Y.; Ohshiro, K.; et al. Curcumin (diferuloylmethane) inhibits constitutive active Nf-kappaB, leading to suppression of cell growth of human t-cell leukemia virus type I-infected T-cell lines and primary adult T-cell leukemia cells. *Int. J. Cancer* **2006**, *118*, 765–772. [CrossRef] [PubMed]

22. Wang, Z.; Zhang, Y.; Banerjee, S.; Li, Y.; Sarkar, F.H. Notch-1 down-regulation by curcumin is associated with the inhibition of cell growth and the induction of apoptosis in pancreatic cancer cells. *Cancer* **2006**, *106*, 2503–2513. [CrossRef] [PubMed]

23. Everett, P.C.; Meyers, J.A.; Makkinje, A.; Rabbi, M.; Lerner, A. Preclinical assessment of curcumin as a potential therapy for b-cll. *Am. J. Hematol.* **2007**, *82*, 23–30. [CrossRef] [PubMed]

24. Li, M.; Zhang, Z.; Hill, D.L.; Wang, H.; Zhang, R. Curcumin, a dietary component, has anticancer, chemosensitization, and radiosensitization effects by down-regulating the MDM2 oncogene through the PI3K/mTOR/ETS2 pathway. *Cancer Res.* **2007**, *67*, 1988–1996. [CrossRef] [PubMed]

25. Lin, Y.G.; Kunnumakkara, A.B.; Nair, A.; Merritt, W.M.; Han, L.Y.; Armaiz-Pena, G.N.; Kamat, A.A.; Spannuth, W.A.; Gershenson, D.M.; Lutgendorf, S.K.; et al. Curcumin inhibits tumor growth and angiogenesis in ovarian carcinoma by targeting the nuclear factor-kappaB pathway. *Clin. Cancer Res.* **2007**, *13*, 3423–3430. [CrossRef] [PubMed]

26. Bachmeier, B.E.; Mohrenz, I.V.; Mirisola, V.; Schleicher, E.; Romeo, F.; Hohneke, C.; Jochum, M.; Nerlich, A.G.; Pfeffer, U. Curcumin downregulates the inflammatory cytokines CXCL1 and -2 in breast cancer cells via NfkappaB. *Carcinogenesis* **2008**, *29*, 779–789. [CrossRef] [PubMed]

27. Kunnumakkara, A.B.; Diagaradjane, P.; Guha, S.; Deorukhkar, A.; Shentu, S.; Aggarwal, B.B.; Krishnan, S. Curcumin sensitizes human colorectal cancer xenografts in nude mice to gamma-radiation by targeting nuclear factor-kappaB-regulated gene products. *Clin. Cancer Res.* **2008**, *14*, 2128–2136. [CrossRef] [PubMed]

28. Milacic, V.; Banerjee, S.; Landis-Piwowar, K.R.; Sarkar, F.H.; Majumdar, A.P.; Dou, Q.P. Curcumin inhibits the proteasome activity in human colon cancer cells in vitro and in vivo. *Cancer Res.* **2008**, *68*, 7283–7292. [CrossRef] [PubMed]

29. Sahu, R.P.; Batra, S.; Srivastava, S.K. Activation of ATM/Chk1 by curcumin causes cell cycle arrest and apoptosis in human pancreatic cancer cells. *Br. J. Cancer* **2009**, *100*, 1425–1433. [CrossRef] [PubMed]

30. Glienke, W.; Maute, L.; Wicht, J.; Bergmann, L. Curcumin inhibits constitutive STAT3 phosphorylation in human pancreatic cancer cell lines and downregulation of survivin/BIRC5 gene expression. *Cancer Investig.* **2010**, *28*, 166–171. [CrossRef] [PubMed]

31. Ali, S.; Ahmad, A.; Banerjee, S.; Padhye, S.; Dominiak, K.; Schaffert, J.M.; Wang, Z.; Philip, P.A.; Sarkar, F.H. Gemcitabine sensitivity can be induced in pancreatic cancer cells through modulation of mir-200 and mir-21 expression by curcumin or its analogue CDF. *Cancer Res.* **2010**, *70*, 3606–3617. [CrossRef] [PubMed]

32. Yang, C.L.; Liu, Y.Y.; Ma, Y.G.; Xue, Y.X.; Liu, D.G.; Ren, Y.; Liu, X.B.; Li, Y.; Li, Z. Curcumin blocks small cell lung cancer cells migration, invasion, angiogenesis, cell cycle and neoplasia through janus kinase-STAT3 signalling pathway. *PLoS ONE* **2012**, *7*, e37960. [CrossRef] [PubMed]

33. Yu, L.L.; Wu, J.G.; Dai, N.; Yu, H.G.; Si, J.M. Curcumin reverses chemoresistance of human gastric cancer cells by downregulating the Nf-kappaB transcription factor. *Oncol. Rep.* **2011**, *26*, 1197–1203. [PubMed]

34. Basha, R.; Connelly, S.F.; Sankpal, U.T.; Nagaraju, G.P.; Patel, H.; Vishwanatha, J.K.; Shelake, S.; Tabor-Simecka, L.; Shoji, M.; Simecka, J.W.; et al. Small molecule tolfenamic acid and dietary spice curcumin treatment enhances antiproliferative effect in pancreatic cancer cells via suppressing sp1, disrupting Nf-κB translocation to nucleus and cell cycle phase distribution. *J. Nutr. Biochem.* **2016**, *31*, 77–87. [CrossRef] [PubMed]

35. Cao, L.; Xiao, X.; Lei, J.; Duan, W.; Ma, Q.; Li, W. Curcumin inhibits hypoxia-induced epithelialmesenchymal transition in pancreatic cancer cells via suppression of the hedgehog signaling pathway. *Oncol. Rep.* **2016**, *35*, 3728–3734. [PubMed]

36. Parsons, H.A.; Baracos, V.E.; Hong, D.S.; Abbruzzese, J.; Bruera, E.; Kurzrock, R. The effects of curcumin (diferuloylmethane) on body composition of patients with advanced pancreatic cancer. *Oncotarget* **2016**. [CrossRef] [PubMed]

37. Sahebkar, A. Curcumin: A natural multitarget treatment for pancreatic cancer. *Integr. Cancer Ther.* **2016**. [CrossRef] [PubMed]

38. Yarla, N.S.; Bishayee, A.; Sethi, G.; Reddanna, P.; Kalle, A.M.; Dhananjaya, B.L.; Dowluru, K.S.; Chintala, R.; Duddukuri, G.R. Targeting arachidonic acid pathway by natural products for cancer prevention and therapy. *Semin. Cancer Biol.* **2016**. in press. [CrossRef] [PubMed]

39. Luthra, P.M.; Lal, N. Prospective of curcumin, a pleiotropic signalling molecule from curcuma longa in the treatment of glioblastoma. *Eur. J. Med. Chem.* **2016**, *109*, 23–35. [CrossRef] [PubMed]

40. Tsai, C.F.; Hsieh, T.H.; Lee, J.N.; Hsu, C.Y.; Wang, Y.C.; Kuo, K.K.; Wu, H.L.; Chiu, C.C.; Tsai, E.M.; Kuo, P.L. Curcumin suppresses phthalate-induced metastasis and the proportion of cancer stem cell (CSC)-like cells via the inhibition of AhR/ERK/SK1 signaling in hepatocellular carcinoma. *J. Agric. Food Chem.* **2015**, *63*, 10388–10398. [CrossRef] [PubMed]

41. Hu, B.; Sun, D.; Sun, C.; Sun, Y.F.; Sun, H.X.; Zhu, Q.F.; Yang, X.R.; Gao, Y.B.; Tang, W.G.; Fan, J.; et al. A polymeric nanoparticle formulation of curcumin in combination with sorafenib synergistically inhibits tumor growth and metastasis in an orthotopic model of human hepatocellular carcinoma. *Biochem. Biophys. Res. Commun.* **2015**, *468*, 525–532. [CrossRef] [PubMed]

42. Diaz Osterman, C.J.; Gonda, A.; Stiff, T.; Sigaran, U.; Valenzuela, M.M.; Ferguson Bennit, H.R.; Moyron, R.B.; Khan, S.; Wall, N.R. Curcumin induces pancreatic adenocarcinoma cell death via reduction of the inhibitors of apoptosis. *Pancreas* **2016**, *45*, 101–109. [CrossRef] [PubMed]

43. Zhao, Z.; Li, C.; Xi, H.; Gao, Y.; Xu, D. Curcumin induces apoptosis in pancreatic cancer cells through the induction of forkhead box o1 and inhibition of the PI3K/Akt pathway. *Mol. Med. Rep.* **2015**, *12*, 5415–5422. [PubMed]

44. Azimi, H.; Khakshur, A.A.; Abdollahi, M.; Rahimi, R. Potential new pharmacological agents derived from medicinal plants for the treatment of pancreatic cancer. *Pancreas* **2015**, *44*, 11–15. [CrossRef] [PubMed]

45. Sinha, D.; Biswas, J.; Sung, B.; Aggarwal, B.B.; Bishayee, A. Chemopreventive and chemotherapeutic potential of curcumin in breast cancer. *Curr. Drug Targets* **2012**, *13*, 1799–1819. [CrossRef] [PubMed]

46. Lao, C.D.; Ruffin, M.T.; Normolle, D.; Heath, D.D.; Murray, S.I.; Bailey, J.M.; Boggs, M.E.; Crowell, J.; Rock, C.L.; Brenner, D.E. Dose escalation of a curcuminoid formulation. *BMC Complement. Altern. Med.* **2006**, *6*. [CrossRef] [PubMed]

47. Vareed, S.K.; Kakarala, M.; Ruffin, M.T.; Crowell, J.A.; Normolle, D.P.; Djuric, Z.; Brenner, D.E. Pharmacokinetics of curcumin conjugate metabolites in healthy human subjects. *Cancer Epidemiol. Biomark. Prev.* **2008**, *17*, 1411–1417. [CrossRef] [PubMed]

48. Cheng, A.L.; Hsu, C.H.; Lin, J.K.; Hsu, M.M.; Ho, Y.F.; Shen, T.S.; Ko, J.Y.; Lin, J.T.; Lin, B.R.; Ming-Shiang, W.; et al. Phase I clinical trial of curcumin, a chemopreventive agent, in patients with high-risk or pre-malignant lesions. *Anticancer Res.* **2001**, *21*, 2895–2900. [PubMed]

49. Li, L.; Braiteh, F.S.; Kurzrock, R. Liposome-encapsulated curcumin: In vitro and in vivo effects on proliferation, apoptosis, signaling, and angiogenesis. *Cancer* **2005**, *104*, 1322–1331. [CrossRef] [PubMed]

50. Bisht, S.; Feldmann, G.; Soni, S.; Ravi, R.; Karikar, C.; Maitra, A.; Maitra, A. Polymeric nanoparticle-encapsulated curcumin ("nanocurcumin"): A novel strategy for human cancer therapy. *J. Nanobiotechnol.* **2007**, *5*. [CrossRef] [PubMed]

51. Antony, B.; Merina, B.; Iyer, V.S.; Judy, N.; Lennertz, K.; Joyal, S. A pilot cross-over study to evaluate human oral bioavailability of BCM-95CG (biocurcumax), a novel bioenhanced preparation of curcumin. *Indian J. Pharm. Sci.* **2008**, *70*, 445–449. [CrossRef] [PubMed]

52. Shaikh, J.; Ankola, D.D.; Beniwal, V.; Singh, D.; Kumar, M.N. Nanoparticle encapsulation improves oral bioavailability of curcumin by at least 9-fold when compared to curcumin administered with piperine as absorption enhancer. *Eur. J. Pharm. Sci.* **2009**, *37*, 223–230. [CrossRef] [PubMed]

53. Anand, P.; Nair, H.B.; Sung, B.; Kunnumakkara, A.B.; Yadav, V.R.; Tekmal, R.R.; Aggarwal, B.B. Design of curcumin-loaded plga nanoparticles formulation with enhanced cellular uptake, and increased bioactivity in vitro and superior bioavailability in vivo. *Biochem. Pharmacol.* **2010**, *79*, 330–338. [CrossRef] [PubMed]

54. Sasaki, H.; Sunagawa, Y.; Takahashi, K.; Imaizumi, A.; Fukuda, H.; Hashimoto, T.; Wada, H.; Katanasaka, Y.; Kakeya, H.; Fujita, M.; et al. Innovative preparation of curcumin for improved oral bioavailability. *Biol. Pharm. Bull.* **2011**, *34*, 660–665. [CrossRef] [PubMed]

55. Kanai, M.; Imaizumi, A.; Otsuka, Y.; Sasaki, H.; Hashiguchi, M.; Tsujiko, K.; Matsumoto, S.; Ishiguro, H.; Chiba, T. Dose-escalation and pharmacokinetic study of nanoparticle curcumin, a potential anticancer agent with improved bioavailability, in healthy human volunteers. *Cancer Chemother. Pharmacol.* **2012**, *69*, 65–70. [CrossRef] [PubMed]

56. Kesharwani, P.; Banerjee, S.; Padhye, S.; Sarkar, F.H.; Iyer, A.K. Parenterally administrable nano-micelles of 3,4-difluorobenzylidene curcumin for treating pancreatic cancer. *Colloids Surf. B Biointerfaces* **2015**, *132*, 138–145. [CrossRef] [PubMed]

57. Margulis, K.; Srinivasan, S.; Ware, M.J.; Summers, H.D.; Godin, B.; Magdassi, S. Active curcumin nanoparticles formed from a volatile microemulsion template. *J. Mater. Chem. B Mater. Biol. Med.* **2014**, *2*, 3745–3752. [CrossRef] [PubMed]

58. Howells, L.M.; Sale, S.; Sriramareddy, S.N.; Irving, G.R.; Jones, D.J.; Ottley, C.J.; Pearson, D.G.; Mann, C.D.; Manson, M.M.; Berry, D.P.; et al. Curcumin ameliorates oxaliplatin-induced chemoresistance in HCT116 colorectal cancer cells in vitro and in vivo. *Int. J. Cancer* **2011**, *129*, 476–486. [CrossRef] [PubMed]

59. Jutooru, I.; Chadalapaka, G.; Lei, P.; Safe, S. Inhibition of NfkappaB and pancreatic cancer cell and tumor growth by curcumin is dependent on specificity protein down-regulation. *J. Biol. Chem.* **2010**, *285*, 25332–25344. [CrossRef] [PubMed]

60. Youns, M.; Fathy, G.M. Upregulation of extrinsic apoptotic pathway in curcumin-mediated antiproliferative effect on human pancreatic carcinogenesis. *J. Cell. Biochem.* **2013**, *114*, 2654–2665. [CrossRef] [PubMed]

61. Li, Y.; Revalde, J.L.; Reid, G.; Paxton, J.W. Modulatory effects of curcumin on multi-drug resistance-associated protein 5 in pancreatic cancer cells. *Cancer Chemother. Pharmacol.* **2011**, *68*, 603–610. [CrossRef] [PubMed]

62. Ning, X.; Du, Y.; Ben, Q.; Huang, L.; He, X.; Gong, Y.; Gao, J.; Wu, H.; Man, X.; Jin, J.; et al. Bulk pancreatic cancer cells can convert into cancer stem cells(CSCs) in vitro and 2 compounds can target these CSCs. *Cell Cycle* **2016**, *15*, 403–412. [CrossRef] [PubMed]

63. Kesharwani, P.; Xie, L.; Banerjee, S.; Mao, G.; Padhye, S.; Sarkar, F.H.; Iyer, A.K. Hyaluronic acid-conjugated polyamidoamine dendrimers for targeted delivery of 3,4-difluorobenzylidene curcumin to cd44 overexpressing pancreatic cancer cells. *Colloids Surf. B Biointerfaces* **2015**, *136*, 413–423. [CrossRef] [PubMed]

64. Osterman, C.J.; Lynch, J.C.; Leaf, P.; Gonda, A.; Ferguson Bennit, H.R.; Griffiths, D.; Wall, N.R. Curcumin modulates pancreatic adenocarcinoma cell-derived exosomal function. *PLoS ONE* **2015**, *10*, e0132845. [CrossRef] [PubMed]

65. Gundewar, C.; Ansari, D.; Tang, L.; Wang, Y.; Liang, G.; Rosendahl, A.H.; Saleem, M.A.; Andersson, R. Antiproliferative effects of curcumin analog l49H37 in pancreatic stellate cells: A comparative study. *Ann. Gastroenterol.* **2015**, *28*, 391–398. [PubMed]

66. Fiala, M. Curcumin and omega-3 fatty acids enhance nk cell-induced apoptosis of pancreatic cancer cells but curcumin inhibits interferon-gamma production: Benefits of omega-3 with curcumin against cancer. *Molecules* **2015**, *20*, 3020–3026. [CrossRef] [PubMed]

67.  Ma, J.; Fang, B.; Zeng, F.; Pang, H.; Zhang, J.; Shi, Y.; Wu, X.; Cheng, L.; Ma, C.; Xia, J.; et al. Curcumin inhibits cell growth and invasion through up-regulation of mir-7 in pancreatic cancer cells. *Toxicol. Lett.* **2014**, *231*, 82–91. [CrossRef] [PubMed]

68.  Duarte, V.M.; Han, E.; Veena, M.S.; Salvado, A.; Suh, J.D.; Liang, L.J.; Faull, K.F.; Srivatsan, E.S.; Wang, M.B. Curcumin enhances the effect of cisplatin in suppression of head and neck squamous cell carcinoma via inhibition of ikkbeta protein of the NfkappaB pathway. *Mol. Cancer Ther.* **2010**, *9*, 2665–2675. [CrossRef] [PubMed]

69.  Sarkar, S.; Dubaybo, H.; Ali, S.; Goncalves, P.; Kollepara, S.L.; Sethi, S.; Philip, P.A.; Li, Y. Down-regulation of mir-221 inhibits proliferation of pancreatic cancer cells through up-regulation of pten, p27(kip1), p57(kip2), and puma. *Am. J. Cancer Res.* **2013**, *3*, 465–477. [PubMed]

70.  Sun, X.D.; Liu, X.E.; Huang, D.S. Curcumin reverses the epithelial-mesenchymal transition of pancreatic cancer cells by inhibiting the hedgehog signaling pathway. *Oncol. Rep.* **2013**, *29*, 2401–2407. [PubMed]

71.  Kunnumakkara, A.B.; Guha, S.; Krishnan, S.; Diagaradjane, P.; Gelovani, J.; Aggarwal, B.B. Curcumin potentiates antitumor activity of gemcitabine in an orthotopic model of pancreatic cancer through suppression of proliferation, angiogenesis, and inhibition of nuclear factor-kappaB-regulated gene products. *Cancer Res.* **2007**, *67*, 3853–3861. [CrossRef] [PubMed]

72.  Parasramka, M.A.; Gupta, S.V. Synergistic effect of garcinol and curcumin on antiproliferative and apoptotic activity in pancreatic cancer cells. *J. Oncol.* **2012**, *2012*, 709739. [CrossRef] [PubMed]

73.  Lin, L.; Hutzen, B.; Zuo, M.; Ball, S.; Deangelis, S.; Foust, E.; Pandit, B.; Ihnat, M.A.; Shenoy, S.S.; Kulp, S.; et al. Novel STAT3 phosphorylation inhibitors exhibit potent growth-suppressive activity in pancreatic and breast cancer cells. *Cancer Res.* **2010**, *70*, 2445–2454. [CrossRef] [PubMed]

74.  Bao, B.; Ali, S.; Banerjee, S.; Wang, Z.; Logna, F.; Azmi, A.S.; Kong, D.; Ahmad, A.; Li, Y.; Padhye, S.; et al. Curcumin analogue CDF inhibits pancreatic tumor growth by switching on suppressor micrornas and attenuating EZH2 expression. *Cancer Res.* **2012**, *72*, 335–345. [CrossRef] [PubMed]

75.  Sureban, S.M.; Qu, D.; Houchen, C.W. Regulation of mirnas by agents targeting the tumor stem cell markers DCLK1, MSI1, LGR5, and BMI1. *Curr. Pharmacol. Rep.* **2015**, *1*, 217–222. [CrossRef] [PubMed]

76.  Bao, B.; Ali, S.; Kong, D.; Sarkar, S.H.; Wang, Z.; Banerjee, S.; Aboukameel, A.; Padhye, S.; Philip, P.A.; Sarkar, F.H. Anti-tumor activity of a novel compound-cdf is mediated by regulating mir-21, mir-200, and pten in pancreatic cancer. *PLoS ONE* **2011**, *6*, e17850. [CrossRef] [PubMed]

77.  Sun, M.; Estrov, Z.; Ji, Y.; Coombes, K.R.; Harris, D.H.; Kurzrock, R. Curcumin (diferuloylmethane) alters the expression profiles of micrornas in human pancreatic cancer cells. *Mol. Cancer Ther.* **2008**, *7*, 464–473. [CrossRef] [PubMed]

78.  Grandhi, B.K.; Thakkar, A.; Wang, J.; Prabhu, S. A novel combinatorial nanotechnology-based oral chemopreventive regimen demonstrates significant suppression of pancreatic cancer neoplastic lesions. *Cancer Prev. Res.* **2013**, *6*, 1015–1025. [CrossRef] [PubMed]

79.  Bisht, S.; Mizuma, M.; Feldmann, G.; Ottenhof, N.A.; Hong, S.M.; Pramanik, D.; Chenna, V.; Karikari, C.; Sharma, R.; Goggins, M.G.; et al. Systemic administration of polymeric nanoparticle-encapsulated curcumin (nanocurc) blocks tumor growth and metastases in preclinical models of pancreatic cancer. *Mol. Cancer Ther.* **2010**, *9*, 2255–2264. [CrossRef] [PubMed]

80.  Padhye, S.; Banerjee, S.; Chavan, D.; Pandye, S.; Swamy, K.V.; Ali, S.; Li, J.; Dou, Q.P.; Sarkar, F.H. Fluorocurcumins as cyclooxygenase-2 inhibitor: Molecular docking, pharmacokinetics and tissue distribution in mice. *Pharm. Res.* **2009**, *26*, 2438–2445. [CrossRef] [PubMed]

81.  Kesharwani, P.; Banerjee, S.; Padhye, S.; Sarkar, F.H.; Iyer, A.K. Hyaluronic acid engineered nanomicelles loaded with 3,4-difluorobenzylidene curcumin for targeted killing of CD44+ stem-like pancreatic cancer cells. *Biomacromolecules* **2015**, *16*, 3042–3053. [CrossRef] [PubMed]

82.  Halder, R.C.; Almasi, A.; Sagong, B.; Leung, J.; Jewett, A.; Fiala, M. Curcuminoids and omega-3 fatty acids with anti-oxidants potentiate cytotoxicity of natural killer cells against pancreatic ductal adenocarcinoma cells and inhibit interferon gamma production. *Front. Physiol.* **2015**, *6*, 129. [CrossRef] [PubMed]

83.  Nagaraju, G.P.; Zhu, S.; Ko, J.E.; Ashritha, N.; Kandimalla, R.; Snyder, J.P.; Shoji, M.; El-Rayes, B.F. Antiangiogenic effects of a novel synthetic curcumin analogue in pancreatic cancer. *Cancer Lett.* **2015**, *357*, 557–565. [CrossRef] [PubMed]

84. Ali, S.; Ahmad, A.; Aboukameel, A.; Ahmed, A.; Bao, B.; Banerjee, S.; Philip, P.A.; Sarkar, F.H. Deregulation of mir-146a expression in a mouse model of pancreatic cancer affecting egfr signaling. *Cancer Lett.* **2014**, *351*, 134–142. [CrossRef] [PubMed]

85. Ranjan, A.P.; Mukerjee, A.; Helson, L.; Gupta, R.; Vishwanatha, J.K. Efficacy of liposomal curcumin in a human pancreatic tumor xenograft model: Inhibition of tumor growth and angiogenesis. *Anticancer Res.* **2013**, *33*, 3603–3609. [PubMed]

86. Nagaraju, G.P.; Zhu, S.; Wen, J.; Farris, A.B.; Adsay, V.N.; Diaz, R.; Snyder, J.P.; Mamoru, S.; El-Rayes, B.F. Novel synthetic curcumin analogues EF31 and UBS109 are potent DNA hypomethylating agents in pancreatic cancer. *Cancer Lett.* **2013**, *341*, 195–203. [CrossRef] [PubMed]

87. Yallapu, M.M.; Ebeling, M.C.; Khan, S.; Sundram, V.; Chauhan, N.; Gupta, B.K.; Puumala, S.E.; Jaggi, M.; Chauhan, S.C. Novel curcumin-loaded magnetic nanoparticles for pancreatic cancer treatment. *Mol. Cancer Ther.* **2013**, *12*, 1471–1480. [CrossRef] [PubMed]

88. Mach, C.M.; Mathew, L.; Mosley, S.A.; Kurzrock, R.; Smith, J.A. Determination of minimum effective dose and optimal dosing schedule for liposomal curcumin in a xenograft human pancreatic cancer model. *Anticancer Res.* **2009**, *29*, 1895–1899. [PubMed]

89. Sharma, R.A.; Euden, S.A.; Platton, S.L.; Cooke, D.N.; Shafayat, A.; Hewitt, H.R.; Marczylo, T.H.; Morgan, B.; Hemingway, D.; Plummer, S.M.; et al. Phase i clinical trial of oral curcumin: Biomarkers of systemic activity and compliance. *Clin. Cancer Res.* **2004**, *10*, 6847–6854. [CrossRef] [PubMed]

90. Garcea, G.; Berry, D.P.; Jones, D.J.; Singh, R.; Dennison, A.R.; Farmer, P.B.; Sharma, R.A.; Steward, W.P.; Gescher, A.J. Consumption of the putative chemopreventive agent curcumin by cancer patients: Assessment of curcumin levels in the colorectum and their pharmacodynamic consequences. *Cancer Epidemiol. Biomark. Prev.* **2005**, *14*, 120–125.

91. Dhillon, N.; Aggarwal, B.B.; Newman, R.A.; Wolff, R.A.; Kunnumakkara, A.B.; Abbruzzese, J.L.; Ng, C.S.; Badmaev, V.; Kurzrock, R. Phase II trial of curcumin in patients with advanced pancreatic cancer. *Clin. Cancer Res.* **2008**, *14*, 4491–4499. [CrossRef] [PubMed]

92. Kanai, M.; Yoshimura, K.; Asada, M.; Imaizumi, A.; Suzuki, C.; Matsumoto, S.; Nishimura, T.; Mori, Y.; Masui, T.; Kawaguchi, Y.; et al. A phase I/II study of gemcitabine-based chemotherapy plus curcumin for patients with gemcitabine-resistant pancreatic cancer. *Cancer Chemother. Pharmacol.* **2011**, *68*, 157–164. [CrossRef] [PubMed]

93. Epelbaum, R.; Schaffer, M.; Vizel, B.; Badmaev, V.; Bar-Sela, G. Curcumin and gemcitabine in patients with advanced pancreatic cancer. *Nutr. Cancer* **2010**, *62*, 1137–1141. [CrossRef] [PubMed]

94. Kanai, M.; Otsuka, Y.; Otsuka, K.; Sato, M.; Nishimura, T.; Mori, Y.; Kawaguchi, M.; Hatano, E.; Kodama, Y.; Matsumoto, S.; et al. A phase I study investigating the safety and pharmacokinetics of highly bioavailable curcumin (theracurmin) in cancer patients. *Cancer Chemother. Pharmacol.* **2013**, *71*, 1521–1530. [CrossRef] [PubMed]

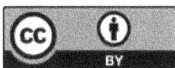

*nutrients*

MDPI

*Review*

# Mangiferin and Cancer: Mechanisms of Action

**Fuchsia Gold-Smith [1], Alyssa Fernandez [2] and Karen Bishop [1,\*]**

[1]  Auckland Cancer Society Research Center, Faculty of Medical and Health Sciences, University of Auckland, Private Bag 92019, Auckland 1142, New Zealand; fgol315@aucklanduni.ac.nz
[2]  Faculty of Medical and Health Sciences, University of Auckland, Private Bag 92019, Auckland 1142, New Zealand; afer098@aucklanduni.ac.nz
\*  Correspondence: k.bishop@auckland.ac.nz; Tel.: +64-9-923-4471

Received: 20 April 2016; Accepted: 22 June 2016; Published: 28 June 2016

**Abstract:** Mangiferin, a bioactive compound derived primarily from Anacardiaceae and Gentianaceae families and found in mangoes and honeybush tea, has been extensively studied for its therapeutic properties. Mangiferin has shown promising chemotherapeutic and chemopreventative potential. This review focuses on the effect of mangiferin on: (1) inflammation, with respect to NFκB, PPARγ and the immune system; (2) cell cycle, the MAPK pathway G$_2$/M checkpoint; (3) proliferation and metastasis, and implications on β-catenin, MMPs, EMT, angiogenesis and tumour volume; (4) apoptosis, with a focus on Bax/Bcl ratios, intrinsic/extrinsic apoptotic pathways and telomerase activity; (5) oxidative stress, through Nrf2/ARE signalling, ROS elimination and catalase activity; and (6) efficacy of chemotherapeutic agents, such as oxaliplatin, etoposide and doxorubicin. In addition, the need to enhance the bioavailability and delivery of mangiferin are briefly addressed, as well as the potential for toxicity.

**Keywords:** mangiferin; cancer; inflammation; NFκB; oxidative stress; cell cycle; combination therapy; nutraceuticals; bioavailability; hallmarks of cancer

---

## 1. Introduction

Cancer has been identified as the leading cause of non-communicable disease mortality globally [1], and is responsible for significant morbidity and costs to healthcare systems. Cancer incidence and mortality has been increasing at a greater rate than population growth alone could account for. The International Agency for Research on Cancer (IARC) reported 14.1 million cases and over 8.2 million mortalities due to cancer in 2012 compared to 10 million cases and six million mortalities in 2000 [2] in a baseline population of 7.1 billion and 6.1 billion, respectively [3]. Much of this increase is due to rising cancer burden in less developed countries (LDCs), with 57% of new cases, and 65% of cancer related deaths occurring in LDCs [2]. When standardized by age, the total number of cases per 100,000 population is greater in more developed countries (MDCs) than LDCs (overall age standardized rate: 268 and 148 respectively) [4]. One exception to this pattern is infection-attributable cancers, which are responsible for 26% of the cancer burden in LDCs but only 8% in MDCs [5].

Cancer is less likely to be identified early or treated successfully in LDCs due to reduced access to screening tools and chemotherapeutic drugs. Previously, cancer has been regarded as a MDC disease. However, through the adoption of a more Westernised lifestyle, cancer incidence has been steadily increasing in LDCs. From the data published by Parkin et al., it can be seen that 40%–45% of cancers can be attributable to lifestyle factors such as diet, smoking status, alcohol consumption and lack of physical activity [6]. Some compounds naturally present in the diet, such as mangiferin in mangoes and honeybush tea, are thought to modulate risk of cancer and retard cancer progression.

Mangiferin (1,3,6,7-tetrahydroxyxanthone-C2-β-D glucoside) [7–11] is a polyphenol [8,11–15] found in many plant species, in particular, those from the Anacardiaceae [7,9,16–20] and Gentianaceae families [7,9,13,17,18,20]. For an extensive breakdown of plant sources of mangiferin and mangiferin content, see Matkowski et al. [21].

Mangiferin is not only present in everyday foods, but utilised in a number of natural medicines. In traditional medicine, different cultures have cultivated and processed mangiferin rich plants for the treatment of a range of illnesses including cardiovascular disease, diabetes, infection and cancer [22–24]. In India, Ayurvedic practitioners [22] have used *Salicia chinesis* (saptarangi) [21,25,26] and *Mangifera indica* (mango), which are two species that contain high levels of mangiferin. *Salicia chinesis* has been used for its hypo-lipidaemic, anti-diabetic, hepatoprotective and antioxidant properties. *Salicia chinesis* has now been over-exploited and research is being conducted into how this plant may be grown in a more sustainable way to meet demands [27]. *Mangifera indica* is used not only in Ayurvedic medicine but also used in Cuba [23], China [21,24] and throughout East Asia [21] for its anti-inflammatory, anti-viral, anti-diabetic and anti-cancer properties. *Mangifera indica*, a member of the Gentianaceae family, contains mangiferin [10,20,21,28–30] in its bark (18.33 g/kg dry weight [31]), leaves [15] (old leaves 36.9 g/kg and young leaves 58.12 g/kg dry weight [31]) and root along with the seed, pulp (0 to 2.65 mg/kg dry weight, depending on the variety [32]) and skin of the fruit [7,8,12,20,33–35] (4.94 g/kg dry weight [31]). However, the concentration of mangiferin in the pulp is unlikely to be sufficient to provide significant health benefits, and can vary greatly depending on variety and the maturity of the fruit [32]. Although somewhat lower than levels found in bark and leaves, the mangiferin in the skin [36] and seed/kernel [31], which are usually considered waste products, may provide a promising sustainable option for mangiferin extraction. To date, these mango by-products have been used to enhance the nutritional density of pasta, biscuits, muffins and pancakes [37–40]. Although the phenolic content of these food items increased 2.8–3.9 fold [37,39], the mangiferin content was not reported. However, in the results detailed in the sections hereafter, the concentrations used or administered varied from 12.5 to 100 µg/mL in in vitro studies [12] and approximately 100 mg/kg body weight in in vivo studies [7]. Clearly, the consumption of such quantities is not achievable by consuming fresh mango pulp, but maybe achievable by adding a leaf, bark, and/or seed extract as a supplement to food, or consuming as a liquid (if palatable).

In Cuba, aqueous extracts of *Mangifera indica* bark have become popular [7,12,41,42] for treatment of not only cancer but gastric and dermatological disorders, AIDS and asthma [43]. Stem bark extracts contain polyphenols, terpenoids, steroids, fatty acids and trace elements alongside mangiferin [21,23]. The natural medicine, Vimang® [7,12,42], produced from aqueous extracts of *Mangifera indica*, contains ~20% mangiferin [23] and is available in tablets, creams and syrups. Vimang® is registered as an "anti-inflammatory phytomedicine" by the Cuban Regulatory Health Authorities and is primarily used by those with multiple and different types of cancer. In China, mango leaves [21,24] and *Dobinea delavayi* (Baill.) leaves [44], which both contain mangiferin, are often used in traditional medicines. The greatest dietary source of mangiferin is Honeybush tea, popular in South Africa and obtained from *Cyclopia sp.* [21]. Honeybush tea leaves have been found to consist of up to 4% mangiferin by dry weight [21].

Research into mangiferin has resulted in the identification of a similar compound, namely mangiferin aglycone or norathyriol, which appears to have greater biological activity in some instances. The compound mangiferin aglycone can be artificially synthesized, bypassing any sustainability concerns surrounding mangiferin. The structure of mangiferin and mangiferin aglycone are shown in Figure 1. Mangiferin aglycone has shown greater biological activity in some targets than mangiferin, possibly due to greater water solubility [28], and the former appears to reduce UV-induced skin cancer [8]. Further studies are required to elucidate the degree of similarity in action of mangiferin and mangiferin aglycone.

A

Mangiferin

B

Mangiferin Aglycone

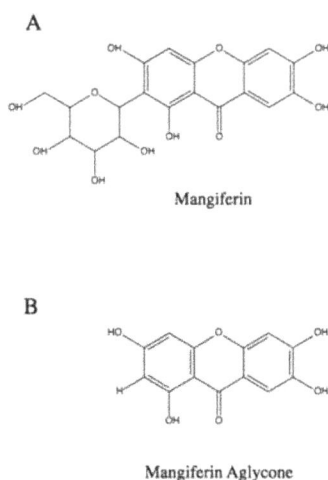

**Figure 1.** The molecular structure of: (**A**) mangiferin [45]; and (**B**) mangiferin aglycone [46].

Evidence suggests that mangiferin could prove to be a useful, inexpensive compound to not only maintain and improve health in the worried well, but also to significantly improve the outlook for those with certain cancers (e.g., breast cancer [41]) and reduce the likelihood of developing cancer. This is of particular relevance to LDCs, where the more expensive chemotherapeutic drugs may be inaccessible, while mangiferin containing plants are abundant. In MDCs, the potential enhanced synergistic effect seen with major chemotherapeutic drugs may allow for lower dosages of drugs, thus reducing toxicity and providing greater selective toxicity to malignant cells, reducing the extent of side effects [47]. However, it is acknowledged that the quantity of fruit required in order to achieve clinically relevant levels of mangiferin may be unreasonably high. For this reason substitution of flour and sugar with mango processing by product [37,39] may prove an additional and useful method of increasing mangiferin intake.

The anti-cancer properties of mangiferin have been extensively studied over the past few decades. This review article seeks to consolidate the most recent research on the anti-neoplastic properties of mangiferin, with a focus on molecular pathways and uses of mangiferin, in conjunction with known chemotherapeutic agents, to aid further research on this topic.

## 2. Molecular Mechanisms of the Anti-Cancer Action of Mangiferin

Mangiferin acts through a myriad of mechanisms to exert anti-inflammatory [11,14,20–24,28,29,42,48], immunomodulatory [8,9,14,19,20,23,24,28,29,49], cell cycle arrest, anti-proliferative, anti-apoptotic [48], anti-oxidative [8,11,14,15,19,20,22–24,28–30,36,42,48–51], anti-genotoxic [30] and anti-viral [11,15,20,48] effects which cumulatively result in anti-tumour activity [9,11,15,19–21,23,24,29,41,50]. Mangiferin has demonstrated broad-spectrum efficacy against an array of different cancers in in vitro and in vivo studies [8,11,12,14,21]. To date, evidence suggests that the side effects of mangiferin vary from mild to non-existent [52]; however, there may be some variation according to source of mangiferin.

### 2.1. Inflammation

The chronic activation of inflammatory processes is widely regarded as an enabling characteristic towards the acquisition of cancer [53]. Approximately 20% of cancers are attributable to chronic inflammation [54], which may be induced by bacterial or viral infections, autoimmune disease, or constant exposure to irritants. Chronic inflammation can drive tumour growth by providing a favourable environment, rich in inflammatory mediators, to enhance cell growth and survival [53,55].

In addition, inflammation involves the production of reactive oxygen species (ROS), which can cause DNA damage, enhancing carcinogenic capabilities [56]. Mangiferin is thought to dampen down the inflammatory response primarily by interference with Nuclear Factor κ-light-chain-enhancer of activated B cells (NFκB) [34].

By reducing inflammation, mangiferin not only provides unfavourable conditions for cancer, but can provide anti-diabetic effects [11,15,19,21,23,24,28,29,50] and reduce risk of cardiovascular disease. Mangiferin also reduces serum glucose levels and lipid levels [8,14,30], further decreasing development and severity of diabetes and cardiovascular disease. Thus, while many medications used to treat these widespread non-communicable diseases may create adverse conditions in the body that may lead to other diseases, mangiferin provides broad spectrum benefits across a range of diseases such as cancers, cardiovascular disease and diabetes [26,33,35,39].

### 2.1.1. Nuclear Factor κ-Light-Chain-Enhancer of Activated B Cells Activity

The transcription factor NFκB regulates many important processes in inflammation, including the expression of pro-inflammatory cytokines, migration molecules, growth factors and other genes involved in proliferation and survival [34]. NFκB is up-regulated during inflammation. Under inflammatory conditions, ligands bind and activate Toll-like receptors (TLRs) and Interleukin-1 Receptors (IL-1R), triggering the Myeloid Differentiation Primary Response Gene 88 (Myd88) to recruit Interleukin-1 Receptor Activated Kinase 1 (IRAK1) to this receptor-signalling complex for phosphorylation [57,58]. Association of IRAK1 with Myd88 allows phosphorylation by IRAK4 and subsequent autophosphorylation. In its phosphorylated form, IRAK1 interacts with Tumour necrosis factor Receptor-Associated Factor 6 (TRAF6) to form a complex, which signals sequentially through Transforming growth factor beta-activated kinase 1/Transforming growth factor beta-activated kinase 1-binding protein 1 and 2 (TAK1/TAB1/TAB2), NFκB Essential Modulator/Inhibitor of NFκB Kinase subunit-β/Inhibitor of NFκB Kinase subunit-α (NEMO/IKK-β/IKK-α) and Inhibitor of κB (IκB)/p50/p65 complexes to ultimately activate NFκB [57]. Recent findings suggest mangiferin inhibits NFκB activation at various steps in the pathway (Figure 2A,B) [11,47]. NFκB can be activated via the classical or alternative pathways. The classical pathway is regulated by the IκB kinase complex and p50, while the alternative pathway is regulated by IKKα and p52 [59].

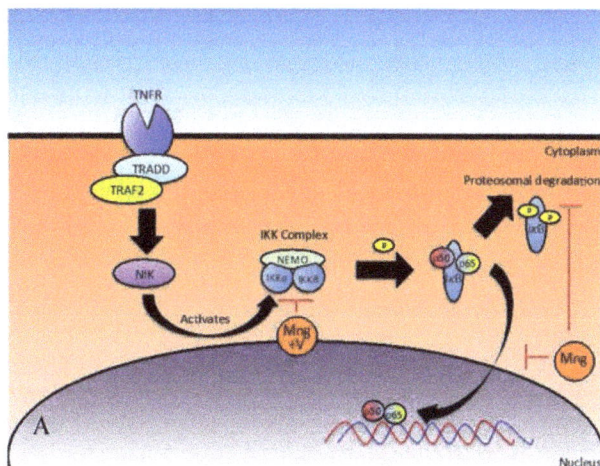

**Figure 2.** *Cont.*

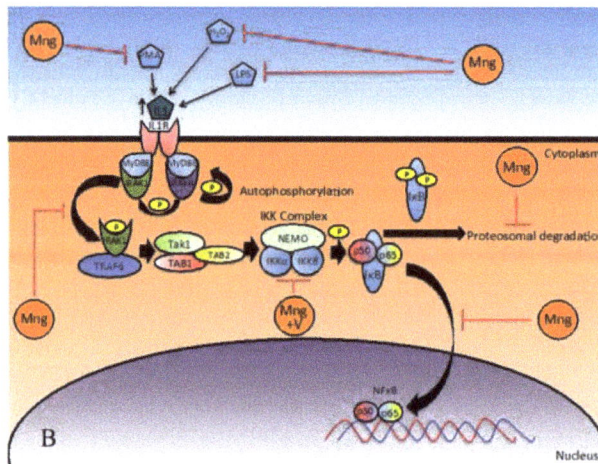

**Figure 2.** Inhibition of NFκB via the (**A**) classical and (**B**) alternative pathways by mangiferin and Vimang (adapted from [11,45,55]) (abbreviations: Mng, mangiferin; V, Vimang®).

Initial Stimulus for NFκB Activation

When studied, it was found that mangiferin blocks Tumour Necrosis Factor (TNF) [8], lipopolysaccharide (LPS), peptidoglycan (PDG) [60], phorbol-12-myristate-13-acetate (PMA) [11] or hydrogen peroxide ($H_2O_2$) mediated NFκB activation by inhibiting ROS production [61]. This effect has been demonstrated in U-937 (lymphoma), HeLa (cervical cancer), MCF-7 (breast cancer) and IRB3 AN27 (human foetal neuronal) cell lines [11]. Jeong et al. [60] demonstrated that the inhibitory effect of mangiferin on NFκB expression when induced by LPS and PDG in peritoneal macrophages was elicited in part by inhibition of IRAK1 phosphorylation and consequently activation. In parallel, mangiferin impedes NFκB activation via inflammatory genes [11,48]. Inhibition of IRAK1 by mangiferin may reduce development of resistance to chemotherapeutic drugs. In particular, triple negative breast cancers have been associated with overexpression of IRAK1, and it is reported that inhibition of IRAK1, through the p38-MCL1 pathway, may reverse paclitaxel resistance [62]. Mangiferin, as a component of combination therapy, will be addressed in Section 4.

Subsequent studies have implicated mangiferin in suppressing the TNF signal transduction pathway [11,48], where under normal conditions, canonic interactions of TNF Receptor (TNFR) with Tumour Necrosis Factor Receptor type-1-Associated Death Domain protein (TRADD), TNFR-Associated Factor 2 (TRAF2) and NCK Interacting Kinase (NIK) along with subsequent phosphorylation and degradation of IκBα initiates NFκB activation (Figure 2A) [11]. To identify the site of action, U-937 cells were transfected with TNFR1, TRADD, TRAF2, NIK, IKK and p65 plasmids. Secreted Embryonic Alkaline Phosphatase (SEAP) was used as a reporter gene for NFκB and expression levels were monitored in treated and un-treated cells. Mangiferin inhibited TNFR1, TRADD, TRAF2, NIK and IKK induced SEAP expression but did not have a significant effect on p65 induced SEAP expression. Consequently, mangiferin must act downstream from IKK [11].

Signal Transduction to Activate NFκB

In a study carried out by García-Rivera et al. on estrogen negative MDA-MB231 breast cancer cells, the efficacy of Vimang® (aqueous extract from *Mangifera indica*) was investigated and compared to treatment with either mangiferin only or gallic acid only (another bioactive present in Vimang®) [41]. At baseline, MDA-MB231 cells, which have a mutated p53 gene, demonstrate high NFκB activity [41]. When cells were pre-treated for 4 h with 200 μg/mL Vimang® or 100 μg/mL of mangiferin, there was no change in IKKα expression, but reduced phosphorylation of IKKα and IKKβ was observed [41]. These proteins must be phosphorylated in order to transduce the signal and activate NFκB, thus mangiferin attenuated signal transduction. These authors also report that time taken for IκB phosphorylation and consequently degradation in response to TNF stimulation was doubled and time taken for IκB resynthesis was significantly reduced [41]. The action of mangiferin on IκB degradation has also been reported in a number of other studies [11,41,47,48,63]. Once IκBα is degraded, its inhibitory effect on the NFκB activation pathway is diminished [63] and thus NFκB can freely bind to DNA, allowing transcription and translation of the respective genes and proteins that it regulates [64]. Additionally, mangiferin and Vimang® were found to reduce phosphorylation and translocation of p65 into the nucleus and impeded NFκB/DNA binding in response to TNF [41]. Other studies have also reported that mangiferin affects IκBα and p65 in this way [8,11,48]. García-Rivera et al. revealed that Vimang®, but not mangiferin alone was found to prevent parallel NFκB transactivation [41], emphasising the beneficial effects provided by other bioactive constituents of this aqueous extract.

It is clear that mangiferin is likely to attenuate NFκB expression in a multifaceted way, [34,47] with additional mechanisms yet to be elucidated.

Consequential Effects of NFκB Downregulation

NFκB is implicit in regulating expression of Cyclooxygenase-2 (COX-2), Intercellular Adhesion Molecule-1 (ICAM-1), B Cell Lymphoma-2 (bcl-2), Interleukin-6 (IL-6), Interleukin-8 (IL-8), C-X-C Chemokine Receptor type-4 (CXCR4), X linked Inhibitor of Apoptosis Protein (XIAP) and Vascular Endothelial Growth Factor (VEGF), which are all involved in inflammation, metastasis, cell survival and angiogenesis [11,29,42,48] (more on COX-2 below). As a downregulator of NFκB, mangiferin consequentially reduces expression of the genes listed above [41] and increases apoptosis [8].

IL-6 and IL-8 are both inflammatory cytokines that enhance cell proliferation. In MDA-MB231 cells, proliferation is conditional on autocrine synthesis of inflammatory cytokines and growth factors [41]. Vimang® and mangiferin have each been found to down-regulate IL-6 and IL-8 production when stimulated by TNF [41], thus reducing the inflammatory response.

2.1.2. Peroxisome Proliferator-Activated Receptor γ (PPARγ)

PPARγ is a nuclear receptor that also functions as a transcription factor, regulating expression of genes involved in cell differentiation and tumourigenesis [65]. Under normal circumstances, when the corresponding ligand binds to PPARγ, transcriptional activation of COX-2 is suppressed through a number of mechanisms [66]. COX-2 is one of the key drivers of chronic inflammation through the production of prostaglandins leading to further activation of inflammatory processes [67], and thus COX-2 overexpression favours cancer progression [29]. PPARγ also has a pleiotropic effect on blood glucose levels. PPARγ agonists such as thiazolidinediones are widely used in management of diabetes and have a hypoglycaemic effect [65]. Hyperglycaemia is regarded as an emerging risk factor for cancer development [65]. Mangiferin, like thiazolidinedione may also act to reduce hyperglycaemia, benefiting diabetics and decreasing cancer risk.

Mangiferin increases mRNA expression of the PPARγ gene [68] and thus decreases transcriptional activation of COX-2. This reduces inflammation and creates a less favourable environment for acquisition and proliferation of malignant cells. Mangiferin also impedes expression of COX-2 [41] via upregulation of TGF-β and downregulation of NFκB. Mangiferin may play a beneficial role in modulating PPARγ and COX-2 regulation as evidenced by in vitro studies in MDA-MB231 breast cancer cells [43].

2.1.3. Immune Response

Cancer cells can sometimes escape detection and avoid the immune system, which would otherwise destroy abnormal cells. Cancer cells not only express immune checkpoint proteins that dampen the immune response, but they may also release cytokines and growth factors that promote tumour cell proliferation and minimize apoptosis. By enhancing a patient's immune response a better outcome can be achieved. In in vivo studies, mangiferin has been found to enhance the number and activity of immune cells [9,10].

Rajendran et al. found that in mice treated with benzo(a)pyrene (B(a)P) to induce lung cancer, dosing with mangiferin influenced the types of immune cells present and concentrations of various immunoglobulins [9]. Mangiferin treatment resulted in higher numbers of lymphocytes and neutrophils [9]. Mangiferin treatment of B(a)P mice increased levels of IgG and IgM immunoglobulins and decreased levels of IgA immunoglobulins, relative to animals only receiving B(a)P treatment [9]. In addition, mangiferin inhibited phagocytic capacity and nitric oxide production of macrophages when stimulated with LPS and IFN$\gamma$ [9]. Thus, with respect to the inflammatory response, less collateral damage is likely to occur. In a later study, it was found that in tumour bearing Swiss mice, mangiferin promoted cytotoxic behaviour of lymphocytes and macrophages against malignant cells, and thus the incidence of fibrosarcoma was reduced [7].

## 2.2. Cell Cycle

Maintenance of a normal cell cycle is essential for homeostasis. It allows cells to be replaced at the same rate as they are lost. Often in cancer, the length of the cell cycle is reduced, allowing aberrant proliferation of malignant cells.

Findings suggest that mangiferin influences the Mitogen Activated Protein Kinase (MAPK) pathway and progression from the $G_2/M$ checkpoint, thus maintaining a more normal cell cycle length, or cell cycle arrest at the appropriate checkpoint [8,13,52].

### 2.2.1. Mitogen Activated Protein Kinase Pathway

The MAPK pathway is frequently implicated in tumourigenesis as it plays a role in processes such as cell proliferation, growth, differentiation, apoptosis and migration [69]. Mangiferin attenuates MAPK signalling [34] by inhibiting MAPKs p38, Extracellular signal-Regulated Kinase (ERK) and c Jun N-terminal Kinase phosphorylation [60]. Li et al. found that mangiferin aglycone, a metabolite of mangiferin, formed through deglycosylationin vivo, also inhibited ERK1/2 when phosphorylation was induced by UVB [70]. In this study, mangiferin aglycone was found to significantly reduce UV-induced skin cancers in mice, primarily through this interaction with ERK [70]. While further study is required, this suggests a beneficial effect against skin cancer.

### 2.2.2. $G_2/M$ Checkpoint

Under normal conditions, cells with mutations are not able to undergo mitosis, as there are a number of checkpoints in the cycle that prevent mutated DNA from replicating [71]. Cancer cells must acquire characteristics that allow them to bypass these checkpoints in order to survive and proliferate [71].

The $G_2/M$ checkpoint occurs during the transition from $G_2$ to mitotic entry. The $G_2$ phase involves rapid growth of a cell as it prepares for mitosis. Cell progression from the $G_2/M$ checkpoint only occurs in the absence of DNA damage signals [72]. DNA damage can be sensed by Ataxia telangiectasia mutated protein (ATM) and Ataxia Telangiectasia and Rad3-related protein (ATR) which signal via Checkpoint kinase 1 (Chk1) and Checkpoint Kinase 2 (Chk2) to cause degradation of M-phase inducer phosphatase 1 (cdc25a), which results in inhibition of the Cyclin-Dependent Kinase 1 (CDK1)-cyclinB1 complex and thus cell cycle arrest [71,72] (see Figure 3). The cdc2-cyclinB1 complex is often overexpressed in malignant cells, enhancing entry into mitosis in eukaryotic cells. Malignant cells may acquire characteristics, which enable them to escape cell cycle arrest regardless of mutations. Chemotherapeutic agents such as etoposide target malignant cells at the $G_2/M$ checkpoint, thus when cell cycle progression is inhibited, the efficacy of etoposide at inducing apoptosis is increased. Mangiferin is thought to induce $G_2/M$ phase arrest [8], reducing proliferation of malignant cells and increasing efficacy of chemotherapeutic agents that target this phase.

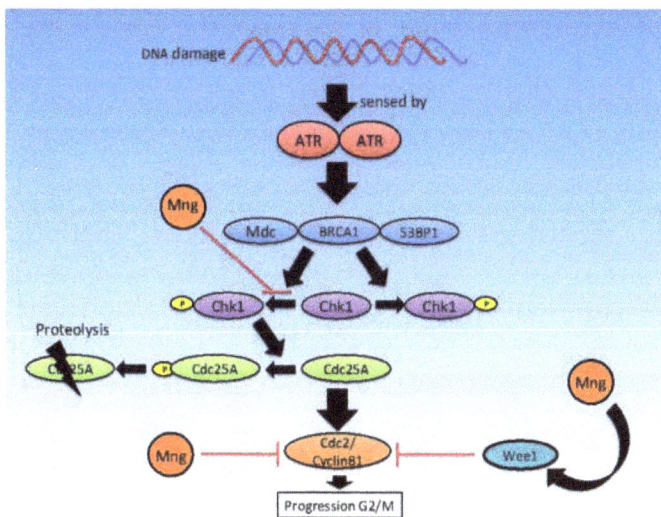

**Figure 3.** Mangiferin affects the molecular events leading to cell cycle $G_2/M$ phase arrest (Figure adapted from [71]).

Mangiferin has been shown to arrest cell cycle progression in a time dependent manner at the $G_2/M$ phase through suppression of the cdc2-cyclin B1 signalling pathway in MCF-7 cells [8]. This was observed through analysis of cell cycle distribution through flow cytometry, where a greater number of cells were found in the $G_2/M$ phase after incubation with mangiferin [13,52]. These findings are in keeping with results from the Peng et al. study in HL-60 cells [8]. Peng et al. [52] also found that in HL-60 leukaemia cells, gene expression of Chk1, cdc25 and Wee1 was elevated when exposed to low concentrations of mangiferin, but at higher concentrations, Chk1 and cdc25 gene expression was reduced at the mRNA level. Mangiferin has been shown to significantly inhibit phosphorylation of ATR, Chk1 and other proteins with anti-proliferative properties such as Wee1, Akt and Erk1/2, while increasing phosphorylation of cdc2 and cyclinB1 [52]. Lv et al. used a Western blot assay to identify a reduction in cdc2 (cdk1) and cyclinB1 [8] protein levels in response to treatment with mangiferin. Findings suggest that inhibition of the ATR-Chk1 stress response DNA damage pathway by mangiferin is responsible for cell cycle arrest.

While $G_2/M$ phase arrest has been identified in response to mangiferin treatment in a number of cancer cell lines (MCF-7, HL-60, BEL-7404 and CNE2) [16,18,35,52,73], further study is required to determine dosages of mangiferin required to elicit an effect. In addition to $G_2/M$ phase arrest, Lv et al. also suggest that mangiferin may induce $G_0/G_1$ cell cycle arrest in MCF7 cells [8].

### 2.3. Proliferation/Metastasis

Under normal circumstances, the rate of cell replication and cell death is matched to maintain homeostasis. In cancer cells, the mediators of these processes may be deregulated, allowing cells to proliferate continuously, exceeding rates of cell death. Cancer cells may develop a more motile phenotype, due to deregulation of cell adhesion pathways. Loss of adhesion allows cells to escape their site of origin and spread to other sites, causing secondary malignancies.

Mangiferin is thought to reduce cell proliferation [16] through modulation of β-catenin and consequently metalloproteinase-7 (MMP-7), MMP-9, and EMT (epithelial to mesenchymal transition) [14]. Through NFκB, mangiferin may influence VEGF-A transcription to modulate angiogenesis. Additionally, in in vivo experiments, mangiferin has shown efficacy at reducing tumour volume in mice [14].

In a variety of breast cancer cell lines, mangiferin has been implicated in reduced cell proliferation (MDA-MB-231, BT-549, MCF-7 and T47D) [8,14] and reduced metastasis (MDA-MB-231 and BT-549) in a dose-dependent manner [14]. In HL-60 cells, Li et al. reinforced that mangiferin reduced proliferation [14]. In contrast, Wilkinson et al. found that mangiferin did not suppress proliferation in MCF-7 cells, while mangiferin aglycone did [74]. This may be a result of differential activation of estrogen receptors [74]. Kim et al. also reported no significant effect on proliferation when HeLa cells were treated with 25–200 µM of mangiferin [36] and Garcia-Rivera et al. found no significant inhibition of proliferation in MDA-MB231 cells when treated with mangiferin, but proliferation was inhibited by Vimang® [41]. Thus, further evidence is required to ascertain an effect.

### 2.3.1. Glycogen Synthase Kinase-3β/β-Catenin

In cancer, aberrant activation of β-catenin is often observed [14]. High levels of expression of β-catenin are associated with proliferation and metastasis. Glycogen synthase kinase -3β (GSK-3β) is capable of phosphorylating and degrading β-catenin [14]. GSK-3β may be inhibited by a number of signals. Mangiferin is hypothesised to suppress the β-catenin pathway [14].

Using a Western blot assay to analyse protein expression in breast cancer cell lines, mangiferin was found to down-regulate β-catenin and decrease levels of inactive GSK-3β, indicating suppression of the β-catenin pathway, which in turn down-regulates MMP-7, MMP-9 and snail expression [14]. Snail can be used as an epithelial/mesenchymal phenotye indicator [14], thus lower levels of snail, which are seen on exposure to mangiferin, favour a more epithelial, less mobile phenotype, while higher expression of snail would indicate a more motile phenotype, allowing malignant cells to metastasise.

### 2.3.2. Matrix Metalloproteinases

Activation of matrix MMPs is a crucial step towards metastasis as these enzymes facilitate cell escape from the initial site of the malignancy, through degradation of the extracellular matrix. As above, mangiferin has been linked to downregulation of NFκB, which in turn influences downstream expression of MMPs [64,75].

In breast cancer, the matrix metalloproteinases MMP-2, -7 and -9 are often up-regulated [14]. Li et al. have demonstrated through a Western blot assay that of these three enzymes, MMP-2 was not significantly affected while MMP-7 and MMP-9 were down-regulated by mangiferin [14]. MMP-7 and -9 strongly promote cancer progression by allowing malignant cells to metastasise [76]. In LNCaP prostate cancer cells, activation of NFκB by TNF-α increases levels of MMP-9 mRNA and protein present in the cell [75]. Mangiferin is capable of attenuating this effect, ultimately reducing metastasis [75]. In addition to this pathway of MMP-9 activation, Xiao et al. (2015) discovered that mangiferin stimulates miR-15b expression, which in turn down-regulates MMP-9 expression in U87 glioma cells [16], thus reducing the capability of malignant cells to escape the extracellular matrix and metastasise. In the study by Jung et al., mangiferin prevented PMA induced MMP-9 expression without influencing other MMP expression in human astroglioma cell lines: U87MG, U373MG and CRT-MG [19]. MMP-1, -2, -3 and -14 expressions were not influenced by mangiferin [19]. Mangiferin is thought to act by suppressing NFκB and AP-1 binding to the promoter region of MMP-9 and prevents phosphorylation of Akt and MAP kinases (see above section) induced by PMA [19]. Jung et al. also suggest that mangiferin acts on MMP-9 suppressors, *Tissue Inhibitor of Metalloproteinase -1* and -2 (*TIMP-1* and -2). TIMP-1 and TIMP-2 mRNA levels were enhanced by the presence of mangiferin, implying another favourable quality of mangiferin [19]. Jung et al. suggest that mangiferin, through these mechanisms, may reduce glioma invasiveness [19]. Overall, published studies indicate that mangiferin may play an important role in reducing expression of MMP-9, limiting cancer invasiveness [16,19].

### 2.3.3. Epithelial to Mesenchymal Transition

EMT involves the loss of adherence and gain of a motile phenotype and resistance to apoptosis, which may allow motile cancer cells to migrate from their site of origin and survive, causing secondary metastases [53]. β-catenin signalling may also play a role in EMT [14]. Mangiferin appears to enhance epithelial characteristics in breast cancer cell lines and thus help protect against metastasis [14].

Li et al. [14] investigated the effect of mangiferin on EMT through analysis of two mesenchymal-like breast cancer cell lines (MDA-MB-231 and BT-549). Mesenchymal characteristics were reduced upon treatment with mangiferin, whereby cells obtained a more epithelial-like morphology. Associated with these physical observations, increased expression of the epithelial phenotype marker, E-cadherin, and decreased expression of mesenchymal phenotype markers, vimentin, snail and slug were seen [14]. In MDA-MB-231 xenograft mice treated with mangiferin, Western blot analysis revealed the same shift in expression in epithelial and mesenchymal markers with lower expression of active β-catenin, MMP-7, MMP-9 and vimentin (mesenchymal markers) and higher expression of E-cadherin (an epithelial marker) [14], reinforcing the in vitro results. While these results are promising in breast cancer cells, investigation in a more diverse range of cell lines is required to determine if these findings may be applicable to a broader range of breast cancer cell lines as well as other cancer cell lines.

### 2.3.4. Angiogenesis

Sustained angiogenesis is widely regarded as an enabling characteristic of cancer, as tumours are unable to survive beyond a certain size without their own blood supply [53]. Angiogenic tumours are able to grow and proliferate using nutrients and oxygen from their own blood supply. The VEGF-A protein is known to stimulate angiogenesis [53]. Both mangiferin and Vimang® extracts have demonstrated inhibitory effects on TNF-induced transcription of VEGF-A in MDA-MB231 cells [41]. However, this experiment was carried out over a short time period. Further investigation over longer time periods and evidence from in vivo/ex vivo studies are required to further determine the effect of mangiferin on angiogenesis.

### 2.3.5. Tumour Volume

Duringin vivo experiments in mice, mangiferin has been found to reduce tumour volume. In C57BL/6J mice inoculated with MCF-7 cells on the neck, a reduction of 89.4% in tumour volume relative to control was seen when mice were medicated with 100 mg/kg of mangiferin. This value was closely comparable to the results obtained from cisplatin treatment (91.5%), an established chemotherapeutic drug [8]. In a similar experiment, the lifespan of these mice was extended at dosages from 10 mg/kg mangiferin and above and 60% of mice survived until the end of the assay period [8], while in the no treatment group, there were no mice surviving after day 40 following MCF-7 inoculation. A high dosage of mangiferin (100 mg/kg) extended lifespan to the same degree as cisplatin, with no significant difference ($p < 0.05$) being observed between these treatments [8]. Dose dependency was observed [8].

These results show that mangiferin can act as a potent chemotherapeutic agent in mice and thus further investigation into mangiferin-based products could benefit treatment of cancer in humans.

### 2.4. Apoptosis

In order to survive and proliferate, cancer cells must be able to evade apoptosis, despite carrying malignant characteristics [53]. Under normal circumstances, either the intrinsic pathway via the mitochondria, or the extrinsic pathway involving death receptors, can induce apoptosis. The intrinsic pathway generally involves increased permeability of the mitochondrial membrane and the release of cytochrome C to activate initiator procaspase-9, while the extrinsic pathway involves Fas Associated Death Domain (FADD) and procaspase-8 [36] (Figure 4). Apoptosis is the preferred pathway of cell death, as necrotic cell death may induce inflammatory changes due to the release of immune-stimulatory molecules. In order to eradicate cancer, many chemotherapeutic agents seek to induce apoptosis in malignant cells. From the peer reviewed literature, it can be concluded that mangiferin has promising apoptosis inducing properties in a number of cell lines and is involved in regulating apoptosis via multiple targets [8,14,36].

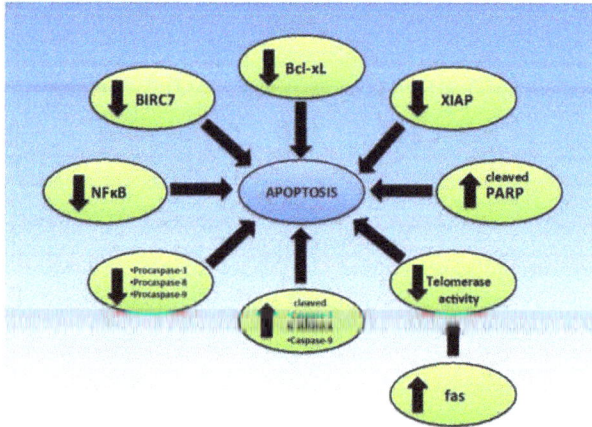

**Figure 4.** Effect of Mangiferin on proteins implicated in apoptosis.

In 2013, two studies were published that demonstrated a dose dependent increase in apoptosis in response to increasing mangiferin concentration in MDAMB-231, BT-549, MCF7 and T47D breast cancer cell lines [8,14]. Kim et al. reported similar findings in HeLa cells in response to treatment with ethanolic extracts of mango skin or flesh [36]. There are a number of suggested mechanisms by which an increase in apoptosis in these cancer cells may be potentiated. As discussed earlier, mangiferin down-regulates the transcription factor NFκB. It is hypothesized that this dampening of NFκB activity is likely to be responsible for increased apoptosis in HL-60 acute myeloid leukaemia (AML) cells, MCF7 cells and HeLa cells [8,13,35,77].

### 2.4.1. Mangiferin and Hesperidin in *Cyclopia* Sp. Extracts

Bartoszewski et al. showed in HeLa cells that treatment with *Cyclopia sp.* tea extracts, which are high in mangiferin and hesperidin, caused up-regulation of TRADD and TNFR superfamily member 25 (TRAMP), which are involved in signalling of the extrinsic apoptotic pathway [77]. However, when compared to mangiferin only and hesperidin only, it would appear that hesperidin is a more potent activator of apoptosis in HeLa cells than mangiferin [77]. Regardless, mangiferin did enhance the activity of hesperidin, even when added in low concentrations. Mangiferin itself caused down-regulation of Baculoviral IAP Repeat Containing 7 (BIRC7), which sensitizes cells to death by the extrinsic apoptotic pathway [77].

### 2.4.2. Bax/Bcl-2

The Bcl-2 protein acts to block programmed cell death while the Bcl-2 associated X protein (Bax) protein favours apoptosis. When the ratio of Bax:Bcl-2 is increased, a cell's sensitivity to apoptosis is increased [78], and consequently malignant cells are less likely to survive. Current literature suggests that the effect of mangiferin on the Bax:Bcl-2 ratio is dependent on cell type, dosage and perhaps the form of mangiferin used [35,79].

Pan et al. found that when CNE2 nasopharyngeal carcinoma cells were treated with mangiferin, the mRNA and protein expression levels of Bcl-2 were consistently down-regulated while Bax was up-regulated [35]. As a consequence, these cells were primed for apoptosis. Bcl-2 was also down-regulated upon treatment with an ethanolic extract of mango skins, which contained mangiferin, mangiferin gallate and isomangiferin gallate [36]. This ultimately resulted in activation of caspase-3, -6, -8 and -9 alongside poly (ADP-ribose) polymerase (PARP) protein [36], favouring cell death. However, Klavitha et al. [22] have found that the reverse applies in the context of excitotoxicity in neurons, whereby mangiferin blocks upregulation of Bax, thus attenuating cell death, making it a promising compound for further research with regard to Parkinson's disease [22]. Furthermore, Bartoszewski et al. demonstrated that on analysis of green fermented *Cyclopia* sp. extracts (in which the primary compounds were mangiferin and hesperidin), there were no significant changes in Bax/Bcl2 mRNA levels or protein levels [77], although Bartoszewski et al. acknowledge that the most likely cause of this disparate finding was low dosage.

In addition to the Bax/Bcl2 ratio, Zhang et al. and Pan et al. reported that apoptosis could be triggered by mangiferin in HL-60 cells due to changes in levels of similar proteins [13,35]. HL-60 cells responded to mangiferin by decreasing levels of Bcl-extra large (Bcl-xL) and XIAP [13,35], resulting in increased apoptosis.

Further experimentation in a wider range of cell lines is required to elucidate what dosage of mangiferin is likely to provide an effect.

### 2.4.3. Intrinsic/Extrinsic Apoptotic Pathway

To identify whether mangiferin was acting on the intrinsic or extrinsic apoptotic pathway, Kim et al. performed a Western blot experiment to assess expression levels of proteins involved in either the intrinsic pathway, extrinsic pathway or both pathways [36]. Results indicated that there was slightly lower expression levels of BH3 interacting domain (Bid), pro-caspase-3 and pro-caspase-8, but increased expression of cleaved, active forms of PARP, caspase-7 and caspase-9 [36], when HeLa cells were treated with an ethanolic extract of mango peel. Consequently, it is likely that the ethanolic extracts of mango pulp and skin influenced both apoptotic pathways, which is crucial for effective apoptosis. Lv et al. further strengthened the evidence for the role of mangiferin in the intrinsic apoptotic pathway by considering cytochrome C [8]. They found that when MCF-7 cells were treated with mangiferin, cytochrome C concentration in the mitochondria was reduced, while a corresponding increase in cytochrome C concentration was observed in the cytosol. This indicates that cytochrome C was released from the mitochondria in response to mangiferin treatment and thus apoptosis may be induced via the mitochondrial pathway [8]. In addition to these findings, increased expression of caspase-3, -8 and 9, and decreased expression of procaspase-3, -8 and -9 expression was noted, suggesting activation of both intrinsic and extrinsic apoptotic pathways [8]. Based on results from their study, du Plessis-Stoman et al. have suggested that mangiferin may favour apoptotic cell death over necrotic cell death, which has potential to reduce inflammation [48].

### 2.4.4. Telomerase

Aside from the study of various pathways of apoptosis, in the literature it is reported that mangiferin can inhibit telomerase activity in K562 human leukaemia cells with dose- and time-dependent behaviour [8,35,80], promoting apoptosis. It has been suggested that this may be due to increased *fas* gene expression and protein levels of fas [8]. Enhanced telomerase activity is found in a variety of cancers and is permissive and required for sustained growth of late cancers. Almost all cancers exhibit some form of telomerase reactivation [81]. By reducing telomerase activity, mangiferin can be used to reduce the progression of existing cancers and create an environment in which malignant cells are unlikely to survive.

Mangiferin has demonstrated pro-apoptotic activity in a number of cancer cell lines including K562 leukaemia, MCF-7 breast cancer and CNE2 nasopharyngeal cells [8,35].

## 2.5. Oxidative Stress

Oxidative stress occurs when the burden of ROS is not balanced by antioxidants and detoxification systems. The presence of these excess reactive species can result in cellular damage, particularly to DNA, lipids and proteins. Over time, oxidative stress increases the risk of developing cancer and may exacerbate inflammation. Mangiferin is thought to play a role in: (1) modulating the Nrf2/antioxidant response element (ARE) detoxification pathway (Figure 5); (2) directly detoxifying reactive species; and (3) activating detoxification enzymes such as catalase.

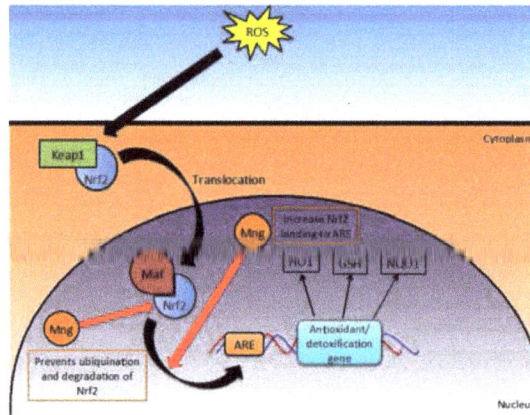

**Figure 5.** Effect of Mangiferin on the Nrf2/ARE Detoxification Pathway.

### 2.5.1. Nrf2/ARE Detoxification Pathway

Under normal conditions, Nrf2 gene transcription is inhibited by Kelch-like ECH-associated protein-1 (KEAP-1). However, oxidative stress, dietary components and synthetic chemicals can induce Nrf2 transcription [18]. Consequently, Nrf2 protein can accumulate in the nucleus where it forms heterodimers with musculoaponeurotic fibrosarcoma (maf) protein. This heterodimer signals through the ARE to initiate transcription of a number of phase II detoxification enzymes [17], such as NAD(P)H: quinine reductases (NQO1), glutathione S-transferase (GSH) and heme oxygenase (HO-1) [18]. HO-1, when activated, can translocate into the nucleus to further activate transcription factors relevant to the stimulus [82]. Ultimately, this pathway provides activation of detoxification enzymes when oxidative stresses are presented. Mangiferin manipulates this pathway in such a way that the survival of healthy cells but not malignant cells is enhanced. Mangiferin modulated this Nrf2/ARE signaling pathway at multiple steps [13,17,18].

While mangiferin does not directly influence Nrf2 transcription rates, Zhao et al. have demonstrated that the half-life of Nrf2 is increased due to impaired ubiquitination and thus degradation of the protein [18], which results in higher levels of the protein being present within the cell. Zhang et al. also reported similar findings in human umbilical cord mononuclear blood cells, where mangiferin increased the quantity of Nrf2 accumulating in the nucleus in a time dependent manner [17]. Protein quantity was assessed by microscopy and verified by Western blotting [17]. Additionally, mangiferin increased the binding of Nrf2 to ARE which in turn was shown to increase downstream production of NQO1 (a prominent antioxidant enzyme) when assessed in a Western blot assay [13,17].

Nrf-ARE signaling can provide protection against agents that are chemotherapeutic to normal cells [13] (more on synergistic effects of mangiferin and chemotheraputics later). Similarly, overexpression of Nrf2 in cancer cells can promote resistance to therapy, through up-regulation of antiapoptotic bcl-xL. Mangiferin seems able to differentiate between malignant cells and healthy cells, promoting Nrf2 activation in healthy cells (human umbilical cord mononuclear blood cells) but not cancerous cells (HL-60). Thus, survival is aided in healthy cells by enhanced efficiency of the Nrf2/ARE detoxification pathway while the development of resistance to chemotherapeutics is not permitted in malignant cells [13]. To date, mangiferin is the only known Nrf2 activator that does not confer protection to malignant cells against chemotherapeutic agents [13], making it a promising agent for cancer therapy.

Downstream effects in the Nrf2/ARE detoxification pathway have been further studied upon treatment with Vimang®. Treatment of MDA-MB231 breast cancer cells with 200–400 µL/mL of Vimang® was found to significantly increase HO-1 transcription. However, when treated with mangiferin alone, there was no significant increase in HO-1 transcription [41]. From this result, one may deduce that the Nrf2/ARE detoxification pathway may not have been activated by mangiferin, as was reported earlier in the HL-60 cancer cell line. It is possible that an alternative bioactive, found in Vimang® may be responsible for the up-regulation of HO-1 transcription in the MDA-MB231 breast cancer cells. Overall, results would suggest that mangiferin may provide some benefit through activation of the Nrf-ARE detoxification pathway.

2.5.2. Elimination of Reactive Species

Reactive species must be eliminated promptly to avoid damage to important biological molecules. This may be done directly by antioxidant species, or by inducing and up-regulating detoxification pathways. Mangiferin is an established antioxidant that is able to neutralize a range of reactive species and influence expression and activity of key detoxification enzymes. By performing these actions, oxidative stress and inflammation are reduced.

Mangiferin is able to directly protect against hydroxyl [28], 2,2-diphenyl-1-picrylhydrazyl (DPPH), superoxide, hydrogen peroxide [51], and peroxynitrite free radicals, lipid peroxides [9,21], hypochlorus acid [28] and heavy metal induced reactive oxygen species [15]. Findings from numerous studies can be used to reinforce the notion that mangiferin has greater or comparative antioxidative capacity to other known antioxidants, such as quercetin, baicalein, catechins, phenylpropanoic acids [21], vitamin C, vitamin E and β-carotene [28]. Alongside its antioxidative potential, mangiferin influences ROS production through modulating Fenton-type reactions. Fenton-type reactions usually involve the production of a hydroxyl radical and the oxidation of $Fe^{2+}$ to $Fe^{3+}$. In the presence of mangiferin, Fenton-type reactions are inhibited by chelating $Fe^{2+}$ ions, reducing production of subsequent ROS [15,29,51]. Additionally, Duang et al. have suggested that mangiferin protects against lipid peroxidation [29]. This protection may in part be responsible for reduced DNA damage and amelioration of cytotoxic action seen in response to ionising radiation in healthy cells [9,83].

Both in vitro and in vivo evidence suggests that mangiferin up-regulates expression of various detoxifying enzymes, resulting in enhanced clearance of ROS. In N2A neuroblastoma cells, Kavintha et al. implicated mangiferin in reducing oxidative stress by providing protection against 1-methyl-4-phenylpyridine ($MPP^+$) induced cytotoxicity, due to its capability to restore glutathione action and reduce expression of superoxide (SOD) and catalase [22]. In addition to these findings, Matkowski et al. also reported that mangiferin influenced SOD, catalase and glutathione peroxidase in such a way that it halts ROS centred apoptotic pathways through dampening endogenous ROS production [21]. Sarker et al. demonstrated the relationship between mangiferin and glutathione levels by showing that mangiferin increased levels of GSH more than 2× the amount observed on treatment with other anti-oxidants [11]. It has been suggested that mangiferin increases GSH levels by up-regulation of γ-Glutamylcysteine Synthetase (γ-GCS), the enzyme controlling the rate limiting step of GSH synthesis [11]. In vivo studies demonstrate a similar pattern of increased detoxification enzyme activity. In experiments using B(a)P-treated mice, B(a)P attenuated SOD and catalase (see below for more on catalase) activity in lymphocytes, polymorphonuclear cells and macrophages [9]. However, mangiferin co-administration provided a protective effect against these events. Rajendran et al. also found that mangiferin reduced the production of $H_2O_2$ in B(a)P treated animals [9]. In animals with lung cancer, enhanced activity of glutathione transferase [48], quinine reductase and uridine 5′-diphosphate-glucuronosyl transferase activity has been demonstrated upon treatment with mangiferin [8]. These events each contribute to a reduction in oxidative stress through increased capacity to deal with assault from reactive species. Sarker et al. further suggest that the ability of mangiferin to reduce oxidative stress may also be linked to NFκB down-regulating capabilities, which reduces TNF-induced reactive oxygen intermediate generation [11].

### 2.5.3. Catalase

Catalase is a detoxification enzyme present in most organisms exposed to oxygen that converts $H_2O_2$ into water and oxygen. $H_2O_2$ can cause oxidative damage if not rapidly converted into less toxic species. Mangiferin may directly increase the efficiency of the catalase enzyme by interacting directly with the enzyme, thus reducing oxidative damage that can be done prior to detoxification of $H_2O_2$ [61]. Increased activity of catalase may modulate downstream signalling pathways that favour an environment that does not promote cancer development and survival. However, not all published findings are consistent with the notion that mangiferin increases catalase activity [11,61].

In silico docking studies using AutoDock and PyMol predict that mangiferin has the capacity to bind to the active site of catalase, but not other oxidase enzymes [61]. The binding of mangiferin to catalase enhanced the activity of catalase by 44% during the in vitro studies conducted by Sahoo et al. [61]. An earlier study by Sarkar et al. reported disparate findings, where mangiferin caused a 0%–23% increase in activity when compared to untreated cells, and did not influence the quantity of enzyme present [11]. In both experiments, U-937 cells were treated alongside other cell lines with 10 µg/mL of mangiferin for 3 h [11].

To further elucidate the effect of mangiferin on catalase activity, Sahoo et al. conducted fluorescent spectrophotometry experiments on catalase in the unbound state (peak at 330 nm, excitation wavelength 280 nm) and subsequently, increasing concentrations of mangiferin were added [61]. As the concentration of mangiferin was increased, the peak at 330 nm decreased in magnitude, suggesting interaction with mangiferin. When the binding constant was calculated ($3.1 \times 10^{-7}$ M$^{-1}$), this indicated a strong binding affinity between catalase and mangiferin [61]. Mangiferin also proved capable of overriding aminotriazole (ATZ) inhibition of catalase in lipid peroxidation assays [61]. Sahoo et al. further demonstrated that direct quenching of $H_2O_2$ by mangiferin was not significant, implying that the entire 44% difference found may be attributable to enhanced activity of the catalase enzyme [61].

It has been suggested that increased catalase activity may dampen excessive activation of MAPK/AKT, which is commonly found in malignant cells [61] (See above for MAKP/AKT). Sarker et al. suggested that high expression of catalase would reduce NFκB levels [11]. However, evidence does not support any change in catalase expression, only in the efficiency of this enzyme [11,61]. Increased catalase activity could reduce oxidative stress and inflammation, thus favouring a chemopreventative environment.

### 2.6. DNA Damage

DNA damage facilitates mutations in the genetic material of a cell. Mutation is required to initiate the development of cancer and also expedites the acquisition of characteristics required for a malignant cell to survive. Thus, a higher susceptibility to DNA damage results in a higher incidence of mutation and the development of cancer [84]. The role of mangiferin with regard to DNA damage is controversial.

Studies have reported that mangiferin is capable of protecting not only DNA [42] but also deoxyribose, phospholipids, polyunsaturated fatty acids and proteins [21]. However, Rodeiro et al. [12] found that when aqueous extracts from *Mangifera indica* bark were applied to lymphocytes and lymphoblastic cells, DNA damage was induced. When this effect was further investigated with the compound mangiferin alone, there was a reduction in DNA damage, thus there is likely to be an alternative compound in the extract that is inducing DNA damage [12]. In addition, Rodeiro et al. found that when DNA damage was induced by γ-radiation, the aqueous extract was protective against DNA damage [12].

Radiation Damage

Ionising radiation has been shown to induce DNA damage. In patients undergoing radiotherapy, many healthy cells acquire collateral damage. Mangiferin and mangiferin aglycone have demonstrated protective effects against radiation damage during in vitro studies [28].

Lei et al. demonstrated that pre-treatment of human intestinal epithelial cells with mangiferin aglycone reduced the percentage of cells with double strand breakages in their DNA by 47% when treated with ionizing radiation [28]. This was more effective than the 40% reduction seen following mangiferin pre-treatment. Currently, there are few radioprotective agents, and these agents tend to be associated with high levels of toxicity [28]. Mangiferin may provide some protection to cancer patients undergoing chemotherapy as well as improve efficiency of anti-cancer treatments.

## 3. Synergistic Effects

The use of many chemotherapeutic agents induces a range of side effects, which can cause serious illness. Mangiferin shows potential to reduce or negate these side effects by selectively targeting malignant cells for cell death and enhancing survival of healthy cells. Mangiferin may potentiate cell death by existing drugs through modulation of NFκB activity [11] and causing cell cycle arrest in malignant cells at the $G_2/M$ checkpoint, leaving cells susceptible to apoptosis induced by chemotherapeutic agents such as etoposide [13]. Through NFκB inhibition, mangiferin is likely to reduce resistance to chemotherapeutic agents in cancer cells [13,48]. Studies using pro-apoptotic agents such as oxaliplatin, etoposide, doxorubicin and paclitaxel have documented additional beneficial effects when co-administered with mangiferin (Table 1).

**Table 1.** Summary of proposed beneficial effects of co-administration of mangiferin alongside chemotherapeutic agents.

| Chemotherapeutic Agent | Cell Line | Reference | Evidence |
|---|---|---|---|
| Oxaliplatin | HeLa, HT29, HL60 | [48] | Reduction in oxaliplatin IC50 values; counteracts resistance to oxaliplatin. |
| Etoposide | HL60, U937 | [11,13] | Reduces oxidative stress. Protects normal cells without reducing sensitivity of HL60 to etoposide [13]. Activity of the drug is enhanced by mangiferin [11]. |
| Doxorubicin | MCF7, U937 | [13,33] | At high concentrations mangiferin can inhibit P-glycoprotein expression and chemosensitise for doxorubicin therapy [33]. Activity of the drug is enhanced by mangiferin [11]. |
| Paclitaxel | Triple negative breast cancer | [60,62] | IRAK1 overexpression confers a growth advantage [62]. Mangiferin may inhibit *IRAK1* activation [60,62]. |
| Cisplatin | U937 | [11] | Inhibits ROS production [8]. Activity of the drug is enhanced by mangiferin; Impedes NFκB activation; Enhanced cell death in the presence of TNF [11]. |
| Vincristine | U937 | [11] | Inhibits ROS production [8]. Activity of the drug is enhanced by mangiferin; Impedes NFκB activation; Enhanced cell death in the presence of TNF [11]. |
| Adriamycin | U937 | [11] | Inhibits ROS production [8]. Activity of the drug is enhanced by mangiferin; Impedes NFκB activation; Enhanced cell death in the presence of TNF [11]. |
| AraC | U937 | [11] | Inhibits ROS production [8]. Activity of the drug is enhanced by mangiferin; Impedes NFκB activation; Enhanced cell death in the presence of TNF [11]. |

*3.1. Pro-Apoptotic Agents*

While mangiferin (at a concentration of 10 μg/mL) does not trigger apoptotic cell death itself [11], it may enhance action of chemotherapeutic pro-apoptotic agents. Sarker et al. [11] demonstrated that this was due to down-regulation of NFκB by transfecting U-937 cells with an IκBα-double negative construct, blocking NFκB activation and also transfecting with a p65 construct and observing cell death after 36 h by MTT assay, using the Live/Dead cell assay. In IκBα-double negative transfected cells, cell death increased by 12% and increased cell death with TNF from 42% to 53%. Cell death in the presence of mangiferin was increased a further 4%. In p65 overexpressing cells, cell death was not observed in response to treatment with TNF or TNF and mangiferin. By considering SEAP as a reporter gene, IκBα-double negative cells were shown to down-regulate NFκB and p65 overexpressing cells up-regulated NFκB. Thus, it was found that down-regulation of NFκB primes cells for cytotoxic agents [11].

Sarkar et al. reported that the activity of the pro-apoptotic agents cisplatin, vincristine, doxorubicin, etoposide, Adriamycin and AraC was enhanced significantly by co-administration of mangiferin in U-937 cells [11]. Unlike other antioxidants, mangiferin was not found to be toxic to the cells, as it only enhanced cell death when exposed to TNF [11].

Oxidative damage induced by chemotherapeutic drugs correlates with the development of secondary malignancies such as acute myeloid leukaemia (AML). Mangiferin reduces oxidative stress induced by these agents and thus reduces likelihood of developing secondary malignancies [13].

By enhancing apoptotic activity against malignant cells upon treatment with chemotherapeutic agents, lower dosages may be required when co-administered with mangiferin, which may reduce the side effects associated with toxicity.

### 3.1.1. Oxaliplatin

Oxaliplatin is a platinum-based anti-neoplastic agent used for the treatment of colon or rectal cancer once metastasised. It is often given in conjunction with other chemotherapeutic agents. Common side effects, occurring in >30% of patients, include nausea, vomiting, fatigue, loss of appetite, mouth sores, low blood count, diarrhoea and peripheral neuropathy [85]. Apoptotic efficacy of oxaliplatin is enhanced by the addition of mangiferin, as mangiferin inhibits NFκB (see above) [13,14,48,77] and is thought to increase the sensitivity of malignant cells to apoptotic cell death [48].

Du Plessis-Stoman et al. demonstrated the positive effect of mangiferin on oxaliplatin action in HeLa cells and HT29 cells through use of $IC_{50}$ assays [48]. When stained with tryptan blue, cells treated with oxaliplatin and mangiferin displayed fewer non-viable cells than those treated with oxaliplatin only, indicating that there was less necrosis, suggesting the apoptotic pathway for cell death was preferred [48]. Co-administration of mangiferin with oxaliplatin increased caspase 3 activation in HeLa and HT29 cell lines relative to cells that only received oxaliplatin, further implicating the apoptotic pathway of cell death was favoured, thus reducing inflammation [48].

Du Plessis-Stoman et al. have suggested that mangiferin only exhibits NFκB inhibition when used with platinum containing complexes, as they found that treatment of normal cells with mangiferin alone resulted in increased NFκB activity [48]. When treated with mangiferin and oxaliplatin, the level of NFκB inhibition was similar to cells treated with oxaliplatin alone. However, in the presence of mangiferin, the oxaliplatin $IC_{50}$ was 3.4 times lower in the cells receiving both treatments [48]. In addition, when assessing changes in cell cycle, mangiferin caused a delay in S-phase only when used in conjunction with oxaliplatin [48]. On treatment with oxaliplatin or mangiferin alone, a $G_2/M$ phase cell cycle arrest was noted.

Both oxaliplatin and mangiferin are implicated in the mitochondrial pathway of apoptosis through reduction of mitochondrial membrane potential. However, cells treated with mangiferin and oxaliplatin did not show a significantly different mitochondrial membrane potential to those treated with oxaliplatin alone [48].

Evidence indicates that mangiferin increases the efficacy of oxaliplatin at inducing cell death in malignant cells.

### 3.1.2. Etoposide

As discussed above (Section 2.5.1 on Nrf2), mangiferin protects against etoposide induced oxidative damage in human umbilical cord blood mononuclear cells by promoting Nrf2 signalling to activate a number of antioxidant enzymes [13]. Side effects such as myelo-suppression are also reduced. As discussed earlier, literature indicated that mangiferin causes $G_2/M$ phase cell cycle arrest. Etoposide targets cells in this phase [86]. In addition, oxidative damage in response to etoposide may result in p53 activation. However, when the effect of mangiferin on etoposide efficacy was studied, HL-60 cells were used, which lack wild type p53, thus further experimentation is required to elucidate this effect [13].

### 3.1.3. Doxorubicin

Louisa et al. (2014) reported that mangiferin increased the efficacy of doxorubicin in MCF-7 [33]. Cells were initially incubated with a low concentration of doxorubicin for 10 days. The apoptotic rate was measured and found to be reduced, indicating the development of drug resistance. Thereafter, cells were treated with mangiferin and at high concentrations mangiferin significantly reduced cell viability through reduced expression of P-glycoprotein, which acts as a multidrug transporter. The efficacy of mangiferin increased in a concentration dependent manner [33]. In this study it was found that mRNA levels associated with multidrug resistance associated protein-1 and breast cancer resistance protein were unaffected by mangiferin, unlike P-glycoprotein [33].

## 4. Bioavailability and Delivery of Mangiferin

Extraction, quantification, solubility and bioavailability of polyphenols, including mangiferin, are of relevance to clinical success. Bioavailability is dependent on bioaccessibility (quantity of compound released from the food matrix), solubility in gastrointestinal fluids, cellular uptake, compound metabolism and efficiency of the circulatory system [87,88]. Like many other polyphenols, the optimal health benefits of mangiferin are not fully realised due to poor water solubility and oral bioavailability (1.2% in rats) [89].

Using HPLC-MS, Hou et al. evaluated the pharmacokinetics (PK) of mangiferin following oral administration (0.1 g. 0.3 g and 0.9 g) in healthy male volunteers [90]. The point of maximum plasma concentration (38.64 ng/mL$^{-1}$) was at approximately 1 h, and was surprisingly low considering the dose of 0.9 g. This outcome supports other published findings such as those reported by [89,91] in rats. Maximal plasma concentrations, both quantity and time, were enhanced when mangiferin was orally administered to rats as a polyherbal formulation, rather than as mangiferin alone [92]. Similarly, Ma et al., in a rat model, found that permeability and plasma concentrations were improved following administration of a phospholipid complex containing mangiferin, relative to administration of mangiferin alone [93]. However, in addition to whole body PK, intratumoral PK, influenced by packing density of solid tumour cells and components of the extracellular matrix, is also important [94], and these challenges could be addressed by co-formulation and innovative delivery modes.

Bioavailability can be influenced by the properties of the food matrix (composition and structure) and hence the oral bioavailability of bioactive compounds, in this case, mangiferin could be improved if the major limiting factors were characterised [88] and modes of delivery designed accordingly. McClements et al. developed a new system for the classification of factors limiting oral bioavailability of nutraceuticals such that the design of food matrices can be optimised for each nutraceutical. The classification system is largely based on bioaccessibility (liberation, solubilisation and interactions), absorption (mucus layer, bilayer permeability and tight-, active- and efflux- transporters), and transformation (chemical degradation and metabolism) [88]. Such a system assists with determining an optimal food matrix design that will maximise oral bioavailability e.g., the encapsulation of a compound with low bilayer permeability or the addition of components that may protect a compound, that is sensitive to metabolism, against enzymes in the gut [88]. Many of these characteristics need to be assessed for mangiferin in order to improve oral bioavailability.

Encapsulation of compounds has improved PK properties in general, and is particularly suitable for compounds such as mangiferin, that are poorly water soluble [50]. Spray-drying formulations can impact on retention of mangiferin in the particle as demonstrated by the comparison of a pectin formulation versus a chitosan polysaccharide, with pectin being found to have a better retention of mangiferin in the particles than a chitosan formulation [50]. Numerous types of nanovehicles have been developed, and many polysaccharide-based nanovehicles have been used for the delivery of anti-cancer drugs, some of which may interact with membrane receptors. (See Caro and Pozo for an overview on the application of polysaccharides as nanovehicles in cancer therapy [95]). Specialised polysaccharide-based nanovehicles may be suitable for the delivery of mangiferin. It is clear that further work is required with respect to improving bioavailability and delivery methods of mangiferin from fruit or supplement to tumour site. The design of a "smart vehicle" for the delivery of mangiferin to the tumour cells, rather than healthy cells, and for avoidance or minimisation of a delivery gradient within the solid tumour, the "smart vehicle" will likely need to be unique to mangiferin and possibly to the cancer type.

## 5. Toxicity

In addition to bioavailability and delivery of bioactive compound to enhance health, it is critical to consider toxicity of the compound. Being a natural compound, mangiferin exhibits minimal toxicity [34] and is generally regarded as non-toxic [28]. Stem-bark extract from *Mangifera indica* has only shown toxicity in animals when injected intra-peritoneally and after acute exposure [12]. Mangiferin's reported toxic dose in mice is 400 mg/kg [28,50]. In experiments involving blood peripheral lymphocytes and hepatocytes of rats, mangiferin did not induce cytotoxicity, genotoxicity or mutagenicity [12]. However, in a more recent study by Prado et al. [96], oral administration of mangiferin in rodents demonstrated low acute and sub-chronic toxicity. Nonetheless, it is still anticipated that there is a wide safety margin for this compound when taken orally [96]. Due to the polyphenolic structure of mangiferin, it is likely to undergo biotransformation in the liver, and for this reason it is suggested that further investigation into the safety of mangiferin metabolites may be required [23].

## 6. Conclusions

Evidence strongly supports the link between mangiferin treatment and modulation of many molecular pathways to prevent the development and progression of cancer. Mangiferin is primarily implicated in down-regulating inflammation, causing cell cycle arrest, reducing proliferation/metastasis, promoting apoptosis in malignant cells and protecting against oxidative stress and DNA damage. Perhaps the most promising anti-proliferative effect observed on treatment with mangiferin was that seen during in vivo experiments where mangiferin reduced tumour volume to a similar extent as treatment with cisplatin. Literature consistently shows that mangiferin enhances the efficacy of pro-apoptotic chemotherapeutic agents, with the most evidence supporting synergistic effects with oxaliplatin, etoposide and doxorubicin. This is of particular interest when we consider that mangiferin exhibits low toxicity and has a wide oral safety margin, unlike other compounds with similar activity. However, the bioavailability and delivery of mangiferin requires further research and development.

Ultimately, there is strong evidence, in a number of pathways, for a protective effect of mangiferin. However, in some cases, there may be variation in effect due to dosage, origin of extract or cell line used. Furthermore, low water solubility as well as low oral bioavailability are two factors that limit clinical use at present, and further research efforts targeting appropriate delivery systems are required in order to improve clinical efficacy. In addition, investigations into in vivo effects are required to determine the significance of these results to human health. Clinical trials in humans could substantially improve our understanding of the macroscopic effects of mangiferin. Additionally, further investigation into mangiferin aglycone, may uncover a more sustainable way of achieving greater efficiency than that observed with mangiferin alone.

**Acknowledgments:** Funding to Fuchsia Gold-Smith from the School of Medicine Foundation. Funding to Karen Bishop from the Auckland Cancer Society Research Center, Auckland, New Zealand.

**Author Contributions:** All authors conceived of the idea, proofread and edited the manuscript. Fuchsia Gold-Smith and Alyssa Fernandez summarised the literature and Fuchsia Gold-Smith wrote the manuscript. Alyssa Fernandez drew the schematic diagrams and Fuchsia Gold-Smith drew the chemical structures. Karen Bishop guided the development of the manuscript and performed the final manuscript edits.

**Conflicts of Interest:** The authors declare no conflict of interest.

## Abbreviations

The following abbreviations are used in this manuscript:

| | |
|---|---|
| AML | acute myeloid leukaemia |
| ARE | antioxidant response element |
| ATM | Ataxia telangiectasia mutated protein |
| ATR | Ataxia Telangiectasia and Rad3-related protein |
| ATZ | aminotriazole |
| Bax | Bcl-2 associated X protein |
| bcl-2 | B Cell Lymphoma-2 |
| bcl-xL | B Cell Lymphoma-extra large |
| B(a)P | benzo(a)pyrene |
| Bid | BH3 interacting domain |
| BIRC7 | Baculoviral IAP Repeat Containing 7 |
| Chk1 | Checkpoint kinase 1 |
| CHk2 | Checkpoint Kinase 2 |
| CDK1 | Cyclin-Dependent Kinase 1 |
| COX | Cyclooxygenase-2 |
| CXCR4 | C-X-C Chemokine Receptor type-4 |
| DPPH | 2,2-diphenyl-1-picrylhydrazyl |
| EMT | Epithelial to Mesenchymal Transition |
| ERK | Extracellular signal-Regulated Kinase |
| FADD | Fas Associated Death Domain |
| GSH | glutathione S-transferase |
| HO-1 | heme oxygenase |
| $H_2O_2$ | hydrogen peroxide |
| IARC | International Agency for Research on Cancer |
| ICAM-1 | Intercellular Adhesion Molecule-1 |
| IκB | Inhibitor of κB |
| IKK-α | Inhibitor of NFκB Kinase subunit-α |
| IKK-β | Inhibitor of NFκB Kinase subunit-β |
| IL-1R | Interleukin-1 Receptors |
| IL-6 | Interleukin-6 |
| IL-8 | Interleukin-8 |
| IRAK1 | Interleukin-1 Receptor Activated Kinase 1 |
| IRAK4 | Interleukin-1 Receptor Activated Kinase 4 |
| KEAP-1 | Kelch-like ECH-associated protein-1 |
| LDC | Less Developed Countries |
| LPS | lipopolysaccharide |
| maf | musculoaponeurotic fibrosarcoma |
| MAPK | Mitogen Activated Protein Kinase |
| MDCs | More developed countries |
| MMP | matrix metalloproteinase |
| MPP⁺ | 1-methyl-4-phenylpyridine |
| MTT | 3-(4,5-dimethyl-2-thiozolyl)-2,5-diphenyl-2H-tetrazolium bromide |
| Myd88 | Myeloid Differentiation Primary Response Gene 88 |

| | |
|---|---|
| NEMO | NFκB Essential Modulator |
| NFκB | Nuclear Factor κ-light-chain-enhancer of activated B cells |
| NIK | NCK Interacting Kinase |
| NQO1 | NAD(P)H: quinine reductases |
| Nrf2 | Nuclear factor erythroid 2-Related Factor 2 |
| PDG | peptidoglycan |
| PK | pharmacokinetics |
| PMA | phorbol-12-myristate-13-acetate |
| PPARγ | Peroxisome Proliferator-Activated Receptorγ |
| ROS | Reactive oxygen species |
| SEAP | Secreted Embryonic Alkaline Phosphatase |
| SOD | superoxide |
| TAB1 | Transforming growth factor beta-activated kinase 1-binding protein 1 |
| TAB2 | Transforming growth factor beta-activated kinase 1-binding protein 2 |
| TAK1 | Transforming growth factor beta-activated kinase 1 |
| TLRs | Toll-like receptors |
| TNF | Tumour Necrosis Factor |
| TNFR | Tumour Necrosis Factor Receptor |
| TRADD | TNFR with Tumour Necrosis Factor Receptor type-1-Associated Death Domain protein |
| TRAF2 | Tumour Necrosis Factor Receptor-Associated Factor 2 |
| TRAF6 | Tumour necrosis factor Receptor-Associated Factor 6 |
| VEGF | Vascular Endothelial Growth Factor |
| XIAP | X linked Inhibitor of Apoptosis Protein |

## References

1. WHO. In Health in 2015 from Millenium Development Goals to Sustainable Development Goals 2015. Available online: http://www.who.int/gho/publications/mdgs-sdgs/MDGs-SDGs2015_chapter6.pdf (accessed on 20 April 2016).
2. Torre, L.; Bray, F.; Siegel, R.; Ferlay, J.; Lortet-Tieulent, J.; Jemal, A. Global cancer statistics 2012. *Cancer J. Clin.* **2015**, *65*, 87–108. [CrossRef] [PubMed]
3. United Nations Department of Economic and Social Affairs. *World Population Prospects: The 2012 Revision, Highlights and Advance Tables*; United Nations: New York, NY, USA, 2013.
4. World Cancer Research Fund International. Comparing More and Less Developed Countries. Available online: http://www.wcrf.org/int/cancer-facts-figures/comparing-more-less-developed-countries (accessed on 12 November 2015).
5. Boon, V.; Carr, J.; Klebe, S. The role of viruses in carcinogenesis. *AMSJ* **2013**, *4*, 11–15.
6. Parkin, D.M.; Boyd, L.; Walker, L.C. The fraction of cancer attributable to lifestyle and environmental factors in the UK in 2010. *Br. J. Cancer.* **2011**, *105*, S77–S81. [CrossRef] [PubMed]
7. Rajendran, P.; Rengarajan, T.; Nishigaki, I.; Ekambaram, G.; Sakthisekaran, D. Potent chemopreventive effect of mangiferin on lung carcinogenesis in experimental Swiss albino mice. *J. Cancer Res. Ther.* **2014**, *10*, 1033–1039. [PubMed]
8. Lv, J.; Wang, Z.; Zhang, L.; Wang, H.L.; Liu, Y.; Li, C.; Deng, J.; Yi, W.; Bao, J.K. Mangiferin induces apoptosis and cell cycle arrest in MCF-7 cells both in vitro and in vivo. *J. Anim. Vet. Adv.* **2013**, *12*, 352–359.
9. Rajendran, P.; Jayakumar, T.; Nishigaki, I.; Ekambaram, G.; Nishigaki, Y.; Vetriselvi, J.; Sakthisekaran, D. Immunomodulatory effect of mangiferin in experimental animals with Benzo(a)pyrene-induced lung carcinogenesis. *Int. J. Biomed. Sci.* **2013**, *9*, 68–74. [PubMed]
10. Hu, X.Y.; Deng, J.G.; Wang, L.; Yuan, Y.F. Synthesis and anti-tumor activity evaluation of gallic acid-mangiferin hybrid molecule. *Med. Chem.* **2013**, *9*, 1058–1062. [CrossRef] [PubMed]
11. Sarkar, A.; Sreenivasan, Y.; Ramesh, G.T.; Manna, S.K. β-D-glucoside suppresses tumor necrosis factor-induced activation of nuclear transcription factor κB but potentiates apoptosis. *J. Biol. Chem.* **2004**, *279*, 33768–33781. [CrossRef] [PubMed]

12. Rodeiro, I.; Delgado, R.; Garrido, G. Effects of a Mangifera indica L. stem bark extract and mangiferin on radiation-induced DNA damage in human lymphocytes and lymphoblastoid cells. *Cell Prolif.* **2014**, *47*, 48–55. [CrossRef] [PubMed]

13. Zhang, B.-P.; Zhao, J.; Li, S.-S.; Yang, L.-J.; Zeng, L.-L.; Chen, Y.; Fang, J. Mangiferin activates Nrf2-antioxidant response element signaling without reducing the sensitivity to etoposide of human myeloid leukemia cells in vitro. *APS* **2014**, *35*, 257–266. [PubMed]

14. Li, H.; Huang, J.; Yang, B.; Xiang, T.; Yin, X.; Peng, W.; Cheng, W.; Wan, J.; Luo, F.; Li, H. Mangiferin exerts antitumor activity in breast cancer cells by regulating matrix metalloproteinases, epithelial to mesenchymal transition, and β-catenin signaling pathway. *Toxicol. Appl. Pharmacol.* **2013**, *272*, 180–190. [CrossRef] [PubMed]

15. Das, S.; Nageshwar Rao, B.; Satish Rao, B.S. Mangiferin attenuates methylmercury induced cytotoxicity against IMR-32, human neuroblastoma cells by the inhibition of oxidative stress and free radical scavenging potential. *Chem. Biol. Interact.* **2011**, *193*, 129–140. [CrossRef] [PubMed]

16. Xiao, J.; Liu, L.; Zhong, Z.; Xiao, C.; Zhang, J. Mangiferin regulates proliferation and apoptosis in glioma cells by induction of microRNA-15b and inhibition of MMP-9 expression. *Oncol. Rep.* **2015**, *33*, 2815–2820. [CrossRef] [PubMed]

17. Zhang, B.; Zhao, J.; Li, S.; Zeng, L.; Chen, Y.; Fang, J. Mangiferin activates the Nrf2-ARE pathway and reduces etoposide-induced DNA damage in human umbilical cord mononuclear blood cells. *Pharm. Biol.* **2015**, *53*, 503–511. [CrossRef] [PubMed]

18. Zhao, J.; Zhang, B.; Li, S.; Zeng, L.; Chen, Y.; Fang, J. Mangiferin increases Nrf2 protein stability by inhibiting its ubiquitination and degradation in human HL60 myeloid leukemia cells. *Int. J. Mol. Med.* **2014**, *33*, 1348–1354. [CrossRef] [PubMed]

19. Jung, J.S.; Jung, K.; Kim, D.H.; Kim, H.S. Selective inhibition of MMP-9 gene expression by mangiferin in PMA-stimulated human astroglioma cells: Involvement of PI3K/Akt and MAPK signaling pathways. *Pharmacol. Res.* **2012**, *66*, 95–103. [CrossRef] [PubMed]

20. Das, J.; Ghosh, J.; Roy, A.; Sil, P.C. Mangiferin exerts hepatoprotective activity against D-galactosamine induced acute toxicity and oxidative/nitrosative stress via Nrf2-NFκB pathways. *Toxicol. Appl. Pharmacol.* **2012**, *260*, 35–47. [CrossRef] [PubMed]

21. Matkowski, A.; Kuś, P.; Góralska, E.; Woźniak, D. Mangiferin—A bioactive xanthonoid, not only from mango and not just antioxidant. *Mini Rev. Med. Chem.* **2013**, *13*, 439–455. [CrossRef] [PubMed]

22. Kavitha, M.; Nataraj, J.; Essa, M.M.; Memon, M.A.; Manivasagam, T. Mangiferin attenuates MPTP induced dopaminergic neurodegeneration and improves motor impairment, redox balance and Bcl-2/Bax expression in experimental Parkinson's disease mice. *Chem. Biol. Interact.* **2013**, *206*, 239–247. [CrossRef] [PubMed]

23. Tolosa, L.; Rodeiro, I.; Donato, M.T.; Herrera, J.A.; Delgado, R.; Castell, J.V.; Gómez-Lechón, M.J. Multiparametric evaluation of the cytoprotective effect of the Mangifera indica L. stem bark extract and mangiferin in HepG2 cells. *J. Pharm. Pharmacol.* **2013**, *65*, 1073–1082. [CrossRef] [PubMed]

24. Zou, T.; Wu, H.; Li, H.; Jia, Q.; Song, G. Comparison of microwave-assisted and conventional extraction of mangiferin from mango (Mangifera indica L.) leaves. *J. Sep. Sci.* **2013**, *36*, 3457–3462. [PubMed]

25. Chellan, N.; Joubert, E.; Strijdom, H.; Roux, C.; Louw, J.; Muller, C.J.F. Aqueous extract of unfermented honeybush (Cyclopia maculata) attenuates STZ-induced diabetes and β-cell cytotoxicity. *Planta Med.* **2014**, *80*, 622–629. [CrossRef] [PubMed]

26. Chavan, J.J.; Ghadage, D.M.; Kshirsagar, P.R.; Kudale, S.S. Optimization of extraction techniques and RP-HPLC analysis of antidiabetic and anticancer drug mangiferin from roots of saptarangi (Salacia chinensis L.). *J. Liq. Chromatogr. Relat. Technol.* **2015**, *38*, 963–969. [CrossRef]

27. Chavan, J.J.; Ghadage, D.M.; Bhoite, A.S.; Umdale, S.D. Micropropagation, molecular profiling and RP-HPLC determination of mangiferin across various regeneration stages of Saptarangi (Salacia chinensis L.). *Ind. Crops Prod.* **2015**, *76*, 1123–1132. [CrossRef]

28. Lei, J.; Zhou, C.; Hu, H.; Hu, L.; Zhao, M.; Yang, Y.; Chuai, Y.; Ni, J.; Cai, J. Mangiferin aglycone attenuates radiation-induced damage on human intestinal epithelial cells. *J. Cell. Biochem.* **2012**, *113*, 2633–2642. [CrossRef] [PubMed]

29. Duang, X.Y.; Wang, Q.; Zhou, X.D.; Huang, D.M. Mangiferin: A possible strategy for periodontal disease to therapy. *Med. Hypotheses* **2011**, *76*, 486–488. [CrossRef] [PubMed]

30. Kaivalya, M.; Rao, B.N.; Satish Rao, B.S. Mangiferin: A xanthone attenuates mercury chloride induced cytotoxicity and genotoxicity in HepG2 cells. *J. Biochem. Mol. Toxicol.* **2011**, *25*, 108–116. [CrossRef] [PubMed]

31. Barreto, J.C.; Trevisan, M.T.; Hull, W.E.; Erben, G.; de Brito, E.S.; Pfundstein, B.; Wurtele, G.; Spiegelhalder, B.; Owen, R.W. Characterization and quantitation of polyphenolic compounds in bark, kernel, leaves, and peel of mango (Mangifera indica L.). *J. Agric. Food Chem.* **2008**, *56*, 5599–5610. [CrossRef] [PubMed]

32. Hewavitharana, A.K.; Tan, Z.W.; Shimada, R.; Shaw, P.N.; Flanagan, B.M. Between fruit variability of the bioactive compounds, β-carotene and mangiferin, in mango (Mangifera indica). *Nutr. Diet.* **2013**, *70*, 158–163. [CrossRef]

33. Louisa, M.; Soediro, T.M.; Suyatna, F.D. In vitro modulation of P-glycoprotein, MRP-1 and BCRP expression by mangiferin in doxorubicin-treated MCF-7 cells. *Asian Pac. J. Cancer Prev.* **2014**, *15*, 1639–1642. [CrossRef] [PubMed]

34. Dou, W.; Zhang, J.; Ren, G.; Ding, L.; Sun, A.; Deng, C.; Wu, X.; Wei, X.; Mani, S.; Wang, Z. Mangiferin attenuates the symptoms of dextran sulfate sodium-induced colitis in mice via NF-κB and MAPK signaling inactivation. *Int. Immunopharmacol.* **2014**, *23*, 170–178. [CrossRef] [PubMed]

35. Pan, L.L.; Wang, A.Y.; Huang, Y.Q.; Luo, Y.; Ling, M. Mangiferin induces apoptosis by regulating Bcl-2 and bax expression in the CNE2 nasopharyngeal carcinoma cell line. *Asian Pac. J. Cancer Prev.* **2014**, *15*, 7065–7068. [CrossRef] [PubMed]

36. Kim, H.; Kim, H.; Mosaddik, A.; Gyawali, R.; Ahn, K.S.; Cho, S.K. Induction of apoptosis by ethanolic extract of mango peel and comparative analysis of the chemical constitutes of mango peel and flesh. *Food Chem.* **2012**, *133*, 416–422. [CrossRef] [PubMed]

37. Ramírez-Maganda, J.; Blancas-Benítez, F.J.; Zamora-Gasga, V.M.; García-Magaña, M.d.L.; Bello-Pérez, L.A.; Tovar, J.; Sáyago-Ayerdi, S.G. Nutritional properties and phenolic content of a bakery product substituted with a mango (Mangifera indica)'Ataulfo'processing by-product. *Food Res. Int.* **2015**, *73*, 117–123. [CrossRef]

38. Yatnatti, S.; Vijayalakshmi, D.; Chandru, R. Processing and Nutritive Value of Mango Seed Kernel Flour. *Curr. Res. Nutr. Food Sci. J.* **2014**, *2*, 170–175. [CrossRef]

39. Ajila, C.M.; Aalami, M.; Leelavathi, K.; Prasada Rao, U.J.S. Mango peel powder: A potential source of antioxidant and dietary fiber in macaroni preparations. *Innov. Food Sci. Emerg. Technol.* **2010**, *11*, 219–224. [CrossRef]

40. Bandyopadhyay, K.; Chakraborty, C.; Bhattacharyya, S. Fortification of Mango Peel and Kernel Powder in Cookies Formulation. *J. Acad. Ind. Res.* **2014**, *2*, 661.

41. García-Rivera, D.; Delgado, R.; Bougarne, N.; Haegeman, G.; Vanden Berghe, W. Gallic acid indanone and mangiferin xanthone are strong determinants of immunosuppressive anti-tumour effects of Mangifera indica L. bark in MDA-MB231 breast cancer cells. *Cancer Lett.* **2011**, *305*, 21–31. [CrossRef] [PubMed]

42. Zhang, B.; Fang, J.; Chen, Y. Antioxidant effect of mangiferin and its potential to be a cancer chemoprevention agent. *Lett. Drug Des. Discov.* **2013**, *10*, 239–244. [CrossRef]

43. Telang, M.; Dhulap, S.; Mandhare, A.; Hirwani, R. Therapeutic and cosmetic applications of mangiferin: A patent review. *Expert Opin. Ther. Pat.* **2013**, *23*, 1561–1580. [CrossRef] [PubMed]

44. Cheng, Z.Q.; Yang, D.; Ma, Q.Y.; Yi, X.H.; Zhou, J.; Zhao, Y.X. A new benzophenone from Dobinea delavayi. *Chem. Nat. Compd.* **2013**, *49*, 46–48. [CrossRef]

45. Xu, G.A. Drug Composition for Treating 2 Type Diabetes and its Chronicity Neopathy. Google Patents EP 2070540 A1, 17 June 2009.

46. Zhang, W.; Li, P.; Gong, Y.; Gao, X. Mangiferin Aglycone Crystal form i and Preparation Method Thereof. Google Patents EP 2716637 A1, 9 April 2014.

47. Ahmad, A.; Padhye, S.; Sarkar, F.H. Role of novel nutraceuticals garcinol, plumbagin and mangiferin in the prevention and therapy of human malignancies: Mechanisms of anticancer activity. In *Nutraceuticals and Cancer*; Springer: New York, NY, USA, 2012; Volume 1, pp. 179–199.

48. Du Plessis-Stoman, D.; du Preez, J.G.H.; Van de Venter, M. Combination treatment with oxaliplatin and Mangiferin Causes Increased Apoptosis and downregulation of NFκB in cancer cell lines. *AJOL* **2011**, *8*, 177–184.

49. Hudecová, A.; Kusznierewicz, B.; Rundén-Pran, E.; Magdolenová, Z.; Hašplová, K.; Rinna, A.; Fjellsbo, L.M.; Kruszewski, M.; Lankoff, A.; Sandberg, W.J.; et al. Silver nanoparticles induce premutagenic DNA oxidation that can be prevented by phytochemicals from Gentiana asclepiadea. *Mutagenesis* **2012**, *27*, 759–769. [CrossRef] [PubMed]

50. De Souza, J.R.R.; Feitosa, J.P.A.; Ricardo, N.M.P.S.; Trevisan, M.T.S.; de Paula, H.C.B.; Ulrich, C.M.; Owen, R.W. Spray-drying encapsulation of mangiferin using natural polymers. *Food Hydrocoll.* **2013**, *33*, 10–18. [CrossRef]

51. Kawpoomhae, K.; Sukma, M.; Ngawhirunpat, T.; Opanasopit, P.; Sripattanaporn, A. Antioxidant and neuroprotective effects of standardized extracts of Mangifera indica leaf. *Thai J. Pharm. Sci.* **2010**, *34*, 32–43.

52. Peng, Z.G.; Yao, Y.B.; Yang, J.; Tang, Y.L.; Huang, X. Mangiferin induces cell cycle arrest at G2/M phase through ATR-Chk1 pathway in HL-60 leukemia cells. *Genet. Mol. Res.* **2015**, *14*, 4989–5002. [CrossRef] [PubMed]

53. Hanahan, D.; Weinberg, R.A. Hallmarks of cancer: The next generation. *Cell* **2011**, *144*, 646–674. [CrossRef] [PubMed]

54. Pikarsky, E.; Porat, R.M.; Stein, I.; Abramovitch, R.; Amit, S.; Kasem, S.; Gutkovich-Pyest, E.; Urieli-Shoval, S.; Galun, E.; Ben-Neriah, Y. NF-κB functions as a tumour promoter in inflammation-associated cancer. *Nature* **2004**, *431*, 461–466. [CrossRef] [PubMed]

55. Vendramini-Costa, D.B.; Carvalho, J.E. Molecular link mechanisms between inflammation and cancer. *Curr. Pharm. Des.* **2012**, *18*, 3831–3852. [CrossRef] [PubMed]

56. Yao, J.; Hu, R.; Gou, Q.L. Inflammation and cancer. *Pharm. Biotechnol.* **2011**, *18*, 372–376.

57. Bhoj, V.G.; Chen, Z.J. Ubiquitylation in innate and adaptive immunity. *Nature* **2009**, *458*, 430–437. [CrossRef] [PubMed]

58. Rhyasen, G.W.; Starczynowski, D.T. IRAK signalling in cancer. *Br. J. Cancer* **2015**, *112*, 232–237. [CrossRef] [PubMed]

59. Tully, J.E.; Nolin, J.D.; Guala, A.S.; Hoffman, S.M.; Roberson, E.C.; Lahue, K.G.; van der Velden, J.; Anathy, V.; Blackwell, T.S.; Janssen-Heininger, Y.M.W. Cooperation between classical and alternative NF-κB pathways regulates proinflammatory Responses in Epithelial Cells. *Am. J. Respir. Cell Mol. Biol.* **2012**, *47*, 497–508. [CrossRef] [PubMed]

60. Jeong, J.J.; Jang, S.E.; Hyam, S.R.; Han, M.J.; Kim, D.H. Mangiferin ameliorates colitis by inhibiting IRAK1 phosphorylation in NF-kappaB and MAPK pathways. *Eur. J. Pharmacol.* **2014**, *740*, 652–661. [CrossRef] [PubMed]

61. Sahoo, B.K.; Zaidi, A.H.; Gupta, P.; Mokhamatam, R.B.; Raviprakash, N.; Mahali, S.K.; Manna, S.K. A natural xanthone increases catalase activity but decreases NF-kappa B and lipid peroxidation in U-937 and HepG2 cell lines. *Eur. J. Pharmacol.* **2015**, *764*, 520–528. [CrossRef] [PubMed]

62. Wee, Z.N.; Yatim, S.M.J.M.; Kohlbauer, V.K.; Feng, M.; Goh, J.Y.; Bao, Y.; Lee, P.L.; Zhang, S.; Wang, P.P.; Lim, E. IRAK1 is a therapeutic target that drives breast cancer metastasis and resistance to paclitaxel. *Nat. Commun.* **2015**, *6*, 8746. [CrossRef] [PubMed]

63. DiDonato, J.A.; Mercurio, F.; Karin, M. NF-kappaB and the link between inflammation and cancer. *Immunol. Rev.* **2012**, *246*, 379–400. [CrossRef] [PubMed]

64. Hoesel, B.; Schmid, J.A. The complexity of NF-kappaB signaling in inflammation and cancer. *Mol. Cancer* **2013**, *12*, 86. [CrossRef] [PubMed]

65. Belfiore, A.; Genua, M.; Malaguarnera, R. PPAR-agonists and their effects on IGF-I receptor signaling: Implications for cancer. *PPAR Res.* **2009**, *2009*, 18. [CrossRef] [PubMed]

66. Vandoros, G.P.; Konstantinopoulos, P.A.; Sotiropoulou-Bonikou, G.; Kominea, A.; Papachristou, G.I.; Karamouzis, M.V.; Gkermpesi, M.; Varakis, I.; Papavassiliou, A.G. PPAR-gamma is expressed and NF-kB pathway is activated and correlates positively with COX-2 expression in stromal myofibroblasts surrounding colon adenocarcinomas. *J. Cancer Res. Clin. Oncol.* **2006**, *132*, 76–84. [CrossRef] [PubMed]

67. Hugo, H.J.; Saunders, C.; Ramsay, R.G.; Thompson, E.W. New Insights on COX-2 in Chronic Inflammation Driving Breast Cancer Growth and Metastasis. *J. Mammary Gland Biol.* **2015**, *20*, 109–119. [CrossRef] [PubMed]

68. Mahmoud-Awny, M.; Attia, A.S.; Abd-Ellah, M.F.; El-Abhar, H.S. Mangiferin mitigates gastric ulcer in ischemia/reperfused rats: Involvement of PPAR-γ, NF-κB and Nrf2/HO-1 signaling pathways. *PLoS ONE* **2015**, *10*, e0132497. [CrossRef] [PubMed]

69. Santarpia, L.; Lippman, S.M.; El-Naggar, A.K. Targeting the MAPK-RAS-RAF signaling pathway in cancer therapy. *Expert Opin. Ther. Targets* **2012**, *16*, 103–119. [CrossRef] [PubMed]

70. Li, J.; Malakhova, M.; Mottamal, M.; Reddy, K.; Kurinov, I.; Carper, A.; Langfald, A.; Oi, N.; Kim, M.O.; Zhu, F.; et al. Norathyriol suppresses skin cancers induced by solar ultraviolet radiation by targeting ERK kinases. *Cancer Res.* **2012**, *72*, 260–270. [CrossRef] [PubMed]

71. Shimada, M.; Nakanishi, M. DNA damage checkpoints and cancer. *J. Mol. Histol.* **2006**, *37*, 253–260. [CrossRef] [PubMed]

72. Mitra, J.; Enders, G.H. Cyclin A/Cdk2 complexes regulate activation of Cdk1 and Cdc25 phosphatases in human cells. *Oncogene* **2004**, *23*, 3361–3367. [CrossRef] [PubMed]

73. Huang, H.; Nong, C.; Guo, L.; Meng, G.; Zha, X.L. The proliferation inhibition effect and apoptosis induction of Mangiferin on BEL-7404 human hepatocellular carcinoma cell. *Chin. J. Dig.* **2002**, *6*, 341–343.

74. Wilkinson, A.S.; Taing, M.W.; Pierson, J.T.; Lin, C.N.; Dietzgen, R.G.; Shaw, P.N.; Gidley, M.J.; Monteith, G.R.; Roberts-Thomson, S.J. Estrogen modulation properties of mangiferin and quercetin and the mangiferin metabolite norathyriol. *Food Funct.* **2015**, *6*, 1847–1854. [CrossRef] [PubMed]

75. Dilshara, M.G.; Kang, C.H.; Choi, Y.H.; Kim, G.Y. Mangiferin inhibits tumor necrosis factor-α-induced matrix metalloproteinase-9 expression and cellular invasion by suppressing nuclear factor-κB activity. *BMB Rep.* **2015**, *48*, 559–564. [CrossRef] [PubMed]

76. Roy, R.; Yang, J.; Moses, M.A. Matrix metalloproteinases as novel biomarker s and potential therapeutic targets in human cancer. *J. Clin. Oncol.* **2009**, *27*, 5287–5297. [CrossRef] [PubMed]

77. Bartoszewski, R.; Hering, A.; Marsza, M.; Hajduk, J.S.; Bartoszewska, S.; Kapoor, N.; Kochan, K.; Ochocka, R. Mangiferin has an additive effect on the apoptotic properties of hesperidin in Cyclopia sp. tea extracts. *PLoS ONE* **2014**, *9*, e92128. [CrossRef] [PubMed]

78. Salakou, S.; Kardamakis, D.; Tsamandas, A.C.; Zolota, V.; Apostolakis, E.; Tzelepi, V.; Papathanasopoulos, P.; Bonikos, D.S.; Papapetropoulos, T.; Petsas, T. Increased Bax/Bcl-2 ratio up-regulates caspase-3 and increases apoptosis in the thymus of patients with myasthenia gravis. *In Vivo* **2007**, *21*, 123–132. [PubMed]

79. Kavitha, M.; Manivasagam, T.; Essa, M.M.; Tamilselvam, K.; Selvakumar, G.P.; Karthikeyan, S.; Thenmozhi, J.A.; Subash, S. Mangiferin antagonizes rotenone: Induced apoptosis through attenuating mitochondrial dysfunction and oxidative stress in SK-N-SH neuroblastoma cells. *Neurochem. Res.* **2014**, *39*, 668–676. [CrossRef] [PubMed]

80. Cheng, P.; Peng, Z.; Yang, J.; Song, S. The effect of mangiferin on telomerase activity and apoptosis in Leukemic K562 cells. *Zhong Yao Cai* **2007**, *30*, 306–309. [PubMed]

81. Shay, J.W.; Wright, W.E. Role of telomeres and telomerase in cancer. *Semin. Cancer Biol.* **2012**, *21*, 349–353. [CrossRef] [PubMed]

82. Foresti, R. *Anti-Inflammatory and Antioxidant Activities of Nrf2/HO-1 Activators: In Vitro Studies in Microglia and Retinal Cells*; Univesity of Catania: Paris, France, 2014.

83. Menkovic, N.; Juranic, Z.; Stanojkovic, T.; Raonic-Stevanovic, T.; Šavikin, K.; Zdunić, G.; Borojevic, N. Radioprotective activity of Gentiana lutea extract and mangiferin. *Phytother. Res.* **2010**, *24*, 1693–1696. [CrossRef] [PubMed]

84. Valko, M.; Izakovic, M.; Mazur, M.; Rhodes, C.J.; Telser, J. Role of oxygen radicals in DNA damage and cancer incidence. *Mol. Cell. Biochem.* **2004**, *266*, 37–56. [CrossRef] [PubMed]

85. Chemocare.com. Oxaliplatin. Available online: http://www.chemocare.com/chemotherapy/drug-info/oxaliplatin.aspx (accessed on 2 September 2016).

86. Schonn, I.; Hennesen, J.; Dartsch, D.C. Cellular responses to etoposide: Cell death despite cell cycle arrest and repair of DNA damage. *Apoptosis* **2010**, *15*, 162–172. [CrossRef] [PubMed]

87. Carbonell-Capella, J.M.; Buniowska, M.; Barba, F.J.; Esteve, M.J.; Frígola, A. Analytical methods for determining bioavailability and bioaccessibility of bioactive compounds from fruits and vegetables: A review. *Compr. Rev. Food Sci. Food Saf.* **2014**, *13*, 155–171. [CrossRef]

88. McClements, D.J.; Li, F.; Xiao, H. The Nutraceutical Bioavailability Classification Scheme: Classifying Nutraceuticals According to Factors Limiting their Oral Bioavailability. *Ann. Rev. Food Sci. Technol.* **2015**, *6*, 299–327. [CrossRef] [PubMed]

89. Han, D.; Chen, C.; Zhang, C.; Zhang, Y.; Tang, X. Determination of mangiferin in rat plasma by liquid-liquid extraction with UPLC-MS/MS. *J. Pharm. Biomed. Anal.* **2010**, *51*, 260–263. [CrossRef] [PubMed]

90. Hou, S.; Wang, F.; Li, Y.; Li, Y.; Wang, M.; Sun, D.; Sun, C. Pharmacokinetic study of mangiferin in human plasma after oral administration. *Food Chem.* **2012**, *132*, 289–294. [CrossRef] [PubMed]

91. Liu, Y.; Xu, F.; Zeng, X.; Yang, L.; Deng, Y.; Wu, Z.; Feng, Y.; Li, X. Application of a liquid chromatography/tandem mass spectrometry method to pharmacokinetic study of mangiferin in rats. *J. Chromatogr. B* **2010**, *878*, 3345–3350. [CrossRef] [PubMed]

92. Kammalla, A.K.; Ramasamy, M.K.; Inampudi, J.; Dubey, G.P.; Agrawal, A.; Kaliappan, I. Comparative Pharmacokinetic Study of Mangiferin After Oral Administration of Pure Mangiferin and US Patented Polyherbal Formulation to Rats. *AAPS PharmSciTech* **2015**, *16*, 250–258. [CrossRef] [PubMed]

93. Ma, H.; Chen, H.; Sun, L.; Tong, L.; Zhang, T. Improving permeability and oral absorption of mangiferin by phospholipid complexation. *Fitoterapia* **2014**, *93*, 54–61. [CrossRef] [PubMed]

94. Al-Abd, A.M.; Aljehani, Z.K.; Gazzaz, R.W.; Fakhri, S.H.; Jabbad, A.H.; Alahdal, A.M.; Torchilin, V.P. Pharmacokinetic strategies to improve drug penetration and entrapment within solid tumors. *J. Control Release* **2015**, *219*, 269–277. [CrossRef] [PubMed]

95. Caro, C.; Pozo, D. Polysaccharide Colloids as Smart Vehicles in Cancer Therapy. *Curr. Pharm Des.* **2015**, *21*, 4822–4836. [CrossRef] [PubMed]

96. Prado, Y.; Merino, N.; Acosta, J.; Herrera, J.A.; Luque, Y.; Hernández, I.; Prado, E.; Garrido, G.; Delgado, R.; Rodeiro, I. Acute and 28-day subchronic toxicity studies of mangiferin, a glucosyl xanthone isolated from Mangifera indica L. stem bark. *J. Pharm. Pharm. Res.* **2015**, *3*, 13–23.

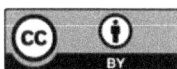

**MDPI**

*Commentary*

# Malignant Mesothelioma and Delivery of Polyphenols

**Karen S. Bishop [1],\*, Andrea J. Braakhuis [2] and Lynnette R. Ferguson [2]**

[1] Auckland Cancer Society Research Center, FM & HS, University of Auckland, Private Bag 92019, Auckland 1142, New Zealand

[2] Discipline of Nutrition and Dietetics, FM & HS, University of Auckland, Private Bag 92019, Auckland 1142, New Zealand; a.braakhuis@auckland.ac.nz (A.J.B.); l.ferguson@auckland.ac.nz (L.R.F.)

\* Correspondence: k.bishop@auckland.ac.nz; Tel.: +64-9-923-4471

Received: 31 May 2016; Accepted: 31 May 2016; Published: 2 June 2016

Malignant Mesothelioma (MM) is a rare form of cancer that affects the thin cell wall lining of the body's internal organs and structures. MM has a particularly poor outcome following standard treatment options. MM is found in the pleura, the peritoneum, and more rarely in the heart. MM is known only to be caused by exposure to asbestos fibres either directly, or through someone who was exposed, and this risk may be modified by genotype [1]. The disease develops through a multistep process resulting from chronic inflammation, DNA damage and dysregulation of the immune system. Benvenuto and colleagues from the University of Rome recently published an article of great public interest in the *Nutrients* Special Issue: Polyphenols for Cancer Treatment or Prevention, wherein they present current knowledge on the properties of polyphenols and protective effects against asbestos-mediated MM [2].

Polyphenols are commonly found in edible plants, are known to improve the immune function, reduce chronic inflammation [2], modify aberrant intraperitoneal cytokine levels [3] and reduce growth of cancer cells [2]. Benvenuto *et al.* list the various subclasses of polyphenols and their sources, and in addition, highlight the fact that a reduction in chronic inflammation may be the key to the prevention and/or stunted progression of MM [2].

Interestingly, Benvenuto *et al.* [2] provide a "profile" of up and down regulated cytokines for healthy subjects *vs.* asbestos exposed *vs.* MM patients. Upon further refinement, such profiles may be useful as a biomarker for MM risk and progression.

Despite the health benefits associated with polyphenols, the bioavailability of many polyphenol bioactives limits their effect. Problems with poor absorption, fast-metabolism and food preparation techniques, amongst others, remain to be solved. Importantly, Benvenuto *et al.* [2] have summarised the relevant published literature and suggest administering polyphenols to the serous cavity, so as to avoid problems associated with bioavailability and to deliver a clinically relevant dose to the tumour site. The location of MM tumours makes intratumoral administration feasible.

Bioavailability is a common problem whether we are considering the action of drugs or the clinical application of bioactives in foods. Granja and colleagues, from the University of Porto, Portugal, in a recent publication in the same *Nutrients* Special Issue, also recognise the need to improve stability and bioavailability of food bioactives that have shown promising anti-cancer activity *in vitro*. They reviewed published data and summarised various delivery systems for the polyphenol (−)-Epigallocatechin-3-gallate (EGCG). EGCG is most commonly associated with green tea, and is believed to work in synergy with various anti-cancer drugs [4]. Granja *et al.* [4] provide an overview of the nanotechnologies employed to overcome the poor pharmacokinetic and pharmacodynamics of this promising anti-cancer agent. In particular, gold nanoparticles; biodegradable, polymeric nanoparticles, functionalised with cell surface specific antibodies; as well as nanoliposomes [4], hold much promise for the delivery or co-delivery (with FDA approved anti-cancer drugs) of polyphenols as anti-cancer

*Nutrients* **2016**, *8*, 335

agents. Further research is required, but such an approach is likely to solve many of the challenges surrounding absorption and bioavailability of polyphenols to aid in the prevention and treatment of numerous cancers, as well as their treatment related side-effects.

**Conflicts of Interest:** The authors declare they have no conflict of interest.

## References

1. Tunesi, S.; Ferrante, D.; Mirabelli, D.; Andorno, S.; Betti, M.; Fiorito, G.; Guarrera, S.; Casalone, E.; Neri, M.; Ugolini, D.; *et al.* Gene–asbestos interaction in malignant pleural mesothelioma susceptibility. *Carcinogenesis* **2015**, *36*, 1129–1135. [CrossRef] [PubMed]
2. Benvenuto, M.; Mattera, R.; Taffera, G.; Giganti, M.G.; Lido, P.; Masuelli, L.; Modesti, A.; Bei, R. The Potential Protective Effects of Polyphenols in Asbestos-Mediated Inflammation and Carcinogenesis of Mesothelium. *Nutrients* **2016**, *8*, 275. [CrossRef]
3. Miller, J.M.; Thompson, J.K.; MacPherson, M.B.; Beuschel, S.L.; Westbom, C.M.; Sayan, M.; Shukla, A. Curcumin: A Double Hit on Malignant Mesothelioma. *Cancer Prev. Res. (Phila Pa)* **2014**, *7*, 330–340. [CrossRef] [PubMed]
4. Granja, A.; Pinheiro, M.; Reis, S. Epigallocatechin Gallate Nanodelivery Systems for Cancer Therapy. *Nutrients* **2016**, *8*, 307. [CrossRef] [PubMed]

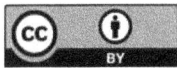

![nutrients logo] *nutrients*

MDPI

*Review*

# Epigallocatechin Gallate Nanodelivery Systems for Cancer Therapy

**Andreia Granja, Marina Pinheiro * and Salette Reis**

UCIBIO/REQUIMTE, Department of Chemical Sciences, Faculty of Pharmacy, University of Porto,
Rua de Jorge Viterbo Ferreira, 228, 4050-313 Porto, Portugal; bio11041@fe.up.pt (A.G.); shreis@ff.up.pt (S.R.)
* Correspondence: mpinheiro@ff.up.pt; Tel.: +351-220-428-672

Received: 23 March 2016; Accepted: 12 May 2016; Published: 20 May 2016

**Abstract:** Cancer is one of the leading causes of morbidity and mortality all over the world. Conventional treatments, such as chemotherapy, are generally expensive, highly toxic and lack efficiency. Cancer chemoprevention using phytochemicals is emerging as a promising approach for the treatment of early carcinogenic processes. (−)-Epigallocatechin-3-gallate (EGCG) is the major bioactive constituent in green tea with numerous health benefits including anti-cancer activity, which has been intensively studied. Besides its potential for chemoprevention, EGCG has also been shown to synergize with common anti-cancer agents, which makes it a suitable adjuvant in chemotherapy. However, limitations in terms of stability and bioavailability have hampered its application in clinical settings. Nanotechnology may have an important role in improving the pharmacokinetic and pharmacodynamics of EGCG. Indeed, several studies have already reported the use of nanoparticles as delivery vehicles of EGCG for cancer therapy. The aim of this article is to discuss the EGCG molecule and its associated health benefits, particularly its anti-cancer activity and provide an overview of the studies that have employed nanotechnology strategies to enhance EGCG's properties and potentiate its anti-tumoral activity.

**Keywords:** green tea; EGCG; cancer; nanotechnology; nanochemoprevention; anti-cancer therapy

## 1. Introduction

Cancer is a disease characterized by an excessive and uncontrolled growth of cells that can metastasize to several organs and eventually cause death of the host [1]. This disease is one of the leading causes of morbidity and mortality all over the world [2]. In 2012, approximately 14.1 million new cases were diagnosed and 8.2 million cancer-related deaths occurred worldwide [3]. By 2025, 19.3 million new cases are expected to emerge each year [4]. The costs associated with cancer are also a major matter of concern. In 2013, the total healthcare expenditure associated with cancer in the US was $74.8 billion [1]. Conventional treatments for the disease include surgery, hormone therapy, radiation and chemotherapy [1]. Chemotherapy is the main treatment for most cancers in advanced stage [5]. This therapeutic has, however, several limitations such as high costs, lack of efficiency and elevated toxicity, causing various side effects, including anemia, exhaustion, nausea and hair loss, which greatly impacts quality of life [5–7]. Therefore, it is essential to explore and develop novel strategies to minimize the undesirable effects of chemotherapy and increase its anti-cancer efficacy [5].

The use of natural compounds, such as phytochemicals has emerged as a potential strategy for cancer management. These compounds are of great interest due to their high spectrum of biological activity, low cost and minimal side effects [8,9]. One popular phytochemical with great potential is found in green tea, which is a healthy beverage consumed worldwide and produced from the leaves of *Camellia sinensis* [8,10]. (−)-Epigallocatechin-3-gallate (EGCG) is the most abundant and the most biologically active catechin in green tea and its role in cancer treatment has been intensively studied [11].

EGCG chemopreventive and chemotherapeutic activity has been demonstrated in several *in vitro* and *in vivo* animal studies [12–16]. The results have also been corroborated by various epidemiological and preclinical studies, which demonstrated a correlation between green tea regular consumption and cancer prevention and the inhibition of tumor progression [17–21]. In addition, EGCG offers several advantages over conventional therapies since it is widely available and inexpensive to isolate from green tea, it can be administered orally and it has an acceptable safety profile [22]. Despite its enormous potential as an anti-cancer agent, EGCG has a short half-life, low stability and low bioavailability, greatly limiting its use in clinical settings [8,23]. In a study developed by Nakagawa *et al.* [24] EGCG levels detected in plasma corresponded to only 0.2%–2% of the ingested amount. In addition, the effective anti-tumoral concentration of EGCG *in vitro* is generally an order of magnitude higher than the levels measured *in vivo*, which restricts its effectiveness [8]. Moreover, EGCG lacks target specificity [23]. Therefore, a strategy that increases EGCG stability and bioavailability and simultaneously targets cancer cells is necessary. Recently, the concept of nanochemoprevention was introduced [25]. This strategy consists of the use of nanotechnology to improve the pharmacokinetic and pharmacodynamic of chemopreventive agents in order to prevent, slow-down or revert cancer [25]. EGCG encapsulation into a specific nanocarrier can increase its solubility and bioavailability, protect it from premature degradation, prolong its circulation time and induce higher levels of target specificity due to the possibility of nanoparticle (NP) surface functionalization [25]. Several studies have already implemented this strategy encapsulating EGCG into different types of nanoparticles for cancer treatment [25].

The aim of this article is to provide a critical review of the EGCG molecule and its associated health benefits with a special focus on its anti-cancer activity. In addition, an overview of the applications that used nanotechnology strategies to deliver EGCG to cancer cells will also be given.

## 2. EGCG

### 2.1. Source and Chemical Structure

Green tea is composed of different chemical compounds, such as amino acids, vitamins, inorganic elements, carbohydrates, lipids, caffeine and tea polyphenols [26]. Polyphenols constitute about 30% of the dry weight of green tea leaves and are the main compound responsible for its health promoting effects [27]. Catechins form the major group of polyphenols found in green tea and comprise different molecules such as (−)-Epicatechin (EC), (−)-Epicatechin-3-gallate (ECG), (−)-Epigallocatechin (EGC), and (−)-Epigallocatechin-3-gallate (EGCG) [28]. The chemical structures of catechins are represented in Figure 1.

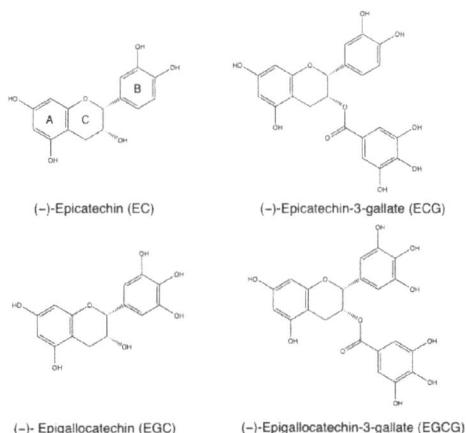

**Figure 1.** Chemical structure of (−)-Epicatechin (EC), (−)-Epicatechin-3-gallate (ECG), (−)-Epigallocatechin (EGC) and (−)-Epigallocatechin-3-gallate (EGCG).

These molecules are composed of a polyphenolic structure that allows electron delocalization, enabling the quenching of free radicals [29]. Catechins are characterized by a dihydroxyl or trihydroxyl substitution on the B ring, a meta-5, 7-dihydroxyl substitutions on the A ring and, in the case of the galloylated catechins ECG and EGCG, the trihydroxyl substitutions on the D ring [29]. EGCG is the major catechin and the most biologically active compound, accounting for 50%–80% of the total catechins in green tea [5,12]. This molecule has a trihydroxyl substitution on the B ring and a gallate moiety esterified at carbon 3 on the C ring [28]. These structural characteristics contribute to its increased anti-oxidant and iron-chelating activities [28]. Tea catechins, particularly EGCG, have several pharmacological and biological properties, such as anti-oxidant, free radical scavenging [30,31], anti-bacterial [32,33], anti-viral [34–36], anti-diabetic [37–40], cardioprotective, anti-atherosclerotic, anti-inflammatory [41–46], anti-obesity [47], neuroprotective [48–50] and anti-carcinogenic effects [12–21]. The latter, in particular, has been intensively studied [12–21].

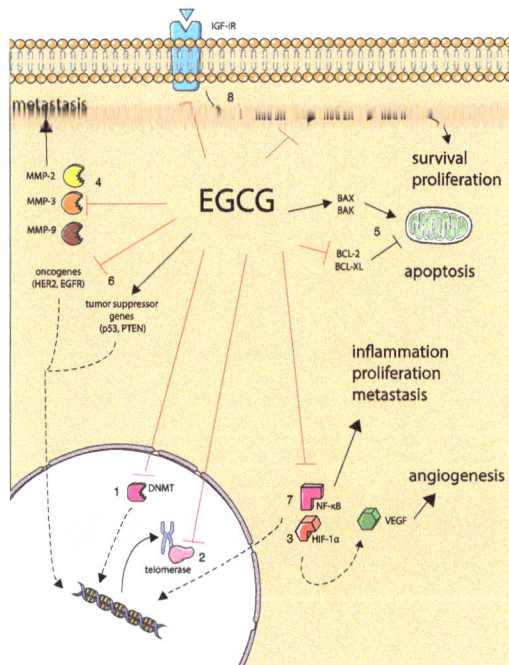

**Figure 2.** Cancer-related cell mechanisms modulated by EGCG: (**1**) Inhibition of DNA hypermethylation by direct blocking of DNA methyltransferase (DNMT); (**2**) Repression of telomerase activity; (**3**) Inhibition of angiogenesis by repression of transcription factors Hypoxia-inducible factor 1-α (HIF-1α) and Nuclear factor kappa B (NF-κB); (**4**) Blocking of cell metastasis by inhibition of Matrix metalloproteinases (MMPs) -2, -9 and -3; (**5**) Promotion of cancer cell apoptosis by induction of pro-apoptotic proteins BCL-2-associated X protein (BAX) and BCL-2 homologous antagonist killer (BAK) and repression of anti-apoptotic proteins B-cell lymphoma 2 (BCL-2) and B cell lymphoma-extra large (BCL-XL); (**6**) Induction of tumor suppressor genes *p53* and *Phosphatase and tensin homolog* (*PTEN*) and inhibition of oncogenes *Human epidermal growth factor receptor 2* (*HER2*) and *Epidermal growth factor receptor* (*EGFR*); (**7**) Inhibition of NF-κB and subsequent events of cell inflammation, proliferation, metastasis and angiogenesis; and (**8**) Anti-proliferative activity by inhibition of Mitogen-activated protein kinases (MAPK) pathway and Insulin-like growth factor I receptor (IGFIR).

*2.2. Anti-Cancer Activity*

EGCG has been shown to play a significant role as an anti-cancer agent. Cancer is a disease characterized by an abnormal growth of cells, which generates excessive cell proliferation over cell death [51]. This imbalance culminates in the formation of a group of cells that can invade tissues and metastasize to distant regions, causing morbidity and, eventually, death of the host [51]. Cancer is associated with multiple changes in gene expression, which affect the normal mechanisms of cell division and differentiation [51]. The factors that trigger these alterations are not clearly defined in most cases, however, it is established that both external (such as an unhealthy diet, chemicals, tobacco and radiation) and internal (such as inherited genetic mutations and immune conditions) factors may have an impact in the onset of the disease [51]. EGCG's anti-tumoral effects have been demonstrated both in cell culture and animal experiments and in epidemiological and clinical studies [12–21].

EGCG is involved in numerous signaling pathways and biological mechanisms related with cancer development and progression (Figure 2), discussed in more detail below.

2.2.1. DNA Hypermethylation

DNA methylation is a biochemical modification that consists of the addition of a methyl group to a cytosine within a CpG site, a process that is performed by the enzyme DNA methyltransferase (DNMT) [52]. Hypermethylation usually inhibits the binding of the transcription factors to the promoter region, which induces gene silencing [53]. This process occurs frequently during cancer development with inhibition of cell cycle regulator, receptor and apoptotic genes [54]. It has been demonstrated that EGCG has the ability to directly block DNMTs, and consequently, restore the expression of these genes, which may have an impact on cancer progression [55].

2.2.2. Telomerase Activity

Telomeres are regions localized at the end of eukaryotic chromosomes responsible for DNA protection and genomic stability [56]. Telomerase is a reverse transcriptase responsible for telomere preservation [56]. These enzymes were found to be upregulated in various types of tumors [57]. Different studies demonstrated the capacity of EGCG to inhibit telomerase activity in different cancer cell lines including lung carcinoma [58], cervical cancer [59], leukemia and adenocarcinoma cells [60], thus emphasizing its potential to block the development and progression of these tumors.

2.2.3. Angiogenesis

Tumor angiogenesis is one of the hallmarks of cancer with a huge impact on tumor progression [61]. It consists of the recruitment of blood vessels to the tumor site, to assure oxygen and nutrient supply [62]. Angiogenesis is stimulated by several different factors, including Vascular Endothelial Growth Factor (VEGF) [63]. Various studies described that EGCG can significantly inhibit VEGF expression through repression of transcription factors Hypoxia-inducible factor 1-$\alpha$ (HIF-1$\alpha$) and Nuclear factor kappa B (NF-$\kappa$B), thus suppressing angiogenesis [64–66]. *In vivo* studies using nude mice also corroborated this capacity, showing an inhibition of vascularity and tumor growth and proliferation after treatment with EGCG [65,67].

2.2.4. Metastasis

Another cancer hallmark is cell metastasis, which is an extension of cell invasion [62]. After invasion, cancer cells can pass through the extracellular matrix and enter into the bloodstream, being able to disseminate and create a new niche in another location, forming a metastatic focus [61]. To metastasize, tumor cells have to degrade the basement membrane and the stroma, which is possible through the secretion of specific proteases called Matrix metalloproteinases (MMPs) [61]. Inhibition of these MMPs has been revealed to inhibit metastasis and tumor growth in mouse xenograft models [61]. EGCG has demonstrated ability to prevent cancer cell metastasis, due to inhibition of matrix MMPs -2, -3 and -9, which play an important role in metastasis, via direct binding and gene expression repression [68–71].

### 2.2.5. Cancer Cell Apoptosis

Apoptosis is the process of programmed cell death that often culminates in the activation of cysteine-aspartic proteases (caspases), which are responsible for the cleavage of intra-cellular proteins triggering sequential events that will culminate into induction of cell death [72]. Two main pathways can induce this event: extrinsic and intrinsic pathway [72]. In the extrinsic pathway, apoptosis is triggered by the binding of death ligands to death receptors, which induces intra-cellular signaling mechanisms that activate caspases [72]. In the intrinsic pathway, activation of pro-apoptotic proteins BCL-2-associated X protein (BAX) and BCL-2 homologous antagonist killer (BAK) promotes the release of proteins from the mitochondria leading to the formation of the apoptosome and culminating in the activation of caspases [72]. The regulation of this pathway is done by apoptosis inhibitors, such as B-cell lymphoma 2 (BCL-2) and B cell lymphoma-extra large (BCL-XL), which antagonize with BAX and BAK [72]. The apoptotic pathways described above are often downregulated in cancer [72,73]. As a consequence, apoptosis has been widely studied as a target for anti-cancer therapies [72]. Different studies have demonstrated that EGCG can inhibit the expression of the anti-apoptotic proteins BCL-2 and BCL-XL and induce the expression of apoptotic proteins BAX and BAK, with subsequent activation of caspases in several types of cancers [73–76]. In addition, EGCG has revealed ability to induce $H_2O_2$ production [77], block cell cycle progression [78] and inhibit NF-κB [79,80], events which will also induce apoptosis.

### 2.2.6. Tumor Suppressor Genes and Oncogenes Expression

Tumor suppressor genes are genes that reduce the probability of a normal cell to become a tumor cell [81]. These genes are usually associated with cell cycle arrest and apoptosis induction triggered by DNA damage [81]. Mutations in tumor suppressor genes severely increase the probability of cancer development [81]. In fact, their inactivation has been observed in several types of tumors [81]. EGCG has revealed capacity to increase the expression of tumor suppressor gene *p53* [82,83] and *Phosphatase and tensin homolog (PTEN)* [84] and cyclin-dependent kinase inhibitors *p21* and *p27* [83,85] in different cancer cell lines, including breast, pancreas and prostate cancer. Oncogenes are mutated genes that have influence on the development of cancer [86]. There are several types of oncogenes, whose function is usually associated with cell proliferation, such as *Epidermal growth factor receptor (EGFR)* and *Human epidermal growth factor receptor 2 (HER2)*. These genes are frequently overexpressed in several types of cancers [87,88]. Some studies revealed that EGCG is able to inhibit the activation of HER2 and EGFR in different cancer cells lines, such as, lung, thyroid, breast cancer and squamous-cell carcinoma [89–92].

### 2.2.7. NF-κB Activation and Nuclear Translocation

NF-κB is a family of transcription factors activated by numerous stimuli, amongst them free radicals, inflammatory signals, cytokines, carcinogens, UV-light and tumor promoters [93]. After activation, NF-κB migrates to the nucleus and induces the expression of genes responsible for the suppression of apoptosis, inflammation, proliferation and metastasis [93]. Different studies showed that EGCG can efficiently inhibit the activation and nuclear translocation of this transcription factor, preventing the subsequent events related to cancer progression in different types of tumor cell lines, including epidermoid carcinoma cells [94], bladder [95], breast, and head and neck [96] cancer cells.

### 2.2.8. Anti-Proliferative Activity

EGCG revealed anti-proliferative ability on cancer cells by inhibiting mitogenic signal transduction pathways. Mitogen-activated protein kinases (MAPK) are protein kinases involved in the cytoplasmic phase of the signaling pathway initiated by the binding of growth factor to a transmembrane receptor [97]. These pathways are responsible for cell survival and proliferation and are highly related to cancer development [97]. EGCG has proven its ability to inhibit MAPK pathway in different cancer cell types, such as colon [98], endometrial [99] and leukemia [100]. In addition EGCG was shown to directly bind and inhibit Insulin-like growth factor I receptor (IGFIR) activity, which is one of the receptors than can lead to activation of the MAPK pathway and plays an important role in cell proliferation [101,102].

### 2.2.9. Protein Binding

The anticancer effects of EGCG may be explained in part due to its capacity to bind directly to several proteins involved in different cell mechanisms such as proliferation, apoptosis and metastasis. Suzuki *et al.* showed that EGCG can bind to plasma protein fibrinogen and cell adhesive proteins fibronectin and laminin [103,104]. These interactions may be related to the capacity of EGCG to inhibit metastasis [105]. EGCG has also been shown to directly bind to Fas, triggering Fas-mediated apoptosis [106]. This may be one of the main mechanisms by which EGCG induces apoptosis in cancer cells [106]. Tachibana *et al.* identified 67-kDa laminin receptor as a mediator of EGCG anticancer effects (67LR) [107]. Ermakova *et al.* [108] demonstrated that EGCG binds to vimentin, a protein responsible for mitosis, locomotion and structural integrity, and inhibits its phosphorylation, decreasing cell proliferation. The same authors found other relevant proteins inhibited by EGCG via direct binding such as the chaperone protein glucose-regulated protein 78 (GRP78), whose anti-apoptotic effects are related to chemotherapeutic drug resistance [109], IGFIR, highly associated with cell proliferation and cancer development [102] and the tyrosine kinases Fyn [110] and ZAP-70 [111]. Other EGCG-binding proteins were also identified such as Ras-GTPase-activating protein SH3 domain-binding protein 1 (G3BP1) [112] and peptidyl prolyl cis/trans isomerase (Pin1) [113], both involved in oncogenic cell signaling pathways.

### 2.2.10. *In Vivo* Experiments

Inhibition of tumorigenesis by EGCG was also demonstrated *in vivo* in mice models for different types of cancer, including breast [13], lung [14], intestine [15], skin [16] and prostate [114].

### 2.2.11. Clinical Studies

Different clinical studies have corroborated the *in vitro* results. Patients with papilloma virus-infected cervical lesions were treated with 200 mg capsules of EGCG or green tea extracts and the treatment demonstrated effectiveness, with a 69% response rate [115]. Bettuzzi *et al.* demonstrated that daily administration of 600 mg of EGCG was effective in treating premalignant lesions in men with high-grade prostate intraepithelial neoplasia [18]. Consistent with this, McLarty *et al.* developed a phase II clinical trial in prostate carcinoma patients demonstrating a significant reduction in the levels of different cancer-related biomarkers in serum after oral administration of 800 mg of EGCG [116]. On the other hand, in a phase II study after administration of daily doses of EGCG to 42 androgen independent prostate cancer patients, only limited antineoplasic activity was detected [117].

### 2.2.12. Epidemiological Data

Different epidemiological studies have addressed the effects of green tea and particularly EGCG, in prevention and treatment of cancer, further supporting the *in vitro* and *in vivo* results. A prospective cohort study with over 8000 individuals found that daily consumption of green tea delayed cancer onset [17]. Additionally, a follow up study with stages I and II breast cancer patients, determined lower recurrence rate and longer disease-free period after daily consumption of green tea [17]. Green tea daily consumption has also demonstrated a preventive effect against prostate cancer [19]. A prospective cohort study also revealed that green tea consumption is inversely associated with distal gastric cancer occurrence among women [20]. In this study, participants who consumed five or more cups per day had 49% less risk of having gastric tumors in the distal portion compared with the ones who drank less than 1 cup per day [20]. More recently, the protective role of green tea against stomach cancer was also demonstrated in a meta-analysis, where a reduction of 14% in the risk of stomach cancer with high green tea consumption was determined [21]. On the other hand, there are also many studies where weak or no association between cancer risk and green tea consumption was found as reported by Zhou *et al.* [118], Lin *et al.* [119] and Sasazuki *et al.* [120] For a more detailed review on this subject, see [121]. These differences in results may be explained in part by the low levels of EGCG present in the blood following green tea consumption, which may be insufficient to induce a chemopreventive effect [121].

The vast majority of these studies highlight the importance of EGCG in cancer and the pertinence of exploiting it in anti-tumoral therapy. Conventional treatments against cancer often consist of the administration of cytostatic drugs, which present several limitations. One of the most relevant is the lack of precision, which implies that only a small part of the drug reaches the tumor region, reducing the efficacy of the drug and causing systemic toxicity [122]. Another drawback is the fact that the drugs are also toxic to healthy cells, including bone marrow and gastrointestinal cells [122]. All these factors contribute to the well-known side effects associated with chemotherapy such as nausea, fatigue and hair loss [122]. EGCG can be used as an adjuvant in chemotherapy [123] lowering the doses of the cytostatic drugs used in chemotherapy and, consequently, the associated toxicity and side effects.

## 3. Nanotechnology and Nanochemoprevention

Nanotechnology is an interdisciplinary field that comprises the areas of biology, engineering, chemistry and medicine and relies on the use of nanosystems, which are man-made devices with at least one dimension in the range of 1–100 nanometers [124]. Nanotechnology is currently being studied and implemented in diagnosis and treatment of cancer, with the development of nanosensor devices and nanovectors [124]. Nanovectors include nanoparticles (NPs) for loading drugs or imaging agents and subsequent delivery and targeting to tumor cells [124]. A wide variety of different nanoparticles may be applied to develop anti-cancer drug delivery systems, including liposomes, magnetic NPs, polymeric NPs, among many others [124]. The potential of nanoparticles as anti-cancer drug delivery systems is enormous since they increase the absorption, solubility and bioavailability of the drug, protect it from premature degradation and extend its circulation time [23,124,125]. In addition, NPs can increase drug retention in tumor tissues, due to the enhanced permeability and retention effect (EPR), facilitate intra-cellular penetration, increase target specificity due to the possibility of surface functionalization and minimize drug toxic effects [23]. Furthermore, they enable oral administration of the drug, which is the preferred delivery route in terms of patient compliance and convenience [126].

Chemoprevention is a promising strategy that consists of the use of natural and synthetic compounds, such as EGCG, as a strategy for cancer prevention, slowdown or reversion [124]. Despite its potential, the efficiency of this approach is still limited due to toxicity and ineffective systemic delivery and bioavailability [25]. To overcome these limitations, Siddiqui *et al.* [25] introduced the concept of nanochemoprevention, which consists of the use of nanotechnology to improve the pharmacokinetic and pharmacodynamic of chemopreventive agents in order to manage cancer. In addition to chemopreventive applications, EGCG may also have a relevant role as an adjuvant in chemotherapy. Indeed, EGCG has already been shown to synergize with common anti-cancer agents such as doxorubicin, tamoxifen and paclitaxel in multiple cell lines [123]. Several studies reported in the literature have already applied nanotechnology strategies, using different types of nanoparticles as delivery vehicles of EGCG to target different types of cancer both *in vitro* and *in vivo*. These reports are discussed below in more detail grouped according to the type of nanoparticle used. The main strategies followed are schematically represented in Figure 3.

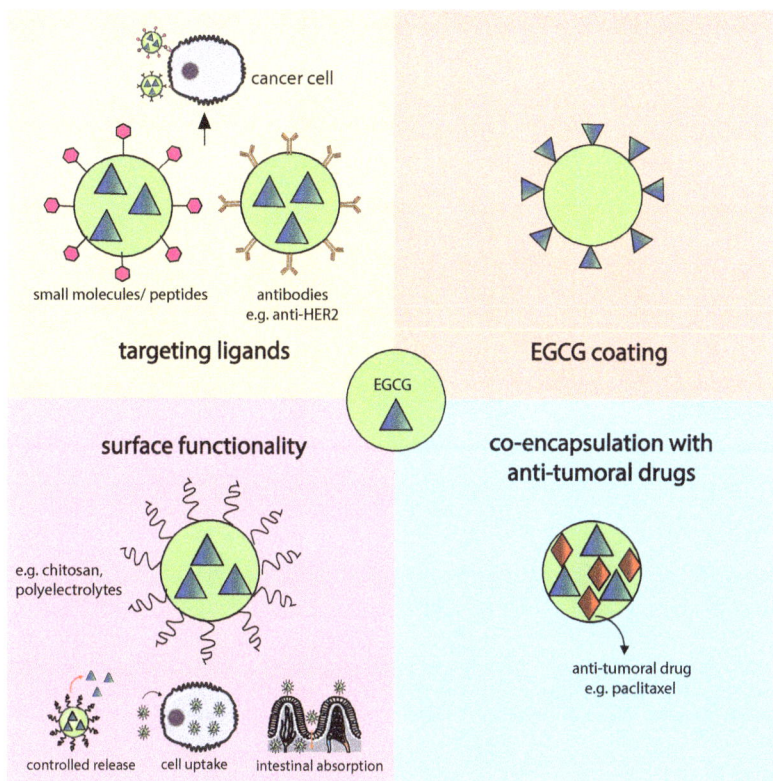

**Figure 3.** Summary of EGCG delivery approaches for cancer therapy reported in the literature: (**1**) incorporation of ligands (small molecules, peptides and antibodies) at the surface of the nanoparticle to target specific cancer cell receptors or antigens; (**2**) use of EGCG as a capping agent; (**3**) surface functionalization with specific polymers to enhance drug release properties, cell uptake and intestinal absorption; and (**4**) co-encapsulation with common cytostatic drugs such as paclitaxel.

### 3.1. Gold Nanoparticles

Gold nanoparticles present unique physicochemical properties, such as small size, plasmon resonance, capacity to bind amine and thiol groups, high atomic number and biocompatibility [127]. Synthesis of these NPs usually involves the reduction of Au (III) derivatives, such as Chloroauric acid ($HAuCl_4$) [127]. Generally, an aqueous solution of $HAuCl_4$ is mixed with an aqueous solution of a reducing agent, which leads to the reduction of $Au^{3+}$ and formation of gold nanoparticles [127]. Polyphenols may act as both reducing and capping agents of this process as reported by Nune *et al.* [128]. This approach avoids the use of an additional synthetic chemical reagent, which makes it a green chemistry process [128].

Due to their distinctive properties, gold NPs have been exploited in several biomedical applications as biosensors, contrast agents, drug delivery vehicles and anti-tumoral agents [125,129]. Gold NPs are suitable anti-cancer agents mainly due to their small size, which enables them to penetrate in the tissues and accumulate in the tumor site and their optical properties, which allow their use in photothermal anti-cancer therapies [125].

Several reports have described the effect of gold NPs in conjugation with EGCG for cancer treatment. The main results of these studies, including nanoparticle type, size, zeta potential, loading capacity (LC) encapsulation efficiency (EE) and *in vitro* and *in vivo* evaluation are summarized in Table 1.

**Table 1.** Gold nanoparticles used as EGCG nanocarriers for cancer therapy.

| Composition | Size (nm) | Zeta Potential (mV) | LC (%) | EE (%) | Route of Administration | *In Vitro/In Vivo* Results | Reference |
|---|---|---|---|---|---|---|---|
| Gold (EGCG/pNG 50 μM: 1.5 ppm) | 20–1200 | +21 ± 5 | N/A | N/A | Oral Intra-tumoral or intra-peritoneal | High cytotoxicity towards bladder cancer cells (MBT-2) Marked reduction in tumor volume in bladder cancer xenograft model further accentuated via the intra-tumoral and intra-peritoneal administration route | [130] |
| Gold (EGCG/pNG 50 μM: 2.5 ppm) | 64.7 | −3.36 | 27 | N/A | intra-tumoral | High cytotoxicity towards B16F10 murine melanoma cells Reduction in tumor volume in a mouse melanoma model | [125] |
| Gold | 25.55 ± 7.26 | N/A | N/A | N/A | N/A | Retention of EGCG's anti-oxidant activity Induction of apoptosis in neuroblastoma SH-SY5Y-CFP-DEVD-YFP cells | [131] |
| Gold | 45 | +43 | N/A | N/A | N/A | High toxicity towards EAC cells and protection of normal mouse hepatocytes | [11] |

Hsieh *et al.* [130] coated gold NPs with EGCG (EGCG-pNG) through an ultrasonication process and tested their effect in the treatment of bladder cancer both *in vitro* and *in vivo*. Their results showed that this strategy induced high levels of cytotoxicity in bladder cancer cells (MBT-2) without affecting the viability of normal cells (Vero cells). Treatment with EGCG-pNG was shown to induce apoptosis through triggering the intrinsic apoptotic pathway via the activation of caspases-3 and -7. *In vivo* tests confirmed these results. C3H/HeN mice subcutaneously implanted with MBT-2 cells revealed a significantly higher reduction in tumor volume after oral administration of EGCG-pNG in comparison with free EGCG. In addition, NPs were also administered via intra-tumoral and intra-peritoneal. These previous two administration routes were more effective than oral administration in suppressing tumor growth. In a more recent work, the same group [125] tested the efficiency of similar NPs against melanoma both *in vivo* and *in vitro*. *In vitro* results showed that gold NPs induced 4.91 times higher levels of apoptosis in B16F10 murine melanoma cells compared to non-encapsulated EGCG. Apoptosis was caused by activation of a mitochondrial-mediated pathway. This nanocarrier also demonstrated a high biocompatibility, inducing low damage to human red blood cells. *In vivo* results demonstrated that intra-tumoral injection of EGCG NPs induced a reduction in the tumor volume of a mouse melanoma model compared with the control treatment. This ability to inhibit tumor growth was 1.66 times higher when EGCG was encapsulated compared to free EGCG.

Sanna *et al.* [131] synthesized gold NPs using a similar process to the one described by Nune *et al.* [128]. EGCG-conjugated gold nanoparticles revealed high stability in simulated biological fluids and were able to retain EGCG's anti-oxidant activity [131]. In addition, the nanoparticles were efficient in inducing apoptosis (through activation of caspase-3) in neuroblastoma SH-SY5Y-CFP-DEVD-YFP cells in a concentration dependent-manner after 72 h of exposure. The authors concluded that the efficiency of EGCG was maintained after adsorption to the surface of gold NPs. The same chemical process for the synthesis of gold NPs was replicated recently by Mukherjee *et al.* also with encouraging results [11]. EGCG-conjugated gold NPs revealed higher anti-oxidant activity, cellular internalization and cytotoxicity towards tumor cells than EGCG in a free form. At the same dose (20 μg/mL), EGCG NPs induced 30% more cell death in Ehrlich's Ascites Carcinoma (EAC) cells than native EGCG. Apoptosis was induced due to an increase in lipid peroxidation and in the levels of ROS. A reduction in the levels of anti-oxidant enzymes, such as glutathione was observed as well as an inhibition of the nuclear translocation of the transcription factor NF-κB and subsequent activation of its downstream survival molecules. On the other hand, in normal primary mouse hepatocytes, EGCG NPs promoted an increase in the levels of anti-oxidant enzymes, protecting the cells against tumor-induced cellular damage. The results revealed that these NPs are able to induce tumor cell apoptosis and simultaneously protect hepatocytes against undesirable effects.

### 3.2. Polymeric Nanoparticles

Polymeric NPs present important characteristics, which make them suitable for biomedical applications, such as biocompatibility, biodegradability, with the possibility of controlling the rate of polymer degradation, mechanical strength, and high structure versatility [132,133].

Several polymers, natural or synthetic, can be employed to produce polymeric NPs, the most common include polycaprolactone (PCL), polylactic acid (PLA), poly (lactic-co-glycolic acid) (PLGA), chitosan and gelatin [134]. PLA and PLGA are approved and recognized as safe by the US Food and Drug Administration (FDA) for human applications and are metabolized in the organism into biodegradable biocompatible monomers (lactic and glycolic acid) [134]. Intravenous injection of PLGA and PLA usually leads to their rapid clearance by the immune system [25]. To increase their circulation time, NPs are frequently coated with PEG, also approved by the FDA, which stabilizes and avoids their recognition by the immune system [25]. Chitosan is a natural polymer characterized by its non-toxic, non-immunogenic and mucoadhesive properties in the gastrointestinal tract, which makes it suitable for oral routes of administration [126]. Gelatin is intensively used in food and medical products and it is also a non-toxic biodegradable polymer [134]. It is characterized by its mechanical, thermal and swelling properties, which are highly dependent on the degree of crosslinking [134]. Several groups have already encapsulated EGCG into different polymeric NPs for cancer therapy. The main findings from these studies are shown in Table 2.

**Table 2.** Polymeric nanoparticles used as EGCG nanocarriers for cancer therapy.

| Composition | Size (nm) | Zeta Potential (mV) | LC (%) | EE (%) | Route of Administration | *In Vitro/In Vivo* Results | Reference |
|---|---|---|---|---|---|---|---|
| PLGA-PEG | 80.53 ± 15 | N/A | N/A | 9.61 ± 0.7 | N/A | Increased cytotoxicity towards PSMA-positive LNCaP prostate cancer cell line | [135] |
| PLGA | 127.2 ± 12 | −24.5 ± 1.89 | N/A | 6 | N/A | Increase in DNA damage levels of oxaliplatin- and satraplatin-treated lymphocytes from colorectal and healthy cancer patients | [132] |
| PLGA-casein | 190–250 | −41 ± 3.4 | N/A | 76.8 ± 9.1 | N/A | Inhibition of NF-κB signaling Enhanced cytotoxicity towards breast cancer cells (MDA-MB-231 cell line and patient-derived cells) | [136,137] |
| PLA-PEG | 260 | −7.92 | N/A | N/A | Intra-tumoral | High induction of apoptosis in prostate cancer PC3 cell line; inhibition of angiogenesis Significant decrease in tumor size in prostate cancer xenograft model | [25] |
| Chitosan | 150–200 | N/A | N/A | 10 | Oral | Higher inhibiton of tumor growth in prostate cancer xenograft model Inhibition of cancer cell proliferation and angiogenesis. | [126] |

Table 2. *Cont.*

| Composition | Size (nm) | Zeta Potential (mV) | LC (%) | EE (%) | Route of Administration | *In Vitro/In Vivo* Results | Reference |
|---|---|---|---|---|---|---|---|
| Chitosan | N/A | N/A | N/A | N/A | Oral | High cytoxicity against Mel 928 human melanoma cells Inhibition of tumor growth in melanoma xenograft model | [138] |
| CPP-chitosan | 245.3 ± 18.3 | 32.4 ± 6.1 | N/A | 71 | N/A | Higher stability in simulated GI tract conditions Maintenance of EGCG anti-tumoral activity against gastrointestinal cancer cell line BGC823 | [139] |
| Gelatin | 200 | N/A | N/A | 20–70 | N/A | Sustained release of EGCG Ability to inhibit HGF in MDA-MD-231 breast cancer cell line | [8] |

Sanna *et al.* [135] designed EGCG-loaded PLGA-PEG NPs for treatment against prostate cancer. In this study, the function of the NPs was enhanced with a prostate-specific membrane antigen (PSMA) ligand (DCL). These NPs allowed a greater control of the rate of release of EGCG relative to that of free EGCG. Encapsulation and functionalization with DCL increased the cytotoxicity of the NPs towards LNCaP prostate cancer cell line, which were PSMA-positive. On the other hand, no significant inhibition of cell growth inhibition was detected in HUVECs (human umbilical vein endothelial cells). These results suggest that PLA-PEG-DCL EGCG-loaded NPs were able to efficiently kill PSMA-positive prostate cancer cells without influencing the viability of normal cells.

Alotaibi *et al.* [132] also prepared PLGA NPs for EGCG encapsulation. The DNA damage effect of these NPs was tested against lymphocytes of healthy and colorectal cancer patients pretreated with oxaliplatin of satraplatin. The obtained results suggest that encapsulated EGCG significantly intensified DNA damage levels in a dose-dependent way. In contrast, free EGCG promoted a reduction in DNA damage. The authors suggested that this catechin might alternate between an anti-oxidant (bulk form) and a pro-oxidant (encapsulated form) state.

Narayanan *et al.* [136] synthesized PLGA-casein NPs constituted by a core and a shell, where paclitaxel and EGCG, respectively, were entrapped. This organization enabled a sequential and controlled release of both drugs. Nanocarriers revealed a longer circulatory lifespan and increased biocompatibility both *in vitro* and *in vivo*. In a more recent study, the same authors tested the chemotherapeutic effect against breast cancer cells (MDA-MB-231 cells and patient-derived tumor cells) [137]. With that purpose some of the NPs were functionalized with antibodies specific for the cell surface receptors anti-EGFR and anti-HER2. The results showed an enhanced cellular uptake by MDA-MB-231 cells and a higher rate of apoptosis compared with individually encapsulated paclitaxel and EGCG. Both results were improved when NPs were functionalized with anti-EGFR. This therapy also showed an inhibitory effect in the protein levels of NF-κB, a signaling molecule activated by paclitaxel that may interfere with chemotherapy effectiveness, promoting angiogenesis, metastasis and drug resistance. Combination treatment functionalized with both EGFR and HER2 antibodies towards breast cancer samples from patients also showed significantly higher anti-tumoral activity.

Siddiqui *et al.* [25] reported the use of PLA-PEG NPs to encapsulate EGCG. The efficiency of NPs against human prostate cancer was determined both *in vitro* and *in vivo*. The *in vitro* results showed that EGCG NPs induced the same extent of cellular death in human prostate cancer PC3 cells as non-encapsulated EGCG with an over 10-fold dose advantage. These NPs promoted an increase in pro-apoptotic molecules, such as BAX and a decrease in anti-apoptotic molecules, such as BCL-2 confirming the ability that the NPs have to retain EGCG's biological activity even at very low concentrations. Furthermore, EGCG-loaded NPs were also able to efficiently inhibit angiogenesis. This data was validated by *in vivo* results where it was observed that treatment with EGCG NPs induced a significant decrease in the tumor volume of athymic nude mice injected with androgen-responsive 22Rv1 cells with a 10-fold lower dose. More recently the same group [126], developed an EGCG nanocarrier specifically designed for oral administration using water-soluble chitosan. In this study, chitosan NPs revealed stability in an acidic environment, inducing a very slow release of EGCG in simulated gastric juice and a faster release in neutral pH (simulated intestinal fluid). The *in vivo* results determined in a prostate cancer xenograft model showed a significantly higher inhibition of tumor growth compared with both control and free EGCG-treated groups. This inhibition was found to be dose-dependent. Other relevant *in vivo* results include: inhibition of serum prostate cancer marker PSA; activation of DNA damage-related protein PARP; activation of mitochondrial pathway of apoptosis, with increase in the levels of pro-apototic protein BAX, decrease in the levels of anti-apoptotic protein BCL-2 and activation of caspases -3, -8 and -9, inhibition of cell proliferation markers (Ki-67 and PCNA) and angiogenesis markers (CD31 and VEGF). This oral nanoformulation with EGCG also demonstrated efficiency against melanoma cells [138]. After treatment with EGCG-encapsulated chitosan NPs, a higher cytotoxic effect against Mel 928 human melanoma cells was observed with regulation of intrinsic apoptotic pathways and induction of cell cycle arrest with a dose advantage over free EGCG. These results were supported by the *in vivo* tests performed in a melanoma xenograft model where it was shown that oral administration of encapsulated EGCG was able to inhibit tumor growth and induce the intrinsic apoptotic pathway and cell cycle arrest.

Hu *et al.* [139] reported the use of genipicin-crosslinked caseinophosphopeptide (CPP)–chitosan NPs for encapsulation of EGCG. Cross-linking of the NPs with genipicin increased the stability of the nanocarriers at different pH values, and at simulated gastric and intestinal fluid (SGF and SIF). Alterations in the crosslinking degree of the NP enabled the modulation of the release profile of EGCG. This release rate was found to be higher in the SIF than in the SGF, which is appropriate for an oral delivery system. *In vitro* test with gastrointestinal cancer cell line BGC823 demonstrated that encapsulated EGCG retained its anti-tumoral activity.

Shutava *et al.* [8] synthesized gelatin-based NPs with or without a coating of polyelectrolytes polystyrene sulfonate/polyallylamine hydrochloride produced through the layer-by-layer technique. Gelatin NPs revealed a more sustained release of EGCG as compared with uncoated NPs. Encapsulated EGCG maintained its biological activity, being able to inhibit hepatocyte growth factor (HGF) and subsequent activation of cell signaling pathways responsible for cell invasion in breast cancer cell line MDA-MD-23.

### 3.3. Liposomes

Liposomes are vesicles forming a membrane-like phospholipid bilayer enclosing an aqueous compartment [140]. These structural properties enable the encapsulation of both lipophilic and hydrophilic drugs [141]. In addition, liposomes are biodegradable and present minimal levels of toxicity [140]. Few studies have used these nanocarriers for delivery of EGCG to cancer cells. Results are summarized in Table 3.

Fang *et al.* [142] developed liposomal formulations with EGCG and other catechins for topical and intra-tumoral administration to treat BCC (basal cell carcinoma) in female nude mice. The authors concluded that intra-tumoral injection of liposomes was the most effective route to reach cancer cells, promoting a great amount of EGCG deposition in tumor tissues. The same group reported the use of liposomal formulations for BCCs treatment *in vivo* after intra-tumoral administration [140]. Nanoencapsulation significantly increased EGCG stability compared to free drug, which, according to the authors, may indicate that liposomes protect EGCG from oxidation and degradation. The synthesized liposomes also enabled higher EGCG accumulation in tumor tissues and induced higher levels of BCC cell death compared to the non-encapsulated EGCG treatment at lower concentrations [140].

**Table 3.** Liposomes used as EGCG nanocarriers for cancer therapy.

| Composition | Size (nm) | Zeta Potential (mV) | LC (%) | EE (%) | Route of Administration | *In Vitro/In Vivo* Results | Reference |
|---|---|---|---|---|---|---|---|
| Liposomes | 157.4 ± 2.9 | −7.2 ± 0.7 | N/A | 36.3 ± 5.7 | Topic and intra-tumoral | Great amount of EGCG deposition in tumor tissues in BCC model in female nude mice | [142] |
| | 268.9 ± 16.7 | −66 ± 2.2 | | 89.7 ± 0.4 | | | |
| Liposomes | 104.6–378.2 | −0.9 ± 0,4 | N/A | 99.6 ± 0.1 | Intra-tumoral | Higher EGCG accumulation in BCCs cells and higher apoptosis induction compared to free EGCG | [140] |
| | | −36.1 ± 1.7 | | 84.6 ± 3.8 | | | |
| Chitosan-coated liposomes | 85 ± 6.6 | 16.4 ± 2.8 | 3 | 90 | N/A | High anti-proliferative and pro-apoptotic effects in MCF7 breast cancer cell line | [23] |
| Liposomes | 126.7 ± 4.3 | −37.5 | N/A | 60.21 ± 1.59 | N/A | MDA-MB-231 breast cancer cell apoptosis and cell invasion inhibition | [141] |

In work published by de Pace *et al.* [23], EGCG was encapsulated in the hydrophilic core of nanoliposomes formed by cholesterol and phosphatidylcholine and coated with 0.2% of chitosan. *In vitro* results demonstrated that these NPs significantly enhanced EGCG stability and prevented its premature degradation in both PBS and cell culture mediums, when compared to free EGCG which was degraded much faster. In addition, nanoencapsulation promoted a more extended release and a higher EGCG content in MCF7 breast cancer cells compared to free EGCG. Differences in EGCG cellular content were also detected after treatment with both chitosan-coated and non-coated nanoliposomes suggesting that chitosan increases cell absorption. A dose of 10 mM of chitosan-coated liposomes also revealed significant anti-proliferative and pro-apoptotic effects with a decrease of 40% of MCF7 cells' proliferation compared with native EGCG and induction of 27% of MCF7 cell apoptosis.

More recently, Ramadass *et al.* [141] developed a liposomal co-delivery system comprising EGCG and paclitaxel for invasive cancer therapy using MDA-MB-231 breast cancer cell line. The results proved that this synergistic combination was effective in inducing cancer cell apoptosis and inhibiting cell invasion, which was demonstrated by an increase in caspase-3 activity and a decrease in MMP expression. These effects were higher in comparison with both paclitaxel and EGCG individual effects.

### 3.4. Other Type of NPs

A large variety of other different materials can be used for the design of nanoparticles. Encapsulation of EGCG for the purpose of cancer therapy using different materials, including carbohydrates, transition metals, inorganic materials and lipids are summarized in Table 4.

**Table 4.** Nanoparticles designed with various materials used as EGCG nanocarriers for cancer therapy.

| Composition | Size (nm) | Zeta Potential (mV) | LC (%) | EE (%) | Route of Administration | *In Vitro/In Vivo* Results | Reference |
|---|---|---|---|---|---|---|---|
| Maltodextrin-gum arabic | 120 ± 28 | −12.3 ± 0.8 | N/A | 85 ± 3 | N/A | Higher reduction in cell viability in Du145 human prostate cancer cells | [143] |
| Ruthenium | 73.59 | −17.9 | N/A | N/A | Intra-tumoral | Induction of cancer cell apoptosis, oxidative stress and inhibition of migration Tumor growth inhibition in liver cancer xenograft model | [144] |
| Ca/Al-NO3 LDH | N/A | +30.6 | N/A | N/A | N/A | Enhanced anti-tumoral activity of EGCG in PC3 prostate cancer cell line | [5] |

Rocha *et al.* [143] reported the encapsulation of EGCG into carbohydrate NPs composed of gum arabic and maltodextrin, whose properties enables them to protect the drug from oxidation. This nanocarrier promoted a reduction in cell viability in Du145 human prostate cancer cells and an induction of caspase-3 activation, and hence, apoptosis. These effects were higher comparing to free EGCG at low concentrations.

Zhou *et al.* [144] developed an anti-liver cancer therapy based on ruthenium NPs loaded with luminescent ruthenium complexes using EGCG as reducing and capping agent. Functionalization with EGCG was performed due to its high affinity to 67LR overexpressed in Hepatocellular carcinoma cells (HCC). *In vitro* results showed that the synthesized NPs had high specificity to liver cancer cells (SMMC-7721 HCCs) and their route of internalization was endocytosis mediated by 67LR. These NPs induced high levels of cytotoxicity, cell migration inhibition and induction of oxidative stress in HCC, while no harmful effects were detected in normal L-02 cells. The *in vivo* assay performed in a liver tumor xenograft model showed that intra-tumoral injection of EGCG functionalized nanocarriers could significantly inhibit tumor growth.

In a recent study developed by Shafiei *et al.* [5] EGCG was incorporated in Ca/Al-NO3 Layered double hydroxide (LDH) NPs using co-precipitation and ion-exchange techniques. The *in vitro* results revealed a higher anti-tumoral activity of the EGCG-LDH nanohybrid in a prostate cancer cell line (PC3), with a five-fold dose advantage over native ECGC and a longer release period compared to physical mixture of LDH and EGCG.

In these studies different types of nanoparticles were used including gold, polymeric, liposomes, metallic and carbohydrate-based. The majority of the studies have focused on polymeric NPs and liposomes, possibly due to their beneficial properties such as biocompatibility. A wide range of sizes was found varying from 20 to 1200 nm, although the majority of NPs were smaller than 250 nm. Different zeta potentials were also found, varying from positive (+30) to negative (−41). Encapsulation efficiencies were in general high, above 60%. EGCG anticancer activity was tested mainly in breast and prostate cancer models. Overall, the different types of nanoparticles promoted an enhancement of EGCG's bioavailability, stability and release profile as well as improvement of its anticancer activity compared to free catechin. In some studies, surface functionalization increased some of these characteristics particularly the release profile and the bioavailability. Moreover, the use of targeting ligands described on some of the works, contributed to increase EGCG specificity and anti-tumoral activity. Two of the studies have addressed an interesting topic, which is the combination of EGCG with common cytostatic drugs, demonstrating their synergistic effect, which is encouraging for future chemotherapy approaches. Most studies, however, have not revealed whether the nanoparticles could protect EGCG from degradation and oxidation. This would be particularly relevant since this compound is very susceptible to oxidation, specially in alkaline environments [145,146]. Future studies should address this issue and evaluate the capacity that different nanoparticles have to protect EGCG from oxidation and premature degradation.

## 4. Conclusions

EGCG is the major bioactive component in green tea with many health benefits, including anti-cancer activity, which has been demonstrated in *in vitro* and *in vivo* models and corroborated by some clinical and epidemiological studies. Despite that, this catechin is still not currently used in clinical settings due to its limited bioavailability and stability. In order to overcome these limitations, several studies have been developed applying the concept of nanochemoprevention, the use of nanotechnology to improve the pharmacokinetic and pharmacodynamic of chemopreventive agents to manage cancer. In these studies, different types of nanoparticles including gold, polymeric, metallic, carbohydrate-based and liposomes were used as delivery vehicles of EGCG. In the majority of these studies, the size of the nanoparticles was below 250 nm and encapsulation efficiencies were higher than 60%. The results revealed that EGCG nanoparticles promoted prolonged circulation time in blood, increased cell internalization in tumor sites and inhibited tumor growth both *in vitro* and *in vivo* predominantly in breast and prostate cancer models. Surface functionalization was employed to enhance drug release, cell uptake and intestinal absorption. The use of targeting ligands further increased cancer cell specificity and improved the anti-tumor effects of EGCG. Some studies reported the combination therapy of EGCG with cytostatic agents, emphasizing the synergistic effect of the two compounds. These advances in EGCG nanodelivery systems highlight the importance of nanotechnology in the enhancement of EGCG anti-cancer activities and hold great promise for upcoming clinical applications. With this approach, it is expected that, in the future, EGCG could be commercially produced by nutraceutical and dietary supplement industries as innovative supplements for cancer prevention. In addition, when combined with conventional cytostatic drugs, EGCG may provide a useful contribution to cancer treatments. This synergistic association is expected to increase the effectiveness of the drug and decrease the administered doses, hence, minimizing its adverse side effects, which will greatly improve the efficiency of future cancer therapies and the quality of life of cancer patients.

**Acknowledgments:** This work received financial support from the European Union (FEDER funds) and National Funds (FCT/MEC, Fundação para a Ciência e Tecnologia and Ministério da Educação e Ciência) under the Partnership Agreement PT2020 UID/MULTI/04378/2013-POCI/01/0145/FEDER/007728. MP thanks FCT (Fundação para a Ciência e Tecnologia) and POPH (Programa Operacional Potencial Humano) for her Post-Doc grant SFRH/BPD/99124/2013.

**Author Contributions:** Marina Pinheiro and Salette Reis conceived the searching strategy, the structure and the information eligible for the review; Andreia Granja conducted the research, analyzed the information and wrote the paper; and Marina Pinheiro and Salette Reis revised the subsequent drafts and approved the manuscript for submission.

**Conflicts of Interest:** The authors declare no conflict of interest.

## References

1. Cancer Facts & Figures 2016. American Cancer Society. Available online: http://www.cancer.org/research/cancerfactsstatistics/cancerfactsfigures2016/ (accessed on 7 February 2016).

2. Stewart, B.W.; Wild, C.P. *World Cancer Report 2014. International Agency for Research on Cancer*; World Health Organization: Geneva, Swizerland, 2014.

3. Worldwide Cancer Statistics. Cancer Research UK. Available online: http://www.cancerresearchuk.org/health-professional/cancer-statistics/worldwide-cancer#heading-Zero (accessed on 20 January 2016).

4. CDC—Global Cancer Statistics. Available online: http://www.cdc.gov/cancer/international/statistics.htm (accessed on 21 January 2016).

5. Shafiei, S.S.; Solati-Hashjin, M.; Samadikuchaksaraei, A.; Kalantarinejad, R.; Asadi-Eydivand, M.; Abu Osman, N.A. Epigallocatechin gallate/layered double hydroxide nanohybrids: Preparation, characterization, and *In vitro* anti-tumor study. *PLoS ONE* **2015**, *10*, e0136530. [CrossRef] [PubMed]

6. Morgan, G.; Ward, R.; Barton, M. The contribution of cytotoxic chemotherapy to 5-year survival in adult malignancies. *Clin. Oncol. J. (R. Coll. Radiol.)* **2004**, *16*, 549–560. [CrossRef]

7. Siddiqui, M.; Rajkumar, S.V. The high cost of cancer drugs and what we can do about it. *Mayo Clin. Proc.* **2012**, *87*, 935–943. [CrossRef] [PubMed]

8. Shutava, T.G.; Balkundi, S.S.; Vangala, P.; Steffan, J.J.; Bigelow, R.L.; Cardelli, J.A.; O'Neal, D.P.; Lvov, Y.M. Layer-by-layer-coated gelatin nanoparticles as a vehicle for delivery of natural polyphenols. *ACS Nano* **2009**, *3*, 1877–1885. [CrossRef] [PubMed]

9. Nyamai, D.W.; Arika, W.; Ogola, P.E.; Njagi, E.N.M.; Ngugi, M.P. Medicinally Important Phytochemicals: An Untapped Research Avenue. *Res. Rev. J. Pharmacogn. Phytochem.* **2016**, *4*, 35–49.

10. Xiao, L.; Mertens, M.; Wortmann, L.; Kremer, S.; Valldor, M.; Lammers, T.; Kiessling, F.; Mathur, S. Enhanced *in vitro* and *in vivo* cellular imaging with green tea coated water-soluble iron oxide nanocrystals. *ACS Appl. Mater. Interfaces* **2015**, *7*, 6530–6540. [CrossRef] [PubMed]

11. Mukherjee, S.; Ghosh, S.; Das, D.K.; Chakraborty, P.; Choudhury, S.; Gupta, P.; Adhikary, A.; Dey, S.; Chattopadhyay, S. Gold-conjugated green tea nanoparticles for enhanced anti-tumor activities and hepatoprotection—Synthesis, characterization and *in vitro* evaluation. *J. Nutr. Biochem.* **2015**, *26*, 1283–1297. [CrossRef] [PubMed]

12. Rahmani, A.H.; Al Shabrmi, F.M.; Allemailem, K.S.; Aly, S.M.; Khan, M.A. Implications of green tea and its constituents in the prevention of cancer via the modulation of cell signalling pathway. *BioMed Res. Int.* **2015**, *2015*. [CrossRef] [PubMed]

13. Thangapazham, R.L.; Singh, A.K.; Sharma, A.; Warren, J.; Gaddipati, J.P.; Maheshwari, R.K. Green tea polyphenols and its constituent Epigallocatechin gallate inhibits proliferation of human breast cancer cells *in vitro* and *in vivo*. *Cancer Lett.* **2007**, *245*, 232–241. [CrossRef] [PubMed]

14. Xu, Y.; Ho, C.T.; Amin, S.G.; Han, C.; Chung, F.L. Inhibition of tobacco-specific nitrosamine-induced lung tumorigenesis in A/J mice by green tea and its major polyphenol as antioxidants. *Cancer Res.* **1992**, *52*, 3875–3879. [PubMed]

15. Ju, J.; Hong, J.; Zhou, J.; Pan, Z.; Bose, M.; Liao, J.; Yang, G.; Liu, Y.Y.; Hou, Z.; Lin, Y.; *et al.* Inhibition of intestinal tumorigenesis in Apcmin/+ mice by (−)-Epigallocatechin-3-gallate, the major catechin in green tea. *Cancer Res.* **2005**, *65*, 10623–10631. [CrossRef] [PubMed]

16. Lu, Y.P.; Lou, Y.R.; Xie, J.G.; Peng, Q.Y.; Liao, J.; Yang, C.S.; Huang, M.T.; Conney, A.H. Topical applications of caffeine or (−)-Epigallocatechin gallate (EGCG) inhibit carcinogenesis and selectively increase apoptosis in UVB-induced skin tumors in mice. *Proc. Natl. Acad. Sci. USA* **2002**, *99*, 12455–12460. [CrossRef] [PubMed]

17. Fujiki, H. Two stages of cancer prevention with green tea. *J. Cancer Res. Clin. Oncol.* **1999**, *125*, 589–597. [CrossRef] [PubMed]

18. Bettuzzi, S.; Brausi, M.; Rizzi, F.; Castagnetti, G.; Peracchia, G.; Corti, A. Chemoprevention of human prostate cancer by oral administration of green tea catechins in volunteers with high-grade prostate intraepithelial neoplasia: A preliminary report from a one-year proof-of-principle study. *Cancer Res.* **2006**, *66*, 1234–1240. [CrossRef] [PubMed]

19. Kurahashi, N.; Sasazuki, S.; Iwasaki, M.; Inoue, M.; Tsugane, S. Green tea consumption and prostate cancer risk in Japanese men: A prospective study. *Am. J. Epidemiol.* **2008**, *167*, 71–77. [CrossRef] [PubMed]

20. Sasazuki, S.; Inoue, M.; Hanaoka, T.; Yamamoto, S.; Sobue, T.; Tsugane, S. Green tea consumption and subsequent risk of gastric cancer by subsite: The JPHC Study. *Cancer Causes Control.* **2004**, *15*, 483–491. [CrossRef] [PubMed]

21. Kang, H.; Rha, S.Y.; Oh, K.W.; Nam, C.M. Green tea consumption and stomach cancer risk: A meta-analysis. *Epidemiol. Health* **2010**, *32*, e2010001. [CrossRef] [PubMed]

22. Singh, B.N.; Shankar, S.; Srivastava, R.K. Green tea catechin, Epigallocatechin-3-gallate (EGCG): Mechanisms, perspectives and clinical applications. *Biochem. Pharmacol.* **2011**, *82*, 1807–1821. [CrossRef] [PubMed]

23. De Pace, R.C.C.; Liu, X.; Sun, M.; Nie, S.; Zhang, J.; Cai, Q.; Gao, W.; Pan, X.; Fan, Z.; Wang, S. Anticancer activities of (−)-Epigallocatechin-3-gallate encapsulated nanoliposomes in MCF7 breast cancer cells. *J. Liposome Res.* **2013**, *23*, 187–196. [CrossRef] [PubMed]

24. Nakagawa, K.; Okuda, S.; Miyazawa, T. Dose-dependent incorporation of tea catechins, (−)-Epigallocatechin-3-gallate and (−)-Epigallocatechin, into human plasma. *Biosci. Biotechnol. Biochem.* **1997**, *61*, 1981–1985. [CrossRef] [PubMed]

25. Siddiqui, I.A.; Adhami, V.M.; Bharali, D.J.; Hafeez, B.B.; Asim, M.; Khwaja, S.I.; Ahmad, N.; Cui, H.; Mousa, S.A.; Mukhtar, H. Introducing nanochemoprevention as a novel approach for cancer control: Proof of principle with green tea polyphenol Epigallocatechin-3-gallate. *Cancer Res.* **2009**, *69*, 1712–1716. [CrossRef] [PubMed]

26. Yamamoto, T.; Juneja, L.R.; Chu, sDjong-C.; Kim, M. *Chemistry and Applications of Green Tea*; CRC Press: Boca Raton, FL, USA, 1997.

27. Ahmad, N.; Mukhtar, H. Green tea polyphenols and cancer: Biologic mechanisms and practical implications. *Nutr. Rev.* **1999**, *57*, 78–83. [CrossRef] [PubMed]

28. O'Grady, M.N.; Kerry, J.P. Using antioxidants and nutraceuticals as dietary supplements to improve the quality and shelf-life of fresh meat. In *Improving the Sensory and Nutritional Quality of Fresh Meat*; Woodhead Publishing Limited: Cambridge, UK, 2009; pp. 356–386.

29. Velickovic, T.C.; Gavrovic-Jankulovic, M. *Food Allergens: Biochemistry and Molecular Nutrition*; Springer: New York, NY, USA, 2014.

30. Nakagawa, T.; Yokozawa, T. Direct scavenging of nitric oxide and superoxide by green tea. *Food Chem. Toxicol.* **2002**, *40*, 1745–1750. [CrossRef]

31. Ho, C.T.; Chen, Q.; Shi, H.; Zhang, K.Q.; Rosen, R.T. Antioxidative effect of polyphenol extract prepared from various Chinese teas. *Prev. Med. (Baltim.)* **1992**, *21*, 520–525. [CrossRef]

32. Betts, J.W.; Wareham, D.W. *In vitro* activity of curcumin in combination with Epigallocatechin gallate (EGCG) *versus* multidrug-resistant Acinetobacter baumannii. *BMC Microbiol.* **2014**, *14*, 172. [CrossRef] [PubMed]

33. Steinmann, J.; Buer, J.; Pietschmann, T.; Steinmann, E. Anti-infective properties of Epigallocatechin-3-gallate (EGCG), a component of green tea. *Br. J. Pharmacol.* **2013**, *168*, 1059–1073. [CrossRef] [PubMed]

34. Huang, H.C.; Tao, M.H.; Hung, T.M.; Chen, J.C.; Lin, Z.J.; Huang, C. (−)-Epigallocatechin-3-gallate inhibits entry of hepatitis B virus into hepatocytes. *Antivir. Res.* **2014**, *111*, 100–111. [CrossRef] [PubMed]

35. Calland, N.; Albecka, A.; Belouzard, S.; Wychowski, C.; Duverlie, G.; Descamps, V.; Hober, D.; Dubuisson, J.; Rouillé, Y.; Séron, K. (−)-Epigallocatechin-3-gallate is a new inhibitor of hepatitis C virus entry. *Hepatology* **2012**, *55*, 720–729. [CrossRef] [PubMed]

36. Weber, C.; Sliva, K.; von Rhein, C.; Kümmerer, B.M.; Schnierle, B.S. The green tea catechin, Epigallocatechin gallate inhibits chikungunya virus infection. *Antivir. Res.* **2015**, *113*, 1–3. [CrossRef] [PubMed]

37. Munir, K.M.; Chandrasekaran, S.; Gao, F.; Quon, M.J. Mechanisms for food polyphenols to ameliorate insulin resistance and endothelial dysfunction: Therapeutic implications for diabetes and its cardiovascular complications. *Am. J. Physiol. Endocrinol. Metab.* **2013**, *305*, E679–E686. [CrossRef] [PubMed]

38. Babu, P.V.A.; Liu, D.; Gilbert, E.R. Recent advances in understanding the anti-diabetic actions of dietary flavonoids. *J. Nutr. Biochem.* **2013**, *24*, 1777–1789. [CrossRef] [PubMed]

39. Iso, H. The relationship between green tea and total caffeine intake and risk for self-reported type 2 diabetes among japanese adults. *Ann. Intern. Med.* **2006**, *144*, 554–562. [CrossRef] [PubMed]

40. Panagiotakos, D.B.; Lionis, C.; Zeimbekis, A.; Gelastopoulou, K.; Papairakleous, N.; Das, U.N.; Polychronopoulos, E. Long-term tea intake is associated with reduced prevalence of (type 2) diabetes mellitus among elderly people from Mediterranean islands: MEDIS epidemiological study. *Yonsei Med. J.* **2009**, *50*, 31–38. [CrossRef] [PubMed]

41. Khurana, S.; Venkataraman, K.; Hollingsworth, A.; Piche, M.; Tai, T.C. Polyphenols: Benefits to the cardiovascular system in health and in aging. *Nutrients* **2013**, *5*, 3779–3827. [CrossRef] [PubMed]

42. Osada, K.; Takahashi, M.; Hoshina, S.; Nakamura, M.; Nakamura, S.; Sugano, M. Tea catechins inhibit cholesterol oxidation accompanying oxidation of low density lipoprotein *in vitro*. *Comp. Biochem. Physiol. C Toxicol. Pharmacol.* **2001**, *128*, 153–164. [CrossRef]

43. Kuriyama, S.; Shimazu, T.; Ohmori, K.; Kikuchi, N.; Nakaya, N.; Nishino, Y.; Tsubono, Y.; Tsuji, I. Green tea consumption and mortality due to cardiovascular disease, cancer, and all causes in Japan: The Ohsaki study. *JAMA* **2006**, *296*, 1255–1265. [CrossRef] [PubMed]

44. Geleijnse, J.M.; Launer, L.J.; Van der Kuip, D.A.M.; Hofman, A.; Witteman, J.C.M. Inverse association of tea and flavonoid intakes with incident myocardial infarction: The Rotterdam Study. *Am. J. Clin. Nutr.* **2002**, *75*, 880–886. [PubMed]

45. Yang, Y.C.; Lu, F.H.; Wu, J.S.; Wu, C.II.; Chang, C.J. The protective effect of habitual tea consumption on hypertension. *Arch. Intern. Med.* **2004**, *164*, 1534–1540. [CrossRef] [PubMed]

46. Geleijnse, J.M.; Launer, L.J.; Hofman, A.; Pols, H.A.; Witteman, J.C. Tea flavonoids may protect against atherosclerosis: The Rotterdam Study. *Arch. Intern. Med.* **1999**, *159*, 2170–2174. [CrossRef] [PubMed]

47. Diepvens, K.; Westerterp, K.R.; Westerterp-Plantenga, M.S. Obesity and thermogenesis related to the consumption of caffeine, ephedrine, capsaicin, and green tea. *Am. J. Physiol. Regul. Integr. Comp. Physiol.* **2006**, *292*, R77–R85. [CrossRef] [PubMed]

48. Lim, H.J.; Shim, S.B.; Jee, S.W.; Lee, S.H.; Lim, C.J.; Hong, J.T.; Sheen, Y.Y.; Hwang, D.Y. Green tea catechin leads to global improvement among Alzheimer's disease—Related phenotypes in NSE/hAPP-C105 Tg mice. *J. Nutr. Biochem.* **2013**, *24*, 1302–1313. [CrossRef] [PubMed]

49. Mandel, S.A.; Amit, T.; Weinreb, O.; Youdim, M.B.H. Understanding the broad-spectrum neuroprotective action profile of green tea polyphenols in aging and neurodegenerative diseases. *J. Alzheimers Dis.* **2011**, *25*, 187–208. [PubMed]

50. Rigacci, S.; Stefani, M. Nutraceuticals and amyloid neurodegenerative diseases: A focus on natural phenols. *Expert Rev. Neurother.* **2015**, *15*, 41–52. [CrossRef] [PubMed]

51. Ruddon, R.W. *Cancer Biology*; Oxford University Press: New York, NY, USA, 2007.

52. Mikeska, T.; Craig, J.M. DNA methylation biomarkers: Cancer and beyond. *Genes* **2014**, *5*, 821–864. [CrossRef] [PubMed]

53. Jones, P.A.; Baylin, S.B. The fundamental role of epigenetic events in cancer. *Nat. Rev. Genet.* **2002**, *3*, 415–428. [PubMed]

54. Baylin, S.B. DNA methylation and gene silencing in cancer. *Nat. Clin. Pract. Oncol.* **2005**, *2* (Suppl. 1), S4–S11. [CrossRef] [PubMed]
55. Fang, M.Z.; Wang, Y.; Ai, N.; Hou, Z.; Sun, Y.; Lu, H.; Welsh, W.; Yang, C.S. Tea polyphenol (−)-Epigallocatechin-3-gallate inhibits DNA methyltransferase and reactivates methylation-silenced genes in cancer cell lines. *Cancer Res.* **2003**, *63*, 7563–7570. [PubMed]
56. Gavory, G.; Farrow, M.; Balasubramanian, S. Minimum length requirement of the alignment domain of human telomerase RNA to sustain catalytic activity *in vitro*. *Nucleic Acids Res.* **2002**, *30*, 4470–4480. [CrossRef] [PubMed]
57. Kim, N.W.; Piatyszek, M.A.; Prowse, K.R.; Harley, C.B.; West, M.D.; Ho, P.L.; Coviello, G.M.; Wright, W.E.; Weinrich, S.L.; Shay, J.W. Specific association of human telomerase activity with immortal cells and cancer. *Science* **1994**, *266*, 2011–2015. [CrossRef] [PubMed]
58. Sadava, D.; Whitlock, E.; Kane, S.E. The green tea polyphenol, Epigallocatechin-3-gallate inhibits telomerase and induces apoptosis in drug-resistant lung cancer cells. *Biochem. Biophys. Res. Commun.* **2007**, *360*, 233–237. [CrossRef] [PubMed]
59. Yokoyama, M.; Noguchi, M.; Nakao, Y.; Pater, A.; Iwasaka, T. The tea polyphenol, (−)-Epigallocatechin gallate effects on growth, apoptosis, and telomerase activity in cervical cell lines. *Gynecol. Oncol.* **2004**, *92*, 197–204. [CrossRef] [PubMed]
60. Naasani, I.; Seimiya, H.; Tsuruo, T. Telomerase Inhibition, Telomere Shortening, and Senescence of Cancer Cells by Tea Catechins. *Biochem. Biophys. Res. Commun.* **1998**, *249*, 391–396. [CrossRef] [PubMed]
61. Sledge, G.; Miller, K. Exploiting the hallmarks of cancer. *Eur. J. Cancer* **2003**, *39*, 1668–1675. [CrossRef]
62. Roudsari, L.C.; West, J.L. Studying the influence of angiogenesis in *in vitro* cancer model systems. *Adv. Drug Deliv. Rev.* **2015**, *97*, 250–259. [CrossRef] [PubMed]
63. Byrne, A.M.; Bouchier-Hayes, D.J.; Harmey, J.H. Angiogenic and cell survival functions of vascular endothelial growth factor (VEGF). *J. Cell. Mol. Med.* **2005**, *9*, 777–794. [CrossRef] [PubMed]
64. Wang, H.; Bian, S.; Yang, C.S. Green tea polyphenol EGCG suppresses lung cancer cell growth through upregulating miR-210 expression caused by stabilizing HIF-1α. *Carcinogenesis* **2011**, *32*, 1881–1889. [CrossRef] [PubMed]
65. Gu, J.-W.; Makey, K.L.; Tucker, K.B.; Chinchar, E.; Mao, X.; Pei, I.; Thomas, E.Y.; Miele, L. EGCG, a major green tea catechin suppresses breast tumor angiogenesis and growth via inhibiting the activation of HIF-1α and NFκB, and VEGF expression. *Vasc. Cell* **2013**, *5*, 9. [CrossRef] [PubMed]
66. Li, X.; Feng, Y.; Liu, J.; Feng, X.; Zhou, K.; Tang, X. Epigallocatechin-3-gallate inhibits IGF-I-stimulated lung cancer angiogenesis through downregulation of HIF-1α and VEGF expression. *J. Nutr. Nutr.* **2013**, *6*, 169–178.
67. Shankar, S.; Ganapathy, S.; Hingorani, S.R.; Srivastava, R.K. EGCG inhibits growth, invasion, angiogenesis and metastasis of pancreatic cancer. *Front. Biosci.* **2008**, *13*, 440–452. [CrossRef] [PubMed]
68. Isemura, M.; Saeki, K.; Kimura, T.; Hayakawa, S.; Minami, T.; Sazuka, M. Tea catechins and related polyphenols as anti-cancer agents. *Biofactors* **2000**, *13*, 81–85. [CrossRef] [PubMed]
69. Garbisa, S.; Biggin, S.; Cavallarin, N.; Sartor, L.; Benelli, R.; Albini, A. Tumor invasion: Molecular shears blunted by green tea. *Nat. Med.* **1999**, *5*, 1216. [CrossRef] [PubMed]
70. Demeule, M.; Brossard, M.; Pagé, M.; Gingras, D.; Béliveau, R. Matrix metalloproteinase inhibition by green tea catechins. *Biochim. Biophys. Acta* **2000**, *1478*, 51–60. [CrossRef]
71. Zhen, M.; Huang, X.; Wang, Q.; Sun, K.; Liu, Y.; Li, W.; Zhang, L.; Cao, L.; Chen, X. Green tea polyphenol Epigallocatechin-3-gallate suppresses rat hepatic stellate cell invasion by inhibition of MMP-2 expression and its activation. *Acta Pharmacol. Sin.* **2006**, *27*, 1600–1607. [CrossRef] [PubMed]
72. Koff, J.; Ramachandiran, S.; Bernal-Mizrachi, L. A Time to Kill: Targeting Apoptosis in Cancer. *Int. J. Mol. Sci.* **2015**, *16*, 2942–2955. [CrossRef] [PubMed]
73. Shankar, S.; Suthakar, G.; Srivastava, R.K. Epigallocatechin-3-gallate inhibits cell cycle and induces apoptosis in pancreatic cancer. *Front. Biosci.* **2007**, *12*, 5039–5051. [CrossRef] [PubMed]
74. Leone, M.; Zhai, D.; Sareth, S.; Kitada, S.; Reed, J.C.; Pellecchia, M. Cancer prevention by tea polyphenols is linked to their direct inhibition of antiapoptotic Bcl-2-family proteins. *Cancer Res.* **2003**, *63*, 8118–8121. [PubMed]
75. Sonoda, J.I.; Ikeda, R.; Baba, Y.; Narumi, K.; Kawachi, A.; Tomishige, E.; Nishihara, K.; Takeda, Y.; Yamada, K.; Sato, K.; *et al.* Green tea catechin, Epigallocatechin-3-gallate, attenuates the cell viability of human

non-small-cell lung cancer A549 cells via reducing Bcl-xL expression. *Exp. Ther. Med.* **2014**, *8*, 59–63. [CrossRef] [PubMed]

76. Yang, W.H.; Fong, Y.C.; Lee, C.Y.; Jin, T.R.; Tzen, J.T.; Li, T.M.; Tang, C.H. Epigallocatechin-3-gallate induces cell apoptosis of human chondrosarcoma cells through apoptosis signal-regulating kinase 1 pathway. *J. Cell. Biochem.* **2011**, *112*, 1601–1611. [CrossRef] [PubMed]

77. Yang, G.Y.; Liao, J.; Li, C.; Chung, J.; Yurkow, E.J.; Ho, C.T.; Yang, C.S. Effect of black and green tea polyphenols on c-jun phosphorylation and $H_2O_2$ production in transformed and non-transformed human bronchial cell lines: Possible mechanisms of cell growth inhibition and apoptosis induction. *Carcinogenesis* **2000**, *21*, 2035–2039. [CrossRef] [PubMed]

78. Ahmad, N.; Cheng, P.; Mukhtar, H. Cell cycle dysregulation by green tea polyphenol Epigallocatechin-3-gallate. *Biochem. Biophys. Res. Commun.* **2000**, *275*, 328–334. [CrossRef] [PubMed]

79. Fatemi, A.; Safa, M.; Kazemi, A. MST-312 induces G2/M cell cycle arrest and apoptosis in APL cells through inhibition of telomerase activity and suppression of NF-κB pathway. *Tumour Biol.* **2015**, *36*, 8425–8437. [CrossRef] [PubMed]

80. Singh, M.; Singh, R.; Bhui, K.; Tyagi, S.; Mahmood, Z.; Shukla, Y. Tea polyphenols induce apoptosis through mitochondrial pathway and by inhibiting nuclear factor-kappaB and Akt activation in human cervical cancer cells. *Oncol. Res.* **2011**, *19*, 245–257. [CrossRef] [PubMed]

81. Pflaum, R.K. Tumor Suppressor Genes; Nova Publishers, Hauppauge, NY, USA, 2007.

82. Thakur, V.S.; Gupta, K.; Gupta, S. Green tea polyphenols increase p53 transcriptional activity and acetylation by suppressing class I histone deacetylases. *Int. J. Oncol.* **2012**, *41*, 353–361. [PubMed]

83. Hastak, K.; Agarwal, M.K.; Mukhtar, H.; Agarwal, M.L. Ablation of either p21 or Bax prevents p53-dependent apoptosis induced by green tea polyphenol Epigallocatechin-3-gallate. *FASEB J.* **2005**, *19*, 789–791. [CrossRef] [PubMed]

84. Liu, S.; Wang, X.J.; Liu, Y.; Cui, Y.F. PI3K/AKT/mTOR signaling is involved in (−)-Epigallocatechin-3-gallate-induced apoptosis of human pancreatic carcinoma cells. *Am. J. Chin. Med.* **2013**, *41*, 629–642. [CrossRef] [PubMed]

85. Liang, Y.C.; Lin-Shiau, S.Y.; Chen, C.F.; Lin, J.K. Inhibition of cyclin-dependent kinases 2 and 4 activities as well as induction of Cdk inhibitors p21 and p27 during growth arrest of human breast carcinoma cells by (−)-Epigallocatechin-3-gallate. *J. Cell. Biochem.* **1999**, *75*, 1–12. [CrossRef]

86. Ozols, R.F. *Ovarian Cancer*; BC Decker Inc: Hamilton, ON, Canada, 2003; Volume 1.

87. Iqbal, N.; Iqbal, N. Human epidermal growth factor receptor 2 (HER2) in cancers: Overexpression and therapeutic implications. *Mol. Biol. Int.* **2014**. [CrossRef] [PubMed]

88. Milanezi, F.; Carvalho, S.; Schmitt, F.C. EGFR/HER2 in breast cancer: A biological approach for molecular diagnosis and therapy. *Expert Rev. Mol. Diagn.* **2008**, *8*, 417–434. [CrossRef] [PubMed]

89. Ma, Y.C.; Li, C.; Gao, F.; Xu, Y.; Jiang, Z.B.; Liu, J.X.; Jin, L.Y. Epigallocatechin gallate inhibits the growth of human lung cancer by directly targeting the EGFR signaling pathway. *Oncol. Rep.* **2014**, *31*, 1343–1349. [PubMed]

90. Lim, Y.C.; Cha, Y.Y. Epigallocatechin-3-gallate induces growth inhibition and apoptosis of human anaplastic thyroid carcinoma cells through suppression of EGFR/ERK pathway and cyclin B1/CDK1 complex. *J. Surg. Oncol.* **2011**, *104*, 776–780. [CrossRef] [PubMed]

91. Masuda, M.; Suzui, M.; Lim, J.T.E.; Weinstein, I.B. Epigallocatechin-3-gallate inhibits activation of HER-2/neu and downstream signaling pathways in human head and neck and breast carcinoma cells. *Clin. Cancer Res.* **2003**, *9*, 3486–3491. [PubMed]

92. Pianetti, S.; Guo, S.; Kavanagh, K.T.; Sonenshein, G.E. Green tea polyphenol Epigallocatechin-3 gallate inhibits Her-2/neu signaling, proliferation, and transformed phenotype of breast cancer cells. *Cancer Res.* **2002**, *62*, 652–655. [PubMed]

93. Aggarwal, B.B.; Shishodia, S. Molecular targets of dietary agents for prevention and therapy of cancer. *Biochem. Pharmacol.* **2006**, *71*, 1397–1421. [CrossRef] [PubMed]

94. Ahmad, N.; Gupta, S.; Mukhtar, H. Green tea polyphenol Epigallocatechin-3-gallate differentially modulates nuclear factor kappaB in cancer cells *versus* normal cells. *Arch. Biochem. Biophys.* **2000**, *376*, 338–346. [CrossRef] [PubMed]

95.  Qin, J.; Wang, Y.; Bai, Y.; Yang, K.; Mao, Q.; Lin, Y.; Kong, D.; Zheng, X.; Xie, L. Epigallocatechin-3-gallate inhibits bladder cancer cell invasion via suppression of NF-κB-mediated matrix metalloproteinase-9 expression. *Mol. Med. Rep.* **2012**, *6*, 1040–1044. [PubMed]

96.  Masuda, M.; Suzui, M.; Lim, J.T.E.; Deguchi, A.; Soh, J.W.; Weinstein, I.B. Epigallocatechin-3-gallate decreases VEGF production in head and neck and breast carcinoma cells by inhibiting EGFR-related pathways of signal transduction. *J. Exp. Ther. Oncol.* **2002**, *2*, 350–359. [CrossRef] [PubMed]

97.  Seger, R.; Krebs, E.G. The MAPK signaling cascade. *FASEB J.* **1995**, *9*, 726–735. [PubMed]

98.  Cerezo-Guisado, M.I.; Zur, R.; Lorenzo, M.J.; Risco, A.; Martín-Serrano, M.A.; Alvarez-Barrientos, A.; Cuenda, A.; Centeno, F. Implication of Akt, ERK1/2 and alternative p38MAPK signalling pathways in human colon cancer cell apoptosis induced by green tea EGCG. *Food Chem. Toxicol.* **2015**, *84*, 125–132. [CrossRef] [PubMed]

99.  Park, S.B.; Bae, J.W.; Kim, J.M.; Lee, S.G.; Han, M. Antiproliferative and apoptotic effect of Epigallocatechin-3-gallate on Ishikawa cells is accompanied by sex steroid receptor downregulation. *Int. J. Mol. Med.* **2012**, *30*, 1211–1218. [PubMed]

100. Ly, B.T.K.; Chi, H.T.; Yamagishi, M.; Kano, Y.; Hara, Y.; Nakano, K.; Sato, Y.; Watanabe, T. Inhibition of FLT3 expression by green tea catechins in FLT3 mutated-AML cells. *PLoS ONE* **2013**, *8*, e66378. [CrossRef] [PubMed]

101. Adhami, V.M.; Siddiqui, I.A.; Ahmad, N.; Gupta, S.; Mukhtar, H. Oral consumption of green tea polyphenols inhibits insulin-like growth factor-I-induced signaling in an autochthonous mouse model of prostate cancer. *Cancer Res.* **2004**, *64*, 8715–8522. [CrossRef] [PubMed]

102. Li, M.; He, Z.; Ermakova, S.; Zheng, D.; Tang, F.; Cho, Y.Y.; Zhu, F.; Ma, W.Y.; Sham, Y.; Rogozin, E.A.; *et al.* Direct inhibition of insulin-like growth factor-I receptor kinase activity by (−)-Epigallocatechin-3-gallate regulates cell transformation. *Cancer Epidemiol. Biomark. Prev.* **2007**, *16*, 598–605. [CrossRef] [PubMed]

103. Sazuka, M.; Itoi, T.; Suzuki, Y.; Odani, S.; Koide, T.; Isemura, M. Evidence for the interaction between (−)-Epigallocatechin gallate and human plasma proteins fibronectin, fibrinogen, and histidine-rich glycoprotein. *Biosci. Biotechnol. Biochem.* **1996**, *60*, 1317–1319. [CrossRef] [PubMed]

104. Suzuki, Y.; Isemura, M. Inhibitory effect of Epigallocatechin gallate on adhesion of murine melanoma cells to laminin. *Cancer Lett.* **2001**, *173*, 15–20. [CrossRef]

105. Suzuki, Y.; Isemura, M. Binding interaction between (−)-Epigallocatechin gallate causes impaired spreading of cancer cells on fibrinogen. *Biomed. Res.* **2013**, *34*, 301–308. [CrossRef] [PubMed]

106. Hayakawa, S.; Saeki, K.; Sazuka, M.; Suzuki, Y.; Shoji, Y.; Ohta, T.; Kaji, K.; Yuo, A.; Isemura, M. Apoptosis induction by Epigallocatechin gallate involves its binding to Fas. *Biochem. Biophys. Res. Commun.* **2001**, *285*, 1102–1106. [CrossRef] [PubMed]

107. Tachibana, H.; Koga, K.; Fujimura, Y.; Yamada, K. A receptor for green tea polyphenol EGCG. *Nat. Struct. Mol. Biol.* **2004**, *11*, 380–381. [CrossRef] [PubMed]

108. Ermakova, S.; Choi, B.Y.; Choi, H.S.; Kang, B.S.; Bode, A.M.; Dong, Z. The intermediate filament protein vimentin is a new target for Epigallocatechin gallate. *J. Biol. Chem.* **2005**, *280*, 16882–16890. [CrossRef] [PubMed]

109. Ermakova, S.P.; Kang, B.S.; Choi, B.Y.; Choi, H.S.; Schuster, T.F.; Ma, W.Y.; Bode, A.M.; Dong, Z. (−)-Epigallocatechin gallate overcomes resistance to etoposide-induced cell death by targeting the molecular chaperone glucose-regulated protein 78. *Cancer Res.* **2006**, *66*, 9260–9269. [CrossRef] [PubMed]

110. He, Z.; Tang, F.; Ermakova, S.; Li, M.; Zhao, Q.; Cho, Y.Y.; Ma, W.Y.; Choi, H.S.; Bode, A.M.; Yang, C.S.; *et al.* Fyn is a novel target of (−)-Epigallocatechin gallate in the inhibition of JB6 Cl41 cell transformation. *Mol. Carcinog.* **2008**, *47*, 172–183. [CrossRef] [PubMed]

111. Shim, J.H.; Choi, H.S.; Pugliese, A.; Lee, S.Y.; Chae, J.I.; Choi, B.Y.; Bode, A.M.; Dong, Z. (−)-Epigallocatechin gallate regulates CD3-mediated T cell receptor signaling in leukemia through the inhibition of ZAP-70 kinase. *J. Biol. Chem.* **2008**, *283*, 28370–28379. [CrossRef] [PubMed]

112. Shim, J.H.; Su, Z.Y.; Chae, J.I.; Kim, D.J.; Zhu, F.; Ma, W.Y.; Bode, A.M.; Yang, C.S.; Dong, Z. Epigallocatechin gallate suppresses lung cancer cell growth through Ras-GTPase-activating protein SH3 domain-binding protein 1. *Cancer Prev. Res. (Phila.)* **2010**, *3*, 670–679. [CrossRef] [PubMed]

113. Urusova, D.V.; Shim, J.H.; Kim, D.J.; Jung, S.K.; Zykova, T.A.; Carper, A.; Bode, A.M.; Dong, Z. Epigallocatechin- gallate suppresses tumorigenesis by directly targeting Pin1. *Cancer Prev. Res. (Phila.)* **2011**, *4*, 1366–1377. [CrossRef] [PubMed]

114. Liao, S.; Umekita, Y.; Guo, J.; Kokontis, J.M.; Hiipakka, R.A. Growth inhibition and regression of human prostate and breast tumors in athymic mice by tea Epigallocatechin gallate. *Cancer Lett.* **1995**, *96*, 239–243. [CrossRef]

115. Ahn, W.S.; Yoo, J.; Huh, S.W.; Kim, C.K.; Lee, J.M.; Namkoong, S.E.; Bae, S.M.; Lee, I.P. Protective effects of green tea extracts (polyphenon E and EGCG) on human cervical lesions. *Eur. J. Cancer Prev.* **2003**, *12*, 383–390. [CrossRef] [PubMed]

116. McLarty, J.; Bigelow, R.L.H.; Smith, M.; Elmajian, D.; Ankem, M.; Cardelli, J.A. Tea polyphenols decrease serum levels of prostate-specific antigen, hepatocyte growth factor, and vascular endothelial growth factor in prostate cancer patients and inhibit production of hepatocyte growth factor and vascular endothelial growth factor *in vitro*. *Cancer Prev. Res. (Phila.)* **2009**, *2*, 673–682. [PubMed]

117. Jatoi, A.; Ellison, N.; Burch, P.A.; Sloan, J.A.; Dakhil, S.R.; Novotny, P.; Tan, W.; Fitch, T.R.; Rowland, K.M.; Young, C.Y.F.; *et al.* phase II trial of green tea in the treatment of patients with androgen independent metastatic prostate carcinoma. *Cancer* **2003**, *97*, 1442–1446. [CrossRef] [PubMed]

118. Zhou, Y.; Li, N.; Zhuang, W.; Liu, G.; Wu, T.; Yao, X.; Du, L.; Wei, M.; Wu, X. Green tea and gastric cancer risk: Meta-analysis of epidemiologic studies. *Asia Pac. J. Clin. Nutr.* **2008**, *17*, 159–165. [PubMed]

119. Lin, Y.; Kikuchi, S.; Tamakoshi, A.; Yagyu, K.; Obata, Y.; Kurosawa, M.; Inaba, Y.; Kawamura, T.; Motohashi, Y.; Ishibashi, T. Green tea consumption and the risk of pancreatic cancer in Japanese adults. *Pancreas* **2008**, *37*, 25–30. [CrossRef] [PubMed]

120. Sasazuki, S.; Tamakoshi, A.; Matsuo, K.; Ito, H.; Wakai, K.; Nagata, C.; Mizoue, T.; Tanaka, K.; Tsuji, I.; Inoue, M.; *et al.* Green tea consumption and gastric cancer risk: An evaluation based on a systematic review of epidemiologic evidence among the Japanese population. *Jpn. J. Clin. Oncol.* **2012**, *42*, 335–346. [CrossRef] [PubMed]

121. Wang, H.; Zhou, H.; Yang, C.S. Cancer prevention with green tea polyphenols. In *Cancer Chemoprevention and Treatment by Diet Therapy*; Springer: Dordrecht, The Netherlands, 2013; pp. 91–119.

122. Selvamuthukumar, S.; Velmurugan, R. Nanostructured lipid carriers: A potential drug carrier for cancer chemotherapy. *Lipids Health Dis.* **2012**, *11*, 159. [CrossRef] [PubMed]

123. Lecumberri, E.; Dupertuis, Y.M.; Miralbell, R.; Pichard, C. Green tea polyphenol Epigallocatechin-3-gallate (EGCG) as adjuvant in cancer therapy. *Clin. Nutr.* **2013**, *32*, 894–903. [CrossRef] [PubMed]

124. Siddiqui, I.A.; Adhami, V.M.; Ahmad, N.; Mukhtar, H. Nanochemoprevention: Sustained release of bioactive food components for cancer prevention. *Nutr. Cancer* **2010**, *62*, 883–890. [CrossRef] [PubMed]

125. Chen, C.C.; Hsieh, D.S.; Huang, K.J.; Chan, Y.L.; Hong, P.D.; Yeh, M.K.; Wu, C.J. Improving anticancer efficacy of (−)-Epigallocatechin-3-gallate gold nanoparticles in murine B16F10 melanoma cells. *Drug Des. Dev. Ther.* **2014**, *8*, 459–473.

126. Khan, N.; Bharali, D.J.; Adhami, V.M.; Siddiqui, I.A.; Cui, H.; Shabana, S.M.; Mousa, S.A.; Mukhtar, H. Oral administration of naturally occurring chitosan-based nanoformulated green tea polyphenol EGCG effectively inhibits prostate cancer cell growth in a xenograft model. *Carcinogenesis* **2014**, *35*, 415–423. [CrossRef] [PubMed]

127. Jain, S.; Hirst, D.G.; O'Sullivan, J.M. Gold nanoparticles as novel agents for cancer therapy. *Br. J. Radiol.* **2012**, *85*, 101–113. [CrossRef] [PubMed]

128. Nune, S.K.; Chanda, N.; Shukla, R.; Katti, K.; Kulkarni, R.R.; Thilakavathy, S.; Mekapothula, S.; Kannan, R.; Katti, K.V. Green nanotechnology from tea: Phytochemicals in tea as building blocks for production of biocompatible gold nanoparticles. *J. Mater. Chem.* **2009**, *19*, 2912. [CrossRef] [PubMed]

129. Nie, L.; Liu, F.; Ma, P.; Xiao, X. Applications of gold nanoparticles in optical biosensors. *J. Biomed. Nanotechnol.* **2014**, *10*, 2700–2721. [CrossRef] [PubMed]

130. Hsieh, D.S.; Wang, H.; Tan, S.W.; Huang, Y.H.; Tsai, C.Y.; Yeh, M.K.; Wu, C.J. The treatment of bladder cancer in a mouse model by Epigallocatechin-3-gallate-gold nanoparticles. *Biomaterials* **2011**, *32*, 7633–7640. [CrossRef] [PubMed]

131. Sanna, V.; Pala, N.; Dessi, G.; Manconi, P.; Mariani, A.; Dedola, S.; Rassu, M.; Crosio, C.; Iaccarino, C.; Sechi, M. Single-step green synthesis and characterization of gold-conjugated polyphenol nanoparticles with antioxidant and biological activities. *Int. J. Nanomedicine* **2014**, *9*, 4935–4951. [PubMed]

132. Alotaibi, A.; Bhatnagar, P.; Najafzadeh, M.; Gupta, K.C.; Anderson, D. Tea phenols in bulk and nanoparticle form modify DNA damage in human lymphocytes from colon cancer patients and healthy individuals treated

*in vitro* with platinum based-chemotherapeutic drugs. *Nanomedicine (Lond.)* **2013**, *8*, 389–401. [CrossRef] [PubMed]

133. Elsabahy, M.; Wooley, K.L. Design of polymeric nanoparticles for biomedical delivery applications. *Chem. Soc. Rev.* **2012**, *41*, 2545–2561. [CrossRef] [PubMed]

134. Kumari, A.; Yadav, S.K.; Yadav, S.C. Biodegradable polymeric nanoparticles based drug delivery systems. *Colloids Surf. B. Biointerfaces* **2010**, *75*, 1–18. [CrossRef] [PubMed]

135. Sanna, V.; Pintus, G.; Roggio, A.M.; Punzoni, S.; Posadino, A.M.; Arca, A.; Marceddu, S.; Bandiera, P.; Uzzau, S.; Sechi, M. Targeted biocompatible nanoparticles for the delivery of (−)-Epigallocatechin 3-gallate to prostate cancer cells. *J. Med. Chem.* **2011**, *54*, 1321–1332. [CrossRef] [PubMed]

136. Narayanan, S.; Pavithran, M.; Viswanath, A.; Narayanan, D.; Mohan, C.C.; Manzoor, K.; Menon, D. Sequentially releasing dual-drug-loaded PLGA–casein core/shell nanomedicine: Design, synthesis, biocompatibility and pharmacokinetics. *Acta Biomater.* **2014**, *10*, 2112–2124. [CrossRef] [PubMed]

137. Narayanan, S.; Mony, U.; Vijaykumar, D.K.; Koyakutty, M.; Paul-Prasanth, B.; Menon, D. Sequential release of Epigallocatechin gallate and paclitaxel from PLGA-casein core/shell nanoparticles sensitizes drug-resistant breast cancer cells. *Nanomedicine* **2015**, *11*, 1399–1406. [CrossRef] [PubMed]

138. Siddiqui, I.A.; Bharali, D.J.; Nihal, M.; Adhami, V.M.; Khan, N.; Chamcheu, J.C.; Khan, M.I.; Shabana, S.; Mousa, S.A.; Mukhtar, H. Excellent anti-proliferative and pro-apoptotic effects of (−)-Epigallocatechin-3-gallate encapsulated in chitosan nanoparticles on human melanoma cell growth both *in vitro* and *in vivo*. *Nanomedicine* **2014**, *10*, 1619–1626. [CrossRef] [PubMed]

139. Hu, B.; Xie, M.; Zhang, C.; Zeng, X. Genipin-structured peptide-polysaccharide nanoparticles with significantly improved resistance to harsh gastrointestinal environments and their potential for oral delivery of polyphenols. *J. Agric. Food Chem.* **2014**, *62*, 12443–12452. [CrossRef] [PubMed]

140. Fang, J.Y.; Lee, W.R.; Shen, S.C.; Huang, Y.L. Effect of liposome encapsulation of tea catechins on their accumulation in basal cell carcinomas. *J. Dermatol. Sci.* **2006**, *42*, 101–109. [CrossRef] [PubMed]

141. Ramadass, S.K.; Anantharaman, N.V.; Subramanian, S.; Sivasubramanian, S.; Madhan, B. Paclitaxel/Epigallocatechin gallate coloaded liposome: A synergistic delivery to control the invasiveness of MDA-MB-231 breast cancer cells. *Colloids Surf. B Biointerfaces* **2015**, *125*, 65–72. [CrossRef] [PubMed]

142. Fang, J.Y.; Hung, C.F.; Hwang, T.L.; Huang, Y.L. Physicochemical characteristics and *in vivo* deposition of liposome-encapsulated tea catechins by topical and intratumor administrations. *J. Drug Target.* **2005**, *13*, 19–27. [CrossRef] [PubMed]

143. Rocha, S.; Generalov, R.; Peres, I.; Juzenas, P. Epigallocatechin gallate-loaded polysaccharide nanoparticles for prostate cancer chemoprevention. *Nanomedicine (Lond.)* **2011**, *6*, 79–87. [CrossRef] [PubMed]

144. Zhou, Y.; Yu, Q.; Qin, X.; Bhavsar, D.; Yang, L.; Chen, Q.; Zheng, W.; Chen, L.; Liu, J. Improving the Anticancer Efficacy of Laminin Receptor-Specific Therapeutic Ruthenium Nanoparticles (RuBB-Loaded EGCG-RuNPs) via ROS-Dependent Apoptosis in SMMC-7721 Cells. *ACS Appl. Mater. Interfaces* **2015**. [CrossRef] [PubMed]

145. Janeiro, P.; Oliveira Brett, A.M. Catechin electrochemical oxidation mechanisms. *Anal. Chim. Acta* **2004**, *518*, 109–115. [CrossRef]

146. Dube, A.; Ng, K.; Nicolazzo, J.A.; Larson, I. Effective use of reducing agents and nanoparticle encapsulation in stabilizing catechins in alkaline solution. *Food Chem.* **2010**, *122*, 662–667. [CrossRef]

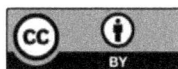

nutrients

MDPI

*Review*

# The Potential Protective Effects of Polyphenols in Asbestos-Mediated Inflammation and Carcinogenesis of Mesothelium

**Monica Benvenuto** [1,†], **Rosanna Mattera** [1,†], **Gloria Taffera** [1], **Maria Gabriella Giganti** [1], **Paolo Lido** [2], **Laura Masuelli** [3], **Andrea Modesti** [1] and **Roberto Bei** [1,*]

[1] Department of Clinical Sciences and Translational Medicine, University of Rome "Tor Vergata", Rome 00133, Italy; monicab4@hotmail.it (M.B.); rosannamatter@gmail.com (R.M.); g.taffera@gmail.com (G.T.); giganti@med.uniroma2.it (M.G.G.); modesti@med.uniroma2.it (A.M.)

[2] Internal Medicine Residency Program, University of Rome "Tor Vergata", Rome 00133, Italy; paulshore@virgilio.it

[3] Department of Experimental Medicine, University of Rome "Sapienza", Rome 00164, Italy; Laura.masuelli@uniroma1.it

[*] Correspondence: bei@med.uniroma2.it; Tel.: +39 06 7259 6522

[†] These authors contributed equally to this work.

Received: 24 March 2016; Accepted: 4 May 2016; Published: 9 May 2016

**Abstract:** Malignant Mesothelioma (MM) is a tumor of the serous membranes linked to exposure to asbestos. A chronic inflammatory response orchestrated by mesothelial cells contributes to the development and progression of MM. The evidence that: (a) multiple signaling pathways are aberrantly activated in MM cells; (b) asbestos mediated-chronic inflammation has a key role in MM carcinogenesis; (c) the deregulation of the immune system might favor the development of MM; and (d) a drug might have a better efficacy when injected into a serous cavity thus bypassing biotransformation and reaching an effective dose has prompted investigations to evaluate the effects of polyphenols for the therapy and prevention of MM. Dietary polyphenols are able to inhibit cancer cell growth by targeting multiple signaling pathways, reducing inflammation, and modulating immune response. The ability of polyphenols to modulate the production of pro-inflammatory molecules by targeting signaling pathways or ROS might represent a key mechanism to prevent and/or to contrast the development of MM. In this review, we will report the current knowledge on the ability of polyphenols to modulate the immune system and production of mediators of inflammation, thus revealing an important tool in preventing and/or counteracting the growth of MM.

**Keywords:** malignant mesothelioma; inflammation; immune system; ROS and RNS; polyphenols; asbestos

---

## 1. Introduction

Malignant Mesothelioma (MM) is a rare primary tumor arising from the mesothelial cell linings of the serous membranes, most commonly involving the pleural and peritoneal spaces [1]. The development of MM consists of a multi-step process driven by cellular DNA damage and tumor cell promotion, in which genetically modified mesothelial cells are prone to grow, and tumor progression, in which mesothelial cells develop a more aggressive phenotype and eventually acquire the ability to metastasize and invade other tissues. The immune system's involvement in the development of MM is complex and multifaceted and is likely to involve both the innate and adaptive immune systems [2–4]. A chronic inflammatory response orchestrated by mesothelial cells contributes to the development and progression of mesothelial cells into MM [2–4].

Cisplatin and antifolate-based combination chemotherapy represent the standard first-line treatment for advanced and unresectable MM patients [5]. However, taking into account the poor outcome and toxicity of chemotherapy, novel approaches based on targeting abnormally activated signaling pathways in MM cells were employed to improve survival in MM patients, as described in the review by Remon *et al.* [5]. Clinical trials have employed antiangiogenic and vascular disrupting agents, PI3K/AKT/mTOR pathway inhibitors, heat shock protein S90 inhibitors and arginine depletory molecule, and immunotherapy. However, although some of these clinical trials sustain further studies, the absolute response rates (RRs) are limited compared to other tumors [5].

The knowledge of MM pathophysiology might influence novel approaches [6–9].

The evidence that: (a) multiple signaling pathways are aberrantly activated in MM cells [10]; (b) asbestos-mediated chronic inflammation through the release of reactive oxygen species (ROS), nitrogen species (RNS) and cytokines has a key role in MM carcinogenesis [11]; (c) the deregulation of the immune system might favor the onset of MM [9]; and (d) a drug might have a better efficacy when injected into a serous cavity, thus bypassing biotransformation and reaching an effective dose [12], have prompted investigations to evaluate the effects of polyphenols for the therapy and prevention of MM. Dietary polyphenols possess pleiotropic properties capable of being able to (a) inhibit cancer cell growth by targeting multiple signaling pathways; (b) reduce inflammation and (c) modulate immune response [13–17].

The ability to reduce chronic inflammation might represent a key mechanism to contrast the development and/or to prevent MM. Accordingly, the local or systemic administration of polyphenols might reduce the production of pro-inflammatory molecules by targeting signal transduction pathways or ROS and RNS. In addition, the pro-oxidant activity of polyphenols could be a strategy to kill cancer cells and thus to limit tumor growth [14].

In this review we will report the current knowledge on the ability of polyphenols to modulate the immune system and production of mediators of inflammation in MM, thus revealing an important tool to prevent and/or to counteract the growth of MM.

## 2. Polyphenols

Polyphenols, a large group of phytochemicals ubiquitously found in plants, are secondary metabolites that perform functions in the host's defense against pathogens, ultraviolet radiation, and signal transduction [18]. Polyphenols are present in food and beverages of plant origin, such as fruits, vegetables, cereals, spices, legumes, nuts, olives, tea, coffee, and wine [19]. These compounds exhibit anti-inflammatory, antimicrobial, anticancer, and immunomodulatory activities, and thus are beneficial for human health [20].

Polyphenols have a characteristic phenolic structure and are classified according to the number of phenol rings that they contain and by the structural elements that bind these rings to one another. The main classes of polyphenols are flavonoids, phenolic acids, stilbenes, and lignans [18,21].

Among flavonoids, the most important subclasses are flavonols, flavones, flavan-3-ols, anthocyanins, flavanones, and isoflavones. The flavonoid subclasses dihydroflavonols, flavan-3,4-diols, chalcones, dihydrochalcones, and aurones are minor components of our diet [22].

Quercetin, kaempferol, and myricetin, found mostly in fruits, edible plants, wine, and tea, are the main flavonols [18]. The most abundant flavones in foods are apigenin (parsley, celery, onion, garlic, pepper, chamomile tea) and luteolin (Thai chili, onion leaves, celery) [20]. The flavan-3-ol subclass includes a wide range of compounds with different chemical structures that can be divided in monomers, (+)-catechin, (−)-epicatechin, (+)-gallocatechin, (−)-epigallocatechin, (−)-epicatechin-3-O-gallate, (−)-epigallocatechin-3-O-gallate, and polymers (proanthocyanidins) and are found mainly in fruits, berries, cereals, nuts, chocolate, red wine, and tea [20]. The most abundant anthocyanins (cyanidin, pelargonidin, delphinidin, peonidin, petunidin, and malvidin) are found mainly in berries, cherries, red grapes, and currants [23]. Flavanones are present in citrus fruit and the most important are hesperetin and naringenin and their correspondent glycated forms (naringin (naringenin-7-*O*-neohesperidoside), neohesperidin (hesperetin-7-*O*-neohesperidoside), narirutin (naringenin-7-*O*-rutinoside), and hesperidin (hesperetin-7-*O*-rutinoside)) [21,24]. Daidzein, genistein, and glyciten are the most common members of isoflavones, found mainly in soybeans, soy products, and leguminous plants [25].

Among phenolic acids, the hydroxybenzoic acids (protocatechuic acid and gallic acid) are found in few edible plants, while hydroxycinnamic acids (caffeic acid, ferulic acid, *p*-coumaric acid, and sinapic acid) are found in fruits, coffee, and cereal grains [18].

The main member of stilbenes is resveratrol (3,5,4′-trihydroxystilbene) and is present in grapes, berries, plums, peanuts, and pine nuts [21]. Lignans (ecoisolariciresinol, matairesinol, medioresinol, pinoresinol, and lariciresinol) are found in high concentration in linseed and in minor concentration in algae, leguminous plants, cereals, vegetables, and fruits [18]. Curcumin (1,7-bis-(4-hydroxy-3-methoxyphenyl)-1,6-heptadiene-3,5-dione), a member of the curcuminoid family, is another polyphenol compound found in turmeric, a spice produced from the rhizome of *Curcuma longa* [26].

Polyphenols have important anti-inflammatory effects by regulating innate and adaptive immunity through the modulation of different cytokines and also by acting as an immune surveillance mechanism against cancer through the regulation of apoptosis [14]. Polyphenols also possess anti-oxidant and pro-oxydant activities [27–30] and are able to modulate multiple targets involved in carcinogenesis through simultaneous direct interaction or modulation of gene expression [13]. It is worth nothing that these compounds are able to inhibit the growth of cancer cells without having an adverse effect on normal cells. In this way, polyphenols play selectively an antitumor role in cancer [14]. However, despite promising results obtained from *in vitro* studies, the use of polyphenols as anticancer agents is yet limited in clinical practice due to their low bioavailability in the human body, which affects the effective dose delivered to cancer cells. In fact, polyphenols have a poor absorption and biodistribution and a fast metabolism and excretion in the human body. Only nano- or micromolar concentrations of polyphenols and polyphenol metabolites are found in plasma (0–4 μM after an intake of 50 mg of aglycone equivalents) [31]. Several mechanisms limit the bioavailability of polyphenols, including their metabolism in the gastrointestinal tract and liver, their binding on the surfaces of blood cells and microbial flora in the oral cavity and gut, and regulatory mechanisms that prevent the toxic effects of high compound levels on mitochondria or other organelles [32]. In addition to endogenous factors, dietary factors can affect the bioavailability of polyphenols, such as food matrix and food preparation techniques [33]. Promising strategies for improving the *in vivo* anticancer effects of polyphenols are the combination of polyphenols, or polyphenols and conventional cancer treatments, and the intratumoral administration of polyphenols, in order to bypass biotransformation and reach an effective dose directly available at the site of tumor [22]. Several pre-clinical and Phase I and Phase II clinical trials are employing intratumoral administration to deliver different therapeutics such as drugs, viral-based cancer vaccines, immune cell-based vaccines, cytokines, DNA, bacterial products, nanoparticles, and natural compounds to the tumor site [34–39]. Thus, intratumoral delivery of cancer therapeutics could be a more efficient route of administration for several agents in easily accessible tumors, such as MM. An intratumoral route of administration is able to prevent the occurrence of systemic side effects and makes the therapeutic agents directly available at the tumor site, allowing for the highest concentration close to tumor cells [40].

## 3. Asbestos Fibers and MM

MM was broadly observed in the mid-to-late 1960s among workers whose asbestos exposure began 30–40 years earlier [41]. Accordingly, the development of MM has been linked to exposure to asbestos fibers [1]. Although the use of asbestos has by now been prohibited in 55 countries, the occurrence of asbestos-related diseases cannot decrease due to: the long latency period of MM, the continued use of asbestos in Third World Countries and the continued occupational exposure in Western Countries, such as the US and Europe [5,42].

Thermo-resistant magnesium and calcium silicate fibers were usually used as insulating materials in buildings and are deposited in the alveoli upon inhalation. Asbestos fibers are genotoxic, causing random chromosome breaks [43]. Asbestos is classified into two major categories (amphibole and serpentine) [43]. There are five members of the amphibole category: crocidolite (blue asbestos), amosite (brown asbestos), tremolite, anthophyllite, and actinolite. The serpentine class is made up of only one member (chrysotile, white asbestos) [43]. The International Agency for Research on Cancer (IARC) classifies asbestos as a Group I carcinogen, because of the ability of chrysotile, crocidolite, and amosite to induce lung cancer or MM [44]. Fiber translocation into the pleural cavity can occur across the alveolar surface or via pulmonary lymph flow [45].

Although the link between MM and asbestos is well established, other carcinogenic or co-carcinogenic events must be involved in MM development because only 10% of all MM cases occur in asbestos-exposed subjects [46].

## 4. Chronic Inflammation Affects MM Development

### 4.1. Overproduction of ROS and RNS

A key immune-mediated involvement in asbestos-related carcinogenesis is superimposed on the fibers' damage to the mesothelium integrity. Mesothelial cells offer the first defense against chemical and biological injuries by building a mechanical barrier and also by activating inflammation through the release of ROS, RNS, and cytokines [47–51]. In fact, mesothelial cells express on their luminal surface a sialomucins veil that electrostatically repels bacteria, viruses, and chemicals and mechanically decreases their adherence to the mesothelial layer [47]. In addition, serous spaces are surrounded by several defensive molecules including lysozyme, IgA immunoglobulins, and complement factors [47]. Mesothelial cells damaged by asbestos fibers release inflammatory mediators that maintain an inflammatory environment [48–50].

Asbestos induces free radical production by mesothelial cells through the iron content of the asbestos fibers which increases the hydroxyl radical formation from hydrogen peroxide through iron catalysed reactions and by inflammatory cells such as pulmonary alveolar macrophages and neutrophils [52]. Kinnula *et al.* reported that inflammatory cells are the essential cells responsible for the free radical-mediated mesothelial cell injury during asbestos exposure *in vivo* [53,54]. During the respiratory burst, leukocytes produce multiple ROS, including hydroxyl radical, superoxide anions, and hydrogen peroxide [55]. Hansen *et al.* reported that the geometry and/or chemical composition of asbestos is important for the release of superoxide anions by leucocytes during frustrated phagocytosis [56,57]. Indeed, crocidolite and amosite induced significant ROS generation by neutrophils with a peak at 10 min, whereas that of chrysotile was ~25% of the crocidolite/amosite response [58].

Leukocytes and mesothelial cells are also able to overexpress nitric oxide synthase (NOS) in response to a variety of stimuli [52]. Inflammatory cytokines and oxidant stress can each augment iNOS expression and activity in pulmonary alveolar epithelial cells [52]. The inhalation of either chrysotile or crocidolite asbestos fibers was shown to induce the production of nitric oxide in bronchoalveolar lavage cells and the formation of nitrotyrosine within the lungs and pleura [59]. The majority of MM was found to express high levels of iNOS, while its expression was occasionally found in non-neoplastic healthy mesothelium [60]. Thus, RNS might have an important role in asbestos-mediated mesothelioma oncogenesis [52]. Peroxynitrite can be produced by the reaction of ROS with RNS. The overproduction of ROS and RNS in the inflammatory microenvironment can cause DNA damage to mesothelial cells, thus leading to the development of MM [61].

Macrophages are recruited and activated to clear away asbestos fibers [48]. Vitronectin captures crocidolite asbestos and enhances fiber phagocytosis by mesothelial cells via integrins [62]. Yang *et al.* provided the mechanistic rationale that associates asbestos-mediated mesothelial cell necrosis to the chronic inflammatory reaction that is, in turn, linked with asbestos-mediated tumorigenesis [63].

The authors reported that exposure of mesothelial cells to crocidolite asbestos induces them to activate poly(ADP-ribose) polymerase, to secrete hydrogen peroxide, to deplete ATP, and to secrete high-mobility group box 1 protein (HMGB1) into the extracellular space. This latter stimulates macrophages to secrete tumor necrosis factor-$\alpha$ (TNF-$\alpha$) and the inflammatory response associated with asbestos-mediated carcinogenesis [2].

The asbestos-mediated chronic inflammation can increase the genotoxic damage due to the secretion of free radicals [48].

In addition, several studies have shown that asbestos fibers induce the activation of EGFR (Epidermal growth factor receptor) and thus MAPK (Mitogen-activated protein kinase) pathway and AP-1 (Activator protein-1), leading to cell proliferation [43] (Figure 1).

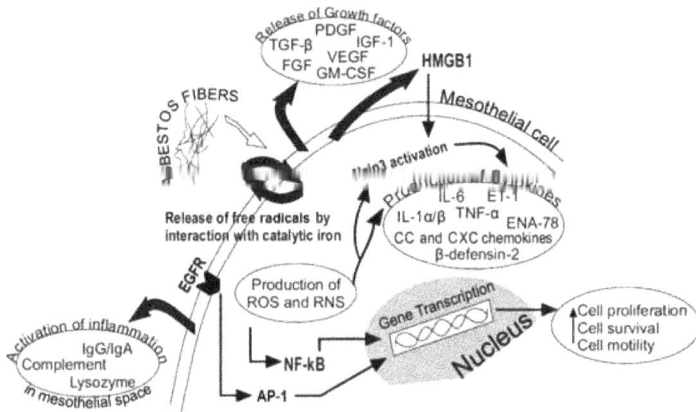

**Figure 1.** The asbestos-mediated long-lasting inflammation in mesothelial cells. Biological responses of mesothelial cells to asbestos fiber injury. Abbreviations: ROS, Reactive Oxygen Species; RNS, Reactive Nitrogen Species; HMGB1, High-Mobility Group Box 1 Protein; PDGF, Platelet-Derived Growth Factors; FGF, Fibroblast Growth Factor; IGF-1, Insulin-Like Growth Factor-1; VEGF, Vascular Endothelial Growth Factor; TGF-$\beta$, Transforming Growth Factor-$\beta$; GM-CSF, Granulocyte/Macrophage-Colony Stimulating Factor; IL-6, Interleukin-6; ET-1, Endothelin-1; IL-1 $\alpha/\beta$, Interleukin-1 $\alpha/\beta$; TNF-$\alpha$, Tumor Necrosis Factor-$\alpha$; ENA-78, Epithelial Neutrophil Activating Protein-78; NF-$\kappa$B, Nuclear Factor-kB; EGFR, Epidermal Growth Factor Receptor; AP-1, Activator Protein-1.

### 4.2. Inflammasome Activation and Cytokines Secretion

It was reported that exposure to asbestos induces mesothelial cell necrosis and the release of HMGB1 into the extracellular space [2]. HMGB1 is a key mediator of chronic inflammation in MM, leading to Nalp3 inflammasome activation, macrophages accumulation, interleukin (IL)-1$\beta$ and TNF-$\alpha$ secretion, and thus to activation of the NF-$\kappa$B pathway, which increases cell survival and tumor growth after asbestos exposure [50]. A recent study reported that HMGB1 localization was regulated by its acetylation. In fact, HMGB1 is localized in the nucleus to stabilize nucleosomes when it is in the nonacetylated form. When HMGB1 is hyperacetylated, it is actively secreted into the extracellular space. The authors indicated that HMGB1 hyperacetylation could be a sensitive and specific biomarker to discriminate MM patients from asbestos-exposed individuals and from healthy unexposed controls. They demonstrated that hyperacetylated HMGB1 was significantly higher in MM patients compared with asbestos-exposed individuals and healthy controls, and did not vary with tumor stage [4].

Accordingly, asbestos fibers induce NLRP3 priming and activation, thus leading to increased transcription of pro-inflammatory cytokines [63,64]. The inflammasome is a constituent of the inflammation machinery which includes NOD-like receptors (NLRs) whose activation induces the activation of caspase-1 and of the mature form pro-inflammatory cytokines, such as IL-1$\beta$ and

IL-18 [65,66]. It was reported that the NLRP3 inflammasome is necessary for early inflammatory responses to asbestos, but it is not indispensable for asbestos-induced MM [64]. Hillegass *et al.* linked NLRP3 activation to the release of several pro-inflammatory cytokines (IL-1β, IL-6 and IL-8) and the vascular endothelial growth factor (VEGF) by fiber-stimulated human mesothelial cells *in vitro* [63]. They showed that mesothelial cells secrete IL-1β in response to asbestos/erionite and that through an autocrine stimulation they undergo transformation [63]. In addition, the authors demonstrated that treatment of MM tumor-bearing SCID mice with IL-1R (Interleukin-1 receptor) antagonist (Anakinra) decreased the levels of IL-8 and VEGF in peritoneal lavage fluid, thus indicating that IL-1 has a key role in regulating the production of other cytokines, thus affecting the tumorigenesis of mesothelial cells [63]. A combination of IL-1β and TNF-α and erionite, or at least two cytokines together without erionite, for at least four months, induced transformation of the immortalized, non-tumorigenic human mesothelial cell line (MeT-5A) *in vitro* [67].

Accordingly, the release of cytokines driving inflammation represents a hallmark of exposure to asbestos. Mesothelial inflammatory processes were reported to occur both in animal models and in the lungs of patients exposed to asbestos. The production of different cytokines by mesothelial cells indicates the particular transcriptional aptitude of mesothelial cells [68]. A cytokine network is established in the serous membranes after mesothelial cell injury. Among the other cytokines, chemokines produced by mesothelial cells can recruit leukocytes [68] (Figure 1). Driscoll *et al.* showed that alveolar macrophages release TNF-α and IL-1 in rats exposed to crocidolite fibers [69]. In addition, crocidolite enhanced the production of mitochondrial-derived hydrogen peroxide which in turn contributes to crocidolite activation of NF-κB and increased MIP-2 (Macrophage Inflammatory protein-2) gene expression in rat alveolar Type II cells [70]. Recently, Acencio *et al.* performed an *in vitro* experiment to determine the acute inflammatory response of mesothelial cells damaged by asbestos fibers. They showed that mesothelial cells exposed to either crocidolite or chrysotile produced high levels of IL-6, IL-1β, MIP-2 and that these cytokines, when acting together with asbestos, increased cell death of pleural mesothelial cells [49]. Indeed, they showed that anti-IL-1β and anti-IL-6 antibodies significantly inhibited necrosis and apoptosis of mesothelial cells exposed to crocidolite [49]. High levels of cytokines, including transforming growth factor beta (TGF-β), IL-6, IL-1 and TNF-α were produced during MM development in an *in vivo* mouse model by the MM cells and/or tumor infiltrating leukocytes [71]. TNF-α, IL-6, TGF-β, and IL-10 have been shown to participate in cancer initiation and progression [72]. TGF-β counteracts proliferation and differentiation of different immune cells, thus inducing immunosuppression and favoring cancer cell growth [73]. IL-1β may confer a proliferative advantage to cancer cells through autocrine mechanisms [74]. The pro-inflammatory cytokines IL-1β, IL-6, IL-8, and VEGF promote tumor angiogenesis [75].

Fox *et al.* investigated the expression of CC and CXC chemokine genes I response to cytokines in MM and mesothelial cell cultures derived from two different mouse strains (BALB/*c* and CBA/CaH). They found that monocyte chemoattractant protein-1 (MCP-1)/JE, GRO-α/KC and RANTES were expressed in mouse MM and mesothelial cells, whereas MIP-1α and MIP-2 were infrequently expressed in these cell lines. MCP-1 was up-regulated in response to TNF-α and other cytokines [76]. MCP-1 and RANTES have been shown to induce cell growth and to act as monocyte attractants [77]. GRO-α/KC mRNA was overexpressed in cancer cells [76].

*In vivo* human studies were performed as well. The study of the RENAPE (French Network for Rare Peritoneal Malignancies) aimed to evaluate the intraperitoneal levels of IL-6, IL-8, IL-10, TNF-α, and sICAM (soluble intercellular adhesion molecule) in patients with pseudomyxoma peritonei and peritoneal mesothelioma. They found that cancer patients had significantly higher intraperitoneal cytokine levels than non-cancer patients. Cytokines peritoneal levels were significantly higher in peritoneal fluids compared with matched sera, thus indicating the cytokines production from either peritoneal cells or immune cells. In addition, they found a correlation between cytokine peritoneal levels and aggressiveness of peritoneal surface malignancies [78].

Comar *et al.*, employing Luminex Multiplex Panel Technology, measured the serum levels of a large panel of cytokines and growth factors from workers previously exposed to asbestos (Asb-workers). They found that interferon (IFN)-α, EOTAXIN, and RANTES were highly expressed in Asb-workers while IL-12(p40), IL-3, IL-1α, MCP-3, β-NGF (nerve growth factor), TNF-β, and RANTES were highly produced in MM patients [79].

Xu *et al.* found that the amount of CCL3 in the serum of healthy subjects potentially exposed to asbestos was significantly higher than for the control group. In addition, they observed that the pleural plaque, benign hydrothorax asbestosis, and lung cancer patients had serum CCL3 levels similar to that of healthy subjects potentially exposed to asbestos. They detected the CCL3 chemokine in the serum of nine of the 10 patients diagnosed with MM and three patients with MM showed very high CCL3 levels [80]. The elevated levels of CCL3 are very likely produced by macrophages chronically interacting with asbestos fibers [80].

### 4.3. Innate Immunity and Cytokines in the Development of MM: MM-Driven Immunoediting

The activation of an adaptive immune response and/or cell proliferation by inflammasome effectors is dependent on the cell type and tissue microenvironment [81]. The creation of a local cytokine-based microenvironment is employed by MM to avoid the apoptic immune response. IL-1β and IL-18 released by epithelial cells promote a Th2 response and recruitment of suppressive immune cells in the absence of IL-12 rather than activating Th1 and Th17 cells. In addition, the release of growth factors will favor angiogenesis and tumor invasiveness [81]. Indeed, IL-1β promotes carcinogenesis and induces the invasive potential of malignant cells by favoring the expression of matrix metalloproteinases, VEGF, chemokines, growth factors, and TGF-β in chronic inflamed tissue [82]. However, inflammasome's activation in dendritic cells (DCs) and macrophages can bias Th1, Th17 immune response ability to reduce tumor growth in the presence of an appropriate microenvironment [81]. We recently demonstrated that macrophages and CD4+ T-cells were polarized by MM to produce IL-17, and that this cytokine exerts multiple tumor-supporting effects on both cell growth and invasiveness [83].

Many MM-derived factors can skew monocyte development through the recruitment of tumor-supporting cells, as reported by the presence of myeloid-derived suppressor cells (MDSCs) in murine models of MM. Employing a mouse model of transplanted diffuse MM, it was reported that MDSCs arise simultaneously with the recruitment of inflammatory cells in tumor foci. The presence of MDSCs came before the accumulation of macrophages and regulatory T lymphocytes which suppress T-cell function [84]. The cytokine profile three weeks after MM injection induced a tumor microenvironment that suppressed immune surveillance and antitumor immunity. At that stage, high expression levels of CXCL12, a chemotactic factor for MDSC, CCL9, and CXCL5, were observed [84]. Veltman *et al.* demonstrated that BALB/c mice carrying MM have PMN-MDSCs that induce immunosuppressive activity by releasing ROS via a cyclooxygenase-2 (COX-2)-dependent mechanism, which then induces T-cell immunosuppression [85]. The same authors inoculated mice with MM cells and treated them with celecoxib, a COX-2 inhibitor. They observed that treatment of tumor-bearing mice with the celecoxib prevented the local and systemic expansion of all MDSC subtypes [86]. However, a recent study by Yang *et al.* also reported that aspirin (a COX inhibitor) exerted a protective effect against MM growth through a COX-2-independent mechanism. In fact, the authors demonstrated that aspirin inhibited MM growth in a xenograft model by inhibiting the activities of HMGB1. The authors concluded that aspirin could be administered to people who were exposed to asbestos or erionite to prevent or delay MM development and progression [87].

Tumor-associated macrophages (TAMs) represent a major link between inflammation and cancer [88]. M1 macrophages have immunostimulatory Th1-activating properties while M2 cells have poor antigen-presenting capacity and suppress Th1 adaptive immunity [88]. Prostaglandin E2 (PGE2), TGF-β, IL-6, and IL-10 promote M2 macrophage polarization. Inhibition of the antitumor responses is achieved not only by the secretion of immunosuppressive cytokines but also by the selective recruitment of naive T-cells, trough CCL18, and of Th2 and Treg, through CCL17 and CCL22 [88]. The majority of TAMs in MM have the M2 phenotype. By retrospectively reviewing 667 tumor specimens of patients with MM it was found that, within the tumors, macrophages comprised 27% of the tumor area and had an immunosuppressive phenotype [89]. Hegmans *et al.* detected in pleural effusion of MM patients several cytokines involved in immune suppression and angiogenesis, including TGF-β. In addition, they demonstrated that human MM tissue contained a high number of Foxp3+ CD4+ CD25+ regulatory T-cells and when the CD25+ regulatory T-cells were depleted in an *in vivo* mouse model, mice survival increased [90]. The expression profile of cytokines and chemokines in mice transplanted with MM cells was consistent with M2-polarized cells [91]. They found elevated IL-10 and IL-10RA expression as well as expression of CXCL13, CCL22, CCL24, and their respective receptors [91]. In a recent report by Napolitano *et al.*, it was also observed that mice with germline BAP1 (BRCA1-associated protein-1) mutations (BAP1$^{+/-}$ mice) exposed to low-dose asbestos fibers had alterations in the peritoneal inflammatory response. In fact, BAP1$^{+/-}$ mice showed higher levels of pro-tumorigenic M2 macrophages and lower levels of M1 macrophages, cytokines (IL-6, leukemia inhibitory factor), and chemokines (MCP-1, keratinocyte-derived chemokine). Thus, these mice showed higher MM incidence after exposure to very low doses of asbestos, doses that rarely induced MM in wild-type mice. The authors suggested that patients with this mutation have an increased risk of developing MM, even after a minimal exposure of asbestos, due to alterations of the inflammatory response [92].

Asbestos induces partially functional decreases in T helper (Th) cells, natural killer (NK) cells, and cytotoxic T lymphocytes (CTLs) in patients with MM [93]. To elucidate the antitumor immune interference of asbestos caused to CD4+ T-cells, Maeda *et al.* established an *in vitro* T-cell model of long-term and low-level exposure to chrysotile asbestos from a human adult T-cell leukemia virus-1-immortalized human polyclonal CD4+ T-cell line (MT-2). They observed a decreased expression of CXCR3, IFN-γ, and CXCL10/IP10 in the MT-2 cell line, thus suggesting that exposure to asbestos may impair the antitumor immune responses [94]. They also found that chrysotile asbestos reduces the chemokine receptor CXCR3 expression in human peripheral CD4+ T-cells, thus suggesting that immune response might be impaired in patients with asbestos-related disease because the low expression of CXCR3 might reduce chemotaxis [95]. In addition, in a recent report, the same authors showed that an asbestos-induced apoptosis-resistant subline (MT-2Rst), which was established from a human adult T-cell leukemia virus-immortalized T-cell line (MT-2Org) by continuous exposure to asbestos chrysotile-B, produced high levels of TGF-β1 through phosphorylation of p38 MAPK, and acquire resistance to inhibition of cell growth by TGF-β1 [96]. It was observed that asbestos can trigger a cascade of biological events including the increase of IL-10 expression and Bcl-2 overexpression in human T-cell leukemia virus-immortalized T-cell line and that CD4+ T lymphocytes from MM patients had significant up-regulation of Bcl-2 expression thus affecting their survival. The Bcl-2 up-regulation might affect the Treg population thus contributing to immunosuppression in cancer patients [97] (Figure 2).

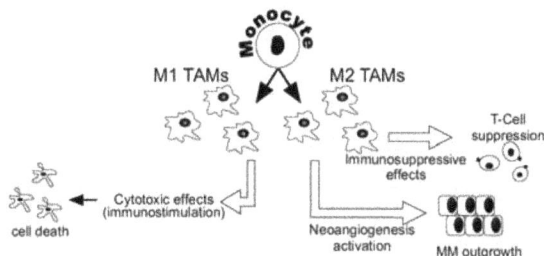

**Figure 2.** Role of the innate immunity in the development of MM. Tumor-associated macrophages (TAMs) represent a major link between inflammation and cancer. The majority of TAMs in MM have the M2 phenotype. M2 TAMs have poor antigen-presenting capacity, suppress T-cells adaptive immunity, and support MM growth.

## 5. Effects of Polyphenols in MM

### 5.1. Effects of Polyphenols on ROS in MM

Epidemiological studies indicate the existence of an inverse correlation between the consumption of polyphenols and the incidence of various chronic diseases and cancer. In fact, polyphenols possess anti-oxidant activities and thus are able to protect cells from oxidative stress, providing an anti-inflammatory effect [98–100]. For instance, flavonoids are able to scavenge ROS generated by neutrophils and macrophages and to impair ROS production by inhibiting NADPH oxidase, xanthine oxidase, and myeloperoxidase [27,29,30]. In addition, polyphenols modulate the activity of ROS-generating enzymes, such as COX and lipoxygenase (LOX) [30,101,102]. Furthermore, polyphenols inhibit NO production from activated macrophages [103,104] and also inducible nitric oxide synthase (iNOS) protein and its mRNA expression [105].

However, polyphenols also possess a pro-oxidant activity, depending on their concentration and chemical structure, cell type, or experimental conditions (pH, redox stress) [106,107]. The pro-oxidant effect of polyphenols is important in cancer cells, since this effect leads to oxidative breaking of DNA, inhibition of cell growth and apoptosis [14]. In fact, in the last few years the use of pro-oxidants against cancer is an emerging topic in research, since it has been observed that ROS contribute to the cytotoxic activity of some chemotherapeutics and that cancer cells are more susceptible to ROS than normal cells [107].

As for MM, asbestos produces ROS and RNS, that act as second messengers to drive initiation and progression of MM-carcinogenesis, through genetic alterations, activation of the survival pathways, stimulation of matrix metalloproteinases (MMP), and angiogenic signaling. Furthermore, ROS mediate extrinsic and intrinsic pathways of apoptosis, necrosis, and autophagy, thus ROS production is also used as a therapy for MM, to limit tumor growth [51]. In this way, polyphenols, which also possess pro- and anti-oxidant properties, are a promising tool to treat MM.

Several studies have explored the ability of different polyphenols as pro-oxidant agents in MM. It has been demonstrated that curcumin (40 µM) increased ROS production in HMESO cells *in vitro*, leading to caspase-1 activation and pyroptotic cell death of MM cells [108].

Satoh *et al.* demonstrated that the flavan-3-ol epigallocatechin-3-gallate (EGCG) induced ROS production and impaired the mitochondrial membrane potential and these effects were responsible for the induction of apoptosis in MM cells *in vitro*. In fact, the treatment of MM cells with ROS scavengers, such as tempol and catalase, inhibited the apoptosis induced by EGCG [109]. A similar effect was reported by Ranzato *et al.* They demonstrated that EGCG induced both apoptotic and necrotic cell death in MM cells. In particular, it has been shown that EGCG had a pro-oxidant effect and induced cell death by the release of $H_2O_2$ outside of cells [110]. Similarly, a recent study showed that EGCG, when added to culture medium, induced $H_2O_2$ formation and decreased proliferation both in MM cells and MET5A cells (normal cells). Due to EGCG instability that causes $H_2O_2$ formation in culture medium, ECGC was added to cells in presence of catalase (CAT) and exogenous superoxide dismutase (SOD). In this way, EGCG decreased cell proliferation only in MM cells and induced mitochondrial apoptosis [111].

The increased levels of ROS induce the nuclear translocation and activation of Nrf2 (nuclear factor E2-related factor 2) in MM. Normally, Nrf2 is sequestered in cytosol by its inhibitor Keap-1 (Kelch-like ECH-associated protein 1); when MM arises, the ROS levels increase and one or multiple cysteines bind to Keap-1, which undergoes a conformational change releasing Nrf2. Next, Nrf2 translocates to the nucleus and activates the transcription of downstream genes, as HO-1. The high levels of Nrf2 create an anti-oxidant environment which is resistant to MM-therapy. It has been demonstrated that the combined treatment of clofarabine and resveratrol inhibited the Nrf2 pathway by reducing nuclear localization of Nrf2 and by decreasing Nrf2 and HO-1 protein levels *in vitro*. Lee *et al.* hypothesized that resveratrol with clofarabine decreased the chemoresistance of MM, modulating the levels of proteins activated by ROS, as Nrf2 [112]. In addition, the same authors demonstrated that the combined treatment of clofarabine and resveratrol increased the nuclear expression of phospho-p53. Hence, p53 induced the expression of pro-apoptotic proteins, as Bax, Puma, and Noxa [113]. Faraonio *et al.* indicated the possibility of crosstalk between p53 and Nrf2. p53 could prevent the generation of an anti-oxidant environment counteracting the effect of Nrf2 and inducing apoptosis [114].

A recent study by Pietrofesa *et al.* reported the *in vitro* ability of LGM2605 (a synthetic lignan secoisolariciresinol diglucoside) to reduce asbestos-induced cytotoxicity and ROS generation and to induce phase II anti-oxidant enzymes stimulated by Nrf2 (HO-1 and Nqo1) in murine peritoneal macrophages. LGM2605 acted as a direct free radical scavenger and anti-oxidant in a dose-dependent manner. They hypothesized the possible use of this synthetic lignan as a chemopreventive agent in the development of asbestos-induced MM [115].

Kostyuk *et al.* have conducted several studies on the efficacy of different polyphenols in preventing asbestos-induced injury of peritoneal macrophages and red blood cells. They demonstrated that quercetin and rutin were able to reduce peritoneal macrophages injury caused by asbestos and to scavenge ROS. They suggested that quercetin and rutin could be promising drug candidates for a prophylactic asbestos-induced disease [116]. Similarly, in another study they explored the efficacy of the main polyphenolic constituents of green tea extract, (−)-epicatechin gallate (ECG) and (−)-epigallocatechin gallate (EGCG). They observed that ECG and EGCG had a protective effect against chrysotile and crocidolite-induced cell injuries in peritoneal macrophages, and this effect was attributed to the scavenger properties towards the superoxide anion and the ability of polyphenols to chelate iron ions [117]. They also concluded in a comparative study that the protective effect increased in the following series: rutin < dihydroquercetin < quercetin < ECG < EGCG [118].

Effects of polyphenols on ROS in MM are summarized in Table 1.

**Table 1.** Effects of polyphenols on ROS production and scavenging in MM.

| Polyphenols | Cell Type | Effects on ROS | Ref. |
| --- | --- | --- | --- |
| Curcumin | H-MESO cells | ↑ ROS<br>↑ Caspase-1<br>↑ Pyroptotic cell death | [108] |
| EGCG | ACC-meso 1, Y-meso 8A, EHMES-10, EHMES-1, MSTO-211H, REN, MM98, BR95, E198 cells | ↑ ROS<br>↑ $H_2O_2$ outside of cells<br>↑ Apoptosis and necrosis<br>↓ Cell proliferation | [109–111] |
| Resveratrol (+Clofarabine) | MSTO-211H cells | ↓ Nrf2 pathway<br>↑ p53 phosphorylation<br>↑ Pro-apoptotic proteins | [112,113] |
| LGM2605 (a synthetic lignan) | Murine peritoneal macrophages | ↓ ROS<br>↓ Cytotoxicity<br>↑ Phase II anti-oxidant enzymes | [115] |
| Quercetin + Rutin | Peritoneal macrophages of Wistar rats | ↓ ROS<br>↓ Peritoneal macrophages injury by asbestos | [116] |
| EGCG + ECG | Peritoneal macrophages of Wistar rats | ↓ ROS<br>↓ Peritoneal macrophages injury by asbestos | [117] |

↓: decrease; ↑: increase.

*5.2. Effects of Polyphenols on Mediators of Inflammation in MM*

Inflammation plays a critical role in the process of carcinogenesis by regulating the different stages of initiation, promotion, progression, and metastasis, and also the responses to therapies [119]. In this regard, it has been observed that the tumor microenvironment is infiltrated by innate and adaptive immune cells, such as macrophages, neutrophils, mast cells, myeloid-derived suppressor cells, dendritic cells, NKcells, and T and B lymphocytes that communicate to each other through the production of cytokines [119].

Polyphenols possess the ability to directly modulate innate and also adaptive immune cells that infiltrate the tumor. In fact, it has been demonstrated that different polyphenols, such as genistein, EGCG, curcumin, and resveratrol, are able to modulate these immune cells to enhance an antitumor response or to suppress the immune escape of tumors [14].

In addition, it has been demonstrated that polyphenols possess the ability to control the inflammatory process by inhibiting the secretion of pro-inflammatory cytokines (IL-1$\beta$, IL-2, IL-6, IFN-$\gamma$, TNF-$\alpha$) and chemokines [20]. The inhibition of the production of these cytokines also led to inhibition of ROS, since cytokines trigger ROS production [120]. Several studies have reported this ability of polyphenols. For instance, curcumin and different flavonoids, such as flavones, EGCG, and flavonols, are able to inhibit the secretion of TNF-$\alpha$, IL-6, IL-1$\beta$, IL-8, and IFN-$\gamma$ from various cell types [121–129].

By the activation of different transcription factors, such as NF-$\kappa$B, AP-1, STAT-3, SMAD, and caspases, cytokines can promote or inhibit tumor progression [119]. It has been demonstrated that polyphenols, such as resveratrol, flavones, flavonols, EGCG, anthocyanins, isoflavones, and curcumin, are able to modulate NF-$\kappa$B [130–138]. Curcumin, resveratrol, and EGCG also inhibit STAT-3 activation [139–142].

Inflammation, and thus the production of inflammasome, has an essential role in the development of MM [143]. As previously described, the active inflammasome induces the activation of caspase-1 and mature form of pro-inflammatory cytokines IL-1$\beta$ and IL-18 and thus the inflammatory cell death pyroptosis [144].

In this regard, the anti-inflammatory effect of polyphenols, by regulating innate and adaptive immunity through the modulation of different cytokines, chemokines, and transcription factors could be a promising strategy to contrast development of this type of cancer [14].

Miller *et al.* has observed that curcumin was able to kill MM cells *via* pyroptosis without the classical inflammasome-related cytokines, IL-1$\beta$ and IL-18. They observed that curcumin increased the concentration of caspase-1 but did not increase IL-1$\beta$ and IL-18 expression. Furthermore, they observed a higher concentration of pro-IL-1$\beta$, indicating a block of the maturation of cytokine. Curcumin treatment increased the expression of NLRP3, which alone induces a decreased NF-$\kappa$B expression. Curcumin reduced the inflammasome-related gene expression, NF-$\kappa$B, TLR and IL-1 pathway. In addition, curcumin down-regulated the expression of MYD88, NLRC4, and TXNIP and up-regulated HSP90AA1 (heat shock protein 90 kDa alpha class A member 1), IL-12, IL-6. Hence, curcumin has an anti-inflammatory effect on MM cells by blocking cytokine processing of IL-1$\beta$ and genes involved in the NF-$\kappa$B pathway [108].

Wang *et al.* demonstrated that curcumin also suppressed MM cell growth *in vitro* and *in vivo* (oral administration) and enhanced the efficacy of cisplatin. In particular, curcumin inhibited cell growth through activation of p38 kinase, caspases 9 and 3, increased pro-apoptotic protein Bax levels, stimulated PARP cleavage, and induced apoptosis. In addition, curcumin stimulated expression of novel transducers of cell growth suppression, such as CARP-1, XAF1, and SULF1 proteins [145].

It has been shown that the activated NF-$\kappa$B and high levels of the activated phosphorylated STAT-3 are present in MM. Cioce *et al.* showed that butein (3,4,2′,4′-tetrahydroxychalcone), a natural inhibitor of NF-$\kappa$B and STAT-3, inhibits the migration of MM cells and strongly affects the clonogenicity of MM cells *in vitro* by inhibiting the phosphorylation of STAT-3, the nuclear localization of NF-$\kappa$B and the interaction of NF-$\kappa$B and phospho-STAT-3. Different genes involved in cancer progression of pro-angiogenic cytokines (VEGF) and of IL-6 and IL-8 were also down-regulated. Furthermore, they showed that butein was able to severely affect tumor engraftment and to potentiate the anticancer effects of pemetrexed in mouse xenograft models *in vivo*. Intraperitoneal treatment with butein was safe, since butein does not significantly affect the viability of human untransformed mesothelial cells *in vitro* or the survival of tumor-free mice *in vivo* [146].

The activation of STAT-3 is associated to PIAS-3 expression levels in MM cell lines. PIAS-3 specifically interacts with phospho-STAT-3 and decreases the STAT-3 DNA-binding capacity and transcriptional activity. The overexpression of PIAS-3 can inhibit STAT-3 transcriptional activity and induces apoptosis *in vitro* [147]. Dabir *et al.* demonstrated that an inverse correlation between PIAS-3 and STAT-3 is present in MM cells. In fact, they showed that high levels of phospho-STAT-3 and low levels of PIAS-3 are present. Furthermore, they observed that treatment with curcumin (1.0 μM) was able to increase PIAS-3 levels and thereby decreased STAT-3 phosphorylation and cell viability in MM cells [148].

Flaxseed lignans, enriched in secoisolariciresinol diglucoside (SDG), have been investigated for the prevention of asbestos-induced peritoneal inflammation in a mouse model of accelerated MM development that recapitulates many of the molecular, genetic, and cell-signaling features of human MM after asbestos injection. Mice were supplemented with a diet containing lignans seven days before an intraperitoneal injection of crocidolite asbestos and three days after asbestos exposure; they were evaluated for abdominal inflammation, pro-inflammatory/pro-fibrogenic cytokine release, WBC gene expression changes, and oxidative and nitrosative stress in peritoneal lavage fluid. The results showed that dietary lignan administration diminished acute inflammation by decreasing the number of WBCs and the release of IL-1β, IL-6, HMGB1, and TNF-α pro-inflammatory cytokines and pro-fibrogenic active TGF-β1. Furthermore, lignan acted as an anti-oxidant by decreasing mRNA levels of inducible nitric oxide synthase, and thus nitrosative and oxidative stress, and by increasing the expression of the Nrf2-regulated anti-oxidant enzymes, HO-1, Nqo1 and Gstm1 [42].

In a preliminary study, Martinotti *et al.* demonstrated that the combined treatment with EGCG, ascorbate, and gemcitabine (AND) synergistically affected the viability of MM cells [149]. Next, the same authors showed that AND treatment increased DAPK2 (Death-Associated Protein Kinase 2), a calcium- and calmodulin-dependent regulator of apoptosis and tumor suppressor, and TNSFR11B expression. The TNSFR11B gene encodes a cytokine receptor belonging to the TNF receptor family, called osteoprotegerin (OPG). OPG acts as receptor for RANK ligand, inhibiting RANK-dependent activation of NF-κB. Furthermore, they observed a decreased expression of TNFAIP3 (tumor necrosis factor-α-induced protein 3), an inhibitor of NF-κB activation and TNF-mediated apoptosis, typically up-regulated in inflammation and in tumors. In this study, they found a down-regulated TNFAIP3 expression because AND treatment decreased p65 subunit of NF-κB. Hence, the combined treatment induced a non-inflammatory apoptosis [150].

The transcription factor Specificity protein 1 (Sp1) is highly expressed in different cancers and is associated with poor prognosis. Sp1 modulates the expression of oncogenes and tumor suppressors, as well as genes involved in proliferation, differentiation, the DNA damage response, apoptosis, senescence, and angiogenesis and it is also implicated in inflammation and genomic instability [151].

Lee *et al.* showed that resveratrol decreased the Sp1 expression and down-regulated Sp1-dependent gene expression in MM. They observed a decreased tumor volume and an increased number of caspase-3-positive cells after intraperitoneal treatment with resveratrol [152]. In another study, it has been demonstrated that the combined treatment of clofarabine and resveratrol decreased levels of Sp1, p-Akt, c-Met, cyclin D1, and p21 [153].

Similarly, Chae *et al.* found that 20–80 μM quercetin suppressed the Sp1 expression and modulated the target genes, as cyclin D1, Mcl-1 (myeloid cell leukemia), and survivin in MM. Furthermore, quercetin induced apoptosis through the Bid, caspase-3, and PARP cleavage, the up-regulation of Bax, and down-regulation of Bcl-xL in MSTO-211H cells [154].

In another study, the same authors focused on the anticancer effects of honokiol (HNK), a pharmacologically active component found in the traditional Chinese medicinal herb, *Magnolia* species. It has been observed that HNK inhibited MM cell growth, down-regulated Sp1 expression and Sp1 target transcription factors, including cyclin D1, Mcl-1, and survivin, and induced the apoptosis by increasing Bax, reducing Bid and Bcl-xL and activating caspase-3 and PARP [155].

Kim *et al.* found that licochalcone A (LCA), a natural product derived from the Glycyrrhiza inflata, regulated the cell growth and down-regulated the Sp1 expression in MSTO-211H and H28 cell lines. Furthermore, LCA down-regulated the expression of Sp1 downstream genes, as cyclin D1, Mcl1 and survivin. Like quercetin and honokiol, LCA increased Bax and decreased Bcl-2 expression, inducing the mitochondrial apoptotic pathway [156].

Lee *et al.* demonstrated that hesperidin, a flavanone presents in citrus fruits, inhibited the cell growth and down-regulated the SP1 expression in MSTO-211H cells. Hesperidin significantly suppressed mRNA and protein levels of Sp1 and regulated the expression of p27, p21, cyclin D1, Mcl-1, and survivin. Furthermore, hesperidin induced the apoptosis pathway through cleavages of Bid, caspase-3, and PARP, and up-regulation of Bax and down-regulation of Bcl-xL [157]. Similarly, the same authors showed that cafestol and kahweol, two diterpenes present in the typical bean of *Coffea Arabica*, induced apoptosis and suppressed the Sp1 protein levels in MSTO-211H cells. These compounds modulated the expression of genes regulated by Sp1, including cyclin D1, Mcl-1, and survivin. Furthermore, the cafestol treatment induced the cleavage of Bid, caspase-3, and PARP, and the kahweol treatment up-regulated Bax and down-regulated Bcl-xL [158].

The effect of a novel mixture containing lysine, proline, ascorbic acid, and green tea extract has been investigated by Roomi *et al.* in MM cell line MSTO-211H. They demonstrated that this mixture was able to inhibit MMP secretion and invasion and thus is a promising candidate for therapeutic use in the treatment of MM [159].

Effects of polyphenols on mediators of inflammation in MM are summarized in Table 2.

**Table 2.** Effects of polyphenols on production of mediators of inflammation in MM.

| Polyphenols | Cell Type or Animal Model | Effects on Inflammation | Ref. |
|---|---|---|---|
| Curcumin | H-MESO, NCI-2052, NCI-H2452, MSTO-211H, and NCI-H28 cells | ↑ Caspase-1 <br> ↑ pro-IL-1β and block of maturation of IL-1 β <br> ↑ NLRP3 <br> ↓ NF-κB, TRL, and IL-1 pathways <br> ↑ PIAS-3 <br> ↓ p-STAT-3 | [108,148] |
| Butein | MSTO-211H, NCI-H28, NCI-H2052 | ↓ NF-κB, p-STAT-3 <br> ↓VEGF <br> ↓ IL-6, IL-8 | [146] |
| Flaxseed Lignans | MM-prone Nf2$^{+/mut}$ mice | ↓ IL-1β, IL-6, HMGB1, TNF-α, TGF-β1 <br> ↑ Nrf2-regulated anti-oxidant enzymes | [42] |
| EGCG + Ascorbate + Gemcitabine (AND) | REN cells | ↑ DAPK2 <br> ↑ TNSFR11B <br> ↓ TNFAIP3 <br> ↓ NF-κB pathway | [150] |
| Resveratrol | MSTO-211H cells | ↓ Sp1, p21, p27, cyclin D1, Mcl-1 <br> ↓ survivin <br> ↑ Apoptosis | [152] |
| Resveratrol + Clofarabine | MSTO-211H cells | ↓ Sp1, p-Akt <br> ↓ c-Met, cyclin D1, p21 | [153] |

Table 2. *Cont.*

| Polyphenols | Cell Type or Animal Model | Effects on Inflammation | Ref. |
|---|---|---|---|
| Quercetin | MSTO-211H cells | ↓ Sp1, cyclin D1, Mcl-1, survivin<br>↑ Apoptosis | [154] |
| Honokiol | MSTO-211H cells | ↓ Sp1<br>↓ cyclin D1, Mcl-1, survivin<br>↑ Apoptosis | [155] |
| Licochalcone A | MSTO-211H and H28 cells | ↓ Sp1<br>↓ cyclin D1, Mcl-1, survivin<br>↑ Apoptosis | [156] |
| Hesperidin | MSTO-211H cells | ↓ Sp1<br>↓ p27, p21, cyclin D1, Mcl-1, survivin<br>↑ Apoptosis | [157] |
| Cafestol and kahweol | MSTO-211H cells | ↓ Sp1, cyclin D1, Mcl-1, survivin<br>↑ Apoptosis | [158] |

↓: decrease; ↑: increase.

## 6. Conclusions

The immune system, and in particular inflammation, has an essential role in the development of MM. A long-lasting inflammatory response orchestrated by mesothelial cells contributes to the initiation, promotion, and progression of mesothelial cells into MM. Polyphenols possess important anti-inflammatory properties by regulating innate and adaptive immunity through the modulation of different mediators of inflammation and also by acting as an immune surveillance mechanism against cancers through the regulation of apoptosis. Furthermore, polyphenols possess a pro-oxidant activity, which could be used against cancer. In fact, in the last few years the use of ROS-generating agents against cancer is an emerging strategy to kill cancer cells, since it has been observed that ROS contribute to the cytotoxic activity of some chemotherapeutics and that cancer cells are more susceptible to ROS than normal cells.

Accordingly, the local or systemic administration of polyphenols might reduce the production of pro-inflammatory molecules by targeting signal transduction pathways or ROS and RNS in order to prevent MM. On the other hand, the administration of polyphenols might also induce MM cell death to limit tumor growth.

Furthermore, MM is a tumor arising from the mesothelial cell linings of the serous membranes, thus the local administration of polyphenols in the serous cavity might be a better strategy to treat MM, because in this way polyphenols could bypass biotransformation and could reach an effective dose directly available at the site of tumor.

Thus the use of polyphenols might represent a promising strategy to contrast the development and/or to prevent MM.

**Acknowledgments:** This study was supported by a grant from Ricerche Universitarie Sapienza (C26A14T57T). We thank Evelyn Carpenter for help in English language editing. Rosanna Mattera is a recipient of the Sapienza PhD program in Molecular Medicine.

**Author Contributions:** All authors of this paper have directly participated in the planning or drafting of this manuscript and have read and approved the final version submitted.

**Conflicts of Interest:** The authors declare no conflict of interest.

## References

1. Carbone, M.; Ly, B.H.; Dodson, R.F.; Pagano, I.; Morris, P.T.; Dogan, U.A.; Gazdar, A.F.; Pass, H.I.; Yang, H. Malignant mesothelioma: Facts, myths, and hypotheses. *J. Cell Physiol.* **2012**, *227*, 44–58. [CrossRef] [PubMed]

2. Yang, H.; Rivera, Z.; Jube, S.; Nasu, M.; Bertino, P.; Goparaju, C.; Franzoso, G.; Lotze, M.T.; Krausz, T.; Pass, H.I.; *et al.* Programmed necrosis induced by asbestos in human mesothelial cells causes high-mobility group box 1 protein release and resultant inflammation. *Proc. Nat. Acad. Sci. USA* **2010**, *107*, 12611–12616. [CrossRef] [PubMed]

3. Jube, S.; Rivera, Z.S.; Bianchi, M.E.; Powers, A.; Wang, E.; Pagano, I.; Pass, H.I.; Gaudino, G.; Carbone, M.; Yang, H. Cancer cell secretion of the DAMP protein HMGB1 supports progression in malignant mesothelioma. *Cancer Res.* **2012**, *72*, 3290–3301. [CrossRef] [PubMed]

4. Napolitano, A.; Antoine, D.J.; Pellegrini, L.; Baumann, F.; Pagano, I.; Pastorino, S.; Goparaju, C.M.; Prokrym, K.; Canino, C.; Pass, H.I.; *et al.* HMGB1 and its hyperacetylated isoform are sensitive and specific serum biomarkers to detect asbestos exposure and to identify mesothelioma patients. *Clin. Cancer Res.* **2016**. [CrossRef] [PubMed]

5. Remon, J.; Lianes, P.; Martinez, S.; Velasco, M.; Querol, R.; Zanui, M. Malignant mesothelioma: New insights into a rare disease. *Cancer Treat. Rev.* **2013**, *39*, 584–591. [CrossRef] [PubMed]

6. Faig, J.; Howard, S.; Levine, E.A.; Casselman, G.; Hesdorffer, M.; Ohar, J.A. Changing Pattern in Malignant Mesothelioma Survival. *Transl. Oncol.* **2015**, *8*, 35–39. [CrossRef] [PubMed]

7. Testa, J.R.; Cheung, M.; Pei, J.; Below, J.E.; Tan, Y.; Sementino, E.; Cox, N.J.; Dogan, A.U.; Pass, H.I.; Trusa, S.; *et al.* Germline BAP1 mutations predispose to malignant mesothelioma. *Nat. Genet.* **2011**, *43*, 1022–1025. [CrossRef] [PubMed]

8. Astoul, P.; Roca, E.; Galateau-Salle, F.; Scherpereel, A. Malignant pleural mesothelioma: From the bench to the bedside. *Respiration* **2012**, *83*, 481–493. [CrossRef] [PubMed]

9. Izzi, V.; Masuelli, L.; Tresoldi, I.; Foti, C.; Modesti, A.; Bei, R. Immunity and malignant mesothelioma: From mesothelial cell damage to tumor development and immune response-based therapies. *Cancer Lett.* **2012**, *322*, 18–34. [CrossRef] [PubMed]

10. Menges, C.W.; Chen, Y.; Mossman, B.T.; Chernoff, J.; Yeung, A.T.; Testa, J.R. A phosphotyrosine proteomic screen identifies multiple tyrosine kinase signaling pathways aberrantly activated in malignant mesothelioma. *Genes Cancer* **2010**, *1*, 493–505. [CrossRef] [PubMed]

11. Albonici, L.; Palumbo, C.; Manzari, V. Role of inflammation and angiogenic growth factors in malignant mesothelioma. In *Malignant Mesothelioma*; Belli, C., Ed.; InTech: Rijeka, Croatia, 2012.

12. Bajaj, G.; Yeo, Y. Drug delivery systems for intraperitoneal therapy. *Pharm. Res.* **2010**, *27*, 735–738. [CrossRef] [PubMed]

13. Benvenuto, M.; Fantini, M.; Masuelli, L.; de Smaele, E.; Zazzeroni, F.; Tresoldi, I.; Calabrese, G.; Galvano, F.; Modesti, A.; Bei, R. Inhibition of ErbB receptors, Hedgehog and NF-kappaB signaling by polyphenols in cancer. *Front. Biosci.* **2013**, *18*, 1290–1310.

14. Ghiringhelli, F.; Rebe, C.; Hichami, A.; Delmas, D. Immunomodulation and anti-inflammatory roles of polyphenols as anticancer agents. *Anticancer Agents Med. Chem.* **2012**, *12*, 852–873. [CrossRef] [PubMed]

15. Gonzáles, R.; Ballester, I.; López-Posadas, R.; Suárez, M.D.; Zarzuelo, A.; Martínez-Augustin, O.; de Medina, F.S. Effects of flavonoids and other polyphenols on inflammation. *Crit. Rev. Food Sci. Nutr.* **2011**, *51*, 331–362. [CrossRef] [PubMed]

16. Santangelo, C.; Vari, R.; Scazzocchio, B.; di Benedetto, R.; Filesi, C.; Masella, R. Polyphenols, intracellular signalling and inflammation. *Ann. Ist. Super. Sanità* **2007**, *43*, 394–405. [PubMed]

17. Cuevas, A.; Saavedra, N.; Salazar, L.A.; Abdalla, D.S. Modulation of immune function by polyphenols: Possible contribution of epigenetic factors. *Nutrients* **2013**, *5*, 2314–2332. [CrossRef] [PubMed]

18. Manach, C.; Scalbert, A.; Morand, C.; Rémésy, C.; Jiménez, L. Polyphenols: Food sources and bioavailability. *Am. J. Clin. Nutr.* **2004**, *79*, 727–747. [PubMed]

19. Scalbert, A.; Manach, C.; Morand, C.; Rémésy, C.; Jiménez, L. Dietary polyphenols and the prevention of diseases. *Crit. Rev. Food Sci. Nutr.* **2005**, *45*, 287–306. [CrossRef] [PubMed]

20. Marzocchella, L.; Fantini, M.; Benvenuto, M.; Masuelli, L.; Tresoldi, I.; Modest, A.; Bei, R. Dietary flavonoids: Molecular mechanisms of action as anti- inflammatory agents. *Recent Patent Inflamm. Allergy Drug Disc.* **2011**, *5*, 200–220. [CrossRef]

21. Crozier, A.; Jaganath, I.B.; Clifford, M.N. Dietary phenolics: Chemistry, bioavailability and effects on health. *Nat. Prod. Rep.* **2009**, *26*, 1001–1043. [CrossRef] [PubMed]

22. Fantini, M.; Benvenuto, M.; Masuelli, L.; Frajese, G.V.; Tresoldi, I.; Modesti, A.; Bei, R. *In vitro* and *in vivo* antitumoral effects of combinations of polyphenols, or polyphenols and anticancer drugs: Perspectives on cancer treatment. *Int. J. Mol. Sci.* **2015**, *16*, 9236–9282. [CrossRef] [PubMed]

23. Bei, R.; Masuelli, L.; Turriziani, M.; Li Volti, G.; Malaguarnera, M.; Galvano, F. Impaired expression and function of signaling pathway enzymes by anthocyanins: Role on cancer prevention and progression. *Curr. Enzym. Inhib.* **2009**, *5*, 184–197. [CrossRef]

24. Tomás-Barberán, F.A.; Clifford, M.N. Flavanones, chalcones and dihydrochalcones-nature, occurrence and dietary burden. *J. Sci. Food Agric.* **2000**, *80*, 1073–1080. [CrossRef]

25. Cassidy, A.; Hanley, B.; Lamuela-Raventos, R.M. Isoflavones, lignans and stilbenes-origins, metabolism and potential importance to human health. *J. Sci. Food Agric.* **2000**, *80*, 1044–1062. [CrossRef]

26. Prasad, S.; Tyagi, A.K.; Aggarwal, B.B. Recent developments in delivery, bioavailability, absorption and metabolism of curcumin: The golden pigment from golden spice. *Cancer Res. Treat.* **2014**, *46*, 2–18. [CrossRef] [PubMed]

27. García-Lafuente, A.; Guillamón, E.; Villares, A.; Rostagno, M.A.; Martínez, J.A. Flavonoids as anti-inflammatory agents: Implications in cancer and cardiovascular disease. *Inflamm. Res.* **2009**, *58*, 537–552. [CrossRef] [PubMed]

28. Izzi, V.; Masuelli, L.; Tresoldi, I.; Sacchetti, P.; Modesti, A.; Galvano, F.; Bei, R. The effects of dietary flavonoids on the regulation of redox inflammatory networks. *Front. Biosci.* **2012**, *17*, 2396–2418. [CrossRef]

29. Edwards, S.W. The O-2 Generating NADPH Oxidase of Phagocytes: Structure and Methods of Detection. *Methods* **1996**, *9*, 563–577. [CrossRef] [PubMed]

30. Cotelle, N. Role of flavonoids in oxidative stress. *Curr. Top. Med. Chem.* **2001**, *1*, 569–590. [CrossRef] [PubMed]

31. Manach, C.; Williamson, G.; Morand, C.; Scalbert, A.; Rémésy, C. Bioavailability and bioefficacy of polyphenols in humans. I. Review of 97 bioavailability studies. *Am. J. Clin. Nutr.* **2005**, *81*, 230S–242S. [PubMed]

32. Ginsburg, I.; Kohen, R.; Koren, E. Microbial and host cells acquire enhanced oxidant-scavenging abilities by binding polyphenols. *Arch. Biochem. Biophys.* **2011**, *506*, 12–23. [CrossRef] [PubMed]

33. Bohn, T. Dietary factors affecting polyphenol bioavailability. *Nutr. Rev.* **2014**, *72*, 429–452. [CrossRef] [PubMed]

34. Masuelli, L.; Fantini, M.; Benvenuto, M.; Sacchetti, P.; Giganti, M.G.; Tresoldi, I.; Lido, P.; Lista, F.; Cavallo, F.; Nanni, P.; *et al.* Intratumoral delivery of recombinant vaccinia virus encoding for ErbB2/Neu inhibits the growth of salivary gland carcinoma cells. *J. Transl. Med.* **2014**, *12*. [CrossRef] [PubMed]

35. Masuelli, L.; Marzocchella, L.; Focaccetti, C.; Lista, F.; Nardi, A.; Scardino, A.; Mattei, M.; Turriziani, M.; Modesti, M.; Forni, G.; *et al.* Local delivery of recombinant vaccinia virus encoding for neu counteracts growth of mammary tumors more efficiently than systemic delivery in neu transgenic mice. *Cancer Immunol. Immunother.* **2010**, *59*, 1247–1258. [CrossRef] [PubMed]

36. Galanis, E.; Russell, S. Cancer gene therapy clinical trials: Lessons for the future. *Br. J. Cancer* **2001**, *85*, 1432–1436. [CrossRef] [PubMed]

37. Forsyth, P.; Roldán, G.; George, D.; Wallace, C.; Palmer, C.A.; Morris, D.; Cairncross, G.; Matthews, M.V.; Markert, J.; Gillespie, Y.; *et al.* A phase I trial of intratumoral administration of reovirus in patients with histologically confirmed recurrent malignant gliomas. *Mol. Ther.* **2008**, *16*, 627–632. [CrossRef] [PubMed]

38. Roberts, N.J.; Zhang, L.; Janku, F.; Collins, A.; Bai, R.Y.; Staedtke, V.; Rusk, A.W.; Tung, D.; Miller, M.; Roix, J.; *et al.* Intratumoral injection of Clostridium novyi-NT spores induces antitumor responses. *Sci. Transl. Med.* **2014**, *6*. [CrossRef] [PubMed]

39. Fujiwara, S.; Wada, H.; Miyata, H.; Kawada, J.; Kawabata, R.; Nishikawa, H.; Gnjatic, S.; Sedrak, C.; Sato, E.; Nakamura, Y.; *et al.* Clinical trial of the intratumoral administration of labeled DC combined with systemic chemotherapy for esophageal cancer. *J. Immunother.* **2012**, *35*, 513–521. [CrossRef] [PubMed]

40. Masuelli, L.; Pantanella, F.; la Regina, G.; Benvenuto, M.; Fantini, M.; Mattera, R.; Di Stefano, E.; Mattei, M.; Silvestri, R.; Schippa, S.; *et al.* Violacein, an indole-derived purple-colored natural pigment produced by *Janthinobacterium lividum*, inhibits the growth of head and neck carcinoma cell lines both *in vitro* and *in vivo*. *Tumour Biol.* **2016**, *37*, 3705–3717. [CrossRef] [PubMed]

41. Price, B.; Ware, A. Time trend of mesothelioma incidence in the United States and projection of future cases: An update based on SEER data for 1973 through 2005. *Crit. Rev. Toxicol.* **2009**, *39*, 576–588. [CrossRef] [PubMed]

42. Pietrofesa, R.A.; Velalopoulou, A.; Arguiri, E.; Menges, C.W.; Testa, J.R.; Hwang, W.T.; Albelda, S.M.; Christofidou-Solomidou, M. Flaxseed lignans enriched in secoisolariciresinol diglucoside prevent acute asbestos-induced peritoneal inflammation in mice. *Carcinogenesis* **2016**, *37*, 177–187. [CrossRef] [PubMed]

43. Chew, S.H.; Toyokuni, S. Malignant mesothelioma as an oxidative stress-induced cancer: An update. *Free Radic. Biol. Med.* **2015**, *86*, 166–178. [CrossRef] [PubMed]

44. Otsuki, T.; Maeda, M.; Murakami, S.; Hayashi, H.; Miura, Y.; Kusaka, M.; Nakano, T.; Fukuoka, K.; Kishimoto, T.; Hyodoh, F.; *et al.* Immunological effects of silica and asbestos. *Cell. Mol. Immunol.* **2007**, *4*, 261–268. [PubMed]

45. Miserocchi, G.; Sancini, G.; Mantegazza, F.; Chiappino, G. Translocation pathways for inhaled asbestos fibers. *Environ. Health* **2008**, *7*. [CrossRef] [PubMed]

46. Tunesi, S.; Ferrante, D.; Mirabelli, D.; Andorno, S.; Betti, M.; Fiorito, G.; Guarrera, S.; Casalone, E.; Neri, M.; Ugolini, D.; *et al.* Gene-asbestos interaction in malignant pleural mesothelioma susceptibility. *Carcinogenesis* **2015**, *36*, 1129–1135. [CrossRef] [PubMed]

47. Jantz, M.A.; Antony, V.B. Pathophysiology of the pleura. *Respiration* **2008**, *75*, 121–133. [CrossRef] [PubMed]

48. Carbone, M.; Bedrossian, C.W. The pathogenesis of mesothelioma. *Semin. Diagn. Pathol.* **2006**, *23*, 56–60. [CrossRef] [PubMed]

49. Acencio, M.M.; Soares, B.; Marchi, E.; Silva, C.S.; Teixeira, L.R.; Broaddus, V.C. Inflammatory cytokines contribute to asbestos-induced injury of mesothelial cells. *Lung* **2015**, *193*, 831–837. [CrossRef] [PubMed]

50. Carbone, M.; Yang, H. Molecular pathways: Targeting mechanisms of asbestos and erionite carcinogenesis in mesothelioma. *Clin. Cancer Res.* **2012**, *18*, 598–604. [CrossRef] [PubMed]

51. Benedetti, S.; Nuvoli, B.; Catalani, S.; Galati, R. Reactive oxygen species a double-edged sword for mesothelioma. *Oncotarget* **2015**, *6*, 16848–16865. [CrossRef] [PubMed]

52. Kamp, D.W.; Weitzman, S.A. The molecular basis of asbestos induced lung injury. *Thorax* **1999**, *54*, 638–652. [CrossRef] [PubMed]

53. Kinnula, V.L.; Aalto, K.; Raivio, K.O.; Walles, S.; Linnainmaa, K. Cytotoxicity of oxidants and asbestos fibers in cultured human mesothelial cells. *Free Radic. Biol. Med.* **1994**, *16*, 169–176. [CrossRef]

54. Kinnula, V.L.; Raivio, K.O.; Linnainmaa, K.; Ekman, A.; Klockars, M. Neutrophil and asbestos fiber-induced cytotoxicity in cultured human mesothelial and bronchial epithelial cells. *Free Radic. Biol. Med.* **1995**, *18*, 391–399. [CrossRef]

55. Moslen, M.T. Reactive oxygen species in normal physiology, cell injury and phagocytosis. *Adv. Exp. Med. Biol.* **1994**, *366*, 17–27. [PubMed]

56. Hansen, K.; Mossman, B.T. Generation of superoxide (O2-.) from alveolar macrophages exposed to asbestiform and nonfibrous particles. *Cancer Res.* **1987**, *47*, 1681–1686. [PubMed]

57. Shukla, A.; Gulumian, M.; Hei, T.K.; Kamp, D.; Rahman, Q.; Mossman, B.T. Multiple roles of oxidants in the pathogenesis of asbestos-induced diseases. *Free Radic. Biol. Med.* **2003**, *34*, 1117–1129. [CrossRef]

58. Funahashi, S.; Okazaki, Y.; Ito, D.; Asakawa, A.; Nagai, H.; Tajima, M.; Toyokuni, S. Asbestos and multi-walled carbon nanotubes generate distinct oxidative responses in inflammatory cells. *J. Clin. Biochem. Nutr.* **2015**, *56*, 111–117. [CrossRef] [PubMed]

59. Tanaka, S.; Choe, N.; Hemenway, D.R.; Zhu, S.; Matalon, S.; Kagan, E. Asbestos inhalation induces reactive nitrogen species and nitrotyrosine formation in the lungs and pleura of the rat. *J. Clin. Investig.* **1998**, *102*, 445–454. [CrossRef] [PubMed]

60. Soini, Y.; Kahlos, K.; Puhakka, A.; Lakari, E.; Säily, M.; Pääkkö, P.; Kinnula, V. Expression of inducible nitric oxide synthase in healthy pleura and in malignant mesothelioma. *Br. J. Cancer* **2000**, *83*, 880–886. [CrossRef] [PubMed]

61. Reuter, S.; Gupta, S.C.; Chaturvedi, M.M.; Aggarwal, B.B. Oxidative stress, inflammation, and cancer: How are they linked? *Free Radic. Biol. Med.* **2010**, *49*, 1603–1616. [CrossRef] [PubMed]

62. Wu, J.; Liu, W.; Koenig, K.; Idell, S.; Broaddus, V.C. Vitronectin adsorption to chrysotile asbestos increases fiber phagocytosis and toxicity for mesothelial cells. *Am. J. Physiol. Lung Cell. Mol. Physiol.* **2000**, *279*, L916–L923. [PubMed]

63. Hillegass, J.M.; Miller, J.M.; MacPherson, M.B.; Westbom, C.M.; Sayan, M.; Thompson, J.K.; Macura, S.L.; Perkins, T.N.; Beuschel, S.L.; Alexeeva, V.; *et al.* Asbestos and erionite prime and activate the NLRP3 inflammasome that stimulates autocrine cytokine release in human mesothelial cells. *Part. Fibre Toxicol.* **2013**, *10*, 39. [CrossRef] [PubMed]

64. Chow, M.T.; Tschopp, J.; Möller, A.; Smyth, M.J. NLRP3 promotes inflammation-induced skin cancer but is dispensable for asbestos-induced mesothelioma. *Immunol. Cell Biol.* **2012**, *90*, 983–986. [CrossRef] [PubMed]

65. Petrilli, V.; Dostert, C.; Muruve, D.A.; Tschopp, J. The inflammasome: A danger sensing complex triggering innate immunity. *Curr. Opin. Immunol.* **2007**, *19*, 615–622. [CrossRef] [PubMed]

66. Westbom, C.; Thompson, J.K.; Leggett, A.; MacPherson, M.; Beuschel, S.; Pass, H.; Vacek, P.; Shukla, A. Inflammasome modulation by chemotherapeutics in malignant mesothelioma. *PLoS ONE* **2015**, *10*, e0145404. [CrossRef] [PubMed]

67. Wang, Y.; Faux, S.P.; Hallden, G.; Kirn, D.H.; Houghton, C.E.; Lemoine, N.R.; Patrick, G. Interleukin-1beta and tumour necrosis factor-alpha promote the transformation of human immortalised mesothelial cells by erionite. *Int. J. Oncol.* **2004**, *25*, 173–178. [PubMed]

68. Antony, V.B. Immunological mechanisms in pleural disease. *Eur. Respir. J.* **2003**, *21*, 539–544. [CrossRef] [PubMed]

69. Driscoll, K.E.; Maurer, J.K.; Higgins, J.; Poynter, J. Alveolar macrophage cytokine and growth factor production in a rat model of crocidolite-induced pulmonary inflammation and fibrosis. *J. Toxicol. Environ. Health* **1995**, *46*, 155–169. [CrossRef] [PubMed]

70. Driscoll, K.E.; Carter, J.M.; Howard, B.W.; Hassenbein, D.; Janssen, Y.M.; Mossman, B.T. Crocidolite activates NF-kappa B and MIP-2 gene expression in rat alveolar epithelial cells. Role of mitochondrial-derived oxidants. *Environ. Health Perspect.* **1998**, *106*, 1171–1174. [CrossRef] [PubMed]

71. Bielefeldt-Ohmann, H.; Fitzpatrick, D.R.; Marzo, A.L.; Jarnicki, A.G.; Himbeck, R.P.; Davis, M.R.; Manning, L.S.; Robinson, B.W. Patho- and immunobiology of malignant mesothelioma: Characterisation of tumour infiltrating leucocytes and cytokine production in a murine model. *Cancer Immunol. Immunother.* **1994**, *39*, 347–359. [CrossRef] [PubMed]

72. Landskron, G.; de la Fuente, M.; Thuwajit, P.; Thuwajit, C.; Hermoso, M.A. Chronic inflammation and cytokines in the tumor microenvironment. *J. Immunol. Res.* **2014**, *2014*. [CrossRef] [PubMed]

73. Caja, F.; Vannucci, L. TGFβ: A player on multiple fronts in the tumor microenvironment. *J. Immunotoxicol.* **2015**, *12*, 300–307. [CrossRef] [PubMed]

74. Zitvogel, L.; Kepp, O.; Galluzzi, L.; Kroemer, G. Inflammasomes in carcinogenesis and anticancer immune responses. *Nat. Immunol.* **2012**, *13*, 343–351. [CrossRef] [PubMed]

75. Naldini, A.; Carraro, F. Role of inflammatory mediators in angiogenesis. *Curr. Drug Targets Inflamm. Allergy* **2005**, *4*, 3–8. [CrossRef] [PubMed]

76. Fox, S.A.; Loh, S.S.; Mahendran, S.K.; Garlepp, M.J. Regulated chemokine gene expression in mouse mesothelioma and mesothelial cells: TNF-α upregulates both CC and CXC chemokine genes. *Oncol. Rep.* **2012**, *28*, 707–713. [CrossRef] [PubMed]

77. Rollins, B.J. Inflammatory chemokines in cancer growth and progression. *Eur. J. Cancer* **2006**, *42*, 760–767. [CrossRef] [PubMed]

78. Vlaeminck-Guillem, V.; Bienvenu, J.; Isaac, S.; Grangier, B.; Golfier, F.; Passot, G.; Bakrin, N.; RodriguezLafrasse, C.; Gilly, F.N.; Glehen, O. Intraperitoneal cytokine level in patients with peritoneal surface malignancies. A study of the RENAPE (French Network for Rare Peritoneal Malignancies). *Ann. Surg. Oncol.* **2013**, *20*, 2655–2662. [CrossRef] [PubMed]

79. Comar, M.; Zanotta, N.; Bonotti, A.; Tognon, M.; Negro, C.; Cristaudo, A.; Bovenzi, M. Increased levels of C-C chemokine RANTES in asbestos exposed workers and in malignant mesothelioma patients from an hyperendemic area. *PLoS ONE* **2014**, *9*, e104848. [CrossRef] [PubMed]

80. Xu, J.; Alexander, D.B.; Iigo, M.; Hamano, H.; Takahashi, S.; Yokoyama, T.; Kato, M.; Usami, I.; Tokuyama, T.; Tsutsumi, M. Chemokine (C-C motif) ligand 3 detection in the serum of persons exposed to asbestos: A patient-based study. *Cancer Sci.* **2015**, *106*, 825–832. [CrossRef] [PubMed]

81. Terlizzi, M.; Casolaro, V.; Pinto, A.; Sorrentino, R. Inflammasome: Cancer's friend or foe? *Pharmacol. Therap.* **2014**, *143*, 24–33. [CrossRef] [PubMed]

82. Dinarello, C.A. Why not treat human cancer with interleukin-1 blockade? *Cancer Metastasis Rev.* **2010**, *29*, 317–329. [CrossRef] [PubMed]

83. Izzi, V.; Chiurchiù, V.; Doldo, E.; Palumbo, C.; Tesoldi, I.; Bei, R.; Albonici, L.; Modesti, A. Interleukin-17 produced by malignant mesothelioma-polarized immune cells promotes tumor growth and invasiveness. *Eur. J. Inflamm.* **2013**, *11*, 203–214.

84. Miselis, N.R.; Lau, B.W.; Wu, Z.; Kane, A.B. Kinetics of host cell recruitment during dissemination of diffuse malignant peritoneal mesothelioma. *Cancer Microenviron.* **2010**, *4*, 39–50. [CrossRef] [PubMed]

85. Veltman, J.D.; Lambers, M.E.; van Nimwegen, M.; Hendriks, R.W.; Hoogsteden, H.C.; Hegmans, J.P.; Aerts, J.G. Zoledronic acid impairs myeloid differentiation to tumour-associated macrophages in mesothelioma. *Br. J. Cancer* **2010**, *103*, 629–641. [CrossRef] [PubMed]

86. Veltman, J.D.; Lambers, M.E.; van Nimwegen, M.; Hendriks, R.W.; Hoogsteden, H.C.; Aerts, J.G.; Hegmans, J.P. COX-2 inhibition improves immunotherapy and is associated with decreased numbers of myeloid-derived suppressor cells in mesothelioma. Celecoxib influences MDSC function. *BMC Cancer* **2010**, *10*, 464. [CrossRef] [PubMed]

87. Yang, H.; Pellegrini, L.; Napolitano, A.; Giorgi, C.; Jube, S.; Preti, A.; Jennings, C.J.; de Marchis, F.; Flores, E.G.; Larson, D.; *et al.* Aspirin delays mesothelioma growth by inhibiting HMGB1-mediated tumor progression. *Cell Death Dis.* **2015**, *6*, e1786. [CrossRef] [PubMed]

88. Sica, A.; Allavena, P.; Mantovani, A. Cancer related inflammation: The macrophage connection. *Cancer Lett.* **2008**, *267*, 204–215. [CrossRef] [PubMed]

89. Burt, B.M.; Rodig, S.J.; Tilleman, T.R.; Elbardissi, A.W.; Bueno, R.; Sugarbaker, D.J. Circulating and tumor-infiltrating myeloid cells predict survival in human pleural mesothelioma. *Cancer* **2011**, *117*, 5234–5244. [CrossRef] [PubMed]

90. Hegmans, J.P.; Hemmes, A.; Hammad, H.; Boon, L.; Hoogsteden, H.C.; Lambrecht, B.N. Mesothelioma environment comprises cytokines and T-regulatory cells that suppress immune responses. *Eur. Respir. J.* **2006**, *27*, 1086–1095. [CrossRef] [PubMed]

91. Miselis, N.R.; Wu, Z.J.; van Rooijen, N.; Kane, A.B. Targeting tumor-associated macrophages in an orthotopic murine model of diffuse malignant mesothelioma. *Mol. Cancer Ther.* **2008**, *7*, 788–799. [CrossRef] [PubMed]

92. Napolitano, A.; Pellegrini, L.; Dey, A.; Larson, D.; Tanji, M.; Flores, E.G.; Kendrick, B.; Lapid, D.; Powers, A.; Kanodia, S.; *et al.* Minimal asbestos exposure in germline BAP1 heterozygous mice is associated with deregulated inflammatory response and increased risk of mesothelioma. *Oncogene* **2016**, *35*, 1996–2002. [CrossRef] [PubMed]

93. Nishimura, Y.; Kumagai-Takei, N.; Matsuzaki, H.; Lee, S.; Maeda, M.; Kishimoto, T.; Fukuoka, K.; Nakano, T.; Otsuki, T. Functional alteration of natural killer cells and cytotoxic T lymphocytes upon asbestos exposure and in malignant mesothelioma patients. *BioMed. Res. Int.* **2015**, *2015*. [CrossRef] [PubMed]

94. Maeda, M.; Nishimura, Y.; Hayashi, H.; Kumagai, N.; Chen, Y.; Murakami, S.; Miura, Y.; Hiratsuka, J.; Kishimoto, T.; Otsuki, T. Reduction of CXC chemokine receptor 3 in an *in vitro* model of continuous exposure to asbestos in a human T-cell line, MT-2. *Am. J. Respira. Cell Mol. Biol.* **2011**, *45*, 470–479. [CrossRef] [PubMed]

95. Maeda, M.; Nishimura, Y.; Hayashi, H.; Kumagai, N.; Chen, Y.; Murakami, S.; Miura, Y.; Hiratsuka, J.; Kishimoto, T.; Otsuki, T. Decreased CXCR3 expression in CD4+ T cells exposed to asbestos or derived from asbestos-exposed patients. *Am. J. Respira. Cell Mol. Biol.* **2011**, *45*, 795–803. [CrossRef] [PubMed]

96. Maeda, M.; Chen, Y.; Hayashi, H.; Kumagai-Takei, N.; Matsuzaki, H.; Lee, S.; Nishimura, Y.; Otsuki, T. Chronic exposure to asbestos enhances TGF-β1 production in the human adult T cell leukemia virus-immortalized T cell line MT-2. *Int. J. Oncol.* **2014**, *45*, 2522–2532. [CrossRef] [PubMed]

97. Miura, Y.; Nishimura, Y.; Katsuyama, H.; Maeda, M.; Hayashi, H.; Dong, M.; Hyodoh, F.; Tomita, M.; Matsuo, Y.; Uesaka, A.; *et al.* Involvement of IL-10 and Bcl-2 in resistance against an asbestos-induced apoptosis of T cells. *Apoptosis* **2006**, *11*, 1825–1835. [CrossRef] [PubMed]

98. Feskanich, D.; Ziegler, R.G.; Michaud, D.S.; Giovannucci, E.L.; Speizer, F.E.; Willett, W.C.; Colditz, G.A. Prospective study of fruit and vegetable consumption and risk of lung cancer among men and women. *J. Natl. Cancer Inst.* **2000**, *92*, 1812–1823. [CrossRef] [PubMed]

99.  Bazzano, L.A.; He, J.; Ogden, L.G.; Loria, C.M.; Vupputuri, S.; Myers, L.; Whelton, P.K. Fruit and vegetable intake and risk of cardiovascular disease in US adults: The first National Health and Nutrition Examination Survey Epidemiologic follow-up study. *Am. J. Clin. Nutr.* **2002**, *76*, 93–99. [PubMed]

100. Mennen, L.I.; Sapinho, D.; de Bree, A.; Arnault, N.; Bertrais, S.; Galan, P.; Hercberg, S. Consumption of foods rich in flavonoids is related to a decreased cardiovascular risk in apparently healthy French women. *J. Nutr.* **2004**, *134*, 923–926. [PubMed]

101. Chang, H.W.; Baek, S.H.; Chung, K.W.; Son, K.H.; Kim, H.P.; Kang, S.S. Inactivation of phospholipase A2 by naturally occurring biflavonoid, ochnaflavone. *Biochem. Biophys. Res. Commun.* **1994**, *205*, 843–849. [CrossRef] [PubMed]

102. Kang, H.K.; Ecklund, D.; Liu, M.; Datta, S.K. Apigenin, a non-mutagenic dietary flavonoid, suppresses lupus by inhibiting autoantigen presentation for expansion of autoreactive Th1 and Th17 cells. *Arthritis Res. Ther.* **2009**, *11*, R59. [CrossRef] [PubMed]

103. Chi, Y.S.; Kim, H.P. Suppression of cyclooxigenase-2 expression of skin fibroblasts by wogonin, a plant flavones from Scutellaria radix. *Prostaglandins Leukot. Essent. Fat. Acids* **2005**, *72*, 59–66. [CrossRef] [PubMed]

104. Liang, Y.C.; Huang, Y.T.; Tsai, S.H.; Lin-Shiau, S.Y.; Chen, C.F.; Lin, J.K. Suppression of inducible cyclooxygenase and inducible nitric oxide synthase by apigenin and related flavonoids in mouse macrophages. *Carcinogenesis* **1999**, *20*, 1945–1952. [CrossRef] [PubMed]

105. Hamalainen, M.; Nieminen, R.; Vuorela, P.; Heinonen, M.; Moilanen, E. Anti-inflammatory effects of flavonoids: Genistein, kaempferol, quercetin, and daidzein inhibit STAT-1 and NF-kappaB activations, whereas flavone, isorhamnetin, naringenin, and pelargonidin inhibit only NF-kappaB activation along with their inhibitory effect on iNOS expression and NO production in activated macrophages. *Mediat. Inflamm.* **2007**, *2007*. [CrossRef]

106. Halliwell, B. Are polyphenols antioxidants or pro-oxidants? What do we learn from cell culture and *in vivo* studies? *Arch. Biochem. Biophys.* **2008**, *476*, 107–112. [CrossRef] [PubMed]

107. León-Gonzáles, A.J.; Auger, C.; Schini-Kerth, V.B. Pro-oxidant activity of polyphenols and its implication on cancer chemoprevention and chemotherapy. *Biochem. Pharmacol.* **2015**, *98*, 371–380. [CrossRef] [PubMed]

108. Miller, J.M.; Thompson, J.K.; MacPherson, M.B.; Beuschel, S.L.; Westbom, C.M.; Sayan, M.; Shukla, A. Curcumin: A double hit on malignant mesothelioma. *Cancer Prev. Res.* **2014**, *7*, 330–340. [CrossRef] [PubMed]

109. Satoh, M.; Takemura, Y.; Hamada, H.; Sekido, Y.; Kubota, S. EGCG indices human mesothelioma cell death by inducing reactive oxygen species and autophagy. *Cancer Cell Int.* **2013**, *13*, 19. [CrossRef] [PubMed]

110. Ranzato, E.; Martinotti, S.; Magnelli, V.; Murer, B.; Biffo, S.; Mutti, L.; Burlando, B. Epigallocathechin-3-gallate induces mesothelioma cell death via H2 O2-dependent T-type Ca2+ channel opening. *J. Cell. Mol. Med.* **2012**, *16*, 2667–2678. [CrossRef] [PubMed]

111. Valenti, D.; de Bari, L.; Manente, G.A.; Rossi, L.; Mutti, L.; Moro, L.; Vacca, R.A. Negative modulation of mitochondrial oxidative phosphorylation by epigallocatechin-3 gallate leads to growth arrest and apoptosis in human malignant pleural mesothelioma cells. *Biochim. Biophys. Acta* **2013**, *1382*, 2085–2096. [CrossRef] [PubMed]

112. Lee, Y.J.; Im, J.H.; Lee, D.M.; Park, J.S.; Won, S.Y.; Cho, M.K.; Nam, H.S.; Lee, Y.J.; Lee, S.H. Synergistic inhibition of mesothelioma cell growth by the combination of clofarabine and resveratrol involves Nrf2 downregulation. *BMB Rep.* **2012**, *45*, 647–652. [CrossRef] [PubMed]

113. Lee, Y.J.; Park, I.S.; Lee, Y.J.; Shim, J.H.; Cho, M.K.; Nam, H.S.; Park, J.W.; Oh, M.H.; Lee, S.H. Resveratrol contributes to chemosensivity of malignant mesothelioma cells with activation of p53. *Food Chem. Toxicol.* **2014**, *63*, 153–160. [CrossRef] [PubMed]

114. Faraonio, R.; Vergara, P.; Di Marzo, D.; Pierantoni, M.G.; Napolitano, M.; Russo, T.; Cimino, F. p53 suppresses the Nrf2-dependent transcription of antioxidant response genes. *J. Biol. Chem.* **2006**, *281*, 39776–39784. [CrossRef] [PubMed]

115. Pietrofesa, R.A.; Velalopoulou, A.; Albelda, S.M.; Christofidou-Solomidou, M. Asbestos Induces Oxidative Stress and Activation of Nrf2 Signaling in Murine Macrophages: Chemopreventive Role of the Synthetic Lignan Secoisolariciresinol Diglucoside (LGM2605). *Int. J. Mol. Sci.* **2016**, *17*, 322. [CrossRef] [PubMed]

116. Kostyuk, V.A.; Potapovich, A.I.; Speransky, S.D.; Maslova, G.T. Protective effect of natural flavonoids on rat peritoneal macrophages injury caused by asbestos fibers. *Free Radic. Biol. Med.* **1996**, *21*, 487–493. [CrossRef]

117. Kostyuk, V.A.; Potapovich, A.I.; Vladykovskaya, E.N.; Hiramatsu, M. Protective effects of green tea catechins against asbestos-induced cell injury. *Planta Med.* **2000**, *66*, 762–764. [CrossRef] [PubMed]

118. Potapovich, A.I.; Kostyuk, V.A. Comparative study of antioxidant properties and cytoprotective activity of flavonoids. *Biochemistry* **2003**, *68*, 514–519. [PubMed]

119. Grivennikov, S.I.; Greten, F.R.; Karin, M. Immunity, inflammation, and cancer. *Cell* **2010**, *140*, 883–899. [CrossRef] [PubMed]

120. Valko, M.; Leibfritz, D.; Moncol, J.; Cronin, M.T.; Mazur, M.; Telser, J. Free radicals and antioxidants in normal physiological functions and human disease. *Int. J. Biochem. Cell Biol.* **2007**, *39*, 44–84. [CrossRef] [PubMed]

121. Cohen, A.N.; Veena, M.S.; Srivatsan, E.S.; Wang, M.B. Suppression of interleukin 6 and 8 production in head and neck cancer cells with curcumin via inhibition of Ikappa beta kinase. *Arch. Otolaryngol. Head Neck Surg.* **2009**, *135*, 190–197. [CrossRef] [PubMed]

122. Wang, Y.; Yu, C.; Pan, Y.; Yang, X.; Huang, Y.; Feng, Z.; Li, X.; Yang, S.; Liang, G. A novel synthetic mono-carbonyl analogue of curcumin, A13, exhibits anti-inflammatory effect *in vivo* by inhibition of inflammatory mediators. *Inflammation* **2011**, *35*, 594–604. [CrossRef] [PubMed]

123. Serafini, M.; Peluso, I.; Raguzzini, A. Flavonoids as anti-inflammatory agents. *Proc. Nutr. Soc.* **2010**, *69*, 273–278. [CrossRef] [PubMed]

124. Hirano, T.; Higa, S.; Arimitsu, J.; Naka, T.; Shima, Y.; Ohshima, S.; Fujimoto, M.; Yamadori, T.; Kawase, I.; Tanaka, T. Flavonoids such as luteolin, fisetin and apigenin are inhibitors of interleukin-4 and interleukin-13 production by activated human basophils. *Int. Arch. Allergy Immunol.* **2004**, *134*, 135–140. [CrossRef] [PubMed]

125. Chen, P.C.; Wheeler, D.S.; Malhotra, V.; Odoms, K.; Denenberg, A.G.; Wong, H.R. A green tea-derived polyphenol, epigallocatechin-3-gallate, inhibits IKappaB kinase activation and IL-8 gene expression in respiratory epithelium. *Inflammation* **2002**, *26*, 233–241. [CrossRef] [PubMed]

126. Shin, H.Y.; Kim, S.H.; Jeong, H.J.; Kim, S.Y.; Shin, T.Y.; Um, J.Y.; Hong, S.H.; Kim, H.M. Epigallocatechin-3-gallate inhibits secretion of TNF-alpha, IL-6 and IL-8 through the attenuation of ERK and NF-kappaB in HMC-1 cells. *Int. Arch. Allergy Immunol.* **2007**, *142*, 335–344. [CrossRef] [PubMed]

127. Ahmed, S.; Marotte, H.; Kwan, K.; Ruth, J.H.; Campbell, P.L.; Rabquer, B.J.; Pakozdi, A.; Koch, A.E. Epigallocatechin-3-gallate inhibits IL-6 synthesis and suppresses transsignaling by enhancing soluble gp130 production. *Proc. Natl. Acad. Sci. USA* **2008**, *105*, 14692–14697. [CrossRef] [PubMed]

128. Rasheed, Z.; Anbazhagan, A.N.; Akhtar, N.; Ramamurthy, S.; Voss, F.R.; Haqqi, T.M. Green tea polyphenol epigallocatechin-3-gallate inhibits advanced glycation end product-induced expression of tumor necrosis factor-alpha and matrix metalloproteinase-13 in human chondrocytes. *Arthritis Res. Ther.* **2009**, *11*, R71. [CrossRef] [PubMed]

129. Park, H.H.; Lee, S.; Son, H.Y.; Park, S.B.; Kim, M.S.; Choi, E.J.; Singh, T.S.; Ha, J.H.; Lee, M.G.; Kim, J.E. Flavonoids inhibit histamine release and expression of proinflammatory cytokines in mast cells. *Arch. Pharm. Res.* **2008**, *31*, 1303–1311. [CrossRef] [PubMed]

130. Sun, C.; Hu, Y.; Liu, X.; Wu, T.; Wang, Y.; He, W.; Wei, W. Resveratrol downregulates the constitutional activation of nuclear factor-kappaB in multiple myeloma cells, leading to suppression of proliferation and invasion, arrest of cell cycle, and induction of apoptosis. *Cancer Genet. Cytogenet.* **2006**, *165*, 9–19. [CrossRef] [PubMed]

131. Manna, S.K.; Mukhopadhyay, A.; Aggarwal, B.B. Resveratrol suppresses TNF-induced activation of nuclear transcription factors NF-kappaB, activator protein-1, and apoptosis: Potential role of reactive oxygen intermediates and lipid peroxidation. *J. Immunol.* **2000**, *164*, 6509–6519. [CrossRef] [PubMed]

132. Kim, G.Y.; Kim, K.H.; Lee, S.H.; Yoon, M.S.; Lee, H.J.; Moon, D.O.; Lee, C.M.; Ahn, S.C.; Park, Y.C.; Park, Y.M. Curcumin inhibits immunostimulatory function of dendritic cells: MAPKs and translocation of NF-kappaB as potential targets. *J. Immunol.* **2005**, *174*, 8116–8124. [CrossRef] [PubMed]

133. Garcia-Mediavilla, M.V.; Crespo, I.; Collado, P.S.; Esteller, A.; Sanchez-Campos, S.; Tunon, M.J. Anti-inflammatory effect of the flavones quercetin and kaempferol in Chang Liver cells involves inhibition of inducible nitric oxide synthase, cyclooxygenase-2 and reactive C-protein, and down-regulation of the nuclear factor kappaB pathway. *Eur. J. Pharmacol.* **2007**, *557*, 221–229. [CrossRef] [PubMed]

134. Nicholas, C.; Batra, S.; Vargo, M.A.; Voss, O.H.; Gavrilin, M.A.; Wewers, M.D.; Guttridge, D.C.; Grotewold, E.; Doseff, A.I. Apigenin blocks lipopolysaccharide-induced lethality *in vivo* and proinflammatory cytokines

expression by inactivating NF-kappa B through the suppression of p65 phosphorylation. *J. Immunol.* **2007**, *179*, 7121–7127. [CrossRef] [PubMed]

135. Romier, B.; van de Walle, J.; During, A.; Larondelle, Y.; Schneider, Y.J. Modulation of signaling nuclear factor-kappaB activation pathway by polyphenols in human intestinal Caco-2 cells. *Br. J. Nutr.* **2008**, *100*, 542–551. [CrossRef] [PubMed]

136. Lin, R.W.; Chen, C.H.; Wang, Y.H.; Ho, M.L.; Hung, S.H.; Chen, I.S.; Wang, G.J. (−)-Epigallocatechin gallate inhibition of osteoclastic differentiation via NF-kappaB *Biochem. Biophys. Res. Commun.* **2009**, *379*, 1033–1037. [CrossRef] [PubMed]

137. Laua, F.C.; Josepha, J.A.; McDonald, J.E.; Kalt, A.W. Attenuation of iNOS and COX2 by blueberry polyphenols is mediated through the suppression of NF-κB activation. *J. Funct. Foods* **2009**, *1*, 274–283. [CrossRef]

138. Kim, J.W.; Jin, Y.C.; Kim, Y.M.; Rhie, S.; Kim, H.J.; Seo, H.G.; Lee, J.H.; Ha, Y.L.; Chang, K.C. Daidzein administration *in vivo* reduces myocardial injury in a rat ischemia/reperfusion model by inhibiting NF-κB activation. *Life Sci.* **2009**, *84*, 227–234. [CrossRef] [PubMed]

139. Bharti, A.C.; Donato, N.; Aggarwal, B.B. Curcumin (diferuloylmethane) inhibits constitutive and IL-6-inducible STAT3 phosphorylation in human multiple myeloma cells. *J. Immunol.* **2003**, *171*, 3863–3871. [CrossRef] [PubMed]

140. Chakravarti, N.; Myers, J.N.; Aggarwal, B.B. Targeting constitutive and interleukin-6-inducible signal transducers and activators of transcription 3 pathway in head and neck squamous cell carcinoma cells by curcumin (diferuloylmethane). *Int. J. Cancer* **2006**, *119*, 1268–1275. [CrossRef] [PubMed]

141. Wung, B.S.; Hsu, M.C.; Wu, C.C.; Hsieh, C.W. Resveratrol suppresses IL-6- induced ICAM-1 gene expression in endothelial cells: Effects on the inhibition of STAT3 phosphorylation. *Life Sci.* **2005**, *78*, 389–397. [CrossRef] [PubMed]

142. Masuda, M.; Suzui, M.; Weinstein, I.B. Effects of epigallocatechin-3- gallate on growth, epidermal growth factor receptor signaling pathways, gene expression, and chemosensitivity in human head and neck squamous cell carcinoma cell lines. *Clin. Cancer Res.* **2001**, *7*, 4220–4229. [PubMed]

143. Kadariya, Y.; Menges, C.W.; Talarchek, J.; Cai, K.Q.; Klein-Szanto, A.J.; Pietrofesa, R.A.; Christofidou-Solomidou, M.; Cheung, M.; Mossman, B.T.; Shukla, A.; Testa, J.R. Inflammation-Related IL-1β/IL-1R Signaling Promotes the Development of Asbestos-Induced Malignant Mesothelioma. *Cancer Prev. Res.* **2016**, *9*, 406–411. [CrossRef] [PubMed]

144. Miao, E.A.; Rajan, J.V.; Aderem, A. Caspase-1-induced pyroptotic cell death. *Immunol. Rev.* **2011**, *243*, 206–214. [CrossRef] [PubMed]

145. Wang, Y.; Rishi, A.K.; Wu, W.; Polin, L.; Sharma, S.; Levi, E.; Albelda, S.; Pass, H.I.; Wali, A. Curcumin suppresses growth of mesothelioma cells *in vitro* and *in vivo*, in part, by stimulating apoptosis. *Mol. Cell. Biochem.* **2011**, *357*, 83–94. [CrossRef] [PubMed]

146. Cioce, M.; Canino, C.; Pulito, C.; Muti, P.; Strano, S.; Blandino, G. Butein impairs the protumorigenic activity of malignant pleural mesothelioma cells. *Cell Cycle* **2012**, *11*, 132–140. [CrossRef] [PubMed]

147. Dabir, S.; Kluge, A.; Dowlati, A. The association and nuclear translocation of the PIAS3-STAT3 complex is ligand and time dependent. *Mol. Cancer Res.* **2009**, *7*, 1854–1860. [CrossRef] [PubMed]

148. Dabir, S.; Kluge, A.; Kresak, A.; Yang, M.; Fu, P.; Groner, B.; Wildey, G.; Dowlati, A. Low PIAS3 expression in malignant mesothelioma is associated with increased STAT3 activation and poor patient survival. *Clin. Cancer Res.* **2014**, *20*, 5124–5132. [CrossRef] [PubMed]

149. Martinotti, S.; Ranzato, E.; Burlando, B. *In vitro* screening of synergistic ascorbate-drug combinations for the treatment of malignant mesothelioma. *Toxicol. Vitro* **2011**, *25*, 1568–1574. [CrossRef] [PubMed]

150. Martinotti, S.; Ranzato, E.; Parodi, M.; Vitale, M.; Burlando, B. Combination of ascorbate/ epigallocatechin-3-gallate/gemcitabine synergistically induces cell cycle deregulation and apoptosis in mesothelioma cells. *Toxicol. Appl. Pharmacol.* **2014**, *274*, 35–41. [CrossRef] [PubMed]

151. Beishline, K.; Azizkhan-Clifford, J. Sp1 and the 'hallmarks of cancer'. *FEBS J.* **2015**, *282*, 224–258. [CrossRef] [PubMed]

152. Lee, K.A.; Lee, Y.J.; Ban, J.O.; Lee, Y.J.; Lee, S.H.; Cho, M.K.; Nam, H.S.; Hong, J.T.; Shim, J.H. The flavonoid resveratrol suppresses growth of human malignant pleural mesothelioma cells through direct inhibition of specificity protein 1. *Int. J. Mol. Med.* **2012**, *30*, 21–27. [PubMed]

153. Lee, Y.J.; Lee, Y.J.; Im, J.H.; Won, S.Y.; Kim, Y.B.; Cho, M.K.; Nam, H.S.; Choi, Y.J.; Lee, S.H. Synergistic anti-cancer effects of resveratrol and chemotherapeutic agent clofarabine against human malignant mesothelioma MSTO-211H cells. *Food Chem. Toxicol.* **2013**, *52*, 61–68. [CrossRef] [PubMed]

154. Chae, J.I.; Cho, J.H.; Lee, K.A.; Choi, N.J.; Seo, K.S.; Kim, S.B.; Lee, S.H.; Shim, J.H. Role of transcriptor factor Sp1 in the quercetin-mediated inhibitory effect on human malignant pleural mesothelioma. *Int. J. Mol. Med.* **2012**, *30*, 835–841. [PubMed]

155. Chae, J.I.; Jeon, Y.J.; Shim, J.H. Downregulation of Sp1 is involved in honokiol-induced cell cycle arrest and apoptosis in human malignant pleural mesothelioma cells. *Oncol. Rep.* **2013**, *29*, 2318–2324. [PubMed]

156. Kim, K.H.; Yoon, G.; Cho, J.J.; Cho, J.H.; Cho, Y.S.; Chae, J.I.; Shim, J.H. Licochalcone A induces apoptosis in malignant pleural mesothelioma through downregulation of Sp1 and subsequent activation of mitochondria-related apoptotic pathway. *Int. J. Oncol.* **2015**, *46*, 1385–1392. [CrossRef] [PubMed]

157. Lee, K.A.; Lee, S.H.; Lee, Y.J.; Baeg, S.M.; Shim, J.H. Hesperidin induces apoptosis by inhibiting Sp1 and its regulatory protein in MSTO-211H cells. *Biomol. Ther.* **2012**, *20*, 273–279. [CrossRef] [PubMed]

158. Lee, K.A.; Chae, J.I.; Shim, J.H. Natural diterpenes from coffee, cafestol and kahweol induce apoptosis through regulation of specificity protein 1 expression in human malignant pleural mesothelioma. *J. Biomed. Sci.* **2012**, *19*, 60. [CrossRef] [PubMed]

159. Roomi, M.W.; Ivanov, V.; Kalinovsky, T.; Niedzwiecki, A.; Rath, M. Inhibition of malignant mesothelioma cell matrix metalloproteinase production and invasion by a novel nutrient mixture. *Exp. Lung Res.* **2006**, *32*, 69–79. [CrossRef] [PubMed]

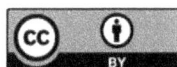

MDPI AG

St. Alban-Anlage 66

4052 Basel, Switzerland

Tel. +41 61 683 77 34

Fax +41 61 302 89 18

http://www.mdpi.com

*Nutrients* Editorial Office

E-mail: *nutrients*@mdpi.com

http://www.mdpi.com/journal/nutrients

www.ingramcontent.com/pod-product-compliance
Lightning Source LLC
Chambersburg PA
CBHW051700210326
41597CB00032B/5324